NEW
FAMILY
MEDICAL
GUIDE

Better Homes and Gardens®

NEW
FAMILY
MEDICAL
GUIDE

Edited by
Edwin Kiester, Jr.

Illustrations by
Kelly Solis-Navarro
and
Evanell Towne

Other Better Homes and Gardens®
Health and Medical Books:
Woman's Health and Medical Guide
After-40 Health and Medical Guide
New Baby Book

BETTER HOMES AND GARDENS® BOOKS
Editor: Gerald M. Knox
Art Director: Ernest Shelton
Managing Editor: David A. Kirchner

Associate Art Director (Managing): Randall Yontz
Associate Art Director (Creative): Linda Ford,
    Neoma Alt West
Copy and Production Editors: Nancy Nowiszewski,
    Lamont Olson, Mary Helen Schiltz,
    David A. Walsh
Assistant Art Directors: Faith Berven,
    Harijs Priekulis
Graphic Designers: Mike Burns, Alisann Dixon,
    Mike Eagleton, Lynda Haupert, Deb Miner,
    Lyne Neymeyer, Bill Shaw, D. Greg Thompson

Editor in Chief: Neil Kuehnl
Group Editorial Services Director: Duane L. Gregg
Executive Art Director: William J. Yates

General Manager: Fred Stines
Director of Publishing: Robert B. Nelson
Director of Retail Marketing: Jamie Martin
Director of Direct Marketing: Arthur Heydendael

NEW FAMILY MEDICAL GUIDE
Copy and Production Editor: Lamont Olson
Graphic Designer: Harijs Priekulis

The publishers are grateful to the following
    individuals and companies for assistance in the
    preparation of this book:
Barbara Behrens, R.N.; Philip Gelpi, M.D.;
    Walter Vogel, M.D.; Cutter Laboratories;
    Journal of Psychosomatic Research.

FOREWORD

When the Better Homes and Gardens® *Family Medical Guide* was first published in the early 1960s, tuberculosis was a major cause of illness and death. Children routinely endured the discomforts of measles and mumps, risking their potentially damaging consequences, and heart disease was rampant. At the same time, it was the age of medical miracles. In the most dramatic example, polio vaccine in a single stroke had virtually eradicated one of the most feared of all diseases.

Health-conscious Americans needed a reliable and authoritative guide through this maze of old problems and new solutions. The eminent science writer and editor, Donald G. Cooley, enlisted a nationally recognized corps of medical specialists from prominent hospitals and universities to provide it. Specially commissioned artwork was researched and executed by the distinguished medical illustrator, Paul Zuckerman. The contributors to the Better Homes and Gardens *Family Medical Guide* were assigned one simple objective: to explain in lucid, everyday terms and with clear illustrations how the body works, what can go wrong, and how to repair it.

One aim was to inform and enlighten the public. Another was to assist the busy physician, who didn't always have the time and communications skills to explain things for himself. How well they succeeded can be measured. The *Family Medical Guide* quickly became a best seller and has sold more than 5 million copies.

Two decades later, the picture of American health and sickness is vastly different. Tuberculosis is rare. Immunizations have almost wiped out the classic childhood diseases. Heart disease is declining. Yet Americans remained concerned about their health. Sales of running shoes and simple diets attest that we seek prevention as well as cure.

The Better Homes and Gardens *New Family Medical Guide* seeks to meet these new needs. Aimed at a different generation with different concerns, it is totally revamped in word and picture. But in a larger sense it is unchanged. The objective is still to explain the human body, its functions and malfunctions, without cant or technical language, and to help—not replace—the physician. The broader goal is better health for all Americans.

Throughout its history, the roster of contributors to the *Family Medical Guide* has read like a who's who of medicine. Many past contributors have retired or passed on after a lifetime of accomplishment; it is no longer possible to list all their names. The equally distinguished present group appears overleaf. The contributions of all have been invaluable, both to the *New Family Medical Guide* and to healthier Americans.

ACKNOWLEDGMENTS

Edwin Kiester, Jr., editor of the Better Homes and Gardens® *New Family Medical Guide,* is also co-author with Sally Valente Kiester of the Better Homes and Gardens® *New Baby Book*. His articles on medicine, science, and other subjects have appeared in many magazines. Former editor-at-large of *Today's Health,* published by the American Medical Association, he also has been a top editor at *Parade, True,* and *Change* magazines.

L. Fred Ayvazian, M.D. Chief, Pulmonary Section, Veterans Administration Medical Center, East Orange, New Jersey; Professor of Medicine, College of Medicine and Dentistry of New Jersey; Professor of Clinical Medicine, New York University Medical Center.

Robert A. Bagramian, D.D.S., Dr. P.H. Professor and Chairman of Community Dentistry, School of Dentistry; Professor of Dental Public Health, School of Public Health, University of Michigan.

Arthur E. Baue, M.D. Donald Guthrie Professor and Chairman, Department of Surgery, Yale University School of Medicine; Chief of Surgery, The Yale-New Haven Hospital, New Haven, Connecticut.

Philip W. Brickner, M.D., F.A.C.P. Director, Department of Community Medicine, Saint Vincent's Hospital and Medical Center of New York; Associate Professor of Clinical Medicine, New York Medical College.

William D. Carey, M.D. Staff Physician, Cleveland Clinic Foundation; Member, American Association for the Study of Liver Disease, American Society of Gastrointestinal Endoscopy, and American Gastroenterological Association.

William H. Crosby, M.D., F.A.C.P. Colonel, Medical Corps, United States Army. Department of Hematology, Walter Reed Army Institute of Research; Professor of Medicine, Uniformed Services University; Clinical Professor of Medicine, George Washington University, Washington, D.C.

Michael Eliastam, M.D., M.P.P. Assistant Professor of Medicine and Surgery, Stanford University School of Medicine; Director of Emergency Services, Stanford University Hospital.

Richard G. Farmer, M.D., F.A.C.P. Chairman, Division of Medicine, and Head, Department of Gastroenterology, Cleveland Clinic Foundation; Past President, American College of Gastroenterology; Member, National Commission on Digestive Diseases.

Robert D. Fazzaro, M.D. Director, Respiratory Therapy Services, Millville Hospital, Millville, New Jersey.

ACKNOWLEDGMENTS continued

John Stirling Meyer, M.D. Chief, Cerebrovascular Research, Veterans Administration Medical Center, Houston, Texas; Professor of Neurology, Baylor College of Medicine; Former Member, Advisory Council, National Institute of Neurological and Communicative Diseases and Stroke; Chairman, Stroke Committee, President's Commission on Heart Disease, Cancer, and Stroke; Diplomate, American Board of Neurology and Psychiatry, Inc.

Gerald P. Murphy, M.D., D.Sc. Professor of Surgery, State University of New York at Buffalo; Director, Roswell Park Memorial Institute.

William L. Proudfit, M.D. Clinical Emeritus Consultant, Cleveland Clinic Foundation; Formerly Head, Department of Clinical Cardiology, Cleveland Clinic Foundation.

Aldo A. Rossini, M.D. Associate Professor of Medicine and Director of Diabetes and Metabolism, Division of Endocrinology and Metabolism, University of Massachusetts Medical Center, Worcester, Massachusetts.

Gloria E. Sarto, M.D., Ph.D. Professor and Assistant Chairman, Department of Obstetrics and Gynecology, Northwestern University Medical School and Prentice Women's and Maternity Center of Northwestern Memorial Hospital, Chicago, Illinois.

Clark T. Sawin, M.D. Professor of Medicine, Tufts University School of Medicine; Chief, Endocrine-Diabetes Section, Veterans Administration Medical Center, Boston, Massachusetts.

Michael B. Shimkin, M.D. Professor Emeritus of Community Medicine and Oncology, School of Medicine, University of California at San Diego, La Jolla, California.

Lester F. Soyka, M.D., F.A.A.P. Professor of Pharmacology and Pediatrics and Chairman, Department of Pharmacology, University of Vermont College of Medicine; Chairman, Section of Clinical Pharmacology and Therapeutics, American Academy of Pediatrics.

William J. Spanos, Jr., M.D. Assistant Professor of Radiotherapy and Assistant Radiotherapist, the University of Texas System Cancer Center, M.D. Anderson Hospital and Tumor Institute; Assistant Professor, University of Texas Medical School, Houston, Texas.

Bruce E. Spivey, M.D. Professional Chairman, Department of Ophthalmology, Pacific Medical Center, San Francisco; President, Pacific Medical Center, San Francisco; Executive Vice President, American Academy of Ophthalmology.

Patti Tighe, M.D. Associate Professor and Director of Education, Department of Psychiatry, Pritzker School of Medicine, University of Chicago.

James F. Toole, M.D., L.L.B. Professor of Neurology and Chairman of Department of Neurology, Bowman-Gray School of Medicine, Wake Forest University, Winston-Salem, North Carolina; Member, Advisory Council, National Institute of Neurological Diseases and Stroke.

Julia A. Walsh, M.D. Associate in Medicine, Harvard Medical School and Peter Bent Brigham Hospital, Boston.

Jess R. Young, M.D. Head, Department of Peripheral Vascular Disease, Cleveland Clinic Foundation.

TABLE OF CONTENTS

TABLE OF CONTENTS

TABLE OF CONTENTS

LIST OF ILLUSTRATIONS

CHAPTER 1   PHILIP W. BRICKNER, M.D., F.A.C.P.

A PREVENTIVE APPROACH TO HEALTH

To feel well, to be effective, and to meet life's challenges, you must understand yourself, be psychologically confident and stable, and physically vigorous.

In order to achieve these goals, which obviously are in your own interests, common sense, good judgment, and prudence are necessary. Being well is primarily your responsibility. The health professions and your doctor are available to help, but you make the basic decisions which, in large part, lead either to health or disease.

The appetites we all have as biological creatures, and which give zest to life, we must learn to control. The alternative is allowing our desires to control us. One definition of a mature person is one who is in control of his or her impulses, and who thus can use mind and body rationally.

But this is hard to achieve. The temptations we face are strong, and they are enhanced by the huckstering world we live in, by lack of facts, and often by a wish to hide from reality.

Being fit requires a positive program aimed at improving health, a program that includes eating properly, resting properly, getting enough exercise, minimizing the stresses and frictions of life, and avoiding harmful substances. It also means being prepared for interruptions in health. Finding and working with a doctor and being ready financially for possible illness are part of that preventive approach.

Many of these topics are covered at length in succeeding chapters of this book. In this chapter we look at the elements that promote good health and prevent illness.

KNOWING YOUR BODY

Good health begins with awareness of your body. You need to sense how your body usually functions so that you can detect variations from normal. The other chapters describe the ordinary workings of the body, but variations within these outlines can be infinite. Many of these differences are unimportant in themselves. You only need to be aware of them so that you can detect change. Your physician should be alerted to such changes so that he or she can help you recognize significant ones.

It is also important to be aware of your medical history. The illnesses of earlier years may have bearing on your health today. Keep a thorough record and make certain that your doctor has the information. As you know, certain diseases are family connected. Therefore, a family health history, concerning your grandparents, parents, siblings, and other close relatives, is valuable. Maintain an accurate record of this material for your doctor.

NUTRITION AND VITAMINS

The foods we eat and the liquids we drink contain the building blocks for construction and maintenance of a healthy body. Chapter 19 explains the essentials of nutrition, such as what nutrients are present in what foods and how the body uses them. Here we will discuss the importance of nutrition in keeping healthy.

Healthy adults who eat a normal American diet are almost invariably well-nourished. That normal diet contains ample vitamins, making supplementary vitamins unnecessary. Obviously there are special needs for infants and children, pregnant women and nursing mothers, and people who are ill. These require advice from a physician.

Recommendations about diet are widespread. They can be found regularly in newspapers and magazines, on the backs of cereal boxes, in advertising circulars, and on radio and television. We are all subjected to a barrage of diet information, much of it self-serving, some of it misleading. The consequence is often anxiety and confusion, sometimes even bodily harm.

Using common sense and good judgment based on facts is the only requirement for planning proper nourishment.

Basic nutrition. The appropriate amounts of proteins, carbohydrates, fats, vitamins, and trace elements, all in sufficient quantity, are present in any prudent diet. All these elements are needed, as chapter 19 explains. But sometimes people who are misguided adopt diets that overemphasize one element or another. The Food and Nutrition Board of the National Research Council has concluded:

"We are aware of no convincing evidence of unique health benefits accruing from consumption of a large excess of any one nutrient."

Any claims that excessive amounts of foods or vitamins will cure diseases are likely to be wrong, and should be looked at with skepticism. False beliefs of this nature simply delay proper diagnosis and treatment.

Calories are the fuel that the machinery of the body needs to operate. If we take in too few calories we lose weight, and if we continue to do so, the result is illness and starvation. Consuming too many calories, on the other hand, produces obesity and may lead to disease. The balance is not difficult to maintain. Use of a simple bathroom scale is sufficient to tell us whether we are taking in too many calories or not enough.

What ideal weight should we strive for? Guidelines for reasonable weight for adults are related to height and body build. Those published by the U.S. Department of Agriculture are shown in a chart in chapter 19, but they are only a rough measure. There is no need to seek compulsively to remain within these figures.

An average woman engaged in a normal amount of physical activity needs about 2,000 calories daily. Men, because they have larger frames, require about 2,700. This rough guide varies widely, depending on age and energy expenditure. Active, growing teenagers need more calories, and sedentary elderly people need fewer. The variables of illness, pregnancy, and lactation require a doctor's guidance, as do the needs of growing children.

Proteins are the materials used by the body to form most of the molecules needed in biological activity. Growth and development of the individual, virtually all biological functions, and the basic structure of all cells require protein.

The quality and amount of protein we eat is therefore of major importance. The bulk of protein in the American diet comes from meat, fish, eggs, milk, and milk products. Other food sources are certain fruits, nuts, beans, vegetables, and grains. At least one-third of daily protein intake should be derived from animal sources, including eggs and dairy products. That is because certain vital materials, the so-called essential amino acids, cannot be obtained in a purely vegetarian diet (see chapter 19).

How much we eat each day should vary with individual taste, energy demand, health, and age. About 15 percent of the calories in a proper diet should be protein.

Carbohydrates. Almost half of the calories in the typical American diet come from carbohydrates, found in grains and root vegetables. Sugar is a pure carbohydrate. By and large, carbohydrates are inexpensive, easily digested, and serve as a major source of energy for all bodily activity.

Carbohydrates are necessary to a balanced diet. Despite poorly informed comments to the contrary, it is important to include substantial amounts in the foods you eat. Potatoes, bread, pasta, and certain root vegetables are good examples.

There has been concern expressed about the hazards of using sugar. Although excessive use of sugar is unwise, eating reasonable amounts is acceptable. Sugar occurs naturally in many substances. When added during cooking it makes certain foods taste better. Giving children heavily sugared packaged cereal is excessive, but unless sugar is prohibited by your doctor, it is reasonable to enjoy your share of cookies and cake.

Fats contain basic materials essential to good health. They are found widely in the food chain and contribute about 35 percent of the calories in a sound diet. Fats are stored in the body and serve as a reservoir to be drawn upon when needed. They are carriers of fat-soluble vitamins, and they provide much of the taste and flavor in our foods.

The relationship of disease to certain fatty substances such as cholesterol remains controversial in scientific circles, and should not be regarded as proven. While prudence may dictate that we limit our intake of high-cholesterol foods such as beef or eggs, there is no proof that by so doing we will improve our health. Cholesterol itself is a normal component of the body, related closely to vitamin D and to major hormones.

Vitamins are naturally occurring chemical compounds necessary for proper functioning of the body. Quantities required are small and are obtained easily from the foods we eat. Only in peculiar conditions of illness, bizarre diets, or the special needs of infancy, childhood, pregnancy, and lactation are vitamin supplements useful.

If vitamin pills and capsules are eaten by people on normal diets the substances are simply wasted, excreted in the stool and urine. Indeed, certain vitamins taken in excess can cause physical symptoms and illness.

It is important to realize that a large manufacturing and advertising industry is devoted to the promotion of vitamin use. There are widespread claims that doses of these substances are necessary for good health, attractive appearance, sexual potency, and treatment of disease. For normal, healthy people who eat a balanced diet, these claims are likely to be false.

Fad diets. Extensively promoted and advertised weight loss diets, including those written by physicians, should be looked at with caution. Some are based on acceptable scientific principles, but others are not thought through carefully and may be hazardous.

Before starting on a crash diet, take time to decide whether your own good judgment has been used. If in doubt, check with your doctor.

EXERCISE

Keeping your body fit pays off with increased vigor and appetite for life. We should value exercise for the pleasure it provides, the companionship it may offer, and the calories it can lose for us. However, exercise in itself does not prolong life, and it may shorten life if we use bad judgment.

A sensible exercise program is designed to fit conditions of age and body. Obviously, an 18-year-old man is likely to be more robust physically than an 80-year-old woman, yet an exercise program is feasible for each.

For people who are not in trim when the exercise program starts, the key element is a gradual increase in effort. The muscles, tendons, and joints of mature adults usually have lost some of youth's flexibility. Unless they are slowly brought into shape, injury can result from sudden use. Beyond this, sudden maximum effort by the untrained body places a strenuous demand on the heart. It may not be able to pump blood fast enough to meet the body's demands, or satisfy its own need for blood through the coronary arteries.

Good judgment dictates a graduated exercise program. Walking and swimming are excellent forms of exercise to start with, and safe (assuming you know how to swim). Pace and time should be slowly increased to the point of maximum satisfaction. Roughly an hour of vigorous activity a day for average adults is a reasonable goal. Beyond this, the exercise program becomes a goal in itself, rather than simply part of daily life.

Exercise is beneficial for all body components. The heart and lungs, of course, are stimulated by a properly planned program to function at a more efficient level. Muscles, joints, and even bones become stronger.

After illness, the careful use of exercise to regain strength is appropriate when planned with a physician. This is a common concern of patients with coronary artery disease who have had heart attacks. Research has shown that coronary patients, if guided properly, can achieve vigorous activity safely, depending on the extent of heart muscle damage.

REST AND SLEEP

No one knows how much sleep the human body requires. Elaborate experiments have shown that, removed from the stimulus of the clock or the sun, people still sleep about eight hours out of 24. But whether this amount is learned behavior or biologically dictated is not known.

We do know that regular amounts of restful sleep are as important for good health as food and exercise. Experiments also have shown that when people are kept awake for long periods, they lose their capacity to perform simple tasks. We all know from experience that we do not think as clearly when sleepy. We also know that chronically fatigued people are more vulnerable to illness. The body-building mechanisms of sleep may be related to the levels of certain chemicals and hormones, which have been demonstrated to vary with the clock (see chapter 16, "The Hormones and Endocrine Glands"). Regardless of the explanation, regular hours of sleep must be built into a health program. We should not sleep only when there is nothing else to do.

Adequate rest is obviously important in maintaining normal health. Persistent attempts to work excessive hours are self-defeating. An exhausted mind and a tired body cannot carry out first-quality tasks. If overwork is taken to an extreme, our body machinery simply breaks down.

STRESS AND EMOTIONS

Psychological stability is essential to health. We put ourselves at risk when we place excessive emotional stress upon ourselves. Although it is true that we achieve nothing in life unless we make rigorous demands upon our abilities and use our skills and experience fully, it is equally true that there are limits to the pressures we can tolerate.

Preventing psychological breakdown requires a realistic assessment of our abilities and the nature of the tasks we face. To maintain equilibrium demands that each of us have a good level of self-understanding, and the willingness to seek professional counseling when we need it.

SMOKING, DRUGS AND ALCOHOL

People ingest a variety of foreign substances. Some are clearly more harmful than others (see chapter 33, "Drugs and Medicines"). Avoiding misuse of these substances is important in maintaining health.

Smoking

Cigarette smoking is hazardous. Any controversy was effectively ended by the publication of the U.S. Surgeon General's Report on Smoking and Health in 1964. Evidence of the hazards continues to grow, revealing that:
• Cigarette smokers have substantially higher rates of death and disability than their non-smoking counterparts. This means that smokers tend to die earlier and have more days of disability than comparable non-smokers.
• A substantial number of early deaths and excess disability cases would not have occurred if those affected had never smoked.
• Fetal injury can occur if pregnant women smoke.

It is established that the most common type of lung cancer occurs most frequently in cigarette smokers. Emphysema and chronic bronchitis, two forms of potentially disabling lung disease, are clearly made worse by smoking. Further, coronary disease is associated with cigarette smoking. The nicotine that enters the bloodstream with each puff stimulates the heart, and a heart already burdened by illness is forced repeatedly to beat harder uselessly.

Pipe or cigar smokers face lesser risks, according to careful studies. Pipe smokers face a small increased incidence of cancer of the mouth and throat. Beyond this, pipes and cigars are benign, as long as the smoker does not inhale. If tobacco smoke from any source is inhaled, health hazards rise.

Effects on others. Smokers must realize that the fumes they produce can be hazardous to persons around them. This is not simply a question of social amenity and common courtesy to non-smokers. People who suffer eye and throat irritation from the smoke of others quite properly have a right to feel abused. Non-smokers who are ill with heart or lung disease can be made sicker by inhaling smoke-filled air.

This matter is a public issue, recognized for years by the airlines, and more recently by legislators who have adopted regulations limiting the rights of smokers in public areas. Many states and cities have concluded that the personal habits of smokers should be controlled so others are not forced to inhale polluted air.

In addition, the psychological impact of smoking on an impressionable child should be considered. The image of maturity and wisdom in the eyes of a child is, of course, likely to be a beloved and respected adult. Children are great imitators. Rational parents who do not wish their children to smoke should not smoke themselves.

Why do people smoke? The reasons people give for smoking are various, imaginative, and clever. They reflect fully the human capacity for self-delusion. An opinion sample taken a few years ago among 1,200 hospital employees revealed the following ingenious defenses for smoking:
• "Polluted air is more hazardous to the lungs than smoking, yet no one urges that we stop breathing."
• "I've been smoking so long that the damage has already been done."
• "The pleasure I get, which is certain, outweighs the health hazard, which is uncertain."
• "We don't stop the use of alcohol or automobiles, yet they are more dangerous than cigarettes."
• "You can prove anything by statistics."

Stopping smoking. The decision to stop will be effective only when based on strong motivation. The beneficial result must be worth the pain. This is a tough challenge for any confirmed smoker, and fully deserves the help of family and friends. The support groups that exist in many communities can be useful. Behavior modification methods work for many people. For some, there is no way to stop except to stop abruptly.

Drug Abuse

People ingest potent chemicals in liquid, solid, and gaseous forms through every orifice of the body and by penetrating the skin. This is often done for a defensible and approved purpose under a physician's direction, but using drugs to alter one's psychological mood is widespread.

Drugs that change mood have been taken since man has been able to put hand to mouth. Although the use and abuse of manufactured drugs is largely an event of the last 100 years, our ingenuity as a species has allowed us to extract active substances from plants for centuries. Coffee, tobacco, and alcohol are commonly used examples. While each of these can be hazardous, we do have the advantage of understanding clearly how they work on the body, and the ability to measure the quantity of active chemical agent we absorb. Further, we are protected against contamination by foreign material because these three products are sold legitimately, subject to governmental control and inspection. None of these protections apply to drugs purchased or sold illegally. We are at the mercy of the pusher.

Because the human capacity for self-delusion about the value and safety of drugs is so widespread, and because with money and determination people can obtain whatever they wish, we must assume that drug abuse will remain a problem in our society.

If you are tempted to use these chemicals, at a minimum you should have some understanding of drug effects and hazards.

What is abuse? Drug abuse is non-medical use of drugs for the purpose of altering the user's mood, producing novel experiences, or changing his perception of himself and the world around him.

To understand drug abuse, we must recognize that ingesting these chemicals alters our connection with reality. An artificial and distorted image of the world is imposed upon our minds. In essence, we dream our lives away.

Physical effects. Generally, drugs are sought for their effect upon the psyche. Physical effects also may occur, however. These range from virtually unnoticeable increases in heart rate and blood pressure after taking stimulants to extreme changes in consciousness level—and perhaps death—from overdose of depressants.

Classification of Drugs

A vast number of drugs affect the mind and are subject to abuse. One way to classify them is by their major effect, although there are numerous areas of overlap. The confusion is magnified when people take several drugs simultaneously.

Narcotics relieve pain, but are abused for the highly pleasurable sensation that may accompany their prime use. Taking any narcotic carries the risk of addiction. Addiction means that withdrawal from the drug (stopping its use) produces discomfort and sometimes an uncontrollable compulsion to take more.

Drugs such as morphine, Demerol,® and codeine are of great value for their pain-killing effects, but of great risk when abused.

Opium and heroin use is almost entirely illegal, although a few scientific investigations are taking place.

Methadone is legally supplied to heroin addicts in organized programs designed to wean them away from the more hazardous drug. The results vary, but one unfortunate consequence has been the appearance of methadone on the illegal market. Another legitimate use of methadone, when mixed with other approved drugs, is the control of certain kinds of pain in cancer patients.

Sedatives. A large number of substances are used to depress brain function. These include barbiturates and other sleep inducers, tranquilizers, inhalants such as gasoline and glue, and alcohol. The latter is of major importance, and is discussed at length elsewhere in this chapter.

All of these, of course, can be used for legitimate purposes. Sleeping pills, taken under a doctor's direction, are sometimes useful. The value of tranquilizers is more debatable, but they have occasional medical value. Gasoline and volatile glues, of course, have purposes totally outside medicine. And yet this diverse group has important elements in common:
• Addiction potential.
• Withdrawal symptoms physically more dangerous than those associated with narcotics.
• Production of calmness followed by sleep, and by death from failure to breathe when taken in excessive amounts.
• Increased hazard when mixed, especially the combination of alcohol and other sedatives. The effect of each is multiplied significantly.

It is a tribute to the ease with which human beings fool themselves that some of these drugs are taken for their excitatory effect. Sniffing glue, for instance, produces a brief jag, but then somnolence. Alcohol, although it loosens inhibitions, also depresses bodily functions, so that desire cannot be fulfilled, and is instead subdued by sleep.

Stimulants. Amphetamines and cocaine were once in vogue for treatment of physical disorders. Cocaine was used as a local anesthetic in the care of eye diseases, and amphetamines were used to suppress appetite in obese people. When abused, a common effect is a rapid onset of euphoria and grandiose thinking. The immediate danger is a potential for aggressive, violent behavior, followed by the possibility of psychosis. This form of insanity is similar to classical paranoid schizophrenia, with delusions of persecution and hallucinations. Return to normal may occur within a week, but some people remain disturbed.

Hallucinogens. A vast number of substances cause hallucinations. These include marijuana and similar drugs, LSD, and a group of abused substances with names that shift and change as fads come and go.

Marijuana causes feelings of relaxation and ease, similar to alcohol intoxication. Emotions are enhanced and all seems more profound.

The hazards of marijuana, hashish, and THC, depend, first of all, on the circumstances in which users place themselves. To be out of control or in a borderline state of judgment requires a proper environment for safety.

Beyond this, carefully controlled scientific studies have shown that heavy use of marijuana distorts perceptions and interferes moderately with fine hand coordination. Possibly it hampers immediate memory and intellectual function, and decreases levels of male sex hormone. The question of damage to chromosomes and the genetic structure of future children of users remains unclear. It is certain that use of marijuana by pregnant women poses a risk to the fetus.

LSD is usually taken by mouth. It causes a marked change in the user's sense of the surrounding world. Feelings of unreality, changes in color, size, and shape of familiar objects, and other delusions abound. Poor judgment follows.

The common psychosis of LSD use, with delusions, usually lasts up to 48 hours. It abates spontaneously, but occasionally an episode can last for weeks. More severe episodes of psychosis with homicidal or suicidal behavior have occurred rarely, apparently caused by highly believable hallucinations. Convulsions are rare.

The most well-known hazard is the so-called "bad trip." This is manifested by uncontrollable fear and panic, with a belief that insanity is impending.

Other drugs used for hallucinogenic effects include several chemical structures known by their initials (DMT, DET, DOM). Others are peyote and mescaline, obtained from cactus, and medications such as atropine and sco-

polamine, which in proper dosage can be taken safely for clinical purposes, but are abused for their side effects.

Beyond the ability to cause hallucinations, all these substances accelerate the heart rate, increase blood pressure, and diminish appetite.

Pregnant women must recognize the possibility that any of these drugs taken without proper medical advice may cause harm to the fetus.

Complications of injection. Beyond the physical and psychological effects, specific diseases and health problems may result from the injection of drugs. Puncturing the skin may allow bacteria to enter the body. Because drug users do not always observe sterile technique, infection is commonplace. The consequences range in severity from abscess formation, a painful but treatable matter, to potentially fatal diseases such as tetanus and bacterial endocarditis (inflammation of the lining of the heart).

Certain forms of hepatitis, a virus disease of the liver, are transmitted by shared needles or syringes. A microscopic quantity of contaminated blood from a hepatitis carrier is sufficient to cause disease when injected into other people (see chapter 20, "The Digestive System").

Veins used as injection sites may become inflamed and allow clotted blood to deposit. Clots can break off as solid matter (emboli), flow through the bloodstream into the heart, and plug a blood vessel in the lung. Obviously, this can be life-threatening.

Drugs obtained from pushers (illicit sellers) are an unknown. It is not possible to judge accurately the quantity, quality, or purity. As a result, users are frequently misled either through the purchase of inert or contaminated material, chemicals that are improperly labeled, or dosages measured inaccurately. The danger of death from overdose is obvious.

Alcohol

Drinking of alcohol is a common social custom in the Western world, including the United States. Drinking has long been associated with festive occasions, and has even had a place in medicine (see chapter 20, "The Digestive System"). When misused, however, alcohol can produce personal and social consequences of grave import. We all realize the potential damage of alcohol abuse, but often we fail to grapple effectively with this issue in our lives. It is vital that we each preserve for ourselves full opportunity to make intelligent and educated choices about the use of alcohol, so that we can avoid unfortunate results based on ignorance. In order to exercise proper self-control, we need to have a clear understanding of the results of drinking on our physical and emotional health, on our families, our associates at work, and on the society we live in.

Who is an alcoholic? Is excessive drinking a disease or is it the result of a moral defect? This is a hotly debated issue in the medical and social service communities. In any case, we must define the term "alcoholism" before we can obtain a genuine understanding of the problem, which may lead to treatment and cure.

Anyone who repeatedly drinks alcoholic beverages to the point of loss of control is an alcoholic. Note that this definition covers a wide range of people, including skid-row derelicts, housewives, blue collar workers, executives, and elected officials. It may well include friends, family members, and you.

It is a paradox that we often drink to obtain the supposed stimulating effect of alcohol when in fact alcohol depresses body function. There is loss of inhibition but decreased ability to act out our wishes.

How many alcoholics? About seven percent of the people in the U.S. are considered problem drinkers, and some 100,000 people die in this country yearly from alcohol-related causes. This is a singular tragedy, because most of these deaths can be prevented. As pointed out by Joseph Califano when he was secretary of the U.S. Department of Health, Education and Welfare:

> "No other disease exacts such a fearful economic cost. Billions of dollars in direct health care costs, in lost productivity and unemployment, in auto accidents, violent crimes, fires, social service costs. Informed estimates put the economic costs of problem drinking at more than $40 billion each year. Put another way, we all pick up the tab for the three-martini lunch, and the tab is $40 billion."

There are roughly 10 million adult Americans with a drinking problem, including about two million women. The adolescents who drink too much number several million.

Warning Signs of Alcoholism

The urge to drink in tense situations.
Inappropriate behavior when drinking.
Drinking when alone.
Drinking early in the day.
The need to drink in order to function.
Gradual increase in regular alcohol intake.
Mixing drinking and driving.

Consequences of Drinking

The abuse of alcohol leads to a number of problems, but among the most apparent are disease, injuries, suicides, and violence to others, including murder.

Injury. Because drinking causes loss of judgment, people injure themselves more easily when drunk than sober. This is a major issue in industry, and applies particularly to drivers. The toll of injury and death from automobile accidents caused by drinking is more than notable. Remember. "If you drive, don't drink. If you drink, don't drive."

Suicide. There is a high suicide rate among alcoholics compared to the general population. The reasons are unclear, but either depression leads to drinking and ends in self-destruction, or alcoholism itself creates suicidal wishes.

Violence to others. Investigation of people who commit major criminal acts against others shows a high incidence of alcoholism. Murder, assault, rape, and child beating in significant proportion are included. The loss of personal control caused by drinking is in part responsible.

Disease. Alcohol, when ingested and metabolized by the body, forms by-products that can damage major organs. The pleasure of feeling well is lost, and life-span is decreased.

The liver is a key target. Alcohol can cause fatty changes that enlarge the liver, leading in some cases to scarring of the organ. This condition is called cirrhosis and results in jaundice, bleeding, and death (see chapter 20, "The Digestive System").

Heart disease is also a major consequence of alcoholism. A poisoning effect takes place in the heart muscle, resulting in disordered heart action (see chapter 3, "The Heart and Circulation"). A different and more common cardiac problem, coronary artery disease, also is more frequent among alcoholics.

Cancer occurs more commonly among heavy drinkers than in the general population. Malignancies of the esophagus, stomach, liver, and lungs increase. These are among the least curable of cancers.

Alcohol also can damage the brain. Decrease of intellectual ability, with loss of memory and ability to concentrate, is common among alcoholics.

In addition, specific types of insanity may occur, as well as loss of control over eye muscles controlled by the brain. Easily recognized early symptoms of heavy drinking, such as tremors and convulsions, may lead to delirium tremens, or DTs, a disorder which may include hallucinations and which has a fatality rate of up to 20 percent.

Drinking in pregnancy. Any ingestion of alcohol by a pregnant woman causes a measurable risk to the fetus. The accompanying table, prepared by Dr. Ruth Little, makes the point.

Level of Alcohol Use and Risks to Fetus

"Regular" Social Drinking
(2 or more drinks daily)

  Intrauterine growth retardation

  Increased risk of birth defects

  Behavioral effects in the newborn and infant

  Increased risk of stillbirth

  Decreased placental weight

"Binge" Drinking
(5 or more drinks on occasion)

  Structural brain abnormalities

Very Heavy Drinking
(a quart of alcohol daily)

  Fetal alcohol syndrome

The full-blown fetal alcohol syndrome causes poor growth of the fetus and the newborn. Abnormalities of head and face structure, joint, limb, and heart abnormalities, and mental deficiency are part of the picture.

Drinking presents a danger to the pregnant woman, too. The combination of a few drinks and the swaybacked posture of pregnancy may make her unsteady on her feet, leading to the possibility of a dangerous fall.

Treatment of Alcohol Problems

Help is available for the treatment of alcoholism. The essential prerequisite is motivation on the part of the alcoholic to stop drinking.

Alcoholics Anonymous (AA). AA is the single most effective alcoholism recovery program in terms of numbers of people who have been helped to stop drinking. AA defines itself as a "worldwide fellowship of men and women who help each other maintain sobriety and who offer to share their recovery experience freely with others who may have a drinking problem."

The only requirement for membership is a desire to stop drinking. The organization stresses that it does not furnish the initial motivation for alcoholics to stop drinking or try to control its members. It does not provide "drying out treatment," nursing services, or hospital treatment. Nor does it offer spiritual or religious services, engage in education or propaganda about alcohol, provide social services, or domestic or vocational counseling. It accepts no money for its services, and no contributions from non-AA sources.

AA meetings take place in virtually all areas of this country.

Professional counseling. Psychologists, psychiatrists, pastors, and other professionally trained therapists may be an asset to alcoholics. This is likely when drinking is a result of personal strain that can be relieved by counseling. As in any other form of treatment, the first step is self-awareness. Once this has been accomplished, methods other than getting drunk can be sought to solve the problems of life. The counseling process may include participation by family members.

Federal and state programs. Through the Veterans Administration (VA) and state mental hospitals, thousands of people with drinking problems receive help each year. At the VA, eligible veterans get treatment for acute episodes of drinking and long-term follow-up counseling, both without charge. At the state hospital level, the bulk of care is simple confinement, but some institutions provide group therapy and educational resources.

Voluntary and proprietary hospitals. Most hospitals lack cohesive treatment programs for alcoholics. Although many hospital beds are occupied by alcoholics, institutions usually concentrate on treating the medical complications of drinking rather than the underlying cause. There are exceptions, however. Some major voluntary hospitals have developed in-patient units for alcoholics, associated with comprehensive treatment programs. A number of institutions run for profit also cater specifically to people with drinking problems. Before seeking help at any proprietary program, always obtain references from knowledgeable people. Your physician, clergyman, or even the local Better Business Bureau may have important information.

YOUR PHYSICIAN

As part of a sound health program, it is important to have a physician who knows you and your situation. An understanding between patient and doctor must be consistent and long-term in order to achieve the following goals:

- Patient and family education on how to stay healthy and fit.
- Application of preventive medical techniques, including immunizations.
- Family counseling.
- Regular physical assessment.
- Availability during acute illness.
- Treatment as needed.

Finding a doctor. We all want a physician who is both competent and responsive. Word of mouth from trustworthy friends and relatives is a likely basis for referral. Another useful source of information is the local hospital of good reputation where lists of available staff physicians are often maintained.

Large-scale group practices, such as the Kaiser-Permanente program in the Western states, and the Health Insurance Plan (HIP) in the East, supply family physicians.

Hospital out-patient departments, conducted by most large inner-city institutions, serve the needs of many people. Health maintenance organizations (HMOs) guide people in staying healthy and treat them when sick.

When seeking a new medical contact, a preliminary visit to the doctor is valuable. This permits you to evaluate the physician, judge whether you and he or she are compatible, and ask questions about such matters as fees, hospital affiliation, house calls, and telephone hours. At the same time, the doctor has a chance to learn whether you take a responsible attitude toward maintaining your health, and whether you will be someone he or she finds comfortable to work with.

When to see the doctor. Routine visits to the physician's office should be planned to meet the age and health status of each person.

Pregnant women, for instance, and healthy infants require regular appointments for assessment. Without close observation, the incidence of miscarriage, stillbirth, and failure of babies to thrive increases.

During childhood, adolescence, and adulthood, when most people are healthy, a base-touching visit to the doctor should be scheduled on a regular basis, the interval depending on physician's advice. Contact should be frequent enough to allow doctor and patient to know each other. Perhaps once each year is a sound schedule. Beyond this, people become strangers.

The value of these visits when in good health includes the opportunity for the doctor to find hidden diseases and begin early treatment. In addition, regular review of personal habits— use of alcohol, tobacco, drugs, medications, eating, and exercise—can help avoid potential harmful effects.

When to call the doctor. During illness, no matter how mild, you will begin to wonder whether a telephone call to the doctor will be useful. Should the call be made? When?

In people whose basic health is normal, minor symptoms, such as those of the common cold, should not require urgent contact with a doctor. On the other hand, if the patient already is chronically ill, new symptoms should be viewed with concern.

Parts of the body are especially vulnerable. A quick call to the doctor is important after a head injury, eye damage, or other accidents. Some communities have a paramedical service to handle such cases (see chapter 35, "First Aid"). A doctor also should be called for chest pain, which may indicate a heart attack, and for marked shortness of breath.

The general rule: When in doubt, call.

The value of asking questions. Unless you are fully informed, you cannot effectively take responsibility for maintaining your own health. A basic knowledge of the human body, through standard educational opportunities, is available to all of us. Reliable magazines and books like this one are useful. However, when more complex issues arise, such as those related to fertility, pregnancy, lactation, care of infant and child, or diagnosis and treatment of disease, asking questions of your doctor is the key to understanding.

Common areas of confusion concern diet, medications, and preparation for medical tests. Unless you comprehend the instructions, everybody's effort is wasted, and prospects for good health are diminished. Don't hesitate to ask, and be certain that you understand what you are told. You have a right to know, not simply an abstract right, but a practical one, necessary for you to participate properly in any treatment plan.

When in doubt, ask.

Patient rights and responsibilities. You have a right to ask questions, to receive answers, and to understand every aspect of treatment and diagnosis. You need this information in order to care for yourself properly. Your doctor should cooperate happily with you in providing it. Most doctors prefer working with well-informed patients because the likelihood of successful treatment is enhanced.

You have responsibility as well to yourself. In an important sense, your doctor is your partner in preserving your health. Be open and frank. If medications and treatment are prescribed, if advice about health habits is offered, it is useless to pretend that you will cooperate if you have no such intention. Your doctor is of value to you only if you carry out intelligently and consistently the health care plan you have worked out together.

It is also your responsibility to avoid obvious risks to health. You have yourself to blame, for instance, if you are injured in an automobile accident while not wearing a seat belt. Similar obvious tasks include safety-proofing the house if infants or young children are present. Stairs should be protected by gates, medication enclosed in proper containers, cleaning materials and other potentially poisonous substances kept out of reach of children.

For people of advanced age, side rails may be necessary on beds, and supports may be placed at the bathtub to avoid falls.

MEDICATIONS

The use of any medication, prescription or nonprescription, must be taken seriously. The chemicals contained in drugs have great potential both for good and harm. The instructions of the prescribing physician should be understood and followed with care. By all means, ask questions if you are uncertain about any aspect of drug treatment.

When to use medications. Many routine ailments are curable without drugs of any kind. It is not in your interest, for example, to insist that your doctor prescribe antibiotics for simple upper respiratory infections. Illnesses such as the common cold are caused by viruses. Penicillin and other antibiotics do not affect them, and may provoke side effects. (On the other hand, a doctor may prescribe an antibiotic to avoid possible bacterial complications in viral illnesses.) To take potent drugs pointlessly is risky and foolish. You are likely to face more hazard from the treatment than the disease.

Once a medication is prescribed, be certain that you understand the instructions clearly. Obviously, this means knowing the exact dosage and the frequency and length of treatments. It also includes such simple questions as whether to take drugs before or after meals. Some drugs are absorbed properly only when the stomach is empty. Others need to be taken with food, or should follow a meal.

Some medications, such as antibiotics, are commonly used only for the duration of the illness. But if prescribed for a specific length of time, they should be continued even if symptoms disappear. Others need to be taken for prolonged periods, and some must be taken for a lifetime, such as digitalis for heart treatment and insulin for diabetes mellitus. Therefore, be sure that you understand whether drug prescriptions are to be renewed.

Medications are to be used only for the patient. Never assume that a pill or capsule prescribed for a friend or neighbor is right for you, and don't believe that you do a favor for friends by giving them your drugs. The chance of doing harm is simply too great.

Side effects and drug allergies. Make sure that your doctor knows your history of problems with medications, including allergic reactions, before prescriptions are written. It is sensible to keep a record on your person of allergies and other side effects from previous treatments. When seeing a new doctor, one of the first points you should make is to enter this information on your new medical record. This is the best way to avoid inadvertent use of medicines that are wrong for you.

Medication control. Medicine bottles should be labeled clearly with the name of the drug, the patient and the doctor, the dosage and frequency. This information may be unexpectedly useful if questions arise later.

Drugs can become outdated, so ask the pharmacist to date the label if he or she does not automatically do so. Otherwise you may take deteriorated or ineffective medicine.

You should be able to obtain from your doctor or druggist information prepared by the drug manufacturer about prescribed drugs. In some cases, printed materials are included with the drugs. This can be useful in understanding the value, proper handling, and potential dangers of the prescription. Books are available for laymen describing commonly used medications.

Safety precautions. When people take more than one medication, possibility of error exists. If a patient has poor vision or is mentally confused by illness, even greater potential for harm arises. Drug containers should have large, easy-to-read labels, or color coding. It may help to place daily doses in separate glasses or receptacles and use check-off lists. If necessary, medication should be taken under supervision.

Pregnant women should be especially cautious. No medication can be taken safely without clearance from a doctor. The fetus may be injured. The same precaution applies to breast-feeding mothers, because chemicals may enter the milk.

Protecting babies and young children from accidental drug ingestion is a high priority. Accidental poisoning remains a leading cause of death in preschool years. Be certain that medications are properly sealed or have childproof caps, and keep them safely out of reach. Remember, pills and capsules may look colorful, glittering, and attractive to children. Keep temptation out of the way.

Never refer to a child's medicine as "candy" or try to coax him or her into taking it with comments about how good it tastes. This only creates confusion, and may lead to disaster.

Sleeping pills, sedatives, and tranquilizers. The tendency to feel that there is a pill to solve every problem has led many of us to depend on sedatives, tranquilizers, and similar drugs. Our bodies and minds are structured to survive the stress of daily life without the use of chemicals. In an important sense, the use of drugs that obliterate our direct connection with reality is a weak way of avoiding important issues. Problems are not solved, merely avoided temporarily.

These drugs can be dangerous. Dependency, even addiction, may occur. Overdoses may cause death, particularly if taken with alcohol, when even small amounts can be fatal.

Under ordinary circumstances these drugs should be avoided, and certainly never used without a physician's advice. Under unusual and temporary circumstances, or during illness, there may be reason for them. Basically, it pays to remember that nature is on your side. You can solve the problem, you can sleep, and you can do so without being drugged.

HOSPITALIZATION
AND HEALTH INSURANCE

Part of a good health program is to be ready for emergencies, including the financial ones, of sudden illness. In the complex world of modern medicine, it is essential that you have insurance to cover major expenses. Hospitalization now costs several hundred dollars per day in some institutions, and considerably more in special units such as intensive care.

Hospital expense insurance through Blue Cross plans or commercial insurance carriers can be obtained through your place of work or by individual contract. A local insurance agent is a basic source of information if necessary.

An additional plan to cover doctor fees, the cost of registered nurses, and other benefits is also worth considering. This, too, may be available as an employee benefit through Blue Shield or other carriers, or it may be obtained privately.

In addition to these plans, a form of overall coverage usually known as a major medical policy may be a valuable benefit. This fills in the gaps in other coverages.

Medicare. This is federally funded comprehensive health insurance under the sponsorship of the Social Security system. It is available to almost all people over the age of 65, and to persons totally and permanently disabled. Part A of Medicare covers hospital cost of a semi-private room. Part B covers physicians' fees and has some other benefits. Be certain to obtain both parts when you apply.

Medicaid. This form of health insurance, sponsored by most states, is available to people whose income places them below established levels. Most people eligible for welfare benefits may also obtain Medicaid coverage. Check with your local welfare office.

General rules. Obtain copies of your insurance papers and read them carefully. Understand the benefits you are entitled to, be aware of the exclusions and of the deductible provisions that may apply. If in doubt, ask questions. After you become ill it is too late to make changes.

CHAPTER 2   MICHAEL M. KABACK, M.D.

MEDICAL
GENETICS

We all begin life with our future partially programmed. In every cell of our bodies we carry specialized material called genes, a legacy from each of our parents. These genes influence and sometimes dictate many aspects of what we are and will become. They determine what kind of body build we have, the color of our eyes, whether our hair is curly or straight. There is controversy over whether they shape our intelligence, too.

Genes have an important impact on lifelong health. Genetics, the study of the genes and their role in the development of organisms, is a rapidly expanding area of research, and not all the answers are known about its influence on our medical history. It is suspected, for instance, that genes partially determine not only how our cells develop but when they wear out. Heredity may explain why members of one family develop cataracts, diabetes, or arthritis at age 60, while members of another family are not afflicted until 90. Our genes probably play some part in cancer, heart disease, perhaps even our susceptibility to the common cold.

In other chapters, the hereditary aspects of certain diseases and abnormalities are discussed. This chapter discusses medical genetics, the study of conditions present at birth or evident shortly afterwards that affect the health and welfare of the child.

GENETICS AND INFANCY

Every parent wonders before a child is born, "Will my baby be normal?" Usually the newcomer turns out to be 100 percent perfect in the eyes of the parents (although a more exacting and unbiased eye might detect a trifling or easily correctable imperfection of little consequence).

Relatively few prospective parents or couples contemplating marriage have the slightest reason to undergo exhaustive tests and genetic studies to assess the potential liabilities of offspring. However, there is reasonable cause for concern if a couple has already borne an infant with a birth defect, or if an obviously hereditary trait recurs in direct bloodlines. In addition, there are other times when, because of parental age, ethnic background, or certain reproductive problems such as three or more spontaneous miscarriages, consultation with a physician can be helpful.

Often the conversation itself is enough. The family physician or obstetrician can give answers that are often comforting. For example, the doctor can assure the brother of a person with hemophilia, a hereditary inability of the blood to clot, that he cannot transmit the disease to his offspring. The doctor can assure a couple that cerebral palsy due to premature birth or birth injury is not hereditary. Diagnosis and treatment of the most frequent forms of congenital disease are within the physician's area of competence. The small number of patients who need special help can be referred to genetic counselors and specialists.

About 3,000 disorders, too many and too rare to be enumerated, have been identified as hereditary. Probably most diseases have a genetic component, if all the facts were known, but there are still great gaps in knowledge. Medical geneticists cannot give hard and fast answers to every question. Sometimes answers are immensely consoling, sometimes qualified. Often, risks can be stated only in rather cold terms of mathematical odds. But in almost every instance, a more informed basis can be reached upon which decisions about having children can be made.

Congenital or Hereditary

A congenital abnormality is one that is present at birth. It is not necessarily hereditary, which means not necessarily transmitted by germ cells of the parents.

Accidental birth defects are not inherited and almost certainly will not be repeated in subsequent offspring. Among the causes of such accidents are birth injury, infections of the mother with German measles or toxoplasmosis during pregnancy, or her exposure during early pregnancy to drugs, toxins, or radiation, which may harmfully alter the environment of the fetus in the womb at a critical stage of development. Cerebral palsy, some forms of epilepsy, and certain types of retardation usually have an accidental cause.

Hereditary birth defects are transmitted by parental germ cells. Mathematical odds for or against repetition can usually be calculated.

Some birth defects are thought to result from extremely complex interactions of genes and environment. The more complex the genetics of a particular defect (cleft palate, heart abnormalities), the less likely it is to be repeated in offspring. Parents of a baby with a cleft palate can be told that odds are 20 to 1 against another baby with the same condition. That calculates to a five percent risk, only slightly greater than the overall risk for all birth defects combined in the general baby population.

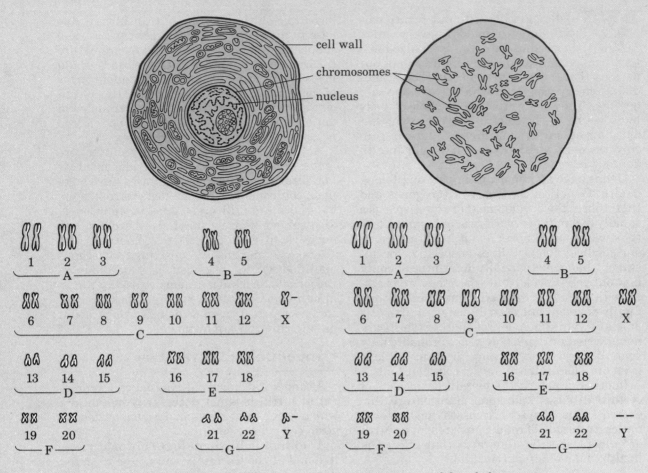

cell wall

chromosomes

nucleus

normal male karyotype

normal female karyotype

CHROMOSOMES

Chromosomes determine the heredity of every organism. The "package" of chromosomes of any organism, when analyzed, is called its karyotype. Top drawings show delicate filaments in every cell nucleus (left) that contract, segment, and form "arms," as in close-up at right. Center drawings show normal human karyotypes, each of which contains 23 pairs of chromosomes. Researchers usually classify the pairs in descending order of size and position of the arms. The 23rd pair of chromosomes determines sex. The drawing at left shows a normal male karyotype, containing a large X chromosome in the 23rd pair, and a small Y chromosome. The right drawing of a normal female karyotype has two large X chromosomes. The lower drawing shows a "banded" karyotype of a normal male. When the chromosomes are prepared and chemically stained, they can be seen under a microscope. Each pair has a unique pattern of staining (banding).

"banded" karyotype

Family susceptibility. A third category includes diseases that are not strictly hereditary but appear to have a hereditary component. They involve an inborn susceptibility or weakness that may be triggered into full-blown disease if the person is exposed to certain factors in the environment. However, some who are susceptible never develop disease. These are the diseases we usually mean when we refer to those that "run in families." Geneticists sometimes speak of the "two-hit" theory, meaning that the person is "hit" at birth with a weakened gene, but no disease will develop until a second "hit" occurs.

Thus diabetes tends to recur in families, but a potential middle-aged diabetic may never develop the disease if he or she stays physically fit and eats a well-balanced diet. Women with two or more close female relatives who had breast cancer are three times more likely to develop the disease than other women, but not every woman in this group is affected. Pernicious anemia patients inherit a predisposition to premature degeneration of the stomach membranes, and psoriasis patients inherit a tendency to excessively rapid turnover of epidermal cells.

In the future, medical genetics may play a greater role in preventive medicine by informing us early of hereditary vulnerabilities against which medical defenses may be built. Moreover, research advances in genetic engineering and gene therapy portend a future where gene replacement may be possible for selected disorders.

GENETIC BLUEPRINTS

All the directions for the structure and functioning of our bodies are contained in our chromosomes, which are composed primarily of structural protein and DNA (deoxyribonucleic acid). The DNA contains the genes. These are molecules and parts of molecules; heredity is a chemical phenomenon.

Chromosomes are threadlike particles in the nucleus of every cell. When stained and prepared, they can be seen under a microscope. Human beings normally have 46 chromosomes, comprised of 23 pairs. One chromosome in each pair comes from the mother through the egg cell. The other chromosome of each pair comes from the sperm of the father. At the time of conception, these two sets of 23 chromosomes each combine into a single cell, which develops into the new human being.

Heredity is encoded in DNA within the chromosomes. Long DNA molecules consist of

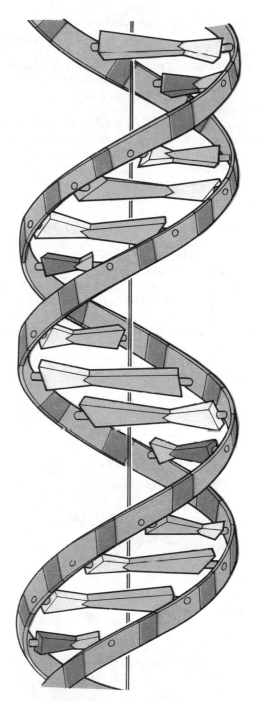

THE DOUBLE HELIX

The long molecule of DNA (deoxyribonucleic acid) that contains the human genetic code resembles a spiral stairway. The sides or rails are chains of sugar (ribose) and phosphate molecules. The steps or rungs are built of molecules of thymine, cytosine, adenine, and guanine repeated thousands of times in different sequences.

two intertwining chains coiled around a common axis, something like a spiral ladder, with thousands of connecting "rungs" or steps. The rungs are built of four rather simple chemical units, repeated thousands upon thousands of times in different sequences along the length of the chain.

A gene is a very small cluster of these units, constituting the rungs and sides of a particular tiny portion of the long DNA molecule. A gene or gene combination is a unit of heredity, specifying a particular trait, such as whether an organism will have blue or brown eyes. Collectively, genes determine whether an organism will have the organs and functions of a mouse or a man.

How can an infinitesimal group of molecules have such omnipotence? The "one gene, one enzyme" concept holds that a gene directs the assembly of an enzyme, which is a chemical catalyst essential for some body process. If a gene is defective, its associated enzyme is defective or lacking. The effect may be harmless and not apparent, or it may impose a major derangement of some body process.

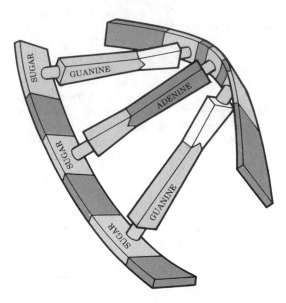

A CLOSEUP OF DNA

The DNA "ladder" shows distinctive features. Guanine always links with cytosine, thymine with adenine, to form "rungs" attached to sugar-phosphate chains, but there are different sequences of bases encoded with genetic information.

CYTOSINE   GUANINE

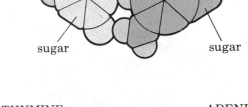

sugar   sugar

THYMINE   ADENINE

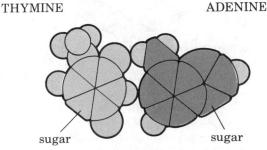

sugar   sugar

SCHEME OF A GENE

Pairs of DNA bases compose the structure of the molecule. A gene is thought to be a tiny segment of DNA in which a cluster of several base pairs activates a process of heredity, singly or in conjunction with other genes.

Gene-containing DNA imprints the genetic code upon a slightly different nucleic acid, RNA (ribonucleic acid). Forms of RNA direct the cell to manufacture specific enzymes and other proteins by linking amino-acid building blocks (at least 22 different types) in inviolable sequences. A seemingly insignificant error, such as a "wrong" amino acid in a chain of many hundreds, may have far-flung effects.

Sickle-cell trait, present in 1 in 10 American blacks, is a classic instance of a hereditary defect in the amino-acid chain (see chapter 6, "The Blood"). The hemoglobin, or oxygen-carrying red blood cell protein, of these persons contains only one "incorrect" amino acid in its sequence. The trait is benign, but a double dose, inherited from both parents, produces full-blown sickle-cell disease, a form of anemia that can be serious indeed.

How Traits Are Inherited

One of the 23 pairs of human chromosomes constitutes the sex chromosomes, designated XX in the female and XY in the male. The other 22 pairs are called autosomes and are identical in male and female. Sexual reproduction makes human variation possible by drawing upon the unique traits of parents in random ways. Whether a fetus is male or female, for instance, is a matter of chance, depending on whether a sperm carrying an X or Y fertilizes an egg. If a sperm carrying a Y chromosome unites with a maternal X (the female sex chromosome is always X), the offspring will be XY and male. An X-carrying sperm produces a girl. Thus if you predict a boy or a girl, you have a 50 percent chance of being right (or wrong). With other traits, too, genetic counselors often must state the probability of their appearance in terms of mathematical odds.

Some traits appear to be determined multigenically, which means two or more genes in combination influence whether they recur. There are other complexities and unknowns in predicting whether a trait will appear, but in general, a single gene influences a single trait. In common genetic languages, genes (and the traits they shape) are thought of as "recessive" or "dominant."

One might think of a recessive gene as "weak," unable to generate its specific enzyme, producing too little of it, or an abnormal molecule. But if it is paired with a normal gene, the latter takes over the job of influencing that particular trait and no abnormal symptoms appear. However, if recessive genes are transmitted from both parents—a "double dose"—the disorder appears in the offspring. If only one parent has a recessive gene, he or she is a carrier, but offspring will be normal. Carriers of such recessive traits are completely unaffected and their carrier state has implications only for their children.

In the case of a dominant gene, the "dose" transmitted from one parent overrides the effects of a normal matching gene from the other parent.

Most inherited metabolic diseases are transmitted recessively. The most common in the United States are sickle-cell disease and cystic fibrosis, a disease of young people in which the mucous glands are defective (see chapter 8, "The Lungs").

Dominant hereditary disorders are quite rare. They include Huntington's disease, a progressive disorder of the nervous system, and achrondoplasia, a form of dwarfism. A number of other uncommon degenerative nervous system diseases also are transmitted by dominant genes.

Conditions such as hemophilia (the so-called "bleeder's disease"), color-vision deficiency or "color blindness," and certain forms of muscular dystrophy are sex-linked. The trait is determined by the X chromosomes received from the mother. The mother is a carrier but is not affected by the disease herself. Only male offspring are affected. Statistically, half the sons of a carrier mother will be affected, and half the daughters will be carriers.

Members of a family with recessive disorders should know that both parents of an affected child are almost invariably normal. Each is a carrier, contributing the recessive gene in equal measure. Neither is more to blame than the other. Usually, both partners are completely unaware that they are carriers. Generations may have passed without the disorder's appearing in full form. And with a different partner, the disease might not have appeared now, either.

Fortunately, relatively simple tests can often be performed to determine whether other family members also carry the recessive trait. These tests can be invaluable in allaying anxieties about their own reproduction or aiding those found to be "at risk." When a recessively transmitted disease does appear in a family, it is important for other members to have these tests performed.

In cases of a dominantly transmitted disorder, only those manifesting the disease can pass it on to their offspring. Unaffected family members and their children are disease-free. However, some persons may have the dominant gene but be affected only mildly. Their offspring remain at risk. When a dominantly transmitted disease appears in a family, it is important for other family members to have a careful evaluation by a medical geneticist.

Genetic Disorders in Ethnic Groups

There are more than 100 recognized genetic disorders that occur predominantly in specified population groups. This is easily understood if we recognize that over the centuries people of ethnic, religious, racial, or national backgrounds have tended to marry and reproduce with individuals of the same ancestry. Since each of us carries a few recessive traits, certain of these genes have tended to become "inbred" within certain population groups, while other traits may be more prevalent in another group. Double doses of recessive genes and the diseases they can cause are

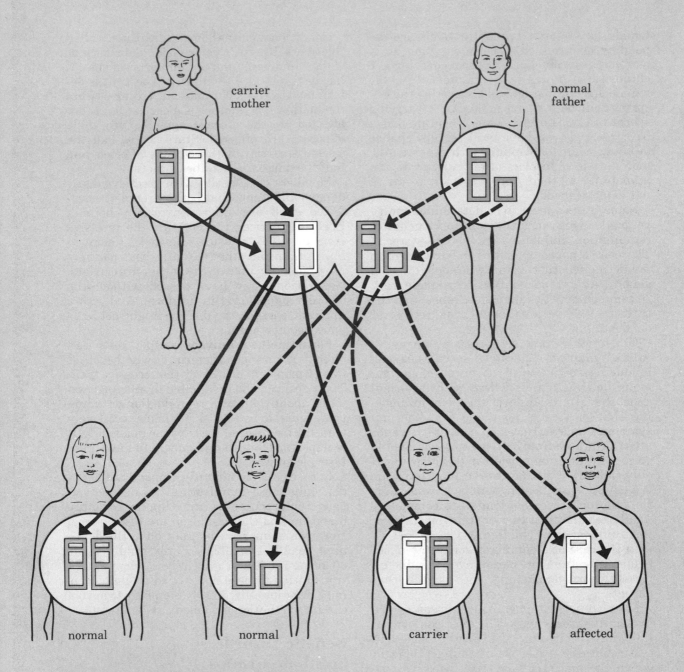

carrier mother

normal father

normal

normal

carrier

affected

SEX-LINKED DISORDERS

The pattern of transmission of a sex-linked disorder like classic hemophilia begins with a carrier mother. Rectangles within the circles above represent X (female) chromosomes; the hemophiliac chromosome is yellow. Squares are Y (male) chromosomes. A normal X chromosome cancels the effect of a hemophiliac X chromosome in female carriers, who are not affected by the disease but can transmit it. The Y

chromosome gives no protection to males who inherit a hemophiliac X chromosome (lower right). A male who receives a normal X from the mother plus a Y is not affected, nor is a daughter who receives normal X chromosomes from both parents. For chart of how Queen Victoria, a hemophilia carrier, transmitted the disease to several European ruling families see chapter 6, "The Blood."

thus much more likely to occur. Of course, none of these disorders are absolutely restricted to a particular group. Tay-Sachs disease in infants of European Jewish ancestry, sickle-cell anemia in American blacks, and beta-thalassemia (another serious blood disorder) in persons of Mediterranean heritage are among the best known examples of such disorders in the United States. Many others are recognized in subpopulations throughout the world.

Recent technological developments make it possible to determine the carriers of such traits by simple blood tests. In this way, two persons of Jewish ancestry, for example, can learn if they both are carriers for the Tay-Sachs gene before they have children. If neither partner or only one carries the gene, there is no risk to their offspring. In about 1 in 750 Jewish couples, however, both are carriers. Through genetic counseling, these couples can be helped to have only unaffected children, if they choose. Similar capabilities are becoming available for sickle cell anemia and thalassemia as well.

What the Odds Mean

If a child has a recessively transmitted disease, chances that a subsequent child of the same parents will have the disease are 1 in 4. Looked at positively, this means a 75 percent chance that the next child will be healthy. If a disorder is dominantly transmitted, there is a 50 percent chance that each child will be affected, about the same chance as boy or girl determination.

A sex-linked disorder carries its own odds. The chances are 50–50 that a son will be affected by the condition. The disease-free son cannot transmit the disease to his children. Likewise, chances are 50–50 that a daughter will carry the gene, making her offspring vulnerable although she herself is not affected. Daughters who do not inherit the gene are not carriers and neither their sons nor daughters will be affected.

A statement of odds is not overly reassuring but gives a basis for hard decisions. No matter what the odds are on paper, it is quite possible that a given hereditary defect of either type will appear in none of the children of a couple, or in very rare instances it may appear in all of them. If a coin is tossed and comes down heads, chances that the next toss will come down tails are not increased. They are still 50–50. Each toss is "a whole new ball game." So with parenthood, an adventure not without risks, and not without rewards.

DIAGNOSIS AND COUNSEL

If supposed hereditary diseases or birth defects are a cause for worry, the first step is accurate diagnosis, which often need go no further than the family physician. But rare and complex hereditary conditions require careful detective work, detailed knowledge of genetics, and exacting discrimination. There are, for example, several forms of hereditary deafness and muscular dystrophy.

Newborn Screening

For certain treatable hereditary disorders, it is possible to screen every newborn infant to determine whether he or she is affected, even with no family history. In some states a screening test (involving only a tiny blood sample) is mandatory. Early diagnosis can lead to simple treatment that is often life-saving. This is particularly true of such metabolic disorders as phenylketonuria (PKU), methylmalonic acidemia (an inability to break down certain amino acids), and galactosemia (an inborn error of milk-sugar metabolism), in which the tiny body is unable to metabolize certain substances which then accumulate and can cause mental retardation or death. Relatively simple dietary or replacement therapies can offset the disease's effects before damage is done, giving the child, in most instances, full potential for a normal life.

Hypothyroidism, which stems from a deficiency of thyroid hormone and which is a major cause of mental and growth retardation, also can be treated effectively if detected early. Probably, as research continues and our capability to treat hereditary diseases grows, many more disorders may be detected by screening in the newborn period.

Fetal Diagnosis

Several kinds of tests and studies, rapidly increasing in number and sophistication, help greatly to evaluate a variety of genetic factors in the developing fetus, often quite early in pregnancy, and to establish the facts as a sound basis for counseling. Although no test can absolutely guarantee a normal child, certain pregnancies, at increased risk for particular types of genetic disorders, might be candidates for such examinations. This new area of medical genetics, called prenatal diagnosis, has expanded enormously since 1970.

Ultrasound. This technique involves the use of high-frequency sound waves to obtain a visual-echo image of the fetus within the uterus from early stages of development (see chapter 32, "X Rays and Radiology"). By electrically examining the reflected echoes picked up by a sound transducer placed on the mother's abdomen, certain characteristics of the fetal anatomy can be determined. This is particularly important when such conditions as hydrocephalus (fluid accumulation in the brain) or severe dwarfing disorders are suspected.

Enormous progress is being made in the use of ultrasound, with steadily improving clarity of the fetal images. There is no known hazard to the mother or fetus from ultrasound testing.

Ultrasound also helps determine whether a multiple birth can be expected, the stage of fetal development, and the placement of the placenta within the uterus.

Amniocentesis is the withdrawal, through a hollow needle inserted into the mother's womb, of a sample of amniotic fluid in which the fetus "swims." The fluid contains fetal cells, which can be grown in culture, and other products, which are studied for chromosomal or chemical abnormalities that may indicate the presence of certain birth defects. About 100 genetic diseases can now be diagnosed in this way.

The procedure is a relatively simple one, usually undertaken about the 16th week of pregnancy. The prospective mother lies on her back with local anesthesia. A very thin needle is inserted through the abdominal wall into the uterine cavity. Only a small amount of the fluid is needed, which is rapidly replaced by the mother's body. Analyzing the sample takes about two weeks.

Although considered safe in competent hands, amniocentesis is not trivially resorted to. It is invaluable if there is a substantial risk of abnormality, as in a woman who has previously borne a child with genetic disease. Many specialists consider it particularly important if the mother is of advanced maternal age (over 35) because older women face a much greater risk of giving birth to an infant with Down's syndrome (formerly called mongolism) and other chromosome abnormalities.

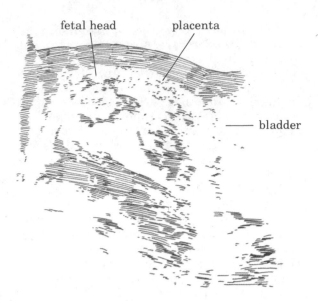

fetal head   placenta

bladder

ULTRASOUND

Echo patterns of high-frequency sound focused on the abdomen of a pregnant woman give a fuzzy but unmistakable picture of the developing fetus. This ultrasonic scan, taken at 14 weeks, shows the position of the fetal head, along with the placenta and the mother's bladder. White areas within the uterus represent amniotic fluid, in which the baby is suspended. The scan helps determine whether the fetus is developing normally and whether a multiple birth is expected.

Sex of the fetus is also readily determined by amniocentesis, and this knowledge can have more than mere curiosity value. Often, the news can be immensely heartening. Hemophilia is a genetic disease that afflicts only males. If the fetus is found to be female, the baby will not have hemophilia. When a previous son has been affected, such information can greatly allay a family's anxiety.

The AFP test. Another test using amniotic fluid involves the measurement of alpha-fetoprotein (AFP). AFP, a fetal blood protein present throughout fetal development, has been shown to be dramatically elevated in the amniotic fluid when the formation of the brain or spinal cord of the fetus has somehow been interrupted early in development. The AFP test is often recommended in families where previous children have had such abnormalities, or where other family members have been affected. In the near future, it may be possible to measure the AFP factor in the mother's blood in early pregnancy to determine whether she is at increased risk for such a defect in her fetus. Such a screening test

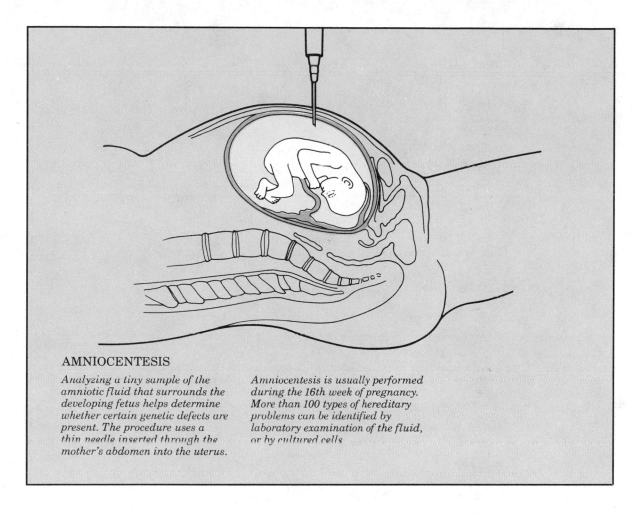

AMNIOCENTESIS

Analyzing a tiny sample of the amniotic fluid that surrounds the developing fetus helps determine whether certain genetic defects are present. The procedure uses a thin needle inserted through the mother's abdomen into the uterus.

Amniocentesis is usually performed during the 16th week of pregnancy. More than 100 types of hereditary problems can be identified by laboratory examination of the fluid, or by cultured cells.

could be applied to all pregnant women and greatly increase the detection rate of such defects during fetal life.

Chromosome studies. A number of birth defects can be diagnosed by identifying abnormalities of structure or number of chromosomes, using the amniotic fluid obtained by amniocentesis. Many such defects are not hereditary but "developmental" or environmental, which means something happens to disturb the fusion of normal parental chromosomes in the fertilized egg.

The most common chromosomal birth defect that can be diagnosed by amniocentesis cell studies is Down's syndrome. The affected child has abnormal features, mental retardation, and abnormalities of many systems of the body. The child carries an extra chromosome (in position 21, see page 38) caused by a defect in separation of chromosomes called nondisjunction. The parents practically always have normal chromosomes, so the defect is not truly hereditary. Chances that a subsequent child will be normal are quite good, except that there is a striking association between Down's syndrome and the age of the mother. The risks of bearing a Down's syndrome child, regardless of family history, go up sharply after age 35.

A different, quite rare form of Down's syndrome affects infants of young as well as older mothers. This form also has a distinctive chromosome abnormality. One pair of chromosomes carries an extra part from another chromosome, a phenomenon called translocation. This form of the disorder may be hereditary. One of the parents can carry the chromosomal rearrangement in a "balanced form" and not be affected by it. If the mother carries the rearrangement there is a 15 to 20 percent chance that each of her children will have Down's syndrome. If the father carries the rearrangement, then the risk is about 5 to 10 percent with each pregnancy.

Differences in two seemingly identical diseases underline the importance of fine discrimination when doing genetic studies.

DOWN'S SYNDROME

The chromosome arrangement of a female infant shows the extra chromosome characteristic of Down's syndrome, or mongolism, a form of retardation. The extra bit of genetic material is in position 21, and is known as Trisomy 21 (arrow). Banding, in which each chromosome stains in a unique way, allows specific identification of the extra chromosome as a 21.

TRANSLOCATION

When a pair of chromosomes carries an extra part from another chromosome, the phenomenon is called translocation. Above, a portion of chromosome 22 has been "translocated" to chromosome 9. The male with this arrangement is a victim of chronic myologenous leukemia. Previously, it was believed the condition was caused by the absence of one of the 22 chromosomes. Banding techniques enabled researchers to discover the true cause, the transfer of materials as indicated by arrows.

In addition, such chromosome rearrangements may lead to increased spontaneous pregnancy losses. Families in which three or more pregnancies have been lost spontaneously may benefit from chromosome tests in order to rule out a chromosomal rearrangement in either parent.

Pedigrees

Accurate interpretation of genetic factors may require that facts be obtained by pedigree studies, painstaking investigations of the health histories of blood relatives through parents, siblings, cousins, aunts, grandparents, and beyond. Pedigrees can give insight into patterns of inheritance of a trait and give a basis for prediction. It is vital, of course, that this information be accurate. This is not always easy if relatives live at great distances or if vital statistics records in their communities are sketchy. Many pedigree studies are done by researchers in genetic aspects of disease and often are not strictly necessary in a family situation.

TREATMENT

An increasing number of genetic disorders can be treated. Approaches include modifications of diet or hormone replacement to prevent mental retardation and offset certain metabolic errors. Children with cystic fibrosis may have fewer symptoms when treated with pancreatic enzymes and mist inhalations although no definite therapy is available yet. Hemophilia can be treated by victims themselves with home transfusions of the needed clotting factor. As we learn more about the fundamental nature of human genetic disorders, our ability to devise effective treatment programs increases accordingly. Unfortunately, however, effective therapies or cures are not available as yet for many hereditary disorders.

In spite of this, many patients with hereditary conditions can benefit from medical intervention and guidance.

If tests performed in early pregnancy reveal that the fetus is afflicted with a serious and untreatable hereditary disorder, the parents then have a choice, strictly their own, of terminating pregnancy or of completing pregnancy and having the child with the abnormal condition. For many families, the opportunity to have fetal testing performed has provided an option that has enabled them to have children unaffected with the condition for which they were at risk—children who might otherwise not have been conceived or born.

If the chances that some serious genetic condition will recur can only be stated mathematically, say one chance in four, the risks are real but not so overwhelming as to be totally unacceptable to every couple. In some instances genetic counseling can provide other options including artificial insemination. Again, not a perfect solution, but one that can enable families to make informed decisions about their future offspring.

Genetic diseases vary in implications and handicaps. Many developmental birth defects have no known genetic basis. Not a few worries about supposed hereditary traits arise from misconceptions. Medical counsel can bring the facts to light. There is reason to hope that genetic disease may some day be treated and cured by "gene therapy." Intensive research in genetic manipulation is exploring some astonishing possibilities: use of harmless viruses to carry correct genetic information into cells, taking samples of a sick person's cells, transferring correct genetic information to the cells, growing them in tissue culture and returning them to the donor, transferring whole chromosomes by cell fusion. Such possibilities sound like science fiction, but serious investigators pursue them.

WHERE TO SEEK HELP

In matters of inherited disorders, the first source of help is the family physician. If he or she recognizes that special skills are needed, patients can be referred to reliable laboratory and counseling centers. Some services are evaluation centers where a team of specialists determines an infant's medical problem and recommends treatment in consultation with the family physician and the parents. Another type of service is a birth defects treatment center, usually established in a teaching hospital or in affiliation with the medical school of a university. Few communities are far away from laboratory and counseling services in large towns and cities. Persons or families who wish to know where genetic counseling is available can request a free list of such services in the United States and Canada from the medical department of the National Foundation-March of Dimes, P.O. Box 2000, White Plains, New York, 10602

CHAPTER 3   WILLIAM L. PROUDFIT, M.D.

THE HEART AND CIRCULATION

The human heart is a specially adapted hollow mass of muscle about the size of a fist. Located almost dead center in the chest, it is canted slightly from right to left. The heart is roughly pear-shaped, with the base of the pear at the top, suspended from blood vessels, with the tapered end at the bottom. Alas for Saint Valentine, it bears little resemblance to the shape on greeting cards.

In legend and romantic ballad, the heart is the source of human courage and the seat of the emotions. Its actual function is simpler but perhaps more important than that. The heart muscle is the center of the circulatory system, squeezing or contracting to force blood through a closed system of flexible tubes (arteries) and thus provide life-sustaining oxygen and nutrients to all the cells of the body. The blood is then collected from the tissues by small blood vessels that empty into larger veins, which return the blood to the heart for recirculation.

The heart beats 72 times a minute, 24 hours a day. Its ceaseless, spontaneous thumping is beyond our conscious control, regulated by nerves and chemicals circulating in the blood. The amount of work the heart performs is prodigious. Each beat propels two to three ounces of blood into the arteries—four to six quarts a minute, 8,600 quarts a day. The heart beats 104,000 times a day, 38 million times a year. The power in one minute of beating is said to be enough to lift an 80-pound weight one foot in the air. That means raising one ton 41 feet every 24 hours.

Despite these superlatives, the heart does not work itself to death. Unlike the muscles of the arms and legs, it does not require exercise for proper function or to keep working well, and it does not wear out with age. The heart is a model of operating at a proper pace. It works continually, but rests between beats. The contraction or working phase consumes only about 40 percent of the heart cycle, so the muscle is resting more than half the time. People do not die of broken hearts in the literal sense.

The heart is well protected against damage, too. It rests on the strong muscles of the diaphragm, with the lungs surrounding most of the remaining external surface. The ribs and spine comprise a stout case around it. Even in severe chest injuries the heart is seldom damaged. A good thing, too, for the heart is truly the "heart" of life. When it stops, we stop.

ANATOMY OF THE HEART

The heart in some primitive animals is a simple tube, but in higher forms of life it is more complex because there are two circulatory systems, each with its own pump. The pumps are adjacent to each other and normally beat together in perfect harmony. One system is called the pulmonary circulation. It carries blood to and from the lungs, where it receives oxygen and gives up carbon dioxide. The second system, called systemic circulation, supplies the remainder of the body with oxygen-laden blood, picking up carbon dioxide and waste products from the tissues and nutrients from the digestive system.

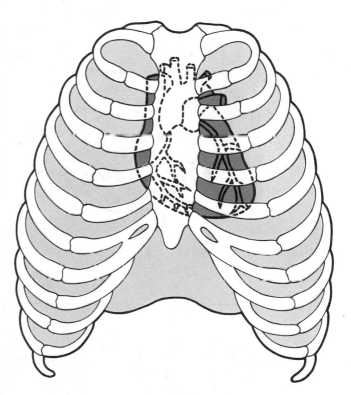

WHERE THE HEART IS

Encased by the rib cage and resting on the diaphragm, the heart is located almost in the center of the chest, directly behind the breastbone. The heart tapers to the left, and the tapered end, or apex, is where the beat is felt, so that we mistakenly think of the heart as being on the left side of the body. Because of its protection, the heart is seldom damaged, even in crushing injuries.

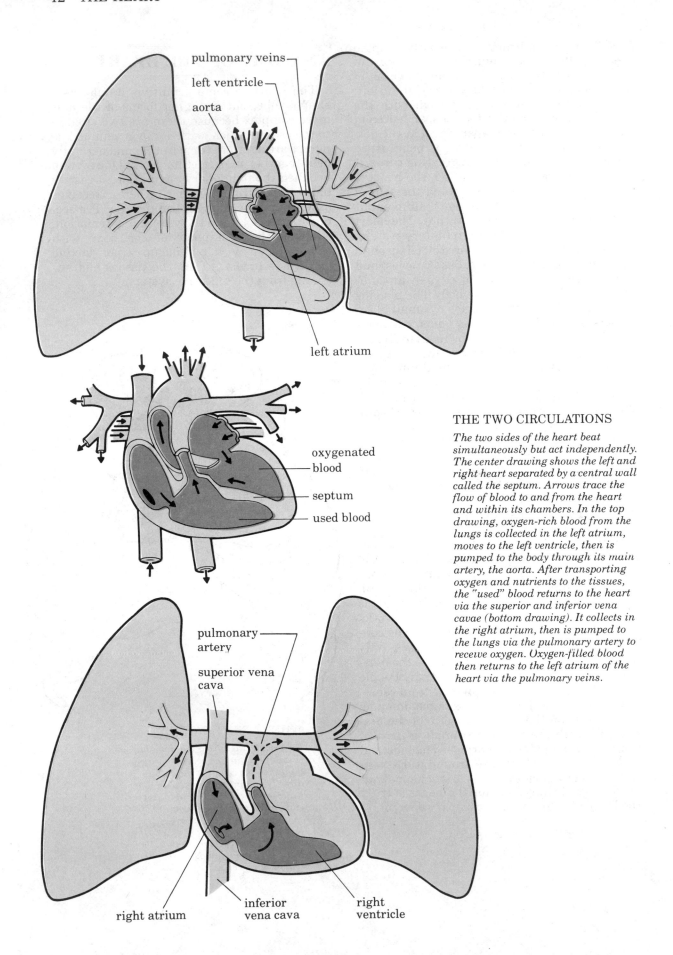

pulmonary veins
left ventricle
aorta
left atrium

oxygenated
blood
septum
used blood

THE TWO CIRCULATIONS

The two sides of the heart beat simultaneously but act independently. The center drawing shows the left and right heart separated by a central wall called the septum. Arrows trace the flow of blood to and from the heart and within its chambers. In the top drawing, oxygen-rich blood from the lungs is collected in the left atrium, moves to the left ventricle, then is pumped to the body through its main artery, the aorta. After transporting oxygen and nutrients to the tissues, the "used" blood returns to the heart via the superior and inferior vena cavae (bottom drawing). It collects in the right atrium, then is pumped to the lungs via the pulmonary artery to receive oxygen. Oxygen-filled blood then returns to the left atrium of the heart via the pulmonary veins.

pulmonary
artery
superior vena
cava

right atrium
inferior
vena cava
right
ventricle

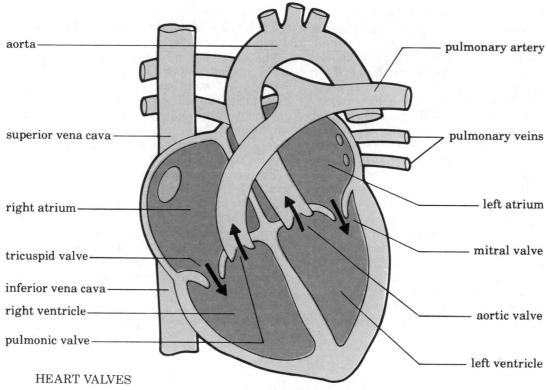

aorta

superior vena cava

right atrium

tricuspid valve

inferior vena cava

right ventricle

pulmonic valve

pulmonary artery

pulmonary veins

left atrium

mitral valve

aortic valve

left ventricle

HEART VALVES

The four valves of the heart regulate the direction blood flows within the heart and into the circulation. The mitral and tricuspid valves open so that collected blood may pour from the left and right atria into the ventricles. Then the valves close to *prevent backflow. When the heart contracts, the pulmonic valve opens to permit blood to be pumped to the lungs. Simultaneously, the aortic valve opens to admit blood to the systemic circulation.*

It would be easy to understand the circulation if a simple design were applicable, but the maker did not have this learning experience in mind during the design period. The illustration on page 42 shows that the heart is divided into four compartments, two above and two below. The upper compartments are the atria, the lower are the ventricles. The atria serve primarily as reservoirs, the ventricles as pumps. A central wall called the septum divides the heart into the right side (pulmonary circulation) and the left (systemic). A system of valves connects the chambers, each opening and closing as blood moves from one to another, just as the valves in an automobile engine seal off a cylinder to allow compression.

The circulatory flow begins with the return of blood from the tissues of the body via two large veins, the superior vena cava and inferior vena cava. These empty into the thin-walled right atrium, the heart's upper right compartment. The right atrium is primarily a collection point, although it does

have some ability to contract. From here the blood, under low pressure, pours downward through the tricuspid valve (named for its three cusps, or leaflets) into the more muscular right ventricle.

The ventricle pumps the blood out through the pulmonic valve into the large pulmonary artery, under increased but still relatively low pressure. This artery divides into branches supplying each lung, and these subdivide repeatedly, finally becoming microscopic vessels called capillaries, which lie in contact with the air sacs (alveoli) of the lungs. Here the important work of gas exchange takes place (see chapter 8, "The Lungs"). Oxygen inhaled through the respiratory system passes to the blood; carbon dioxide is transferred the other way, to be exhaled into the outside world. Now rich in oxygen, the blood travels through veins of ever-increasing size and finally flows into the left atrium.

The left atrium, like the right, is primarily a reservoir. When it is full, the blood is pumped into the left ventricle below, moving through the two-leaflet mitral valve. The left ventricle has a thick wall, measuring more than half an inch in an adult, capable of exerting high pressure on the blood it contains. The pressure closes the mitral valve and opens the aortic valve, which leads into the aorta, the body's main artery. The "blood pressure" of which we speak represents the pressure in the aorta. From the aorta blood flows into the arteries of progressively decreasing size until microscopic capillaries are reached. Here the reverse of the lung action takes place. Oxygen and nutrients are passed through the thin capillary walls to the tissues, and carbon dioxide and waste products make the reverse trip. The capillaries then unite to form minute veins, which combine into larger veins until, completing the circuit, they terminate in the two large veins, the vena cavae.

STRUCTURES OF THE HEART

The heart lies in a sac called the pericardium. Its shape is the shape you would get if you punched your fist into an air-filled balloon, except that the balloon in this case is empty of air and contains only a small amount of fluid, which serves as a lubricant between the two layers. The part of the sac nearest the heart muscle is attached to it.

The heart muscle itself is myocardium. The walls of the hollow chambers vary considerably in thickness. The right ventricle has a much thinner wall than the left. It is adapted to pumping large volumes of blood at low pressure. The thicker-walled left ventricle is more efficient at high pressure. All the chambers of the heart are lined with tough, smooth tissue called endocardium.

Endocardium also forms the valves. The tricuspid and mitral valves, which separate

aortic valve (open)   mitral valve (open)

HOW THE VALVES WORK

Seen from above, the valves between the heart's upper and lower chambers look like this. The aortic valve, opening to the general circulation, has three cusps or leaflets that fold back to allow the blood to enter, then form a tight seal against backflow. The mitral valve, which controls flow on the heart's left side, has only two cusps which form a curved-line junction.

aortic valve (closed)   mitral valve (closed)

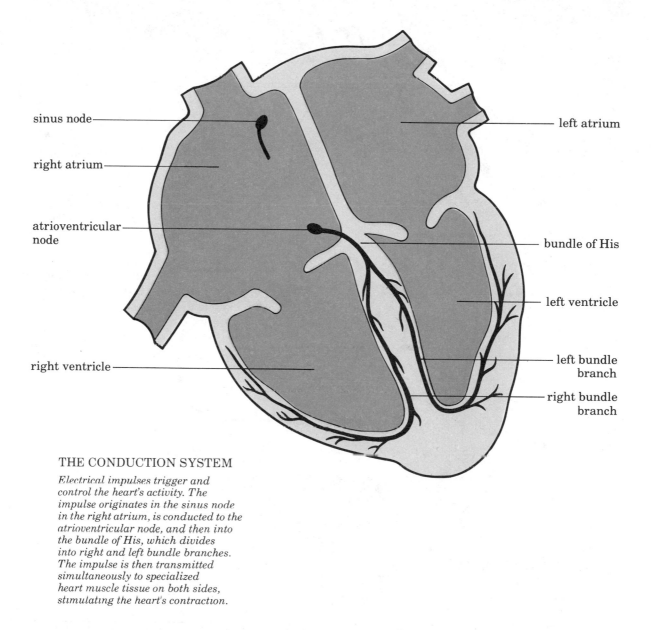

sinus node

right atrium

atrioventricular node

right ventricle

left atrium

bundle of His

left ventricle

left bundle branch

right bundle branch

THE CONDUCTION SYSTEM

Electrical impulses trigger and control the heart's activity. The impulse originates in the sinus node in the right atrium, is conducted to the atrioventricular node, and then into the bundle of His, which divides into right and left bundle branches. The impulse is then transmitted simultaneously to specialized heart muscle tissue on both sides, stimulating the heart's contraction.

the upper chambers from the lower chambers, are almost paper-thin, but strong. They are held in place when the heart contracts by thin strands of tissue, the chordae, which are connected to papillary muscles in the ventricle walls. The pulmonic and aortic valves leading into the blood vessels each have three leaflets or cusps, which open when the heart contracts and close when it rests, preventing blood from returning to the ventricles from the pulmonary arteries and aorta. The three-leaflet valve is a model of efficient design, as the Renaissance artist Leonardo da Vinci noted. Da Vinci drew diagrams of these valves showing how they function better than a two-cusp or four-cusp design.

The heart has a conduction system that initiates and distributes the electrical impulses which coordinate the heart's beating. We cannot see the structures of this system in humans, but we understand how it works. An electrical impulse is formed in a structure in the right atrium called the sinus node. It is conducted through the two atria in a more or less uniform manner and eventually reaches the atrioventricular (AV) node near the base of the two atria. After a brief pause, the impulse is passed into a short conduit called the bundle of His, which divides into two branches, the right and left bundle branches. These supply the impulse simultaneously to the two ventricles via specialized tissue connecting with the heart muscle cells. The arrival in the ventricles stimulates their contraction, what we know as the heartbeat.

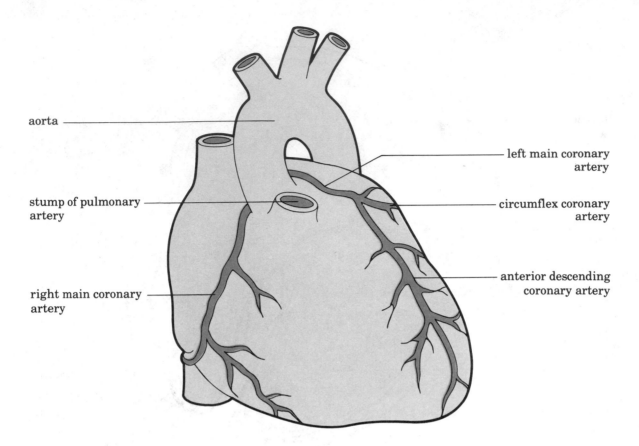

aorta

stump of pulmonary
artery

right main coronary
artery

left main coronary
artery

circumflex coronary
artery

anterior descending
coronary artery

CORONARY ARTERIES

The heart's own blood supply is received via the coronary arteries, so-called because they are said to resemble a crown. The right main coronary artery supplies the right ventricle and part of the left ventricle. The left main coronary artery has two large branches, the anterior descending artery and the circumflex artery, which circles around the back of the heart. Consequently, it is often said that there are three coronary arteries. In this drawing, the pulmonary artery has been cut away to show the left main coronary artery.

Although great volumes of blood pass through it, the heart muscle does not draw nourishment from this supply. That task is handled by the heart's own blood vessels, called the coronary circulation. The word "coronary" means "crown," but this designation is not entirely appropriate. Although the arteries do surround the base of the ventricle, the "prongs" of the crown—the major branch arteries—point downward.

The coronary arteries usually arise from two openings immediately above the aortic valve. The right coronary artery circles halfway around the heart and then usually turns downward toward the lower tip, or apex, of the heart, supplying the right ventricle and, more importantly, the portion of the left ventricle that rests on the diaphragm. The left coronary artery divides after a short distance into the anterior descending and circumflex branches.

Because the left main coronary artery before branching is less often affected by severe disease than the other arteries, it is sometimes said that there are three main coronary arteries: the right, the anterior descending, and the circumflex. Branches of these main arteries penetrate the heart muscle at right angles and divide into small vessels that supply the capillaries. The blood is collected into coronary veins, which empty into the right atrium.

HOW THE HEART WORKS

Two of the main properties of heart muscle are automaticity and rhythmicity. Automaticity is the ability of the heart to beat without external stimulation, and rhythmicity is the tendency of the beating to be regular. However,

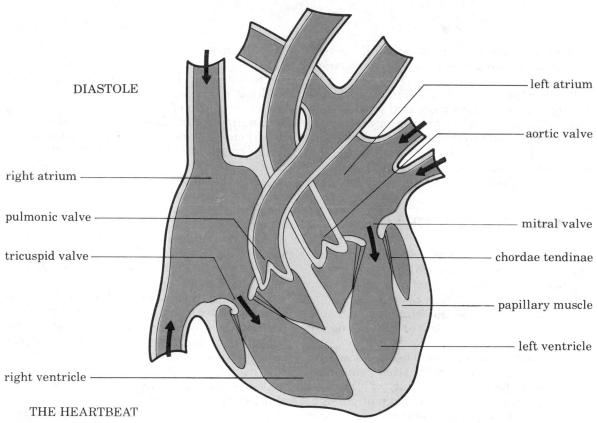

DIASTOLE

left atrium

aortic valve

right atrium

pulmonic valve

mitral valve

tricuspid valve

chordae tendinae

papillary muscle

left ventricle

right ventricle

THE HEARTBEAT

The two phases of the heartbeat are called diastole and systole. During diastole, the heart is relaxed and the ventricles are filling with blood from the atria. The tricuspid and mitral valves have opened, controlled by the chordae tendinae, small, tendon-like cords attached to the papillary muscles of the heart walls. In systole, the heart muscle contracts, the pulmonic and aortic valves open, and blood is forced into circulation.

the basic beat is more rapid in some parts of the heart than others. The sinus node beats fastest and usually controls the heart. Its electrical impulse, transmitted through the conduction system, stimulates the ventricular muscle to contract at just the proper interval after contraction of the atria, so that the maximum amount of blood can be pumped with each stroke. An automatic adjustment system correlates the strength of the contraction to the amount of blood entering the chambers.

The part of the beat during which the heart relaxes and the ventricles are filling is called the diastole. The period of contraction is the systole. The blood pressure differs between the two, which is why the doctor speaks of systolic and diastolic blood pressure. In a blood pressure reading of 120/80, the higher figure represents the pressure during contraction, and the lower figure is the reading at rest.

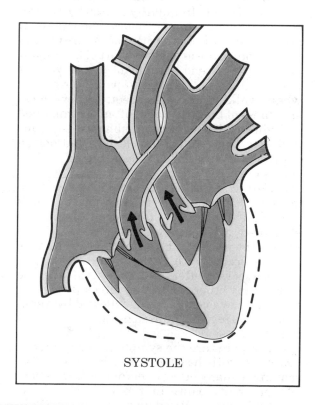

SYSTOLE

Both figures record the number of millimeters a column of mercury is raised by the force of the pumped blood.

There is little flow into the coronary arteries during contraction, so most of the blood flow occurs during the resting phase, or diastole. If the blood pressure in the aorta is too low or the resting phase is too short (when there is an extremely rapid heart rate), normal coronary arteries may not supply enough blood.

EXAMINING THE HEART

Symptoms. The symptoms of an illness are usually the reason for seeking medical care. In problems of the heart, they may also be the principal diagnostic clues. Some heart symptoms are highly specific and may indicate disease when all diagnostic examinations are normal.

The principal symptoms of heart disease are pounding of the heart (palpitation), shortness of breath (dyspnea), swelling of the legs (edema), fainting (syncope), and pain. Cough, spitting up blood, and weakness may occur also. None of these symptoms, of course, occurs only in heart disease. Shortness of breath, for example, is more frequently caused by a condition not related to the heart. "Shortness of breath" is also difficult to define. Many normal people consider themselves short of breath but are able to ascend a flight of stairs without resting, and feel no need to pause for breath when walking on the street. Others have shortness of breath at rest, often accompanied by light-headedness and numbness of the arms and legs. This is hyperventilation syndrome, a sign of nervous tension resulting in unconscious overbreathing.

Swelling of the legs is common in people in good health, especially in hot weather, but it may be a sign of heart failure. In those cases shortness of breath almost always accompanies the swelling. Fainting in heart disease usually occurs with little or no warning, so that the person often injures himself when he falls. Many other conditions can cause sudden fainting, however. Fainting followed by weakness, sweating, and nausea usually stems from nervous tension.

Chest pains are the symptoms most persons associate with heart disease, but these, too, may have many other explanations. Dull aching or sharp pains in the left side of the chest are rarely caused by heart disease. Pain lasting more than 15 minutes usually is caused by some other condition. Occasionally, momentary severe chest pains may result from premature contractions of the heart, but these are of no serious significance.

On the other hand, pain precipitated by walking and relieved in a few minutes by rest is characteristic of angina pectoris (meaning "strangling in the chest"), and usually stems from heart disease, especially disease of the coronary arteries. The pain strikes anywhere in the upper half of the body, but most commonly is felt in the center of the chest. Use of the arms or a strong emotion often precipitates the pain, and cold weather or eating may bring it on more quickly. Dreams sometimes initiate chest pains, or it may occur when the individual first lies down at night. Mild shortness of breath, nausea, and sweating may accompany the pain.

Listening to the heart. When a doctor listens to the heartbeat, he or she often gets important clues to heart disease. The sounds are better heard than described. Medical students learn to recognize them from tapes, not books. It is usually said that the normal adult heart makes paired sounds described as a noise like "lubb-dupp." The thudding "lubb" represents the closing of the mitral and tricuspid valves and the beginning of the ventricular contraction. The higher-pitched "dupp" represents the clicking shut of the aortic and pulmonic valves. A third sound of any sort may indicate heart disease.

Heart noises include swishing, whooshing, clicking, crackling, and even breathing sounds. They may be harsh and noticeable or faint. Some are classified as murmurs, prolonged noises occupying a part of the heart cycle, but murmurs may also be heard in normal people. Loud systolic murmurs, occurring during the contraction phase, usually indicate heart disease but softer murmurs often are normal and are almost universal in children. Diastolic murmurs, occurring during the resting phase, always indicate heart disease, although it may not be serious. Rubbing sounds over the heart may be a sign of inflammation of the pericardium, or pericarditis. Crackling sounds over the lower part of the lungs in the back may indicate congestion, a clue to inefficient action of the heart.

Besides these extraneous noises, the heartbeat may be rapid and irregular, but this is seldom a specific sign of heart disease.

The electrocardiogram. If heart disease is suspected, an electrocardiogram may be performed in the doctor's office to record electrical activity within the heart muscle. With the person lying down or resting in a chair, a set of electrodes, or "leads," are affixed to several parts of the body and attached to a machine, where moving pens trace out the electrical rhythm on a moving strip of paper. The leads to the arms and legs are identified as 1, 2, 3, R, L and F; those to the chest usually V-1 to V-6.

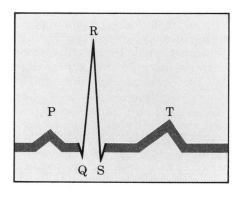

THE ELECTROCARDIOGRAM

The path of electrical impulse through the heart can be traced by an electrocardiogram or ECG. The distinctive waves and spikes are given alphabetical designations. Above, the P wave represents electrical stimulation of the atrium. The QRS complex shows the spread of electrical activity through the ventricles. The T wave is the recovery of the ventricle after stimulation.

Positioning is important because limb leads are most useful in diagnosing irregularities of heart rhythm and certain types of heart attacks, while the chest leads are more helpful in diagnosing problems of enlargement of the heart and other types of heart attacks.

The line traced by the movements of the pen follows a readily interpreted pattern. The sharp spikes and smoother curves of the electrocardiogram are named for letters of the alphabet from P to T. The P wave is a small deflection representing the electrical activity of the upper chambers of the heart (atria). Although there are two chambers, there is only one wave because the electrical events occur simultaneously in the two chambers. If the rhythm is abnormal, the P wave is abnormal, either in shape or frequency. The first downward deflection after the P wave is called the Q wave, the first upward wave is the R wave, and the downward deflection following

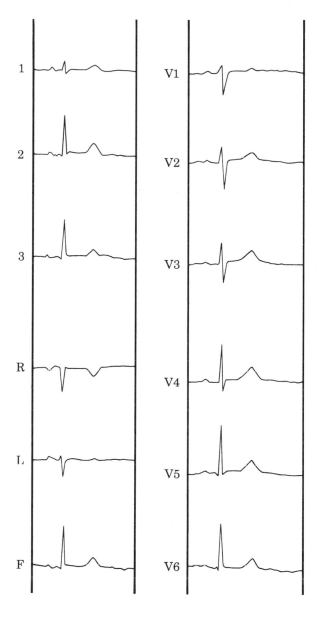

NORMAL HEART WAVES

To measure the heart's electrical activity, five to ten wires are attached to small metal plates (electrodes) at various points on the body. The number of contact points depends on whether all combinations of wires ("leads") are recorded simultaneously or in sequence. The leads from the arms and legs are designated 1, 2, 3, R, L, and F. The six placed on the chest are V-1 through V-6. Each lead produces a distinctive tracing. The normal patterns are shown above.

the R wave is called an S wave. Sometimes this group of three is called the QRS complex. It represents electrical transmission through the ventricles. The usually smaller rounded wave after the QRS complex is the T wave. Abnormalities of the QRS complex are more specific than those of the T waves.

The electrocardiogram, often referred to as ECG or EKG, may be normal even though heart disease is present. Since it records only the heart's electrical activity, it may be essential in diagnosing disturbances of the heart rhythm, and it provides important clues to other conditions, but is not infallible in disclosing heart disease.

An office electrocardiogram, moreover, records electrical activity only during the brief period of examination. Sometimes a fleeting, intermittent disturbance of heart rhythm is suspected, yet cannot be captured by ordinary means. In such cases a continuous tape recording of the electrocardiogram for 12 to 24 hours may be required. To achieve this a person may wear a miniature recording device as he or she goes about daily activity. Or a disturbance may be suspected only when the heart is stressed. Then an ECG may be taken during and after exercise performed on a two-step staircase, a calibrated bicycle, or a treadmill.

X ray of the chest is most useful in determining the size of the heart, or in showing enlargement of one or more chambers, which gives a clue to the presence or severity of certain anatomical defects. The X ray will also show the lungs and the arteries supplying the lungs, and disclose congestion or increased circulation.

The echocardiogram is a painless test using sound waves to gain information about the interior of the heart. A blunt probe that emits a sound wave is applied to the surface of the chest over the heart. The echocardiograph measures the time required for the wave to strike a portion of the heart and be reflected back to the probe. Sometimes a movable probe or several probes are used. Fluid in the sac around the heart (pericardial fluids), valve defects, abnormalities during contraction, and variations in chamber size or wall thickness can be disclosed by this method.

Radioactive substances also are used to investigate coronary disease. The amount of material taken up by the heart muscle or passed through the chambers may be measured. Sometimes this method is combined with electrocardiographic exercise testing.

Catheterization. For some conditions only catheterization of the heart will yield the information needed for proper treatment, especially when surgery is required. Catheterization means insertion of a tiny flexible tube through the circulation to obtain an accurate "road map" of blood flow. It is particularly important for repair of most congenital heart defects, in valve problems, or in surgical treatment of coronary artery disease.

Either or both sides of the heart may be catheterized, depending on the problem. The procedure is carried out with local anesthesia and the patient is unaware of the passage of the flexible catheter through the circulation. A small incision is made in the arm or groin and the catheter is inserted or it is threaded over a wire that has been inserted through the skin into a vessel. If a vein is used, the right side of the heart is studied. If an artery is used, the left side of the heart is investigated. Pressures in the various chambers may be measured, the pressure waves in the chambers recorded, the output (the amount of blood pumped) of the heart determined, and photographs of the chambers or coronary arteries obtained. The risk of this procedure is slight, and the importance of the information it produces usually outweighs that risk.

Other clues to heart disease. Besides the symptoms above, there are two other serious conditions common to several types of heart disease.

Congestive heart failure occurs when the heart's output is not enough to meet the demands of the body. Sometimes the output may be normal but the demands excessive. This occurs in such unusual conditions as toxic thyroid, thiamin chloride deficiency (vitamin B_1), and abnormal connections between a major artery and vein. More commonly, congestive heart failure occurs because the heart pumps inadequately due to disease in the muscle or pericardium, or because of narrowing of a valve.

In all of these conditions the body retains sodium (salt), which causes retention of excess water. The fluid accumulates most obviously in the lungs and in the legs. Shortness of breath occurs because of the fluid, and the person may be unable to lie down, or may awaken with acute breathing difficulty, usually relieved by sitting up for 5 to 15 minutes. Sometimes the shortness of breath persists longer at night and is accompanied by wheezing and cough, a condition known as cardiac asthma. These are signs of serious heart disease and are indications for intensive treatment. Response to treatment usually is good. Sodium in the form of salt or baking soda is restricted, and a drug called digitalis or a derivative is given. Diuretics (drugs to promote the loss of fluids) are prescribed. In severe cases medication to relax the blood vessels and lower the blood pressure may be used. It is important to determine the cause of congestive heart failure and to correct the cause if possible.

The blood clot is another serious complication of several types of heart disease. A clot (thrombus) tends to form in the heart if blood flow in a chamber is extraordinarily sluggish or if the endocardium or valves are inflamed. This may result from narrowing of the mitral valve associated with irregularity of heartbeat. Or it may stem from bacterial infection of a valve, severe impairment of pumping action, acute damage to the endocardium as a result of a heart attack, or a bulge (aneurysm) of the left ventricle resulting from a previous heart attack. Clots in the heart may break off and flow to any part of the body where they may lodge in smaller arteries and obstruct circulation, causing damage or even death. Such a clot is called an embolus. The most serious are those going to the brain, though often the clots are small and cause no permanent disability. Anticoagulants and surgery offer protection against recurrences.

TYPES OF HEART DISEASE

Heart disease may be classified in several ways but a common method is by cause.

Abnormalities of Rhythm

Abnormalities of the heart rhythm (arrhythmias) are common. In fact the majority of apparently healthy people have a type of rhythm disturbance called premature contraction, although few are aware of it. The abnormality may be discovered only by tape recording the electrocardiogram for 12 hours or more if it occurs rarely. Premature contractions may occur in either the atrium or ventricle. Some persons have only occasional irregularity but others have periods in which every other beat is premature. A spot in an atrium or ventricle discharges electrically without waiting for the impulse to be received from the sinus node. There is a pause following this discharge, then normal rhythm is restored. Some people are aware of the irregularity and say that their heart "stops," or "turns

flip-flops," or "skips." Occasionally a momentary sharp pain may be experienced at the precise moment of the irregularity. Premature contractions are rarely important except for the symptoms experienced, if any. Treatment is seldom required, but drugs may be prescribed if symptoms are bothersome.

Atrial paroxysmal tachycardia is an irregularity in which the atria beat about 180 times a minute, two to three times the normal rate. The ventricles respond to each beat. The rhythm is regular. Attacks begin and end abruptly, lasting from a few seconds to hours. There is usually no obvious heart disease. Attacks occur more commonly in young people than in the elderly and often disappear in middle or old age. Sweating, weakness, and palpitation may accompany the attacks. Sometimes the attacks may be stopped by forceful breath-holding, voluntary gagging, immersing the face in ice cold water for 30 seconds or less, or pressing on a nerve center near the angle of the jaw. Occasionally medical treatment is required, and may be needed to prevent episodes from occurring frequently.

Atrial flutter is marked by an atrial rate of about 300 beats per minute. The ventricles respond to alternate atrial contractions, so the pulse rate is about 150 per minute and usually is regular. Attacks begin and end suddenly, but tend to be longer than those of atrial paroxysmal tachycardia. Heart disease may be present. Drugs can be used to slow the ventricular rate until the attack terminates. Electric shock across the chest during brief anesthesia will end an attack.

Atrial fibrillation may also occur in the presence or absence of organic heart disease. Rheumatic disease of the mitral valve is particularly likely to cause these extremely rapid and incomplete contractions of the atria. They may be temporary or permanent. Fibrillation starts suddenly, although the patient may not be aware of it. The rate is variable, usually 120 to 160 beats per minute, and the rhythm is irregular. The rate can be controlled by drugs. Electric shock may be used to restore normal rhythm, but if rhythm has been irregular for a year or more, shock treatment may fail. Atrial fibrillation and atrial flutter may be caused by a severe thyroid condition.

Ventricular tachycardia is usually associated with organic heart disease. A small area in one ventricle starts beating spontaneously at a rapid rate, with slightly irregular rhythm. The atrial rhythm does not change. The output of blood from the heart may decrease severely. Marked weakness, sweating,

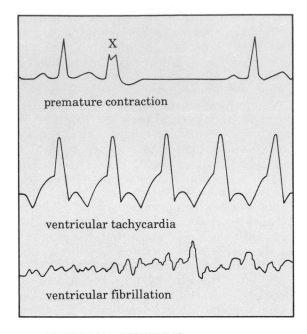

ABNORMAL RHYTHMS

Three types of disturbed ventricular rhythms produce these distinctive electrocardiogram tracings. The top line depicts premature contraction of a ventricle (marked X), a common abnormality sometimes described as "skipping a beat." In ventricular tachycardia (center line), the heart rate is rapid and the rhythm is slightly irregular. The width of the QRS complex is increased. The bottom line shows ventricular fibrillation, a very serious abnormality. It is characterized by irregular and extremely rapid contractions, and is fatal unless corrected quickly.

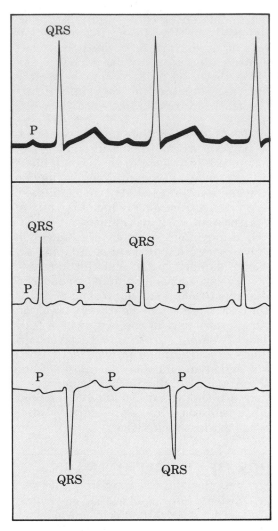

CONDUCTION DEFECTS

When the electrical impulse is not properly transmitted through the heart, any of the above conduction defects may occur, showing an electrocardiogram pattern that differs from the normal tracing on page 49. Top line shows delay in the transmission of the P wave to the ventricle. In the center line, only alternate P waves stimulate the ventricle to contract, as depicted by the QRS complex. The bottom line shows complete heart block. No relation exists between the P wave, which normally touches off the electrical impulse, and the QRS complex, which represents ventricular contraction.

and even fainting may occur if the rate is rapid. Some attacks end spontaneously but often drug treatment or an electric shock is required to end them.

Ventricular fibrillation usually is fatal unless stopped by treatment in a matter of minutes. It may occur as a complication of ventricular tachycardia or arise spontaneously. Although there is electrical activity in the ventricles, the contraction of the heart is uncoordinated and the aortic valve does not open. No heart sounds can be heard. The flow of blood stops and unconsciousness occurs in five to eight seconds unless the irregular rhythm ends. External massage of the heart accompanied by mouth-to-mouth breathing (see page 53) will maintain circulation temporarily, and external electric shock will restore normal rhythm in many cases. Organic heart disease is usually responsible for ventricular fibrillation, so the outlook may not be good unless the basic problem can be corrected or the tendency to recur can be reduced with drug treatment.

Ventricular asystole is similar to ventricular fibrillation, except there is no electrical activity in the ventricle, so the beat stops. The outlook is poor. Occasionally a vigorous blow over the heart will restore beating. External heart massage and artificial respiration may maintain life until normal rhythm can be restored. Sometimes a temporary electrical pacemaker may be used and a permanent unit installed later if the response has been good.

Heart block occurs when transmission of the electrical impulse from the atrium to the ventricles through the conduction system is partially or completely blocked. In partial block some impulses are transmitted while others are not. Sometimes alternate beats are blocked, causing a slow heart rate, or there may be a total block of all impulses so that the atria and ventricles beat at different rates, the ventricle at about half the normal rate. This is called complete heart block, and it is a serious abnormality because the ventricles may develop fibrillation or asystole unless controlled by impulses coming from above. If the rate of ventricle contractions can be increased, the outlook is good. This may be done with drugs, but much more effectively with an artificial pacemaker.

"Sick sinus-node syndrome" refers to improper function of the sinus node, the structure in the right atrium where the electrical impulse starts. The person may experience episodes of slow heart rate or contractions may cease temporarily (asystole). Sometimes there are attacks of rapid heart action as well. Sick sinus-node syndrome can be studied electrically by putting an impulse into an area of the right atrium and measuring its transmission.

Bundle branch block is sometimes confused with complete heart block. In this condition, however, the impulse from the atrium reaches the bundle of His normally, but transmission through one of the bundle branches is blocked. The problem is diagnosed by electrocardiogram. The impulse that starts contraction of the ventricles is transmitted throughout the heart but more directly to one ventricle than to the other. The function of the heart is normal, and the condition may occur despite no evident disease of the heart. People who have bundle branch blocks often live normal life-spans without disability if there is no other abnormality. Occasionally the block may progress to complete heart block.

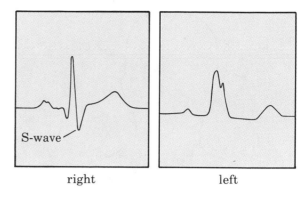

right   left

BUNDLE BRANCH BLOCK

Two types of bundle branch block are detected in these electrocardiograph tracings of lead No. 1. In right bundle branch block, a large S wave is shown. In left bundle branch block, no S wave can be detected. The heart often functions normally despite the block.

A condition sometimes confused with bundle branch block is Wolff-Parkinson-White syndrome. It is of no serious significance but tends to be associated with attacks of rapid heart action, usually atrial paroxysmal tachycardia.

Treatment of arrhythmias. There are three important methods used for treating critical heartbeat irregularities. They are external resuscitation, electric shock treatment, and the artificial pacemaker.

External resuscitation, also called cardiopulmonary resuscitation (see chapter 35, "First Aid"), is often used by trained lay persons and paramedical personnel when someone's heart has stopped and emergency measures are required. It is best performed by two persons, one of whom vigorously compresses the lower breastbone briefly at a rate of one per second, the other of whom forces breath into the nose or mouth every three or four seconds. One trained person can perform both tasks if necessary. Chest compression forces blood out of the heart into the aorta and maintains blood pressure. The forced breathing maintains the oxygen supply to the lungs. External resuscitation can keep the victim alive while he or she is transferred to a medical emergency facility where electric shock treatment is available.

Electric shock treatment usually stops ventricular fibrillation. Large metal paddles are applied to the skin of the chest and a strong

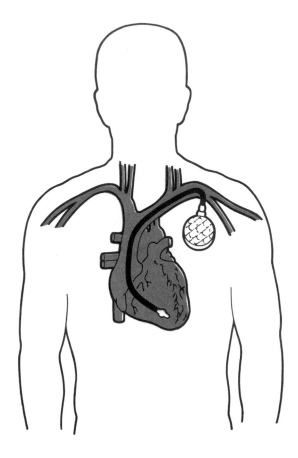

THE PACEMAKER

A battery-powered electrical device called a pacemaker can be implanted in the chest to regulate an erratic heart to beat rhythmically. The generating unit is implanted in the chest, and impulses are transmitted via wires to the right ventricle. Some pacemakers can be left in place up to 10 years, and some may be recharged without removing them.

shock is passed through the heart. The heart muscle reacts by contracting uniformly and normal rhythm is restored. Shock may also be used to stabilize less serious rhythm abnormalities, including atrial flutter, atrial fibrillation, and ventricular tachycardia. A brief anesthesia is then used before the shock is administered because the person is conscious. Electric shock is less risky and more effective than drug treatment in many instances.

An artificial pacemaker is a miniature electrical device installed within the body to stimulate the heart to beat rhythmically. Some pacemakers are developed for specific purposes, but the common type operates at a fixed rate, which usually is adjustable. The pacemaker may stimulate continually or only when the heart rate falls below a certain level. The impulse is transmitted through wires contained in a small tube, the tip of which is wedged into the right ventricle. The generating portion of the unit is buried under the skin of the chest or abdomen. Sometimes a wire is attached to the surface of the heart for stimulation.

An external pacemaker may be used in acute conditions and a permanent unit inserted later if required. Originally the batteries of permanent units lasted a year or two, but improvements have resulted in an estimated battery life of 10 years. Nuclear powered units are being tested. Some pacemakers need not be removed for recharging. Complete heart block is the most common reason for installing a pacemaker, but "sick sinus-node syndrome" is a frequent reason.

Congenital Heart Disease

Heart defects present at birth are called congenital. There are two general types: cyanotic ("blue babies") and non-cyanotic. The non-cyanotic types are more common and most can be corrected surgically. Usually the cause of these defects is not apparent but German measles (rubella) in the early stages of pregnancy is sometimes responsible.

Septal defects are holes in the wall (septum) separating the right and left side of the heart. Defects between the two atria or upper chambers can vary in size and location. Normally, the fetus has an opening between the atria so that blood can pass between them without circulating through the lungs, because fetal lungs contain no air. This opening, called the foramen ovale, closes at birth. Defects in the upper septum are often small and cause no complications throughout life. But if they are large, a considerable amount of blood may be transferred from the left to the right atrium because the pressure is slightly higher in the left. That means the right side of the heart must pump several times as much blood as the left. The vessels of the lungs enlarge to accommodate the additional blood flow. The right side of the heart works harder than the left. Eventually the high blood flow through the lungs may cause changes in the structure and function of the vessels and blood pressure may rise. Irreversible changes in the vessels may develop. X ray and electrocardiogram findings suggest the condition, but catheterization of the heart is necessary for accurate

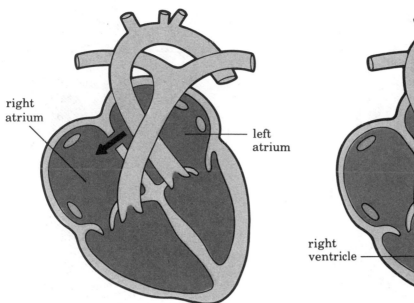

right
atrium

left
atrium

AN ATRIAL DEFECT

*An atrial septal defect, which is an
opening in the wall between the right
and left atria, allows oxygenated and
unoxygenated blood to mix. An
opening is normal in the fetus, but it
should close at birth. Small openings
may do no harm but larger ones may
cause the right side of the heart to
overwork. The defect can be closed
surgically.*

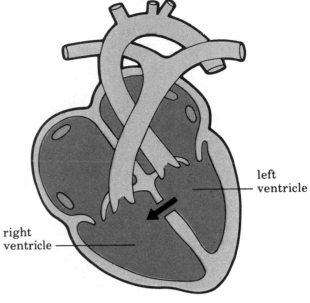

left
ventricle

right
ventricle

VENTRICULAR DEFECT

*An opening between the left and right
ventricles causes abnormal flow out of
the left ventricle. A large opening may
cause heart failure. The defect is
usually present at birth. Small
openings may close as the child grows,
or they can be closed by surgery.*

diagnosis. The treatment is surgical. Small defects are closed by stitches and larger ones eliminated by sewing a patch of synthetic material over the hole. The risk of the operation is minimal.

A defect in the lower atrial septum is less common than in the upper portion and often is associated with an abnormality of the mitral valve. It may be accompanied by a loud murmur. These defects can also be closed although closure is more difficult. Often the mitral valve must be repaired or replaced.

The ventricular septum also may have defects, which allow blood to flow from the left to the right ventricles because of the left's higher pressure. Usually a loud, characteristic murmur discloses the abnormal opening. An unusually large defect may cause heart failure in infancy or childhood but often it is well tolerated. Some of these holes close spontaneously as a child develops and grows and the muscular interventricular septum thickens. If not, or if serious problems arise early in childhood, surgical closure can be done at low risk. The technique is similar to that for septal defects between the atria.

Pulmonic stenosis, narrowing of the pulmonic valve, is the most common important congenital valve defect of the heart. This valve lies at the outflow of the right ventricle and normally has three cusps. The cusps are fused in pulmonic stenosis, with only a small central opening for blood to flow to the lungs. The muscle of the right ventricle enlarges because it must work harder to force blood through the small opening. A characteristic murmur is generated and the electrocardiogram shows evidence of the right ventricle's increased work load. The valve may be opened relatively simply with little risk and good results. Sometimes the muscular tissue just below the pulmonic valve narrows the outflow track of the right ventricle. This, too, may be treated surgically but the procedure is more difficult.

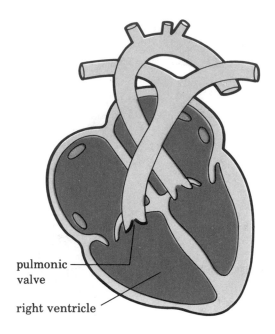

PULMONIC STENOSIS

Narrowing of the pulmonic valve, called pulmonic stenosis, leaves only a small opening for blood to pass to the lungs. The right ventricle must work harder, and blood pressure rises. The defect, usually present at birth, causes a recognizable heart murmur. The valve can be opened by surgery.

pulmonic valve

right ventricle

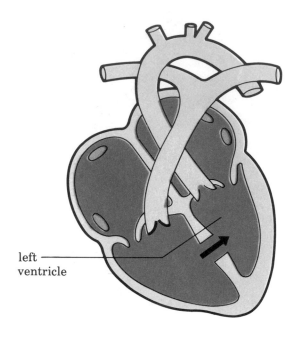

THE "BLUE BABY"

A child looks blue when a narrowed pulmonic valve is combined with a defect in the wall between the ventricles. The narrowed valve limits blood flow to the lungs and the wall defect allows the unoxygenated blood to pass from the right ventricle to the left. Because the blood contains little oxygen, the child's skin and lips have a bluish tinge. Surgery can correct the defect.

left ventricle

"Blue babies" are most commonly victims of a condition called tetralogy of Fallot, named for the French physician who first described it. Tetralogy means there are four defects but only two are essential to understanding the condition: pulmonic stenosis and interventricular septal defect. If pulmonic stenosis is severe the pressure in the right ventricle may exceed that in the left, so blood flows from right to left. The blood in the right ventricle has not been circulated to the lungs and so it is "blue." If the flow is large, the skin and lips have a bluish tinge.

The first surgical treatment for blue babies was the Blalock-Taussig operation, which joins one of the arteries supplying an upper arm to the pulmonary artery supplying the lung. Blood inadequately charged with oxygen then could be circulated back to the lungs to take up more oxygen. The "bluishness" or cyanosis consequently disappeared. Unfortunately, the pressure in the arteries of the lungs often increased and caused vessel changes similar to those of interatrial septal defect. Eventually the cyanosis returned in many instances. A further advance in surgery has made it possible to do a total correction of tetralogy of Fallot in one operation with excellent results.

Patent ductus arteriosus is not a true congenital heart defect but a condition of the arteries. The ductus arteriosus is a vessel through which blood passes from the pulmonary artery to the aorta, the body's main artery, in the baby before birth. Normally it closes soon after birth, but sometimes it remains open, allowing blood to pass from the aorta to the pulmonary artery because of the higher pressure in the aorta. This leakage puts an added burden on the heart, and a characteristic continuous murmur usually can be heard. Cutting the ductus and sewing the two ends together is a relatively simple surgical treatment that repairs the problem.

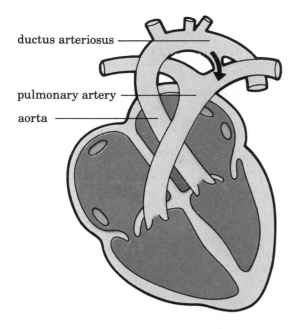

ductus arteriosus

pulmonary artery

aorta

DUCTUS ARTERIOSUS

Patent ductus arteriosus occurs when the blood vessel that links the pulmonary artery and aorta before birth fails to close properly after birth. The leakage puts an additional strain on the baby's heart. The ductus can be severed and closed off in a relatively simple surgical procedure.

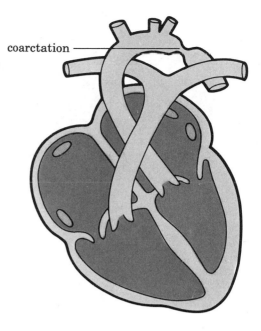

coarctation

A DEFECTIVE AORTA

Coarctation of the aorta, the body's main artery, is a defect present at birth. The aorta narrows just beyond the beginning of the artery that supplies the left arm. Other arteries permit the passage of blood to the abdomen and legs. There may be high blood pressure in the upper part of the body and weak pulses in the lower. Surgery is used to remove the narrowed area and the two ends are joined directly or by a fabric graft.

Coarctation of the aorta is also a congenital arterial defect. The aorta is narrowed severely or completely closed just beyond the beginning of the artery that supplies the left arm. Blood may reach the lower part of the body by way of collateral arteries, which reroute the blood from vessels in and about the neck through the various connecting arteries until it finally empties into the aorta in the lower chest or abdomen. High blood pressure in the upper part of the body draws attention to the possible defect, and the suspicion is confirmed by finding weak or absent pulses in the lower extremities. If the involved portion of the aorta is large and the two cut ends cannot be sewed together directly, the narrowed area of the aorta can be removed and a fabric graft used to bring the two ends together.

Rheumatic Heart Disease

Rheumatic fever is an inflammation resulting from a bacterial infection of the throat by an organism called the hemolytic streptococcus. It is related to scarlet fever, the kidney disorder called Bright's disease or glomerulonephritis, and other conditions caused by delayed reaction to a particular kind of "strep" infection. Symptoms usually begin about two weeks after the initial illness and last several weeks or months. They often include fever plus joint pain and swelling, but may be so mild that the condition is not recognized. The heart is affected in about half the cases, sometimes seriously and even fatally. The victim, usually a child, generally recovers from the acute attack, but recurrences are frequent.

Rheumatic fever was once common and widely feared in the United States. The incidence began to decrease in the 1930s and has continued to decline since. It is still common in less developed countries.

aortic stenosis   mitral stenosis

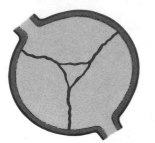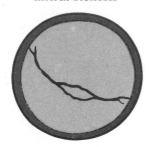

VALVE DISEASE

When the aortic or mitral valves become diseased, scar tissue prevents them from opening or closing normally. At left, aortic stenosis has fused the valve except for a small central portion, shown in the open position. At right, scar tissue has formed along the leaflets of the mitral valve so that only a small area, as shown, can open to permit blood flow.

Rheumatic heart disease develops during rheumatic fever, but often causes no symptoms for a decade or more. In at least half the cases the person cannot recall the earlier episode, because the disorder was mild, misdiagnosed, or forgotten. The disease deforms the valves by scarring them, so the heart must work harder to pump blood.

The valves on the left side of the heart are more frequently affected than those on the right. When the right valves are involved, the valves on the left side are almost always damaged as well. The mitral valve is a more common target than the aortic. Scarring of the valves may prevent proper opening or closing of the valve. In mitral stenosis the lips or cusps of the two leaflets adhere to each other, leaving only a small central opening. The left atrium enlarges because blood pressure increases due to the narrowed opening into the left ventricle. In mitral insufficiency, the valves fail to close properly. When the left ventricle contracts, blood is forced back into the left atrium instead of into the aorta alone. In aortic stenosis, the valve's small opening obstructs blood flow during the contraction. In aortic insufficiency, blood leaks back from the aorta into the left ventricle during the resting phase, when the valve should be closed.

Various combinations of valve defects occur in rheumatic heart disease, and characteristic murmurs are generated by each. In mitral valve disease, atrial fibrillation is a common complication. If the disease is severe, shortness of breath and congestive heart failure may occur. Fainting, pain, and shortness of breath may also strike those with aortic stenosis. Congestive heart failure is a common complication of any form of rheumatic heart disease.

If all rheumatic fever could be prevented, rheumatic heart disease would be eliminated. Similarly, if streptococcal infections were prevented or treated immediately, rheumatic fever would not be a problem. Unfortunately, many streptococcal infections may cause only mild symptoms difficult to notice, and even severe sore throats in children are not always treated aggressively. Rheumatic fever itself also must be treated properly. After an attack, oral penicillin may be administered regularly for years to prevent recurrences.

If rheumatic heart disease has caused severe symptoms, surgery may be necessary. Congestive failure usually responds well to treatment but symptoms tend to recur. Often catheterization of the heart is required before the operation, especially in middle-aged and elderly persons, who constitute the majority of

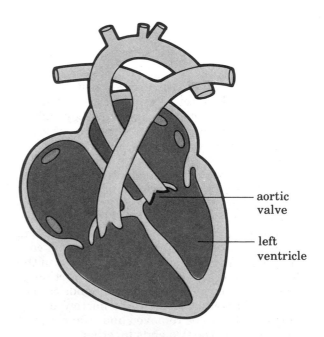

aortic valve

left ventricle

AORTIC VALVE DISEASE

Aortic stenosis narrows the aortic valve leading from the left ventricle to the aorta. The ventricle must work harder to pump blood through the tiny opening, resulting in high blood pressure in the ventricle.

symptomatic patients. Not only can the severity of the valve defect be documented but the coronary circulation can be photographed.

Often calcium is deposited in a scarred valve damaged by rheumatic heart disease. The hardened mineral prevents the valve from opening and closing normally. In rare cases the valve will function quite well if the calcium is removed and the valve opened surgically, but usually the affected valve must be replaced with an artificial substitute (see chapter 31, "Understanding Your Operation").

Early valve operations were done by touch and only mitral stenosis could be treated well. Even then, the results were only fair. Later it became possible to replace temporarily the pumping function of the heart with a heart-lung machine. This device receives "blue blood" from the veins, passes it through oxygenators, and returns the blood to the arterial side of the circulation. The heart can thus be opened and operated on under direct vision while the heart-lung machine does the heart's work.

Open-heart surgery has brought vast benefits. In mitral stenosis the valve can be opened under direct vision more effectively than in the days when the finger was used blindly, and valve replacements can only be performed with a heart-lung machine. Formerly a great deal of blood was required for the heart-lung machine but now only a pint or two may be necessary, sometimes none. Decreased use of blood saves money, avoids possible reactions, and reduces the chance of serum hepatitis (a liver infection) from blood transfusions. Serum hepatitis formerly was a serious complication of heart surgery.

The development of artificial prosthetic valves also has been a great advance. There are two general types. One is made of plastic and metal and the other of human or animal tissue, often combined with a supportive artificial skeleton. Most of the animal valves are taken from pigs, giving them the name porcine valves. Plastic valves may be ball or disc seated in a ring and enclosed in a cage. Ball valves are more commonly used. The great advantage of tissue valves is that "blood thinners" (anticoagulants) that prevent development of clots around the valves are required for only a short time after operation in many cases, in contrast to the permanent requirement in the case of plastic valves. However, plastic valves of modern design should

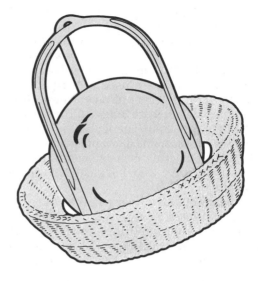

VALVE REPLACEMENT

Thanks to open-heart surgery, diseased or calcified valves of the heart may be replaced with artificial substitutes. The drawing above shows one of several ball-type prosthetic valves. The replacement is installed in the valve opening. Pressure of the blood forces the ball into its cage, allowing blood flow. The ball then returns to the valve seat to shut off the return of blood through the valve.

last almost indefinitely. Porcine valves appear to hold up well for many years but more experience is required for complete evaluation.

Most often a single valve is replaced, but sometimes two or three valves are required. The risk of open-heart surgery has decreased so greatly that it is not much more dangerous than the removal of part of the stomach because of ulcer. Recovery is rapid and long-term results are usually good.

Non-Rheumatic Valve Disease

Besides rheumatic valvular disease, there are several other types, grouped as non-rheumatic defects.

Prolapse (ballooning) of the mitral valve is the most common. The valve closes properly but reopens during the middle of the contraction phase. By this point most of the blood has been pumped out of the left ventricle, so little blood leaks into the left atrium. In mild cases, there is no leak at all; although the valve balloons it does not reopen. When the valve balloons a distinct "click" often is heard. If a leak exists, a murmur follows the click but either the click or the murmur may be absent.

An echocardiogram discloses this abnormality, which is usually minor and only rarely causes serious complications except in the elderly.

The anatomy of the mitral valve includes small threads of tissue called chordae tendinae which connect to the muscular wall of the left ventricle. For reasons unknown these threads sometimes degenerate and rupture, causing severe mitral insufficiency. This condition sometimes develops as a complication of mitral ballooning but often occurs spontaneously. It is relatively rare and surgical treatment is required.

The normal valve tissue is thin but strong. In rare instances, however, it develops a peculiar degeneration and thins further. The valves enlarge and sometimes tear. Either the mitral or aortic valve may be affected, and replacement is required.

Marfan's syndrome is a rare malady that may affect the aortic valve. It is accompanied by multiple defects in the body, particularly in the lens of the eyes and in the joints. Often the wall of the aorta is involved and the aorta greatly increases in size. The first part of the aorta may become so large that the aortic valve does not close properly and aortic insufficiency results. The tissue of the aortic wall degenerates and the middle wall develops microscopic sacs (cystic degeneration). The aortic lining may rupture and blood enter the middle wall, which tears easily because of the small cysts. This separates the aortic wall in such a way that a tube is formed within a tube. This is called a dissecting aneurysm of the aorta, and may also occur in other conditions. Valve replacement may be necessary, as well as repair of the aortic defect.

Aortic stenosis is mentioned under rheumatic heart disease, but more commonly is non-rheumatic. Often it is congenital, in which case the valve has two leaflets instead of three. Sometimes the valve has two leaflets without aortic stenosis, but narrowing of the valve opening is frequent. Symptoms are the same as in rheumatic aortic stenosis: shortness of breath, fainting, pain, and eventual congestive heart failure. It may cause trouble at any age. Sometimes the original defect is mild but calcium deposits gradually build up in the valve and further narrow the opening. Most cardiologists believe that there is also a form of non-rheumatic, non-congenital aortic stenosis, because aortic stenosis often occurs in middle-aged people who have never known of a murmur early in life. The symptoms in all cases are the same as in the rheumatic type. All varieties that cause significant symptoms are best treated surgically.

Disease of the Heart Muscle

The muscle of the heart (myocardium) is responsible for the pumping action. If the entire muscle is severely diseased, the force of contraction is decreased and heart failure results. There are several potential causes of heart muscle damage.

Viral infections sometimes damage the heart muscle. The damage may be difficult to diagnose because the cardiac manifestations may be delayed for days or weeks after the fever of the original illness has subsided, or the symptoms of infection may have been so mild that they are not recalled at a later date. There is no specific treatment other than the measures used to treat congestive heart failure. Permanent damage, even death, may result.

Defects of metabolism within the heart muscle are responsible for some cases of muscle damage. Normally the heart extracts oxygen and nutrients from the blood supplied to it and uses them to provide the energy needed for contractions. This is a complex chemical process, and it is suspected that the chemical reactions in some way go awry. Microscopic examination of the heart muscle does not reveal enough disease to account for the severely impaired heart function. The usual symptom is congestive heart failure, and sometimes there are rhythm irregularities. There may be periods of symptoms separated by long intervals in which the heart seems perfectly healthy. With effective treatment, patients may survive many years. In advanced disease there may be persistent irregularities of rhythm, and blood clots may form in the chambers of the heart.

Alcohol may cause severe damage to the muscle of the heart if consumed in considerable amounts over a long period of time. Any form of alcohol—liquor, wine, or beer—is capable of damage that may persist even after drinking has stopped. Recent studies have shown that even small amounts of alcohol can affect the strength of the heart's contractions, implying that anyone with evidence of a weak heart muscle should avoid drinking.

Hypertension (high blood pressure) puts a strain on the heart (see chapter 4, "Hypertension") because of the increased work demand, but the heart usually tolerates this strain well for many years. However, the muscles of the left ventricle tend to enlarge just as any muscle enlarges when exercised a great deal. Eventually its ability to contract is impaired and heart failure develops. It is almost always possible to control hypertension with drugs.

Subaortic stenosis, which means narrowing under the aortic valve, is a peculiar heart ailment that mimics rheumatic valvular disease yet is different. The left side of the wall (septum) between the ventricles enlarges, narrowing the channel through which blood must flow to reach the aortic valve. Usually there is an abnormality of the mitral valve as well. Treatment with beta blocking drugs to decrease the strength of contraction of the heart muscle can be helpful. An operation is rarely required. In those cases the surgeon may remove part of the overgrown muscle of the septum and sometimes replace the mitral valve as well. The cause of subaortic stenosis is unknown. Some think it is a congenital defect that often goes unrecognized until adult life.

ARTERIOSCLEROTIC
HEART DISEASE

Arteriosclerosis, popularly known as hardening of the arteries, is universal with advancing age. It is not known whether the thickening and hardening of the arterial walls and the loss of their elasticity represents a natural phenomenon or is the result of disease. Under certain conditions arteriosclerosis may even occur in childhood, and there is evidence that the process begins early in life.

Arteriosclerosis does no harm if the process does not decrease the inside diameter of the arteries. In the form called atherosclerosis, the lining membrane (intima) of one or more arteries becomes thickened, and a fatty substance called cholesterol is deposited. As deposits build up, blood must pass through a tube smaller than normal. A clot may form in the narrowed opening and stop blood flow completely.

None of the arteries are spared from the arteriosclerotic process (see chapter 5, "Blood Vessel Disorders" and chapter 11, "Stroke"). Common targets, however, are the coronary arteries controlling the blood supply to the heart. Disease of these arteries is widespread in Western society. It is the leading cause of death in the United States and most of Europe. Although coronary arteriosclerosis is often spoken of as "coronary heart disease," it is technically a condition of the arteries, not of the heart itself, but it is the heart that suffers.

New and Artificial Hearts

The first complete heart transplant was performed in 1966 and hundreds of persons with disabled hearts have received replacements since then (see chapter 31, "Understanding Your Operation"). Patients have survived more than 10 years after receiving a new heart. Some have undergone more than one transplant.

Heart transplant is most commonly considered when all or a large portion of the heart muscle is diseased, and the disease resists treatment. Candidates for transplant are chosen carefully. The overwhelming majority are under 50 years old and are otherwise healthy.

Although a transplant operation sounds heroic, it is not much more difficult for a skilled heart surgeon than replacing two heart valves. Two serious limitations, however, have prevented widespread use: availability of donor hearts and rejection of the new heart by the recipient's immune system. Unlike the kidney, for instance, a live donor may not choose to donate a heart. Moreover, donated hearts cannot be preserved for long periods, as kidneys can. The donor heart must be available from a reasonably young and healthy person who has died from causes not related to the heart, and the recipient must be ready for immediate transplant. If a kidney transplant fails, the recipient may always be returned to the artificial kidney until another operation can be attempted. A heart transplant patient seldom gets a second chance.

Rejection of a transplanted heart occurs because the recipient's immune system identifies the new organ as foreign and acts to repel it. Attempts are made to match tissues of donor and recipient, but it is unlikely that close matching will ever be possible on a large scale. Therefore the recipient is often given medication to suppress the immune response. This in turn leaves him vulnerable to infections, so he requires close supervision by immunologists as well as heart specialists.

A totally artificial heart would be preferable to a transplanted one because it would be available "off the shelf" and rejection would be eliminated. Attempts to design such an organ have been conducted for many years.

Symptoms arise when the narrowed arteries choke off the blood flow to the heart muscle.

Although the basic features of coronary arteriosclerosis are well known, the explanation for them is still debated despite a great deal of research. The fat (cholesterol) deposited in the lining membrane (intima) may be accompanied by clumps of blood platelets (necessary for normal clotting of the blood.) Many cardiologists think that the primary problem is a defect in fat metabolism which leaves fats that accumulate in the lining membrane. About half of the people who have coronary disease show abnormal amounts of fat in the blood. Other cardiologists think that deposits of blood platelets or occasionally blood clots come first and that fats later invade the affected areas. A recent theory is that the problem does not start in the lining membrane but in the middle wall of the artery. The muscle cells in the middle wall migrate into the lining membrane, where they degenerate. Fat is then deposited in the degenerated cells. Obviously, more understanding of the mechanism of arteriosclerosis is necessary if effective prevention and treatment are to be expected.

The risk factors. Statistically, it is known that certain circumstances increase the chances that a person will develop coronary arteriosclerosis. These circumstances are called risk factors. It is important to note that they are not synonymous with causes of coronary artery disease. They are simply characteristics found in large population samples that are associated with increased likelihood of developing the disease. Quite frequently, however, none of the known factors are present, but the disease still strikes. Sometimes the reverse is true.

Usually, several risk factors are listed:

• *Age* is the most obvious risk factor. Coronary disease is more common in the elderly than in the young. It is diagnosed most frequently between the ages of 45 and 55. However, it is not rare under the age of 40, may be encountered under 30, and rarely occurs in the teens.

• *Heredity* is another important factor. If one of your parents had coronary disease before age 50, your risk is significantly increased. Of course, as with any common medical problem, it would not be surprising to have some family history of coronary disease by chance alone.

• *Being male* is a risk factor. Men are more likely to be affected than women before the age of 50 but more women seem to be acquiring the disease early than was true several decades ago. Contraceptive pills apparently cause a slight increase in the development of coronary disease but the pill alone does not account for the change.

• *Obesity* appears to be a factor, but a slight one. There is some evidence that physically active people are less likely to develop coronary disease than sedentary ones.

• *Smoking* is definitely a risk factor. Avoiding cigarettes may be the single most important step toward preventing coronary disease. The increase in smoking among young women may be one explanation for increased coronary disease in females.

• *Stress* is often cited as a risk factor, but stress is difficult to define and measure. What is stressful to one person is not to another. Stress is a universal part of life, so its relationship to a specific disease or event in life may be more apparent than real. Some believe that having a certain personality type—the "Type A" personality—the conscientious, compulsive "doer," strongly increases the likelihood of coronary disease.

• *High blood pressure* (hypertension) is definitely associated with coronary disease as well as other diseases of the blood vessels. So is diabetes (see chapter 17, "Diabetes Mellitus") when it is acquired early in life.

• *Cholesterol.* The relationship between high blood cholesterol and coronary disease has been known for a long time and widely publicized. Nevertheless, the precise link remains unclear. Cholesterol is a natural fatty substance that plays an important role in body metabolism. It is also found in many foods, including eggs, meat, and shellfish. There is no doubt that a group of people who have high blood cholesterol levels have more coronary disease than a group in which the cholesterol level is normal or low. Yet coronary disease does occur in the low-cholesterol group, and many who have high cholesterol levels escape. It has been theorized that the cholesterol level is more important in persons under 50 than in older people.

Even if it were acknowledged that cholesterol is a primary risk factor for coronary disease, the question would remain: What makes it high? Cholesterol is a fat and there is some association between the amount of fat in the diet and the amount of cholesterol that turns up in the blood. But the relationship is not simple. A rigid, low-fat diet does not assure a decrease in the level of blood cholesterol, whether coronary disease is present or not.

Recent research has centered on two types of cholesterol, or lipoproteins. High-density lipoproteins appear to exert a protective effect against arteriosclerosis, but the low-density form appears to be implicated in the fat build-up within the arterial walls. Here, too, however, the apparent benefits of a high level of high-density lipoproteins appear to hold for statistical groups but not for individuals. There is no evidence that increasing the levels of high-density lipoproteins will reverse the course of coronary disease.

It is possible that unknown dietary factors influence the development of coronary disease. One that is being investigated is the amount of fiber in the diet. It is theorized that the substances contained in grains, cereals, seeds, and fruits may help clear excess cholesterol from the body, or perhaps may limit its formation.

The so-called coronary risk factors do not fully explain the occurrence of the disease. Certainly no risk factor has been shown to be a direct cause of disease. What should be done to protect ourselves against coronary disease?

Because heredity, sex, and age are imposed on us, the factors that we might be able to influence are smoking, stress, level of blood fats, and exercise. Although the evils of smoking have been publicized widely for years, the use of cigarettes remains widespread, even though this is an easy risk factor to modify. The number of smokers has decreased only 25 percent in two decades. If this simple change in lifestyle cannot be modified effectively on a mass basis, there may be little hope for changes requiring even more vigorous cooperation.

Stress, if it is a factor, is difficult to change. Stressful circumstances are part of life and even bring out the best qualities of some personalities. Changing our reactions to stress might help prevent the disease, but more research is necessary, both in the relationship, if any, of stress to disease and ways to modify it.

As for modification of diet, certainly the standard American diet contains more fat than necessary. A moderate restriction of dietary fat might be beneficial, but to prove it would require many years of reduction on a large scale. Obesity should be avoided even though it is not a major risk factor. The value of exercise is difficult to determine, but at least a moderate amount of regular, vigorous activity seems advisable.

Vigorous exercise throughout life might decrease the chances of development of coronary disease, but this is difficult to prove.

One of the problems with modifying risk factors is that to be most effective, the change must be undertaken early in life, at an age at which people are not prone to worry about development of disease in "old age," an age that turns out to be as young as the 30s and 40s.

Symptoms of Coronary Disease

In chronic cases of coronary disease, angina pectoris (the chest pain described on page 48) is the most common symptom. A complete description of this condition was first given by William Heberden in England in 1768. Thirty years later Caleb Parry, another English physician, presented a powerful argument for its association with coronary disease, but the idea was not widely accepted until the 1920s.

The chest pain of angina pectoris results when the work demanded of the heart is greater than the blood flow that can be delivered through the coronary arteries. Usually this occurs because the work load is increased by exertion or emotional upset. Sometimes the work load is unchanged and the inadequate flow is caused by a spasm that clamps down one or more arteries.

Walking is the most common activity to bring on the feelings of pain, pressure, tightness, and burning that characterize angina. The amount of exercise required to cause distress may remain the same for years or may increase with the passage of time. Improvement may stem from the development of small arteries (collateral vessels) which detour or reroute blood from one artery or part of an artery to another. These small arteries exist from birth but may increase in size in the presence of disease. In other cases of angina the ability to walk is impaired progressively. Pain may come even at rest, such as when the person first lies down at night. It has been shown that dreams are often responsible for pains during the night.

Heart Attack

The medical term for the common heart attack is myocardial infarction. This means death of heart muscle. Coronary thrombosis (blood clot) is often used to designate the same condition but the two are not synonymous. Myocardial infarction occurs without coronary thrombosis and coronary thrombosis occurs without myocardial infarction. Sometimes a heart attack is spoken of as "a coronary." This is poor English as well as poor medicine.

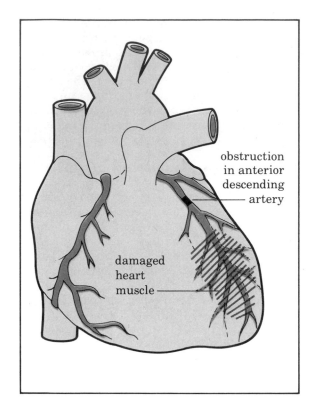

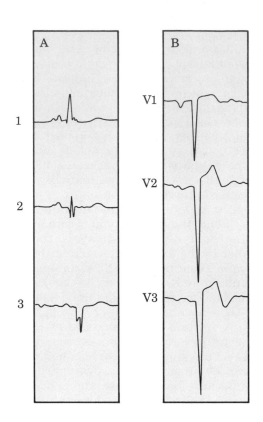

HEART ATTACK

The common heart attack, or myocardial infarction, occurs when one of the coronary arteries becomes blocked. In this illustration the anterior descending artery is blocked. The blood supply is reduced or closed off and the heart muscle that depends on it is damaged or dies. Outlook for the victim depends on the amount of damage and its location. The accompanying electrocardiogram *recorded during the attack shows a typical pattern when compared to the normal tracing on page 49. The three leads in drawing A show deep Q waves in leads 2 and 3, indicating damage to the bottom (inferior) wall of the heart. The three leads in B lack an R or positive wave and indicate an infarction of the front (anterior) wall of the heart.*

Myocardial infarction is caused by an acute reduction of blood flow through an artery. That reduction of flow is often caused by a clot. The drop in flow may be so severe that a portion of heart muscle dies. Chest pain similar to that experienced with angina pectoris is the typical symptom, but it is usually more severe, is not ordinarily precipitated by walking, and is prolonged for hours unless relieved by medication. The pain is often felt in the left arm and shoulder as well and may be accompanied by nausea, vomiting, sweating, and loss of consciousness.

Sometimes there is only mild pain or none at all, and other symptoms are evidence of the heart attack. Sometimes neither pain nor other symptoms occur and the attack is said to have been "silent." The damage may be discovered accidentally later, or even after death from other causes. The electrocardiogram is usually altered in a characteristic way during acute myocardial infarction, and generally some of these changes persist permanently. The death of muscle fibers of the heart releases certain enzymes into the blood, which can be measured. Enzyme levels are usually quite high in an acute heart attack but quickly return to normal.

If it were possible to predict an impending heart attack, early treatment might prevent serious damage. Unfortunately there are no reliable early warning signs. The appearance of pain not relieved by rest or by nitroglycerin (if the drug is available) is usually the first symptom, and this is commonly a sign that the attack is taking place rather than a warning sign of something yet to come.

Sometimes survivors later recall vague pains, feelings of breathlessness, or fatigue for several days preceding the attack. Significantly, a large number of heart attack victims have sought medical help in the month before the attack, a possible indication of awareness of fleeting symptoms. In any case, it is often difficult to predict a potential attack without elaborate procedures performed in a hospital.

The initial symptoms of myocardial infarction may often be so vague that they are ignored or rationalized. Pain in the chest may be written off as indigestion, perspiration blamed on mild fever or a warm day. Although speed is important in obtaining treatment, studies have shown that the average patient delays at least three hours after symptoms begin before seeking aid, and more if the symptoms begin at night. Among victims who are doctors, who presumably should be more aware of the dangers, the interval is even longer.

When myocardial infarction occurs, it is an emergency. Many persons die within minutes, before reaching a hospital or medical aid. About 15 to 20 percent of those who do reach a hospital die despite treatment.

Most major hospitals now include a coronary care unit (see chapter 31, "Understanding Your Operation") to which a victim is immediately transported.

In a coronary care unit experienced nurses are in constant attendance, and expensive equipment is available for monitoring the heart, recording the blood pressure, and measuring pressure in the vessels of the lungs. Other machines can alleviate serious irregularities of heart action, give precise amounts of potentially dangerous but necessary medications, and assist the circulation. The combination of equipment and expert help has reduced the hospital mortality rate from heart attacks.

In addition to heart muscle damage, blood pressure may decrease markedly during a heart attack, plunging the person into a state of shock. This is a serious complication and the victim has a poor outlook. Sometimes a balloon assist device is used to increase and maintain the blood pressure. A catheter tube on which a deflated balloon is mounted is threaded through an artery, usually in the leg, and passed into the aorta, the body's main artery. The balloon can be inflated and deflated alternately to help the pumping of the heart. Inflation of the balloon is timed by the electrocardiogram to occur during the resting phase of the heart cycle, so that the natural and artificial pumps do not compete. The blood pressure often rises markedly and may be maintained at a satisfactory level for hours or days. Unless the heart's total pumping ability is severely impaired, the patient is gradually "weaned" from the balloon pump.

With modern treatment of cardiac irregularities and cardiac resuscitation, the risk of the acute attack has decreased. In general, the risk is proportional to the amount of heart muscle damaged. Formerly, prolonged bedrest was part of the standard treatment, but in recent years the period of inactivity has been short. There may be no period of absolute bedrest in uncomplicated cases. Anticoagulants ("blood thinners") were part of routine treatment for a generation but many cardiologists now doubt their value.

After recovery from an acute heart attack, a scar forms in the region of dead muscle. If the scar is not extensive, the total pumping action of the heart returns to normal, which is the usual outcome. However, damage may be so widespread or there may be scars from previous attacks, so that the heart does not function efficiently as a pump. Heart failure may result. Or, when a large area is damaged, the wall of the heart may bulge, especially during contraction, assuming a dome-shaped appearance called ventricular aneurysm. In acute myocardial infarction, the thin wall of the heart may rupture, but ventricular aneurysms do not rupture because an aneurysm is composed of a strong scar, sometimes lined by blood clot. However, a large aneurysm reduces the heart's blood output because some blood is pumped into the bulge instead of out through the aortic valve. The result may be congestive heart failure. Some aneurysms are removed surgically. The risk of operation is low and the results are good in properly selected patients.

Coronary Insufficiency

A different condition causes more prolonged pain than angina pectoris, yet produces no evidence of damage to the heart muscle as in myocardial infarction. Various terms have been used to describe it, including intermediate syndrome, coronary insufficiency, coronary failure, preinfarction syndrome. The patient usually has typical angina pectoris as well. The prolonged pains usually occur without any apparent cause, lasting for 15 minutes to hours. Sometimes one or more of these pains may strike just before a myocardial infarction ("heart attack"), but more frequently infarction does not follow.

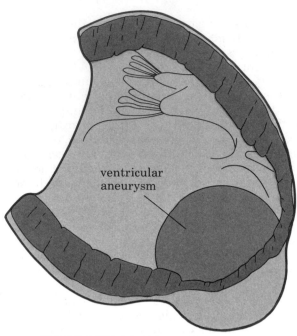

VENTRICULAR ANEURYSM

A ventricular aneurysm is a dome-shaped ballooning of the heart wall. It may develop after a heart attack if a large area of heart muscle has been damaged, as shown in this cross section. Paradoxically, the aneurysm may be stronger than the rest of the heart wall because it is composed of scar tissue. However, the heart may have to work harder because it pumps blood into the balloon-shaped area, and heart failure can result.

Another type of coronary pain has been called the variant form of angina pectoris. Pains are of short duration, as in ordinary angina, but occur without any apparent reason, predominantly and sometimes only at night. This pain has all the characteristics of angina pectoris except that exercise usually does not precipitate it. Certain peculiar changes in the electrocardiogram may be seen during an attack of pain. The cause is a spasm of a coronary artery. The muscular wall of a short segment of a major artery contracts, narrowing the artery to such an extent that not enough blood is supplied to part of the heart muscle. The pulse rate and blood pressure characteristically remain normal, unlike the rises that occur in typical angina pectoris. Occasionally, irregularities of the heart follow, and they sometimes cause fainting. This ailment tends to respond well to drugs.

Diagnosing and Treating Coronary Artery Disease

The diagnosis of coronary artery disease can be simple or difficult. If typical angina pectoris is present, the diagnosis is almost certain for men but not so for women, for unknown reasons. Physical examination is not very helpful and ordinary laboratory studies are of no diagnostic value. The electrocardiogram at rest is normal in about half the cases. When it is abnormal, the change is not necessarily a specific sign of coronary disease. Sometimes there is evidence of a "silent" myocardial infarction, recently or long ago. An electrocardiogram during and after exercise (graded stress test) may show abnormalities highly indicative of coronary disease. The uptake of various radioactive elements by the heart muscle can be helpful.

Finally, however, coronary arteriography may be done. This is a form of catheterization of the heart in which a liquid visible on X ray is injected into the right and left coronary arteries through a catheter. A high speed 35-millimeter movie will show the coronary arteries clearly, and study of the films in slow motion enables careful evaluation. A catheter also can be introduced into the left ventricle through the aortic valve, and an injection into this chamber shows the size and character of contraction of the ventricle (ventriculography). The blood pressure in the left ventricle can also be measured.

The treatment of chronic coronary artery disease aims to decrease the work of the heart and increase the coronary circulation. Neither of these objectives attacks the basic problem, the narrowing or total obstruction of one or more arteries. An ideal treatment would restore the lining membrane of the coronary arteries to normal but no such approach has been developed. Future possibilities are promising because coronary arteriography has shown that severely obstructed areas occasionally tend to return to normal. There is no obvious reason for this improvement.

A class of drugs known as beta blocking agents decreases the work of the heart by impairing the strength of contraction, slowing the pulse rate, and sometimes decreasing the blood pressure. The demand for coronary blood flow diminishes, so the reduced supply provided by the narrowed arteries may be sufficient. Angina may improve markedly or even disappear. Control of hypertension also can improve symptoms by decreasing demand. Limiting physical activity or the speed of activity can do the same. Regular exercise is important but repeatedly precipitating angina by exertion should be avoided. With a program of regular exercise, it is possible to increase the amount of exercise performed before symptoms occur. This benefit appears to result from improvement in the efficiency of the skeletal muscles rather than from any direct effect on the heart.

Drugs called vasodilators (blood vessel expanders) are used to increase the coronary circulation. The best known is nitroglycerin, which usually relieves angina after a minute or two when placed under the tongue. Nitroglycerin also lowers the blood pressure. The drug is destroyed rapidly in the body so that the effect dissipates in about 15 minutes. Because of its fast action and short-term effect, it is sometimes used before performance of an activity likely to precipitate pain, such as hurrying or sexual intercourse. But the short duration of effectiveness is a disadvantage, and chemically related drugs with longer-term action have been developed. The combination of these drugs with beta blocking agents is particularly helpful.

Persons with coronary disease certainly should stop smoking, because it has been demonstrated that the death rate is higher for smokers than for non-smokers. Whether the diet should be changed remains controversial. If the blood fats (cholesterol and triglycerides) are quite high, a diet low in animal fat is generally prescribed. Sometimes medicines are used to lower the fat levels. Changes in the blood fat levels usually are rather modest. Avoidance of alcohol might lower the triglyceride level. Most physicians believe that strenuous dietary measures are not helpful in persons over 50 years old.

Few people are severely disabled by angina although they may be inconvenienced. Some of the anxiety of angina patients stems from the realization that coronary disease is serious and angina serves as a recurrent reminder of the danger.

When a person has suffered one myocardial infarction or is diagnosed as having coronary disease, coronary arteriography often can provide clues about the outlook. There are two main coronary arteries, right and left, but the left divides into two branches, the anterior descending and circumflex arteries, so often it is said that there are three main arteries and many branches. The outlook is related to the number of arteries more than 50 percent narrowed. Narrowing of the left main artery is especially grave. A second factor is the condition of the left ventricle as shown by ventriculography. The outlook is best if the ventricle is normal, but the prognosis is not

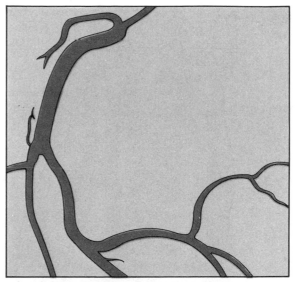

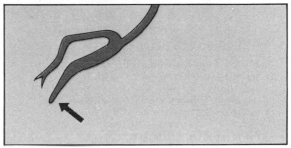

ARTERIOGRAM

Coronary arteriography enables a doctor to inspect the arteries for obstruction. Top drawing shows a normal right coronary artery. Lower drawing shows the same artery totally blocked. The arrow shows the point of obstruction caused by a spasm. An arteriogram is recorded by injecting a radiopaque dye, then taking a rapid sequence of X-ray photos. The blocked artery appears to end because the dye cannot pass the obstruction.

severely affected if the impairment is limited to a small area. However, if impairment is spread throughout the ventricle, outlook is poor. High blood pressure, diabetes, and age over 50 are also adverse factors.

It is not possible to state the outlook for a particular patient, only for groups having certain characteristics, because people die of progression of the condition, not from the symptoms that spur them to seek medical help. If medical science could assure us that the disease would not progress thanks to treatment, the outlook would be excellent. However, treatment is not aimed at the cause because the cause is unknown, so we should expect limited benefits.

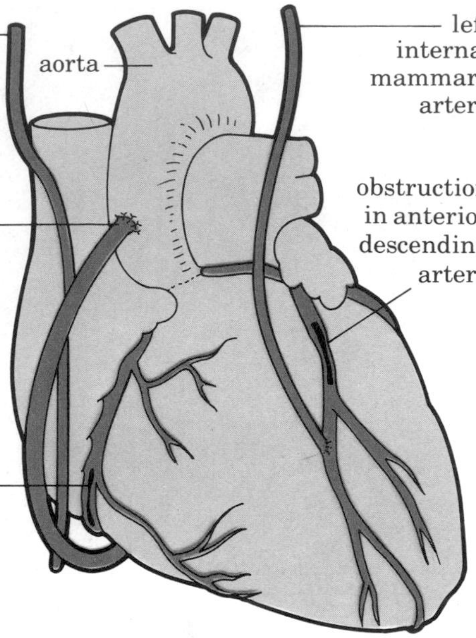

right internal mammary artery

aorta

left internal mammary artery

saphenous vein graft

obstruction in anterior descending artery

obstruction in right coronary artery

BYPASSING A BLOCK

The coronary bypass has become one of the most commonly performed operations. Two types are shown here. At left, a saphenous vein from the leg has been grafted from the aorta to the right coronary artery to bypass the blockage. At right, the internal mammary artery from the chest has been moved and grafted to the anterior descending artery, bypassing a blockage above. Sometimes all three coronary arteries may be bypassed in one operation.

Coronary disease tends to be episodic rather than relentlessly progressive. A person may have angina for five years and then experience a myocardial infarction. After that the angina may disappear or persist for 10 years, when another infarction may occur. Several years later a third infarction may cause death. Another patient may die suddenly at the first sign of heart disease. Still another may have an infarction and live for 30 years without further problems. Statistically, a person who has suffered one infarction faces a greater risk of a second, but the statistic has little meaning in individual cases. Until the cause or causes of coronary disease are identified, an accurate prediction of the future of a particular patient is unlikely.

Coronary Bypass Operations

The coronary bypass operation was introduced in 1967 and has been widely applied since. Like many other operations, it was often done poorly at first and frequently performed on the wrong type of patient. Gradually proper selection of patients has evolved and the operation can be accomplished at low risk with good results.

The original and still the most common bypass operation involves removing a vein from the leg and using a segment or several segments of the vein as conduits between the aorta and one or more of the coronary arteries. The grafts are inserted to bypass the narrowed area of the artery. If the graft remains open, which it does in about 85 to 90 percent of cases, a normal blood flow may reach each artery grafted. In the early developmental stages of the operation, post-operative myocardial infarction occurred in about 5 to 6 percent of cases. This risk has been lowered to 1 or 2 percent. Not all arteries can or should be grafted and not every patient who has coronary disease needs a graft.

Another bypass technique, the internal mammary artery graft, connects one of the arteries inside the chest to a coronary artery. This operation is more difficult but these vessels stay open more often—in about 95 percent of all cases. The left anterior descending artery is most feasible for this type of graft. Often this operation is combined with a vein graft for other arteries.

Properly performed bypass surgery certainly brings relief of angina in properly selected patients. The discussion among heart specialists and surgeons has centered on whether life expectancy is improved. The outlook seems better for patients at highest risk, those who have obstructions of the left main coronary artery or the three principal coronary arteries. Studies of patients who had involvement of two arteries suggest improvement also. In serious narrowing of a single artery, the risk is relatively low so it is difficult to demonstrate decreased risk afterwards.

Bypass surgery does not cure coronary disease but it does deal with the effects. Fortunately, narrowing of the coronary arteries tends to be most severe in the initial part of the artery and the surgeon grafts beyond this region. Graft failures due to obstruction may occur at any time, but most occur early, probably immediately after operation.

A recent development is a technique in which the narrowed portion of an artery can be dilated by a specially designed balloon catheter. This procedure is called angioplasty.

Inflation of the balloon ruptures the lining membrane of the narrowed area of the artery, and some of the material in the lining is carried away by the blood, leaving a much wider pipe through which the blood can flow. Narrowed areas that have been present for a long time tend to accumulate calcium and cannot be dilated, and some coronary arteries do not respond to dilation as well as others. The risk of the treatment is not much less than the risk of bypass surgery, but the procedure is simpler, less expensive, and painless. It appears that the method is helpful in a small percentage of patients, but much more experience will be required before it can be determined how long the beneficial effect lasts.

Bacterial Endocarditis

Bacterial infection of the valves of the heart or, more rarely, of other portions of the endocardium, is called bacterial endocarditis. Bacteria usually enter the blood during an illness, such as a sore throat accompanied by fever, or after a dental or surgical procedure. The bacteria normally are destroyed quickly but if the person has valve disease, the bacteria may set up an infection on the surface of the valve. Untreated bacterial endocarditis is almost invariably fatal. Any diseased valve may be the site for infection. Even normal valves are affected sometimes. Acute infections generally are caused by a virulent organism and may follow operations, especially those of the urinary tract. Even normal valves may then be involved. There is high fever and the responsible organism may be grown in a sample taken from the blood. Subacute bacterial endocarditis is less dramatic. The main symptom is mild intermittent fever which responds temporarily to antibiotics. The fever may last for many months before the diagnosis is made. Endocarditis attacks previously damaged valves or congenitally defective valves. Patients who have artificial valves are susceptible, too. Endocarditis almost always strikes the valves of the left side of the heart. Those on the right side are generally free from infection except for endocarditis encountered in drug addicts in which bacteria are usually introduced via contaminated needles.

Both acute and subacute endocarditis may cause serious damage to the valve affected, either during the infection's active phase or as a result of scarring from the healing process. Most cases respond well to prolonged treatment with antibiotics. In resistant cases, if there is serious valve damage or if the patient has an artificial valve, surgical treatment may be required. Antibiotics given at the time of sore throat with fever, and before and after dental procedures or operations decrease the likelihood of bacterial endocarditis.

Pericarditis

Infection of the membrane that covers the heart is called pericarditis. Acute cases are marked by fever and usually pain in the middle of the chest or slightly to the left of the middle. Deep breathing accentuates the pain. The infection is usually caused by a virus, although in rare instances bacteria may be responsible. A scratchy sound called a pericardial rub is heard in most cases. The electrocardiogram and echocardiogram usually show characteristic abnormalities and the chest X ray may reveal an enlargement of the shadow of the heart because of excessive fluid formed by the pericardium. Occasionally the fluid is so excessive that proper filling of the heart chambers is impaired and the fluid must be removed with a needle or by operation. Viral pericarditis usually subsides without treatment, although sometimes it recurs once or twice. Bacterial pericarditis responds to antibiotics.

Tuberculosis is responsible for a chronic type of pericarditis that is usually painless. The most visible symptom is swelling of the abdomen and legs caused by heart failure. Congestive heart failure results from impaired contractions of the heart and interference with its complete filling with blood because of thickened, diseased tissue and scar surrounding the heart. There is another similar but nontuberculous type of pericarditis of unknown cause. Surgical treatment involves peeling the thickened pericardium from the surface of the heart.

Tumors of the Heart

Tumors of the heart are rare. The most common arises from the interatrial septum, usually on the left side. It is called a myxoma and is usually benign, but nonetheless may cause death if it becomes large enough to obstruct a valve. Because it is more frequent on the left side, the symptoms and physical signs resemble those of mitral stenosis. The tumor can be removed surgically. Malignant tumors, most commonly of the lung or adjacent structures, may invade the heart and sometimes cause cardiac symptoms.

Considering the number of abnormalities that may affect the heart it is remarkable that this wonderful pump works so well in so many people for so long with no care.

CHAPTER 4   HERBERT G. LANGFORD, M.D.

HYPERTENSION (HIGH BLOOD PRESSURE)

Few major causes of death in the Western world can be reasonably and easily treated. The killers of history, such as malnutrition and infectious epidemics, have almost disappeared. Most of the problem diseases of today, such as heart disease and cancer, resist cures. High blood pressure (hypertension) is an exception. It is widespread, and it is a major cause of death and illness, but it *can* be treated.

WHAT IS BLOOD PRESSURE?

Each pumping stroke of the heart propels oxygen-enriched blood into the aorta, the body's main artery. From there the blood travels through gradually smaller arteries until it reaches the arterioles. These small elastic vessels regulate the flow of blood into the capillaries, which nourish the tissues. Between pumping actions the heart rests. The heart's pumping phase is called systole. The resting period is called diastole.

"Blood pressure" refers to the force that the blood is exerting against the arterial walls during both phases. Systolic blood pressure, which is the pressure during the pumping phase, primarily measures the force at the point of entry into the arterial circulation, the aorta. In a blood pressure reading, it is the larger (and the first) of the two numbers. The systolic blood pressure reflects strength of the heart muscle and rigidity of the large arterial walls. Diastolic blood pressure, the pressure during the resting phase, primarily refers to the pressure within the arterioles when the heart is not contracting. It can be affected by constriction (narrowing) of these small vessels. Diastolic blood pressure is the second number in a blood-pressure reading.

Blood pressure is not strictly a matter of the heart's pumping action. It is also affected by hormones secreted by the kidneys (see page 75) and by the sympathetic nervous system, which controls dilation and constriction (expansion and narrowing) of blood vessels.

MEASUREMENT OF

BLOOD PRESSURE

Normally blood pressure is measured indirectly. The examination, using either a mercury or more commonly an aneroid (dial) Baumanometer, is familiar to almost everyone. A cuff is placed around the upper arm and inflated until blood flow in the artery is stopped. Air gradually is let out of the cuff.

Through a stethoscope placed over the artery at the elbow, the person taking the pressure hears a thumping sound. This sound is the systolic pressure, the peak of pressure produced by the heart's contraction. As the pressure in the cuff is reduced, the noise fades. This represents the diastolic pressure and corresponds to the low point of pressure in the arteries.

Both these measurements are expressed in terms of how high the pressure will raise the column of mercury in the Baumanometer. A "blood pressure reading" of 120 over 80 means that the column stands at 120 millimeters of mercury during the pumping phase, and 80 millimeters during the resting phase. The reading is usually written as 120/80.

It is now possible to buy "kits" to measure your blood pressure at home. Coin-operated blood-pressure machines are also found in shopping centers. In general, if a person has regular medical checkups, it is seldom necessary for patients to take their own blood pressure. For some persons, however, periodic home measurement can be helpful in adjusting dosage of blood-pressure medication.

NORMAL BLOOD PRESSURE

Life expectancy is greatest when the blood pressure lies between 100/60 and 130/80. Above 130/80 life expectancy is progressively shortened as blood pressure is increased. Increase in either systolic or diastolic pressure can be responsible.

As a rule, both systolic and diastolic pressure are high at the same time. Occasionally one or the other is elevated alone. All the evidence suggests that either elevation is associated with an increased chance of disease. However, treatment of elevated diastolic pressure (the smaller number) has proven to be of value, while an elevation of systolic pressure (the larger number) is more likely to be an indication of disease than a cause of trouble.

Blood pressure is highly variable. It responds to emotion, exercise, caffeine, and pain. The blood pressure recorded in an apprehensive person in pain may be much higher than the blood pressure in the same person at ease in a doctor's office. The decision to treat high blood pressure is usually made on the reading taken in the office. Usually, the doctor will measure pressure several times and average the results to minimize the variables. The more often a physician takes blood pressure readings before deciding to treat a patient, the better the treatment is likely to be. A single reading taken when a person is in pain clearly could give an incorrect impression.

There is no sharp line between normal and abnormal blood pressure. If you measured the blood pressure of every person in a given geographical area, you would find a gradual change from clearly normal, in which there was no apparent association between blood pressure and early death, to hypertension, in which persons were more likely than others to die at an early age. Sir George Pickering refers to hypertension as a quantitative disease: The higher the pressure, the more disease is present.

For most persons, both systolic and diastolic pressure rise gradually with age. However, there is no truth to the old saying that normal systolic blood pressure represents the number of years of one's age plus 100.

HIGH BLOOD PRESSURE

Malignant hypertension is a rare form of high blood pressure. It gets its name because the blood pressure often will rise suddenly, rapidly, and progressively, with life-threatening consequences. The reasons for the sudden increase are often unknown, although almost any cause of untreated hypertension can culminate in the malignant form.

If the blood pressure goes high enough fast enough, it is a medical emergency. If the patient is not quickly treated with drugs or surgery, bleeding within the small vessels of the eye, brain, and kidney can cause severe damage, even death.

Symptoms of High Blood Pressure

Hypertension causes diseases with symptoms, but hypertension itself usually has no symptoms. People who claim they "can tell when their blood pressure is up" are usually wrong. But constant or recurrent headaches can be a symptom of hypertension. Perhaps a feeling of a "full head" or a little giddiness may be produced by high blood pressure. This may happen in someone who has had recent and rapid increases in blood pressure after stopping antihypertensive therapy.

Many persons with high blood pressure say they feel perfectly well and frequently are surprised when told they have hypertension. Not surprisingly, they sometimes resist treatment because they feel no symptoms. Even serious hypertension may not be discovered until it has been present for many years.

The Damage of Hypertension

The relentless pressure of uncontrolled hypertension damages the walls of both large and small arteries. The result is potential damage to key organs of the body, particularly the heart, brain, and kidneys, as well as the blood vessels themselves. The risks of heart attack and stroke, the two leading causes of death in the United States, rise sharply in a person with elevated blood pressure.

Several kinds of arterial damage can occur. Severe hypertension causes patchy destruction of the small arterioles. Arterioles may leak or burst in the eye, interfering with vision, or in the brain, causing confusion, fits, and coma. Damage to the arterioles in the kidney can interfere with the kidney's ability to rid the body of wastes.

Hypertension also causes the walls of the arteries to thicken. The process narrows the inner diameter of the artery, so the blood flow meets greater resistance, and pressure must be increased to push the blood through. The narrowing of the arterial channel also slows and reduces the blood supply, which is particularly serious in the kidney and may lead to kidney failure.

Uncontrolled high blood pressure over a long period may weaken the arterial walls and cause outpouchings (aneurysms) in the small arteries, especially in the brain. These aneurysms are relatively small, but they may burst and bleed, leading to a stroke.

The heart itself suffers when a person has high blood pressure. More heart muscle is necessary to enable the heart to pump against increased resistance. At first the heart is able to keep up with this demand. Later, probably because the heart muscle outgrows its blood supply, the heart will fail.

The major damage caused by hypertension occurs in association with arteriosclerosis, the process by which the arterial walls harden and lose their elasticity. Hypertension apparently helps to hasten the process called atherosclerosis, in which fatty deposits build up in the arterial walls, further narrowing the channel (see chapter 5, "Blood Vessel Disorders"). The exact relationship between hypertension and atherosclerosis is not known.

Probably hypertension injures the intima, the lining of the arteries, so that clots may form more easily. Perhaps the heightened blood pressure drives the cholesterol into the blood vessel walls.

Smoking also has been shown to accelerate the occurrence of atherosclerosis. It increases the risk of heart attack by further raising the blood pressure. Research has indicated that malignant hypertension in particular is more likely to occur in smokers than in nonsmokers.

Whatever the mechanism, the facts seem clear. A person whose cholesterol level or smoking habits would not lead to atherosclerotic vessel disease without high blood pressure becomes a likely candidate for disease if he or she has high blood pressure.

What Causes High Blood Pressure?

We don't know what causes high blood pressure in most patients. The name given to hypertension of unknown cause is essential hypertension. This name stems from previous fallacious reasoning by the medical profession. Moderately elevated blood pressure was once considered to do no harm and to be "essential" for health. Another incorrect adjective often added is "benign." "Benign essential hypertension" is neither benign nor essential.

Although we don't know the cause of most cases of hypertension, we do know factors that correlate with blood pressure.

Family history. High blood pressure runs in families. People whose parents and siblings have normal blood pressure are unlikely to have high blood pressure. Conversely, people whose families are rife with high blood pressure are likely to become hypertensive. We do not know how the family influence exerts its effect. Perhaps part of it is the common environment. However, the blood pressures of identical twins are likely to resemble each other much more than the blood pressures of fraternal twins, suggesting that heredity is more important than environment. Also, identical twins who were raised apart tend to have similar blood pressures. And in studies of adopted and natural children, blood pressure readings of natural children in a family were similar, but adopted children had little blood pressure resemblance to the rest of the family.

Certain strains of rats have been bred to be much more likely to develop hypertension than other laboratory rats, and studies of these animals may indicate how hypertension works in humans. One particular strain apparently has an inherited tendency to react to salt in the diet by developing hypertension. One abnormality in this rat appears to be a lessened ability of the kidney to excrete salt. Because high blood pressure helps to excrete salt, it is thought that these rats retain salt until the pressure goes up, then become able to excrete salt at the higher blood pressure level. Another strain of rats apparently has an overactive sympathetic nervous system. The sympathetic nervous system causes constriction of the arteries and veins, which raises the blood pressure.

Many people think that the human hereditary tendency towards hypertension may be like one or another of these varieties of rats. The sympathetic nervous system may be overactive or the kidney may be laggard in its salt excretion. Evidence has been offered in support of both of these hypotheses, but there is no proof that either of the mechanisms operates in humans.

Recently, several groups of investigators have shown a difference in the way red cells of hypertensive patients handled sodium, compared to red cells of persons with normal blood pressure. This abnormality appears to be confined to patients with "essential hypertension." Furthermore, it appears to be inherited as a simple dominant trait. The implication is that all the world is divided into two groups: those who are susceptible to hypertension and those who are not. If this implication is borne out by further research, it will have importance for our understanding and perhaps prevention of hypertension.

Obesity. The fatter a person is, the more likely he or she is to have high blood pressure. In the excessively obese, however, an elevated blood pressure reading may be misleading. The blood pressure cuff will not be able to compress the artery adequately, and a higher pressure will be recorded than is actually present.

However, when the pressure of the obese person is measured correctly, a blood pressure elevation remains. Weight correlates with blood pressure. Although there are exceptions, the more obese a person, the higher the blood pressure.

One possible explanation for the relationship between obesity and hypertension is that fat people eat more, including more salt. Therefore, it may be that increased salt intake is a major cause of the high blood pressure of the obese. However, even when the amount of salt changes, the relationship to obesity remains. In an Israeli study, obese patients were induced to lose weight on a diet which included large amounts of dill pickles. Apparently these patients did not reduce their salt intake, for they changed to a higher-salt but lower-caloried food. Nonetheless, when they lost weight, their blood pressure dropped.

The relation of obesity to hypertension could have enormous practical implications. For instance, a teenager with blood pressure that is "high normal" and who is somewhat obese certainly should try to lose weight. There is evidence that not only initial weight but weight gain correlates closely with development of hypertension. Also, it appears likely that most moderately hypertensive and slightly to moderately obese patients could control their blood pressure, at least in part, by reducing.

Sodium and potassium. A great deal of experimental work shows that an increase in intake of sodium chloride (table salt) or an increase in salt retention caused by hormone secretion will cause hypertension in experimental animals. Despite a tremendous amount of research, it is not clear how increased sodium raises blood pressure. One hypothesis says that the increased salt is taken up by the arteries, which then swell and narrow the inner channel. A second theory says that salt causes the body to retain water, which increases the blood volume. The heart pumps more blood and the vessels constrict to keep from being overloaded. A third holds that increased sodium affects the sympathetic nervous system, which again causes arteries to constrict.

In any case, it has been shown that tribes that eat little salt and a great deal of potassium (generally found in fresh fruit) have no hypertension. It is true that they also are thin, frequently diseased, and lack many amenities of modern civilization. The inhabitants of northern Japan, on the other hand, eat a great deal of salt, perhaps twice as much as the average American. Hypertension is probably more prevalent in northern Japan than in the United States. People in areas where little potassium is consumed may have more hypertension than those who live in high potassium intake areas. Potassium may prevent high blood pressure by increasing the excretion of sodium.

Emotions and stress. No concept is more deeply embedded in popular thinking than the idea that hypertension is caused by increased tension or stress. Like most basically erroneous ideas, this one has some basis in truth for its conception. Acute emotional episodes can affect blood pressure. Anger, excitement, and pain can raise the reading. Depression slowly lowers it. However, almost every attempt to find a clear-cut relationship between emotional makeup and blood pressure has failed. Attempts to relate hypertension to increased tension or anxiety, either on the job or at home, have almost uniformly failed. In fact, the blood pressure of the average inhabitant of the executive suite is usually much lower than that of the man or woman working at a menial job. One can change the definitions and say the executive really is under less stress. However, this isn't what most people think.

It is possible, although certainly not proven, that an acute emotional episode in a person with hypertension could raise blood pressure enough to produce an acute vascular problem. If so, the problem would be more likely to be a stroke than a heart attack.

Unless stress and disorganization interfere with taking medication, there is little evidence to suggest that the frequent advice to "avoid stress" helps to combat hypertension. Hypertension is not an excess of tension.

Specific Causes of Hypertension

In a small fraction of the people with high blood pressure, a specific cause can be identified. The medical profession can do something to help some of these people, so doctors are extremely interested in finding them.

Oral contraceptives (estrogen). The blood pressure of patients taking oral contraceptive agents increases on the average of one "point" (one mmHg) a year more than normal. The average means that some patients have no increase in blood pressure, and some have a great deal. The problem seems to be less common when low-estrogen birth control pills are used, but the lesson remains clear: Every woman taking oral contraceptives should have her blood pressure measured at least once a year. A woman who already has borderline hypertension or who has a family history of high blood pressure might want to consider another form of contraception. When use of the pill is stopped, hypertension caused by it will stop, too, although it may take as long as three months to return to normal.

There is some evidence that other estrogens given for menopausal symptoms affect blood pressure. The problem appears to be related to the size of the estrogen dose.

Narrowing of the kidney artery. In 1934, Dr. Harry Goldblatt applied clamps to the kidney arteries of dogs and found that persistent blood pressure elevation could be produced. The same situation occurs in humans. Young women may have narrowed kidney arteries caused by a disease of unknown cause called fibromuscular hyperplasia. Older people with atherosclerosis may have partial clotting of a kidney artery. When the kidney is deprived of its normal supply of blood, it responds by excreting less sodium and secreting the hormone renin, which contributes to blood pressure elevation. Diagnosis of narrowed arteries as the cause of hypertension requires X ray of the arteries (arteriograms) to determine arterial disease. Then the physician must identify the offending kidney by sampling blood from its vein to show that it is secreting an excess of renin.

Surgical repair of the diseased artery or removal of the kidney may produce a dramatic change. However, newer drugs that block renin actions, as well as diuretics, have made it possible to treat many patients without surgery.

Coarctation of the aorta. In this disease the great artery from the heart is narrowed above the kidney (see chapter 3, "The Heart and Circulation"). The blood pressure in the arms is high while blood pressure in the legs is low. The surgeon cures the condition by replacing the narrow artery with a graft.

Adrenal gland tumors. The adrenal gland just above the kidney secretes several hormones which, in excess, can produce hypertension (see chapter 16, "The Hormones and Endocrine Glands"). Too much hydrocortisone, for example, can cause hypertension plus obesity, weakness, easy bruising, and emotional changes. Too much aldosterone causes sodium to be retained and potassium to be excreted. Too much epinephrine (adrenalin) or norepinephrine (noradrenalin) causes fluctuating hypertension, nervousness, and sweating.

These rare diseases usually are diagnosed by measuring blood or urine levels of hormones, and they usually are treated surgically.

Chronic kidney disease. Infection or other disease can destroy much of the kidney, leaving patients susceptible to hypertension. A large intake of salt is more likely to raise blood pressure in these patients than in people with normal kidneys.

Special Tests for Hypertension

A few patients may need special studies to determine the cause of hypertension. Very few will require any more laboratory work than is necessary to determine the likelihood of heart or kidney disease. The usual laboratory tests are electrocardiogram and chest X ray, blood creatinine (elevated in kidney disease), blood sugar and blood potassium (which may be changed by drug treatment), blood cholesterol, and urinalysis.

WHO NEEDS TREATMENT

Just as there is no clear distinction between normal and abnormal blood pressures, there is no unequivocal line above which all persons need treatment and below which none should be treated. A person's blood pressure normally varies a good deal. The average blood pressure, as determined over several visits, helps more than a single blood pressure reading in deciding whether therapy should be started.

A large study by the National Heart, Lung, and Blood Institute has given the best guidance about when high blood pressure should be treated. The finding appears unequivocal. Anyone 50 years of age or older whose diastolic blood pressure is 90 or higher should be treated. The study did not recommend whether the treatment had to be drugs or whether dietary rearrangement could be tried in mild cases. The evidence is less clear for the 30–49 year old group, but it is likely that a diastolic pressure reading of 90 is the point at which a decision on treatment should be made for any age. Anything above that level probably should be treated.

PREVENTION

There is no clear evidence that hypertension can be prevented. However, the person who has a family history of hypertension, has a tendency towards high blood pressure, and is somewhat obese faces a higher risk of developing hypertension. Although it has not been proven that hypertension can be prevented by staying thin, keeping one's salt intake low, and eating a lot of green vegetables, root vegetables, and fruit with high potassium content, it seems reasonable to pursue such a course. In addition, persons at risk for developing hypertension should remember that hypertension interacts with other risk factors. It is more important for these persons not to smoke than for someone who has normal blood pressure. It is also more important for them to restrict fat and cholesterol intake. Exercise may help directly to prevent hypertension, although the evidence is not clear-cut. But exercise certainly helps a person stay thin, and thus indirectly may prevent hypertension.

THERAPY

Doctors still debate the exact level of blood pressure that warrants drug treatment. It is clear that treating severe hypertension in men prolongs their lives and reduces the chance of stroke. It is probable that treatment also helps men with milder hypertension and hypertensive women. Therapy usually must be lifelong. There are occasional exceptions, usually persons who have lost a large amount of weight or have markedly decreased salt intake. However, for most patients, it is important to realize that taking a pill must be a daily act, probably for the rest of their lives.

Treatment and life insurance. Because hypertension can reduce life expectancy, an untreated patient usually can obtain life insurance only by paying high premiums, if it is available at all. However, many companies will accept *treated* patients who have demonstrated that they will take medication faithfully and keep their blood pressure under control. These persons pay a rate only slightly higher than the standard rate. There is probably no greater incentive for taking the medications and modifying the diet.

Diet and Weight Loss

There is renewed enthusiasm for weight loss as treatment for mild hypertension, often in conjunction with drugs, but sometimes as the sole therapy. Part of the lack of enthusiasm for prescribing weight loss in the past has been the difficulty in getting patients to take off pounds. However, the patient who decides to lose weight and to keep it off is the kind of patient doctors would like to have.

The benefit of losing weight may not be confined to the obese. The 10 pounds or so that many of us have gained since age 20 is usually not muscle or bone and certainly is not increased brain weight. It's fat. Therefore, the patient often can lose 10 pounds, even if friends consider him or her relatively thin. We still do not know which persons will respond to weight loss with lowered blood pressure, but it occurs frequently enough that even those who are slightly overweight should try reducing.

Salt Restriction

Salt restriction is also being re-emphasized. Here, too, doctors cannot predict how many patients will benefit. However, almost any physician will be delighted if a hypertensive patient voluntarily restricts salt consumption.

A desirable goal for the hypertensive person is to lower salt intake to four grams or less a day. This can be achieved easily if only fresh foods are used. However, grocery shelves are full of traps for the unwary. Soups, catsup, baking powder, self-rising flour, and tomato juice are examples of foods that are high in salt but are not obvious sources. Chinese and Japanese cooking, so healthful in many ways, may be high in salt because soy sauce and monosodium glutamate are sources of large amounts. All prepared meats are high in salt. Pickles are soaked in brine. Salt, to put it simply, is all around us.

Salt Appetite

One problem in reducing salt intake is that people have a salt appetite. Just like the laboratory rat deprived of salt, or cattle on the range, human beings tend to increase their salt intake if they are salt-deprived. However, it probably takes rather marked deprivation to cause this appetite. Much of our salt intake is habitual.

A person who reduces salt intake initially will find that the food tastes insipid. Part of this problem can be overcome by the generous use of spices, lemon juice, and pepper. In addition, some patients will find that salt substitute, which is primarily potassium chloride, will really replace salt. Others say the bitter taste of potassium chloride makes it unacceptable. However, even if not needed as a salt substitute, potassium chloride mixtures are excellent sources of potassium for the patient who must replace the losses produced by diuretics.

Drug Treatment

Diuretics. We don't know that salt causes hypertension, but getting rid of salt frequently controls hypertension. Most patients are started on a "thiazide-type" diuretic, which is the most efficient if they have normal kidneys. Diuretics have some side effects. The drugs rid the body of potassium as well as sodium, so the patient using them must try to increase consumption of potassium. Citrus fruits, lean meats, leafy and root vegetables are good sources of potassium. The best approach, however, is to reduce salt intake. The patient can then take fewer diuretics and achieve with fewer side effects the same blood pressure reduction that a large dose of diuretics would produce. Diuretics also may increase blood sugar and uric acid, and diabetes may be precipitated or gout may occur.

Drugs that interfere with the sympathetic nervous system. Most other drugs that lower blood pressure work by decreasing sympathetic nervous function. There are two types. Beta-blocking drugs interfere with the function of the nerves' beta fibers. These drugs have become a valuable form of hypertensive therapy. Reserpine, methyldopa, and guanethidine block sympathetic function in various ways, but do not primarily involve the beta fibers. Some patients have no side effects. Others have marked depression, loss of interest in sex, diarrhea, and dizziness on standing. The beta-blocking drugs may unmask asthma or make it difficult to treat.

The sympathetic blocking drugs may lower blood pressure by lessening the degree of sympathetic stimulation of the blood vessels, therefore allowing the vessels to dilate. Also, the secretion of renin is partially under sympathetic control. Less renin is secreted by the kidney when there is less sympathetic stimulation.

Vasodilator drugs directly open the small arteries. The most common are hydralazine and minoxidil. Both are effective, but they usually are used when patients have not responded to the combination of a diuretic and a drug that decreases the action of the sympathetic system. The combination of the three drugs is potent. Almost all hypertensive patients can be controlled with so-called "triple therapy."

Other drugs. An interesting new class of drugs soon may be available to treat hypertension. Normally, the kidney secretes renin, and renin then splits a substance from the blood's plasma proteins, angiotensin I. A "converting" enzyme further changes the substance by removing two amino acids. The result is angiotensin II, a very powerful blood pressure raising substance that may be closely linked with the final cause of hypertension. The new class of drugs stops the conversion of angiotensin I to angiotensin II. Many but not all hypertensive patients appear to improve markedly with these medicines. Extensive tests are being done to see whether the early promise of these drugs will be fulfilled.

Avoiding Side Effects

One of the major reasons that patients stop anti-hypertension medicine is the unpleasant side effects. The side effects can be minimized several ways. The dose of the drug often can be reduced if the patient will reduce salt intake. Obviously the less of the drug used, the less the intensity of the undesired side effects. Secondly, alternative drugs can be tried. We cannot predict which drug will be tolerated by which patient, but almost all cases can be controlled without severe side effects.

Discontinuing Treatment

The greatest handicap to blood pressure control is the natural tendency of patients to feel that they are well, and therefore do not need to continue medication. Treatment usually must be for life. The doctor and the patient together must work out a simple and satisfactory drug combination. The patient must remember that a normal blood pressure on medication does not mean that the medicine is no longer needed. It means the medicine is working. Furthermore, blood pressure does not always increase immediately after stopping medication. A normal blood pressure reading, as determined by a machine in a shopping mall, tells nothing about whether the medication should be continued.

Also, some of the drugs used for treating hypertension must not be stopped suddenly, because the blood pressure may go too high. Even angina pectoris can be precipitated in some patients if they suddenly stop taking medications.

LOW BLOOD PRESSURE

In general, the lower your blood pressure, the longer your life expectancy and the less your chances of cardiovascular disease. Low blood pressure (hypotension) is, in all probability, the healthy state. It is true that people with relatively low blood pressure sometimes feel dizzy when they get up rapidly in the morning, but this temporary dizziness—doctors call it postural hypotension—seems a small price to pay for freedom from more serious problems.

Some people blame low blood pressure for "that tired feeling" or "the Monday morning blahs," or inability to concentrate. A few rare diseases are associated with low blood pressure, but these are specific illnesses and not part of a "fatigue syndrome." There is, however, one common cause of postural hypotension—a hangover.

CHAPTER 5   JESS R. YOUNG, M.D.

BLOOD VESSEL DISORDERS

The heart and circulation constitute a single system. Each thump of the rhythmic heart pushes bright-red, oxygen-laden blood into a network of pipes called arteries. The blood travels through ever-smaller arteries until it reaches the microscopic capillaries that nourish the tissues. Then, having yielded its oxygen and changed in color to dusky red, it returns to the heart through another network of tubes, the veins. The arteries, veins, and heart, along with the lymphatics, are known as the vascular system.

There are more veins than arteries, and they are generally larger in diameter. They have thinner walls, and are equipped with valves to prevent backflow, because the blood in them is moving against the force of gravity. Venous circulation is smooth and even, in contrast to the pulsating movement of arterial circulation, powered by the pump-rest-pump cycle of the heart. Otherwise the vessels are similar in structure (which allows surgeons to substitute a section of healthy vein for a damaged artery). They are made up of three layers—the tough outer casing, the fibrous middle layer, and the smooth inner bore. With disease or age, changes can occur in these layers. The result is a group of conditions loosely grouped as vascular diseases or disorders of blood vessels. Some disorders affect arteries, others affect veins.

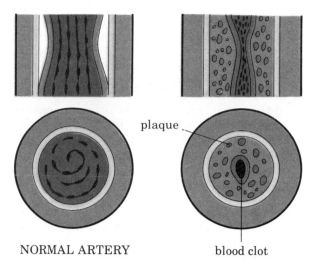

NORMAL ARTERY plaque blood clot

AN OBSTRUCTED ARTERY

The cross section at left shows a normal artery, with its central channel large enough for blood to flow through. At right, the artery has been partly obstructed. Deposits of fats, calcium, and smooth muscle cells have built up in the walls, narrowing the channel and providing a site for formation of a blood clot.

OCCLUSIVE ARTERIAL DISEASE

To "occlude" means to obstruct. The normal inner channel, or lumen, of an artery is smooth and even, and blood flows through it evenly. In occlusive arterial diseases, however, the channel becomes narrowed or blocked and the blood flow is obstructed, with potential damage to the tissues served by these arteries. The obstruction may occur suddenly (spasm), or develop gradually.

Arteriosclerosis Obliterans

(hardened and obstructed arteries)

Arteriosclerosis is the most common form of arterial disease. It is the leading cause of death in the Western world. The term applies to the condition in which the arteries thicken, harden, and lose their elasticity.

This process itself would not necessarily be harmful, but it is usually accompanied by another condition called atherosclerosis. In atherosclerosis, deposits of calcium, fats (especially cholesterol), and smooth muscle cells build up in arteries until they reduce or obstruct the blood flow. The deposits, called plaques, also provide sites where blood clots may form and further obstruct the flow. The combination of hardened arteries with atherosclerotic deposits and obstructed blood flow is known as arteriosclerosis obliterans.

Fortunately, a blocked artery does not always cause destruction of tissue it supplies. If the obstruction develops slowly, a new network of small arteries will develop around the blocked area. This new network—doctors call it collateral circulation—is usually enough to keep the tissues alive, although it may not be sufficient to supply enough blood to muscles during exercise.

The hardening and deterioration of arteriosclerosis can affect any artery in the body. If the arteries that supply the heart are affected, chest pain during exertion (angina pectoris) or a heart attack (myocardial infarction) can occur (see chapter 3). An obstruction in the arteries that lead to the brain can cause a stroke (see chapter 11). If the blockage occurs in the arteries supplying the legs (aorta, iliac, femoral, tibial, and peroneal arteries), walking becomes painful. If the problem isn't treated, gangrene ultimately can result, which could make amputation necessary. Arteriosclerosis obliterans accounts for 90 percent of all cases of occlusive arterial disease of the legs.

Causes. Arteriosclerosis obliterans, like cancer, appears to have many interacting causes. It affects almost all adults in some form, but the location, severity, and rate of development vary greatly. Heredity undoubtedly is important, because some families have a high incidence of early atherosclerosis and the resulting strokes, heart attacks, or gangrene. Even persons in their 20s and 30s may be affected.

The female hormone estrogen appears to provide protection against atherosclerosis. The rate of occurrence increases progressively in men after age 30, but similar increases are not noted in women until after age 50, when estrogen production declines.

A major factor in atherosclerosis appears to be excessive concentrations of blood fats (lipids), particularly cholesterol. The higher amount of blood fats may be related to both heredity and diet. Cigarette smoking, high blood pressure, obesity, diabetes, physical inactivity, and emotional stress also have been linked to the development of atherosclerosis. It seems logical that a disease as variable as atherosclerosis can develop from different combinations of causes in different individuals.

Symptoms. Numbness, tingling of the legs and feet, leg cramps at night, and a feeling of coldness usually are *not* symptoms of the diseases that obstruct arteries, although they are frequently misinterpreted as such. The first symptom is usually a distinctive form of limping known as intermittent claudication. After walking a certain distance, the person develops pain, cramping, or weakness in one or both legs, which disappears within two to five minutes after he stops walking, whether or not

he sits down. Depending on the location of the obstructed artery, the symptoms can occur in the muscles of the arch of the foot, the calf, thigh, buttock, or arm. The pain comes sooner if the patient walks fast or walks uphill. Pain in the arm or leg at rest indicates a worsening of the condition. Resting pain is usually more severe at night, and may be eased by elevating the head of the bed, by hanging the leg over the side of the bed, or by sitting in a chair. Severely painful skin ulcers and gangrene are the final result of severely restricted blood flow to the limb.

Diagnosis. The presence of a blocked or restricted artery, and how severe the problem is can be determined in the doctor's office. The most important finding is the absence or decrease in strength of the leg and foot pulses. A variety of instruments, ranging from simple devices used in the office to more complicated and expensive instruments suitable only for a vascular laboratory, are available for diagnosis. If surgery is contemplated, angiography (X rays taken after injection of dye into the aorta and the thigh artery) is necessary to determine whether surgery is possible and which method of surgical repair is best.

Treatment. The patient who smokes must stop. Nicotine causes spasm (contraction) of the arteries, and is most likely one of the causes of arteriosclerosis.

A good exercise program is important. Leg exercises help improve circulation around the blocked artery. The patient should strive to walk at least an hour every day. He should not stop at the first sign of discomfort, but should walk until he feels that he must stop to rest. Other forms of leg exercises such as jogging, cycling, and swimming are encouraged.

Infections and injuries of the legs and feet should be prevented, because the obstructed artery means they will heal poorly. Many amputations can be avoided with proper care of the toenails, treatment of athlete's foot, and avoidance of extremely hot and cold temperatures. Hot water bottles and heating pads should never be used to warm the feet, no matter how cold they become. Ingrown toenails, corns, and callouses should be treated by a physician or a foot specialist. Shoes should be soft, comfortable, and fit properly. A lotion containing lanolin should be used regularly to help keep the skin supple and prevent infection. The importance of proper foot care in patients with arteriosclerosis cannot be overstressed.

Loss of excess weight is also important for patients with arterial insufficiency. A low-fat diet with a high level of unsaturated fatty acids is advisable. If the person's blood shows persistently high fat levels despite proper diet and weight reduction, a lipid lowering drug may help.

The value of drugs that enlarge or expand the blood vessels is a controversial subject. Many physicians have not found them effective. An ounce of whiskey or brandy, or a glass of wine three or four times daily may be just as effective in dilating the vessels. Having been forbidden nicotine and many desired foods, most patients are relieved to know that alcoholic beverages are permitted in limited quantities.

An operation may be necessary to improve circulation in some patients. Most blood vessel specialists agree that arterial surgery is not recommended for the lameness and calf muscle pain of intermittent claudication except for a few patients whose livelihoods depend on being able to walk considerable distances. Even then, a three- to six-month trial period of diet, weight loss, and exercise may improve circulation enough that an operation will not be necessary. If improvement does not occur, or if the patient develops pain while resting, nonhealing ulcers, or early gangrene, the condition can then be treated surgically.

An operation to remove the deposits of plaque or to bypass the blocked artery may be effective if the arteries beyond the blockage are open and adequate (see chapter 31, "Understanding Your Operation"). If the blockage is in the large arteries of the abdomen, a bypass procedure is performed. A synthetic fabric such as Dacron is generally used for the replacement artery. For blockage in arteries below the groin, the preferred graft is the patient's own leg vein. Other materials are used in this area only if no healthy vein is available. The outcome of surgery depends on many factors such as the site of the blockage, the amount of collateral circulation, and the age and general health of the patient.

Sympathectomy is another form of surgery sometimes used. In this procedure an attempt is made to overcome the narrowing of arterial spasm by cutting certain nerves to the arteries. This may improve the skin circulation, and therefore may help patients who have mild pain at rest, small ulcerations, or minor areas of gangrene. The limping of intermittent claudication and extensive gangrene, however, will not be helped.

Buerger's Disease

Buerger's disease (thromboangiitis obliterans), although relatively rare, ranks second to arteriosclerosis obliterans as a form of occlusive arterial disease. It affects the small and medium arteries and the veins in the arms and legs by causing inflammation, clotting, and blockage. It develops mainly in men 25 to 40 years old. The disease occurs almost exclusively in smokers, and stopping smoking usually brings improvement.

Pain is the outstanding symptom of Buerger's disease. It ranges from the lameness and pain of calf muscles when walking (intermittent claudication) to the severe, steady pain of ulceration and gangrene. Toes and fingers are most commonly affected. About 40 percent of patients have blood clots in the veins at some stage of the disease.

All patients with Buerger's disease should abstain from tobacco in all forms, including chewing tobacco and snuff. This abstinence should be complete and permanent. Even an occasional cigarette may cause a recurrence of the disease. Amputations usually result if the patient cannot stop smoking.

Many patients will improve markedly after they stop smoking, and no further measures will be needed. If sufficient improvement has not occurred within two to three months, the nerve cutting techniques of sympathectomy may help.

ARTERIAL ANEURYSMS

An aneurysm is a ballooned, dilated area of an artery. It can be likened to the ballooning of a weakened spot on an inner tube or tire. Aneurysms can occur anywhere in the circulation, but the segments of the aorta (the body's main artery) that lie in the chest and in the abdomen are common sites.

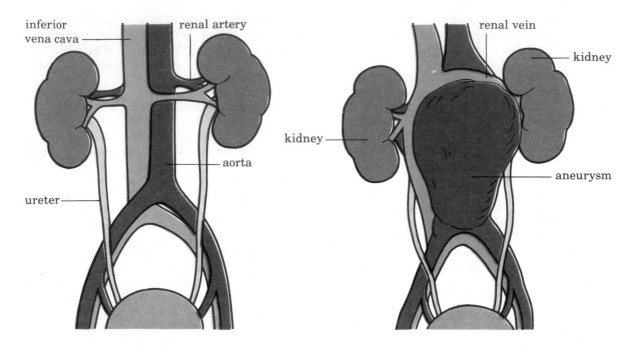

ARTERIAL ANEURYSM

The body's main artery, the aorta, is the most common site for ballooning of a weakened arterial wall, a condition known as aneurysm. The normal structure of aorta, kidneys, and kidney arteries is shown at left. At right, the aorta has ballooned just below the renal arteries, displacing the kidneys, blood vessels, and ureters.

Aneurysms are uncommon in persons under 50, and are 10 times more frequent in men than women. The hardening and loss of elasticity resulting from arteriosclerosis is the major cause of aneurysms. The structural reason for aneurysm formation is damage to the middle layer of the wall of the artery. When only the thin lining and outer fibrous layers remain, the artery begins to dilate or balloon out from the pressure of the pulsating blood flow.

In its early stages, the aneurysm produces no symptoms. Symptoms usually result as it enlarges and exerts pressure on adjacent organs and tissues. In the later stages, symptoms also can be caused by thinning of the aneurysm wall or by leakage of blood through the wall. The location and severity of the symptoms depend largely upon the location and size of the aneurysm.

The most common type of aneurysms occur in the abdominal aorta. They usually start just below the level where the renal arteries branch off to supply the kidneys. The major symptom usually is pain in the upper abdomen or lower back. The pain may extend into the groin and the legs. Pain is an important symptom, because it often indicates rapid enlargement or leaking of the aneurysm. If it is not treated, the aneurysm usually will rupture, causing intense pain and leading to death from loss of blood.

Chest (thoracic) aneurysms usually are discovered on an X ray taken for some other reason. Abdominal aneurysms without symptoms are detected during a physical examination for an unrelated abdominal symptom, but if the patient is obese or if the aneurysm is small, it may not be found. An X ray may show the aneurysm if calcium is present in the aneurysm wall. The use of ultrasound (see chapter 32, "X Rays and Radiology") also has proved valuable. By this method, an image of the aneurysm and its size can be obtained. Not only can the diagnosis be confirmed, but the development of the aneurysm can be followed in patients who are poor risks for surgery.

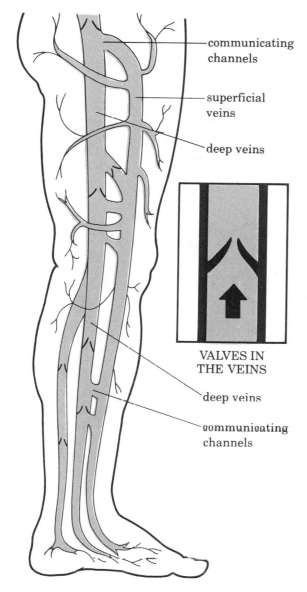

VEINS OF THE LEGS

The main connections between the superficial and deep veins of the legs are behind the knee and in the groin. A series of communicating channels also connects them. The insert drawing shows one of the cup-shaped valves that open to allow blood to flow toward the heart, then close again to prevent backflow. Varicose veins develop when the valves are not working properly, permitting stagnation and pooling of blood. They are most common in superficial veins, which have less muscular support than deep veins.

When an aneurysm is large or is producing symptoms, the preferred treatment is to remove the affected portion of the artery surgically and replace it with a synthetic fabric graft. The decision about whether smaller, symptomless aneurysms should be removed depends on the patient's age and general health. Results of surgery for aneurysms are good, and surgery has been a major factor in reducing the previously high death toll caused by aneurysms that were not treated surgically.

VARICOSE VEINS

More than eight million Americans, six million of them women, suffer from varicose veins. This ailment, often characterized by swollen and all-too-visible bluish "cords in the legs," has been recognized since ancient times. Varicose veins probably date back to the time when prehistoric man learned to stand upright and the blood in the veins of the legs had to flow uphill against gravity from the ankle to the heart.

The veins are the vessels through which blood returns to the heart after the oxygen and nutrients have been distributed to the tissues. Attached to the inside walls of all the main veins are valves. These valves are irregularly spaced, cup-like structures that open as the blood flows upward to the heart, then close to prevent it from dropping back toward the feet. Varicose veins develop when the valves are not working properly.

There are two sets of veins in the legs: superficial and deep. As the names imply, the superficial veins lie near the skin surface, while the deep veins lie far beneath it, next to the arteries and bones. The major connection between the systems is in the area behind the knees and in the groin. The systems also connect by a number of communicating veins.

The muscles of the legs help support the deep veins. In walking or moving, contraction of these muscles helps force the blood along its upward course. The superficial veins are the ones most likely to become varicose because they have the least muscular support.

Causes. Varicose veins develop when the walls of the veins or the valves are weak. Some persons are born with weak veins or valves. In others, disease or injury causes the damage. When the valves can no longer prevent backflow of the column of blood, abnormal pressures dilate the superficial vein system, causing stagnation and pooling of blood.

ARTERIES AND VEINS

Pulmonary arteries carry blood to the lungs to receive oxygen. Blood then returns to the left side of the heart and is pumped to all parts of the body. The arteries are shown in this detailed "road map."

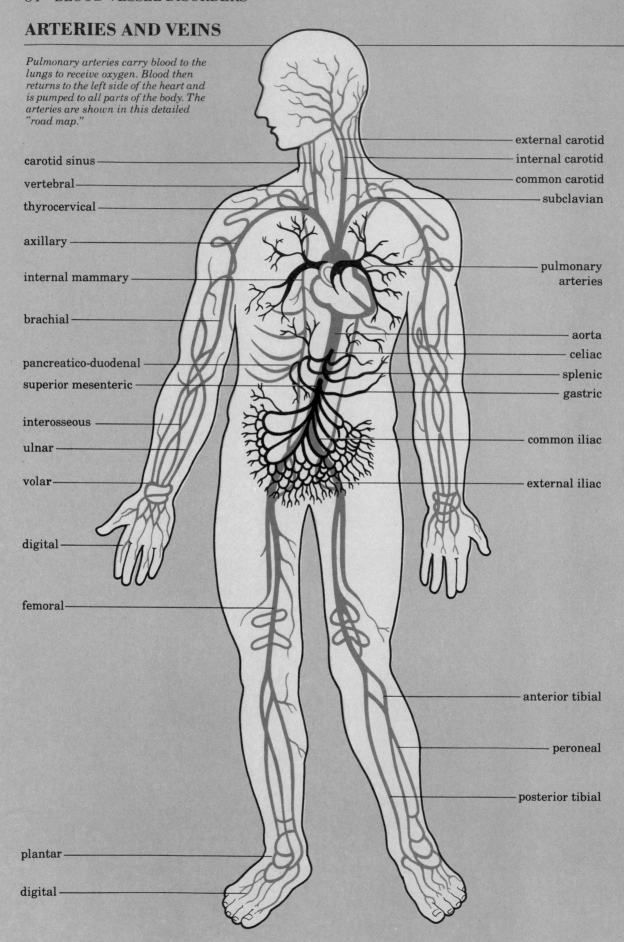

carotid sinus

vertebral

thyrocervical

axillary

internal mammary

brachial

pancreatico-duodenal

superior mesenteric

interosseous

ulnar

volar

digital

femoral

plantar

digital

external carotid

internal carotid

common carotid

subclavian

pulmonary arteries

aorta

celiac

splenic

gastric

common iliac

external iliac

anterior tibial

peroneal

posterior tibial

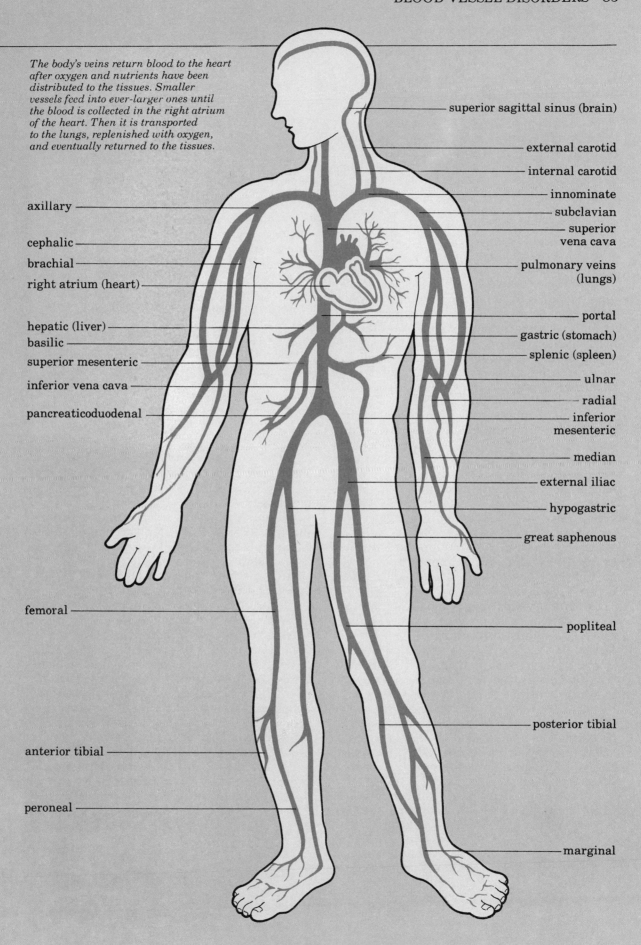

The body's veins return blood to the heart after oxygen and nutrients have been distributed to the tissues. Smaller vessels feed into ever-larger ones until the blood is collected in the right atrium of the heart. Then it is transported to the lungs, replenished with oxygen, and eventually returned to the tissues.

axillary

cephalic

brachial

right atrium (heart)

hepatic (liver)

basilic

superior mesenteric

inferior vena cava

pancreaticoduodenal

femoral

anterior tibial

peroneal

superior sagittal sinus (brain)

external carotid

internal carotid

innominate

subclavian

superior vena cava

pulmonary veins (lungs)

portal

gastric (stomach)

splenic (spleen)

ulnar

radial

inferior mesenteric

median

external iliac

hypogastric

great saphenous

popliteal

posterior tibial

marginal

Heredity is an important factor. Most women and men who suffer from varicose veins have parents or grandparents who have had them. Even in persons born with normal healthy veins, thrombophlebitis (inflammation of the vein with a blood clot; see page 87) can develop and seriously damage the valves and vein wall. Vein valves also can be affected when obesity, pregnancy, or tumors interfere with blood flow in the deep veins. Varicose veins develop in elderly people because the veins tend to lose elasticity with aging, and the muscles supporting them weaken.

Symptoms. Some people with severe varicose veins are never troubled by them, while others with mild cases have many complaints.

A feeling of heaviness in the legs, especially after standing for a long period, is a common early symptom of varicose veins. Other symptoms or signs include feelings of fatigue in the leg muscles, swelling of the ankles at the end of the day, tenderness or soreness along the veins, itching around the ankles, and cramps in the legs at night. Dull leg pain can occur, but severe leg pain should not.

The appearance of legs with varicose veins varies. In a woman with an abundant fat pad under the skin, no varicose veins may be visible in the thigh. In the calf and lower leg, however, masses of veins resembling blue cords may stand out. Another kind of vein is the "spider burst" type. These are tiny, purple veins seen under the skin in multi-legged clusters. They do not have any relationship with varicose veins and are symptomless. At times treatment is attempted to improve the appearance of these "spider" veins, but medically this is rarely necessary.

Complications. When blood reverses its flow and drops back down the varicose veins, it comes to a standstill around the lower legs and ankles. Doctors call this condition venous stasis. Swelling around the ankles is an early sign of venous stasis. When the stasis and swelling continue for long periods, a light brown color may develop in the skin of the lower legs as a result of tiny hemorrhages in the skin. The skin around the lower legs and ankles becomes thin and fragile, and a rash may appear. Leg ulcers or sores that appear in the more advanced stage may heal slowly.

Another complication of varicose veins is rupture of a vein. This can occur when the vein is covered only by a thinned-out layer of skin.

What To Do About Varicose Veins

Persons with varicose veins should follow these recommendations:
- Exercise is beneficial. Walking, jogging, cycling, and swimming enable the muscles of the legs to help push the blood up the veins.
- Sitting with the legs elevated to hip level is helpful. When on a long auto trip, get out of the car and walk for a minute or two every hour.
- Keep your body weight at its recommended level.
- Persons confined to bed by illness or after surgery should wear light elastic hose. Movement of the feet and legs should be encouraged.
- Pregnant women should wear elastic stockings. Operations for varicose veins should not be done during pregnancy, because the veins may improve markedly after delivery.
- Do not cross the legs at the knees. It hampers the flow of blood.

The vein may bleed, but this type of bleeding is easily controlled by applying pressure over the bleeding site.

Patients with varicose veins face a slightly increased risk of blood clots developing in one of the dilated veins. This is not a dangerous type of clotting, however, and usually can be treated at home with rest, elevation of the leg, and a heating pad or warm cloths.

All these complications can be prevented by early care and treatment.

Non-surgical treatment. In the treatment of varicose veins, elastic stockings and sometimes elastic bandages are used to counteract the stagnation of blood flow and swelling. The type of stocking depends on the extent and severity of the varicose veins. For people with mild cases and no complications, a light support hose or panty hose available in any department store may be sufficient. For more severe cases, it may be necessary to purchase a heavier stocking available at a large drugstore or medical supply house. Patients who already have the complications of blood flow stagnation, dermatitis, ulcers, or bleeding, should have heavy elastic stockings made to order. A stocking that reaches the knee is usually enough, but occasionally an above-knee stocking or leotards will be necessary. When in doubt, a physician's advice should be sought before deciding.

At times physicians inject a solution to obliterate a section of the vein. The procedure is not as widely used as it once was because the benefits are likely to be temporary. Today most physicians reserve injections for very small varicose veins, or for small veins that persist after large veins have been removed surgically.

Surgical treatment. An operation for enlarged, varicosed superficial veins means tying them off and removing them, a process known as stripping. Afterwards, the deep veins must carry the blood from the legs to the heart. The operation generally is successful in eliminating symptoms.

As a rule, surgical treatment is not necessary if the patient is willing and able to wear elastic support stockings. Most vein stripping is done for women who do not like the appearance or discomfort of the elastic stockings and are unwilling to wear them.

THROMBOPHLEBITIS

Thrombophlebitis is an inflammation of a vein associated with a clot (*thrombo* means clot, *phleb* means vein, *itis* means inflammation). The term is usually shortened to "phlebitis."

Phlebitis is a relatively common problem. About 70 percent of cases occur in women. This is because more women than men have varicose veins to begin with, because women get pregnant, and because women take birth control pills, all of which increase the likelihood of phlebitis. Other high risk situations incude being bedridden because of surgery or a serious illness, and heart ailments and cancer. Being elderly or obese also increases the risk.

Phlebitis can occur in any vein, but the legs are affected in 95 percent of all cases. There are two kinds of phlebitis: superficial and deep. Superficial phlebitis involves the superficial veins just beneath the skin. At times the superficial vein is a varicose vein. Deep phlebitis involves the deeper veins.

Superficial phlebitis is an annoying condition but not dangerous. Typically there is a sore, reddened, warm area in the calf or thigh. Often a tender cord can be felt beneath the skin. The leg is usually not swollen.

The typical patient is worried when told that she has phlebitis, because she may have heard that clots may break loose and cause death. If the phlebitis is superficial, she can be reassured that the inflammation holds the clot tight and that it does not break loose. Treatment consists of applying warm, moist packs to the inflamed area as often as possible. It is not necessary to remain in bed, but rest, with the leg elevated six to twelve inches, helps to speed healing. Usually after seven to ten days the inflammation disappears.

Deep thrombophlebitis is potentially dangerous. Because the deep veins generally are much larger than the superficial veins, the clots in the veins are larger. They also are more likely to break loose from the vein wall and flow up through the heart to lodge in an artery in the lung. This event is called a pulmonary embolism (see chapter 8, "The Lungs") and can be serious enough to cause death.

The signs and symptoms of deep phlebitis can be mild with slight discomfort and minor swelling, or they can be severe with excruciating pain and massive swelling. The key to early diagnosis is if the problem is suspected by the physician. The diagnosis can be confirmed by X rays of the leg veins after the veins have been injected with dye. New and highly accurate instruments are available to confirm the diagnosis without injections.

Once deep phlebitis is diagnosed, hospitalization is necessary. Anticoagulants, or "blood thinners," are given unless ruled out by complications such as a bleeding ulcer. Anticoagulants are administered intravenously at first, and later by mouth. Rest in bed is necessary for a few days, then over about a week the patient gradually resumes normal walking before discharge from the hospital. Anticoagulants are continued for three to six months. Elastic stockings may be necessary if swelling of the leg persists after the patient resumes her normal activities.

CHAPTER 6   **WILLIAM H. CROSBY, M.D.**

THE BLOOD

oethe, the 19th-century German scientist-philosopher-poet, wrote, "The blood is a peculiar juice." As we learn more about the blood we are continually astounded at its peculiarity. Goethe, 150 years ago, knew that the blood is the only fluid organ, that it circulates to every nook and cranny of the body, that when removed from the body the fluid becomes a solid, and that loss of blood can cause disease and death. But he did not know why people suffer from lack of blood or how the solid clot is formed. He did not know that the blood in a human body contains 25 million *million* blood cells, a population that is continuously replenished as the older cells die. He may have surmised that blood transports the fuels for the chemical fires that warm us and provide the energy by which we move and think. How could he have guessed that the blood is a sort of supplementary nervous system, that it carries messages from place to place, controlling the levels of activity of our vital chemistries?

Year after year information continues to accumulate concerning the functions and malfunctions of this "peculiar juice." We have learned a lot about the blood, but more is unknown than we know.

NORMAL ASPECTS OF BLOOD

Hematology is the study of blood and its associated organs, their structure, their functions and malfunctions, and the diagnosis and treatment of their disorders.

The blood is one of the heaviest organs of the body, second only to the skin in weight. Throughout the whole mammalian kingdom the blood comprises about seven percent of body weight. In an average-size, 150-pound man the volume of blood is about five quarts. The blood is composed of solid particles (the blood cells) and a liquid called plasma. The cells constitute about 40 percent of the five-liter volume and the plasma about 60 percent.

The Blood System

The "blood system" includes several organs in addition to the blood itself.

Bone marrow is the red, pulpy tissue found in the webs of the "flat" bones such as ribs, pelvis, and spine. Red marrow produces blood cells. Yellow marrow in the cylindrical bones of arms and legs is fat, but it can change to active red marrow when the body needs more than the normal number of blood cells. The fatty marrow is a reserve organ, impor-

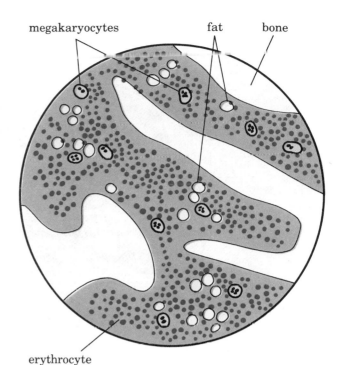

megakaryocytes   fat   bone

erythrocyte

BONE MARROW

The bone marrow in cross section displays the webby structure of the T-bone in a steak. The smooth strips are bone. Between them is the cellular tissue of the marrow where blood cells are manufactured. Empty circles are fat storage cells. Largest cells in the tissue are megakaryocytes (top left), which produce blood platelets. The smaller circles represent developing red cells (erythrocytes) and white cells.

tant because normal blood cells can be produced only in the marrow.

The spleen is an organ about the size and shape of an open hand. It lies in the abdomen behind the lower ribs on the left side. Most of the aged, worn-out blood cells are destroyed by scavenger cells (phagocytes) in the spleen. The spleen also participates in immune reactions, producing antibodies against invading viruses and bacteria, and it manufactures some of the white blood cells called lymphocytes.

Lymphatic tissue is present as small islands in the spleen. It also is found in dozens of lentil-size lymph nodes in the neck, armpits, groin, chest, and abdomen, and there are small masses of lymphatic tissue such as tonsils, adenoids, and the thymus in the chest.

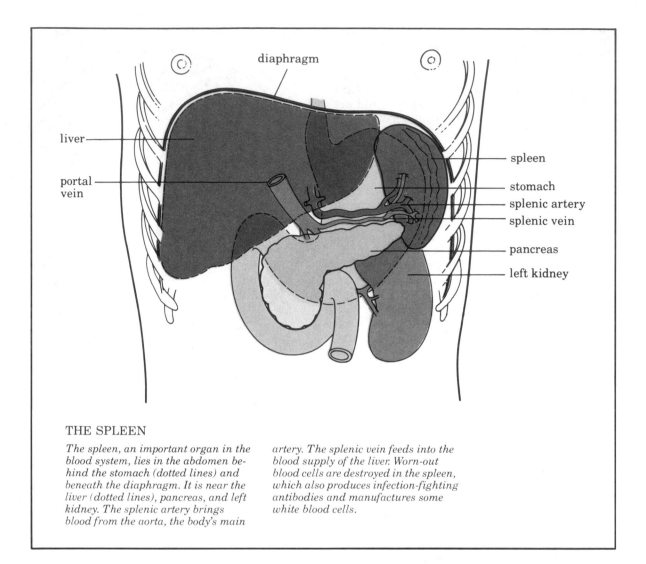

THE SPLEEN

The spleen, an important organ in the blood system, lies in the abdomen behind the stomach (dotted lines) and beneath the diaphragm. It is near the liver (dotted lines), pancreas, and left kidney. The splenic artery brings blood from the aorta, the body's main artery. The splenic vein feeds into the blood supply of the liver. Worn-out blood cells are destroyed in the spleen, which also produces infection-fighting antibodies and manufactures some white blood cells.

Lymphatic tissue also participates in immune reactions. If the spleen is removed, these small organs together with the scavenger cells in the liver become the destroyers of worn-out blood cells.

Reticuloendothelial system is the name given this widely scattered system of lymphatic tissues and scavenger cells.

The blood as a vortex. The volume of the blood remains constant, yet the blood's makeup continually changes. Cells in the blood today were not there last month. Water in the blood today was not there yesterday. This state of dynamic equilibrium resembles a vortex, such as the funnel-shaped swirl of water that forms over the drain as a bathtub empties. The shape of the vortex remains constant, but what about the water that forms the funnel? Try this experiment: Let a drop of ink fall onto the shoulder of the vortex as water drains out of your bathtub. The color "tags" some of the water which is immediately swept down the side of the funnel and down the drain. The shape of the vortex is constant but its constituent water changes continually. So it is with blood. Blood cells die, and they are replaced continually by new cells. As the proteins dissolved in the plasma are put to use, new proteins take their places. The water in the blood disappears as urine and sweat and the mist in our breath, and it, too, is replaced continually. Yet the blood volume neither increases nor decreases and the relative proportions of its constituent parts do not fluctuate.

Controlling blood volume. The temperature of a room in a modern house is kept constant by a heating unit controlled by a thermostat. When heat in the room raises the temperature above the setting on the thermostat, an electric signal from the thermostat shuts off the heating unit. Temperature then gradually falls to the limit set by the thermostat, whereupon another electric signal switches on the heating unit again.

THE LYMPHATIC SYSTEM

The thin lines represent lymph vessels, which collect fluid from the tissue and return it to the blood. Collections of spots in the armpits, groin, spleen, and tonsils are lymph nodes. The nodes are clusters of lymphatic tissue that filter out debris and, when necessary, manufacture antibodies against infection. The arrows show the direction of lymphatic flow.

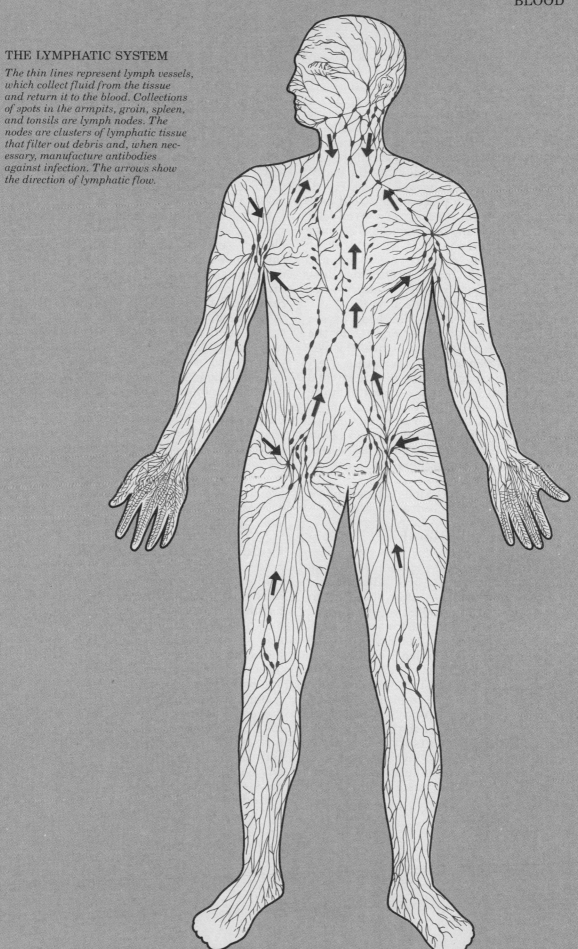

Three components of this feedback system are: (1) A sensor: the thermostat; (2) An effector: the heating unit; (3) Information: the electric signals.

The size of the blood volume (and the mass of blood cells) is maintained by similar feedback systems. Take, for example, the total mass of the red cells in the blood. Red blood cells have a life-span of about 100 to 120 days. At the end of this time they die of old age and are destroyed. A new cell takes the place of each old one. Thus, each day about 1 percent of our red cells live out their time and are replaced. The total mass of red cells in the bloodstream is about two liters, slightly more than two quarts, which means that 20 milliliters of red cells— less than three-quarters of an ounce—are produced each day by the bone marrow.

To maintain these levels, the body uses a sensor in the kidney corresponding to the thermostat. When the concentration of red cells falls below a critical level this ever-vigilant sensor recognizes the deficiency and sends a chemical signal—the hormone erythropoietin—through the bloodstream to the marrow, instructing it to manufacture red cells. When the level of red cells rises above a critical level, the sensor ceases to secrete erythropoietin. Lacking a signal, the marrow's output of red cells subsides.

The production of other kinds of blood cells is under control of similar feedback systems.

Functions of the Blood

The blood is a fluid organ circulating through a system of collapsible tubes. Tough-walled arteries carry blood from the heart at high pressure and thin-walled veins return it. The blood has three important functions: transportation, filling the blood vessels, and the self-sealing function called hemostasis.

Transportation. The surfaces of the body include the skin, the digestive surfaces of the stomach and intestine, the respiratory surface of the lungs, and the excretory surface of the kidneys. The circulation of the blood connects all these with the inner parts of the body where the vital chemistry is working. The blood carries into the body the substances necessary to life, and it carries out the waste products.

Substances transported by the blood can be divided into three classes: solids, liquids, and gases—food, water, and oxygen. Transport is extremely rapid, with materials moving from the surface to the interior in a matter of seconds. Yet speed is essential only for the transport of gases. We can live without food for a number of weeks and we can live without water for a number of days, but we can live without oxygen for only a few minutes. (Try holding your breath.)

Filling the blood vessels. It may seem obvious to say that a function of blood is to fill the blood vessels, but life depends on the fit being a close one. When the blood volume is too large it distends the blood vessels. The heart and lungs cannot operate efficiently. Heart failure can result and the lungs fill with fluid. On the other hand, when the blood volume is too small, heart failure also can result and the lungs also fill with fluid. Heart failure from either cause eventually leads to lung failure.

Hemostasis. The blood is a fluid organ in a system of collapsible tubes, and when one of the tubes is punctured, blood pours out. It is vital that we not lose this blood and the important substances it carries. Thus after a few minutes the rate of blood flow begins to dwindle and finally stops. The blood itself forms a plug in the hole. This self-sealing process is brought about by blood cells called platelets. The process of platelet clumping and blood clotting to form the plug is called hemostasis.

Components of the Blood

Blood is composed of three types of blood cells—red cells, white cells, and platelets—together with the fluid plasma in which the cells are suspended and in which many materials are dissolved: plasma proteins, nutrients including minerals and vitamins, hormones (chemical messengers sent from one organ to another), and salts (blood tastes salty).

Blood cells are formed in the bone marrow. A progenitor cell, or stem cell, divides into two cells. One remains a stem cell that can divide further. The other is a primitive blood cell called a blast. Within four or five days the blasts mature to form blood cells that are then delivered into the bloodstream.

Red blood cells. One form of blast, the erythroblast, matures to become an erythrocyte, or red cell. During maturation these blasts create an enormous amount of the protein hemoglobin, the pigment that gives blood its red color. Just before the red cell is delivered into the blood, it casts off its nucleus. Now the red cell is a sack of protoplasm, or cell sack, without a nucleus, heavily concentrated with hemoglobin. The function of hemoglobin is to carry oxygen from the lungs to all other organs, and the function of the red cell is to carry hemoglobin. The red cells are tiny discs, so small that five million are present in roughly the volume of a pinhead. The average red cell moves completely through the heart and bloodstream about once a minute. During its four-month life-span, a red cell travels almost 100 kilometers (62 miles), continually bumped, crushed, jostled, and squeezed. But when it expires, it is not of injury but of old age.

In its prime, the red cell is equipped with lively chemical machinery to repair its injuries and maintain its vitality. When these chemical reactions run down, it withers. The surface can no longer repel the phagocytes, which ingest all blood cells when their time has come.

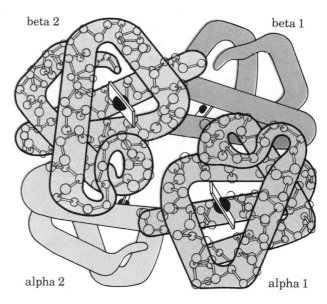

beta 2   beta 1

alpha 2   alpha 1

A HEMOGLOBIN MOLECULE

The complex hemoglobin molecule consists of four amino acid chains, which comprise the "globin" portion of the molecule, and, tucked into the loops of each chain, a small square representing the "heme" portion. An atom of iron is held at the center of each "heme." These four atoms capture oxygen molecules in the lungs and carry them to the muscles, brain, and all other organs. The hemoglobin molecule vastly multiplies the amount of oxygen that can be dissolved and carried in the blood.

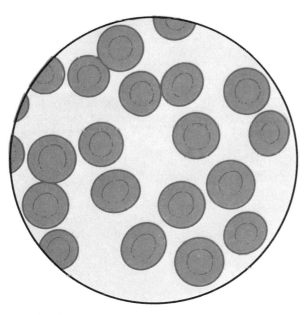

RED BLOOD CELLS

Red blood cells, here magnified 1,000 times, are tiny discs with a slightly concave surface. Their important task is to carry hemoglobin, the protein that transports oxygen from the lungs to all other organs. Hemoglobin gives blood its red color. The red cell prevents the loss of hemoglobin into the urine and tissue. Red cells have a life-span of 100 to 120 days.

The hemoglobin molecule of the red cell is critical to life. It is composed of four globin, long, intertwining chains of amino acids in a globular conformation (see above). Attached to these globin, one per chain, are four molecules of heme, sticking like four little postage stamps. At the center of the heme molecule is an atom of iron, to which oxygen molecules attach themselves to ride from the lungs to the rest of the body. Heme gives the red color to hemoglobin. When it has fulfilled its task of transporting oxygen, hemoglobin is finally destroyed. Its amino acids are used again to make new hemoglobin, but pigment is discarded. After conversion to yellow-brown bile pigment (bilirubin) it is excreted by the liver into the small intestine. Feces are brown because this pigment is present.

The amino acids in the hemoglobin molecule are arranged in two sets of two identical chains: two alpha chains and two beta chains. Each alpha contains 141 amino acids, each beta contains 146; the total for the four chains is

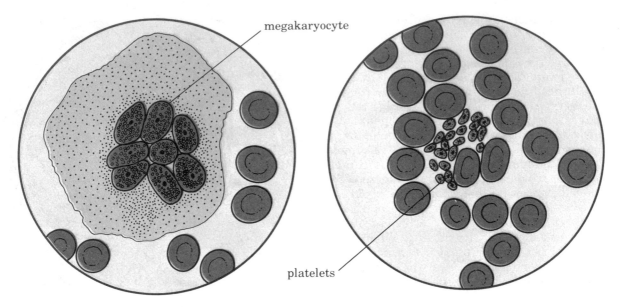

megakaryocyte

platelets

PLATELET PRODUCTION

The megakaryocyte (left) from the bone marrow and its product, the platelets (right), are magnified 1,000 times. The enormous megakaryocyte grows and matures in the marrow.

When platelets are needed it moves into the bloodstream and breaks into platelets. One megakaryocyte may produce 5,000 platelets, which help prevent and stop bleeding.

574. There are 20 different kinds of amino acids in the chains, arranged in an absolutely definite sequence that is genetically determined. When the normal genetic code is disturbed, the results are the diseases called hemoglobinopathies (see page 105).

Normal hemoglobin is called Hemoglobin A. Before birth, the fetal hemoglobin binds oxygen a bit more avidly than does Hemoglobin A, which permits the fetus to capture oxygen from the mother's hemoglobin.

Platelets, the smallest blood cells, are discs so tiny that the volume of a pinpoint could contain about 250,000 of them. The number of platelets is about 1/20th the number of red cells.

Platelets are products of the largest cells in the bone marrow, the megakaryocytes. When these enormous cells become mature, they move into the bloodstream where their cellular tissue fragments into thousands of tiny platelets. The platelets are most important in maintaining the walls of the blood vessels. They plug tiny crevices and help to fill holes or wounds. Injury of the blood platelets provokes a chemical reaction that starts the coagulation of blood. Thus the platelet is the keystone of the blood's hemostatic function. Blood platelets have a life-span of about 10 days. Relatively few are destroyed during hemostasis (see page 92). Most platelets, like most red cells, die of old age.

White blood cells (leukocytes). Red cells and platelets are inhabitants of the blood. They spend their entire career and accomplish their functions within the blood vessels. White blood cells, on the other hand, are only passengers. They ride around doing nothing until a chemical signal attracts them out of the bloodstream. Then they cling to the vessel wall and escape through cracks between the cells to accomplish their important missions outside the bloodstream. Life-span of leukocytes within the blood is relatively brief, averaging only a few hours.

The normal white blood cell count is 5,000 to 10,000 per cubic millimeter (the volume of a pinhead). There are three basic varieties of leukocytes—granulocytes, monocytes, and lymphocytes—and subcategories of each. All are produced in the marrow from corresponding blasts: myeloblasts for granulocytes, monoblasts for monocytes, and lymphoblasts for lymphocytes. Some lymphocytes are also produced in the lymph nodes and spleen.

Granulocytes are somewhat larger than red blood cells. The nucleus of a granulocyte has several lobes and the cell sap contains a sprinkling of small grains, or granules, giving

NEUTROPHILIC GRANULOCYTE

nuclear lobe with clumps of chromatin

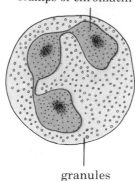

granules

EOSINOPHILIC GRANULOCYTE

bi-lobed nucleus with chromatin clumps

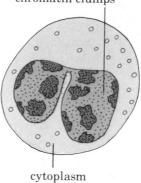

cytoplasm

BASOPHILIC GRANULOCYTE

cytoplasm

nucleus — basophilic granules

SMALL LYMPHOCYTE

nucleus with plaques of nuclear chromatin

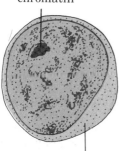

cytoplasm

LARGE LYMPHOCYTE

cytoplasm   granules

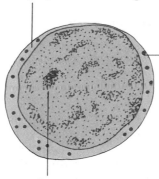

nucleus with plaques of compact chromatin

MONOCYTE

spongy nucleus

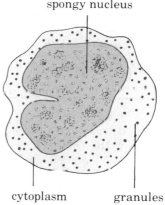

cytoplasm   granules

WHITE BLOOD CELLS

Six types of leukocytes, or white blood cells, from top left, are: neutrophilic granulocyte, eosinophilic granulocyte, basophilic granulocyte, and (lower row) small lymphocyte, large lymphocyte, and monocyte. All are enlarged about 2,500 times. Neutrophils, the most common, combat infection. Lymphocytes deal with immune reactions. Monocytes are scavengers which remove dead or foreign material from the tissue spaces. The function of eosinophils and basophils is uncertain.

the cell its name. These contain chemically active substances concerned with the functions of the cells. Three kinds of granulocytes are identified by how their granules stain on blood smears. Basophilic granulocytes have very dark granules, stained by the dark basic dyes. Eosinophils have red granules stained by the acid dye eosin. Neutrophilic granules are pallid, reacting slightly with either sort of stain.

Neutrophilic granulocytes are the most numerous leukocytes. Their function is to prevent or combat infection. They ingest bacteria and kill them. Neutrophils accumulate in areas of infection, forming a wall to limit spread of infection, and they form pus. Pus, in fact, is a slurry of "used" neutrophils.

Eosinophilic granulocytes remain a mystery. Their numbers increase during allergic reactions, and the blood eosinophil count is high in many parasitic infestations such as hookworm (bloodsuckers on the intestinal wall) and trichinosis (a muscle-worm disease

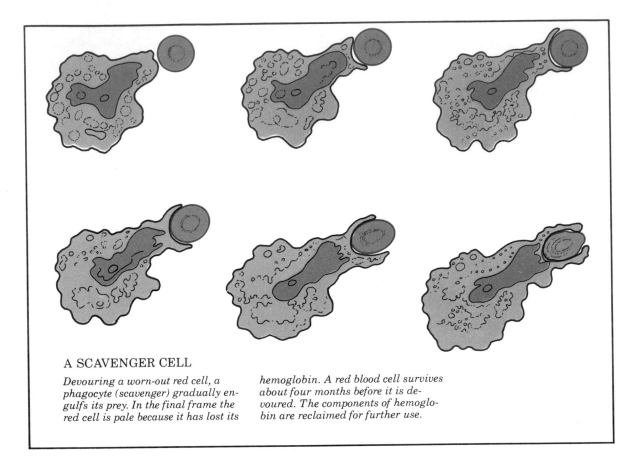

A SCAVENGER CELL

Devouring a worn-out red cell, a phagocyte (scavenger) gradually engulfs its prey. In the final frame the red cell is pale because it has lost its hemoglobin. A red blood cell survives about four months before it is devoured. The components of hemoglobin are reclaimed for further use.

contracted from eating infected, undercooked pork). How the eosinophils function in parasitic disorders is not known.

Basophilic granulocytes contain histamine in their dark-staining granules. This chemical causes an inflammatory reaction, so we guess that the basophil plays some part in inflammation, but its function, too, remains a mystery.

Degranulation is the process by which all granulocytes accomplish their function. The tiny granules release their active chemicals and digestive enzymes either into the cell itself (that's how the neutrophils destroy ingested bacteria) or into the cell's environment (that may be how basophils contribute to inflammatory reactions). The cell is destroyed in the process.

Monocytes, so called because the nucleus is not fragmented ("mono" means "one"), are phagocytes, or scavenger cells. They leave the bloodstream to cruise through the tissue spaces, devouring dead or foreign material, reducing these particles to their component fats, carbohydrates, amino acids, and minerals, and releasing these substances to be reused.

Lymphocytes are the second most common white cells, after the neutrophils. They are at the center of the body's immune system (see chapter 21, "Allergy and The Immune System"). From the lymphocytes are derived the antibodies that defend the body against foreign substances (page 97).

Blood plasma. Blood cells make up about two-fifths of the blood volume. The other three-fifths, the fluid portion in which the cells are suspended, is the plasma, a pale yellow liquid with the consistency of a thin glue. Dissolved in it are the plasma proteins, various salts, and the fats, carbohydrates, minerals, and vitamins needed to nourish the tissues reached by the circulating blood.

The plasma proteins are incredibly diverse. Albumin is present in greatest amounts. Its prime function is to retain water in the blood, offsetting the blood pressure that tends to squeeze water through the capillary walls into the tissues. When there is too little albumin, the legs become swollen with fluid in the tissue spaces. Albumin's ability to "bind" water develops what is called oncotic pressure.

Albumin is a carrier of various body chemicals such as calcium and the bile pigment produced when hemoglobin is destroyed. It also is a source of nutrient protein for growing cells.

Globulin is the name for all of the other plasma proteins. Here is a summary of some of their functions.

Coagulation system. When blood is damaged it turns from liquid to a solid clot, helping to prevent escape of the blood from the body. This occurs when a soluble globulin called fibrinogen is altered to become an insoluble fibrin. The felt-like fibrin mesh entraps all of the cellular elements, forming a solid mass called a coagulum.

But clotting does not happen easily or quickly. Reluctance to clot preserves the fluidity of the blood. We are protected from unnecessary clotting by several safeguards:

• The smooth surfaces of the blood vessels do not damage the clotting mechanism, as roughened surfaces would.

• A complex chain of reactions is essential before fibrinogen is converted to fibrin. One reaction produces an ingredient essential for the second reaction and so forth through a sequence of six preliminary phases. This complexity makes the system relatively difficult to activate.

• Blood is in continual motion. Thus, after injury to the clotting mechanism, the activated globulins are washed away from the site of injury and diluted by uninjured plasma.

• Plasma contains anticoagulants that oppose the activated clotting factors. There is even an enzyme that, when activated, dissolves fibrin clots.

When injury is severe enough to override all of these safeguards the blood does clot. The clots plug holes in blood vessels, diminishing and stopping blood loss. As noted above, platelets also participate in this process.

Immune system. Like the coagulation system, immune reactions are complex (see chapter 21, "Allergy and the Immune System"). In the bloodstream as elsewhere in the body, they center on the relationship between antigen and antibody.

Antigens are intruder molecules, usually protein. An antigen might be part of the membrane on the surface of a bacteria or on a transfused blood cell. It might be contained in pollens or insect venom.

Antigens play a two-part role in immune reactions. When an antigen first appears in the body, it stimulates the immune system to form antibodies. (Hence the name, *anti*body *gen*erator.) This occurs because the phagocytes ingest the antigen and transfer information about its composition to cells of the lymphocytic variety, which in turn are converted to plasma cells that produce the antibody.

When the antigen appears a second time, the antibodies, fortified with information about its makeup, combine with it. These reactions are extremely specific: An antibody can combine only with the antigen that caused its formation, the way a key can fit only one lock. The union neutralizes the antigen. The new combination together with complement injures or destroys the cells or bacteria that carry the antigen, drilling holes in the surface or making the surfaces sticky so that cells clump together or can be ingested and destroyed by phagocytes.

Complement, another complex system of globulins, also helps in the injury and destruction of the antigen targets. It consists of ordinarily inactive enzymes that can be activated by antigen-antibody reactions.

Carrier globulins have the specific job of obtaining a substance in one part of the body and delivering it to another. For example, the iron-binding globulin called transferrin picks up two atoms of iron in the spleen after red cells have been destroyed and delivers the iron to the bone marrow where hemoglobin in new red cells is formed. There are specific carriers for copper and vitamin B_{12}. Certain hormones are transported by specialized globulins. Haptoglobin is a globulin that can bind two molecules of hemoglobin, making a complex too large to escape through the kidney into the urine. It is needed to salvage the components of the few red cells destroyed by bumping and jarring encountered as they circulate. Their hemoglobin is lost into the plasma and would be discarded by the kidneys if it were not captured by haptoglobin. The other transport proteins similarly prevent the small hormones and minerals from escaping through the kidney filter.

Nutrition and Blood

Because the blood is such a large organ and because its cells and proteins must be replaced constantly, considerable quantities of "raw materials" are required. Six grams of protein are needed just for one day's production of hemoglobin, for example, and a similar amount for each day's production of albumin.

The structure of cell surfaces requires fat. Carbohydrate is the fuel that drives the chemical reactions to fabricate the blood cells. The vitamins are essential "lubricants" or catalysts for these metabolic reactions.

Iron metabolism. Red cells require an enormous investment of iron, more than all the other tissues of the body combined. The body takes good care to prevent loss of this essential element. Unlike other nutrient metals, iron cannot be excreted. Excess iron taken into the body, whether by absorption of food, by medication, or by blood transfusion, must be put into storage. Every cell in the body requires a "trace" amount of iron. Iron is in cellular pigments resembling hemoglobin. Some of these pigments move oxygen within the cells and others store a small amount of oxygen. Iron is also essential for the proper action of some cellular enzyme systems.

A small "obligatory" loss of iron occurs in the constant shedding of cells from the skin and coverings of the other surfaces. We lose about one milligram of iron per day of the 4,000 milligrams normally present in the adult human body, but the loss is offset by absorbing one milligram from the 10 to 20 we consume in our daily diet.

Bleeding is another way in which iron is lost. Because blood is rich in iron, heavy bleeding can deplete the supply. To offset the loss, the intestine permits more iron from food to enter, as much as three to six milligrams per day. When iron pills are given, as much as 20 to 30 milligrams can be absorbed.

A small amount of copper is essential for the normal metabolism of iron. Zinc also appears essential. Zinc deficiency results in anemia but the relationship between zinc and iron is not known.

Vitamins and blood formation. Vitamin B_{12} (cobalamin) and folic acid are needed for blood cells to mature normally in the marrow. Vitamin B_{12} is present in all foods of animal origin. It is almost impossible to suffer a dietary deficiency because the daily requirement of one microgram is so minuscule. However, *some* food of animal origin must be eaten in order to prevent deficiency. A completely vegetarian diet (containing no milk, eggs, or fish) can, over a long time, cause vitamin B_{12} deficiency. B_{12} cannot be absorbed without the presence of a substance called intrinsic factor (IF), secreted by the stomach. Vitamin B_{12} deficiency can thus occur when a lack of intrinsic factor prevents proper absorption of the vitamin (see page 107). Fortunately the concentration of B_{12} in blood can be measured, and supplementary B_{12} given if it is deficient.

Folic acid (foliage = green leaves), another of the B-vitamin family, is abundant in the leafy and yellow vegetables of our diet. Folic acid is adequate in a balanced diet, but it is not superabundant. It can be destroyed by prolonged cooking. Folic acid is essential for rapid proliferation of cells. It is good practice to supplement the diet with folic acid during periods of proliferation—such as during pregnancy.

Normal Blood Counts

Just as people can be of different height or have a different shoe size and still be normal, so the blood values of hemoglobin, white cells, platelets, plasma protein, and other components may differ considerably without necessarily being abnormal. The ranges are established by measuring the values in many people known to be normal on the basis of careful evaluation. The results, when plotted on a graph, form a "bell-shaped curve," describing an outline like that of the Liberty Bell. Many of the values are clustered around the highest point of the curve, close to the average of the group. On either side, the frequency of numbers drops off steeply, and at the outer limits of the normal range few numbers are plotted.

The phenomenon of variability creates problems in diagnosis. Take, for example, a 40-year old man. His hemoglobin may measure 14 grams or 18 grams and be considered normal. But suppose at age 35 his hemoglobin had been 16 grams? A value of 14 or 18 now might represent the development of disease. For this reason, physicians hesitate to diagnose on the basis of a single aberration, much less a single test, because tests can be wrong.

Blood Tests

The measurement of substances in the blood encompasses more than tests pertaining to hematology. Remember that one of the three main functions of blood is to transport nutrients, oxygen, hormonal signals, and wastes. The amounts of these substances carried by the blood can be measured to provide clues to the functions and malfunctions of all the body's organs and systems.

NORMAL VALUES FOR BLOOD COUNTS

	Men	Women
Red blood cells (millions per cubic millimeter)	4.7–6.1	4.2–5.4
Hemoglobin (grams per 100 milliliters)	14–18	12–16
Hematocrit (percentage of red blood cells)	42–52%	37–47%
Platelets (per cubic millimeter, both sexes)	130,000 to 400,000	
White blood cells (per cubic millimeter, both sexes)	4,800 to 10,800	

	Range for Both Men and Women
Basophils (percentage of white blood cells)	0– 2%
Neutrophils	40–70%
Eosinophils	0– 7%
Lymphocytes	20–50%
Monocytes	2–10%

Normal blood varies widely in composition. Some cells are so rare that a count of zero in a random sample is considered normal.

For example, blood sugar concentrations might be elevated in patients with diabetes. Waste products in the blood (urea and creatinine, for example) are increased by kidney failure. Blood gases (oxygen and carbon dioxide) reach abnormal levels during certain lung diseases. Quantities of thyroid, adrenal, or pituitary hormones might be increased or decreased in endocrine disease. Moreover, we can measure not only the natural substances but poisons and the concentration of medicines.

Several methods are used to measure the constituents of blood.

Blood cell counters employ diluted blood samples that are sucked through a tiny opening. Each time a cell passes through the opening an electrical current is interrupted. The machine counts these electrical pulses, and, after a measured volume has been tested, the counter prints the total. The machine can be set to count red cells, white cells, or platelets in a given amount of blood. Other machines are able to distinguish the different kinds of white blood cells and report the percentage of each.

The red cell sedimentation rate. The red cell sedimentation rate, when abnormal, is an indication of inflammatory diseases. A test tube filled with blood is allowed to stand motionless, and the red cells slowly sink toward the bottom. At the end of one hour the depth of the column of clear plasma at the top of the tube is measured. In normal blood there is little settling.

Tests of hemostatis. Measurements in test tubes of the speed of clotting of blood plasma provide information about the nature of various bleeding disorders. The clot forms when the dissolved fibrinogen becomes insoluble, visible fibrin. A stopwatch measures the time.

• *Prothrombia time* is the test used to control the dose of anticoagulants sometimes given after heart attack or stroke. When the sample of blood is taken its calcium is neutralized to prevent coagulation. A small amount of plasma is measured into a test tube. Then a tissue extract, thromboplastia, is added, plus the essential calcium. In about 12 seconds a clot forms in a normal solution. The time is prolonged by anticoagulant medication, by liver disease, or by lack of vitamin K.

• *Partial thromboplastia time* is performed in the same way except that a platelet phospholipid is substituted for thromboplastia. Here, clotting time is prolonged by the anticoagulant heparin, by the presence of the serious disorder called disseminated intra-vascular coagulation (see page 113), and in hemophilia (see page 113).

• *Bleeding time* is tested by making a small nick in the skin and timing the interval until the blood spontaneously ceases to flow from the wound. The time usually is less than six minutes, but in some normal people it extends to eight. Bleeding time is prolonged in throm-bocytopenia (see page 111). It also is prolonged after taking a dose of aspirin.

Chemical tests of blood serum components usually employ chemicals called reagents that become brightly colored when they react with the substance to be measured. The depth of color depends on the concentration of the substance being measured.

Multiphasic chemical testing is done with large machines that in one minute can perform a dozen or even two dozen tests simul-taneously on a single small sample of serum. The machine records the results automati-cally, separating the abnormal from the nor-mal. The cost is less than that of a single test performed by hand.

Radioimmunoassay is a procedure used to measure substances present in the blood in amounts too small to be detected by chemical methods. Development of this method was a scientific breakthrough that in 1977 won a Nobel Prize for Dr. Rosalyn Yalow. The es-sential immune reactions involve radio-active antigens or antibodies that, in one way or another, are made to combine with molecules of the substance to be measured. The uncombined radioactivity is removed. The radioactivity remaining is proportional to the concentration of the substance to be measured. Radioimmunoassay is used to test other substances besides blood.

Isotope dilution is a method of measuring blood volume in the circulation. A small, care-fully measured amount of isotope of known specific activity (number of radioactive pulses per minute) is injected into the blood. Within a few minutes the isotope has become uniformly mixed and diluted in the entire volume of the blood. A sample of blood is removed and its specific activity is measured. By comparing the number of radioactive counts in the blood with those in the injection, it is possible to com-pute the extent to which the isotope has been diluted. This extent of dilution is propor-tionate to the blood volume.

Blood grouping is important as a first step to ensure the compatibility of blood transfu-sion. It is how we are able to designate persons as having group A, B, or another group of blood.

Grouping depends upon antigen-antibody reactions. The surfaces of red blood cells have a mosaic of antigens constituting more than two dozen blood-group systems. Some of the sys-tems have alphabetical designations, such as ABO system and MN system. The Rh system was named for the rhesus monkey in which its antibodies were first cultivated, permitting the identification of human blood as Rh-positive or Rh-negative. (About 85 percent of persons have the Rh factor, the other 15 per-cent do not.) Other systems were named for the family in which the system was discov-ered—Kell, Lewis, Diego. All of the systems are genetically determined. With so many antigens the possible combinations make our red cells as individual as our fingerprints.

The ABO blood-group system involves two red-cell antigens, A and B. The surface of a person's red blood cells might carry one anti-gen (group A or group B), or both (group AB), or neither (group O). When one or the other anti-gen is absent the corresponding antibody is present in the plasma. Thus a person of blood group A carries anti-B antibody; a person with group O has both anti-A and anti-B antibodies. Thus A blood cannot be successfully transfused into B or O, B cannot be given to O or A. Type O is the "universal donor" blood that can be transfused into any of the other groups, pro-vided that the minor groups are compatible. AB is the universal recipient and can accept any of the other groups.

Identification of a person's blood group is done by obtaining a pinprick of blood and mix-ing it with a blood-grouping serum containing anti-A antibody and another containing anti-B. When the corresponding antigen is present, the antibodies cause the red cells to form clumps.

Antibodies of the ABO group occur spon-taneously without an immunizing experience. We are born with them. Antibodies of the other blood-group systems do not occur spontane-ously. They appear only after a person has been immunized by exposure to red cells containing a foreign antigen. This can happen, for exam-ple, when an Rh-negative person receives a transfusion of Rh-positive red cells, or when an Rh-negative woman carries an Rh-positive fetus and some fetal red cells cross the placenta into her blood (see page 104). Fortunately, most of the antigens of these "minor" blood-group systems are weakly antigenic. Transfusions can be given without triggering antibodies in the recipient. When antibodies do develop they may be "incomplete" because they cannot cause clumping of red cells that contain the corresponding antigen. Tests are required to demonstrate the incompatibility.

The Coombs test is a standard procedure to determine whether a person's cells are positive or negative for the antigens of each minor blood-group system. The test also is used with the crossmatch of each unit of blood for transfusion to assure compatibility between donor and recipient. And the Coombs test can detect incomplete "autoantibodies" present in a disease called antoimmune hemolytic anemia (see page 104).

Crossmatching is the test of compatibility between recipient and donor before red-cell transfusions are given. Appropriate units of blood are chosen according to the results of ABO blood-grouping tests—group A blood for a group A recipient, for example. Red cells of donor and recipient are washed free of plasma proteins. Then a drop of donor cells is mixed with a drop of recipient serum and vice versa. The mixtures are examined for agglutination, a tight clumping of the red cells, which would mean incompatibility. If none occurs, a Coombs test is performed. If the Coombs test is negative, then the crossmatch testing is negative, and the unit of blood can be successfully transfused into the recipient.

Platelet transfusions and leukocyte transfusions usually are given without antigenic testing.

Blood cultures are done when a person with fever is suspected of having bacteria in the circulation. Samples of blood are injected into culture media and incubated at body temperature. If the culture is positive, bacteria proliferate to form colonies within a day or two. The bacteria are then identified and tested to learn which antibiotics are most effective against them.

Immune testing. Immune testing for infections, past or present, is performed with blood serum to discover specific antibodies that have developed to bacteria and viruses. Some of these antibodies cause bacteria to clump or agglutinate. Others combine with dissolved antigen to form tiny precipitates at the bottom of a test tube.

Serum electrophoresis separates the albumin and globulin components of the serum.

BLOOD GROUPS

	A	B	AB	O
O accepts	○	○	○	●
A accepts	●	○	○	●
B accepts	○	●	○	●
AB accepts	●	●	●	●

● **accepts**
○ **does not accept**

The success of a blood transfusion depends on a careful matching of blood groups. Within the ABO system, O blood can be transfused into any person; AB will accept blood from any other group. A and B accept only their own, plus O. The most common blood type is O.

A drop of serum is placed in an electrical field flowing through a piece of wet paper, a wet starch block, or a gel. The molecules of protein are borne along on the electrical current, the speed depending upon the electrical charges of each molecule. The faster moving ones are carried farthest. After separation the relative amount of each protein is measured.

DISORDERS OF THE BLOOD

The Role of the Marrow

Except for a few lymphocytes, all blood cells are produced in the bone marrow. Production is controlled by feedback systems described on page 90. When more cells are needed the marrow is informed and increases output. The step-up can be evoked by blood loss, excessive blood cell destruction, or by an increased requirement. For example, more white cells are needed during infections.

Normally, part of the marrow consists of fat cells. If increased production is required over a long period, fat storage tissue is converted into functional manufacturing tissue to help with output. In certain diseases fat cells replace functional tissue, resulting in a productive organ too small to meet normal demand, a condition called aplastic anemia. In other diseases, functional tissue is replaced by abnormal cells, scar tissue, or cancer. Sometimes the marrow cells themselves become abnormal, as in leukemia.

The marrow contains its proliferating cells in a delicate scaffolding of fibers and fine blood vessels. This micro-circulation of the marrow is unique. Normal marrow cells cannot develop in the micro-circulation of any other tissue. Disturbance of the scaffolding can disrupt normal proliferation of blood cells.

The Role of the Spleen

At the end of their normal life-span, most red cells and platelets are devoured by phagocytes, usually in the spleen. (Most white cells wander into the tissues to function, and they die on the job.) But the spleen is not an essential organ. When it is removed, its scavenging function can be taken over by other organs with phagocytic cells, especially the liver.

The spleen can malfunction and increase its phagocytic activity to an abnormal degree, resulting in premature destruction of blood cells. The marrow responds to the best of its ability, but production may be inadequate and the number of cells in the blood diminishes.

The spleen also is an organ of the immune system, producing antibodies when challenged by bacteria or other invaders. This function can become perverted so that antibodies are produced against *normal* constituents of the blood, especially the blood cells. These antibodies are called autoantibodies, antibodies against self. They attach themselves to blood cells and can cause them to dissolve. More often they coat the cells in such a way that the cells are attractive to the body's phagocytes and are eaten. The phagocytes of the spleen itself participate, resulting in double jeopardy. The result is called autoimmune disease. Other organs besides the spleen also can generate autoantibodies.

Hypersplenism is the name given to abnormal activities of the spleen.

The Nature of Neoplasms

The program for the construction of a human being is encoded in the genetic information within the parent cells, sperm and ovum. Portions of this information selectively instruct all our cells, in all parts of the body, throughout our lifetime to develop in a preprogrammed way. Undifferentiated cells within the marrow have the capability to become immature examples of any of the types of blood cell. They are genetically coded to receive instructions concerning the rate at which they must proliferate, urging more (or less) proliferation depending upon requirement. They also are encoded with information about the kind of cell that they must become—red cell, granulocyte, megakaryocyte. The process of developing along one line or another is called differentiation, and the changes that take place from the primitive to mature state are called maturation. All cells that follow one set of genetic instructions look and behave alike, provided they receive adequate nutrition and are not disturbed by infections or chemicals or other outside influence.

Neoplasm, a word from the Greek language, means "new tissue." A neoplasm represents a line of cells developing under genetic information different from that established at conception, a scrambling of information that causes cells to develop in an abnormal way. Cancers, of course, are neoplasms, but not all neoplasms are cancers. If we narrow the field to the blood system, leukemia is a neoplasm, but not all neoplasms of the blood system are leukemias.

The garbling of genetic information can affect the proliferating blood cells in several ways:

• The rate of cellular proliferation is controlled by information from feedback systems. The go-no go signals are perceived and obeyed by the proliferating tissue. In one type of neoplasm the tissue seems to become "tone deaf," can't perceive the signals, and produces too much or too little of the corresponding blood cell.

• Instructions concerning design of cells may be garbled. Weird-looking cells are produced, or cells with defective energy systems or surfaces are produced, causing them to die early or live too long.

• Instructions for growth may be garbled so that the cells fail to mature. They remain primitive and die after a protracted infancy.

• Growth patterns may differ from the normal. Normal marrow cells proliferate only in the micro-circulation of the normal marrow. Abnormal cells may be able to proliferate in the spleen, the liver, the skin, or anywhere else with a blood supply.

Red Blood Cell Disorders

Anemia. When the concentration of red cells (and equivalent hemoglobin) is less than normal, the condition is called anemia. It occurs when production of red cells is insufficient to meet requirement. Insufficiency can result from less-than-normal production or greater-than-normal requirement, or from a combination of the two.

Like a fever, anemia is not itself a disease, but a condition. When anemia is discovered, it becomes essential to discover why red cell production is deficient, or what has increased the red cell requirement.

The function of hemoglobin is to transport oxygen, so the symptoms of anemia are those of insufficient oxygen. With lesser degrees of anemia symptoms occur only when the system is stressed by exertion. The anemic person becomes quickly short of breath or easily fatigued. In general, more severe anemia causes more severe symptoms, but people vary greatly in their ability to tolerate anemia. Young people are more tolerant than older ones. Anemic children often show very low hemoglobin without any evident loss of pep. The speed of onset is also a factor. When anemia develops slowly we adapt to it. An anemia steadily worsening over many months might cause little difficulty. The same degree of anemia resulting from rapid bleeding might be incapacitating.

Aregenerative anemia. When the marrow is incapable of producing (or generating) enough red cells for the normal replacement needs, the resulting anemia is called aregenerative. This can result from several causes:
• The volume of productive marrow is lower than normal. This problem is called aplastic anemia or hypoplastic anemia.
• The productive marrow may have been damaged or destroyed by chemicals, medicines, or X ray. (Sometimes this is done deliberately, as in the treatment of leukemia.) Or the person's marrow may be sensitive to a specific medicine or chemical.
• Erythropoietin, the chemical secreted by the kidney that normally stimulates red cell production, may be lacking.
• The body may contain insufficient iron to produce enough hemoglobin.
• The synthesis of hemoglobin may be disturbed. In hereditary Mediterranean anemia (see page 106) globin protein formation is out of control. In lead poisoning, production of the heme pigment is impaired.
• Chronic inflammations and extensive cancers may inhibit production of red cells by means that are not understood.
• The marrow cavities may be filled with abnormal tissue such as bone, fibrous cells, or cancer.
• Neoplastic (abnormal) cells may be incapable of normal red-cell proliferation or maturation.

Hemolytic anemia. Red cells normally live 100 to 120 days. When they are destroyed prematurely, the condition is called hemolytic disease. When the severity of destruction exceeds the marrow's ability to compensate by increased production, the result is hemolytic anemia.

Hemolysis occurs in two ways. In most hemolytic diseases the phagocytes remove and digest abnormal red cells just as they remove normal, aged red cells. This is intracellular hemolysis. In less common forms, the red cells burst in the circulating blood, and their hemoglobin is dissolved in the plasma, a condition called intravascular hemolysis. When intravascular hemolysis is widespread, the plasma turns red and some of the pigment spills into the urine, coloring it red, brown, or black, a condition known as hemoglobinuria.

When large numbers of red cells are destroyed, large amounts of hemoglobin are broken down, too, yielding great quantities of yellow bile pigment. Some of the pigment accumulates in the blood, leading to a faint yellow discoloration of the whites of the eyes. This condition is called hemolytic jaundice.

Hemolysis can result from two sorts of disorder. When something is wrong with the red cell itself we speak of intrinsic defects. When the red cell's environment is at fault we speak of extrinsic hemolysis. There are many diseases of both categories.

Extrinsic hemolytic anemias. These are listed not in terms of frequency but with the simple ones first:

• Crushing. Distance runners, marching soldiers, and even joggers can crush enough red cells in the soles of their feet to cause a brief hemolytic disease. Their urine may turn dark. This is march (or exertional) hemoglobinuria.

• Burning. People with extensive burns can incur hemoglobinuria because the red cells in heat-injured tissues are so damaged that they break open.

• Freezing of hands and feet means freezing of their red cells too. When the red cells thaw they burst.

• Near-drowning draws water into the lungs. This water enters the blood and causes the red cells to burst. This is called drowning hemoglobinuria.

• Chemicals, especially the industrial chemicals arsine and aniline, can destroy red cells.

• Infections. Some infectious agents such as malarial parasites actually enter and destroy the red cell. In the deadly falciparum form of malaria, hemolysis may be so severe that hemoglobin spills into the urine. This is called blackwater fever.

• Immune reactions. There are three main types—blood transfusion reactions, "Rh disease," and a condition known as autoimmune hemolytic disease.

(1) Transfusing blood of an incompatible group into a person causes a reaction between antibodies in his plasma and blood-group antigens on the red cell surface. The red cells are often damaged so severely that they burst. The combination of immune reaction plus hemoglobin destruction can cause serious kidney damage. This is why crossmatching tests are essential before blood transfusions (see page 101).

(2) Hemolytic disease of the newborn (erythroblastosis) usually involves the Rh blood-group system. It occurs when the mother is Rh-negative, lacking the Rh factor, and the father is Rh-positive. The fetus may then be Rh-positive. After the placenta has formed, the Rh-positive red cells of the fetus may leak across the placenta into the mother's Rh-negative blood, causing her immune system to produce antibodies against the "intruders." These antibodies leak back across the placenta and damage or destroy the Rh-positive cells of the fetus.

The hemolytic anemia of "Rh disease" can be mild or severe. A firstborn child is seldom seriously affected. In later children, those not severely damaged can be saved at birth by an exchange transfusion in which the damaged red cells are removed and replaced by Rh-negative cells that cannot be injured by the maternal antibodies still in the baby's bloodstream. Recently it has become possible to administer life-saving transfusions while the fetus is still in the uterus by injecting red cells through the mother's abdomen into the tiny body.

With the discovery of the nature of Rh disease, Rh pregnancies have become rare. They usually occur only in Rh-negative women who have previously been unknowingly transfused with Rh-positive blood, perhaps after an accident, or who have previously miscarried a fetus not known to be Rh-positive. After a first Rh-positive pregnancy, the Rh-negative mother receives injections of anti-Rh antibody to block the development of antibodies in future pregnancies.

(3) Autoimmune hemolytic disease develops when the immune system produces antibodies against its own red blood cells. These antibodies injure red cells and cause their premature destruction. The disease may develop as a complication of lymphoma, or as a part of another autoimmune disease such as lupus erythematosus, or as a temporary complication of an infection such as virus pneumonia or mononucleosis. It also occurs independently of associated disease.

Intrinsic red cell defects. With a few exceptions the intrinsic red cell defects are hereditary. As we learn more of the structure and function of this apparently simple small sack of dissolved hemoglobin, more and more hereditary defects are identified. They include disorders of the cell membrane, abnormalities of the hemoglobin molecule, and malfunctions of the complex chains of chemical reactions that maintain the fabric of the cell and its hemoglobin during the four months of strenuous circulation.

Hereditary spherocytosis is transmitted as an "autosomal dominant" disorder of the red-cell membrane. "Autosomal dominant" means the full-blown disease can be inherited from one affected parent (see chapter 2, "Medical Genetics"). The red cells do not really become spherical, although they are called spherocytes, but their normal disc shape thickens. The deformity tends toward the spherical because the area of the cell membrane is less than normal while the volume in the cell does not correspondingly decrease. Although the affected cells survive an average of only two weeks, the person may show little or no anemia because the marrow can produce seven or eight times the normal number of red cells. The premature destruction of the spherocytes occurs in the spleen. If the spleen is removed, the shape of the cells remains abnormal, yet they survive a normal 100 to 120 days. The disorder usually causes no symptoms aside from mild jaundice and an enlarged spleen, but it can be severe enough to require transfusions and interfere with growth and development of children. Gallstones develop in most of the victims. Removal of the spleen cures the hemolytic disease of hereditary spherocytosis.

Paroxysmal nocturnal hemoglobinuria is another of the red-cell membrane disorders, in this case an acquired disease. The membrane is flawed in such a way that it can bind molecules of complement (see page 97), which cause the red cell to leak and release its hemoglobin. During crises of this disease the patient's urine contains enough hemoglobin to blacken it. For some reason, destruction occurs primarily during sleep so the urine may be discolored only when the patient wakes in the morning. Hence the name nocturnal hemoglobinuria.

Hemoglobinopathy. There is a large family of hereditary disorders of the hemoglobin molecule. Abnormal genetic information governing formation of the four amino acid chains in the molecule substitutes one wrong amino acid. The substitution can completely alter some characteristics of the molecule, such as its solubility, its stability, or its affinity for oxygen.

Sickle-cell hemoglobin is present in 10 percent of American blacks, occurring in about 1 in 400 births. With a sickle-cell gene received from one parent, the individual's red cells contain 25 to 35 percent of sickle-cell hemoglobin and 65 to 75 percent normal hemoglobin A. The cells function normally, causing no distress; this person is a "healthy carrier" of the sickle-cell gene. When genes come from both parents *no* hemoglobin A is formed by the victim. His or her red cells behave abnormally because when its oxygen has been removed by the body's tissues, sickle-cell hemoglobin is slightly less soluble than normal hemoglobin.

The dissolved hemoglobin in the red cells stiffens into needle-shaped crystals, curving the normally pliable disc into an elongated, hard "sickle" shape. The sickle cells have a short life-span of only about two weeks, causing moderate to severe hemolytic anemia.

Sickle-cell anemia is worse than most hemolytic diseases because of its propensity to crisis. With fever, dehydration, insufficient oxygen, or a disturbance of the body's acid balance the number of red cells changing shape greatly increases. They become log-jammed in small blood vessels, completely blocking flow. This, in turn, prevents oxygen from entering so that more red cells stiffen. The tissues suffer from lack of blood flow, pain develops, and areas of tissue may die. Sickle-cell anemia is a great crippler of black children.

The sickle-cell crisis is difficult to treat. The patient needs adequate water to prevent or correct dehydration, and often supplementary oxygen. In severe cases transfusions of normal red blood cells are required to correct the anemia and provide a supply of cells immune to sickling.

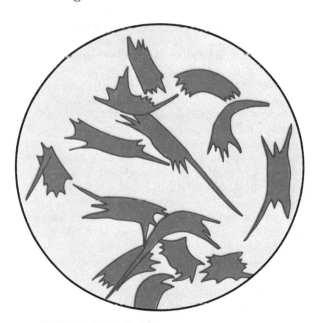

SICKLE CELLS

"Sickle cells" from a person with sickle-cell anemia are illustrated. Normally these red blood cells are concave discs. But when they are stressed by lack of oxygen, lack of water, or fever, the hemoglobin becomes stiff instead of fluid and the cells assume a curved, rigid configuration. When many cells sickle at the same time, a "sickle-cell crisis" occurs.

Hemoglobin Zurich is an example of an amino acid substitution that renders the hemoglobin molecule unstable. (At one time abnormal hemoglobins were named for letters of the alphabet, but there are so many, with new ones being identified every year, that they now are named for the locale of their discovery.) The substitution is near the site on the protein chain where the heme molecule is normally attached. The breakdown called oxidation occurs at this point, resulting in degradation of the hemoglobin molecule. The damaged, useless molecules collect into grains that fuse to the inner surface of the red cell membrane. The injured cell becomes stiff and is soon destroyed by phagocytes.

Hemoglobin Yakima and Hemoglobin Chesapeake are hemoglobins that cannot easily release their molecules of oxygen. As a consequence the feedback system controlling red cell production is stimulated to demand extra red cells. Polycythemia (page 109) results.

The hemoglobins M are a group of hemoglobins with low affinity for oxygen. Such hemoglobin does not take up normal amounts of oxygen in the lungs. Unoxygenated hemoglobin is dark, so hemoglobin-M victims have a bluish complexion, a condition called cyanosis.

Homozygous hemoglobin-C disease causes a mild anemia with pallid red cells. Crystals of hemoglobin form in the red cells and are removed by the spleen, thereby reducing the amount of pigment. Two to three percent of American blacks are carriers of the trait.

Hemoglobin D behaves in most laboratory tests like sickle-cell hemoglobin, but it does not sickle and causes no red cell disorder. The amino acid substitution occurs at an insignificant place on the chain.

Except for sickle-cell disease and homozygous hemoglobin-C disease, the hemoglobinopathies are rare in the U.S.

Thalassemia, or Mediterranean anemia, refers to a group of hereditary disorders of the control of globin synthesis, causing too much or too little synthesis of either the alpha or the beta globin chains. In some cases a wrong kind of chain is produced. In beta-thalassemia deficient amounts of beta chains are produced. In hemoglobin-Lepore thalassemia the beta chain grows longer than the normal 146 amino acids.

When a thalassemia gene is received from only one parent a mild anemia usually results, with red cells that are smaller than normal and that contain less hemoglobin, mimicking iron-deficiency anemia. But when the gene is received from both parents the results are devastating. Homozygous thalassemia (Cooley's anemia) is a severe disease marked by overproduction of red cells but inadequate production of hemoglobin. The hemoglobin-deprived red cells have a brief life-span so that there is hemolytic disease. The overactive marrow crowds its cavity, causing the bones of young victims to swell, weaken, and break. Spleens and livers are massively enlarged. Iron storage disease may damage the heart muscle, sometimes causing heart failure and death. Continual transfusions are necessary to provide enough red cells so that victims' own production ceases and the marrow does not distend the bones. But transfusions may increase the iron overload and further injure the heart. Thalassemia is usually discovered in infancy. It once was thought to be confined to people of Mediterranean ancestry, but variants have been found all over the world. In the United States most cases do occur in Americans of Italian, Greek, Portuguese, or Levantine background.

Enzyme abnormalities of red cells. Enzymes are specialized proteins that facilitate the body's chemical reactions. Red blood cells depend upon several intricate series of enzymatic chain reactions to break down glucose and release the energy stored in the sugar's molecules. This energy is used to maintain hemoglobin in its normally functional condition, to maintain the structure of the red cell's surface, and to keep up the normal concentrations of sodium and potassium. The relatively low sodium and high potassium concentrations in the red cells are maintained by glucose-driven cellular "pumps."

Dozens of enzymes participate in this metabolic effort. Each is susceptible to the same sort of genetic mistakes as is the hemoglobin molecule. Abnormality of a single enzyme can alter the function or survival of the red cells. Each molecule can be genetically disordered in innumerable ways. Year by year new diseases of red cell metabolism are discovered.

G6PD deficiency. More than 15 hereditary abnormalities of the single enzyme glucose-6-phosphate dehydrogenase have been discovered. The most common variety of G6PD deficiency disease occurs in about ten percent of American black men because the genetic code for the enzyme is carried on the X or sex chromosome. Unless a woman inherits an abnormal X chromosome from both parents the disorder, if present, is mild.

Oxygen sustains fire, and it otherwise breaks down substances (as in corrosion) by chemical reactions called oxidation. Hemoglobin normally is protected against oxidation by enzymes that obtain their energy from glucose through the activity of the G6PD enzyme. When G6PD performs inadequately, hemoglobin molecules are destroyed. The debris (detritus) clumps on the cell membrane, damaging it so that the red cells either break up or are destroyed by phagocytes.

In the American variety of G6PD deficiency disease, G6PD behaves normally in young red cells but activity gradually diminishes. Nevertheless, enough activity persists during the life of the cell to protect it against ordinary oxidative stress, the kind involved in normal respiration. Enzyme activity is deficient only with more severe challenges. Certain medicines (some antimalarial and sulfa drugs, for example) or virus infections can provoke an acute hemolytic anemia. Victims of G6PD deficiency are cautioned never to take certain medicines.

G6PD deficiency provides a clear example of an interaction of a defective gene with environment. Unless oxidative stress occurs the disorder is not unmasked.

Other G6PD abnormalities result in more serious deficiency. The red cells are injured even by ordinary breathing, and the patients have chronic hemolytic anemia. One such disorder is called the Mediterranean variant because it was first identified in that area.

More than a dozen other hemolytic disorders have been traced to hereditary abnormalities of red cell enzymes. An additional dozen enzyme deficiencies have been identified that do not appear to interfere with red cell function or life-span.

Nutritional anemias. As noted on page 98, the nutrients iron, vitamin B_{12} (cobalamin), and folic acid are required to form hemoglobin. Lack of any of them can cause anemia. Severe calorie restriction or severe protein deficiency can also result in anemia, but such cases are rare.

Iron-deficiency anemia, the most common nutritional anemia, rarely results from lack of iron in the diet, except when iron requirement is temporarily increased during pregnancy or during the rapid growth of early childhood and adolescence. It is almost always evidence that the body is losing blood. It is most common among young women, a consequence of menstrual bleeding. Most women lose little blood during menstruation, about an ounce or two per period. Perhaps five percent menstruate heavily and require iron tablets or iron supplementation in the diet to prevent anemia.

When iron-deficiency anemia is found in men or in women after menopause, the source of blood loss must be sought. Possible causes range from nosebleed and hemorrhoids to stomach ulcers and cancer of the colon.

Iron-deficiency anemia is characterized by small red cells deficient in hemoglobin. In severe cases the skin may be unhealthy, with cracking at the corners of the mouth, thin nails, hair that sheds easily, and itching. Pica, a craving to eat dirt, paper, ice, laundry starch, or other unusual substances, is a common symptom. The reason for this compulsive appetite, sometimes seen during pregnancy, is not known.

The sure cure for iron-deficiency anemia is to correct the problem causing the blood loss. When that is not possible, the balance can be restored by taking iron tablets with meals. Only rarely is blood transfusion or injected iron necessary.

Vitamin B_{12} deficiency, similarly, is rarely caused by inadequate diet, because B_{12} (cobalamin) is present in all foods of animal origin. Pernicious anemia is the most common cause of B_{12} deficiency, yet it is an uncommon disease. Although not unheard of in young people, it occurs primarily among the elderly.

Vitamin B_{12} cannot be absorbed by the intestine unless combined with a substance called intrinsic factor (IF) secreted by the mucous membrane of the stomach. In pernicious anemia, the mucous membrane becomes thinned and shrinks, and it ceases to secrete IF. The patient becomes anemic because the vitamin is essential for normal blood cell production. The deprived bone marrow contains large cells (megaloblasts) that produce large, short-lived blood cells. The result is a hemolytic anemia.

B_{12} is also necessary for proper functioning of the nervous system, so the first clue to deficiency may be numbness and tingling of hands or feet, staggering gait, or loss of control of bowel and bladder function.

Other rare causes of B_{12} deficiency are injury or loss of that portion of the small intestine (ileum) where B_{12} is absorbed. Intestinal bacteria or tapeworms can consume B_{12} before it can be absorbed.

Once a frightening and debilitating disease, pernicious anemia no longer deserves its unfortunate name. It is no longer pernicious, thanks to a triumph of medical research. In the 1920s, Dr. George Minot demonstrated that adding liver to the diet could correct this invariably fatal anemia. Then it became possible to produce liver extracts, so it was no longer necessary to eat large amounts of the meat. Finally vitamin B_{12} was purified from the liver extracts, allowing it to be given by injection.

Dr. Minot received the Nobel Prize in 1934.

Although injections of B_{12} rapidly correct the anemia, the nerve damage may be irreversible.

Folic acid deficiency usually results from inadequate diet. The daily requirement of folic acid needed for proliferation of cells is about 50 micrograms. (The recommended daily allowance of 400 micrograms is on the safe side.) When diets are low in yellow or leafy vegetables, or vegetables are overcooked, folic acid may be deficient. Heavy drinkers of alcohol have an increased need for folic acid. So do pregnant women, persons with hemolytic anemia whose blood-cell production is increased, and victims of sprue, a disease in which the small intestine absorbs food substances poorly.

The anemia of folic acid deficiency resembles that of pernicious anemia: an abnormal marrow produces large, short-lived red cells. Folic acid tablets rapidly cure the anemia, and in cases of sprue intestinal absorption improves. Folic acid can also correct pernicious anemia, but it does not prevent continuing damage to the nervous system.

Vitamin B₆ deficiency is an extremely rare cause of anemia because the body's need for the vitamin is small compared with the amount in foods. Isoniazid, a medicine used to treat tuberculosis, interferes with the action of B_6. To prevent anemia in tuberculosis victims, B_6 is given along with the medicine. Certain uncommon anemias may be partially improved, but not cured, by enormous doses of B_6, also known as pyridoxine. The reason is not clear. These anemias are called "pyridoxine responsive."

Anemias of endocrine deficiency. A deficiency of hormones—the chemical "messages" produced at one place in the body and carried by the blood to perform their functions in other places—is associated with inadequate red cell production by the marrow and consequent anemia.

Erythropoietin, a hormone produced in the kidney, instructs the marrow to produce red cells. Severe disease or removal of the kidneys can reduce or halt the hormone's output and cause anemia. Erythropoietin is not yet available in medicinal form to correct this.

Removal of the thyroid or spontaneous loss of thyroid activity results in a deficiency of the hormone thyroxin. The accompanying mild-to-moderate anemia can be corrected by proper doses of natural or synthetic thyroid medication.

Pituitary gland destruction by disease or surgery also causes a mild-to-moderate anemia. It is seldom serious enough to be a problem, and can be corrected with a combination of thyroid, adrenal, and testicular hormones.

Pregnancy, with its many hormonal changes, results in a considerable enlargement of the blood volume. Red cell and plasma volume increase. The red cells are diluted and hemoglobin concentration declines. But this dilution is a "false anemia," and does not call for corrective measures. However, the iron and folic acid requirements are increased during pregnancy, and the so-called anemia of pregnancy may be complicated by deficiency of these substances. Most pregnant women should receive supplements of both.

Metabolic anemias. Besides the nutritional anemias, metabolic anemias can occur, including the anemia of kidney failure and anemia of chronic disease.

The anemia of kidney failure, regarded alone, is usually mild to moderate in degree (see chapter 22, "The Kidneys and Urinary System"). It results from a complex mechanism of inadequate red-cell production combined with moderate hemolytic disease. The anemia, however, cannot be corrected except by improving kidney function. The anemia itself is seldom so severe that it compromises the patient's activity.

Anemia of chronic disease is another disorder of complex origin. It is a common complication of chronic infections and inflammatory diseases such as rheumatoid arthritis, and frequently occurs in widespread cancer. In this anemia the responsiveness of the marrow to signals for heightened production is inhibited. Although iron metabolism is not entirely normal, the marrow usually receives enough iron to meet its scaled-down requirement. The anemia is not so severe that it restricts activity. That is fortunate because the anemia cannot be cured except by correcting the underlying disease.

Aplastic anemia. When the productive cells of the marrow diminish, the marrow cavity cannot reduce its volume to the size of the shrunken tissue. The vacant space must be filled with something, and fatty tissue becomes the filler. When doctors discover a marrow with a preponderance of fat cells they call it aplastic. The amount of productive tissue is small, and the blood lacks every sort of cell—red, white, and platelets. The decrease in marrow can be severe, with a life-threatening lack of granulocytes and platelets. Aplastic anemia can be caused by injury to the small blood vessels that sustain the productive marrow, by autoimmune injury to the marrow cells, or by a neoplasm of the marrow cells in which the "new cells" are incapable of adequate response to the body's requirement.

Polycythemia. The polycythemias are disorders resulting in excess red cells, the opposite of anemia. They occur when the feedback system governing red-cell production misbehaves. Reactive polycythemia results when the message incorrectly instructs the marrow to overproduce. Neoplastic polycythemia results when the marrow cells fail to perceive the slowdown signals.

Reactive polycythemia is triggered when insufficient oxygen is perceived by oxygen sensors monitoring the blood in the kidneys. It develops in persons who live at high altitude, or when lung disease interferes with oxygen delivery to the blood, when blood vessels bypass the lungs, when abnormal hemoglobin molecules fail to yield oxygen to the kidney sensors, when blood flow to the kidney is inadequate because of blood vessel narrowing or because of pressure on the kidney. Some tumors of the liver, uterus, and ovaries also cause polycythemia. So may injections of the male hormone testosterone and so do small doses of cobalt.

Reactive polycythemia is actually useful to residents of high-altitude areas and under other conditions of general oxygen deprivation. When the concentration of hemoglobin is increased every drop of blood can carry more oxygen. But otherwise the excess is not useful and may be harmful.

Polycythemia vera results from an abnormality of the marrow that causes it to produce not only too many red cells but also too many white cells and platelets. It is usually a disease of older persons in whom the thick blood and excess of platelets can lead to clotting, causing strokes and heart attacks. These persons are also prone to ulceration and bleeding of the stomach or intestine.

The victim of polycythemia vera is suffused with blood. The face and palms are red, the eyes are bloodshot. Although some sufferers may have no symptoms, headache is a common complaint and so is itching, especially after a hot bath or when the patient is warm in bed. The spleen usually is large although not uncomfortable. In most persons the disease is easily controlled by suppressing the marrow with drugs or by draining off the excess blood. When properly treated, most persons with polycythemia vera have a normal life expectancy. In a small percentage of cases, polycythemia vera eventually develops into leukemia, or the marrow is replaced by fibrous tissue, which causes anemia.

White Blood Cell Disorders

As with other blood cell diseases, diseases of white cells can be divided into three types: too many cells, not enough cells, and the wrong kind of cells.

Leukopenia (not enough white cells) or granulocytopenia (not enough granulocytes) may result from inadequate production of these cells by the marrow or too rapid destruction (by the spleen, for example). The causes of inadequate white cell production are similar to those for inadequate red cell production (see page 103). To understand the impact of leukopenia we must realize that the body's white cell supply includes a large margin for safety. The marrow produces many more leukocytes than we need. Yet sometimes the white cell count can be low in a person who is completely healthy. Nevertheless, it is important to investigate the possible causes of leukopenia in evidently healthy people to be certain that the low count is not caused by some underlying disease.

The dangerous leukopenias are associated with a complete lack of granulocyte production, resulting in a lethal susceptibility to infection. The body cannot form pus, and infections are ineffectually opposed by tissue phagocytes, antibodies, and antibiotics. When the marrow disease is reversible, as it may be after injury by medicines, recovery of granulocyte production usually occurs in time to save the victim's life.

Increased destruction of leukocytes can result from autoimmune diseases in which antibodies are directed against white cells.

Lymphocytopenia. Total absence of antibody-producing lymphocytes results in susceptibility to bacteria. Without antibodies to coat the germs, the granulocytes cannot ingest them.

Leukocytosis, the overproduction of white cells, may be neoplastic (leukemia) or the result of disease. With an infection such as pneumonia, the quantity of granulocytes increases. With whooping cough and infectious mononucleosis, the lymphocytes are increased.

Leukemia. Neoplasms (page 102) of the blood-cell-producing tissues comprise a family called leukemias and lymphomas. The common varieties of leukemia are lymphocytic and granulocytic, acute and chronic.

The cause or causes of leukemia are not well understood. Atomic radiation and heavy doses of X rays have increased the rate of granulocytic leukemia in persons exposed to them.

Certain chemicals like benzol and the antibiotic chloromycetin have caused aplastic anemia that in some persons has developed into granulocytic leukemia. Leukemia, like every neoplasm, represents a disorder of genetic information (see page 102), and it is known that X rays can disrupt chromosomes, the carriers of genetic information. It is not understood why ionizing radiation frequently causes granulocytic leukemia, but never causes lymphocytic leukemia. Certain viruses cause leukemia in animals but not in humans. Babies born with leukemia have healthy mothers. Women with leukemia give birth to healthy babies. In rare cases, identical twins have both developed leukemia, more often than not at about the same age. Despite all this we have no indication of a genetic cause for leukemia.

Acute lymphocytic leukemia is a disease of children, uncommon after the age of 20. The lymphatic tissues, lymph nodes, and spleen enlarge. The marrow is largely replaced by abnormal lymphocytes, and the blood leukocyte count usually is high, with large numbers of abnormal cells. There is anemia, and low platelet counts. The disease progresses rapidly. Untreated children die. But with prompt and aggressive treatment by chemotherapy and radiation, complete remissions can be easily achieved in 90 percent of the cases, without the medicine's destroying the marrow and incurring the subsequent risks of hemorrhage and infection. Acute lymphocytic leukemia is the one variety of leukemia with a good cure rate. Fifty percent of children adequately treated live five years or more free of disease and are presumed cured.

Acute granulocytic leukemia is a disease of adults, uncommon in children. It is often insidious in onset, heralded by symptoms of anemia or unexplained fever. The blood leukocyte count may be high or low but almost invariably the primitive leukemia cells (blasts) are present. Normal granulocytes are decreased; so is the platelet count. The marrow contains characteristic leukemia cells.

This adult variety of leukemia is much more difficult to treat than the childhood type. The drugs used are harsher and can themselves cause death. Repeated treatments are often required. Remissions are usually partial or brief. It is claimed that 80 percent of those who survive the rigorous treatment do achieve remission. Repeated courses of "consolidation" therapy follow. Patients who survive one or two years are exceptional.

It is probable that some young adults have been cured by chemotherapy and by marrow transplantation (page 116).

Chronic lymphocytic leukemia is usually a disease of people over 50. It never occurs in children. It is often a disease of low aggressiveness with long survival. Median life expectancy is five years, and more than a third of the victims live ten years. Chronic lymphocytic leukemia manifests itself by the accumulation of lymphocytes in lymph nodes, spleen, marrow, and blood. As it progresses the problems of anemia and lack of platelets become more insistent. In many patients, the normal lymphocytes that can become antibody-producing plasma cells are suppressed, and the defenses against infection may be lowered. At the same time, autoimmune diseases directed against red cells or platelets can cause serious complications. Treatment with chemotherapy is usually reserved until lymphocyte counts in the blood become high or there is a massive enlargement of nodes or spleen. Early in the disease, response to treatment is usually gratifying. As the disease progresses, it becomes more and more difficult to treat successfully.

Chronic granulocytic leukemia, a disease of adults, is rare in children. It, too, is insidious in onset. The patient usually does not feel ill. He may go to his doctor because of a lump in his left abdomen (an enlarged spleen) or because of fatigue, breathlessness, or other symptoms of anemia. The granulocyte count in the blood is high, but many of the cells are immature, and the marrow is filled with proliferating granulocytic cells. Blood platelet counts usually are normal or elevated. In most patients the leukemia can be controlled with mild chemotherapy, but it is doubtful that this therapy prolongs life. Only about half of the patients live much more than three years after diagnosis. Radiation of the spleen can induce remissions, too, but these patients have an even shorter life expectancy. Median survival is about 20 months. Eventually, the leukemia becomes uncontrollable, becoming, in most patients, an acute granulocytic leukemia that resists treatment.

Myeloma is also an older person's disease, originating in the plasma cells of the marrow. It often causes wasting of the bones, with X rays showing a characteristic "moth-eaten" pattern. Bone pain and fractures result from this destruction. Plasma cells fill the marrow cavity and the counts of normal blood cells are low. Myeloma is usually limited to the marrow. Its cells characteristically do not get into the blood. Normal plasma cells produce plasma proteins, the gamma globulins. Myeloma cells pervert this activity, producing quantities of abnormal gamma globulin and even fragments of gamma globulin. This abundant protein may clog the kidneys, gradually causing kidney failure. Chemotherapy can often inhibit the abnormal production. Radiation can stop the bone erosion, and can be used for pain or when holes appear in weight-bearing bones.

Macroglobulinemia, like myeloma, causes large amounts of abnormal gamma globulin to appear in the plasma. The protein molecules mass together to form "macroglobulins" that cause the plasma to thicken and interfere with platelet function, resulting in easy bleeding. The thick plasma distends the small blood vessels, increases the plasma volume, and puts a heavy burden on the heart to pump the gluey blood. Some patients respond to chemotherapy. The thick plasma can be removed mechanically by plasmapheresis, described on page 116.

Lymphoma and Hodgkin's disease. Lymphomas are neoplasms of the lymphocytic tissues, lymph nodes, and spleen; usually there is also some involvement of the liver and marrow. It has become convenient to separate them into two categories, Hodgkin's disease and non-Hodgkin lymphoma.

Hodgkin's disease, which can occur at any age, was once almost invariably fatal but now is curable in more than half of early cases. It is a disease of the phagocytic cells of the lymph nodes. Usually, at the time of discovery and diagnosis, Hodgkin's disease involves one lymph node or group of nodes, often in the neck. A careful surgical operation called a staging laparotomy may be performed to ascertain if the disease has spread to the nodes in the abdomen. If not, intensive radiation is concentrated on the nodes in the chest, armpits, and neck. If the abdomen is involved, the radiation may be extended to include all the nodes there and in the groin. If the patient also has fever and weight loss, an extended course of chemotherapy is prescribed. When Hodgkin's disease is untreated or not cured, it is progressive. The patient gradually becomes more and more ill and wasted until death.

Non-Hodgkin lymphomas involve lymphocytes or phagocytes. In undifferentiated lymphoma the abnormal cell cannot be identified. Non-Hodgkin lymphomas are further subdivided into "follicular" types, in which the neoplastic cells are grouped in small spheres within the lymph nodes, and "diffuse," in which they are not. At the time of discovery and diagnosis, non-Hodgkin lymphoma has usually spread throughout the body. The dis-

ease is best treated with chemotherapy. In exceptional cases radiation may also be used.

The non-Hodgkin lymphomas vary in how quickly they progress and in how they respond to treatment. The outlook in follicular lymphoma is generally better than in diffuse lymphoma. Even with the best of treatment patients with poorly differentiated lymphocytic lymphoma have a median life expectancy of about 18 months. In histiocytic lymphomas that respond to treatment, 50 to 75 percent live longer than five years.

Platelet Disorders

Platelets have a crucial role in blood clotting and hemostasis, the process that stops bleeding (see page 92). Platelet disorders are associated on the one hand with easy bruising (purpura) and prolonged bleeding, or, on the other hand, with clots forming in the bloodstream: thrombosis and embolism.

Purpura (the Latin word for purple) describes the presence of darkened blood beneath the skin. The blood spots can be large, as in a black eye, when the spot is called an ecchymosis. Scattered pinhead or pinpoint size spots are called petechiae. Sometimes there are blood blisters in the mouth, or spots on the white of the eye.

Purpura represents superficial bleeding from small vessels. The bleeding itself is usually harmless. Senile purpura, the blotches in the tissue-paper-thin skin on the arms of the elderly, is caused by the skin's fragility. Although senile purpura is unsightly, it is not harmful. On the other hand, purpura can be a sign of serious disease when, for example, it results in bleeding from lack of platelets.

Thrombocytopenia (not enough platelets) can result from inadequate production of platelets or from their premature destruction after they enter the bloodstream. The normal platelet count ranges from about 200,000 to 400,000, many more than we need for normal hemostasis. In fact, it is a ten-fold margin of safety, for people with platelet counts as low as 20,000 rarely have serious problems with bleeding, provided the platelets are normal. But persons with platelet counts well below 20,000, and with purpura and spontaneous bleeding, are a great risk. Fatal hemorrhage in the brain is not uncommon.

In patients with inadequate platelet production, the marrow shows a lack of the platelet-producing megakaryocytes. On the other hand when platelets are rapidly destroyed the megakaryocytes are abundant. Platelet production is impaired in aplastic anemia, in leukemia, or as a reaction to toxic chemicals or medicines. Hereditary diseases with few megakaryocytes are rare. Rapid destruction of platelets may occur in infections when platelets stick on bacteria and the combination is devoured by a phagocyte. Diseases that stimulate the clotting system in the circulating blood can rapidly destroy most or all circulating platelets.

The immune thrombocytopenic purpuras result from production of abnormal antibodies directed against the platelets. Sometimes a medicine is the underlying cause. The antibody is directed against the medicine. The medicine-antibody combination sticks to the platelet and injures it, and the combination is then devoured by a phagocyte. Most such immune reactions are temporary, because the offending medicine is withheld, or, as in most childhood cases, the antibody disappears. But in adults these purpuras may become a permanent disease and must be treated with other medicines or by removal of the spleen.

Thrombocytosis (too many platelets) occurs after severe injury, strenuous exercise, surgery, blood loss, or chronic inflammatory disease has stimulated platelet production. The counts return to normal when the stimulus subsides. When platelet production has been temporarily impaired, as by alcohol abuse or vitamin B_{12} deficiency, correction of the impairment causes a temporary "rebound" thrombocytosis.

Thrombocythemia is the exaggerated production of platelets by neoplastic megakaryocytes. A platelet count in the millions may be the cardinal evidence of marrow disease, a sort of megakaryocytic leukemia. Sometimes megakaryocytes can even be found in the blood. Thrombocythemia is also a common phenomenon in polycythemia vera, chronic granulocytic leukemia, and myelofibrosis, all in a family called chronic myeloproliferative diseases. Very high platelet counts are risky. Platelets may clump and block small blood vessels. Clots may form on the clumps and block larger vessels. It is often necessary to reduce the platelet count by inhibiting the marrow with chemotherapy. Sometimes aspirin may be used to make the platelets less sticky.

Platelet disability. Platelets produced in certain neoplastic disorders may be relatively ineffectual. A patient may have a platelet count of 100,000, yet cut him and he bleeds as freely as if his count were 10,000. There are also hereditary disorders with ineffectual platelets. Overuse of certain medicines, including aspirin, may reduce the effectiveness of normal platelets. So do the abnormal plasma proteins in macroglobulinemia (see page 111).

The alteration caused by aspirin is of no consequence in healthy people but may cause severe deterioration in those with low platelet counts or persons susceptible to bleeding, such as hemophiliacs (see page 113).

Thromboembolism. Thrombus is a blood clot. Embolus is a piece of clot (or other debris) carried by the bloodstream from the place it formed to another place where it lodges. A thrombus formed in the veins of the leg may be dislodged and move up the vena cava, the body's principal vein, through the right side of the heart to lodge in the lung. One formed in the left heart and dislodged may be carried into an arm or leg artery or the brain. Thrombotic disease is the most common cause of death in older people. Strokes and heart attacks result from thrombosis (see chapter 3, "The Heart and Circulation," and chapter 8, "The Lungs").

Thrombosis, the formation of blood clots, does not occur under normal circumstances for several reasons: The smooth walls of the vessels repel platelets, the flow of blood dilutes and disperses activated clotting factors, the complexity of the clotting reaction prevents instantaneous coagulation, and the platelets are tough enough to withstand a great deal of buffeting without provoking a hemostatic reaction. But thrombosis does result when these safeguards are overcome in any of the following ways:

• The walls of blood vessels may be roughened by sclerotic deposits that cause turbulence of the circulation and consequent platelet damage—the well-known condition of "hardening of the arteries," or arteriosclerosis. Or sudden crushing injury may damage the normally smooth surface, attracting platelets that accumulate over the injured area.

• Blood flow may be slowed at the site of clogging in a hardened coronary artery or in the sluggish pools in varicose veins, or because of prolonged immobilization. Nowadays patients are told to stand and walk as soon as possible after surgery to prevent stagnation of blood that may result in coagulation and postoperative embolism—once a common and lethal complication of surgery.

• "Hypercoagulability" describes the presence of increased concentration or activity of plasma clotting factors. This occurs, for example, during pregnancy and among women who are heavy smokers and also take oral contraceptives.

• Abnormally high platelet counts increase the possibility of clumping, especially when combined with sluggish blood flow or roughened vessel walls. Sensitive platelets may predispose to thrombosis. In the chronic hemolytic anemia called paroxysmal nocturnal hemoglobinuria, described on page 105, the platelets are susceptible to damage by the same process that destroys the red cells. Thrombosis is the most common cause of death in that disease.

Abnormalities of Coagulation

The complexities of the coagulation system have been discussed on page 97. With one exception, all of the coagulation proteins are essential to normal clotting of the blood. Depletion of any results in a greater tendency to bleed. These clotting factors usually are lacking from birth because of hereditary diseases, but accidents, poisoning, and acquired diseases also may reduce or eliminate some.

Hemophilia. The classic "bleeder's disease," historically famous for its impact on the crowned families of Europe, actually is found in four hereditary forms. Two forms are genetically transmitted as sex-linked abnormalities, meaning that they are passed from unaffected "carrier" mothers to their sons, as happened with the descendants of Queen Victoria. Another form of hemophilia is not sex-linked but is inherited from two carrier parents. The fourth form, known as Von Willebrandt's disease, comes from one affected parent. The latter two diseases affect men and women equally. Except in Von Willebrandt's disease the bleeding-time test (see page 100) is normal, indicating that platelet function is also normal. But coagulation is severely inhibited, and normal clotting does not take place. Although the condition may be discovered in a child at the time of circumcision, the classic "bleeder" usually does not bleed visibly: he does not, as people seem to believe, bleed to death while shaving. Instead, his bleeding is internal, often precipitated by a minor fall, and causes large accumulations of blood in the tissues. Bleeding is particularly common in and around the joints. The pooled blood may force the joints apart, leading to hemophilic crippling.

In times past, the only treatment for hemophiliacs was to replace the lost blood with transfusions of whole blood, a hospital procedure. Now it is possible to separate and freeze-dry the missing factor, and it can be transfused by the patient himself or his family at home. Some patients can learn to anticipate when a bleeding episode is coming on, and to transfuse themselves in advance. Home treatment has enabled many young hemophiliacs to lead nearly normal lives.

Acquired coagulation disorders. Vitamin K is required by the liver for the synthesis of four types of coagulation factors. Lack of vitamin K causes hemorrhagic disease of the newborn. Before the nature of the disease became clear as many as one in 300 newborns died of it. Now supplemental vitamin K is given at birth to tide the baby over until the vitamin can be absorbed from the diet.

Acquired cases of vitamin K deficiency are related to lack of bile, which is essential for absorption of the vitamin. In obstructive jaundice a blocked bile duct prevents bile from entering the intestine. Jaundiced patients may develop hemorrhagic disease if the vitamin is not injected. Patients who can eat no food must also be given vitamin K. In severe liver disease the coagulation factors that depend on vitamin K may be lacking because the liver cells that make the factors are incapacitated, so injecting the vitamin cannot help. Drugs which are used as anticoagulants use vitamin K antagonists. Overdosing causes bleeding.

Disseminated intravascular coagulation is a catastrophic accident in which coagulation factors are activated and used up, platelets are destroyed, and fibrin (clot) is precipitated and then dissolved. The reaction is triggered by the introduction into the bloodstream of some objectionable material: a swarm of bacteria, incompatible blood cells, amniotic fluid from the uterus during delivery of a baby. When this disorder occurs during surgery a severe, uncontrollable bleeding often occurs. If a wound is not present the crisis may pass harmlessly except for a chill, fever, and a drop in blood pressure. Lesser degrees of intravascular coagulation may be recognizable only by laboratory testing.

Acquired anticoagulants. Hemophilic patients with severe deficiency of a particular blood-clotting factor (known as Factor VIII) sometimes produce antibodies against the needed factor, which makes treatment difficult. These antibodies have also occurred in nonhemophiliacs as a sort of autoimmune disease, producing an acquired form of hemophilia. Antibodies against other coagulation factors are less common. Lupus erythematosus is a disease in which acquired anticoagulants are often discovered (see chapter 15, "Arthritis and Related Diseases").

Dysproteinemia. Marrow neoplasms such as myeloma and macroglobulinemia produce large amounts of abnormal plasma protein. Sometimes this protein may coat the surface of blood platelets, making the platelets ineffective. A purpuric disorder results.

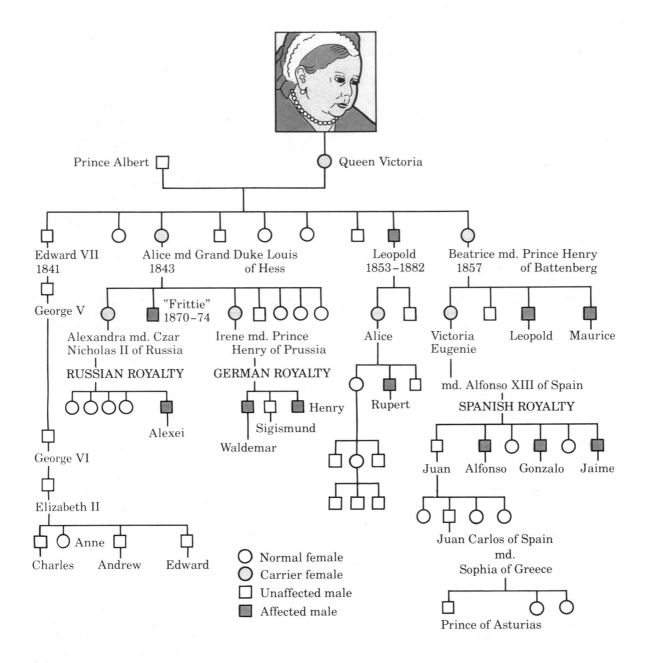

Prince Albert — Queen Victoria

Edward VII 1841 | Alice md Grand Duke Louis of Hess | Leopold 1853–1882 | Beatrice md. Prince Henry of Battenberg

George V

"Frittie" 1870–74

Alexandra md. Czar Nicholas II of Russia
RUSSIAN ROYALTY

Irene md. Prince Henry of Prussia
GERMAN ROYALTY

Alice

Victoria Eugenie
md. Alfonso XIII of Spain

Leopold   Maurice

Alexei

Henry
Sigismund
Waldemar

Rupert

SPANISH ROYALTY

Juan   Alfonso   Gonzalo   Jaime

George VI

Elizabeth II

Charles   Anne   Andrew   Edward

Juan Carlos of Spain md. Sophia of Greece

Prince of Asturias

○ Normal female
◔ Carrier female
□ Unaffected male
■ Affected male

HEMOPHILIA: THE ROYAL CURSE

Through her nine children and many grandchildren, Britain's Queen Victoria, a hemophilia carrier, transmitted the "bleeder's disease" to several royal houses of Europe and affected the course of 19th and 20th century history. Granddaughter Alexandra, princess of Hesse-Darmstadt, married Czar Nicholas II of Russia, and their only son, Alexei, was hemophilic. The "mad monk" Rasputin claimed he could treat the boy's illness and gained influence over Alexandra and through her, the Czar. Rasputin's role is said

to have helped bring on the Russian Revolution, in which Nicholas, Alexandra, Alexei, and their four daughters were executed. Another granddaughter, Victoria Eugenie of Battenberg, married Alfonso XIII of Spain. Two sons, both hemophiliacs, bled to death after minor accidents. A third hemophilic son, Jaime, renounced his right to the throne in favor of brother Don Juan, who was not affected. Alfonso was deposed in 1931 and Don Juan never became king. When the monarchy was restored in 1975, his son Juan Carlos

was crowned. A third granddaughter, Irene, sister of Alexandra, whose brother, "Frittie," died of intracranial bleeding after a childhood injury, carried the disease into the Prussian royal house. Two of her three sons were hemophilic. Of Queen Victoria's four sons, only Prince Leopold was hemophilic. He died of internal bleeding after a fall at age 29. The queen's heir and successor, Edward VII, was free of the disease, so the "curse," as Victoria called it, no longer exists in the British royal family.

TREATMENT OF BLOOD DISEASES

Blood diseases are treated by many kinds of medicines and procedures. These include:

Transfusion

The art of transfusing one person's blood into another who needs it is a triumph of 20th century medicine. A few successful transfusions had been given in earlier times, but the catastrophe caused by blood incompatibility had far outweighed the successes. Only with Karl Landsteiner's discovery of the ABO blood groups in the 1920s was it possible to match donor and recipient and transfuse blood safely and successfully. Even that was fraught with the danger of an occasional disaster until Landsteiner, an Austrian-born biologist, identified the Rh blood group. (He received the Nobel Prize for medicine in 1930.)

Now that transfusion reactions are virtually eliminated, shall we cease to marvel that this life-giving tissue, this peculiar juice, can be transferred from one body to a totally different body without provoking an immune response? Yet, miraculously, we can transfuse not only from one person to another, but time after time, from 100 different donors into a single anemic recipient, thus extending his life for years. The art of transfusion we now take for granted permits surgery that otherwise would be impossible—open-heart surgery, for example—and operations on children with hemophilia. It also allows the aggressive treatment of patients with leukemia and saves the grievously injured who would otherwise bleed to death or die of shock.

Transfusion reactions. Meticulous attention to blood grouping and crossmatching (see page 101) has nearly eliminated the reactions caused by incompatibility. The rare reaction results not from technical fault but from administrative error almost every time. When, by error, incompatible red cells are transfused they are rapidly destroyed and some of their hemoglobin spills into the urine. The clotting system is activated in the bloodstream and the disseminated intravascular coagulation reaction occurs. The patient's blood pressure falls and acute kidney failure may follow.

Less serious incompatibility reactions bring on fever or hives. These are fairly common and not harmful. They result from white cells intermingled with the red cells or from substances in the plasma. Such reactions are prevented by washing the red cells with saline solutions before transfusing them.

The liver disease hepatitis is a risk of blood transfusion that has not been eliminated. Perhaps one in 300 healthy persons is a carrier of hepatitis virus. The recipient of the carrier's blood, about two months later, either falls ill with jaundice, fever, and enlarged liver or, more often, has a "silent" infection that can be detected only by laboratory tests. The hepatitis virus is a tough one, withstanding the rigors of refrigerated storage. The possibility of hepatitis is reduced by testing the donor plasma for the virus, but the test is not sensitive enough to identify every infected unit. The risk is also reduced by not using blood that has been sold by the donor. People who sell their blood are more often carriers of the hepatitis virus than people who donate it.

Iron storage disease can occur in people who, over the years, receive many transfusions. Since there is no normal channel for excretion of iron (page 98), iron given up by transfused red cells must be stored in the body. In time the increasing concentration of iron begins to injure tissue where the iron is stored: liver, pancreas, heart, and endocrine glands.

Blood Fractionation

Nowadays there are relatively few transfusions of whole blood. Instead each unit of blood is divided into its component parts. The plasma and platelets are separated from the red cells. Then the platelets are separated from plasma. The red cells are transfused into patients with anemia. Platelets are used for those with thrombocytopenia. Some of the plasma is frozen while still fresh, thereby preserving the fragile coagulation factors. Or it may be fractionated, divided into its protein components so that gamma globulin can be injected into people who lack antibodies, Factor VIII given to hemophiliacs, and albumin to patients with severe injury or burns.

Platelet transfusion has provided an enormous improvement in the practice of transfusion. Previously many patients with severe thrombocytopenia died of uncontrollable bleeding. Now patients bleeding from lack of platelets can even be operated upon safely. Twenty years ago the results of therapy for adult acute leukemia were horrendous: both disease and treatment destroyed platelet production. Now these patients can be transfused with fresh platelets. The platelets are creamed off almost every unit of blood that is collected. They are concentrated and the platelets from six to 12 units dispensed in a single transfusion. The procedure raises the recipient's platelet count substantially. After treatment for leukemia the patients can be kept from bleeding until the marrow resumes platelet production. Transfused platelets, however, maintain the platelet count for only a few days, after which the transfusion must be repeated. Platelets collected in the blood bank are stored at room temperature and have a "shelf life" of only three to four days. Platelet collection and preservation is arduous and expensive, but it does save lives. Platelets cannot yet be frozen, as some other components can.

White blood cell transfusions are becoming more common. Because white cells in the blood are few and because their life-span is as brief as four hours, the number in one unit of blood is negligible. To obtain a useful quantity of white cells the donor is connected to a machine called a cell separator. Blood from one arm is run through the machine and returned via the other arm after the machine removes the white cells. The white cells are then transfused to the recipient. Platelets can be skimmed off and transfused in the same fashion. The process is called leukopheresis or plateletpheresis. It can also be used to reduce high white cell counts in leukemia or high platelet counts in thrombocythemia.

Frozen red blood cells. When red blood cells are quick-frozen, they can be stored without deterioration for many years, and the technique appears to be ideal for blood banks. It is, however, enormously expensive. The cells must be washed in graduated concentrations of glycerol to protect the cells from destruction during the freezing-thawing procedures. The cells are catalogued and stored at an extremely low temperature ($-80°C$). When ready for use the unit of red cells is carefully thawed and the glycerol is removed by repeated washing. The process may quadruple the cost of a unit of red cells. The frozen blood bank is useful to store red cells of rare blood groups or to maintain supplies against dire emergency (such as when people stop donating during the Christmas season). Presently a store of frozen red cells in a blood bank is a sort of blood banker's status symbol.

Blood Donation

The standard unit of blood is a little less than one pint. In the United States each year about 10 million units of blood are donated to our transfusion services. Shortage of blood is a chronic, disruptive problem. Anemic patients must sometimes wait days for red cells. Surgical operations must be postponed. The reason is that more than 95 percent of our citizens do not get involved. The transfusion service is supplied by less than 5 percent of Americans. A donation entails only the loss of a small amount of time, a split second of discomfort from the needle, loss of one pound of weight, 75 grams of protein, and 200 milligrams of iron.

Autotransfusion

A few weeks before certain surgical procedures a patient may go to the blood bank and donate one or even two units of blood earmarked for his own use during operation. The body, of course, quickly replaces the blood. This sort of self-transfusion blocks the possibility of incompatibility or transmission of infection.

Phlebotomy

Phlebotomy, the opening of a vein, is the name given to the procedure involved in blood donation. Phlebotomy is also used to treat polycythemia. When too much blood or too many red cells are present, one unit at a time is removed until the volume is restored to normal. Thereafter, an occasional phlebotomy is required to maintain the normal volume. Phlebotomy is also used to treat hemochromatosis, a disease in which the intestine absorbs more iron than the body requires. Because storing excess iron eventually damages the storage organs, blood is removed to reduce iron and prevent further damage.

Plasmapheresis

Plasmapheresis is akin to phlebotomy, but only the plasma is retained and the red cells are returned to the donor. Plasmapheresis is helpful when the plasma contains a harmfully high concentration of protein. It can also be used to reduce rapidly a dangerously elevated platelet count. Normal people are plasmapheresed to obtain normal plasma protein components.

Bone Marrow Transplants

Bone marrow transplantation offers the possibility of a cure for leukemia and aplastic anemia. Preparation is rigorous, involving irradiation of the entire body plus chemotherapy to destroy *all* proliferating cells of the blood-forming organs. The danger of overwhelming infection then is great because cellular defenses have been completely destroyed. Young adults are the best candidates for the procedure. Older patients often prove fragile, unable to withstand the shock of the treatment.

During the procedure marrow cells from a carefully matched donor are suspended in plasma and transfused. When all goes well the graft takes, and then precautionary treatment must begin to prevent the transplanted immune system of the donor from generating lethal antibodies against the patient's tissue, the so-called graft-versus-host disease.

The matching of donor and recipient is more difficult than matching for blood transfusion. In blood transfusion the red-cell antigens are matched, in transplantation the white-cell antigens. The Human Leukocytic Antigen (HLA) system is so complex that good matches can usually be found only among brothers and sisters. Identical twins are, of course, the perfect match. Marrow transplantation is risky and still experimental, but it does offer great promise.

Splenectomy

Splenectomy, removal of the spleen, may be performed for any of these reasons:
• Size. The spleen may become so massively enlarged that it limits the patient's mobility, and presses on adjacent organs. More than half of the blood pumped by the heart may be diverted into such a large spleen.
• Destroyer of blood cells. The spleen may destroy so many red cells that it causes anemia or so many platelets that it causes purpura.
• Producer of autoantibodies. Autoimmune diseases often seem centered in the spleen.

The spleen is not an essential organ. Persons without a spleen live in good health. However there is a remote risk of severe infection by pneumococcus bacteria, and the risk is higher in children. Persons without spleens are vaccinated against pneumococcus and admonished to take antibiotics as soon as an infection begins to develop.

Chemotherapy

Poisonous medicines are employed for two hematologic purposes: to kill neoplastic cells in leukemia and lymphoma and to suppress the activity of the immune system in autoimmune diseases. (See Chapter 29, "Cancer.") In general, chemotherapy does not cure blood diseases except in some cases of leukemia and Hodgkin's disease and the rare Burkitt's lymphoma that occurs in African children.

Radiation Therapy

Radiation therapy is used to treat neoplastic diseases by means of high-voltage ionizing irradiation either from an X-ray machine or a radioactive cobalt source. The objective is to destroy the malignant cells with the least possible damage to the normal surrounding tissues. In hematology radiation therapy is used especially to treat the lymphomas. A large proportion of patients with Hodgkin's disease can be cured by radiation. In childhood leukemia the brain is often a "sanctuary" where leukemia cells can escape from chemotherapy. To cure childhood leukemia these cells must be destroyed. Radiation to the brain and spine can accomplish this.

Radiation therapy and chemotherapy are often used in combination.

Radioactive Isotopes

Radioactive isotopes are used to treat neoplasms that can be induced to combine with a radioactive element. In hematology we use radiophosphorus because this element "seeks" the cells of certain leukemias and lymphomas. Radiophosphorus is often successful in controlling chronic leukemia, polycythemia vera, and thrombocythemia. It is not commonly used because of its cost and inconvenience. Patients like it because there are no uncomfortable side effects, and they need treatment once a month or so instead of every day.

Hormones

Hormones in natural or synthetic form are used to treat disease in two ways. One is to replace a lack of hormone. For example, anemia caused by deficiency of thyroid hormone is cured when the hormone thyroxin is taken daily in pill form. The second way is to combat directly certain blood diseases. Hormones of the adrenal cortex such as cortisone or prednisone in large doses suppress the immune system, and are used to treat autoimmune diseases. When cortisone first became available about 1950 it proved capable by itself of producing complete remission in many children with lymphocytic leukemia. It is still used in combination with chemotherapeutic drugs. Prednisone is a part of the formula for the treatment of other leukemias and other kinds of cancer as well. Testosterone, the male sex hormone, in large doses causes polycythemia (see page 109) in normal people. It is used for anemias that do not respond to other treatments, and sometimes it works.

CHAPTER 7   SYLVIA C. JOHNSON, M.D.

THE SKIN

Skin, the most visible organ of the human body, is also the heaviest. From top to toe the outer covering of an average-sized adult weighs about seven pounds, two to three times the weight of the heaviest solid internal organ, the liver. Surprisingly, the skin does not rank first among the organs in surface area. It measures two square yards, much smaller than the convoluted and highly folded surfaces of the circulatory system, the gastrointestinal tract, and the lungs.

If you stand naked before a mirror, you can see virtually the entire surface of your skin. From this perspective, it seems to be an inactive organ, merely a wrapper to keep the inside in and the outside out. The appearance is deceiving. The layers of the skin are full of activity, performing myriad and subtle functions to shield the body from injury and maintain constant internal conditions. That seemingly smooth wrapper is honeycombed with tiny blood vessels, nerve endings, and miniature passageways to the outside world.

In computer jargon, the skin is an interface, the boundary where our space ends and the world's begins. The skin enforces this boundary, but it is not impermeable. It blocks entry of infectious organisms and noxious substances, and holds in water and vital chemicals, but it also allows substances to pass through in both directions, screening them in response to the body's needs. Connective tissue and fatty layers cushion the body against shocks and injuries. The skin's pigment, or coloring matter, protects against the ravages of sunlight. The sun's ultraviolet light stimulates skin to make vitamin D, but this is less important now that vitamin D is added to milk and dairy products.

The skin plays an important role in regulating body temperature, helping to keep it within narrow limits. The thick fatty tissue helps conserve heat. The blood vessels, by constricting and expanding, influence how much heat is lost through the skin. When the outside temperature plunges, the vessels narrow, keeping the heat within the body. When the temperature soars, the vessels dilate and allow heat to pass through the skin. Moisture from the sweat glands also cools the skin through evaporation.

With its vast network of nerves, the skin is a sensory organ that helps us feel touch, pressure, temperature, pain, and itch. Its perceptive powers are extremely sensitive, as a delicate brush with a feather discloses. The skin conveys messages about the external world and from one person to another. Tactile experience during infancy critically affects subsequent development. Touching is the essence of human sexual expression. Blushing, becoming pale, frowning, and sweating are all forms of emotional communication that take place through the skin.

But from a health point of view, perhaps the most important feature of the skin is its sheer visibility. Skin diseases are easily seen and thus can be promptly treated. Potentially serious malignancies can be detected much earlier than in other organs. And the skin is a mirror that reflects changes in other parts of the body. Examining it can provide clues to internal disease.

Visibility, however, is a two-edged sword. Skin diseases are significant not only because they may impair physical health, but because they are often unattractive in appearance. The psychological consequences can be more devastating than the physical ones.

The skin and the psyche are intimately and intricately related. Skin disorders can be both a cause and a consequence of psychological disturbances. Adolescent acne can be psychologically and socially crippling. Itching in certain disorders can be so severe that it drives the victim to suicide. On the other hand, emotionally disturbed people may actually damage their skin by scratching open existing pimples or blemishes or by excoriating skin in such a destructive way that ulcers form.

No simple organ, the human skin, but a vastly complex one.

STRUCTURE OF THE SKIN

The skin is composed of three distinct layers: the epidermis, dermis, and subcutaneous fat. The epidermis normally is the only portion that is visible. It is also the thinnest layer, less than the thickness of a sheet of paper in most areas but even thinner in some places such as the eyelids. The epidermis is composed of several layers of many cells. The dermis, in contrast, contains relatively few cells. Fundamentally fibrous in structure, it is much thicker than the epidermis. In most places the dermis rests on a layer of fat.

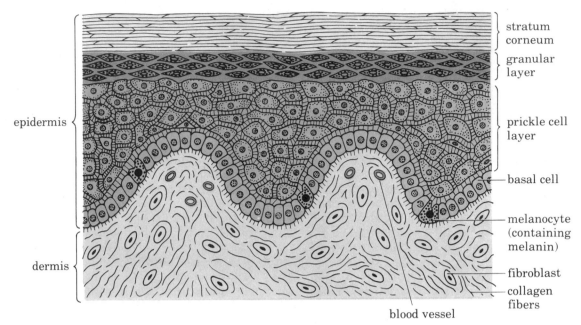

stratum corneum

granular layer

epidermis

prickle cell layer

basal cell

melanocyte (containing melanin)

dermis

fibroblast

collagen fibers

blood vessel

SKIN LAYERS

Layers of the skin are shown in this cross section. Epidermal cells develop at the basal-cell layer and eventually rise to the surface, changing structure and function as they rise. Most are called keratinocytes because they produce the protein keratin. Less numerous melanocytes give skin its color. As cells develop, they differ-entiate into prickle or spinous cells, then accumulate granules to become the granular layer. After 28 days, development stops and cells die, to be sloughed from the stratum corneum, or outer layer. The dermis contains fewer cells and more fiber. It rests on fat and is honeycombed with blood vessels.

Two principal layers make up the epidermis: the stratum corneum (the outermost layer) and the stratum germinativum or Malpighii. The cells that make up most of the epidermis are called keratinocytes because they produce keratin, a protein. New keratinocytes originate at the lowest levels of the epidermis. The lowest level of cells, the basal cells, multiply rapidly and rise progressively to the surface. As they do, the cells undergo changes in their structure and function and eventually die, becoming the dead cells of the stratum corneum. After the basal cells divide they differentiate into prickle or spinous cells, so named because of the conspicuous attachments between the cells as seen under the microscope. Near the surface, the prickle cells abruptly accumulate a dense collection of granules, thereby becoming cells of the granular layer. By this time, keratin has been produced and synthesis within the cells has stopped. Water is lost, and the keratinocytes lose their nuclei and flatten out to form the horny cells of the stratum corneum. The stratum corneum is thus composed mainly of dead keratinocytes and protein (keratin).

This life cycle of a skin cell covers 28 days: two weeks for a basal cell to divide and migrate through the stratum germinativum, and another two weeks for the cell to reach the outermost layer, the stratum corneum. The dead cells of the stratum corneum are constantly being sloughed off. We see them as flaky material after a brisk rubbing with a towel. Normally there is a balance between the loss of dead cells and the formation of new ones.

It is the stratum corneum that endows the skin with its property of being a good barrier. Compact and impermeable to most substances, this outermost layer varies in thickness. It is thickest on the palms and soles, where it is adapted for friction and weight bearing. The stratum corneum has the capacity to absorb much water, as demonstrated by the water-logged appearance of the palms and soles after a bath. On the other hand, prolonged exposure to low humidity produces brittleness and cracking, what we know as dry, chapped skin.

The other major type of epidermal cell is the melanocyte. Melanocytes are much less numerous than keratinocytes, accounting for only about five percent of the total epidermal cell population. Melanocytes are located in the basal layer of the stratum germinativum. Ultraviolet light stimulates them to synthesize pigment granules called melanin. These granules are passed to basal cell keratinocytes and become distributed in the other keratinocytes of the epidermis. White skin and black skin do not differ in numbers of melanocytes. Black skin is darker in part because its melanocytes produce more melanin than those in white skin.

Immediately beneath the epidermis lies a layer of connective tissue known as the dermis. In animals, the dermis is the part of skin that can be tanned into leather. Irregularly rounded elevations of the dermis called dermal papillae project into the lower surface of the epidermis. The dermal connective tissue consists of cells called fibroblasts, the fibrous proteins (collagen, reticulum, and elastin) made by the cells, and a material referred to as ground substance. Besides fibroblasts, other cells turn up occasionally in the dermis, most migrating there from the bloodstream to ingest foreign substances and to help counteract infection. Collagen is the most abundant type of fiber. It is responsible for the skin's mechanical strength. The ground substance, composed of water and a variety of chemical substances, forms a matrix in which are embedded all other dermal components and through which occurs transfer of substances between cells.

Unlike the epidermis, the dermis contains blood vessels, which supply it with nutrients and oxygen and remove metabolic waste products. The dermis also contains lymphatic vessels and nerves, as well as specialized structures called appendages: sweat glands, sebaceous (oil) glands, and hair follicles.

Beneath the dermis the connective tissue becomes more loosely knit and is separated by collections of fat cells. In most parts of the body, this tissue is thicker than the dermis, but in such areas as the eyelids, parts of the ear, and

Fingerprints

During the 13th to 19th weeks of fetal life, a maze of markings develops on the skin. These ridges become increasingly prominent during childhood and remain unchanged throughout life. The swirled patterns that occur on the palms and soles are unique to each individual and can be used as a means of identification. They even permit distinction between identical twins and can help establish paternity.

Fingerprints assume one of three configurations: a whorl, a loop, or an arch. Loops are the most common. Certain diseases caused by chromosomal aberrations (such as Down's syndrome, also known as mongolism) can be recognized by the characteristic patterns of ridging on the palms.

Ridging on the fingertips also helps us to grasp and pick up small objects and to perform delicate manipulations.

the penis, it is absent. There are also differences between the sexes in the amount and distribution of fat, accounting for the more rounded shape of the female torso. Heredity, eating habits, and age also determine where and how much fat is deposited.

GLANDS OF THE SKIN

Within the dermis are three kinds of glands: the eccrine sweat glands, the apocrine sweat glands, and the sebaceous or oil glands. The sebaceous glands open into the hair follicles, and together these form the pilosebaceous apparatus. Most apocrine glands also open into the hair follicle, although occasionally their ducts open directly into the epidermis. Eccrine sweat glands develop independently of hair follicles and their ducts lead directly into the epidermis.

Eccrine Sweat Glands

Eccrine sweat glands are more numerous in man than in any other animal, totaling about three million. They are most dense on the palms and soles, and then, in decreasing order, on the forehead, cheeks, trunk, and the arms and legs. The openings are not visible to the naked eye.

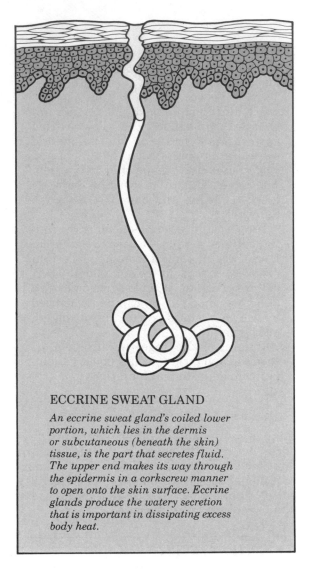

ECCRINE SWEAT GLAND

An eccrine sweat gland's coiled lower portion, which lies in the dermis or subcutaneous (beneath the skin) tissue, is the part that secretes fluid. The upper end makes its way through the epidermis in a corkscrew manner to open onto the skin surface. Eccrine glands produce the watery secretion that is important in dissipating excess body heat.

Along with the dermal blood vessels the eccrine sweat glands play a vital role in regulating body temperature. When the body is hot the eccrine glands release a thin watery solution onto the skin surface, which evaporates to produce cooling. With maximum exertion on a very hot day, more than two quarts of sweat may be produced in an hour. People who lack normally developed sweat glands are susceptible to heat stroke. (Dogs have very few sweat glands. They release heat by panting.)

We perspire for other reasons besides heat. The most important reason is emotional stress—pain, anxiety, fear, anger. This kind of sweating occurs mainly in the palms, soles, and armpits. Eating spicy foods makes some people's faces sweat. This phenomenon is called "gustatory sweating."

Apocrine Sweat Glands

The apocrine glands appear before birth as an outgrowth from the hair follicle just above the budding sebaceous gland. At first the glands are present throughout the body surface. Later, most of them disappear, persisting only in certain areas: the underarms, around the nipples, and in the lower abdomen and genital regions. The glands remain small until puberty, when they enlarge and begin to secrete. In old age, they shrink again in size.

In lower mammals such as rats and mice, the apocrine sweat glands are distributed over the entire surface, and they are believed to function as scent glands for sexual attraction and protection. In humans, apocrine glands apparently perform no useful function, although they may be the site of disease. They also may be a source of unpleasant odor. Freshly produced sweat is odorless. Odor results from its decomposition by bacteria present in apocrine areas.

Sebaceous Glands

Sebaceous or "oil" glands develop as buds from the hair follicles. They are distributed over the entire body surface except for the palms, soles, and the backs of the feet. They are largest and most abundant on the face, scalp, upper chest, and back.

Sebaceous glands produce and secrete sebum, a semi-liquid mixture of lipid (fat) and cellular debris. Sebum spreads over the surface of the hair and outer layer of the skin as a mild lubricant. The main significance of the sebaceous glands is that they are the sites where acne develops.

Sebum production depends on the presence of male hormones called androgens. Newborns have functioning sebaceous glands because of androgens received from the mother through the placenta. Shortly after birth the glands stop functioning and remain at rest until puberty. After puberty androgens are secreted mainly by the testes in males and by the ovaries and adrenal glands in females.

HAIR AND NAILS

Hair grows from structures in the dermis called follicles. New follicles do not form after birth. We are born with our full supply of about five million. At the expanded lower end of each follicle is the hair bulb, which contains the cells of the matrix. The matrix produces the hair shaft, which extends from the follicle above the surface of the skin.

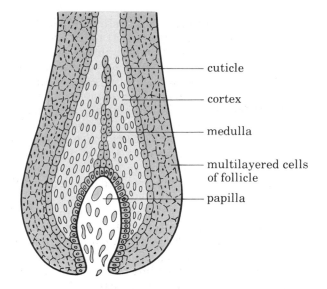

cuticle

cortex

medulla

multilayered cells
of follicle

papilla

THE HAIR SHAFT

*The three components of the hair
shaft, from outside in, are the cuticle,
cortex, and medulla. Surrounding the
hair are several layers of cells in the
follicle that take part in the formation
of the shaft. The papilla is a protrusion of the dermal skin layer from
which the follicle arises.*

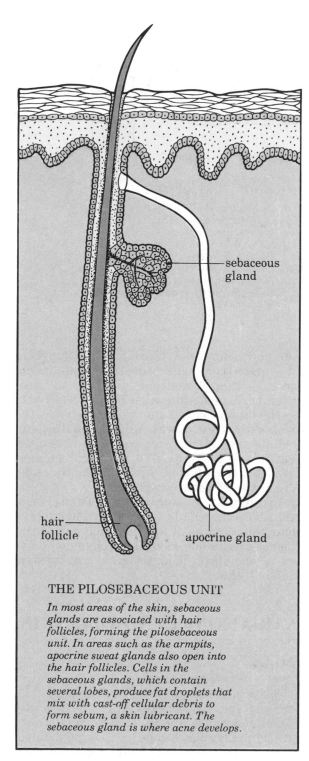

sebaceous
gland

hair
follicle

apocrine gland

THE PILOSEBACEOUS UNIT

*In most areas of the skin, sebaceous
glands are associated with hair
follicles, forming the pilosebaceous
unit. In areas such as the armpits,
apocrine sweat glands also open into
the hair follicles. Cells in the
sebaceous glands, which contain
several lobes, produce fat droplets that
mix with cast-off cellular debris to
form sebum, a skin lubricant. The
sebaceous gland is where acne develops.*

The hair shaft has three components—an
outer cuticle, a cortex, and an inner medulla.
The cuticle is made up of tiny overlapping cells
which protect the cortex. When hair is in good
condition, the cuticle cells lie flat, reflecting
light and giving hair sheen. The cortex is the
main structural part of the hair. It is composed
of tightly packed cells aligned along the long
axis of the hair. The cells of the medulla are
loosely arranged and may even be absent.

The hair shaft is made of keratin, the same
protein present in the stratum corneum. Like
the stratum corneum, hair is dead. In the process of hair formation, the cells of the follicle
manufacture keratin, lose their nuclei, dehy-
drate, and die. The dead cells and the protein
become packed together to form hair.

Two main types of hair are found on human
skin. Terminal hairs are long, coarse, and easily seen. They are most apparent in the scalp,
beard, eyebrows, eyelashes, pubic region, and
under the arms. Most of the hairs on the arms
and legs in men are also terminal hairs. Vellus
hairs are short and fine, visible only on close
inspection. They are present on such areas as
the forehead and eyelids, and replace terminal
hairs on the male scalp when it becomes bald.
Lanugo hair refers to the fine hair that covers
the fetus and disappears in infancy.

Human hair growth is cyclical. It grows for a while, then rests. Individual hairs are pushed out and shed when a new hair begins to grow underneath in the same follicle. Scalp hair grows for an average of four years at a rate of about 15 thousandths of an inch per day. It rests for three months, falling out when the follicle produces a new hair. At any given time, 85 to 90 percent of scalp hairs are in the growing or anagen phase, and 10 to 15 percent are in the resting or telogen phase. Normally 75 to 100 telogen hairs per day are shed by the growth of pushy newcomers.

A man's beard grows in a similar cycle. In contrast, eyebrows and eyelashes grow for only about 10 weeks, then vacation for nine months. That's why it takes so long for eyebrows to reappear after they have been shaved. They grow back faster if plucked rather than shaved, because plucking stimulates follicle activity.

Whether a person is a blonde, brunette, or redhead depends on the kind and amount of pigment in the cortex of the hair shaft. Brown and black pigments (called eumelanin) and yellow and red pigments (called pheomelanin) differ in chemical structure. Hair turns gray as the amount of melanin decreases. Unlike baldness, graying occurs with equal frequency in women and men. The tendency is inherited. The silver threads characteristically appear first in the temples and later spread to the crown and back of the head. The beard and moustache often turn gray before hair on the rest of the body.

The grayness of aging cannot be slowed down or reversed, but it can be concealed by dyeing. Most permanent hair dyes used in the United States contain a chemical called paraphenylenediamine. The dye penetrates through the cuticle of the hair shaft and combines with the protein of the hair cortex. The alteration in color is permanent, and dyed hair can be shampooed without losing its color.

The protein structure and the cross-sectional shape are the same for curly and straight hair. What makes hair curl is not known, although in at least some cases, curly hair is associated with curved follicles.

Nails

Fingernails and toenails are specialized epidermal structures. The major part is the nail plate, which, like hair, is composed of the protein keratin. Nail plate is translucent;

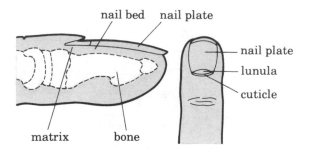

STRUCTURE OF THE NAIL

The matrix, composed of the living cells that produce the dead cells of the nail plate, extends from the end of the nail bed about five millimeters (two-tenths of an inch) beneath the cuticle. The half-moon shaped lunula, seen on most thumbnails and some other nails, is the visible portion of the matrix.

the pink color comes from the blood supply of the underlying nail bed. The small, white crescent-shaped area at the base of most thumbnails and some other nails is referred to as the lunula. This is the visible portion of the matrix, the rest of which lies under the skin behind the cuticle. The matrix is where the nail plate is synthesized. The nail plate is dead, but the cells in the matrix which make it are alive and actively dividing.

In contrast to hair, the growth of nails is continuous. Fingernails lengthen an average of four thousandths of an inch each day, which means a nail would take about eight months to grow one inch. Toenails grow one-third to one-half that fast.

VARIATIONS IN NORMAL SKIN

Moles

Moles are raised, usually discolored (pigmented) spots on the skin. They are generally small and round, and most commonly brown, although they may be black or non-pigmented. More than 95 percent of adults have at least one mole. Some people have only a few, others have hundreds. They may be apparent at birth or become visible during the first few years of life. Moles commonly enlarge from adolescence through the twenties and during pregnancy. They should be removed if they are repeatedly bumped or irritated, if they have an undesirable cosmetic appearance, or if they undergo changes that suggest malignancy.

Moles represent proliferations of nevus cells. These cells have the same developmental origin as melanocytes, the pigment-producing cells of the epidermis. Nevus cells are located in the dermis or along the epidermal-dermal junction. Like melanocytes, they usually produce melanin, giving most moles their brown color. Some nevus cells are less active in melanin production, and the moles which they form are not obviously pigmented.

In rare cases the nevus cells of moles become malignant and develop into melanoma, a form of cancer. Moles are not inherently likely to become malignant, however, and the chance that a mole will give rise to cancer is small. There are two exceptions: One is that certain rare families have an inherited tendency to develop multiple melanomas from moles at a relatively young age. The second exception is that large congenital moles (those that are present at birth) undergo malignant transformation at an unusually high rate. In general, however, most melanomas arise from melanocytes in skin that does not contain nevus cells. The individual nevus cells of a mole are no more prone to malignant change than the melanocytes elsewhere in the skin.

Freckles

Freckles are flat brown spots scattered irregularly over skin that has been exposed to sunlight. The pigment-forming cells in freckles are genetically influenced to synthesize melanin (pigment) more actively than normal after ultraviolet light exposure. The area between them does not tan, but remains a sunburned pink. Freckles are harmless, but they are warning signals to the person who has them that he or she is likely to sunburn more easily than a non-freckled person.

AGING OF THE SKIN

Aging is accompanied by changes in the appearance of the skin that reflect alterations in its structure and function. While decomposition of other organs during aging may critically impair health, aging of the skin, rather than being a serious health problem, usually has mainly cosmetic significance. The skin functions adequately longer than certain other vital organs.

As we grow old, the epidermis becomes slightly thinner. Its keratinocytes begin to vary in size and shape, and some may become so distorted that they resemble cancer cells. The rate at which the cells divide and replace themselves becomes slower, so that wounds take longer to heal. And the number of pigment-producing cells decreases. The skin tans less readily and is more easily damaged by ultraviolet light.

In young people the outer layer of skin (stratum corneum) acts as a barrier to limit the entry of water and chemicals into the epidermis. In the elderly this barrier functions less efficiently. Chemicals penetrate the epidermis more readily and make it more susceptible to damage. Furthermore, chemicals that do enter are removed more slowly by the bloodstream because of less active movement (diffusion) across an altered dermis and because of decreased blood flow.

As we age, the collagen becomes more stable, making the skin of older people more stiff and less pliable. The skin loses elasticity. When you stretch it, it does not "snap back" as rapidly as in youth.

Blood vessels break more easily and skin bruises are more common. This occurs because there is less connective tissue support from the dermis and because the vessels themselves are more fragile.

In many areas of the body, the fat layer beneath the skin decreases. The body is not as well cushioned against outside injury, nor protected against heat loss.

The changes in the dermis and in the subcutaneous tissue contribute to the furrows, deep wrinkles, and sagging of aging skin. But why we develop the fine, superficial wrinkles commonly seen in the skin is not well understood.

Another change that comes with age involves the glands of the skin. Both eccrine and apocrine sweat glands and sebaceous (oil) glands decrease in number and activity. Older people are not able to sweat proficiently and thus may not be able to tolerate hot weather well, although less sweating from apocrine glands also means less underarm odor. Dry skin and dry hair among the elderly are partially the consequences of decreased secretion of sebum, the oily substance produced by the sebaceous glands.

As we become older the skin does not function as well as a sensory organ because the nerve endings in the dermis decrease in number and conduct impulses at a slower rate.

Cosmetic Surgery

Several surgical techniques are used to improve temporarily the appearance of aged skin. Face-lifts are done to take up the slack of sagging skin around the jaws and neck. The procedure is based on the excision of skin at a site where the residual scar will not be readily visible.

During this procedure the skin is incised in the hairline and around the ear. The skin is then separated and lifted up from the underlying muscles and stretched more tautly toward the hairline. Excess skin is cut off, and the skin edges are sewn back together. The resulting scar is masked by the hair and ears.

Improvement in appearance from a face-lift lasts several years. The major complication associated with the procedure is bleeding under the skin, which requires more surgical intervention. Less commonly, part of the facial nerve is severed, although usually at a site where it is not of serious consequence. The operation is expensive—it usually costs several thousand dollars—and the cost is not covered by health insurance.

Blepharoplasty is an operation directed at removal of excessive skin and sometimes fat from the eyelids.

Chemical peels and dermabrasion are procedures used to smooth out fine wrinkles, especially those around the lips. A chemical peel consists of the application of acids to the skin. The resulting inflammation is associated with swelling that makes wrinkles less apparent. The effect is temporary, lasting several months to a year. In dermabrasion the surface of the skin is worn away by a motorized wheel with an abrasive surface. As with chemical peels, subsequent inflammation and swelling contribute to the decrease in visibility of wrinkles. Dermabrasion is also used to make acne scars less conspicuous. If the procedure is done too deeply or repeated too often, the effect can be undesirable. The skin can develop a "pasty" look, and if too much of the surface is destroyed, the skin may lose some of its elasticity and suppleness.

One important purpose of the skin is to help regulate body temperature. It does this partly through contraction and expansion of blood vessels. These reactions occur more slowly in the elderly, and heat regulation is less effective. The reduction in eccrine sweat glands and in the fat layer beneath the skin also contribute to the decrease in the skin's ability to regulate heat.

Several types of benign skin growths commonly appear with age. Among them are cherry angiomas (small, bright red, dome-shaped proliferations of capillaries) and seborrheic keratoses (superficial, warty growths tan to dark brown in color).

Hair. Beyond age 50, most men and a smaller number of women experience noticeable thinning of their scalp hair. How much the hair thins (and when) varies greatly from person to person and is in part genetically determined. Much of it occurs because of the conversion of long, thick, pigmented (terminal) hairs to short, fine, light-colored (vellus) hairs. In addition, hair follicles eventually decrease in number and become less active.

Underarm and pubic hair also become more sparse. In some older men, the hairs of the eyebrows, nostrils, and ears become coarser and longer. Pigment-producing cells in hair follicles become less active and decrease in number at a faster rate than those in the epidermis, turning the hair gray.

Nails. Fingernails and toenails grow more slowly and may develop brittleness, distortion, and ridging. Toenails, particularly, may become very thick.

Sun and aging. Premature aging refers to the appearance at a relatively young age of changes that resemble natural aging but which are caused by too much sun exposure. The appearance of wrinkles and the loss of resiliency of the skin are hastened by sun exposure over many years. Although the effects may look the same as those of natural aging, the underlying changes are different. Another important difference is that although the normal aging process cannot be stopped or slowed, damage to the skin from sun can be minimized by the regular use of sunscreens (see page 129).

SKIN CARE

The first principle of proper skin care is to do no harm. The misguided application of salves or creams, or squeezing and picking at minor pimples or blemishes, can be detrimental. Moisturizers, greasy cleansers, and oil-based cosmetics often precipitate or aggravate acne in some people. Squeezing a pimple, if not done under medical supervision, can inflame it more and even lead to scarring. Frequent, vigorous scrubbing in an attempt to rid the skin of acne can produce excessive irritation.

Certain over-the-counter medications may do more harm than good by causing a rash (allergic contact dermatitis). Notable examples are the lotions and creams that contain diphenhydramine (such as Caladryl) or benzocaine (such as Lanocaine and Solarcaine). These preparations, used to reduce stinging or itching, initially may be soothing but eventually could cause sensitization. An allergy to them should be suspected if an itchy red rash, sometimes with tiny blisters, breaks out where the substance has been applied. There is a small but significant risk that the sensitized person will then react to other medications that chemically cross-react with the original drug (diphenhydramine).

Cleansing

In today's society washing is more a social custom than a practice necessary for healthy skin. How often we should wash depends on the amount of soil and cosmetics to which we have been exposed, and how actively we perspire. Most people consider a daily bath or sponge bath appropriate, but the frequency of bathing is strictly a matter of personal choice. In general, Europeans bathe less often than Americans with no noticeable difference in health.

Water alone dissolves most dirt and adequately removes it from the skin. Oily substances such as grease and cosmetics can be removed more effectively with the help of soap. The oil particles become suspended in the suds. But soap also removes the natural oils of the skin, and regular use of standard soaps can cause excessive skin dryness in some persons. Those persons might be better advised to use special types of cleansers, such as those containing oatmeal, or lipid-free lotions. Superfatted soaps also may be less drying than regular soaps. Superfatted soaps have emollients such as lanolin and oils added. These are designated on the label.

A cold environment of low humidity enhances water loss from the skin, making it dry. Humidifiers are helpful, and bathing and use of soap should be minimized. Water can be replaced in the skin by the proper use of lubricating agents after bathing. During a bath or shower, the outer layer of skin absorbs water. A bath oil, lotion, cream, or ointment, applied immediately after bathing while the skin is still moist, will form a film that traps the water.

Alternatively, a bath oil can be added to the tub water. There are two types of bath oils. The most popular is dispersed throughout the water. The other lies on the surface of the water and coats the body as the person gets out of the tub. Either type is useful to treat dry skin.

Cosmetics for the Face

Besides soap and water or an alternative cleansing agent, what else should be put on the skin? The multimillion dollar cosmetic industry reflects the widespread hope that creams, moisturizers, hormones, vitamins, facial masks, and astringents will benefit our skin. Advertisements claim that regular use of a particular product will help preserve a youthful-looking skin. The truth is that while many of these cosmetics may temporarily improve the appearance and comfort of the skin, none of them bring about lasting change, and they do nothing to stop aging.

Overnight creams and moisturizers can make dry skin feel smoother by coating the irregular surface of a flaking outer layer (stratum corneum). If a moisturizer is applied to the face after it is exposed to water, water loss will be retarded. Moisturizers, cold creams, and other greasy cosmetics should be used sparingly or not at all, however, by persons who are acne-prone.

Astringents are intended to close pores. After their use, the skin may feel tingly and pores may appear less prominent, but only because the astringent has caused mild irritation and swelling of the adjacent skin. The effect is temporary, and no permanent decrease in pore size occurs. Astringents make the face feel cool when the alcohol they contain evaporates.

Most cosmetics will not harm the skin. Specific recommendations about products cannot be made. Choosing makeup and other cosmetics is a matter of personal preference, based on what feels and looks good to you.

Deodorants and Antiperspirants

Antiperspirants and deodorants affect sweat. An antiperspirant reduces perspiration usually through the action of an aluminum salt. A deodorant does not affect the sweating process, but reduces or masks its odor. Apocrine sweat is odorless when it emerges from the gland. Odor occurs when normal skin bacteria decompose the organic contents of the sweat. (Eccrine sweat produces minimal odor because it contains only small amounts of organic material on which bacteria can act.) Most deodorants reduce odor by means of an antibacterial ingredient. A few contain a perfume to mask a disagreeable odor with a more pleasant one. Some preparations have both a deodorant and an antiperspirant action.

Odor associated with sweating is most apparent wherever there are apocrine glands: the armpits, around the nipples and navel, and in the genital region. People are usually most concerned about underarm sweating. In recent years feminine hygiene sprays have been marketed. Not only are these unnecessary, but they can produce irritation and even an allergic reaction when applied to mucous membranes.

Because the purpose of eccrine sweating is to help maintain normal body temperature, no attempt should be made to control it except in areas where moisture creates special problems, such as on the feet, where it may lead to fungus infection (athlete's foot). The eccrine sweating associated with emotional stress, particularly on the palms, soles, and in the armpits, is troublesome if excessive. Preparations available by prescription are helpful in problem areas.

Protection from Sunlight

One of the most important aspects of skin care is to prevent sunburn and avoid chronic overexposure to the sun. Sunburn brings temporary discomfort, and if it is severe enough to cause peeling, it produces an unattractive mottled appearance. More important is that it can damage skin cells. Most of the damage can be repaired, but repeated sunburn eventually causes permanent harm.

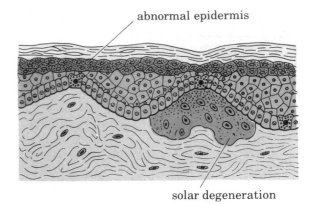

abnormal epidermis

solar degeneration

SKIN DAMAGED BY SUN

Sun-damaged skin seen under the microscope looks like this. Collagen fibers that have been chronically exposed degenerate and stain abnormally. Normal collagen stains red, but damaged fibers are replaced by blue granular material. The abnormality is called solar degeneration.

Many of the changes associated with the normal process of aging, such as wrinkling, dryness, fragility, and thinning of the skin, are accentuated by chronic sun exposure. In addition, too much sun can produce small dilations of blood vessels, a yellowish, pebbly appearance of the skin, flat or slightly raised brown blotches (senile lentigenes, commonly known as "liver spots"), and several kinds of premalignant and malignant lesions.

A look at chronically sun-exposed skin under the microscope shows striking evidence of damage to the protein fibers in the upper dermis. These changes do not occur in skin that is never exposed to the sun, such as on the buttocks.

The main defense of the skin against sun damage is melanin, the pigment that provides color. When sun strikes the skin, it induces the melanocytes to make more of this pigment. Two to three days after exposure, the melanin becomes visible as a tan. Melanin absorbs and scatters ultraviolet light, allowing less to penetrate to the lower epidermis and dermis.

The ability of melanocytes to make melanin is not the same in everyone. The melanocytes in fair-skinned people make less pigment than those in darker-skinned people. Consequently, fair skin is more susceptible to sunburn and the harmful effects of chronic sun exposure.

The importance of melanin in protecting the skin from sun damage is illustrated by a comparison of the relatively healthy-looking facial skin of an older black person with that of a fair-skinned person of the same age. The wrinkles in black skin are caused by aging. Those in fair skin are likely to be more pronounced and numerous because of the added effect of sun exposure. Besides wrinkles, the fair-skinned person may have many of the other skin changes associated with sun exposure, while the black person will have none of these. The greater pigmentation in people of the black race acts as a natural defense mechanism to limit the amount of sunlight that penetrates their skin.

It is extremely important for people who tan poorly and sunburn easily to protect themselves from ultraviolet light. They should especially avoid midday sun, when the sunburn-inducing rays reach the earth in greatest quantity. Wearing a wide-brimmed hat is helpful but not a complete solution because many harmful rays are reflected from the ground.

People who burn upon first exposure to the sun but eventually tan should expose themselves to sun gradually. Starting with a few minutes of exposure will stimulate melanin formation without causing a sunburn. As a protective tan develops, more time may be spent in the sun.

Fortunately, lotions are available that screen out the ultraviolet light rays. Effective sunscreens contain para-aminobenzoic acid (PABA), cinnamates, and benzophenones. The label usually discloses the protective factor, which is a comparison between the amount of sun required to produce redness with and without the application of the sunscreen. People who tan poorly and burn easily should select a sunscreen with a high protective factor. Almost complete protection is provided by creams containing zinc oxide or titanium oxide, but these thick white creams are cosmetically unacceptable to many people.

During the summer months it may be advisable to apply a sunscreen regularly as part of routine morning skin care, to protect against brief but frequent unplanned exposures. Sunscreens should be used in the winter as well, especially when snow covers the ground. Snow enhances sun exposure by reflecting sunlight.

Using a sunscreen slows but does not completely prevent tanning in someone who is genetically able to form melanin. Tanning is still possible because screening is incomplete against the ultraviolet light which causes sunburn and less effective against ultraviolet rays of a longer wavelength which are not as efficient but still active in stimulating melanin formation. Once a tan is present, sun damage is minimized. The light of longer wavelengths may play a supportive role in causing sunburn and chronic damage to the skin, but its effect appears to be relatively small compared to that of the main sunburn-producing spectrum.

Since the adverse effects of sun are cumulative, the use of sunscreens ideally should begin early in childhood. Regular use of a sunscreen can help prevent cosmetically unattractive sun damage, and can help prevent certain types of skin cancer.

Treatment of Sunburn

Even the most careful sunbathers sometimes get too much sun. What can be done for a sunburn once it has occurred?

The sting of a mild sunburn can be partially relieved by applying cool tap water compresses for 20 minutes several times a day. A bland lubricating cream or ointment applied afterwards is soothing, too. Sometimes doctors prescribe a topical corticosteroid, a drug that is applied to the skin to help reduce the inflammation. Most topical anesthetics aren't very effective, and those containing benzocaine can aggravate the problem by causing an allergic rash in sensitive people.

In cases of extreme overexposure to sunlight or sunlamps, it is best to contact a physician immediately, before the worst inflammation appears. If started early, a three-day course of a corticosteroid taken by mouth can almost completely prevent the occurrence of a potentially severe sunburn. An intense sunburn already developed requires continuous cool compresses, topical steroids, and lubricating agents. Aspirin or other analgesics may be necessary to relieve pain. At night, bedsheets should be supported so that they do not rest against the skin. A truly severe sunburn may be accompanied by nausea, fever, chills, and a rapid pulse. Medical attention should be sought.

HAIR CARE

The single most important principle of good hair care is to be gentle. The old ritual of brushing 100 strokes a day should be abandoned, especially by people with long hair. Excessive combing and brushing roughens and wears down the protective outer layer of cells in the cuticle, exposing the cortex. Brush as little as possible, and avoid brushes with stiff bristles. Use a comb with widely spaced, round-tipped teeth made of plastic or bone. Never use one made of metal.

Exposure to sun, wind, and chlorine in swimming pools can damage the hair, causing disulfide chemical bonds to break. (Disulfide bonds hold together the atoms of a molecule.) Blondes are more susceptible to sun damage than brunettes because their hair, like their skin, contains less protective pigment. When possible, cover your head when outdoors for extended periods.

Chemically dyeing, bleaching, curling, and straightening the hair produce minimal damage if done properly. If carried out improperly, however, they can cause significant damage. The cells of the cuticle may lose their smooth, tight-fitting alignment with one another, become ruffled, and stick out.

Shampoos

How often to shampoo depends on the oiliness of a person's scalp and whether dandruff is present. If the scalp is normal, shampoo only often enough to keep the hair looking and feeling clean. If oiliness and scaling are present, more frequent, sometimes daily, shampooing may be needed. Shampoos that contain sulfur and salicylic acid or zinc pyrithione help control mild dandruff. (For information on more severe dandruff associated with an inflamed scalp, see the section on seborrheic dermatitis, page 151.)

In recent years the shampoo industry has promoted the use of "pH-balanced" shampoos. The pH scale from 1 to 14 measures the acidity or alkalinity of a solution. A reading of 7 is neutral, below 7 is acid, and above 7 is alkaline. The pH of "pH-balanced" shampoos is usually 4 to 5, or slightly acidic. The value of "pH-balanced" shampoos has probably been overemphasized. The effect of pH on normal hair is insignificant although using a "pH-balanced" shampoo may be of some benefit for

damaged hair. An alkaline shampoo similar to a regular soap can further harm already damaged hair. In addition, a high pH tends to cause damaged hair to absorb more water, making it appear limp.

Rinses and Conditioners

Rinses applied after washing contain compounds that decrease the electrostatic charge on the surface of hairs. They minimize tangling and make combing and brushing easier, thus reducing damage to the hair.

Conditioners contain similar ingredients, as well as lubricants and protein. A lubricant is a form of oil that coats the hairs and makes them more slippery and easier to comb. Although hair is composed of protein, protein added in the form of a conditioner does not chemically combine with the hair or alter its internal structure in any way. It simply sticks to the surface of the hair shaft and temporarily fills in tiny defects. It washes off with the next shampoo.

Because a conditioner temporarily increases the diameter of the hair shaft, it gives the impression that the hair has more "body." It also tends to make split ends stick together. The main value of a conditioner is that by smoothing out rough places in the cuticle, it reduces friction and tangling between hairs so that they are less susceptible to damage during combing. Rinses and conditioners are especially helpful for long hair.

THE DOCTOR
AND SKIN PROBLEMS

The overwhelming majority of skin problems are minor and do not require professional care. But some skin disorders are troubling both physically and psychologically, and medical intervention is necessary. What can you expect from a dermatologist?

The diagnosis and treatment of skin diseases begins with a conversation. You describe the specific problem to the doctor, telling how long it has lasted, how severe it has been, what treatment you have undertaken. This history usually is followed by a visual examination and close inspection of your skin problem. The doctor will often wish to examine all of your skin, not merely the obviously affected areas.

A complete examination is important for two reasons: (1) Significant lesions, such as skin cancer, that are unrelated to your main complaint may be incidentally discovered and treated. (2) Lesions that you haven't noticed or consider insignificant may in fact be directly or indirectly related to your disease. If the physician does not see these, diagnosis and therapy will be based on incomplete information.

The techniques that are commonly used for further diagnosis of a skin problem are relatively simple. The scale, cellular debris, and seepage from certain eruptions frequently are examined under the microscope. Cultures may be taken. In the case of parasitic infestation, microscopic examination can identify the parasite.

In certain cases, a skin biopsy may be done. This consists of surgically removing a small specimen of skin, most often less than two-tenths of an inch (four millimeters) in diameter. Although not always required, a suture may be used to close the biopsy site. The specimen is then prepared by a laboratory for examination, a process requiring several days.

A useful procedure in the case of suspected allergies to external chemicals is the application of patch tests. The chemicals in question are applied to the skin under tape and left in place for two days. They are then removed and the reactions observed.

Treatment

Once a skin disorder has been diagnosed, treatment will be instituted. Although medication may be given as an injection or as pills, the skin is uniquely accessible for the administration of drugs by direct application. Often surface application works best with the least risk of side effects.

It is important to remember that most medications applied to the skin, whether lotion, cream, ointment, or paste, contain substances that change the function of body cells. Some of them, notably steroids, can be absorbed into the bloodstream. Therefore, they should be used only as prescribed. Application to areas for which they were not intended can cause undesirable and sometimes dangerous side effects. They should not be used for subsequent problems which may have a different cause. Never give them to friends with skin problems that appear similar to your own.

DISEASES OF THE SKIN

Acne Vulgaris

Acne is so common that it affects almost everyone at some time. Outbreaks range from an occasional blackhead or pimple to a festering and scarring process that is long-lasting and emotionally crippling. Although acne flourishes in adolescence and usually diminishes by the late 20s, it can begin late and persist into middle age.

Causes. The acne lesion originates in the sebaceous follicle. In this type of hair follicle, the sebaceous glands are large and have many lobes, while the hair is tiny and inconspicuous. Sebum, the oily substance produced in the follicle, empties into the canal through short ducts from the sebaceous gland. The lining of the follicle has an outer layer of horny cells like the stratum corneum of the visible skin. But these cells are fragile and do not stay together to form a compact layer. Instead, they remain loose within the canal of the follicle. An additional occupant of the canal is a type of bacteria called *Propionibacterium (Corynebacterium) acnes*. The white, cheesy material that can be squeezed out of sebaceous follicles is composed of sebum, keratin (sloughed horny material), and bacteria.

Normally the contents of the follicular canal pass unimpeded to the opening of the follicle and are deposited unnoticed on the skin surface. In acne, for unknown reasons, the horny cells stick together in a solid mass that gradually expands to become what is known as a comedo. The comedo (the plural is comedones) is the primary lesion of acne. At first, it is too small to be seen. Later it enlarges into a visible whitehead. In medical terms, this is known as a closed comedo. Its pore is so tiny that it cannot be seen with the naked eye. Still later, the horny material may expand and dilate the opening of the sebaceous follicle. Now it becomes an open comedo, or blackhead. The dark color is caused by the presence of melanin in the horny cells. Sometimes, rather than becoming a blackhead, the closed comedo may break through the thin walls of the follicular canal and start an inflammation that appears as a pimple (a pustule or red papule). Most pimples probably form from closed comedones too small to be seen except with a microscope.

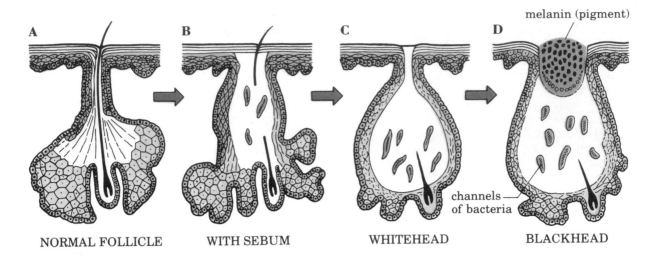

A NORMAL FOLLICLE   **B** WITH SEBUM   **C** WHITEHEAD   **D** BLACKHEAD

melanin (pigment)

channels of bacteria

THE BEGINNING OF ACNE

These four illustrations show the evolution of a comedo, which is the beginning of acne. A normal sebaceous follicle (left) has large, multi-globulated glands and a tiny hair. In drawing B its canal is becoming distended, filling with sebum, horny material, and bacteria.

The closed comedo, or whitehead, in C has a microscopic pore. In D, expansion of the contents has dilated the opening and produced an open comedo, or blackhead. The dark color comes from melanin, pigment made by cells of the upper portion of the follicle.

The usual location of acne on the skin corresponds to the distribution of sebaceous follicles. These are located mainly on the face, chest, upper back, and shoulders.

Why acne affects one person mildly and another severely is not entirely known. Acne has no single cause, but several prerequisites can be identified.

When a boy or girl reaches puberty, changes occur in the sebaceous glands that set the stage for the development of acne. In both sexes the blood level of male hormones (androgens) rises, and the sebaceous glands respond by increasing in size and producing more sebum. Eunuchs (males who have been castrated) do not get acne. But except in rare cases, in which there is overproduction of androgens caused by tumors or enlargement of the adrenals, ovaries, or testes, acne is not caused by hormone "imbalance" in the blood. Normal levels of androgens are enough to play a role in the development of acne in susceptible persons.

Many female patients experience a worsening of acne before a menstrual period. Progesterone, a hormone secreted after ovulation, may in some way influence premenstrual acne, but its exact role is not known.

Bacteria are important in the development of acne. They do not produce a true infection but act indirectly, possibly by altering the sebum or by producing a substance that makes the follicular wall rupture more easily. The role of bacteria is controversial and the subject of investigation. The best evidence of their importance is that certain antibiotics which reduce the acne bacteria also improve the disease.

In addition to the usual type of acne, acne-like lesions can be induced by taking certain drugs. These include medicines that contain iodines and bromides, anti-convulsants, corticosteroids, and a drug active against tuberculosis. Certain industrial chemicals, including chlorinated hydrocarbons, cutting oils, petroleum oil, and coal tar can cause a severe type of acne.

Cleansing. Persons with acne often feel unclean because of the excessive oiliness of their skin. They often wash more frequently than others, hoping that vigorous scrubbing will eventually rid them of the unpleasant-looking lesions. In fact, compulsive washing can be more harmful than beneficial. Certain types of soap, when used excessively, allow comedones to form more easily.

People with acne should wash as often as they feel comfortable, generally once or twice a day. Some soaps made for acne contain abrasive or peeling agents meant to help unseat

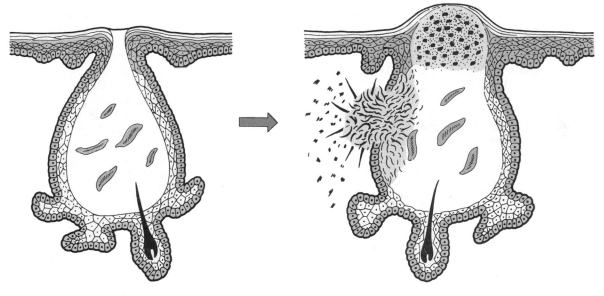

PIMPLE FORMATION

An inflamed pimple occurs when contents of a whitehead, or closed comedo, rupture through the wall of the hair follicle into the dermis. The result is an inflammatory reaction, *seen as a red papule or pustule. If a large portion of the follicle wall is destroyed and swelling is great, a nodule or cyst may form.*

comedones. Most comedones are not so easily removed, however. Soaps cannot reach down into the follicles where the acne process begins, so they do little to prevent the lesions from forming. Abrasive soaps have an irritant effect. They peel the skin surface and make it red by increasing blood flow. In this way they may speed up the clearing of inflammatory lesions.

Cosmetics. Many women unknowingly precipitate acne or make it worse by the use of cosmetics. Any product for the face that contains oil can make acne worse, presumably by aiding in the formation of comedones. These include foundation lotions or creams, greasy cleansers, moisturizers, and night creams. Unfortunately, some cosmetics labeled as "oil-free" do in fact contain oil. Checking the list of ingredients is a more reliable guide to contents. Women often prefer makeup containing oil because it spreads onto the skin more easily and gives a smoother look. The acne-prone woman, however, should avoid oily makeup. If she uses cosmetics at all, she should substitute those with water or other non-oily solvents as a base. Sunscreens, too, should be chosen carefully. Those containing alcohol are better than oily lotions or creams.

Diet. In the past acne patients were admonished against eating chocolate, potato chips, soft drinks, nuts, and "junk foods," which are particularly popular with adolescents. Studies now have shown that diet has little influence on acne. Some acne victims still feel that certain foods sometimes precipitate an outbreak. More likely, the lesion already was being formed when the suspect food was eaten, and the timing was coincidental. Of course, any person who is convinced that he or she breaks out after eating particular foods will feel better avoiding them. In general, the best diet advice for acne patients is to eat a sensible, well-balanced diet.

Emotions. A combination of not enough sleep, psychological tension, and poor diet can adversely affect any disease, including acne. Most people react to acne with some type of emotion, ranging from mild self-consciousness to intense anxiety, depression, and sometimes anger and guilt. These emotional states can in turn aggravate acne, although exactly how they do so is not known.

Mechanical factors. A common observation is that external pressures from articles such as backpacks, head bands, football pads, wide belts, and hockey face guards aggravate acne where they rub. But the friction may not always be so obvious. Some people unconsciously but habitually rest chin or cheek on hand while sitting at a desk or watching television. A person should try to be aware of and avoid any such mechanical stress that can intensify acne.

Treatment. Whether an acne lesion leaves a scar depends on the degree of inflammation. Deep, inflamed cysts are likely to scar. Picking and gouging with the fingernails can make scarring worse. Scars occur because during the healing process the acne lesion is replaced by fibrous tissue that is firmer and more depressed than the surrounding skin. Initially the depressions are red in white people and dark brown in black people. In time, they lighten in color and become less noticeable.

Treatment decreases both the number of active lesions and the severity of inflammation so that the risk of scarring is reduced. Removing scars requires specialized skills and is not always possible or satisfactory. It is much better to prevent scars from forming by treating the acne.

Therapy for acne, determined by the severity of the disease and the types of lesions, falls into two categories: medicines applied to the skin (topical) and medicines taken by mouth (systemic).

Topical medications. Many topical preparations for acne can be bought over the counter (without a prescription). Most contain sulfur, resorcinol, salicylic acid, or benzoyl peroxide, and act by superficially peeling the skin and enhancing blood flow. Increased blood flow helps a pimple heal sooner because products of inflammation are removed faster. Application of carbon dioxide slush and liquid nitrogen works in the same manner.

Two of the most useful preparations applied to the skin are retinoic acid (tretinoin) and benzoyl peroxide. Retinoic acid, available only by prescription, is particularly active against the blackheads and whiteheads of acne. It helps expel existing comedones and interferes with formation of new ones. Because acne pustules and papules are believed to originate from comedones, retinoic acid is used to treat inflammatory acne as well.

Retinoic acid has several possible side effects, however. Initial use may produce redness and scaling. This reaction varies from one person to another, but tends to be more severe in fair-skinned people. The reaction also depends partly on the type and strength of retinoic acid, which is available in different concentrations and as a cream, gel, or solution. In most people the redness subsides after a few weeks of use. Black-skinned people tolerate the preparation well but should be careful not to use so much that it produces excessive irritation. The inflammation may be followed by darkening that persists for a long time.

Skin treated with retinoic acid is more sensitive to sunburn, so users should be cautious in their exposure to sunlight.

Some patients experience a temporary worsening of their acne, even developing new pustules, during the first month of therapy with retinoic acid. The pustules are believed to result from rupture of the walls of follicles which contain minuscule comedones. These lesions usually clear up rapidly, and overall improvement then becomes apparent.

Benzoyl peroxide, usually in concentrations of 5 or 10 percent, is marketed under several different brand names. Some require a prescription. The action of benzoyl peroxide is three-fold: (1) it expels comedones; (2) it induces peeling and stimulates blood flow; (3) it suppresses the growth of bacteria.

Several different antibiotics have been incorporated into solutions that can be applied directly to the skin. These include tetracycline, erythromycin, and clindamycin. Since antibiotics applied to the skin are not significantly absorbed into the circulation, the risk of side effects is minimized. Currently, however, they are less effective than antibiotics taken by mouth, although research eventually may improve them. They are useful when oral antibiotics aren't well tolerated or are not recommended, such as during pregnancy or in certain cases of allergy, and they may be the best treatment for some cases of mild acne. At the other end of the spectrum, patients with severe acne, not adequately controlled by oral antibiotics and other preparations, may benefit by the addition of an antibiotic applied to the skin.

Systemic medications. Severe cases of acne characterized by inflammatory pimples, cysts, and nodules seldom respond satisfactorily to topical medications alone. Antibiotics taken by mouth are then the mainstay of therapy. Improvement is often dramatic, although six weeks to several months of therapy may be required before results can be noticed. Antibiotics reduce the population of the acne-associated bacteria.

Tetracycline is the antibiotic most physicians choose in treating acne, although several others may be used as alternatives. Tetracycline is usually effective, the incidence of side effects is low, and it is relatively inexpensive. To insure adequate absorption, it must be taken on an empty stomach (30 minutes before or two hours after eating). The starting dose varies according to the severity of acne. An average initial dose is one gram per day (usually given as two capsules twice daily), but in severe cases the amount may be higher. After several weeks to months, the dose can usually be reduced, but continuous low-dose therapy over several years is often necessary. Once the acne is brought under control, the objective is maintenance on the lowest effective dose of antibiotic.

Fortunately, taking tetracycline for a long time apparently causes few problems. A small percentage of people develop mild nausea, especially after the first dose in the morning. In rare cases the nausea is bothersome enough that the person cannot tolerate the drug, and alternative therapy must be found.

For women the most common side effect is a yeast infection of the vagina, called monilia or candida vaginitis (see chapter 22, "The Kidneys and Urinary System"). The symptoms are vaginal itching and a whitish discharge. Tetracycline predisposes to this type of infection by suppressing the bacteria that normally live in the vagina, allowing the yeast organisms to flourish. This problem is more common in women who take birth control pills. It is easily treated.

Pregnant women should not take tetracycline. It causes discoloration of developing teeth in the fetus.

Oral contraceptive pills. Some women with severe acne unresponsive to other measures may benefit from estrogen, most easily taken as a birth control pill. Estrogens improve acne by decreasing the size of the sebaceous glands and by reducing sebum production. An oral contraceptive that contains sufficient estrogen must be chosen. At first, new inflammatory lesions may break out, and improvement may not be apparent for two or more months. The effect on sebum production may last only a year or so under continuous therapy. Therefore, birth control pills for acne should be taken for limited periods. Of course, oral contraceptives, especially those containing a high dose of estrogen, are associated with side effects. The patient and her physician should weigh these risks against the potential benefits.

Certain birth control pills should be avoided because they can worsen acne. Most notable are those containing norgestrel, a synthetic hormone with mild androgenic effects.

Acne temporarily worsens in some women when they discontinue the birth control pill. A woman may even develop acne for the first time when she stops taking the pill. The cause of this "rebound" is unknown, but the body seems to perceive stopping the pill as a relative lack of estrogen.

Ultraviolet light. Many people notice that their acne improves in the summer under the sun. One reason is that sun increases blood flow and inflammatory lesions clear faster. A suntan also partially masks lesions so that they aren't as easily seen. And some of the improvement may stem from the relaxation that usually occurs with sunbathing and summer vacations.

It is unlikely that sunshine's ultraviolet rays change the basic process of acne. Probably, benefits come from accelerated clearing of existing acne rather than prevention of new outbreaks. Since we know that ultraviolet light helps bring on the changes of aging and predisposes to skin cancer, it is wise to use moderation in exposure to sunlight and sunlamps.

Acne does not always improve with sun exposure. In some people it gets worse. Women, especially, may develop acne in the summertime, predominantly on the chest, shoulders, and upper arms. The reason for these summer outbreaks is not understood, but increased sweating may play a role.

X rays. X rays improve acne by shrinking the sebaceous glands. They were more commonly used in the past before their potential harmful effects were fully appreciated. Some experienced physicians still occasionally administer restricted doses of X rays in stubborn acne cases. Improvement is temporary, however, and only a limited amount of radiation is safe.

Cosmetic surgery. The appearance of acne scars sometimes can be improved by surgical removal and replacement with a less noticeable scar. Sometimes a small graft of normal skin is taken from behind the ear, or a depressed scar is made more level with the surrounding skin by injecting silicone or a substance called fibrin foam. Chemical peeling agents also can be helpful, at least temporarily. Certain procedures often can flatten elevated scars. Inflamed cysts can be reduced in size quickly by the injection of drugs called corticosteroids, but sometimes the cysts recur.

Dermabrasion is a procedure that planes the scarred skin with a rapidly rotating brush. Improvement of shallow pitted scars can be achieved in carefully selected cases. The procedure usually is restricted to the face.

Rosacea

Acne rosacea, sometimes simply called rosacea, resembles acne vulgaris. Both are characterized by small red papules and pustules on the face. There are important differences, however. Patients with rosacea are typically older—usually at least 35—than patients with common acne. Redness and dilated blood vessels of the nose and central face are characteristic of rosacea. The nose may become enlarged, a condition known as rhinophyma and sometimes called the W. C. Fields nose. Affected individuals should avoid alcohol, caffeine-containing beverages, and spicy foods. These normally stimulate the blood vessels of the skin to dilate, but in rosacea patients even small amounts cause an exaggerated blushing response, leading to permanent redness and dilated blood vessels. Rosacea usually responds to tetracycline treatment.

Eczema

Eczema, sometimes referred to as dermatitis, is not a specific disease but an inflammatory reaction to a variety of stimuli from both inside and outside the body. Eczema can be acute or chronic. In acute eczema, the skin is red, swollen, and often blistered and weeping. Chronic eczema is characterized by scaly, thickened, red or brownish-red skin in which the skin markings are accentuated. In both types, the chief symptom is intense itching.

There are many causes of eczema. Common types include atopic dermatitis, contact dermatitis, dyshidrotic eczema, stasis dermatitis, and lichen simplex chronicus.

Atopic dermatitis usually runs in families, and may be associated with allergies, hay fever, and asthma. When most people use the term eczema, they usually are referring to this disease.

Atopic dermatitis can appear and disappear at any age, but a common pattern is for peaks of activity during infancy, childhood, and early adulthood. Infantile eczema, often beginning about three or four months of age, appears on the scalp, cheeks, and neck, with scattered patches elsewhere. By age two, the rash usually becomes less severe or even disappears. It may recur during childhood from age four to ten, tending to localize in places where the skin flexes—the neck, behind the ears, in front of the elbows, or behind the knees. During adolescence and young adulthood this pattern may become more pronounced.

Atopic dermatitis frequently disappears by age 30, but in some patients the disease remains chronic, sometimes continuing to be widespread, at other times concentrating in a specific area, including the hands and feet.

The skin of a person with atopic dermatitis itches easily, even under normal circumstances. Itching leads to scratching, which is responsible for most of the visible changes in the skin. Itching may be triggered by emotional tension, exercise, extremes of humidity and temperature, friction, or by contact with soap, wool, or other substances. Foods are not thought to be very important in precipitating eczema, although some patients claim to notice a relationship. In rare instances pollens, house dust, or animal dander, through inhalation or contact, aggravate the dermatitis.

A person with atopic dermatitis often develops other medical problems. Breaks in the skin resulting from blisters or scratching can be invaded by bacteria, causing infection. Patients with atopic dermatitis who have cold sores are unusually susceptible to the spread of the cold-sore virus over their skin, a serious illness requiring hospitalization.

The development in the 1950s of corticosteroid drugs that could be applied to the skin revolutionized the treatment of atopic dermatitis, as well as many other skin diseases. Application to the skin of properly selected corticosteroids is the cornerstone of therapy for this disease. The frequent use of moisturizing creams plus antihistamine drugs taken by mouth helps to alleviate itching. Sometimes a change of environment helps.

Contact dermatitis can be either irritant or allergic. Irritant contact dermatitis can occur in anyone who is sufficiently exposed to harsh chemicals. It is caused by direct injury of the skin by contact with the irritant. Allergic contact dermatitis, on the other hand, occurs only in persons who have developed a specific allergy to the responsible substance.

Substances differ in their capacity to cause sensitization and the development of allergic contact dermatitis. Poison ivy, oak, and sumac, which make up a category of plants called *Rhus,* are such potent allergens that in the United States rhus dermatitis is probably responsible for more cases of allergic contact dermatitis than all other substances combined (see below). Other relatively common allergens are nickel (found in jewelry), rubber compounds, paraphenylenediamine (an ingredient in dyes), and chemicals contained in medications (ethylenediamine, neomycin, diphenhydramine, and benzocaine).

Often the source of the allergy is obvious. The pattern of the rash may precisely fit the outline of a particular article of clothing, such as bathing trunks or shoes. It then becomes important to pinpoint the allergy to a specific substance in the garment so that contact with it in other forms can be avoided. Patch testing, done by placing the suspect chemicals under tapes and leaving them in contact with the skin for 48 hours, often helps to identify the responsible allergen.

In other instances, the cause of an allergic contact dermatitis may be difficult to discover. It should be remembered that one or two days usually elapse between the time of contact with an allergen and the appearance of a rash. Considerable detective work may be needed to uncover the offender. An essential step is learning what chemicals are contained in the article of clothing, cosmetic, or other contact thought to be responsible for the rash. It may even be necessary to write the manufacturer to learn the materials used. Fortunately, in the case of cosmetics, federal law now requires that the ingredients be listed on the label.

Cosmetic dermatitis. Often the person who develops an allergic contact dermatitis from a cosmetic is able to determine which one is responsible, especially if the number of cosmetics used has been small. But a person may use the same product for many years without difficulty, then suddenly become hypersensitive to one of its chemicals. Or one or more ingredients may have been changed recently by the manufacturer without the user's being aware of it. Hypoallergenic preparations decrease but do not eliminate the possibility of developing an allergy. Remember that possible culprits also include tweezers and eyelash curlers, and small sponges used to apply rouge or eye shadow, especially if they contain rubber.

The principal site of reaction to a cosmetic does not always coincide with the place where it is applied. Allergy to nail polish, for instance, often appears mainly on the upper eyelids. This is because the skin around the nails is relatively tough and resistant to contact dermatitis compared to the skin of the eyelids, which are often touched unconsciously. Hypersensitivity to shampoo and other products for the hair usually appears primarily on the eyelids, forehead, ears, and neck rather than on the scalp.

Perfumes contained in other cosmetics or used alone are also potential offenders. They can cause not only the usual type of allergic contact dermatitis but also a photo-contact reaction, which is one brought out by exposing the affected area to the sun. The photodermatitis appears as a dark spot with sharply outlined borders corresponding to areas exposed to sunlight. The pigmentation gradually fades within several months.

The first step in dealing with cosmetic dermatitis is to eliminate all cosmetics. Wash the face and shampoo the hair with an unscented soap, and remove all nail products. If the dermatitis subsides promptly, it can be assumed that one of the cosmetics eliminated was responsible. The cosmetics can then be reintroduced one at a time. If a rash recurs, take note of which cosmetic was last used. A reaction to that particular cosmetic can often be confirmed by performing what is called a "usage test." Apply the suspect agent to the skin on the inside of the forearm three times a day for two days and observe the area for redness.

Poison ivy dermatitis. The "poison" in poison ivy, oak, and sumac is an oily substance called urushiol, found in the sap of plants of the *Rhus* family. In the United States urushiol produces an allergic contact dermatitis in about seven out of ten persons exposed to it, and the percentage would probably be higher if more were exposed for longer periods. Some persons are more susceptible than others, but only a very few appear to be completely immune. The first exposure to the plant causes no reaction, which is why many persons falsely believe they are not allergic to it. The initial contact sensitizes the person, however, and another encounter two to three weeks later can produce the characteristic rhus eruption—an acute, red, blistering, oozing, intensely itchy rash in areas the plant has touched. The outbreak often occurs in streaks where branches have brushed across the skin. The rash is spread to other parts of the body by direct transfer of the

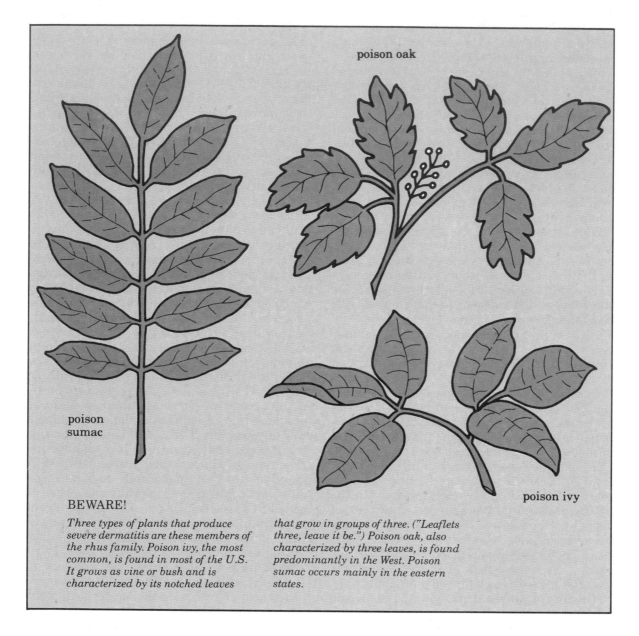

poison oak

poison sumac

poison ivy

BEWARE!

Three types of plants that produce severe dermatitis are these members of the rhus family. Poison ivy, the most common, is found in most of the U.S. It grows as vine or bush and is characterized by its notched leaves that grow in groups of three. ("Leaflets three, leave it be.") Poison oak, also characterized by three leaves, is found predominantly in the West. Poison sumac occurs mainly in the eastern states.

oily substance, usually by the fingers during scratching. The fluid that oozes from the blisters does not cause an allergy, is not contagious, and cannot spread the rash to other areas or to other people.

Sometimes an area of the skin that seemed unaffected at first will erupt later. There are several possible explanations. Different parts of the body vary in the length of exposure to the offending plant. Those with the longest contact usually break out first. Not all skin is equally susceptible. The thick skin of the palms and soles resists penetration by urushiol oil better than the thin skin of the eyelids. The eyelids may redden and swell before the palms develop a rash, even though the hands had more direct and prolonged contact and indeed may have transferred the oil to the eyelids.

Another possible explanation for a delayed reaction is re-exposure by contact with clothing or pets exposed to the plant. A less common source is exposure to oil-bearing smoke from burning plants. The urushiol oil is persistent, and persons have been known to suffer outbreaks in the dead of winter from clothing exposed in the fall.

Obviously, the best "cure" for this sort of dermatitis is prevention. Gardeners, golfers, campers, and other lovers of the outdoors should learn to recognize the offending plants. Poison ivy and poison oak can be identified by their notched leaflets that grow in clusters of three (see above). The poison ivy plant is found throughout the United States except for the extreme southwest. Poison oak is more prevalent on the Pacific coast. Both may appear as either a vine or bush and turn up in backyards as well as deep woods. The poison sumac plant has seven to thirteen leaflets arranged as pairs along a central rib with a single leaflet at the end. It grows in swampy areas throughout the United States.

If exposure to poison ivy or oak is suspected, the skin should be washed promptly with soap and water to remove the plant oils before damage can be done. If a rash develops, the application of cool wet compresses followed by a lotion such as calamine feels soothing and helps dry up the blisters. Antihistamine pills help relieve itching. Be cautious about buying over-the-counter medications to apply to the skin because many contain agents which can make the rash worse by causing their own allergic reaction. Look at the label before buying and especially avoid those that contain diphenhydramine and benzocaine.

If the outbreak is widespread or attacks the face around the eyes, see a physician. Corticosteroids taken by mouth or injection can bring dramatic relief. There may be side effects, however, so corticosteroids are not prescribed in all cases.

For outdoor workers and others who cannot avoid the plants because of their occupation, hyposensitization is a possibility. This means taking daily a small but increasing amount of an extract from the plant to build up tolerance for it. The technique takes several months and is not always successful. It is generally felt to be of limited value.

Hand eczema is usually a contact dermatitis of the irritant type. Less commonly, allergies play a role.

Anyone whose hands are habitually exposed to household or occupational irritants or sensitizers may develop hand eczema. Housewives commonly acquire contact dermatitis caused by soaps, detergents, bleaches, and household cleansers. Bartenders, surgeons, dental hygienists, dentists, and kitchen workers are similarly exposed. The problem usually begins with mild dryness, redness, and scaling, and progresses to fissuring and crusting. Sometimes the fissures become infected. Cold, dry weather can precipitate or aggravate the dermatitis.

Protecting the hands from irritating substances is the basic therapeutic approach. Using long-handled brushes for dishwashing helps decrease contact with soap and water. Cotton gloves dusted with talcum powder should be worn under rubber gloves when exposure to soap and chemicals can't be avoided.

Powdered cotton gloves help absorb perspiration. They also protect the hands from direct contact with rubber, to which some people are allergic. To prevent excessive warmth and sweating, the gloves should not be worn for more than a half-hour. Dishes should be soaked in hot soapy suds for 30 minutes and the water allowed to cool before the gloved hands are immersed.

When bathing infants, wear a pair of cotton gloves *over* the rubber gloves as well as under them so that the baby can be handled without danger of slipping.

When doing dusty or dirty housework, wear cotton gloves. If the fingertips are free of eczema, the tips of the gloves can be cut off to allow air to circulate about the hands to prevent excessive heat and sweating.

Handling certain foods also can irritate inflamed skin. They include raw meats, fruits, especially tomatoes and citrus fruit, and vegetables, particularly onions and garlic. Contact with wool causes itching and irritation for many people.

Coating the hands with a cream helps protect against irritations. Soap and water remove the natural oils, so washing should be minimized. Some persons find it helpful to substitute a superfatted, mild soap or lipid-free cleanser for regular soap because they remove less oil. The best time to apply a hand cream is immediately after washing to replenish oil and to seal in the water absorbed by the stratum corneum. The creams should be kept near the kitchen and bathroom sinks to encourage frequent, habitual use.

For anyone prone to hand eczema, general care of the hands is just as important as medication. When the hands are acutely inflamed, your physician can prescribe a corticosteroid, tar, or other preparation to apply to the skin.

Dyshidrotic eczema. The term dyshidrosis implies that this dermatitis results from faulty sweating, for which there is no convincing evidence. Many affected people do, however, notice excessive sweating of their palms and soles. The cause of dyshidrotic eczema is unknown, but in some people emotional stress triggers it.

Dyshidrotic eczema is characterized by blisters on the palms and soles and between the fingers and toes. There is usually less redness between the blisters than in other types of eczema. The blisters usually spontaneously heal after scales appear in about three weeks. In severe cases painful cracks in the skin occur during this phase. Dyshidrotic eczema tends to be recurrent and chronic. Treatment is similar to that for other types of eczema, but the recurrent nature of the problem can be discouraging.

Stasis dermatitis. Eczema caused by malfunctioning valves of the leg veins is called stasis dermatitis. Often varicose veins are present or there is a history of thrombophlebitis, an inflamed vein containing a blood clot (see chapter 5, "Blood Vessel Disorders"). Blood in the legs is not returned to the heart in the normal fashion, but remains in the veins longer. Gravity causes fluid to move from the veins into the soft tissues of the legs, a condition known as stasis edema.

The skin responds by breaking out in ezcema. The condition can occur anywhere on the lower legs, but most commonly affects the inside of the ankles. The skin becomes itchy, thickened, and darkly pigmented. If the edema is not treated, ulcers may occur.

An essential part of therapy is bedrest with the leg elevated. Wearing support hose is helpful. Prescription medications, including corticosteroids, ease the inflammation, but the problem is likely to recur. Surgical correction of the underlying blood vessel problem may be necessary.

Lichen simplex chronicus. In this disease the itch comes first, and the subsequent scratching eventually produces eczema. Common locations are the ankles, wrists, and back of the neck, where chronic scratching produces lichenification (thickening) and darkening of the skin until it assumes a leathery consistency. Repeated scratching also may enlarge the nerves so that the skin itches more easily, and a vicious itch-scratch cycle is set up. Sometimes the scratching is done unconsciously.

Therapy is aimed at controlling the itch with pills, creams, or ointments, and sometimes local injections of corticosteroids. Once the affected person recognizes that scratching is responsible for the eczema, he often is able to control the scratching impulse.

Psoriasis

The true incidence of psoriasis is unknown, but the disease is estimated to strike one to two percent of all Americans.

Psoriasis occurs because affected skin cells are proliferating too fast. There are too many epidermal cells, and they don't have time to reach full maturity. Psoriatic lesions thus consist of a piling-up of immature cells. The lesions are usually red because the small blood vessels in affected areas are dilated.

The basic cause of the abnormal cell proliferation has not been identified. Genetics apparently plays a role. Although the majority of affected people do not notice any precipitating events, injury to the skin, emotional stress, heavy drinking, or streptococcal throat infections all can bring on or aggravate psoriasis.

A small percentage of patients have an associated arthritis, but the disease only rarely affects the general health. To most psoriasis sufferers, the unsightly skin lesions are a greater burden. They appear as thickened red areas covered by white scale. Although usually there is no discomfort, in some cases the lesions may itch or develop painful fissures. Diseased skin may be confined to the knees and elbows or may cover the entire body. The scalp is often affected, and the scale there may be loose or thick and adherent. Fingernail changes range from mild pitting to severe thickening and deformity. When a person first develops psoriasis, which may be at any time from infancy to old age, there is no reliable way to predict the course the disease will follow.

Sunlight usually has a beneficial effect on psoriatic skin. Most patients spontaneously improve in the summer and get worse during the winter. Further evidence of the sun's benefit is that the face usually is mostly clear, even though there may be extensive psoriasis underneath clothing.

Ultraviolet light exposure is the cornerstore of several treatment regimens for psoriasis. If the disease is widespread, therapy is often carried out best in a hospital or day-care center. One of the oldest treatments, the Goeckerman regimen, is very effective. Coal tar is applied to the affected areas, which are then exposed to artificial ultraviolet light. Patients usually have completely clear skin after three weeks of daily therapy. Once the disease is brought under control, a patient is usually able to manage the disease effectively at home for several to many months. The disadvantage of the Goeckerman treatment is that it is messy and time-consuming. Relapses almost inevitably occur, as with all other forms of psoriasis therapy.

Psoriasis is one disease for which the sun's immediate benefits probably outweigh the long-term potential harm. A person with extensive psoriasis may want to purchase an ultraviolet lamp for home use. Or, for more efficient exposure, he may choose to construct, with the help of an electrician, a walk-in box lined with four-foot fluorescent sunlamps. Use of ultraviolet light at home should be done cautiously and under the guidance of medical personnel. Protective goggles and strict timing of exposures are essential.

Topical corticosteroid medications are widely used to treat psoriasis. A multitude of them are available by prescription. They must be used strictly according to instructions, because they can damage skin if overused or applied to the wrong areas.

Psoriasis of the scalp, when severe, can be a discouraging problem because effective treatment is time-consuming and demands patience and diligence. Once a person understands how to treat scalp psoriasis properly and realizes that it can be helped, he or she usually is sufficiently motivated to keep the condition under control. Treatment consists of removing the scale by applying preparations called keratolytics (often most effective when used under a plastic shower cap), frequent shampooing, and sometimes the application of corticosteroid lotions. Several types of shampoos are helpful, including those containing tars. Persons with light colored hair may prefer non-tar shampoos because tar can discolor their hair.

For severe psoriasis, drugs called antimetabolites may be given. These drugs, also used to treat cancer, prevent the excessive proliferation of the epidermal cells by interfering with cell division. Unfortunately their effect is not limited to the skin. They also affect the metabolism of cells in other organs, such as the bone marrow and gastrointestinal tract. Antimetabolites are therefore potentially dangerous. They must be given in carefully determined doses under close medical supervision. Methotrexate is the most commonly prescribed antimetabolite for psoriasis.

In 1974 a psoriasis treatment known as PUVA was developed. It consists of swallowing a drug called psoralen followed two hours later by exposure to long-wave ultraviolet light (UV-A). The ultraviolet treatments are done in a specially designed cabinet in a doctor's office. After the psoralen reaches the skin, in the presence of ultraviolet light, it becomes photo-activated. It binds with DNA, the large molecule in the nucleus of the cell involved in cell division. In this way the psoralen inhibits DNA synthesis and the reproduction of epidermal cells.

Most dermatologists reserve PUVA treatments for patients who have not responded to the traditional methods, or for older persons with extensive disease who might have difficulty with topical treatment and in whom the benefits outweigh the long-term risk of developing skin cancer, which the treatments appear to increase.

All the treatments for psoriasis help control the disease, but none of them cures it. The distinction is important. A cure in the strict sense means that treatment for a specified time eliminates the disease, and the disease does not recur once treatment is stopped. This is not the case with psoriasis. Even with treatment, psoriasis remains a chronic disease that tends to wax and wane. The type and intensity of treatment must be adjusted to fit its spontaneous course. Accepting the long-term nature of psoriasis is the first step toward effectively dealing with it.

Skin Cancer

Skin cancers are the most common malignant tumors. A recent study estimates there are more than 300,000 new cases a year, nearly three times as many as the most prevalent cancers of other organs. But in contrast to other cancers, skin cancers are readily seen and detected, and thus can be treated promptly.

The two most common types of skin cancer are called basal-cell carcinoma and squamous-cell carcinoma. They account for 29 out of 30 cases of skin cancer, but they are usually discovered while still localized and rarely lead to death. Malignant melanoma, the rarest form, is always potentially fatal unless detected early and treated promptly. In that case complete cure is often possible.

Chronic sun exposure increases the risk of developing the basal-cell and squamous-cell forms of cancer. Persons most susceptible are those who sunburn easily and tan poorly, such as those of Irish, Scottish, or Welsh background, and persons who work outdoors and receive prolonged sun exposure over many years, such as farmers and sailors. Persons who have dark skin or who keep well covered have a lower incidence of skin cancer.

Experimental studies in animals have shown that the wavelengths mainly responsible for skin cancer are the same ones that cause sunburn (UV-B), although long-wave ultraviolet light (UV-A) also may be involved. When melanin (pigment) is not present, ultraviolet light penetrates the cells and injures several components, including DNA.

Usually the DNA damage is repaired, but if it is great enough, the repair mechanisms become overwhelmed and a skin cancer forms.

Although sun exposure is the major cause of these skin cancers, there are several other factors that can make someone susceptible to them. Certain inherited conditions carry the tendency to develop these tumors. X-ray therapy, given in the past for acne and thought to be safe, has been followed years later by the appearance of multiple skin cancers. Exposure to arsenic, formerly used in certain medicines and in agricultural insecticides, increases the likelihood of skin cancer.

Sun exposure also plays some role in the formation of malignant melanomas. The trend toward more leisure time and travel to sunny vacation spots is believed to explain at least partially the increasing occurrence of melanomas in the United States and northern European countries. Significantly, an increasing number of melanomas are found on the back and neck in men and on the lower leg and back in women. It is probably no coincidence that these locations have become increasingly exposed to sun as styles of dress have changed.

Relatively few melanomas occur where skin is almost always covered. Still, a small number of melanomas do occur on the buttocks and female breasts, suggesting that factors other than exposure to sunlight play a role.

Basal-cell carcinoma accounts for more than 75 percent of all skin cancers. The tumor arises when the basal cells of the epidermis proliferate abnormally and invade the dermis. The most common type of basal-cell cancer appears as a small nodule on the skin which eventually ulcerates in the center, intermittently bleeding and forming a crust. Because it usually is painless, the tumor may be neglected for some time. Bleeding and failure of the ulcer to heal usually prompt the person to see a physician.

Although it grows slowly, basal-cell cancer can invade deeply into underlying tissue and bone and be very destructive locally if it is not treated. In contrast to other cancers, however, this tumor rarely spreads to distant sites.

More than 95 percent of basal-cell lesions can be cured with the first treatment. Surgery, destruction of the tissue by high-frequency electricity, freezing with liquid nitrogen (cryotherapy), and radiation are all effective. The choice depends on the patient's age, and the location and size of the tumor. A technique called chemosurgery is especially useful for treating tumors which are recurrent, far-advanced, or in locations close to a vital structure such as the eye. This method of eliminating the tumor is based on microscopic control that usually insures complete removal of the tumor with the least amount of destruction of the surrounding normal tissue.

A person who develops one basal-cell carcinoma has an increased risk of developing additional ones. He or she should be checked at regular intervals by a dermatologist for new lesions and for recurrence of the original tumor. A sunscreen lotion should be used regularly.

Squamous-cell carcinoma, less common than basal-cell carcinoma, arises from uncontrolled growth of the prickle or spinous cells in the epidermis. It may be a small growth with an irregular surface which bleeds, but the appearance varies. If treated early, the outlook is good. If left untreated, squamous-cell cancers eventually will spread to the lymph nodes. The best tactic is to remove the tumor early.

Squamous-cell cancer can arise from what appears to be normal skin, but it most often occurs in skin that has been chronically damaged by sun. This change is called an actinic keratosis. It usually appears as a faint, red, slightly elevated lesion with a sandpaper-like texture. Actinic keratoses can be quite numerous on the face and backs of the hands and forearms of people who have had prolonged sun exposure, especially if they have light complexions and sunburn easily.

Liquid nitrogen may be used to treat actinic keratoses if they are limited in number. When more numerous, a medicine containing 5-fluorouracil may be applied. Sometimes the best approach to numerous lesions in an elderly person is for a doctor to check the lesions periodically for malignant change.

Besides chronic sun exposure, any long-standing irritation or injury to the skin may cause a susceptibility to squamous-cell cancer. Skin damaged by burn scars, skin overlying a bone chronically infected with osteomyelitis, and long-standing ulcerations of the skin are possible sites. Squamous-cell carcinomas arising here or on the genital skin, lips, and inside the mouth have a greater chance of spreading than those in skin damaged by sun alone.

Malignant melanoma causes more deaths in the United States—nearly 8,000 each year—than any other disease that arises in the skin. These deaths are more tragic because most could have been prevented by early diagnosis and treatment of this form of cancer.

Melanomas are classified into three types according to appearance and behavior. Two of the three types spread outward on the surface of the skin before invading downward. This feature allows diagnosis to be made while the malignancy is still curable by surgical removal. These two types, called superficial spreading and lentigo maligna melanomas, together account for about 75 to 80 percent of all melanomas. The third type, nodular melanoma, is the most malignant and tends to invade downward into the skin at an early stage, so the chance for cure is much lower.

Melanomas can occur at any age, but the peak incidence of the most common type is in the late 40s and 50s. Lentigo maligna melanoma, the least common kind, tends to affect older people, the median age being 70. Melanomas can occur anywhere, but the most common location is the back, except for lentigo maligna melanoma, which most often develops on the face from a large, flat tan spot.

What does the early, curable superficial spreading melanoma look like? It usually begins as a brown spot on the skin that first appears during adulthood. The lesion gradually enlarges and assumes characteristic features: an irregular border, variation in color, and an irregular surface. The colors usually are predominantly brown, but shades of brown and black with areas of red, white, and blue are often present. The color changes may not be obvious but can be detected by a doctor using good light and a magnifying glass. Frequently the easiest characteristic for a patient to notice is the irregular border, which is clearly different from the smooth, regular borders of benign moles. Sometimes the patient or a relative notices a melanoma because it stands out as particularly ugly. Obviously, bleeding is a sign that indicates the lesion should be checked by a physician.

Moles acquired after birth have a low chance of becoming malignant (see page 125). In contrast, large moles present at birth, sometimes referred to as bathing trunk or garment congenital nevi, have about a one in ten chance of developing melanoma. The best practice is to attempt to remove these moles surgically during childhood. Many are so large that a plastic surgeon must remove them in stages over a long time. Sometimes complete removal is impossible, in which case they should be examined by a physician for malignant change at least annually. Small moles present at birth have a much lower risk of becoming malignant, but many dermatologists recommend that they, too, be removed.

A definite diagnosis of melanoma is made by examining a biopsy specimen under the microscope. Once melanoma is diagnosed, the type of treatment is determined by how deeply it has invaded the underlying tissue. In the most superficial cases, surgical removal of the melanoma plus a border of normal tissue, sometimes requiring a skin graft, is usually all that is necessary. In more advanced cases, lymph nodes may be removed. Chemotherapy and agents to stimulate the body's immune system are given for deep melanomas or ones that have spread to other parts of the body.

Parasitic Infestation

Pediculosis means an infestation of lice. These parasites feed specifically on human blood. Infestation occurs in three forms, and all are characterized by severe itching.

Head lice (pediculosis of the scalp) are more common in children than adults. Epidemics among school children are not uncommon. The head louse is transferred from one child to another by shared clothing, combs, and brushes. In feeding on the scalp, the lice produce small wheals, temporary skin swellings that itch intensely. Scratching often opens the skin and leads to secondary bacterial infection, or impetigo, which in turn causes lymph glands to swell as they mobilize to fight the infection. Examination of the scalp usually fails to reveal adult lice. Instead, numerous tiny white nits or eggs can be seen firmly attached to the hair shafts, especially on the back of the head and above the ears.

Pubic lice (pediculosis pubis) infest the hairs of the pubic region. The pubic louse is short and squat and has clawlike legs. Because of its resemblance to a crab, infestation with the pubic louse is commonly referred to as "crabs." Occasionally, this type of louse also infests the eyelashes, beard, armpits, and other hairy areas. In affected areas both nits and the animals themselves can be seen. There also may be small, rust-colored specks representing digested and excreted blood. The pubic louse is transmitted from person to person and on clothing, bedding, and towels.

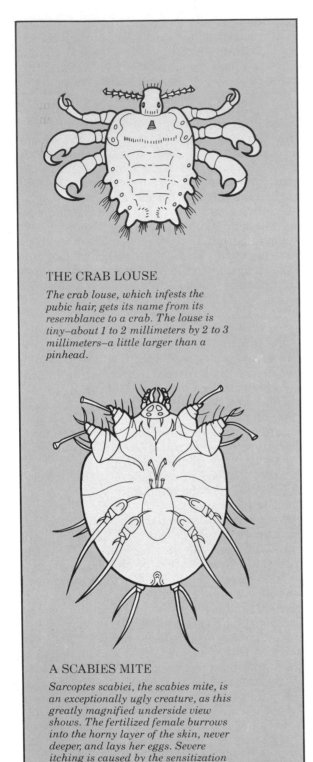

THE CRAB LOUSE

The crab louse, which infests the pubic hair, gets its name from its resemblance to a crab. The louse is tiny—about 1 to 2 millimeters by 2 to 3 millimeters—a little larger than a pinhead.

A SCABIES MITE

Sarcoptes scabiei, the scabies mite, is an exceptionally ugly creature, as this greatly magnified underside view shows. The fertilized female burrows into the horny layer of the skin, never deeper, and lays her eggs. Severe itching is caused by the sensitization of the victim.

Body lice (pediculosis corporis) are not a common louse infestation in the United States. The problem most often occurs in elderly indigents, vagrants, and alcoholics, who seldom bathe or change clothing. In contrast to the head louse and pubic louse, the body louse does not lay eggs in the hair, but in the seams of clothing. It comes out to attack the skin for nourishment in areas that are in constant contact with underwear, such as the waist, shoulders, and upper parts of the back. The louse bites appear as excoriated, red, pimple-like lesions, often arranged in a line. Secondary bacterial infection, including boils, may occur. In long-standing cases chronic scratching results in a brown pigmentation in the skin.

Treatment. Gamma benzene hexachloride (Kwell®), a prescription drug available as a shampoo, cream, or lotion, kills both the lice and nits, but the dead organisms may remain attached to the hairs. They can be loosened by applying a solution of equal parts of white vinegar and water under a towel for an hour, and then removed with a fine-toothed comb. Afterwards, all clothing, bedding, towels, hairbrushes, etc., that might harbor lice or eggs should be laundered. Persons who have had intimate contact with the victim should be informed and treated if symptoms arise.

Scabies is an intensely itchy parasitic infestation caused by a mite, *Sarcoptes scabiei*. The female mite, barely visible to the human eye, burrows a tunnel in the top layer of the skin and lays eggs there. The burrow may resemble a fine, black thread with a minute blister at one end. Burrows are often difficult to see because of overlying redness and crusting caused by scratching. Skin areas most commonly affected are the webs between the fingers, the waistline, underarms, nipples, elbows, buttocks, and penis. The head is almost never involved, except in infants.

Scabies is usually acquired through intimate contact with infested people. In rare instances, the mite that causes scabies in animals (mange) takes up temporary residence on human skin and produces itching.

If you suspect that you have scabies, it is wise to seek medical attention. Self-treatment that fails can confuse the picture and make diagnosis difficult. Once scabies is diagnosed, gamma benzene hexachloride applied from the neck down and left on for 24 hours is usually prescribed. It may be necessary to repeat the application. Intimate contacts should be treated, and all potentially infested clothing, bedding, and linens should be washed in hot water or dry-cleaned. The scabies mite can live for two days without contact with human skin.

Gamma benzene hexachloride applied to the skin can be absorbed into the circulation and is potentially harmful. Other treatments are available for infants, young children, and pregnant women.

Additional medications may be needed to relieve itching, which is usually worse at night. Itching often lasts for a week or more.

Fungal Infections

A distinct group of fungi called dermatophytes has the ability to live in the superficial layer of the epidermis, nails, and hair. Fungal infection can be acquired from three sources: from other people, from the soil, or from animals. Fungi are found everywhere in nature, and everyone is constantly exposed to them. Whether a person becomes infected depends more on inherent susceptibility than on exposure. People who are generally healthy in all other respects may lack the ability to fight off fungus and experience repeated infections.

Warmth and moisture, both in the environment and as local skin conditions, increase the likelihood of acquiring fungal infections. Hence, infections are more common during the summer and in tropical climates. They frequently occur between two skin surfaces where moisture can't easily evaporate, such as between the toes and in the creases of the thigh.

Dermatophyte infection of the skin is commonly referred to as ringworm because the lesions often assume a ring-like shape.

Tinea corporis refers to fungal infection anywhere on the skin except the scalp. The lesions may produce no symptoms or may be mildly itchy. Typically, they are round, light red, and scaling, with a well-defined border. The skin may be clear in the center. When there are only a few lesions, treatment is simple—an anti-fungal cream is applied daily for several weeks. Widespread cases often require an oral medication called griseofulvin.

Athlete's foot (tinea pedis) is the most common of the dermatophyte infections. It primarily affects adults, many of whom are so accustomed to the scaling on their soles and the moist white skin between their toes that they accept the condition as normal. A less common manifestation is blisters on the soles.

There are important reasons for treating athlete's foot. It may cause small fissures in the skin which allow bacteria to enter and set up infections called cellulitis and lymphangitis. And the chronic presence of fungi on the feet provides a source of fungi which can infect other areas, such as the nails, groin, and hands. Once a fungus has infected the toenails, eradication is very difficult.

One of the principles of treating athlete's foot is to eliminate the moisture from the feet, especially between the toes. These areas should be thoroughly dried after bathing and a powder applied regularly. Open shoes or sandals should be worn when possible to expose bare feet to open air. Topical creams or lotions with anti-fungal ingredients can be prescribed.

Tinea cruris ("jock itch") is a fungal infection of the inner surface and upper parts of the thighs, where moisture, warmth, and friction are favorable for the growth of fungus. It is seen most often in men, especially those who also have athlete's foot. Treatment consists of keeping the area dry and the frequent application of an anti-fungal cream or lotion.

Tinea manuum, or fungal infection of the hands, is usually seen as fine scaling with minimal redness over one or both palms. It is almost always accompanied by athlete's foot. Topical treatment alone may be effective, but griseofulvin is sometimes used.

Onchomycosis means fungal infection of the fingernails or toenails. The nails become thickened, white or yellow, and crumbly. The major problems of nail infections are their undesirable appearance and the tendency to catch on stockings and other clothing.

Topical medication is ineffective and griseofulvin is less than satisfactory. Griseofulvin must be taken for five to six months to cure fingernail infection, and sometimes relapse occurs afterwards. Toenails are even more difficult to treat. Medication must be taken for an average of one year, and many cases do not respond even then. Even a high percentage of "cured" cases recur once griseofulvin has been stopped. Therapy is more successful if infected nails are removed, but often when the nails regrow, they again become infected. Many dermatologists feel that treatment of fungal infection of the toenails is not worth the expense and risk of side effects, because results are often disappointing.

Tinea capitis is fungal infection of the scalp. Unlike most other fungus infections, tinea capitis affects more children than adults.

It is quite contagious and may occur in epidemics. The usual appearance is patchy areas of scaling with broken-off hairs or even bald patches. Sometimes a localized painful, boggy, swollen area of inflammation occurs. Often the infecting organisms can be seen by examining the scalp under a special lamp. It can now be cured with griseofulvin.

Tinea versicolor is a common superficial fungal infection caused by the organism *Malassezia furfur*. This is not a dermatophyte but probably a variant of a yeast-like organism found on normal skin. Affected areas show finely scaling, non-inflammatory lesions that are brown, white, or pink and either darker or lighter than normal skin. They are often most noticeable in the summer when failure to tan makes them stand out.

Medications applied to the skin to treat tinea versicolor contain selenium sulfide, salicylic acid, sodium hyposulfite, or various anti-fungal agents. Although the fungus is usually eradicated within several days, the normal skin color does not return until exposed to sun. Relapse or reinfection is common.

Yeast Infections

The yeast *Candida albicans* lives normally in the mouth, gastrointestinal tract, and vagina. Under certain circumstances, its normal relationship can be disturbed and it can cause disease. Predisposing factors include pregnancy, antibiotic and birth control medications, diabetes, and chronic debilitating illness. The major skin requirement for growth of the yeast organism is moisture.

Cutaneous candidiasis appears in several forms. Paronychia is a painful inflammation around the nail involving the cuticle. It is most common in people who frequently immerse their hands in water, such as housewives and dishwashers. Perleche is a moist red area at the corners of the mouth. Since warmth and moisture favor the growth of the yeast organism, a common location for candidiasis is between touching skin surfaces. Monilia intertrigo occurs between the buttocks, in the thigh creases, under female breasts, and under folds of fat. Occasionally the finger webs, especially between the third and fourth fingers, are affected.

Thrush is a yeast infection of the mucous membranes, either the mouth or vagina. Oral thrush is most common in newborns. Vaginal moniliasis may be a complication of pregnancy and medication with oral contraceptives and antibiotics, but it also occurs in other women without predisposing factors. It can be transmitted to a male sexual partner (see chapter 22, "The Kidneys and Urinary System").

To treat most forms of candidiasis effectively means elimination of warmth and moisture. This can be done by applying an absorbent powder, then exposing affected areas to air or a fan several times a day. In the case of infection around the nail, the hands must be protected from water. Medications are available by prescription.

Viral Infections

Warts. Although all warts are caused by the same or at least closely related viruses, warts may vary in appearance depending on their location. Common warts start as pinhead-sized, skin-colored elevations that gradually grow to become larger, raised lesions with a rough surface consisting of numerous tiny projections. Common in children, they are most often located on the backs of the hands but may occur anywhere on the skin.

Filiform and flat warts are most common on the face. Plantar warts are located on the sole (plantar surface) of the foot. They differ from other warts in that calluses usually form over them, and they may be painful because of pressure against nerves during standing or walking.

Condyloma acuminata are warts on the genital skin, most commonly on the penis and around the vaginal and anal areas. They begin as small, isolated bumps but later become grouped together in clusters resembling cauliflower. Condyloma acuminata are also referred to as venereal warts because they are usually acquired through sexual contact.

Susceptibility to the wart virus varies among individuals. The virus is contagious, but except for venereal warts, whether a person becomes infected depends more on the inborn immune system than on the amount of exposure. Recipients of kidney transplants or cancer patients who must take drugs to suppress the immune system have an increased incidence of warts.

The wart virus invades only the uppermost epidermis and does not penetrate into the dermis. This usually allows the warts to be destroyed without scarring—by freezing the cells with liquid nitrogen, zapping them with electric current and then scraping them off, or by applying acids.

The treatment selected depends in part on the location of the warts. Surgical therapy for plantar warts, for instance, may produce a scar that can be painful because of its location on the weight-bearing sole of the foot. If the borders of a plantar wart are well-defined, it can be treated by a technique called blunt dissection, which "shells out" the wart with minimal injury to the surrounding skin. Venereal warts usually are treated with either liquid nitrogen or a strong chemical called podophyllin. The treatment, incidentally, should include sexual partners with warts.

Because most warts eventually heal themselves, a reasonable alternative is to do nothing. (Venereal warts, however, should be treated because they spread more easily than other types.) If you choose to have your warts treated, remember that more than one treatment may be required, and results may be slow. Getting rid of plantar warts in particular is likely to take many weeks.

Molluscum contagiosum consists of one or more firm, dome-shaped bumps which are flesh-colored to pink. They have pearly white centers that usually contain a tiny depression. As the name implies, the disease is contagious, transmitted from person to person by direct contact or spread by the hands from an affected area to another part of the body. Molluscum contagiosum is common in children, usually concentrating on the face, chest, and abdomen. It also occurs frequently on the thighs and in the genital and pubic areas of sexually active young adults.

The lesions usually go away spontaneously but sometimes last for years. They can be removed with a curet, an instrument which contains a loop with sharpened edges attached to a rod-shaped handle, or by applying liquid nitrogen or acids.

Herpes simplex is a virus that causes the common but distressing cold sore. Most people are infected in childhood but usually the person is unaware of the initial infection because it causes no symptoms. Less often, a child, usually between one and five years, will become ill with fever, enlarged lymph nodes, and painful sores in the mouth, with red, swollen gums that bleed easily. Recovery is usually complete within two weeks.

Once a person has been infected by herpes simplex, the virus goes into a latent phase and remains inside the body indefinitely, living inside a nerve near the infected site. At certain times the virus becomes reactivated and causes a cold sore on the outside of the lip.

Less commonly, small grouped blisters occur on other areas of the face. In some people, emotional stress, physical illness such as the common cold, sunburn, or menstruation predictably trigger an outbreak. The cold sores tend to occur repeatedly in the same site.

At present there is no cure for herpes simplex infections, although numerous treatments are often tried. Many different approaches have appeared to be promising, but controlled scientific studies usually have disproven their value. Blisters are thought to heal faster if a local drying agent such as alcohol is applied. Secondary bacterial infection can be prevented by washing the area with an antiseptic solution.

Remember that the blisters of a herpes simplex infection are contagious to others and occasionally may be spread elsewhere on the skin by the hands. Most important in this regard is the eye. Herpes simplex infection of the eye should be suspected if the eye becomes pink and painful in the presence of herpes lesions in other areas (see chapter 12, "The Eyes"). If it does, promptly seek the attention of an ophthalmologist so the infection can be treated before permanent damage occurs. Fortunately, certain medications such as idoxuridine usually are effective against herpes simplex of the eye. Unfortunately, these medications are not as helpful for infections of the skin.

Besides the mouth and face, herpes simplex can also affect the genital area. Such infections are one of the leading causes of venereal disease today (see chapter 22, "The Kidneys and Urinary System," and chapter 28, "Infectious Disease"). Small blisters which quickly break are found on the vulva, vagina, and cervix in women and on the penis in men. The first infection is very painful, especially in women, who may experience such discomfort that urination and even walking and sitting are difficult.

Urination may be less painful if done in a bathtub of warm water. Strong pain medications may be necessary. A topical anesthetic is helpful, and plain petroleum jelly can be used to coat the affected skin surfaces to protect them from irritating friction. Symptoms usually take two weeks to subside.

Recurrent infections can occur after the primary outbreak subsides. Re-exposure to the virus is not necessary, because the virus lives in the nerves of one's own body. Fortunately, the symptoms from recurrent infection are usually mild. Because the blisters harbor the virus, sexual relations should be avoided until they have healed to prevent spreading.

Genital herpes is a special problem to a pregnant woman if present at the time of delivery. The baby can contract a fatal infection by passing through an infected birth canal. In such cases, Cesarean section is usually done.

Shingles (herpes zoster) results from reactivation of the virus that causes chickenpox. A person who has recovered from chickenpox still carries the virus in a latent state in nerve cells along the spinal cord or in the brain. The virus can later be reactivated, migrate to the skin, and cause blisters along a band following a nerve, almost always on one side of the body. Affected people, especially those over 60, may develop associated pain. The pain can be severe and persist for weeks or even months.

Treatment consists of applying cool compresses to help dry up the blisters and prevent bacterial infection. Medication may be needed for relief of pain. Because the virus is present in the lesions, a person with shingles should avoid contact with children who have not had chickenpox and with any other person who is so sick that he or she cannot combat infections normally. When shingles occurs on the face, the virus can affect the eye, which should be cared for by an ophthalmologist.

Bacterial Infections

Impetigo is a common, superficial bacterial infection of the skin caused by streptococcal or staphylococcal bacteria. Children are often affected, with small itchy blisters appearing on the face. The blisters easily rupture and leave yellowish-brown crusts on a red oozing base. Sometimes impetigo occurs on skin where there is another type of rash, a minor cut or abrasion.

Impetigo, especially in children, is contagious. It responds readily to washing with an antibacterial cleanser plus either an antibiotic applied to the skin or one taken internally. The disease is usually uncomplicated, but streptococcal impetigo may occasionally be followed by a kidney disease called glomerulonephritis (see chapter 22, "The Kidneys and Urinary System").

Folliculitis is a mildly painful infection around hair follicles, usually caused by staphylococcus bacteria. Tiny pustules appear at the base of each hair. Common locations are the thighs and buttocks, but folliculitis may occur anywhere there are hairs. Friction and exposure to grease or oil can increase susceptibility to the disorder. Frequent washing with an antibacterial cleanser helps eliminate the infection, but sometimes antibiotics taken by mouth are necessary.

Boils refer to infections that begin around hair follicles but extend outward and downward to form a pocket of pus called an abscess. The cause is usually staphylococcus bacteria. A furuncle is a deep infection around one hair follicle. A carbuncle is infection of a group of adjacent follicles, often draining at multiple sites.

Boils are painful because of the expanding pus within them, which becomes visible when it "comes to a head." Small boils can rupture and heal spontaneously. Large boils need medical attention because incision and drainage, and sometimes an antibiotic and pain medication, are required.

Before you see a doctor, you may apply warm water compresses to the area to hasten the inflammatory process. If the boil does not easily burst, do not squeeze or manipulate it. A rare but serious complication is the seeding of bacteria into the bloodstream and formation of abscesses in other organs, including the brain.

Some people tend to develop recurrent boils. Often they are otherwise healthy, and no reason for their recurrent infections can be found. Careful attention to hygiene with the regular use of antibacterial soap is indicated. Occasionally these people chronically carry staphylococci inside their nostrils, in which case the daily application of an antibacterial ointment to the nose may be helpful.

Pigmentation Problems

Vitiligo is a loss of pigmentation in the skin caused by the disappearance of melanocytes, the cells which make melanin. Why the melanocytes are lost is not known. The loss may occur in only a few small areas or may be extensive. Common sites are the backs of the hands, the face, especially around the mouth and eyes, and the genitalia. Often the distribution of lesions is symmetrical on either side of the body. The involved areas appear white and are most noticeable in dark-skinned individuals.

In rare instances vitiligo is associated with other health problems, such as pernicious anemia and diseases of the thyroid and adrenal glands.

Absence of melanin leaves affected areas unprotected from sunlight, and they sunburn easily. Sunscreens should be used. To improve cosmetic appearance a temporary stain can be painted on the white areas so that they blend with the normal skin. A treatment consisting of a medication called psoralen combined with exposure to long-wave ultraviolet light is sometimes successful in causing pigmentation to return.

Melasma consists of darkened patches on the cheeks and forehead. It occurs mainly in women who take oral contraceptives or who are pregnant, and is sometimes referred to as the "mask of pregnancy." Occasionally melasma affects men or non-pregnant women not on the pill. Exposure to sun is a prerequisite for its development.

Treatment must both prevent further darkening by sunlight and promote lightening of already-darkened areas. A sunscreen that blocks out all light is recommended. Hydroquinone cream will gradually decrease pigmentation, but the dark areas can be more effectively lightened by a prescription preparation containing tretinoin plus a corticosteroid, in addition to the hydroquinone.

Itching

Itching is the most common symptom arising in the skin. Many localized skin diseases are intensely itchy. Itching all over the body in the absence of a specific rash has several benign causes but also may stem from serious illness.

A common cause of itching in older people is dry skin. Itching of this type responds well to skin care that treats the dryness. Pregnant women may develop itching, usually in the last three months of pregnancy, apparently because estrogen interferes with normal excretion of bile in the liver. Psychological stress does not cause itching but can aggravate it by making a person more aware of the sensation. Diseases of the liver and thyroid, kidney failure, and cancer, especially of the lymphatic and blood systems, may be associated with itching. Treatment of itching in these cases often relies upon treatment of the underlying disease.

Anesthetics applied to the skin relieve itching by temporarily deadening the nerves. They may be effective initially but too often they lead to an allergic contact dermatitis, which obviously makes the itching problem worse. Topical preparations containing benzocaine and diphenhydramine should be avoided. If you become allergic to them, you risk reacting in the future to certain other chemically related medications, both those applied to the skin and those taken internally.

Lupus Erythematosus

This complex disease can affect one or several organs of the body (see chapter 15, "Arthritis and Related Diseases"). In its least serious form, the disease is limited to the skin. Skin lesions of the disease have a variety of forms, but the most common is the discoid lesion. This appears as a well-defined red to violet elevation which, if untreated, heals with a scar. The appearance of discoid lesions is so characteristic that usually they can be identified easily by a dermatologist. The lesions usually occur on the face, but can occur on the scalp and particularly on the ears, and on sun-exposed skin such as the chest. Sometimes there is mild swelling and redness across the bridge of the nose and on both cheeks, referred to as a "butterfly rash."

Although the same type of lesion occurs in the form of lupus erythematosus that affects internal organs, most patients with discoid lesions have only skin involvement.

Patients with discoid lupus erythematosus should see a physician regularly for two reasons. First, it is important to make sure that the disease has remained limited to the skin. If the disease involves internal organs, it can almost always be detected by a history, physical examination, and laboratory tests. Second, proper medical management helps control discoid lesions and prevent disfigurement. Treatment consists of sunscreens, corticosteroids (locally injected or applied), and sometimes antimalarial drugs. Patients with skin lupus and especially those with systemic lupus erythematosus should avoid the sun as much as possible.

Pemphigus and Pemphigoid

These two diseases are characterized by blisters. In pemphigus blisters occur in the epidermis because cells lose their adhesion to one another. Only a thin layer of cells remains to form the roofs of the blisters, so that they easily rupture. The majority of patients with pemphigus develop blisters in the mouth as well as on the rest of the skin. These are painful and may interfere with eating.

The blisters in bullous pemphigoid form at a lower level in the skin, just beneath the epidermis at its junction with the dermis. They are larger than in pemphigus and tend to remain intact longer.

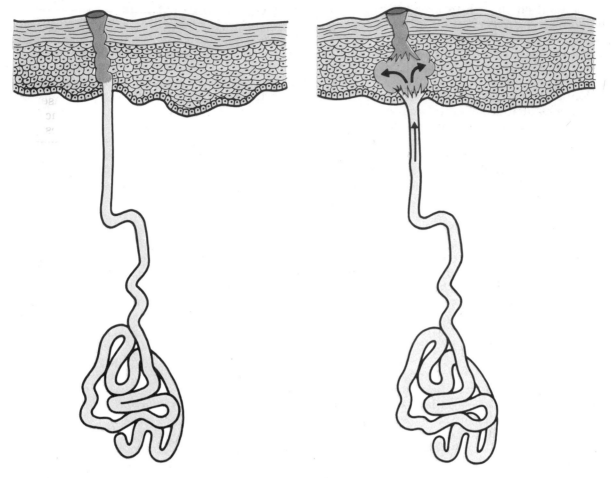

HEAT RASH

"Prickly heat" results from entrapment of sweat in layers of the skin close to the surface. The sweat is trapped if the sweat duct outlets are blocked. At left, a normal gland can deliver sweat to the surface of the skin. At right, rupture of a duct in the *prickle-cell layer of the epidermis means sweat produced by the gland cannot escape and a minute pimple forms. Relatively few of the three million eccrine sweat glands are affected at one time.*

Although pemphigus affects mainly middle-aged persons and bullous pemphigoid occurs primarily in the elderly, both occasionally appear in childhood. They are uncommon but serious diseases. Treatment includes corticosteroids and antimetabolic drugs.

Common Benign Conditions

Heat rash (miliaria) results when eccrine sweat ducts are blocked so that trapped sweat cannot reach the surface of the skin. The sweat duct ruptures below the point of obstruction. The depth of the obstruction determines the type of lesion. When the sweat pores are blocked only within the stratum corneum, tiny clear bubble-like blisters are produced. If the obstruction is deeper, redness surrounds the blisters.

Heat rash breaks out when sweat glands react to a hot environment, fever, or prolonged exertion. When clothing or high humidity impedes evaporation, the accumulation of water apparently injures the cells lining the sweat duct. Sunburn is another common cause.

Lowering the surrounding temperature is the key to treatment. Once sweating stops, the rash clears spontaneously, usually over the course of several days. More inflamed rashes require one to three weeks to clear. Loose clothing should be worn or the affected skin should be exposed to air.

Pityriasis rosea is a common disease that consists of multiple scaling patches, usually affecting young people during the spring and fall. It is self-limited, lasting six to eight weeks. Often a "herald patch" precedes by a few days to two weeks the appearance of other similar, smaller lesions. The lesions are pink to salmon-colored, oval, scaly, and have a crinkly surface. They may resemble ringworm. They are commonly located on the back and chest, where their arrangement resembles a fir tree. The rash usually is not itchy, but a few persons itch intensely.

Most patients feel well, but some will have a run-down feeling. The cause, though unproven, is thought to be a virus.

Dandruff and seborrheic dermatitis both stem from an increased production of scales on the scalp. Simple dandruff is noninflammatory, but seborrheic dermatitis is characterized by scaling and redness, not only in the scalp, but also in the eyebrows, the creases behind the ears, and on each side of the nose. The eyelashes may be involved, and red scaly patches often are present on the chest. In severe cases, red patches also occur in the armpits and groin.

The word seborrheic refers to the tendency for this rash to occur where sebaceous (oil) glands are numerous and active. Involved areas often appear greasy, but no increase or abnormality in sebaceous gland function has been demonstrated. What is known to be abnormal is that the epidermis makes cells at a faster rate than normal, and the abundant immature cells are sloughed off as scales.

Seborrheic dermatitis is a chronic condition that can be controlled but not cured. The first line of therapy is frequent use of a special shampoo to slow down the production of scales and wash away those already formed. Effective preparations contain selenium sulfide, zinc pyrithione, and sulfur and salicylic acid. Tar shampoos are helpful but may stain light-colored hair. If the scalp is very red, a physician may prescribe a steroid solution or spray. Seborrheic dermatitis on the face, chest, and other areas responds readily to a variety of topical medications, including several forms of hydrocortisone cream.

Seborrheic keratoses are common benign lesions that occur almost anywhere on the skin but most frequently on the face, chest, and back. They are *not* related to seborrheic dermatitis. (The name seborrheic in this case refers to the somewhat greasy appearance of the lesions.) Typical seborrheic keratoses are brown or black, have a waxy, slightly elevated surface, and vary in size from a tenth of an inch to three-fourths of an inch or more. They are so superficially located that they appear to be "pasted on" the skin. They often can be partially scraped off with a fingernail. Seborrheic keratoses need not be treated, but if they are itchy or of objectionable appearance, they can be removed easily in a variety of ways.

Cysts (wens) are cavities within the skin that are filled with the fatty secretion sebum, the protein keratin, and cells. They usually occur on the chest, back, face, and scalp. There are two types, epidermal cysts and pilar (sebaceous) cysts, which look alike but display different structures when examined under the microscope. Cysts are painless unless they become infected. They are harmless but can be removed for cosmetic reasons if desired.

Very tiny (less than one tenth of an inch in diameter) epidermal cysts called milia appear mainly on the face, especially on the eyelids, cheeks, and forehead. They are firm, white to yellow, and smooth, resembling whiteheads except that they have no opening to the surface. Milia usually arise without apparent cause but may follow skin injury such as burns or certain skin disorders characterized by blister formation. They can be removed by cutting into the tops and removing the contents.

Canker sores. Most people at some time have had small isolated sores inside the mouth, but about 20 percent of the population experiences the recurrent, painful types known as aphthous stomatitis. Local skin injury, allergy, infectious agents, hormonal imbalance, and emotional and physical stress have been implicated in this problem, but the cause has not been firmly established.

Several topical treatments are available for the relief of pain. Tetracycline compresses are sometimes successful. Corticosteroids taken by mouth during the very early phase of symptoms may halt the attacks or hasten healing. None of these treatments works in every case, and a better therapy awaits clarification of the cause.

Hives. A typical hive is an itchy, well-circumscribed, small pink swelling in the skin. The pink color is caused by dilation of the small blood vessels in the dermis, and the swelling occurs because fluid escapes through the walls of the vessels and collects around the vessels. Occasionally hives become very large. When the reaction occurs in the deeper dermis or underlying tissue, it is called angioedema.

Each individual hive lasts less than 24 hours, although new hives can continue to crop up for many days or even longer. Single acute episodes of hives are common. They are often an allergic reaction to a food, drug, or insect bite (see chapter 21, "Allergy and the Immune System"). Particular foods that seem to induce hives in some persons include shellfish, nuts, chocolate, and tomatoes. Sometimes food additives appear to be responsible, especially salicylates (the chemical contained in aspirin) or a yellow dye called tartrazine. Allergy to penicillin often shows up as hives. Hives that continue for more than six weeks are classified as chronic.

Keeping a diary of the relationship of hives to internal and external exposures is a first step in trying to track down the offender, but often the exact cause cannot be identified. In rare instances hives may accompany a serious disease such as hepatitis, lupus erythematosus, or malignant tumors. A doctor can evaluate the underlying disease and prescribe a drug, usually an antihistamine, to relieve itching and help eliminate the attacks.

Hives in themselves are not dangerous unless the allergic response is so intense that it causes swelling around the larynx and interferes with breathing. Insect bites in particular can produce this serious complication, called anaphylaxis. Emergency care is necessary. A person who knows he or she is susceptible to such attacks should carry an emergency kit containing the drug epinephrine. Epinephrine can be self-administered by injection or by aerosol spray.

Lichen planus is a disease of unknown cause that affects the skin and sometimes the inside of the mouth. Small itchy, angular, purplish bumps may appear anywhere on the skin, but they particularly attack the insides of the wrists. In the mouth, where they can be painful, the lesions appear as a lacelike network of fine white lines. Lichen planus usually lasts several months but can be chronic and persist for years. Treatment is aimed at relief of itching.

Ichthyosis refers to the fish-like scales of dry skin occurring in this inherited disorder. There are several types of ichthyosis, the most serious being apparent at birth. The most common and least severe type, ichthyosis vulgaris, usually appears in infancy and is inherited from a parent. Some victims also have atopic dermatitis or a family history of this disorder. Tiny bumps tend to develop around the hair follicles on the upper arms and thighs, a condition known as keratosis pilaris. In its mildest form, ichthyosis may be noticed only as dry skin. There is no "cure," but emollients such as eucerin applied after a shower or bath help. In recent years progress has been made in treating severe forms of ichthyosis with a drug called cis-retinoic acid.

Keloids are thick, rubbery, elevated scars that occur after injury to the skin or surgical incisions. The skin of the chest and back is quite susceptible to keloid formation. Keloids are especially common in blacks. There is no way to predict whether the skin of a particular person will form keloids unless he or she has had a previous wound. Sometimes keloids can be satisfactorily reduced in size by local injection of corticosteroids.

Drug eruptions. Allergic reactions to drugs often appear as a rash. Antibiotics are among the most common offenders, but almost any drug can produce a rash. Drug rashes assume many different appearances. They usually appear within a week after the person starts taking the drug, but sometimes don't show up until after it has been stopped. Once the medication has been discontinued, the rash continues to develop for a few days and lasts two to three weeks.

Erythema multiforme may be caused by drugs, but has other causes as well. It is characterized by distinctive lesions in concentric circles, resembling a target. It may occur anywhere, but usually is found on the hands, feet, forearms, legs, and sometimes inside the mouth. Although most patients recover completely, the problem in rare instances can be fatal. Besides drugs, two other causes of erythema multiforme are herpes simplex infections (cold sores) and a certain type of pneumonia. Recurrent cold sores in some people are regularly followed by attacks of erythema multiforme.

HAIR DISORDERS

Common Baldness

(male pattern baldness)

A man may view the loss of his crowning glory as an event of major cosmetic significance. It probably is not very reassuring to know that balding is part of the normal aging process and occurs in several species of monkeys, apes, and chimpanzees as well as humans. During balding, the hair follicles become smaller and the hairs they produce change from coarse dark terminal hairs to soft, thin, unpigmented vellus hairs. Hair loss occurs in a characteristic pattern. It tends to affect the parts of the scalp around the temples first, and later involves the crown. Eventually, the two areas may merge.

A scientific term for common baldness is androgenetic alopecia. This term encompasses the two major factors in this type of hair loss—the male hormones or androgens and a hereditary predisposition. We know that minimum levels of male hormones are necessary for baldness because men castrated before puberty don't lose their hair. The precise relationship between androgens and baldness is being investigated. It is thought that the smaller hair follicles in the frontal scalp metabolize hormones to a more active form faster than unaffected follicles. But it is not known why androgen causes the hair follicles to become smaller in this situation when at the same time it stimulates growth of the beard and axillary and pubic hair. Although we know that genes play a role in baldness, the exact inheritance pattern is not clear.

Men as a group vary greatly in how much hair they lose and how fast. What to expect in any individual is difficult to predict, but family history is a useful guide. In general, early, extensive hair loss suggests an unfavorable outlook. On the other hand, thinning of the hair first noticed after age 40 is quite unlikely to evolve rapidly into significant baldness. About 5 percent of white males show the first sign of baldness before age 20. Some men who notice early frontal recession show only very slow extension of the baldness thereafter. One or two percent will develop extensive baldness by age 30. By age 60 about 80 percent show at least some evidence of hair loss. Baldness is not related to hair color or texture.

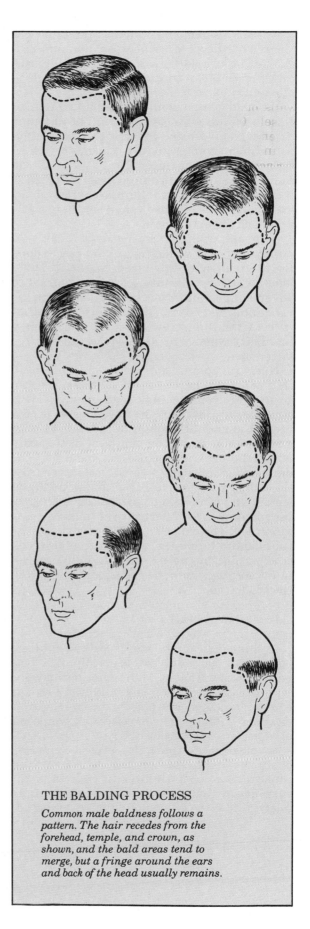

THE BALDING PROCESS

Common male baldness follows a pattern. The hair recedes from the forehead, temple, and crown, as shown, and the bald areas tend to merge, but a fringe around the ears and back of the head usually remains.

154 SKIN

Women also may lose their hair as they get older, but the process begins later and progresses less rapidly. In women thinning usually occurs all over the head, although it is most marked on the crown.

For bald men, it would be helpful if our society placed less emphasis on a full head of hair as a sign of attractiveness. The population density of hairs on the scalp is no more a reflection of health or masculinity than is the number of hairs on the male chest. Variation in hair density is a normal human characteristic, and acceptance of this is the best therapeutic approach for many men.

Short of changing society's standards or one's own negative feelings, what can be done for the man with advanced baldness? There is no totally satisfactory solution. Contrary to advertising claims, no magic salve can be rubbed on, and no treatments can be given that will start the hair growing again. Much money has been wasted by those who pursue this false hope.

Hair transplantation is the only approach that will alter the pattern of baldness. The procedure is expensive and time-consuming. It is suitable only for men who have an area of hair growth abundant enough to serve as a donor site. Usually this is on the back of the scalp above the neck. Plugs of hair about half the diameter of a pencil in size are removed from the donor site. The resulting holes gradually shrink and form inconspicuous scars. Plugs of the same size are taken from the bald scalp and discarded. The donor plugs are then fitted into the holes in the bald area, where they grow just as they did in the old site. Usually several hundred plugs must be transplanted to fill in the bald area.

Alopecia Areata

In this condition the hair is lost in a localized spot, most commonly on the scalp. It affects both and women. Men sometimes develop it in the beard. When the bald spot first becomes noticeable it is usually the size of a dime or quarter. There are no associated symptoms or visible inflammation.

In most cases the hair returns spontaneously after several months. The new hair sometimes appears lighter in color than the surrounding hair. The condition may recur. In a few people the bald spot enlarges to include much of the scalp. In rare cases all the scalp hair is lost, and in unusually rare instances even the eyebrows and eyelashes disappear. The younger the age of onset and the more extensive the hair loss, the worse the prognosis for regrowth of hair.

The cause of alopecia areata is not known. In some cases it appears to result from severe emotional stress.

Treatment is not necessary for most cases because spontaneous regrowth usually occurs. Although injections of corticosteroids temporarily stimulate regrowth, they do not alter the natural course of the disease. Steroid pills also stimulate regrowth, but when they are discontinued, the hair falls out unless the disease has remitted of its own accord. Because of potential serious side effects, long-term steroid medication is not warranted. A wiser approach for extensive cases is the purchase of a wig.

Temporary Hair Loss

Telogen effluvium is the scientific term for temporary hair loss due to a synchronization of the growth cycles of scalp hair. Illness, rapid and large weight loss, high fever, certain drugs, pregnancy, and discontinuing birth control pills can cause hairs to stop growing and prematurely enter the resting phase (telogen) of the growth cycle. As new hairs grow in, the resting hairs are displaced from the follicles and fall out, a normal process. Because an unusually large number of hairs stop growing and fall out at once, the hair loss may be alarming. Within a few months, however, the growth of new hairs becomes apparent, and the normal proportion of growing and resting hairs is restored.

Excessive Hair Growth

Excessive hair growth (hirsutism) in women may be caused by an abnormal increase in androgen production from an endocrine disorder or tumor of the ovary or adrenal gland. The excessive hair growth in these cases is often accompanied by acne and menstrual irregularities.

Some normal women have dark hairs on the face, abdomen, thighs, and around the nipples. This is in part genetically determined. A woman can feel some assurance that her hair growth is normal if her mother and sisters have a similar pattern.

Once underlying medical problems have been ruled out, how can a woman get rid of unsightly hairs? The simplest way is shaving. Shaving does *not* make hair coarser. The bristly quality of the regrowing hairs stems from loss of the gently tapering ends. Chemical hair removers (depilatories) dissolve hair, but they may irritate the skin. Tweezing out hairs usually is reserved for the eyebrows because it is time-consuming and painful. In some salons waxing is used to remove hairs. Warm wax is applied to the skin and allowed to cool. The wax then is quickly pulled away from the skin, taking with it the hairs in that area. The process is no more painful than removing an adhesive bandage, although the area may remain red for a half-hour afterwards. Bleaching may be a satisfactory alternative for some people, but bleached hair may look unnatural and unattractive in dark-skinned women.

Electrolysis is the one method of hair removal that can be permanent. A very fine needle is inserted into the hair follicle and an electric current applied to destroy the hair root. The hair then can be removed easily. The follicles are briefly swollen afterwards. Occasionally tiny, firm red bumps appear, usually lasting several weeks.

Although hair follicles that are producing growing hairs may be destroyed with a single treatment, follicles with hairs in other stages of development usually require several treatments before they are sufficiently damaged to prevent future hair growth. Since a hair-bearing area always contains some hairs in the resting phase, electrolysis must be done over several months to achieve permanent hair removal. Success depends on the skill of the electrologist applying the treatment and on the patience of the woman receiving it. She must be willing to follow through with the necessary number of treatments.

NAIL DISORDERS

Since nails grow from an epidermal structure (the matrix), any skin disease that affects the epidermis can affect the matrix and alter the nails. In these cases, successful treatment of the underlying diseases will correct the nail problem. However, there will be a delay in the return of the nails to normal appearance, because nail plate changes lag behind the matrix defects which produced them. Remember that a fingernail takes about 5½ months to grow out completely.

Two diseases often associated with nail changes are psoriasis and eczema. In psoriasis, the most common changes are pitting and crumbling of the nail plate, separation of the nail plate from the nail bed, and accumulation of yellowish keratin under the nail. Eczema can cause inflammation around the margins of the nail and cross ridging of the nail plate.

The cells in the matrix undergo active division as they make the nail plate and are therefore sensitive to any conditions that affect the metabolism of the body. Serious illness and certain drugs (antimetabolites) may interfere temporarily with the formation of the nail plate. For that period it becomes thinner and a depression appears.

Many people, especially women, complain of brittle nails that break easily and grow slowly. Almost never in Americans is this a reflection of poor nutrition. Nails are made of a protein called keratin, but adding protein to the diet in the form of gelatin or other foods will not increase incorporation of protein into the nails. Fingernails may become thinner naturally with age so that they break more easily. Rate of growth also decreases. There is no cure for these natural events. The cause of brittle nails in young women is not known.

CHAPTER 8   **ROBERT D. FAZZARO, M.D.**
L. FRED AYVAZIAN, M.D.

THE LUNGS

Just as a fire needs oxygen to burn, the human body also needs a continuous supply of this essential element for the process of combustion that goes on constantly in every cell. We ordinarily do not think of body metabolism as combustion, yet that is what it is: the controlled burning of carbohydrates, fats, and proteins to provide energy. The job of the respiratory system is to furnish the oxygen that combines with these fuels in each of the billions of cells, and to carry away the waste product of carbon dioxide.

And so we breathe—14 times a minute, a pint of air per breath, more than 10,000 quarts of air a day. Not all that comes in, of course, is oxygen. Only about one-fifth of the air we breathe is this life-sustaining element. But it makes up an important part of our bodies and our lives. At any given moment, half the body's weight is oxygen. The overwhelming portion, incidentally, is not in the form of a gas, the way we usually think of oxygen.

We loosely use the word "respiration" to describe the process of taking in oxygen and letting out carbon dioxide. To be scrupulously accurate, respiration refers to the ultimate exchange that takes place in the cells themselves, the delivery of oxygen and the removal of carbon dioxide. This gas transfer, as it is scientifically known, is at the heart of human life. If oxygen did not arrive, if the carbon dioxide were not removed, our lives would be abruptly shortened. The exchange must take place in every cell, including those distant from the oxygen-rich atmosphere that surrounds us. Obtaining that oxygen and starting it on its all-important trip through the body begins with those critical organs, the lungs.

A LOOK AT THE LUNGS

Although central to the vital and complex processes of all body cells, the lungs are mechanically simple in form, function, and principle.

They are cone-shaped, gray in color, and weigh a little more than a pound each. The normal lungs of a healthy male have a capacity of nearly 10 quarts. (Those of females are slightly smaller.) Lungs are hardy organs. If one is diseased and removed, the respiratory process continues adequately without it.

Each of the two lungs is contained within its own chest cavity. This "double" cavity, the thorax, consists of the space bounded by the ribs (and their attached muscles) and by the diaphragms, those specialized dome-like muscles that run laterally across the body and on which the lungs rest. The term "cavity" implies emptiness but the thorax actually is completely filled with the lungs, the heart, and other vital structures.

The exterior of the lung is covered by a thin, glistening membrane called the visceral pleura. The inner surfaces of the chest cavity and diaphragms are lined by a similar membrane, the parietal pleura. Under normal circumstances these two membranes are in contact, so that lung and chest wall glide smoothly against each other during the motion of respiration. Lubricating fluids minimize the friction and make the work of breathing easier.

The tops of the lungs extend about one inch above the collarbone. Between them lies their outlet to (and inlet from) the outside world, the windpipe or trachea. The trachea is a hollow tube about four to five inches long, and is composed of C-shaped rings of cartilage that give it stability. Connected to the mouth and pharynx at the upper end and to the airways of the lungs below, the trachea is interrupted only by the voice box, or larynx, located in the Adam's apple portion of the neck. Food and air pass down the pharynx until they reach the tracheal opening. From there the esophagus, or gullet, leads to the digestive system, and the larynx to the airways. The epiglottis, a kind of trapdoor, holds the larynx open for breathing and closes it for swallowing. Occasionally it closes imperfectly and we choke or "swallow the wrong way."

If you could look at a cross section of the respiratory system, it would resemble a tree and its branches, with the trachea as the trunk. Indeed, the branching that occurs where the trachea divides and connects the two lungs is often referred to as the bronchial tree. About one-third of the way down from the apex of the lungs, the trachea divides into two main branches. The branch to the right almost continues the line of the trachea itself, while the left side branches at a more acute angle.

As tree branches grow smaller and smaller in their reach for sunlight, so the bronchi decrease in size. The mainstream bronchi divide into airways known as the lobar bronchi. There are three lobes in the right lung—the upper, middle and lower—and two on the left—the upper and lower—separated by two

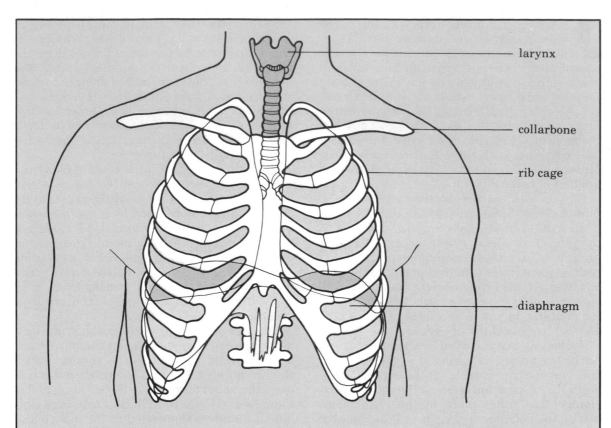

larynx

collarbone

rib cage

diaphragm

LOCATING THE LUNGS

The lungs lie within the flexible rib cage. They normally have only one fixed attachment (at the larynx) and thus have considerable range of motion. The bases of the lungs rest above the diaphragm, the principal muscle of breathing.

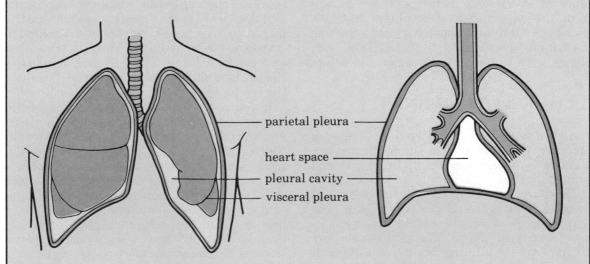

parietal pleura

heart space

pleural cavity

visceral pleura

THE PLEURAL CAVITY

Each lung is surrounded by a glistening membrane, the visceral pleura. The inner surface of the chest has a similar membrane, the parietal pleura. Lubricated by fluids, these membranes glide smoothly against each other when we breathe. Normally there is no space between them, but entry of bacteria, penetrating wounds, or disease may separate the pleura. Drawing at right shows the relationship of the heart to the pleural spaces.

Several important changes occur in the air passages in the transition from trachea to respiratory bronchioles. The prominent rings of cartilage in the larger tubes disappear at the outer level of the terminal bronchioles. The inner surface of the tracheal wall is lined by tall column-like cells with whiplike fingers called cilia that protrude into the tracheal space. They extend through the larger airways to the respiratory bronchioles.

Embedded in the walls of the large airways are cells and glands that secrete mucus and other semi-liquids. These continue through the terminal bronchioles. Between them, the cilia and the secreting glands lubricate and cleanse the bronchial tree. Mucus is moved by the millions of cilia, beating rhythmically together to form a constantly moving "escalator" that sweeps mucus up from the respiratory bronchioles and alveoli to the throat, carrying along foreign substances that have made their way into the bronchial system. From the throat the mucus is swallowed or expectorated as sputum.

The escalator of cilia does not extend to the smaller air sacs. A system of cells known as macrophages protects and cleans at this level. Debris or infectious agents that escape the cilia brigade are engulfed by macrophages and removed to the lymphatic system to be filtered away.

The larger airways contain a layer of smooth muscle that progressively thins and discontinues near the peripheral airways. This smooth muscle is controlled by the autonomic (involuntary) nervous system. Its normal function is unclear but it plays a major role in asthma.

Inside the Lung

The interior wall of the lung has a surface like a sponge. It is composed of more than 300 million tiny alveoli, each scarcely more than a pinhead in diameter, and each open to the atmosphere at one end. The combined surface area of these sacs is so great that if they were flattened out, they would cover a tennis court. The alveolar walls are only a single cell thick, and immediately beneath them, also encased in a wall of single-cell thickness, is the capillary bed of the lungs.

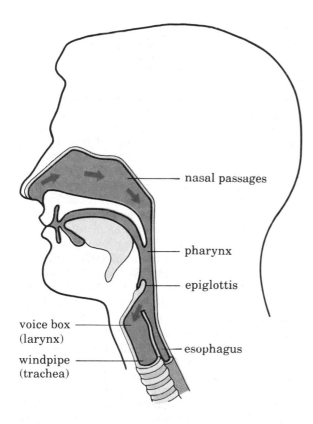

nasal passages

pharynx

epiglottis

voice box (larynx)

windpipe (trachea)

esophagus

THE PATHWAY OF AIR

Inhaled air is warmed and moistened in the nasal passages, then passes down the pharynx. The epiglottis, a kind of trapdoor, opens to permit air intake through the voice box (larynx) into the windpipe (trachea). It closes to confine swallowed food to the esophagus and to prevent it from entering the lungs.

thin layers of visceral pleura. Only a few cells constitute the barriers between lobes, yet the lobes are truly distinct and can be separated in the same way that one segment of an orange can be peeled from another. This is important if it becomes necessary to remove a portion of the lung by surgery.

Each of the five lobes is supplied by a lobar bronchus. The bronchi then branch further into segmental bronchi, ten on the right and nine on the left. The segmental bronchi continue to divide into smaller and smaller airways, finally narrowing to a millimeter or less in diameter, about the thickness of a broomstraw. There are 50 to 80 terminal bronchioles in each lobe, and each of them divides into two respiratory bronchioles. Each respiratory bronchiole further divides into two to eleven alveolar ducts. Finally, clustered like grapes on each duct, are tiny pouchlike air sacs called alveoli. It is here that the vital gas transfer takes place.

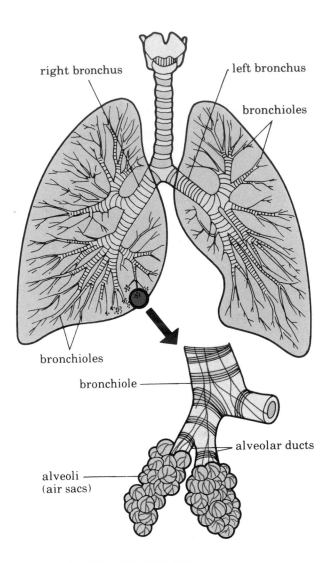

right bronchus

left bronchus

bronchioles

bronchioles

bronchiole

alveolar ducts

alveoli
(air sacs)

INSIDE THE LUNGS

The bronchial tree (top drawing) actually does resemble a tree and its branches. Right and left bronchi enter the respective lungs, then branch into smaller and smaller air tubes called bronchioles, which are much more numerous than shown. The lower drawing is a greatly magnified closeup of the tiniest bronchioles and alveolar ducts which terminate in the alveoli, blind globular air sacs. The bronchioles and alveolar ducts contain smooth muscle. The millions of alveoli are microscopic air cells where the important work of gas exchange takes place. A thin sheet of moving blood picks up oxygen from air in the alveoli and deposits carbon dioxide to be exhaled from the body.

Here in these millions of microscopic junction points the respiratory and circulatory systems come within a postage stamp's thickness of each other and make their important trade. The critical capillary vessels are so small in diameter that there is only room for the red blood cells to flow in single file. They are packed so densely around each alveolus that they resemble a moving sheet of blood more than a collection of blood-containing vessels.

There is a physical principle in the universe called the law of diffusion, and the trade that takes place in the alveoli is one of its outstanding applications. The law of diffusion states that particles move from areas of heavy concentration to areas of lesser concentration. There is such a small amount of carbon dioxide in the fresh air we take into our lungs that carbon dioxide carried in the blood moves readily across the capillary and alveolar walls and into the lungs to be exhaled into the atmosphere. Meanwhile, oxygen makes the opposite trip, diffusing through the walls into the oxygen-depleted capillary blood. Entering the capillary bed, the blood is dusky in color, oxygen-poor and carbon dioxide-rich. Leaving the capillaries it is bright red, oxygen-filled, and ready to be pumped by the heart to every cell of the body.

A remarkable substance in the blood called hemoglobin (see chapter 6, "The Blood") plays a critical role in this process. Hemoglobin has the important ability to bind oxygen molecules to itself and transport them through the bloodstream. And it can receive carbon dioxide and bring it to the lungs to be discarded.

How We Breathe

In the musical comedy *My Fair Lady,* Professor Henry Higgins sang of the two phases of respiration: "Breathing in and breathing out." Technically, these are known as inspiration and expiration. We commonly use the terms "inhale" and "exhale" instead.

Inspiration is accomplished by muscular activity of the chest wall and diaphragm. The chest wall muscles are attached to the ribs in such a way that their contraction causes the chest to enlarge to hold more air. The diaphragm is dome-shaped interwoven sheaths of muscle fibers attached to the inner circumference of the lower ribs. These muscles also separate the chest and abdominal cavities. When the diaphragm contracts, the domes flatten, and the volume of the thorax increases. The chest wall and diaphragm thus act like a bellows. As the chest cavity enlarges, the enclosed lungs also must expand, bringing in air

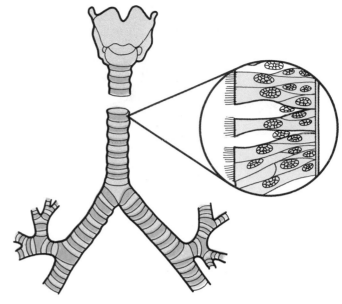

CLEANSING THE LUNGS

Billions of hair-like cilia (seen in the closeup) sweep bacteria and other foreign bodies from the respiratory tract by rhythmically beating back and forth, moving like a field of grain in a light breeze. Air passages are lined with cilia, which form a kind of escalator to move material up and out.

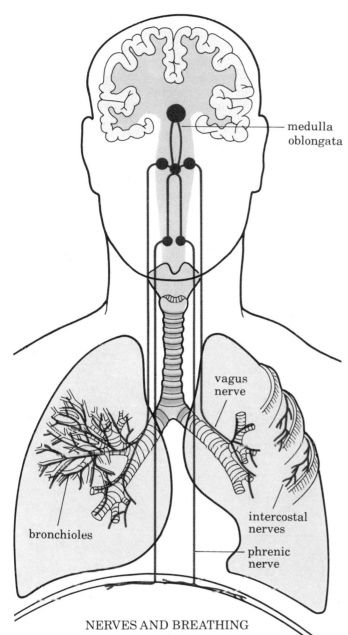

NERVES AND BREATHING

Respiration is controlled by the nervous system, as the schematic drawing shows. Excessive carbon dioxide in the blood triggers the breathing control center in the medulla oblongata. This portion of the brain sends out nerve impulses that cause us to inhale automatically. The phrenic nerve to the diaphragm is the principal nerve of breathing. Branches of the vagus nerve regulate contraction and relaxation of bronchioles in the lungs. The intercostal nerves control muscles that elevate ribs. The connections are much more complex than in this simplified drawing.

through the nose and mouth, down the trachea, into the bronchi and small airways, and ultimately into each of the alveoli.

Expiration is quite different, the result of an important quality of lung tissue known as elasticity. Like rubber, the lungs resist stretching. But when stretched and then released, they snap back to their original configuration. Inspiration stretches the lungs. As the diaphragm and chest wall relax after inspiration, the lung is free to settle back to its "resting" position. As it does, it expels the air that entered during inspiration. Expiration is a passive occurrence. It does not depend on muscle activity, but only on the recoil of elastic lung tissue. Under circumstances of disease or heavy normal exertion, however, several "accessory" groups of muscles, including rib and abdominal muscles, are called on to assist in expiration.

How breathing is regulated. The continuous and largely involuntary breathing cycle is under the control of the nervous system. We can temporarily override that system to speed up breathing or hold our breath, but ultimately the nervous system takes over again.

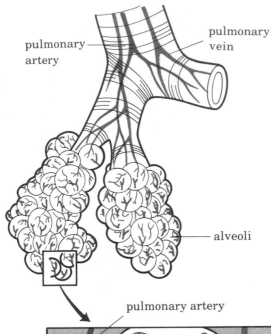

pulmonary artery

pulmonary vein

alveoli

The respiratory control center in the brain stem receives a variety of signals conveyed via nerves from sensors strategically located in muscles, arteries, and lung tissue.

The levels of oxygen and carbon dioxide in blood are the primary factors that regulate rate and depth of breathing. Nerve cells sensitive to the concentration of the gases in blood are located in at least two large arteries of the body—the aorta (leaving the heart) and carotid arteries (supplying the brain). Elevated carbon dioxide and depressed oxygen levels are sensed and relayed to the respiratory control center. The response is more or fewer impulses to the respiratory muscles, which in turn increase or decrease rate and depth of breathing according to the need. Exercise calls for increased oxygen and decreased carbon dioxide, while sleep requires the opposite. The respiratory center observes a normal "awake but resting" rhythm during most of the less active period of the day.

The same arterial sensors also respond to acid levels in the blood. Small increases in acid greatly increase breathing. Another factor that affects the breathing rate is the degree of stretch in respiratory muscles and lung tissue.

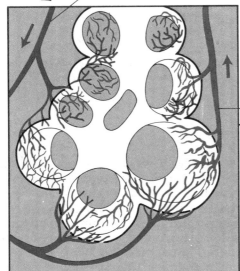

pulmonary artery

pulmonary vein

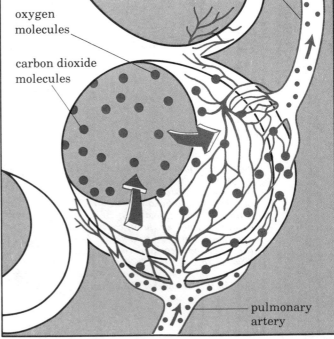

oxygen molecules

carbon dioxide molecules

pulmonary vein

pulmonary artery

THE GAS EXCHANGE

The heart of respiration is shown in these three drawings. At top, the pulmonary artery brings blood loaded with carbon dioxide from the veins to the alveoli. The pulmonary vein returns it, enriched by oxygen, to the heart. The middle drawing shows the microscopic blood vessels in the thin walls of the air-filled alveoli. Bottom drawing of an air cell shows how oxygen molecules diffuse into the blood and carbon dioxide molecules diffuse out of it.

Testing the Lungs

The lungs are hidden from direct view, but physicians have several methods of determining how efficiently they are functioning or why they are malfunctioning. These techniques range from taking a simple medical history to space-age optical instruments that can look deep into the lung itself. Here are the most common and most important:

Radiography. The chest X ray holds an unusual place in diagnosis and treatment. Today we take X rays for granted, but innovations in chest radiography have revolutionized the subject. A considerable number of lung diseases are detectable on X-ray film long before they give rise to symptoms. Lung cancer, for example, often is discovered on chest X ray taken for unrelated conditions. Moreover, X ray is frequently the most useful way to follow the course of many chest diseases. There is no better method of monitoring antibiotic therapy for pneumonia or the shrinkage of a lung tumor following drug therapy.

Chest X-ray technique has been simplified and made safer with recent advances in equipment. The principle of radiology is much like that of photography except that X-ray beams are much more potent than unmodified sunlight. Instead of bouncing off objects, they penetrate all but the densest substances, such as lead. The chest X ray is taken by having the patient place his or her chest next to a photographic plate. The patient sometimes stands, sometimes lies flat, depending on the view wanted. The X-ray beam is then briefly directed at the chest. The beam penetrates the chest and continues until it reaches the photographic plate. The different chest tissues, such as the lung, chest wall, heart, and bone, block the X rays to varying degrees. These show up on developed film as shadows of different density.

A skilled radiologist can read a great deal from a chest X ray. The film can sharply outline the bones, the size and contour of the heart, scarred and calcified lesions from former infections, lymph glands, branching of blood vessels out to their finest ramifications, levels of the diaphragm, excessive breathing and lung volume in emphysema, deposits characterized by occupational exposure, and many more details. As useful as the chest

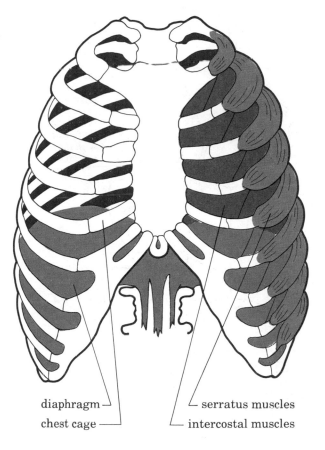

diaphragm — serratus muscles
chest cage — intercostal muscles

MUSCLES OF BREATHING

Contraction of the diaphragm is the basis of breathing. It causes the chest cage to expand, and thus the lungs, held to the chest's inner surface, must also expand. The intercostal muscles between the ribs and the serratus muscles arising from the ribs help the contraction and expansion, but most of the work is done by the diaphragm.

X ray is, it is not without risk (see chapter 32, "X Rays and Radiology"). To minimize this risk, X rays should be taken only by those intimately familiar with radiographic techniques, only with the newest equipment, and only when there is a valid indication of need. It has become clear that the risks of radiation are cumulative. The total lifetime accumulation is what determines ultimate toxicity. Unfortunately such toxicity is frequently displayed as the development of cancer. Until recently it was not uncommon to see chest X rays offered to healthy, asymptomatic, nonsmoking individuals to search for tumors or infections. This is now deplored because of the unnecessary radiation administered and because such screening does not turn up enough disease to justify its cost.

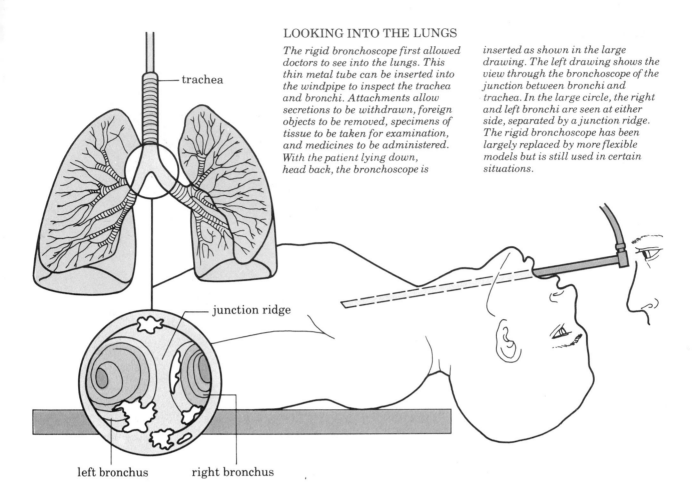

LOOKING INTO THE LUNGS

The rigid bronchoscope first allowed doctors to see into the lungs. This thin metal tube can be inserted into the windpipe to inspect the trachea and bronchi. Attachments allow secretions to be withdrawn, foreign objects to be removed, specimens of tissue to be taken for examination, and medicines to be administered. With the patient lying down, head back, the bronchoscope is inserted as shown in the large drawing. The left drawing shows the view through the bronchoscope of the junction between bronchi and trachea. In the large circle, the right and left bronchi are seen at either side, separated by a junction ridge. The rigid bronchoscope has been largely replaced by more flexible models but is still used in certain situations.

trachea

junction ridge

left bronchus   right bronchus

Computerized tomography (see chapter 32) now offers a refinement of the chest X ray. It involves minutely scanning the lungs "slice by slice," feeding standard photographed images into a computer for reassembly and analysis through a series of cross-section views. With greater refinement and precision, these computerized axial tomogram scans (CAT scans) sharply separate and delineate the chest structures.

Bronchoscopy. Perfected at the beginning of the 20th century, the bronchoscope for the first time enabled a physician to see inside the respiratory system. This rigid, illuminated, pencil-thick tube, equipped with a magnifying eyepiece at one end, is passed through the mouth into the trachea for direct examination of the larynx, trachea, and central bronchi. Bronchoscopy usually is done under local or general anesthesia. The patient is seated or lying down with head tilted back to straighten the line of the pharynx and windpipe to receive

the instrument like a sword-swallower. The technique allows closer inspection of abnormalities detected on X rays, the investigation of bleeding from the lungs, or removal of objects aspirated into the lungs.

Since the 1960s the rigid bronchoscope has been supplemented by an even more delicate instrument of Japanese invention. It converts the rigid hollow metal cylinder into a thin, flexible, and malleable tube, but retains the light source and an optical system capable of projecting an image around a twisting path. The thousands of tiny fibers compacted in a fiberoptic bronchoscope a centimeter in diameter extend the physician's range to the outer reaches of the lungs. A system of wires and pulleys enables the top of the scope to turn in two directions. Smaller instruments can be threaded into the tube to allow for irrigation, suction, delivery of oxygen or medication, or to snip tissue for microscopic examination, all under the safety of direct visual examination. With the flexible fiberoptiscope, general anesthesia is rarely necessary, and even the very ill can tolerate passage of the tiny tube through the nose or mouth with little discomfort and without contorting the neck.

Biopsy. For a precise diagnosis of a suspected lung problem, it may be necessary to obtain tissue for microscopic examination. This is accomplished by open chest surgery, usually a short incision between two ribs, under general anesthesia. The procedure normally is safe, except for patients with chronic lung or heart disease. "Needle" biopsy—inserting a long cutting needle through the skin, between the ribs, and into the lung—also is used to obtain tissue. The procedure involves little discomfort because the lung itself cannot feel pain.

Thoracentesis. The parietal pleura lining the inner wall of the thorax and the visceral pleura lining the lung normally are in direct contact with each another. Sometimes, fluid accumulates between these membranes, moving the lung away from the chest wall. The fluid may be removed by inserting a needle through the skin and chest wall under local anesthesia, a procedure known as thoracentesis. Special needles can drain fluid and sever a piece of pleural membrane for microscopic examination, important in suspected tuberculosis and cancer. Accumulated fluid, although usually painless, always indicates an abnormal condition, so it is important to drain the fluid and find its cause.

THE FIBEROPTIC "SCOPE"

Simpler bronchoscopy is possible with a flexible fiberoptic device capable of projecting an enlarged image around a twisting path. The equipment necessary for fiberoptic bronchoscopy includes the scope, a portable light source, and local anesthetics to make the process painless. The patient remains awake as the bronchoscope is inserted through the nose. Sometimes the passage of the tube causes a patient to cough, but usually is not painful.

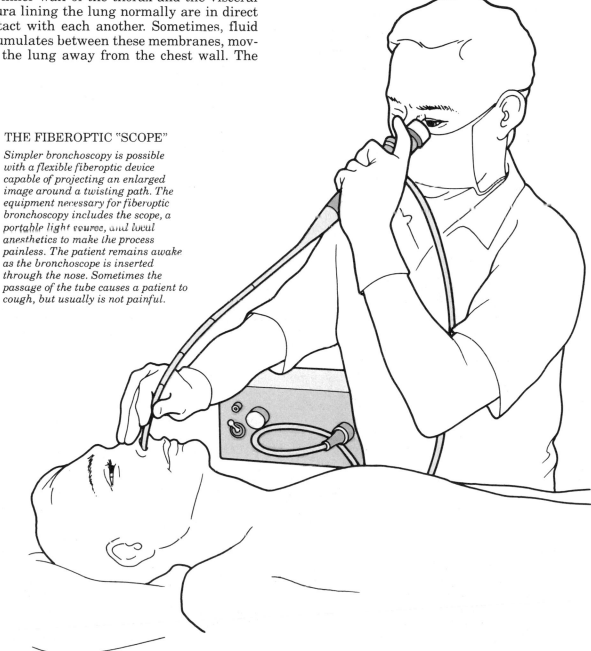

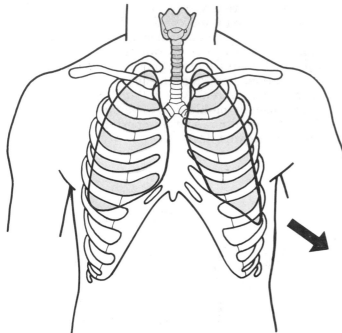

THORACENTESIS

A variety of diseases cause fluid to accumulate in the pleural cavity. An important procedure in such cases is the removal of the fluid for diagnosis and therapy. This is done with a hollow needle (lower right) and is known as thoracentesis.

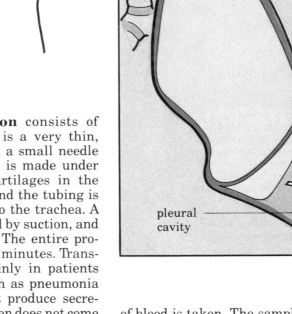

pleural
cavity

Transtracheal aspiration consists of threading a catheter, which is a very thin, flexible plastic tube, through a small needle into the trachea. A puncture is made under local anesthesia between cartilages in the neck just below the larynx, and the tubing is threaded a short distance into the trachea. A specimen of mucus is obtained by suction, and the tube is removed quickly. The entire procedure requires less than five minutes. Transtracheal suction is used mainly in patients suffering from infections such as pneumonia and tuberculosis who cannot produce secretions by coughing. The specimen does not come into contact with the pharynx or oral cavity, which normally contain other germs that can confuse diagnosis.

Pulmonary function tests. Since the ultimate task of respiration is to deliver oxygen to the cells via the circulatory system and carry away carbon dioxide, sampling the blood offers the best gauge of how efficiently the lungs are performing.

The arterial blood-gas test measures dissolved gases and acidity in a sample of arterial blood. As recently as 1960, drawing blood from the arteries was considered a radical procedure. In reality it is relatively free of pain and complications, because the arterial system can seal itself immediately after a small, clean puncture. A needle is simply inserted into the artery at the wrist or midarm where the blood vessels can be seen clearly, and about an ounce

of blood is taken. The sample is then exposed to special electrodes that analyze it for oxygen, carbon dioxide, and acid content. The levels of each indicate the efficiency of oxygen delivery and carbon dioxide removal.

Other common tests of pulmonary function include the measurements of lung volumes and timed expiratory volumes. Lung volumes are measured either by filling the lungs with the inert gas helium (by having the patient inhale it from a tank) or by having the patient breathe while seated in an airtight compartment called a plethysmograph or body box. Measurements are made with the patient sealed in the box, which is similar to a telephone booth. Although they are safe, body boxes frighten some patients, which limits their use.

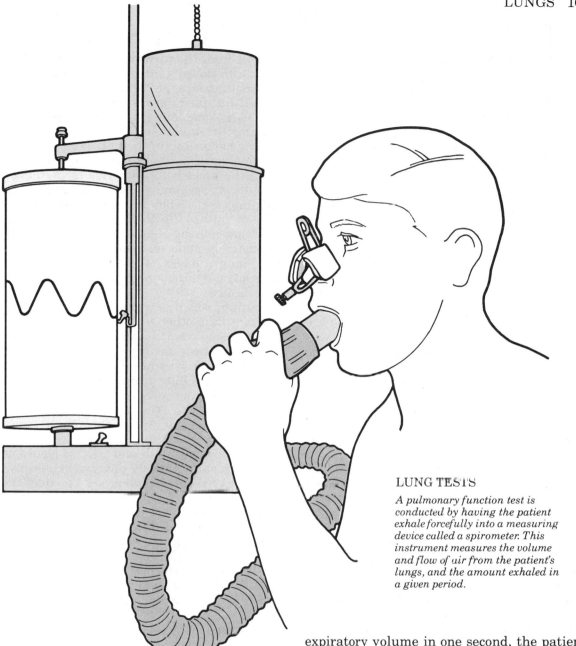

LUNG TESTS

A pulmonary function test is conducted by having the patient exhale forcefully into a measuring device called a spirometer. This instrument measures the volume and flow of air from the patient's lungs, and the amount exhaled in a given period.

The most important measurements of lung volume are tidal volume, vital capacity, residual volume, and total lung capacity.

Tidal volume represents the amount of gas moved during each cycle of inhalation and exhalation while the person is resting. Vital capacity and residual volume are measured by fully expanding the lungs with air and then expelling it as completely as possible. The volume exhaled is the vital capacity; the amount remaining in the lung is the residual volume. Total lung volume is the sum of the vital capacity and the residual volume.

These values are determined by a spirometer, which can also measure the amount exhaled in a given period. In the test for forced

expiratory volume in one second, the patient fills the lungs and then blows the air out as rapidly as possible. The amount expelled in the first full second is measured and recorded. The amount exhaled at other intervals can also be timed. The time required for total expiration is also a useful measurement. Measurements of forced flow are particularly important in testing for obstructive categories of lung disease (see page 172).

The flow-volume curve, a less routine test, helps to disclose obstructions of the larynx, trachea, and large airways. The test is made by comparing air flow from the mouth with simultaneously measured lung volume.

Symptoms of Lung Disease

When the lungs are not functioning properly, the most common symptom is breathlessness, technically known as dyspnea. The feeling of "not getting enough air" is the most prominent feature of lung disease, but it is not limited to lung problems. Dyspnea also may be present in disorders of the heart, blood, muscles, and nervous system.

Why people feel breathless is not known. Apparently, some undefined mechanism enables the body to recognize when its lungs are not supplying enough oxygen, causing a lag in metabolism that can result in frightening symptoms. Surprisingly, a person's sensation of breathlessness might not match how efficiently the lungs are functioning, as documented by lung tests. Moreover, the level of lung trouble that produces breathlessness varies from individual to individual. Persons who display the same degree of abnormality on tests may differ widely in degree of disability or distress.

In the condition known as primary hyperventilation, patients experience breathlessness, yet no underlying lung disease can be detected. They gulp air in deep, rapid breaths until acid and mineral levels in the blood become disturbed and produce numbness and tingling of the lips, muscle spasms, dizziness, and fainting. The so-called hyperventilation syndrome appears to be a psychological problem, and there are indications it runs in families. The best treatment appears to be reassurance and psychiatric counseling.

Cough is one of the most common human symptoms. Everyone coughs intermittently or chronically. But like breathlessness, cough is not always an indication of lung disease. It can be triggered by conditions ranging from a bad cold to the aftermath of a hearty bout of laughter.

A cough is primarily a defensive weapon against an irritating or infective environment. The throat, trachea, and large airways are studded with nerves sensitive to irritation. When stimulated by infection or an airborne irritant, these nerves send impulses to the cough center of the brain. The message to cough is relayed to the muscles that produce the cough, primarily those of expiration, especially in the abdominal wall. The cough mechanism is a forceful expiration against a closed upper airway. Pressure builds behind the closure, until a sudden release results in a high-velocity expulsion of air, not unlike the controlled explosion that occurs in the barrel of a gun. The throat-clearing blast loosens secretions from the airways and propels them, along with the irritant, out of the airway into the mouth to be expectorated.

Sputum, the mixture of mucus, pus, cellular debris, and other material expelled in clearing the throat, tells many tales about what is happening in the respiratory system. Its color, consistency, and odor all provide hints about the underlying condition of the lungs. Samples of sputum are vital in diagnosing lung infections. They are studied microscopically or cultured in the laboratory in search of disease-causing organisms, or examined for distinctively abnormal cells that could indicate lung tumors. Blood in the sputum (hemoptysis) frequently indicates serious lung disease.

Sputum, which originates in the lungs, is different from other secretions such as saliva or postnasal drip. Its occasional presence in a cough is not necessarily a sign of lung disease. But the chronic presence of cough with sputum *is* a warning of lung disorders.

Chest pain is not necessarily an indicator of lung disease. The skin, muscles, bones of the chest, the heart, or the esophagus can cause the pain. The parietal pleura is highly pain-sensitive, but the lungs and visceral pleura do not sense pain. Various pulmonary diseases can attack the parietal pleura and produce the pains of pleurisy, a sharp localized chest pain that worsens with coughing, sneezing, or deep breathing. To avert the pain many persons voluntarily restrict or "splint" their breathing on the affected side. In cases of deep, burning chest pain under the breastbone, the culprit is usually inflammation of the trachea, a common accompaniment of influenza.

Respiratory Assistance

When disease-weakened lungs are not strong enough to supply oxygen and eliminate carbon dioxide, and thus not strong enough to sustain life, a machine must help out. There are several types of breathing-assistance equipment to help keep respiration going during this crucial period.

The essential requirement of breathing assistance is an airtight connection between the trachea and the gas source, which may provide room air, oxygen-enriched air, or pure oxygen.

The seal is made by either of two methods. In endotracheal intubation a flexible tube is inserted into the trachea through the mouth or nose. The inner tip is surrounded by a doughnut-shaped rubber balloon. When inflated, the balloon firmly anchors the tube and seals it into an airtight system. The second method, surgical tracheostomy, consists of inserting a short tube into the trachea through a small slit in the neck. The incision is usually just above the breastbone. Here, too, an inflated balloon anchors the tube and makes an airtight junction with the trachea.

If breathing support appears to be required for only a short time (as with acute, severe pneumonia), endotracheal intubation is preferred over tracheostomy. On the other hand, endotracheal intubation for more than five to seven days can cause pressure damage to the larynx or tracheal wall. Because the tube passes between the vocal cords and makes direct contact with them, voice changes can occur. Furthermore, the endotracheal tube makes swallowing difficult and is uncomfortable for an alert patient.

Once the tube is in place, it is attached to a ventilator. The machine drives gas into the lungs during inspiration and allows it to escape during expiration. Commonly used ventilator models deliver oxygen-enriched gas while a triggering device permits the patient to breathe at his own tempo. The pace can be regulated for the individual patient.

A new mechanism can deliver oxygen to the less-ill patient. The air we breathe contains 21 percent oxygen. It is possible to adjust the concentration from 21 to 100 percent. For certain patients who don't need hospitalization, it can be delivered by a portable system using a loose fitting plastic face mask or double-pronged plastic tubing inserted into the nostrils. A lightweight oxygen container is slung from the shoulder like a purse. The amount of oxygen is tailored to the body's need during exertion. Portable oxygen has allowed ill persons previously sentenced to a bed or chair to lead a near-normal life.

Despite its central role in pulmonary care, oxygen is not a cure-all. If given for long periods at high concentrations, it can damage lung tissue and other body organs. In emphysema or chronic bronchitis patients, oxygen can depress respiration or further aggravate respiratory failure. For this reason physicians prescribe oxygen with the same care that they prescribe drugs.

A special form of physical therapy also is used to assist breathing. Doctors call it postural drainage with percussion. During infections, the lung often cannot clear itself of secretions. The physician may then lower the patient's head, elevate the feet, or tilt the body into various positions with the aid of props and pillows to drain the lungs by force of gravity. He supplements these changes of posture with percussion, clapping the chest wall by hand or with a mechanical vibrator to loosen the secretions clogging the airways.

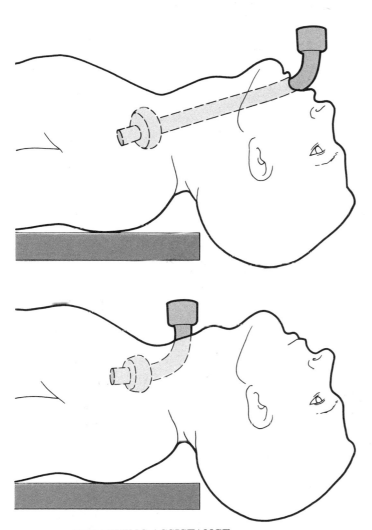

BREATHING ASSISTANCE

When disease-weakened lungs are not strong enough for normal respiration, a machine must help. Two methods of providing an airtight connection to a breathing-assistance device are shown. In endotracheal intubation (top) a flexible tube is inserted into the trachea through the mouth or nose. In surgical tracheostomy (below) the tube is inserted through a slit in the neck. Endotracheal intubation is preferred for short periods. Tracheostomy is used when aid is needed for a week or more.

PORTABLE OXYGEN AND AEROSOL MEDICATION

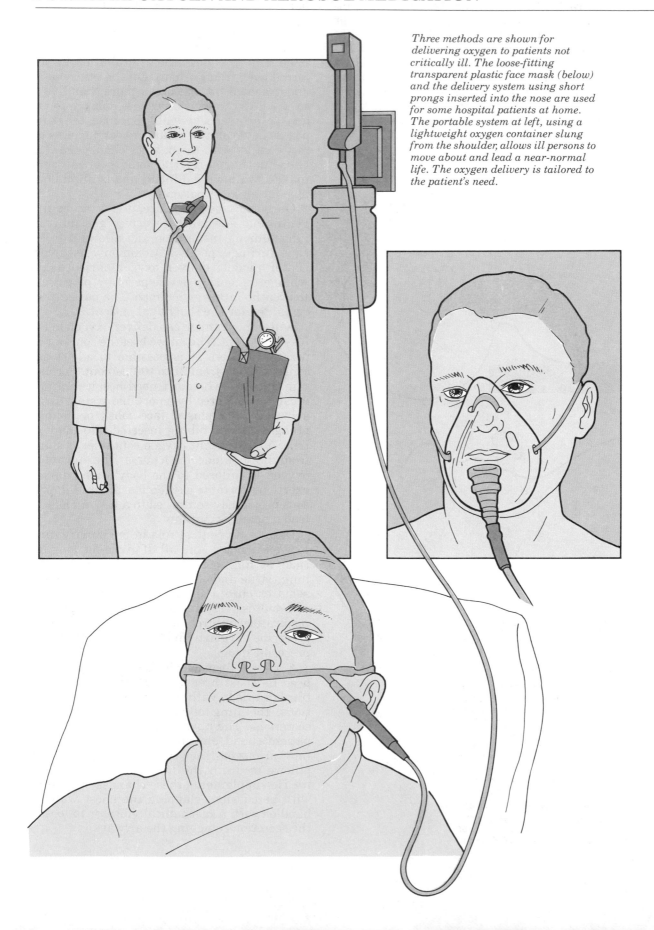

Three methods are shown for delivering oxygen to patients not critically ill. The loose-fitting transparent plastic face mask (below) and the delivery system using short prongs inserted into the nose are used for some hospital patients at home. The portable system at left, using a lightweight oxygen container slung from the shoulder, allows ill persons to move about and lead a near-normal life. The oxygen delivery is tailored to the patient's need.

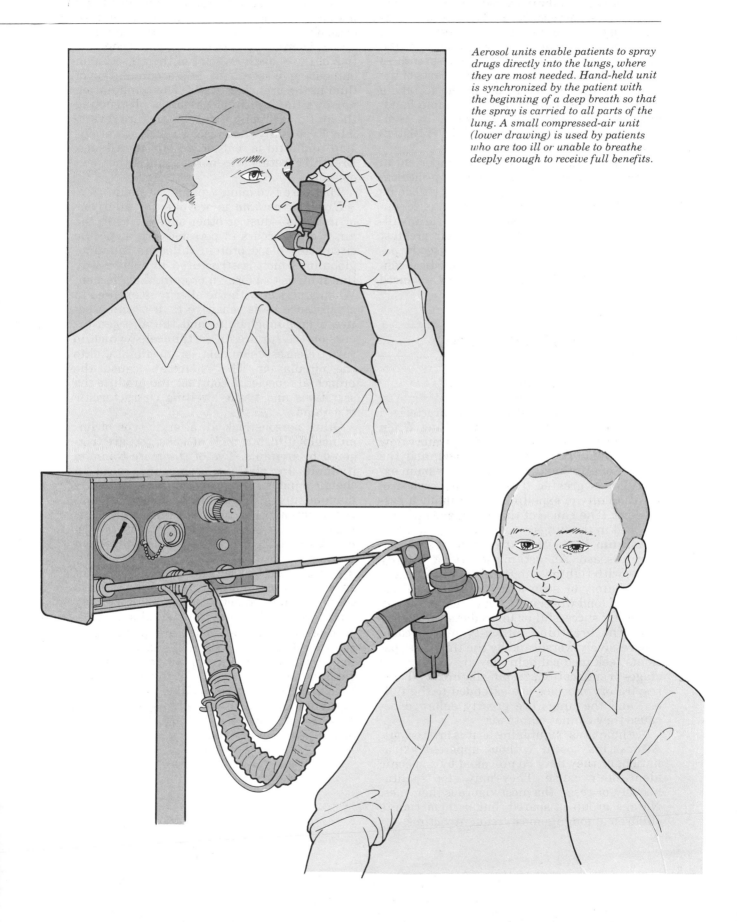

Aerosol units enable patients to spray drugs directly into the lungs, where they are most needed. Hand-held unit is synchronized by the patient with the beginning of a deep breath so that the spray is carried to all parts of the lung. A small compressed-air unit (lower drawing) is used by patients who are too ill or unable to breathe deeply enough to receive full benefits.

Drugs can be administered directly into the lung with an aerosol spray. The simplest supplies a jet of air pumped by a hand-held bulb. The patient synchronizes the squeeze of the bulb with the beginning of a deep breath so that the drug is carried to distant parts of the lung. For persons too ill or unable to take a breath deep enough to use the simple hand-held device, aerosol units driven by compressed air or by small artificial ventilators are substituted.

Aerosol drugs are particularly important in asthma because the muscle-relaxing medication can be placed directly where it will do its job with minimal side effects. Pocket-size containers of aerosol anti-asthma drugs are available and extremely effective. Their greatest disadvantage is that they are overused by patients who panic or try to delay medical consultation, which can lead to a more advanced attack.

DISEASES OF THE LUNG

Obstructive Lung Diseases

Obstructive lung diseases are characterized by resistance to air flow within the lung. When tested, victims show low forced expiratory flow and volume. The lung is enlarged, and the volume of air remaining after a maximum exhalation is greater than normal because of the difficulty of expelling air, normally a passive act. The cause of the enlargement is air trapped in the lungs.

Asthma is the most treatable obstructive lung disease. An asthmatic attack usually starts with tightness in the chest and a cough, immediately or soon followed by breathlessness and loud wheezing. Home treatment may be totally successful or unpredictably ineffective. The breathing difficulty may become progressively worse, and by the time most patients seek medical help they are in the early stages of suffocation, gasping for breath. Their respiratory muscles are extended to the fullest, and the lungs are greatly enlarged because they cannot empty air.

Asthma is as frightening as it is mysterious. Attacks may occur without apparent explanation, or they may be provoked by a specific identifiable cause. They may stop spontaneously, or resist the most vigorous therapies. No age group is spared, but asthma counts children among its most frequent victims.

Asthma is caused by intermittent dramatic increases in the lung's resistance to air flow (see chapter 21, "Allergy and the Immune System"). There are three main reasons: contraction of the smooth muscles of the airways, an outpouring of secretions, and accumulation of fluid in the bronchial walls. The combination narrows the bronchial passages, obstructing the air flow. Happily, these changes are reversible. Eventually the muscles relax, secretions stop, and fluid is reabsorbed into the tissues. Breathing returns to normal until the next episode.

There are two main types of asthma:

• *Extrinsic asthma* is provoked by allergens or irritants—dust or other substances in the air. It often occurs in persons with a specific circulating blood protein called an immunoglobulin, which is structured in such a way that it binds to a foreign protein, the allergen. When a person with the allergy is exposed to a substance he is sensitive to, a reaction between immunoglobulin and the allergen occurs on the surfaces of certain cells, which in turn releases chemicals, or mediators, into the circulation. The chemicals cause the bronchial muscles to contract and produce the secretions and tissue swelling characteristic of asthma.

Other persons lack an allergic type of immunoglobulin, but their attacks, too, are triggered by irritants. Two of the more common irritants are platinum compounds used in chemical industries and by-products of plastics manufacturing. Muscle contraction and mucus secretion occur, but the exact sequence is unclear. It is possible the irritants act on nerves that trigger a reflex muscle contraction in the airways.

• *Intrinsic asthma* appears to occur without an external asthma-provoking irritant. It is possible that the reaction is caused by a poorly understood, hidden environmental substance or represents airways that are particularly sensitive to a combination of substances. Intrinsic asthma is more common in adults than children and is more difficult to treat. Its victims sometimes have grapelike growths in the nasal lining (called nasal polyps), and attacks may be worsened by use of aspirin and other anti-inflammatory drugs.

The chief difference between an asthma victim and others is that the asthmatic's air passages are unusually sensitive. Many of us have minor breathing difficulty in smoggy air or when dust or other irritants are stirred up, but the magnitude of this difficulty is small compared to that of persons with asthma.

The view that the asthmatic's air passages are different is supported by the fact that even everyday events lead to attacks. Emotional crises have long been known to induce asthma. It is now known that cold temperatures and exercise do, too. Interestingly, certain types of activity are more likely to trigger an attack than others. Running, for example, is more asthma-producing than swimming. Respiratory infections also appear to underlie asthmatic attacks. Even non-asthmatics apparently have more sensitive airways for several weeks following viral infections.

The treatment of asthma has recently made great strides. Drugs that relax airways, known as bronchodilators, are the mainstay. They can be administered orally or in aerosol form by the victims themselves in mild or moderate attacks. When the attack is severe, the drugs are given intravenously. The major side effects of bronchodilators are nervousness and gastrointestinal upsets, but these usually respond to adjustments in dosage.

The anti-inflammatory drugs called corticosteroids also are effective, but they cause serious complications if given in large, prolonged doses. However, corticosteroids can be obtained in aerosol form and sprayed directly into the lungs, bypassing organs where side effects commonly occur. Chromalyn sodium, a powder which can be inhaled into the lung, also stabilizes the cells responsible for secreting the chemicals that indirectly cause attacks of asthma.

For persons whose attacks are triggered by a known allergen, avoiding exposure to the allergen is obviously desirable. When this is not possible, hyposensitization injections (to pollens, dusts, foods) may be useful, especially in children. These injections are described in chapter 21. Despite asthma's discomfort, the outlook for asthmatics is good and their expected life-span is normal.

Bronchitis, an inflammation of the air passages of the lung, may result from acute infection, chemical irritation, or other causes. The most prevalent type, chronic bronchitis, is said to exist in anyone having cough and expectoration for at least three months a year for two consecutive years.

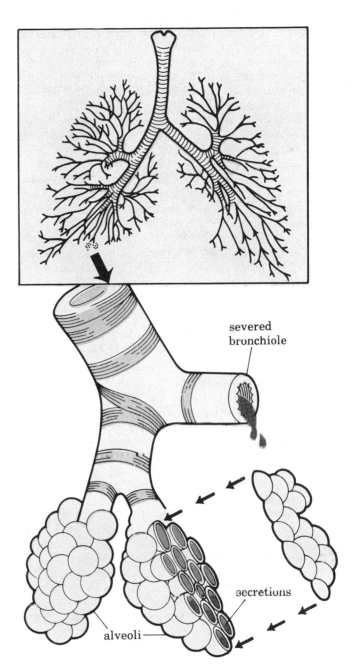

BRONCHITIS

Cough and spitting are characteristic symptoms of bronchitis. The closeup view of a section of the bronchial tree shows dripping from a cut-off bronchiole. The lower drawing, an exploded view of the alveoli, shows secretions in air cells that normally contain only air.

Many environmental substances cause bronchitis or make it more severe, but cigarette smoking is overwhelmingly the most important. In fact, many bronchitis victims diagnose their problem, calling their condition "smoker's cough." Chronic bronchitis occasionally does arise in certain industries and occupations, but even here its victims are primarily smokers.

Like asthma, the underlying problem in bronchitis is obstructed air flow. Unlike asthma, however, the obstruction is caused mainly by greatly increased mucus secretion because of irritation and thickened bronchial wall linings. Unfortunately, these problems are considerably less reversible than asthma's muscle contraction. Bronchitis victims are especially vulnerable to infection because the overabundant secretions are fertile soil for bacterial growth. Once established, infection initiates a vicious cycle by increasing the secretions which, in turn, favor bacterial growth.

Cough and sputum are the prime symptoms of chronic bronchitis. The cough is most prominent in the early morning. Normal pulmonary secretions are scant, clear, and watery; the sputum ("phlegm") in bronchitis is thick and cloudy. As the disease progresses, shortness of breath appears, first during exertion and later at rest, too. A late and serious complication is heart failure caused by the increased work necessary to pump blood through a severely diseased lung with reduced blood oxygen. Cough and sputum increase during episodes of infection. In advanced cases, these episodes overwhelm the lungs' reserves and lead to respiratory failure. The patient may need mechanical breathing help until the acute infection subsides.

Therapeutically, the greatest benefit occurs if the patient stops smoking. Cough and sputum production diminish and may cease. Other treatment is directed at preventing infection and providing breathing support. At the first sign of increased cough or "phlegm" many physicians prescribe oral antibiotics and use physical measures to loosen secretions. Bronchodilators are of less benefit than they are in treating asthma.

Emphysema takes its name from the Greek word for "inflation." Like other obstructive lung diseases it is characterized by greatly enlarged lungs. It is an increasingly common disease, one that strikes many more men than women, especially those between 50 and 70 years of age.

The first symptom of emphysema is progressively worsening breathlessness. Cough is typical, wheezing less so. There is litle sputum. At first the lungs are of normal size, but gradually they enlarge to great dimensions.

Tests reveal breathing obstruction, but the cause is different than in asthma or bronchitis. Emphysema destroys so much tissue that the lung loses its normal stiffness and air passages have a tendency to collapse from lack of support. The tendency is most pronounced on exhaling. In forced expiration the airways may close completely, causing increased resistance to flow and trapping air in the lungs.

The breathing difficulty of emphysema results from lung destruction and scarring, primarily in the branches of the airways that end in the respiratory bronchiole and the alveolar sacs, a single unit of which is known as the acinus. Panacinar (throughout the acinus) emphysema affects mainly the alveoli, whereas centrilobular emphysema (involving the central acinus) predominantly destroys the bronchiole itself, which lies at the center of the acinus. Paraseptal emphysema attacks lung tissue at the outer edge of the lung just under the pleural surface. In all three, destruction is complete, involving both alveolar tissue and blood vessels. The naked eye can detect the grossly empty spaces where tissue has been ravaged.

As in bronchitis, cigarette smoking is an unequivocal cause of emphysema. But the chance discovery in Scandinavia of a rare inherited protein disorder has led to a greater understanding of the background of emphysema. Most people have a level of an anti-enzyme in their blood that inhibits the action of the enzymes that dismantle structural proteins. This anti-enzyme is known as antitrypsin. In the 1960s patients with extremely low levels of antitrypsin were found to have an unusual incidence of emphysema. This was true even of young nonsmokers. It is known that the body's white blood cells contain large amounts of anti-protein enzymes. When there is infection in the lungs, large numbers of white cells are brought in to battle the bacteria. These white cells release anti-protein enzymes which break down the protein of the bacteria. Normally, the structural protein of

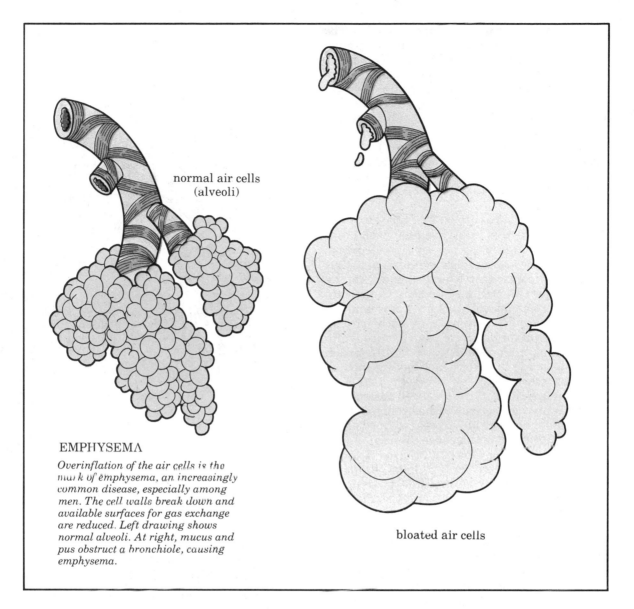

normal air cells
(alveoli)

bloated air cells

EMPHYSEMA

Overinflation of the air cells is the mark of emphysema, an increasingly common disease, especially among men. The cell walls break down and available surfaces for gas exchange are reduced. Left drawing shows normal alveoli. At right, mucus and pus obstruct a bronchiole, causing emphysema.

the lung is protected from harm by antitrypsin, which prevents white cell enzymes from destroying lung tissue. Without adequate antitrypsin, protection drops and repeated infections over the years gradually destroy lung tissue. How smoking is involved is unclear. It may hasten development of emphysema by promoting recurrent infection.

Severe antitrypsin deficiency is rare. It causes emphysema in less than one percent of the American population. The great majority of emphysema patients have no protein abnormality. For them smoking appears to be the predominant cause.

As with bronchitis, the first step in treatment is to stop smoking. Bronchodilators and antibiotics may make breathing easier. Some doctors prescribe exercises to teach victims to slow the respiratory rate. Persons who have emphysema are encouraged to remain active and to learn to deal with the disability rather than stay in bed.

One reason that treatment is similar for bronchitis and emphysema is that most patients have a combination of the two. Pure bronchitis or emphysema is the exception, not the rule. Some doctors make no attempt to differentiate between them, but lump the conditions together as "chronic obstructive lung disease," often shortened to COLD.

Cystic fibrosis is primarily a children's disease, the result of an inborn defect of the glands affecting the respiratory and digestive systems (see chapter 27, "Taking Care of Your Child"). Its symptoms frequently show up soon after birth. Mucus secreted by the lungs is abnormally thick and sticky, and cannot be cleared by the normal movement of cilia. The accumulated secretions are a breeding ground for recurrent bronchial infections. The digestive system is affected, too, because of inadequate secretion of digestive enzymes.

In past years, cystic fibrosis victims frequently died in infancy, weakened by repeated infections or succumbing to respiratory difficulties. Because of improved care, including breathing support, survival is steadily increasing. Research also has identified mild forms of the disease that do not become evident until adulthood.

Cystic fibrosis is treated similarly to other chronic obstructive lung diseases, with bronchodilators, antibiotics to quell infections, physical therapy, and breathing assistance. Research is concentrated on the genetics of the disease (see chapter 2, "Medical Genetics"). Cystic fibrosis qualifies as an autosomal recessive disorder, meaning that both parents are carriers of the defective gene but are symptom-free themselves. In affected families, each child has a one in four risk of having the disease at birth.

Bronchiectasis is the localized destruction and deformity of sections of the bronchial tree. The bronchi enlarge into a cigar-shaped or cylindrical form. Sometimes the ailment is limited to a segment or lobe of a lung, sometimes it occurs throughout both lungs. Bronchiectasis usually starts after childhood damage from serious pneumonia or another disease. Before immunization and antibiotics, whooping cough and tuberculosis were frequent culprits. Because of the decline of these diseases, bronchiectasis is now less common.

The two major symptoms of bronchiectasis are cough and heavy sputum production. Severe sufferers may cough 24 hours a day. More typically the cough is worse in the morning or after the victim shifts body position. Paroxysms of cough may raise ounces of foul-smelling, occasionally blood-streaked mucus and pus. In rare instances significant bleeding may occur suddenly. A routine X ray may show only outlines of the thickened bronchi, but if certain "opaque" dyes are injected into the airways, an abnormally filled tracheobronchial tree appears. The fiberoptic bronchoscope can be used to examine the airways directly.

Treatment aims to reduce the amount of sputum and remove that which remains. Antibiotics help to cut down infected secretions while drainage and percussion dislodge the thick sputum. In cases of persistent, serious bleeding, it is sometimes necessary to remove the affected area surgically.

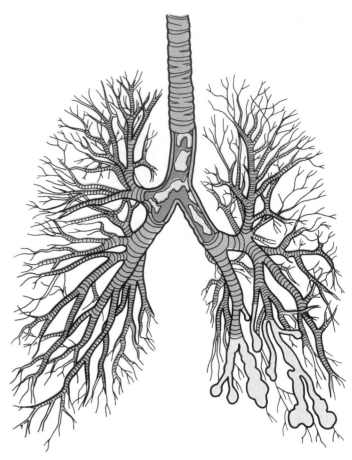

BRONCHIECTASIS

Destruction and deformity of bronchiectasis usually starts after childhood damage from serious pneumonia or other disease. Obstructive foreign bodies and infections that produce abscesses and pus also can be responsible. The dilated, pus-filled outpouchings of the diseased bronchial tree at right contrast sharply with the normal bronchial tree at left. Since development of immunization and antibiotics, bronchiectasis is much less common.

Restrictive Lung Diseases

Restrictive lung diseases are characterized by sharply reduced lung volumes. If the victim fully expands his lungs, both the amount he can exhale and the amount remaining in the lungs are abnormally low. Unlike obstructive diseases in which the lungs become enlarged, restrictive diseases reduce lung size. Forced expiratory flow is reduced, too, but in restrictive diseases, the percentage of air forcibly exhaled in one second remains normal—about

80 percent. In obstructive diseases, the one-second exhalation represents a significantly lowered fraction of the lungs' total volume. In restrictive disorders, too, diseases of the nerves, muscles, and chest walls, as well as the lungs themselves, can be responsible for breathing impairment.

Pulmonary fibrosis is a general term describing a thickening and deformity of the alveolar walls ("fibrous" tissue being the tissue of scars). It may arise from a virtually endless list of diseases: viral, bacterial, fungal, and parasitic infections, a large number of environmental and occupational pollutants, some forms of chronic heart disease, and several diseases of unknown origin.

Regardless of cause, in pulmonary fibrosis scar tissue replaces normally elastic lung tissue. The stiffer lung requires much more energy for expansion. Eventually, lung volumes shrink. By a mechanism not well understood, the body recognizes the increased work required to breathe and takes steps to limit the energy drain. The rate of breathing increases, but the amount of air moved in each breathing cycle decreases. As a consequence, patients in advanced stages of the disease appear to be panting even at rest.

The first signs of fibrosis are shortness of breath, dry cough, and a peculiar swelling of the tips of fingers and toes around the nail beds. This rounded swelling is called clubbing because of the club-like or spooned appearance. It occurs in other lung diseases and in congenital heart diseases. Listening to the lungs, a physician often hears "crackling" sounds, like cellophane being crumpled and uncrumpled. The chest X ray shows undersized lungs marked by small indistinct shadows representing thickened and scarred alveolar walls.

Many cases of fibrosis are of unknown origin (idiopathic) and research is aimed at identifying their cause. The only widely used medical treatment is the administration of anti-inflammatory drugs called corticosteroids, which are thought to limit scar formation. A significant percentage of patients treated with these drugs do show improved lung functions, especially in the early stages when tissue is more inflamed than scarred.

Nerve diseases. Proper breathing requires the muscular power of the chest wall and diaphragm, controlled by healthy nerves and muscles. Many disorders of the nervous system can impair these controls. Among diseases of the peripheral nerves affecting the respiratory muscles, perhaps the most notorious is the "ascending" paralysis of Guillain-Barre (the neurologic disease that occurred as a possible reaction to the swine influenza immunization program of 1976). Its consequences can be so severe that mechanical breathing assistance is required. Poliomyelitis is well-known to result in respiratory failure. Much of what is known about mechanical aids to respiration was learned during the "iron lung" days of polio epidemics. Fortunately, this disease is now rare because of wide use of vaccination. More commonly, some types of muscular dystrophy make effective cough impossible because of respiratory muscle weakness. As a result, its victims accumulate secretions and suffer repeated serious infections. Probably the most prevalent neuromuscular (concerning both nerves and muscles) problem affecting respiration is spinal cord injury. In general, the higher in the spinal cord the damage occurs, the more severe the respiratory impairment. When the cord is damaged high in the neck, nerve impulses to both diaphragm and chest wall are interrupted, and mechanical breathing aid is needed to sustain life.

Skeletal deformities of the spine and thorax interfere with breathing because of bony stiffness of the chest wall and limited expansion of the rib cage. The effect is like fitting a tight girdle around a normal chest. The most common of these abnormalities is kyphoscoliosis. Kyphosis is the curvature of the upper spine, commonly called hunchback. Scoliosis, a curvature of the lower spine, is less noticeable unless severe. Usually, the two occur together. They may be caused by birth injury or by nerve or bone diseases, but many cases have no obvious cause. Only severe cases impair breathing.

A second type of common chest wall deformity involves the sternum, the shield-like bone located between the breasts. Sometimes, this bone protrudes abnormally from the chest (pigeon breast) or is deeply indented (funnel chest). Pigeon breast (pectus carinatum) seldom affects normal breathing. Funnel chest (pectus excavatum) is mostly a cosmetic concern, but a severe defect can cause disability if it interferes with action of the heart or if it restricts the volume of air the lungs can handle. These deformities may run in families. The defect usually is apparent at birth and may improve or worsen with age. In the rare cases where breathing is impaired, surgery may be necessary to correct the defect.

Infectious Diseases of the Lung

Viruses commonly cause respiratory infections. These organisms are ultra-small parasites with incomplete metabolic systems. To survive and reproduce, they must enter host cells and commandeer the metabolic machinery.

A huge number of different viruses cause a gamut of respiratory diseases. The common cold is an infection of the upper respiratory tract caused by many different viruses (see chapter 28, "Infectious Diseases"). Cold symptoms are familiar to everyone: nasal congestion, watery eyes, and sore throat. Fortunately, colds are self-limiting. As in most viral infections, there is no specific medication. The treatment consists of rest and fluids to prevent the dehydration of fever. Vaccination is effective in certain types of viral infections but has been impractical against the common cold because of the number of viruses involved. To be effective a vaccine would have to protect against more than 80 viral species.

Most upper respiratory viral infections are more nuisance than serious. However, many viruses have the potential to cause serious illness in the lower respiratory tract (lungs and trachea) such as pneumonia.

Epiglottitis is an inflammation of the epiglottis, the flap-like structure over the opening of the trachea that acts as a valve to prevent food from entering the airways during swallowing. Viral or bacterial infection can cause the epiglottis to swell and obstruct the airway. Tracheostomy may be needed to assure proper breathing until the infection subsides. Swelling of the epiglottis is predominantly a childhood condition but it occurs in adults as well.

Laryngitis can be caused by viruses. It is an inflammation of the vocal cords, producing hoarseness or loss of voice.

Tracheobronchitis is a viral infection of the trachea and large airways, often producing cough and chest pain.

Pneumonia is any infection of the air spaces of the lung, whether viral or bacterial. It is the least common location for viral respiratory infections and the most difficult to treat.

Viral pneumonias are caused by many types of viruses but the most common is the influenza virus. Viral pneumonias differ from those caused by bacteria because they are preceded not only by upper respiratory symptoms but symptoms elsewhere as well. These include stuffy nose, sore throat, watery eyes, headache, muscle aches, fever, and severe fatigue. The lung infection itself is marked by chest pain, shortness of breath, cough, and high fever. Shaking chills are not as common as with bacterial pneumonias. Viral pneumonia sometimes strikes otherwise healthy persons, but prime targets are chronically ill patients with heart or lung disease. Incidence is also higher in late pregnancy. In rare cases, patients may be so ill that they require breathing support. Most, however, particularly if they previously were healthy, endure relatively mild illness and recover spontaneously without seeing a physician.

At present there is no practical medication to combat viral pneumonia. As with the common cold, treatment usually consists of bed rest, fluids, and analgesics such as aspirin. Occasionally, antibiotics are used when a simultaneous bacterial infection is suspected.

Influenza can be devastating although it is frequently mild. Typically, "flu" begins with sudden weakness and fatigue accompanied by sore throat, nasal stuffiness and headache. Fever, dry cough, and chest pain follow. Although there is a wide spectrum of severity, most patients must remain in bed for the duration of illness.

As headlines repeatedly tell us, flu occurs in periodic worldwide epidemics. At about 10-year cycles the Influenza-A virus undergoes spontaneous changes, mutations in its genetic characteristics. Why and how this happens is unknown. During any viral infection the victim develops resistance to the offending virus so that if exposed again he is immune to reinfection. This "memory" response is related to the chemical structure of the infecting virus. After each epidemic of influenza the infected segment of the population becomes immune to future reinfection with the same virus if it remains unchanged. By periodically changing its structure, the influenza organism bypasses the immune defenses of previous victims. In effect, the "flu" virus is continually in the process of changing to new types capable of reinfecting the same persons.

Flu, of course, does not occur only in periodic epidemics. Each winter there are local outbreaks or isolated cases. But in spite of the virus' periodic changes, effective vaccines against each prevalent strain usually can be developed. Vaccine is especially important for the elderly and chronically ill, in whom influenza produces the severest disease and complications.

Mycoplasmal infections. An organism known as *Mycoplasma pneumoniae,* classified somewhere between viruses and bacteria and sharing properties of both, also infects the respiratory tract. In the lungs it causes a pneumonia resembling viral pneumonia and Legionnaires' disease (see page 180). This usually mild illness differs from viral infections because it can be treated with antibiotics.

Bacteria cause a variety of respiratory diseases, the most important of which are pneumonia and lung abscess. These organisms enter the normally germ-free lower respiratory tract by a number of routes. They may be present in the atmosphere, suspended in minute particles of moisture known as droplet nuclei. These particles may be inhaled and deposited deep in the lungs. Infections in other parts of the body shed bacteria into the bloodstream which find their way into the lungs.

But bacteria's most common entry route is by aspiration, the process of sucking substances into the lungs during inhalation. In all of us, small amounts of nasal and throat secretions regularly enter the trachea, bypassing the usual defenses. These secretions normally contain large quantities of bacteria. When these are disease-causing organisms, aspiration delivers their infectious power into the air spaces.

Persons with depressed levels of consciousness are particularly prone to aspirate and therefore are likely targets for bacterial pneumonia and related diseases. These persons include Skid Row denizens in an alcoholic stupor, institutionalized persons under medication, and anesthetized hospital patients. The hospital recovery room has been established partially to guard against aspiration among postoperative patients.

Once bacteria reach a suitable site in the lungs, they begin to multiply and provoke an inflammatory reaction. The air spaces fill with bacterial products, pus, and inflammatory fluid. The disease may be distributed along airways (broncho-pneumonia) or in specific lobes (lobar pneumonia). Under treatment, this material is converted into liquid and expelled from the lung, usually without damage to underlying tissue. Occasionally an especially harsh bacteria such as the staphylococcus can cause permanent damage. Such infections, known as necrotizing pneumonias, produce small areas of destroyed, "liquefied" lung replaced by pus. This is known as a lung abscess. It leaves behind an empty defect or a fibrous scar.

The symptoms of bacterial pneumonia are sputum-producing cough, fever, chills, and chest pain. The sputum occasionally may be blood streaked. Chest pain indicates that the pneumonia involves the pleural lining. Lung abscesses appear on X ray as round masses containing both fluid (pus) and air. They resemble a balloon inflated partially by water and partially by air, with a sharp horizontal "fluid level" between. Blood and sputum tests usually are necessary to identify the offending bacteria.

The treatment of bacterial pneumonias is one of the major success stories of modern medicine. Although they vary in their susceptibility, all the pneumonia-causing bacteria are susceptible to antibiotics. Treatment is often supplemented with physical therapy. Patients with other underlying chronic lung disease may suffer temporary respiratory failure. Postural drainage and chest percussion help eliminate the inflammatory material.

A percentage of severe pneumonias claim lives despite antibiotics, so preventive measures are important. A vaccine has been perfected to defend against one common bacteria, and is particularly recommended for the elderly and chronically ill.

Tuberculosis has been a scourge of mankind since pre-Biblical days. The lungs of Egyptian mummies show unmistakable evidence of its ravages, and sculptures left by the Maya Indians are shaped with the specific deformity of tuberculosis of the spine. "TB" is far less a threat than in days past, thanks to dramatic advances in treatment and prevention, but it still disables and claims lives.

The offending organism, *Mycobacterium tuberculosis,* is readily recognized under the microscope by its distinct, rod-shaped appearance, clubbed at both ends. It is usually spread by inhalation of droplet nuclei. Although the lungs are most commonly involved, TB can spread to any organ in the body. The disease can persist for months or years. If undetected, it can be fatal rapidly. It can also smolder for life.

When the tuberculosis bacteria make their way into the lungs, they trigger an immune reaction. White blood cells surround each invader, walling it off in a tiny protective capsule. Before this defense can be completed, however, the organism is transported via lymphatic channels into lymph nodes of the chest, and from there is spread by the bloodstream throughout the body. Then the body's defenses throw the same kind of barrier around the bacteria. In the lungs the central tissues of these collections eventually die and are converted into a material of cheese-like consistency. This process is called caseation.

The encapsulated lesions are called tubercles. The tubercle may heal spontaneously or eventually "break down" and release still-living germs (and caseous material) through air passages or into the bloodstream. The material that enters the airways is coughed up but can infect other areas of the respiratory tract. When large collections of caseation empty they leave behind air-filled cavities that are visible on X ray. Bacteria sealed off in other organs retain their infectious potential, too. Poor health, chronic diseases, or other factors that reduce the body's defenses can reactivate them. Most persons contain the organisms effectively and never develop active disease. A minority, however, eventually fall victim to active tuberculosis.

The early stages of TB usually are surprisingly free of symptoms. Cough, weight loss, fever, and night sweats come much later when the disease has become established. There also may be chest pain and accumulation of fluid. Sometimes the sputum is blood streaked. A chest X ray may show that air spaces left by caseation have consolidated or formed cavities, especially in the upper portions of the lungs. Function of the lung is not seriously affected during early stages of the disease, but progressive destruction ultimately leads to fibrosis and breathing difficulty.

Tuberculosis is diagnosed by finding tuberculosis organisms (tubercle bacilli) in the sputum or other body fluids and tissues. A test to demonstrate past exposure, indicating that walled-off organisms may still be in place, involves injecting a small amount of tuberculin, a purified protein extract of tuberculosis organisms, into the skin of the forearm. A previously infected individual reacts with prominent inflammation at the site of the injection.

Persons who have not been exposed do not react, because their immune systems have no memory for the tuberculosis organism. A positive skin test indicates only past exposure to tuberculosis; it does not mean active infection. The chest X ray and tuberculin skin test are the best screening procedures for previous tuberculosis exposure, and isolating the tubercle bacillus is the final diagnostic proof.

Before the late 1940s tuberculosis was a disabling chronic infection. Treatment was only moderately effective. Both the incidence and death rates were high. All over the country, hundreds of tuberculosis sanitariums housed patients for "rest cures" often lasting for years. This changed abruptly with the discovery of a group of antibiotics specifically effective against the tubercle bacillus without serious side effects. Today prolonged hospitalization is not necessary for most TB victims. The drugs are given by mouth so they can be administered at home. A patient with moderately advanced disease might be hospitalized for only two to three weeks, long enough to render him noninfectious, then returned home and to normal activity. He continues medicines for one to two years, after which most patients are cured. With prolonged multiple drug treatment, the cure rate is close to 100 percent.

Some patients with a positive tuberculin test are treated even if no tuberculosis organisms are found in the sputum. Such patients carry a life-long risk of reactivating their walled-off infections. Therapy for one year with the antituberculous drug isoniazid greatly reduces the probability that the infections will later develop active disease.

Legionnaires' disease. In July 1976, a respiratory illness struck a group of conventioning American Legionnaires at the Bellevue-Stratford Hotel in Philadelphia. The epidemic affected 182 persons and 29 died. The initial search for the cause was highly publicized but no known organism seemed to explain the outbreak. Scientists from the U.S. Center for Disease Control eventually were able to classify the disease as infectious by transmitting the illness to guinea pigs with tissue taken from the human victims. Later, they also identified the cause as a newly discovered bacteria which has since been named *Legionella pneumophilia*. It had not been discovered earlier because it did not stain by the usual laboratory techniques and did not grow in standard culture media.

THE DECLINE OF TUBERCULOSIS

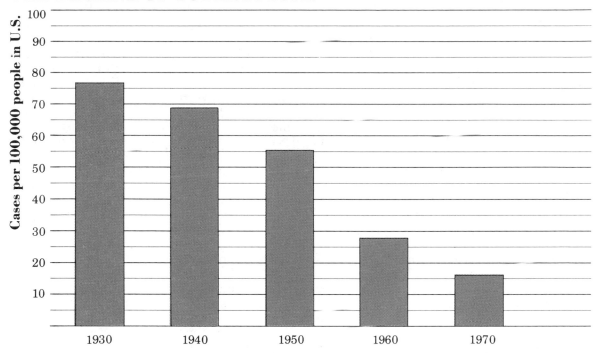

The incidence of tuberculosis has declined markedly in the United States since 1930. This graph shows the number of active cases per 100,000 people plotted over five decades. Despite this marked im- provement, tuberculosis is still an important cause of death and disability, particularly in certain population groups and in Third World countries.

The discovery explained several mysterious earlier epidemics of unknown disease. Tissue and blood specimens saved at the time were reexamined and *Legionella pneumophilia* was identified. Since then, a large number of individual cases of Legionnaires' disease have been reported from all over the world. While the scientific achievement of isolating and characterizing the new bacterium is stunning, the realization that it has been causing disease in our midst for some time is humbling to the medical scientist and clinician.

Whether Legionnaires' disease attacks isolated individuals or groups, its course is similar. Patients are severely ill with cough, shaking chills, diarrhea, chest pain, and poor appetite. Almost all develop high fever. The X-ray findings mimic a variety of other pneu- monias, leading to mistaken diagnosis. Now that the peculiar staining and growth char- acteristics of Legionella are established, the diagnosis is commonly made. Fortunately this organism can be checked by the antibiotic erythromycin and most patients recover completely.

The disease appears to be spread by inhaling droplets from contaminated water sources, such as air conditioners and cooling towers. The organism also has been found in natural streams. If the water-borne hypothesis holds, it may be possible to prevent Legionnaires' disease by chemical treatment of potential water sources.

Fungi are organisms slightly more complex than bacteria that live in soil and rarely cause disease, except in persons already ill from other causes. A few types of fungi, however, can trigger diseases which affect the lung. In the United States the most common fungus-caused respiratory diseases are called histo- plasmosis, blastomycosis, coccidioidomycosis, and aspergillosis. Each is named for the fun- gus that causes the disease. Together they ac- count for about 100,000 illnesses a year.

Most of the fungi, except for Aspergillus, which is distributed worldwide, seem to prefer the soils of certain geographic areas. *Histo- plasma* and *Blastomyces* are found in the Mis- sissippi and Ohio River valleys and in certain mid-Atlantic states. *Coccidioides immitis* is peculiar to the arid regions of California, Arizona, southern Utah, Nevada, New Mexico and west Texas.

Often fungi are found in the droppings of birds and fowl. The fungal spores may lie dormant in the dust of barns, chicken coops, open fields, or even playgrounds until stirred up by human movement or activity. A wave of respiratory fungal infections followed some of the open-air rock music festivals of the 1960s and 1970s.

Once they are airborne, the spores enter the body by being inhaled into the lungs. As in tuberculosis, however, they are quickly spread by the bloodstream to all parts of the body. In acute cases, the symptoms—fever, cough, and chest pain—resemble those of influenza or a bacterial lung infection. More stubborn cases resemble tuberculosis and in the past were often mistaken for it. There is progressive lung involvement along with weight loss, fatigue, weakness, fever, and cough. There may be lung scarring. The rare cases which spread beyond the lungs can cause serious illness and require hospitalization, particularly if the eyes become involved.

No treatment is entirely satisfactory because the most effective drug has serious side effects. Fortunately, most fungal infections are self-limiting, curing themselves within a few weeks without specific medication.

Pulmonary Embolism

During each cycle of circulation, all blood carried by the veins passes through the lungs, where it acquires oxygen. Sometimes, solid materials form in the veins and are swept along through the vessels until they reach the lungs (see chapter 6, "The Blood"). A single particle (embolus) of solid material can flow along ever-narrowing pulmonary arteries until the vessels are too small to pass further. Lodging in the opening of an artery, the embolus can completely or partially block the blood flow. Very large emboli can completely block the blood flow from the heart's right ventricle and can be abruptly fatal. Smaller emboli clog smaller arteries. They cause pain and a blood-streaked cough, but the victim usually recovers.

The most common source of blood clots are the veins in the legs. Often clots develop there during an illness or injury requiring prolonged bed rest and inactivity. That is the main reason surgical patients are directed to dangle their feet or walk with support as soon as possible after an operation. Clots also occur in otherwise healthy persons during long periods of sitting. They are not uncommon in cross-country truck drivers, and may occur in elderly persons during long automobile trips. (Elderly passengers should stop to exercise every hour or two during a long drive.) With a resumption of activity, the clots may break loose and migrate to the lungs to lodge as emboli.

Clots in the legs, a condition called thrombophlebitis, may have no symptoms or may cause local swelling and pain (see chapter 5, "Blood Vessel Disorders"). The first warning that they have moved to the lungs may be chest pain, cough, shortness of breath, and blood-spitting. Once an embolus is suspected, diagnostic efforts are aimed at demonstrating either the origin of the clots or their location in the lungs.

To detect clots in the legs, an opaque dye is injected, and X rays reveal clots as dye-free areas in the affected veins. The procedure is called venography. In seeking lung emboli, the contrast dye is injected into the pulmonary artery, a procedure called pulmonary angiography. The other test commonly used to diagnose an embolus is the lung scan, in which a harmless dose of a radioactive substance is injected into an arm vein to disclose the pattern of the pulmonary circulation. Obviously the danger of pulmonary embolus is interference with oxygenation. This is important in diagnosis because low arterial oxygen is typical for the condition.

Most commonly, leg clots or pulmonary emboli are treated with bed rest and drugs that inhibit blood-clotting, known as anticoagulants. Bed rest appears to reduce the risk of dislodging clots and their subsequent movement to the lungs. Anticoagulants, given either by mouth or injection, prevent enlargement of the clots and can help slightly in dissolving them.

It was formerly believed that anticoagulant treatment had to continue for several months. Prolonged treatment is potentially dangerous because it promotes bleeding, and is costly to administer because frequent blood tests are needed to monitor anticoagulation levels. Current treatment calls for shortening the anticoagulant therapy. Very low doses of anticoagulant may be administered to prevent lung emboli in patients who have conditions that predispose them to clot formation.

Occasionally, the segment of vein containing the clot may be surgically sealed off from the rest of the circulation. This technique is used for patients who cannot tolerate the usual amounts of blood thinner.

LUNG CANCER DEATHS INCREASE

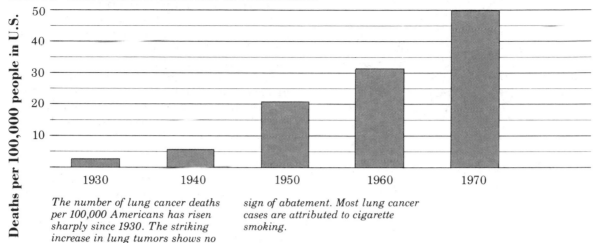

The number of lung cancer deaths per 100,000 Americans has risen sharply since 1930. The striking increase in lung tumors shows no sign of abatement. Most lung cancer cases are attributed to cigarette smoking.

Lung Cancer

Over the last decade great progress has been made in the prevention and treatment of several important cancers. Lung cancer is a disappointing exception. The lung cancer death rate for men has increased more than 25 times since 1935. The number of lung cancer cases has more than doubled for both men and women. Five-year survival rates are not improving significantly. Perhaps the grimmest aspect is that most of these cancer cases would not have occurred if the victims had not been cigarette smokers.

Cigarette smoking is unequivocally identified as the main factor behind the rise of lung cancer. Only 10 percent of all lung cancer patients are nonsmokers. Certain industrial substances such as asbestos, nickel, chromium, arsenic, radon, and halogenated ethers also cause lung cancer, but smoking is clearly the most important risk factor.

As in other organs, cancer in the lung represents the uncontrolled growth of a nucleus of abnormal cells (see chapter 29, "Cancer"). It is believed that cancer cells arise in the cellular lining membrane of the airways, provoked by certain irritants, the most potent being cigarette smoke. Not all smokers, however, develop tumors, which means that other factors must contribute.

Once tumor cells establish their presence they increase in number by cell division. Only after the initial cluster of cells has been present for years is the tumor large enough to be visible on a chest X ray. By this time tumor cells may have dislodged from the growth and spread through the lymphatic system or bloodstream to the liver, brain, or bone.

Typically, lung cancer victims have no complaints while the tumor is small. The luckiest persons are those whose cancers are accidentally discovered when a chest X ray is taken for unrelated reasons. For the less fortunate, the first clue may be weight loss and general fatigue. Still others may bleed from the tumor and expectorate bloody sputum. The first evidence commonly results from spread of the cancer beyond the lungs, such as hoarseness of voice because the nerve to the larynx is involved, or a stroke because of spread to the brain. Chest pain is also a common first clue, usually the result of involvement of the chest wall.

A chest X ray is usually the first step in diagnosis, but the shadows pictured may be confused with infection. Other tests inspect the sputum, which is specially stained and viewed under the microscope. A significant percentage of abnormal tumor cells sometimes can be discerned. A bronchoscope may be used for visual inspection, and chest surgery or needle biopsy may be performed to obtain tissue.

Tumors found in the earliest stages can be removed surgically, often with good results. Lung tumors that have spread require radiotherapy or drug therapy. Radiotherapy involves administering several types of X rays which are more destructive to tumor cells than to normal body cells. Unfortunately, the amount of radiotherapy a patient can tolerate is limited. Drug therapy involves administer-

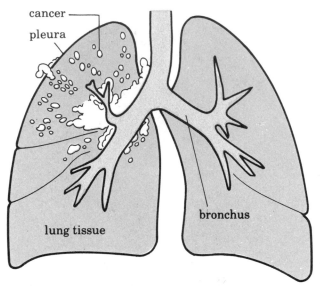

SPREAD OF LUNG CANCER

Drawing shows a primary cancer of the main bronchus, with infiltration into the lung tissue, extension through the pleura, and invasion of neighboring lymph nodes, which permit the malignancy to spread to other organs of the body. Cancer originating in the stomach, uterus, breast, pancreas, prostate, or thyroid often spreads to the lungs.

ing certain drugs that are more effective in poisoning tumor cells than healthy cells. New drugs are tested constantly to find those with maximum effect against tumors and minimum normal cell damage.

Granulomatous Lung Diseases

The body mobilizes various defenses against infections and other foreign substances. One of them involves lymphocytes, white blood cells which become sensitized to specific chemical substances. When these specialized cells recognize their target chemical in the body they incite an inflammatory reaction which inactivates the foreign substance, or at least walls it off by surrounding the site of infection with a group of inflammatory cells. The resulting microscopic growth is called a granuloma, and diseases characterized by granuloma formation are called granulomatous diseases.

The prototype of the granulomatous lung diseases is tuberculosis. Certain fungal diseases also provoke granuloma formation, as do certain neoplastic diseases. But in some granulomatous diseases, no foreign substances can be identified.

Sarcoidosis is a generalized granulomatous disease that tends to occur among young adults and is especially prominent among blacks. It typically involves the lungs but can affect any organ in the body, most commonly the lymph nodes, skin, eyes, joints, heart, and liver.

In the lungs, the severity of sarcoidosis covers a wide spectrum. Most cases are mild, with few or no symptoms. Sarcoidosis may be discovered by X rays done for unrelated reasons. A typical X ray shows enlarged lymph nodes with little or no abnormality of the lung itself. Even with X ray abnormalities many persons have no significant complaints. Those with only lymph-node involvement will spontaneously revert to normal within one to two years.

More seriously affected persons complain of shortness of breath and dry cough, and may have complaints that stem from other organs being affected. Their chest X rays show numerous granulomata with or without lymph-node enlargement. Lung tests disclose reduced lung volumes. Most cases are successfully treated with anti-inflammatory drugs; some patients recover spontaneously. The rest must limit their exercise and work. A few suffer progressive lung scarring and are incapacitated.

The cause of sarcoidosis is not known. No infectious agent or other foreign body has been convincingly linked to it. The most popular theory is that this disease represents a disturbance of the body's immune system, but the underlying condition which triggers the immune reaction is not known.

The greatest recent advance in sarcoidosis has been in diagnosis. The fiberoptic bronchoscope enables doctors to obtain lung tissue to detect the microscopic granulomas of this disease.

Sarcoidosis is by far the most common noninfectious granulomatous disease but it is not the only one. Wegener's granulomatosis is marked by lung and kidney involvement. Until recently no effective treatment was known, but certain antitumor drugs combined with steroids have greatly improved the outlook. Eosinophilic granuloma is marked by involvement of lungs, bone, and central nervous system. As in sarcoidosis and Wegener's, its cause is not known.

Diseases of the Pleura

The lung and the inner chest wall are lined by a thin layer of cells collectively known as the pleura. The linings are separated from each other only by a thin film of lubricating fluid. A variety of diseases, some originating in the respiratory system and others originating elsewhere in the body, can cause abnormal fluids and even air to accumulate in the space separating the pleural surfaces. The general term for fluid accumulation in the pleural cavity is pleural effusion.

Pneumothorax means the presence of air in the pleural cavity. Often it occurs in paraseptal emphysema (see page 174) located high in the lungs just under the pleural surface. This is most common in the young and seems unrelated to smoking. Patients lack the usual symptoms of emphysema, but their emphysema-damaged air spaces may spontaneously rupture and leak air into the pleural space. The ruptures occur during severe exertion or at rest.

Effusions are further subdivided according to their composition. Hemothorax denotes a blood-filled pleural cavity, usually the result of chest injury or pulmonary embolus. Pus in the pleural space, called empyema, is rare since the advent of effective antibiotic drugs. Other effusions contain neither blood or pus. They are clear to deep yellow in color. Transudative effusions contain only small amounts of protein and may be considered a filtrate of blood. They are associated with heart or kidney failure. Exudates contain larger amounts of protein and other large molecules, and except for the absence of red blood cells, more closely resemble the composition of blood plasma. They usually indicate infection or tumor.

A number of other lung diseases can result in pneumothorax, including the more typical emphysema of older patients. Injury to the chest wall also can precipitate pneumothorax, as in puncture of the lung by foreign bodies or by fractured ribs. In rare cases, the punctured lung acts as a one-way valve, admitting air into the pleural cavity during inhalation but not allowing escape when the victim exhales. Great pressures may build up in the chest cavity on the side of the puncture, and this pressure compresses and interfaces with the opposite lung and with the pumping action of the heart. This rare form of "tension" pneumothorax is a medical emergency.

The treatment of the pleural disease varies with the cause. Except where large amounts of fluid cause shortness of breath or where tension pneumothorax threatens life, pleural disease is generally not an emergency. When rapid and complete removal of gas or liquid is deemed necessary, a plastic tube is surgically placed into the pleural space and constant suction is applied. More often, fluid is removed with a small needle (see page 165). Often a second needle is used simultaneously to obtain a tiny piece of pleural tissue (pleural biopsy). The combination can help in diagnosing the underlying condition.

When effusions recur, an irritative drug may be inserted into the pleural cavity. The resulting inflammation causes the pleural linings to adhere to one another and eventually form scar tissue. This closes the normal pleural space, preventing further accumulation of pleural fluid.

Environmental and Occupational Hazards

Air pollution. Air pollution results from the discharge of substances into the atmosphere during combustion of industrial, domestic, and automotive fuels.

In sheer quantity, the most important pollutant is carbon monoxide. A staggering 100 million tons is produced annually in the United States. The potential danger of this colorless, odorless gas is well known. Its use for suicide is not uncommon. Massive exposure to carbon monoxide causes death by occupying the sites in red blood cells that are normally used to carry oxygen. Its more subtle dangers are poorly appreciated. Monoxide is associated with the development of atherosclerosis and with decreased survival rates for heart attack victims. It also has been shown to predispose to premature births and increased infant mortality.

Another important pollutant gas is sulfur dioxide, typically produced by the burning of coal or oil. Unlike carbon monoxide, sulfur dioxide makes its presence known by irritating the eyes and throat. Local episodes of sulfur dioxide pollution combined with airborne particles have been held responsible for acute increase in the death rate among people with chronic heart and lung disease. Although it has been shown that sulfur dioxide adversely affects chronic lung patients, it has *not* been shown to cause obstructive lung disease.

Another combustion product, nitrogen dioxide, has led to emphysema-like changes in experimental animals. Like sulfur dioxide, it contributes to a higher death rate of lung patients during times of heavy smog pollution.

Ozone is an irritant gas formed when other pollutant gases (usually from auto exhaust) are exposed to the sun's rays. Ozone has also been implicated as a cause of chronic lung disease.

The most important of the nongaseous substances in polluted air is tiny particles of metallic lead that come predominantly from motor vehicle exhaust. The dangers of ingested lead are well known. Although inhaling lead particles has not been demonstrated to cause harm, the increased lead in the atmosphere inevitably makes its way into the human food chain via incorporation into plant and animal life. Efforts to reduce lead in the atmosphere are under way, the most important being a move to discontinue the use of leaded gasoline.

Smoking. It is impossible to overstate the detrimental effects of smoking on health. A large number of factors combine to shorten the lives of cigarette smokers. Smokers have an increased risk of heart attack, and those smokers who do suffer heart attacks are less likely to survive than nonsmokers. Smokers also run an increased risk of stroke. The tendency of cigarettes to induce chronic obstructive lung disease has already been mentioned, as has the greatly increased incidence of lung cancer in smokers. And pregnant women who smoke are more likely to have premature or stillborn infants.

The exact mechanisms of these harmful effects are unknown. Cigarette smoke is known to consist of about 10 percent particulate matter, 15 percent carbon dioxide, and 5 percent carbon monoxide. The remainder of its composition is harmless nitrogen, oxygen, and water vapor. Clearly, the cancer-promoting agent lies among the thousands of organic compounds that can be isolated in the tars of cigarette smoke, but which one (or ones) is responsible, and how it causes damage, is not known. Interestingly, pipe and cigar smoke are not significantly different from cigarette smoke. Cigar and pipe smokers suffer less disease because they do not inhale smoke as deeply. But while their rates of lung cancer and lung disease are lower than those of cigarette smokers, they remain more vulnerable than nonsmokers.

The effects of marijuana smoking on lung disease are not known. Recent data indicate that most marijuana cigarettes have more tar

Protecting Your Lungs

- Stop smoking, especially if:
  You work with substances that may cause lung damage or tumors.
  You have hypertension or heart disease.
  You are pregnant.
  You use birth control pills.
- If you must smoke:
  Cut down on the number of cigarettes smoked.
  Smoke only a small part of each cigarette.
  Use filtered, low-tar, low-nicotine cigarettes.
  Consider contraceptive methods other than pills.
- If you have allergic asthma, avoid allergens and irritants.
- If you are over 65 or have a chronic illness, ask your physician about vaccination against pneumonia and influenza.
- If you already have chronic lung disease, notify your physician when fever, increased cough, or increased breathlessness occur.
- If you have been exposed to tuberculosis, notify your doctor or local public-health agency.

than the average tobacco cigarette. Since marijuana smoke is deeply inhaled and held in the lungs, it is possible that chronic users will suffer some or all the consequences of cigarette smoking.

Asbestos-related lung diseases. A great many dust particles find their way in and out of the lungs in normal daily life. Certain dusts have the ability, once deposited in the lungs, to cause scarring or fibrosis of lung tissue and result in a form of restrictive impairment. In the United States, probably the most important of these particles is asbestos.

Because asbestos resists heat and corrosion and is structurally strong, this fibrous mineral is widely used in industry. Workers are exposed during mining and separation of fiber, shipping of asbestos or asbestos products, and during installation of asbestos products as insulating materials in construction. A great reservoir of workers received exposure in shipyards during World War II. During the refurbishing and refitting of ships, the insulation frequently was torn out and replaced, releasing great volumes of microscopic asbestos particles into the atmosphere. The contamination affected everyone in the area, not just workers directly involved. Unfortunately the grave risks of asbestos were realized only after it became widely used.

Asbestos causes a variety of lung problems. The first to be recognized was restrictive lung disease caused by widespread lung scarring, the result of heavy exposure for many years. The first symptoms are shortness of breath and "clubbing" of the fingers. A chest X ray shows thick shadows concentrated in the lower lung regions. Later it was recognized that such persons are at heightened risk for lung cancer, a risk that is greatly increased if they also are cigarette smokers.

Pleural disease also strikes asbestos workers. This takes the form of calcified scars known as plaques and occasionally as fluid accumulation in the pleural cavity. Calcification is plainly seen on X ray. The most dreaded of the asbestos-related lung diseases is a malignant pleural growth known as mesothelioma. The treatment of this form of cancer has been unsuccessful. Equally frightening, mesotheliomas have occurred in persons exposed only briefly to asbestos, such as the wives of asbestos workers who have handled their husbands' work clothes.

The definitive answer to the asbestos problem is not yet available. In view of the potential dangers of even brief exposure, it is difficult to set safe limits. It is clear, however, that those regularly exposed to asbestos must stop smoking. It is possible that many of the functions of asbestos in industry will be fulfilled by other materials.

Silicosis. Silicon is one of the most common elements in the earth's crust. It usually is found in the form of silicon dioxide, also known as silica. Quartz, sand and sandstones, flint, granite, and other hard stones have high silica content. Silicosis results from repeated exposure to free crystals of silica deposited in the lungs. Persons at high risk for silicosis include sandblasters, hardrock tunnelers, quarry workers, stone cutters, foundry workers, and makers of refractory materials.

The mechanism of lung scarring by silica is better understood than the scarring by asbestos. Silica is a potent killer of lung macrophages. As repeated generations of macrophages ingest silica particles and are killed by these particles, they release inflammatory chemicals that eventually provoke a scar tissue response.

There are no clear signs of early silicosis. The first indication is usually an abnormal chest X ray, with scattered pinpoint punctures throughout the lung. This stage of disease, causing neither symptoms nor functional disability, is called simple silicosis. Fortunately, most patients never proceed beyond this stage. In a few, however, a complication known as conglomeration occurs. The small nodules enlarge and blend into large areas of destruction. Patients become breathless and may approach respiratory failure. It is unclear why some patients progress to this stage while others do not. In rare instances the coexistence of tuberculosis may incite the conglomerate phase. It is also possible that silicosis predisposes to the development of tuberculosis.

There is no specific therapy for silicosis. Standards for limiting silica particle concentration in the workplace are well established.

Coal miner's lung ("black lung") shares many of the features of silicosis. It is caused by the inhalation of coal dust, which collects in the lung in local formations known as coal macules. This state of disease is simply a chest X ray finding without symptoms or disability. As in silicosis, there is a progressive form known as progressive massive fibrosis which leads to disability, sometimes death.

Great progress has been made in establishing safe working levels of coal dust. As in all occupational diseases, prevention is much easier than treatment.

Chemical irritants. A large number of gases used in industrial processes irritate the respiratory system. They include ammonia, hydrogen chloride, chlorine, sulfur dioxide, nitrogen dioxide, and phosgene. The soluble gases, such as chlorine and ammonia, cause upper respiratory irritation marked by chest pain and cough. The nonsoluble gases, such as nitrogen dioxide and phosgene, reach the alveoli and small airways where they cause an outpouring of fluid into the lungs, known as pulmonary edema. Great amounts of alveolar fluid interfere with breathing.

It may be necessary to treat these exposures with supplemental oxygen. Occasionally, steroids are used to treat cases of massive pulmonary edema.

Hypersensitivity lung diseases are caused by an immune reaction directed against certain organic substances inhaled into the lung. In farmer's lung particles of fungus growing in moldy hay are shaken into the air when the hay is stirred up, then are inhaled deeply into the lung where they are attacked by the body's immune defenses. Fever, chills, and breathlessness follow several hours later. Similar diseases are incited by other fungi, or organic substances such as animal danders or feathers. Only a small percentage of those exposed develop the disease.

CHAPTER 9   JAMES F. TOOLE, M.D.

THE BRAIN AND NERVOUS SYSTEM

It is almost a cliche to say that the most marvelous and complicated structure on earth is the human brain. In an age of increasingly sophisticated computers, its ability to send, receive, and interpret messages still cannot be matched by any complex of electronic circuitry. The brain and the nervous system of which it is a part distinguish animals from plants, and, depending on the degree of evolution, separate humans from creatures of lower intelligence. It is the nervous system that enables us to walk, eat, have emotions like love or anger, feel pain, and contemplate our world. It is the brain that allows us to communicate with God, and some believe that it is the seat of the soul. Without a functioning brain a person is in a coma and is said to be a "vegetable." With a brain but without nerve or muscle function, as occurs in some diseases, the person can think but cannot move or communicate.

If we were able to look at the nervous system without the intervening skeleton, organs, and body tissue, it would resemble a ghost, a figure of gossamer threads precisely defining the human figure. Nerve fibers extend to every cubic millimeter of the body, carrying sensory information from the receptors to the brain, then carrying messages from the brain to the muscles and organs. But the system has not always been so complicated. The nerve cells collected in the nervous system evolved over hundreds of millions of years. At first, in the lower animals, the simple cell networks that transmit information to one another were adjacent, but eventually the cells moved to locations distinct from one another, joined by tiny cellular tubes called dendrites and axons. More and more cells have been added to form the extremely complicated human network that we subdivide into the brain, spinal cord, and peripheral nerves. About five million years ago the first human-like animals walked the earth. Studying their ancient skulls, anthropologists have been able to trace the evolution of the brain into its present form. There is no reason to suspect that this process of evolution has ceased.

THE NERVE UNIT

The basic unit of the nervous system is called a neuron or nerve cell. By most estimates, there are 40 billion neurons in the human body, 12 billion in the brain alone, although others place the figure in the hundreds of billions. The individual cell resembles a drop of liquid that has been splashed on a hard surface and sprayed out in various directions.

The cell body is the central blob. Extending from it are short branched fibers called dendrites because of their resemblance to tree roots. There is another long single fiber called an axon, which ends in a brush-like tip. Electrical impulses are carried to the cell body and away from it via these branches.

What we call a "nerve" is a mixed bundle of dendrites and axons. It may have the diameter of a bit of twine, or be as thin as the web of a spider. Each fiber is an extension of a cell body that may lie a great distance away. The sciatic nerve, which runs from the spine to the toes, is several feet long.

When nerve cells die they are not replaced. The number we are born with is the most we will ever have. An elderly person has millions fewer neurons than when he or she was born. The original supply was so generous that thousands can be lost without much impairment of function if the losses are not concentrated in a particular nerve center.

A limited amount of nerve repair is possible. All the metabolic processes of a neuron are directed by the cell body, and as long as this vital part is intact, the neuron functions. If a nerve fiber is cut or injured, the part attached to the cell body remains alive, but the part beyond the injury gradually withers away unless the live part can extend itself through the injured component to reach its original destination. In favorable situations severed nerves can be rejoined by a surgeon.

Each axon is covered with a white insulating material called myelin. The "white matter" of nerve tissue is largely myelin-covered fibers, and "gray matter" is the unmyelinated cell bodies and dendrites. Myelin is essential to healthy nerve function. Breakdown of the myelin sheath is characteristic of some disorders known as demyelinating diseases (see page 214).

HOW THE SYSTEM WORKS

Although nerve cells are close to each other, they do not touch. Instead there is a tiny gap where the axon of one cell approaches the dendrites of another. This gap is called a synapse. A cell may synapse with many other cells. Synapses are the junctions where the neurochemical process takes place that is the basis of all animal behavior.

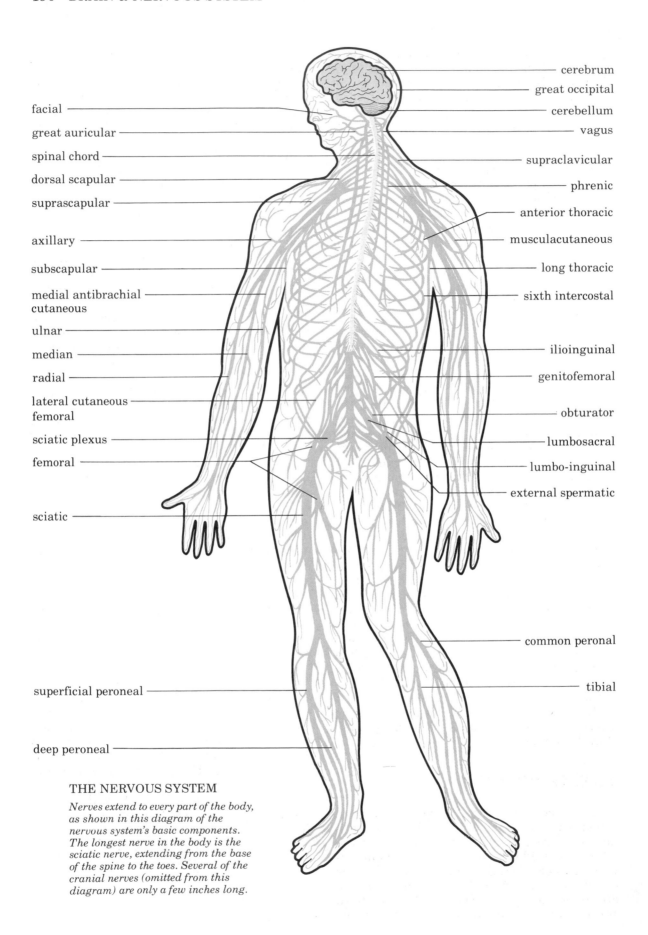

facial

great auricular

spinal chord

dorsal scapular

suprascapular

axillary

subscapular

medial antibrachial
cutaneous

ulnar

median

radial

lateral cutaneous
femoral

sciatic plexus

femoral

sciatic

superficial peroneal

deep peroneal

cerebrum

great occipital

cerebellum

vagus

supraclavicular

phrenic

anterior thoracic

musculacutaneous

long thoracic

sixth intercostal

ilioinguinal

genitofemoral

obturator

lumbosacral

lumbo-inguinal

external spermatic

common peronal

tibial

THE NERVOUS SYSTEM

*Nerves extend to every part of the body,
as shown in this diagram of the
nervous system's basic components.
The longest nerve in the body is the
sciatic nerve, extending from the base
of the spine to the toes. Several of the
cranial nerves (omitted from this
diagram) are only a few inches long.*

When a nerve cell body is excited to action, an electrical impulse is triggered which travels along the axon at speeds up to 270 miles an hour. When the electrical impulse reaches the end of the axon, it causes minute quantities of chemicals called neurotransmitters to be released from tiny globules (packets or vesicles) stored at the end of each axon. These substances cross the synapse and combine with small receptor molecules in the protein membrane of the adjacent cell, initiating a response in the second neuron. Simultaneously, enzymes in the receptor break down the transmitter and inactivate it, so that the sequence can be repeated again within milliseconds. The neuron's response to these events may take one of two forms: (1) The cell membrane may become electrically depolarized, setting off an impulse that is conducted along the length of the cell's dendrites and axons and then transmitted to another cell. (2) The receptor protein may start a sequence of chemical events that triggers a physiological response, such as secretion of a hormone or contraction of a muscle. Of course, many thousands of cells acting together bring about the coordinated response.

The chemistry of brain function is one of the most rapidly changing areas of scientific research. At one time only a few neurotransmitters, such as epinephrine and acetylcholine, were known.

More recently it has been recognized that many neurotransmitters act within the brain, and others are being steadily identified. It is also known that neurotransmissions are closely allied to activities of the endocrine system, which chemically regulates certain body functions, although at a slower tempo than the nervous system (see chapter 16, "The Hormones and Endocrine Glands").

Because of the vast population of cells with specialized functions within the nervous system, a variety of neurotransmitter substances is necessary. Each cell can be stimulated by only a specific type of neurotransmitter, which activates its specific function.

There are general classes or groupings of these neurotransmitters. The first is the monoamines, including dopamine, norepinephrine, serotonin, acetylcholine, and histamine. The second group is the amino acids—gamma aminobutyric acid, glutamic acid, glycine, and tyrosine. The third is the peptides or polypeptides, which are secreted by cells in the brainstem, hypothalamus, or pituitary stalk and which are used to release circulating hormones. These include adrenocorticotropin (ACTH), angiotensin, oxytocin, vasopressin, somatostatin, thyrotropin releasing factor, lactate hormone, and a newly recognized class

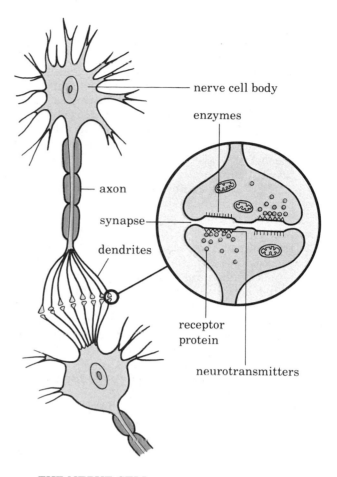

THE NERVE CELL

The basic unit of the nervous system is the nerve cell, or neuron, of which we have at least 40 billion. Its main parts are the cell body, where the cell's activity originates, the dendrites, which branch out from the cell body, and the axon, a long single fiber that reaches out toward other nerve cells. Dendrites are excited by impulses from other nerve cells or from external stimuli. Their message is carried to the cell body, which sends its impulse along the axon to another cell. The impulse is transmitted to other cells at a gap called a synapse (enlarged view), where the nerve cells approach each other but do not touch. An individual nerve cell may synapse with many other cells.

of pain-regulating substances known as the enkephalins. These neuropeptides excite, inhibit, or modulate the environment in which adjacent cells reside. Some are released into the circulating blood and exert their influence at a great distance from the secreting cells. All neurotransmitters are manufactured within the cell. Research has led to the identification of specialized pathways and locations within the nervous system where these neurosecretory cells abound.

Many investigators now believe that many neurological disorders and even some conditions we classify as psychological problems are abnormalities of function in the neurotransmitter. It is recognized that the tremors of Parkinson's disease (see page 209) result from a lack of dopamine, needed for normal coordinated activity and fine movements. Depression may stem from a disorder of the secretion of norepinephrine, produced in the locus ceruleus area of the brainstem, which is believed to affect wakefulness, dreaming, and mood. Huntington's disease (page 209) may be related to concentrations of gamma aminobutyric acid.

Although it is recognized that each receptor can be activated by only the one neurotransmitter that fits into it precisely, it is also known that certain similarly shaped substances can serve as substitutes. That may explain the effects of drugs, both those prescribed by physicians and those used illicitly to produce hallucinations or "highs" (see chapter 33, "Drugs and Medicines"). It also leads to the possibility of specifically designed substitutes that could counteract neurotransmitter deficiencies.

WHAT THE SYSTEM DOES

All of our senses feed information into the nervous system. The things our eyes see, tongue tastes, nose smells, ears hear, and skin feels are sensed with special nerve endings, conducted to the nerve cell body via dendrites, and sent from the cell to the brain by axons. Depending on previous experience, the brain may conclude that what it perceives represents danger, pleasure, or some other effect. The response may be fear, anger, joy, or pain. That response may be conscious or unconscious. Some people react consciously in one way but emotionally in another. This occurs, for example, when a person seemingly wants to do something but "his heart is not in it." The fact is that the "conscious" cells of the brain require something that the "emotion" cells do not and the heart has nothing to do with it. What we call personality, intelligence, moods, imagination, desires, and all activities such as walking, eating, crying, and laughing come from the brain.

Important regulatory functions go on without our paying attention to them, functions such as breathing, heartbeat, digestion, and regulation of body temperature (shivering or perspiration). These, too, are under the jurisdiction of the nervous system.

In order to accomplish all of these activities, the nerve endings distributed throughout the body sense changes in the environment. As might be expected, a variety of cells is involved. The cells for memory differ from those that control walking and vision, for instance. There are specialized receptors that detect light, sound, vibration, chemical change in air or water, and pressure. These transducers accept incoming signals and carry them as electrical signals to the cell body. The axon carries electrical impulses away from the cell body, triggering a response.

Electricity travels over a continuous wire at a speed of 186,000 miles a second. The greatest speed at which nerve impulses travel is less than 300 miles an hour. Therefore, it takes about a tenth of a second for nerve impulses to warn us, and another split second to act upon the information.

The nerve impulses for seeing, hearing, smelling, and tasting are all the same. The differences are where the axons end in the nervous system. Barely detectable or highly stimulating sensations are the result of varying the frequency of nerve impulses, not their amplitude.

Communication between sensory and motor nerves occurs through networks of indescribable complexity to complete a circuit. A red light at a street corner does not excite an invariable response to step on the brakes. A visual impression of color must be interpreted by the brain before impulses are channeled to motor tracts and nerves, which activate leg and foot muscles to apply the brakes. The complicated assessment of stored information which leads to a decision takes place in the interneurons.

The simplest stimulus-response circuit is a spinal reflex, because it does not involve the brain. A familiar example is the knee-jerk reflex. A tap on the muscle tendon just below the kneecap sends an impulse over sensory nerves

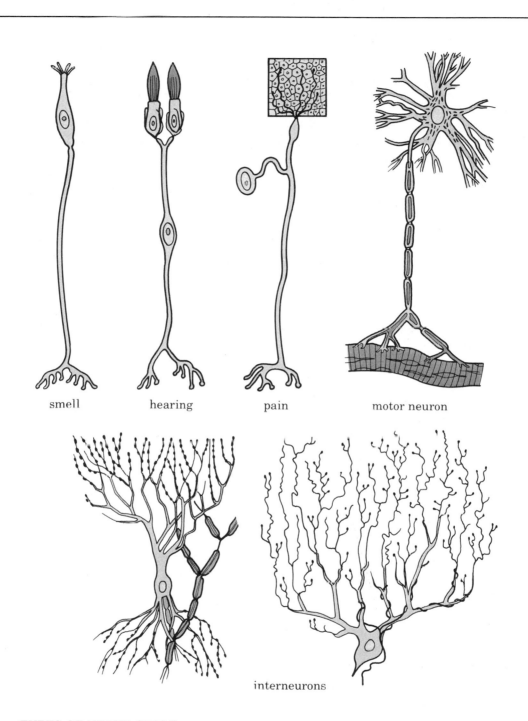

smell   hearing   pain   motor neuron

interneurons

TYPES OF NERVE CELLS

Nerve cells are differentiated according to their function. Sensory neurons have a variety of forms, as shown at top. Each of these performs a single function. Motor neurons (top right) have only one form. The interneurons in the lower row have a network of axons and dendrites connecting to a single cell body and do not extend beyond the local region. The interneuron at left is from the cerebellar cortex; the one at right is from the cerebral cortex. The structure of nerve cells also varies according to their placement in the body.

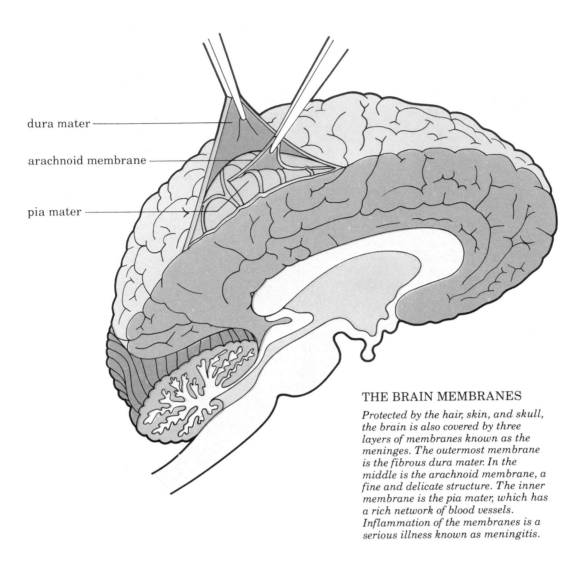

dura mater

arachnoid membrane

pia mater

THE BRAIN MEMBRANES

Protected by the hair, skin, and skull, the brain is also covered by three layers of membranes known as the meninges. The outermost membrane is the fibrous dura mater. In the middle is the arachnoid membrane, a fine and delicate structure. The inner membrane is the pia mater, which has a rich network of blood vessels. Inflammation of the membranes is a serious illness known as meningitis.

to the spinal cord, where motor nerves respond with impulses that move the muscle. Similarly, light stimulates the retina of the eye and the impulse causes an automatic adjustment of the iris muscles to change the size of the pupil. Tests of these and other reflexes give physicians clues about neurological disorders.

Few reflexes of the human nervous system are as simple as the reflexes of lower organisms, reflexes that do a great deal of the organism's "thinking" for it. There are, for instance, important reflexes concerned with human bowel activity, but emotions, training, social taboos, and conditioning can modify pure reflex actions. The nervous system is equipped with countless switches, functions, and evaluation centers that channel ceaseless torrents of nerve impulses toward the proper decision and action.

The neurons are exceedingly sensitive to changes in their environment. Brain temperature must be kept constant, and the brain must not be disturbed by the buildup of metabolites or a shortage of oxygen or glucose. The system is delicately balanced, and even a minor head injury can quickly disturb brain function.

Fortunately, the highly durable skull protects the brain from injury. The brain and spinal cord are covered with three layers of membrane, the dura mater or outer layer, the arachnoid or middle, and the pia mater, the layer next to the nerve cells themselves.

The nerve cells are protected and nurtured by surrounding neuroglia cells. The circulating blood brings nutrients to the neuroglia which ingest and transport them to the neurons. The neuroglia are also able to accept or reject substances in the blood, setting up a barrier that protects the brain from possible harm from toxic substances circulating in the blood. This blood-brain barrier is extremely selective about what it allows to penetrate the zone of the brain cells. Oxygen and glucose diffuse freely. So do some toxic substances such as alcohol, sedatives, and some other drugs, but in general the brain is isolated from proteins and fats that circulate in the blood.

THE NERVOUS SYSTEM

Strictly speaking, the nervous system is a unified and coordinated network of interrelated nerve cells, but for convenience it is usually classified into three parts. The first is the brain, including the right and left hemispheres of the cerebrum. It also includes the brainstem, which carries messages to and from the cerebral hemispheres, and the cerebellum, which controls balance and coordinates movements. The second part is the spinal cord, which carries messages between the brain and the body. The third part includes the peripheral nerves and muscles.

The hemispheres, cerebellum, and brainstem are contained in the skull, and the spinal cord is contained in the vertebrae, while the peripheral nerves run free in soft tissues of the body. The peripheral nerves have two major divisions: the autonomic, with its sympathetic and parasympathetic subdivisions, and the sensorimotor somatic nerves. Each of these major neural structures has many visible divisions and microscopic subdivisions.

Technically speaking, muscles are not part of the nervous system, but because the brain cannot carry out any actions without them, the two are usually considered as a unit.

The Brain

The brain weighs about three pounds and is of jelly-like consistency. The brain amounts to only about 2.5 percent of body weight, but it receives 15 percent of the blood supply and 25 percent of the oxygen consumed by the body. There are various estimates of the numbers of cells the brain contains, but the important point is that the cells are far more individualized in structure and function than cells in any other part of the body.

Cerebrum. Because of its wrinkled, convoluted appearance, the brain is often likened to a cauliflower set on a stalk. The cerebrum is the flower's bud. It is the major portion of the brain, occupying almost the entire part of the skull above the eyes. The surface is irregular with furrows (sulci) between mounds (convolutions).

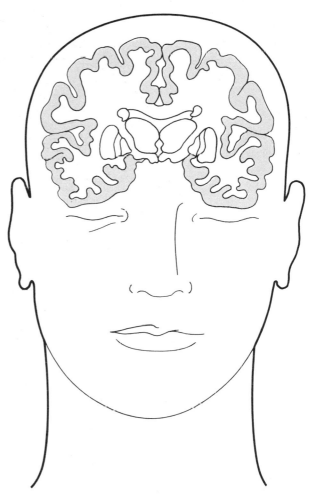

THE CEREBRUM

The highly developed cerebrum sets man apart from the lower animals. As shown here, it occupies most of the skull above the eyes. The convolutions and folds allow more cells to be packed into a confined area. The shaded area represents the cortex, the so-called higher centers where thinking takes place. Most of the interior sections of the brain deal with transmission of messages throughout the body, but are no less important for normal function.

This folded arrangement allows more neurons to be incorporated into the constricted space of the skull than would otherwise be the case. A fissure running from front to back divides the cerebrum into two hemispheres, which are linked by nerve fibers. Other fissures divide each hemisphere into four lobes, and the lobes are further divided into gyri or convolutions. Each area has a specific name and function and is connected with the other areas by axons and dendrites.

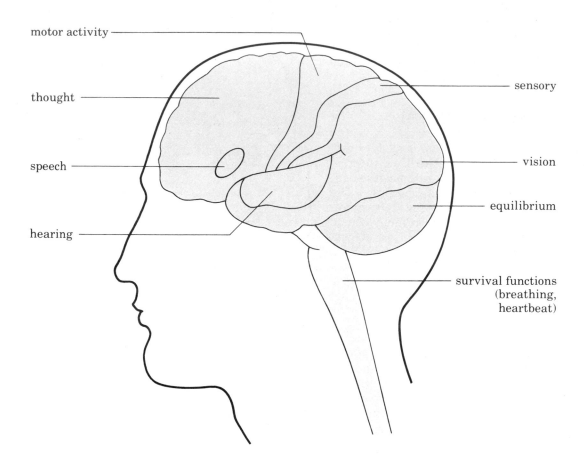

motor activity

thought

speech

hearing

sensory

vision

equilibrium

survival functions
(breathing,
heartbeat)

THE BRAIN CENTERS

Specialized functions have their own distinct areas of control within the brain. The drawing above shows that functions such as speech and equilibrium are located in different areas. In general, functions on one side are duplicated on the opposite side of the brain.

Beneath the meninges is the cortex, the outer surface of the hemispheres, composed of nerve cell bodies. Because it has no myelin, it is gray in color (gray matter). Beneath this outer covering of gray matter is the white matter, which consists of the nerve filaments that carry messages to and from the brain. The cortex interprets information and could be called the brain's thinking part or information processor. It is the development of the cortex that sets humans apart from other animals.

The four lobes of the hemispheres are named frontal, temporal, parietal, and occipital. Each has special functions that in many cases are represented in a similar position in the other hemisphere, but certain activities, including speech, handwriting, and reading, are located on only one side, known as the dominant side. The dominant hemisphere is usually that opposite the hand used for writing. Because most people are right-handed, the left hemisphere is usually the dominant one. Left-handed people often have what is called mixed dominance, meaning that some functions normally concentrated in the dominant hemisphere are divided between left and right. A left-handed person who writes from his right hemisphere may possibly speak from his left hemisphere. As a rule, music, geographic sense, and recognition of faces are in the nondominant hemisphere. Besides speech, handwriting, reading, arithmetic, and recognition of parts of the body are usually in the dominant hemisphere. It is sometimes said that the dominant hemisphere is the logical or organized side of the brain, the nondominant one the artistic side.

The back of the brain (the occipital lobe) deals with vision. This part of the brain records information that the optical system of the eye has collected and focused on the retina. This screen at the back of the eye is made up of central nervous system cells. Visual information that begins as light is converted here into electrical impulses, which pass from the retina along the optic nerve to the brain. The nerves partially cross each other on the floor of the skull, so that information from the left side of the environment passes across to the right side of the brain, and vice versa. The crossover enables us to obtain a single visual image. The impulses triggered in the nerve cells of the retina are perceived as color, light, and darkness. These cells also allow us to distinguish an object's distance, its contour, texture, color, and most important, whether it represents danger. Color blindness (more accurately termed color deficiency) is a defect of the development of the nervous system retinal cells (see chapter 12, "The Eyes").

Another function of the cerebrum is the olfactory sense, the sense of smell. Chemicals in the air stimulate tiny receptors in the upper part of the nose ("the smell patch") which send their messages through dendrites to the frontal lobe of the brain. Chemicals in liquid are perceived as taste by nerve receptors in the mouth. These messages are correlated with other impulses to give us the impressions we think of as delicious or unappetizing.

Hearing is the translation of air waves by the eardrum into mechanical impulses, which are converted into electrical impulses by the auditory nerve. This nerve carries its impulses into the brainstem and up through it to the temporal lobes of the brain, where they are recorded and interpreted.

Cerebellum. How do athletes and circus performers keep their balance in awkward, dangerous positions where falling or tripping could mean failure or even death? How, for that matter, do we manage to bend over without pitching forward? How do we manage to walk on an even keel? To maintain balance is one task of the cerebellum, a mass of ribbed tissue that lies at the back of the head behind the brain stem.

Balance involves the integration of several kinds of information that discloses whether the body is in proper alignment with the environment: vision, the vestibular apparatus in the inner ear (see chapter 13, "Ear, Nose, and Throat"), and impulses caused by the effects of gravity coming from the extremities and the skin. These three sets of data are fitted together by the cerebellum. Outgoing impulses

from the cerebellum adjust the tension of various muscles to keep the body in balance. Gravity tells all of us on earth which way is down by pulling on our clothes and other objects attached to our bodies, by causing our arms to hang down rather than float loosely in space, and by stimulating the vestibular apparatus in the inner ear. Loss of gravity, as experienced by astronauts, causes a feeling of weightlessness.

Besides equilibrium, the cerebellum is involved in muscular coordination and the automatic execution of fine movements.

The basal ganglia are gray concentrations of cell bodies surrounded by white matter deep in each cerebral hemisphere. These collections of gray matter are divided into subgroups consisting of the caudate, putamen, lenticular nucleus, and optic thalamus. Collectively they are called the basal ganglia. Each has a special function and receives nerve impulses coming from the lower parts of the nervous system. They modulate these and send the resulting electrical signals to the appropriate part of the cerebral hemisphere. In addition they secrete neurotransmitters. Our conception of the role of the basal ganglia, especially in relation to their secretions, is one of the most rapidly changing in neurobiology.

The brainstem is sometimes compared to the stalk of the cauliflower. It lies beneath the cerebrum, almost in the center of the skull, and connects the higher brain centers with the spinal cord. The brainstem deals with important basic and involuntary functions. It is divided into several sections. The hypothalamus (see chapter 16, "The Hormones and Endocrine Glands") regulates the flow of hormones throughout the body by its secretions to the pituitary gland, which lies directly beneath it. Growth, puberty, metabolism, and reproduction come under its sway.

In the upper brainstem, or midbrain, just below the basal ganglia, are a series of cell groups prominent in the secretion of neurotransmitters. The most important is the substantia nigra, which secretes dopamine, without which parkinsonism develops (see page 209). The body of Luys nearby is responsible for control of certain body movements. The midbrain proper contains the reticular activating system, which regulates sleep, wakefulness, and coma. The major nerve controlling eye movement, the third cranial nerve, is also located here.

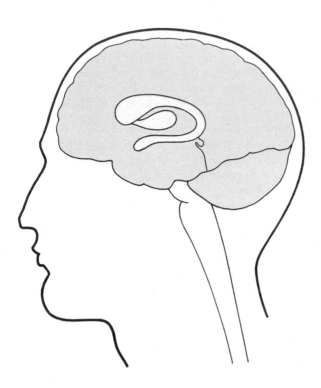

THE BASAL GANGLIA

The nuclei of the basal ganglia at the base of the brain are shown in yellow in this drawing. The ganglia are important in the production and secretion of certain neurotransmitters, the chemical substances that allow communication between nerve cells. When secretion of neurotransmitters is impaired, tremor disorders such as Parkinson's disease and Huntington's disease can result.

Below the midbrain is the pons, the Latin word for bridge, so called because it links the upper with the lower brainstem. It contains other nerves controlling eye and facial movements. It is also a major relay station for integration of reflex and voluntary movements with the cerebellum.

The lowest part of the brainstem is the medulla, whose cell groups deal with many automatic and involuntary functions. It regulates heartbeat, breathing, intestinal activity, swallowing, and other "vegetative" functions of the body.

Spinal Cord

This nerve tissue is about the diameter of a clothesline and weighs only two ounces. It is enclosed in the bony vertebral column of the back. Except for the 12 pairs of cranial nerves that connect directly with the brain, all the nerves of the body enter or leave the spinal cord through openings in the vertebrae.

A cross section of the spinal cord reveals white tissue on the outside and a gray, H-shaped mass of cells in the center. Sensory impulses of many kinds enter the outside white matter of the spinal cord and travel upward far enough to trigger spinal reflexes at various levels or travel to the brain. Motor impulses travel downward from nerve cells in the brain to reach spinal cells which relay messages to various muscles, organs, glands, and blood vessels.

On each side of the body are 31 spinal nerves distributed evenly in segments down the cord. The "incoming" sensory nerve fibers bring signals from the skin, internal organs, joints, and muscles, and enter the back of the cord and connect with gray matter of the rearward (posterior) horns of the H. In the forward (anterior) horn are the motor nerve cells, which send impulses to the muscles.

Peripheral Nerves

Sensory nerves carry impulses to the central nervous system while motor nerves carry them away from it to bring about action. A sensory nerve warns that a finger is resting on a hot stove, and motor nerves direct muscles to contract and jerk the hand away.

Some nerves are composed entirely of motor or sensory fibers, but others contain both kinds. Cell bodies of sensory nerves lie just outside the spinal cord, and those of motor nerves lie within it. From these areas, fibers run out to connect with body tissues, muscles, organs, glands, blood vessels, and skin.

Cranial Nerves

In addition to the spinal nerves there are 12 pairs of cranial nerves that connect directly with the brain. They are called cranial nerves because they arise from the brain within the skull.

(1) The olfactory nerve senses smell. The nerve endings lie in the membranes of the upper nasal air passages and carry impulses to the base of the frontal lobe of the cerebrum of the same side.

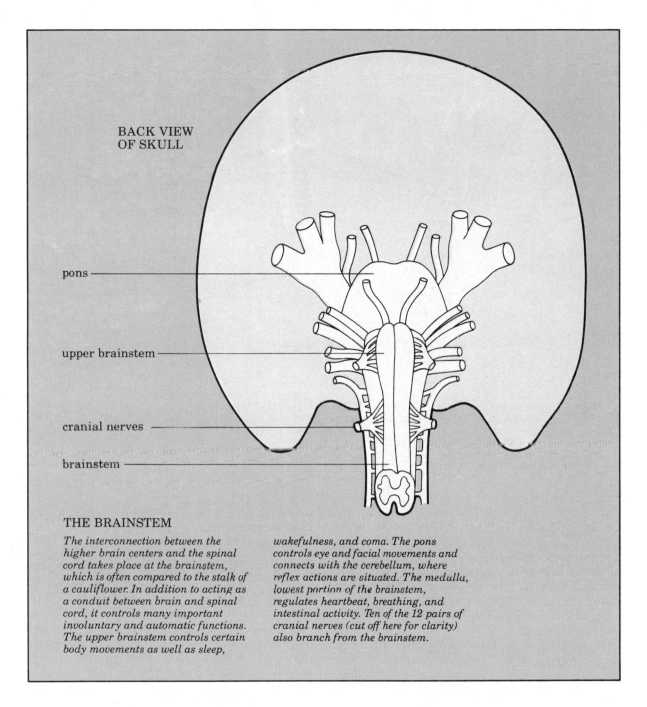

BACK VIEW
OF SKULL

pons

upper brainstem

cranial nerves

brainstem

THE BRAINSTEM

The interconnection between the higher brain centers and the spinal cord takes place at the brainstem, which is often compared to the stalk of a cauliflower. In addition to acting as a conduit between brain and spinal cord, it controls many important involuntary and automatic functions. The upper brainstem controls certain body movements as well as sleep,

wakefulness, and coma. The pons controls eye and facial movements and connects with the cerebellum, where reflex actions are situated. The medulla, lowest portion of the brainstem, regulates heartbeat, breathing, and intestinal activity. Ten of the 12 pairs of cranial nerves (cut off here for clarity) also branch from the brainstem.

(2) The optic nerve detects light and color. Its endings are in the retina, where light causes a chemical reaction that results in an electrical impulse to the brain. Light from the right half of the environment goes to the left half of each eye, where the two retinas detect it and their optic nerves carry the impulse into the skull. Near the pituitary gland the nerves divide so that all impulses from the right half of space go to the left optic thalamus and cerebral hemisphere. Within the hemisphere the fiber pathway goes to the occipital lobe where vision is registered by the brain.

(3, 4, and 6) These three motor nerves control the muscles that make the eyes move synchronously up, down, and to the sides.

(5) The trigeminal nerve senses pain, temperature, and touch for the face. It also controls the movement of the jaw.

(7) The facial nerve carries sensation of taste from the tongue and is responsible for movements of the muscles of the face.

(8) The acoustic and vestibular nerves sense sound (hearing) and position of the head in space. The vibrations in air we call sound make the tympanic membrane in the ear vi-

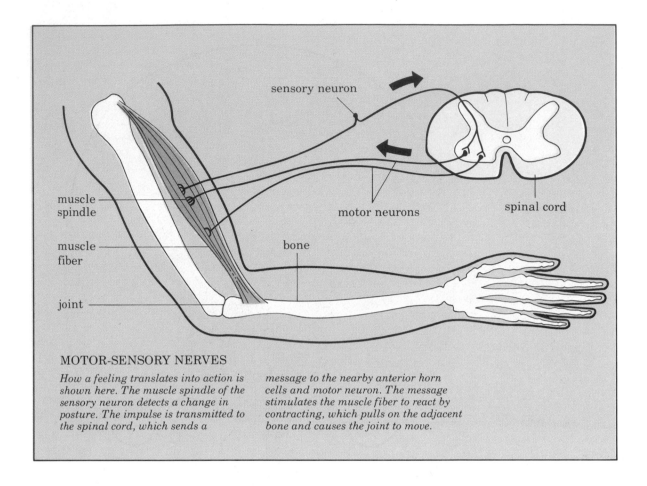

MOTOR-SENSORY NERVES

How a feeling translates into action is shown here. The muscle spindle of the sensory neuron detects a change in posture. The impulse is transmitted to the spinal cord, which sends a message to the nearby anterior horn cells and motor neuron. The message stimulates the muscle fiber to react by contracting, which pulls on the adjacent bone and causes the joint to move.

brate. This activates the small bones in the middle ear, which in turn stimulate the nerve endings of the inner ear. Impulses travel to the medulla and then up to the temporal lobe of the opposite cerebral hemisphere. The vestibular part of the inner ear senses acceleration (movement) and static position, and is an essential part of the complex system that helps us maintain our balance.

(9 and 10) The glossopharyngeal and the vagus nerves sense taste and changes in our digestive, respiratory, and cardiac systems, and regulate their function without our being aware of it.

(11) This spinal accessory nerve helps move the head on the neck by supplying muscles that connect head and neck.

(12) The hypoglossal nerve controls movement of the tongue. Without it there is no swallowing or speech.

The Autonomic System

In addition to the voluntary motor nerves which respond to the brain's commands, an involuntary or automatic system of which we are not conscious functions at all times, even while we sleep. This system regulates our bodily environment, maintaining temperature, oxygen, nutrients, and blood pressures at proper levels. This system also prepares us for emergencies. It has two complementary parts, the sympathetic and parasympathetic.

Sympathetic nerve trunks lie on either side of the bony spinal column. They connect with spinal nerves, and extend fibers to various organs of the chest and abdomen. Parasympathetic trunk lines originate in the brain and the sacral part of the spinal cord. In general, both divisions reach and control the same organs—lungs, heart, liver, spleen, stomach, pancreas, adrenal glands, kidneys, colon, intestines, sex glands, and bladder—but cause opposite effects.

For example, sympathetic impulses speed the heart and stomach and bowel action. Parasympathetic nerves do just the opposite. One set of impulses causes the muscle coat of blood vessels to constrict, the other causes it to dilate. Interplay between the two systems normally keeps body processes at a steady rate of activity, like stepping on the accelerator to climb a hill and applying brakes on the downhill side to maintain even speed.

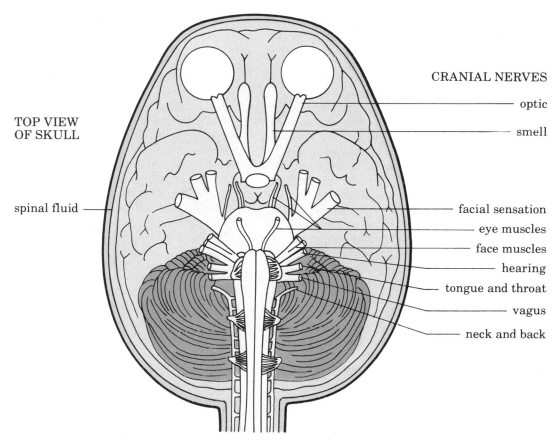

CRANIAL NERVES

TOP VIEW
OF SKULL

optic

smell

spinal fluid

facial sensation

eye muscles

face muscles

hearing

tongue and throat

vagus

neck and back

THE CRANIAL NERVES

Twelve pairs of cranial nerves connect directly from the brain without passing through the spinal cord. They relate primarily to the senses and to facial movements. Three of the pairs control movement of the eyes.

The autonomic system performs another function. For instance, it is more important that the heart pump enough blood into the muscles when we have to run away from danger than for the blood to go to the viscera for peaceful, normal digestion of food. Autonomic adjustments in such a situation speed the heart and suppress digestion which can later be resumed comfortably after we have escaped the threat.

It would be a mistake to think of the nervous system as an entirely independent electrical switchboard. The central nervous system and the endocrine (hormone-producing) systems are intimately associated. For instance, when danger threatens, nerves stimulate the adrenal glands to pour epinephrine into the blood and prepare the muscles for action upon order from the brain. But some special nerve cells also secrete neurohormones that in some respects act in a similar fashion. We may think of the nervous system as a rapid-acting electrical system, and hormones as a more deliberate-acting chemical system. The two systems are not independent but complementary.

HOW THE BRAIN DEVELOPS

When an ovum is fertilized by a sperm to start a new life, one of the first tissues to develop in the embryo is the nervous system. Skin, eye, and nervous system all grow from the same early collection of cells, the ectoderm. Therefore, throughout life, skin, eye, and brain have a special relationship and have many diseases in common. For example, some babies are born with a red mark on the side of the face called a hemiangioma. This is usually accompanied by a similar mark on the brain.

Other examples are abnormalities in which the nervous system does not go through all the stages of prenatal development. These include hydrocephalus (water on the brain), meningomyelocele (defects in the closure of the spinal cord or vertebral column), and the all too common abnormalities that we call mental retardation, in which the brain does not have the number of nerve cells or the connections between them that allow it to think properly. In many cases the skin is also abnormally developed, as in Down's syndrome (mongolism), tuberous sclerosis, and phenylketonuria.

At birth the largest part of the human being is the head, and most of that is the brain. Man is the only animal in which the brain exceeds the rest of the body in size at birth, which says something about the remarkable evolution of the human brain. A baby is born with almost its full complement of brain cells, but development of the connections between the cells continues until about age six or eight. During infancy the skull surrounding the brain is very soft and the cranial bones have not yet fused. As the brain grows, the skull expands. In some cases the skull sutures close or calcify too soon. In this condition, called craniostenosis, the skull cavity becomes too small for the developing brain, increasing the pressure within the head. Various distortions of head shape can occur, and it may be necessary to remove the sutures so the brain can continue to grow. A rare abnormality of a similar nature is twins who are joined together at the head. When this happens the news media are invariably involved while surgeons attempt to separate the enjoined, or Siamese, twins.

As the baby grows outside the mother's uterus, the environment becomes extraordinarily important in teaching the brain how to respond. At first the baby sees only mother and father, and the brain learns to respond to their voices and faces because they represent pleasure. It likes to be fed and it likes to have a clean bottom. The newborn knows no fear and theoretically could be placed in water, close to the edge of a high wall, or near fire without fear or anxiety. But the infant quickly learns that certain things cause pain, and this is how the brain develops fear.

Later, the child is old enough to go to school, which is nothing but a place where the brain is taught information. As much information as can be crammed into the growing, developing brain is tendered in the 12 or more years before the child customarily graduates. At about this age, the brain is said to be fully developed, and the personality has been set by the interaction of the individual brain plus all of the environmental stimuli ever received, each of which is thought to be stored somewhere, perhaps able to be recalled under special circumstances. These unconscious experiences become the motivation and the drives that make all of us operate on a daily basis. Brain functions are divided into the things we think about (consciousness), things we can recall if we choose to do so (preconsciousness), and the things within our brain not subject to recall (unconsciousness). One example is dreams. Another is the ordinary experiences of daily life, which we remember for a day or two but which evidently are gone forever after that.

EXAMINING THE
NERVOUS SYSTEM

The nervous system has so many functions that it is practically impossible to test them all. Every movement of the human body theoretically can be affected in some way by a neurological disorder so that with one lesion a person might, for example, lose the ability to type or play the piano. Another lesion might cause loss of balance, and a third might produce weakness of the legs or arms. Some persons with a brain disorder become unusually forgetful, others undergo changes in personality, and still others have defects of vision. No wonder examination of the nervous system is the most complicated in medicine.

The key to a successful examination is to find out from the patient and family what is malfunctioning. This clinical interview is a detailed consideration of all the abnormalities that the patient and family have noted, coupled with knowledge of what part of the nervous system is most likely to cause the malfunction. A mechanic uses a similar process in trying to learn what part of an automobile is not working properly. He does not examine the entire automobile but spends his time on the parts suggested by the driver. In the case of the nervous system, the driver is both the patient and family members who observe how the patient is malfunctioning.

Tests with simple instruments can glean important information about the health of the nervous system. A neurologist uses a pin, cotton, and a tuning fork to test sensation, a rubber hammer to test reflexes, a key to test skin reflex responses in the abdominal wall and in the feet, a stethoscope to hear abnormal circulatory sounds, and an ophthalmoscope to examine the retina, often the first organ to give evidence of a neurological disturbance.

Disease of the nervous system often is part of a disease that affects the whole body. Diabetes, arteriosclerosis, high blood pressure, and certain infectious diseases all have neurological effects. Other diseases are specific to the nervous system. Doctors cannot always tell from symptoms alone whether the disease is part of an overall process that includes effects on the brain, or whether it is a local process involving only the brain. Therefore, every patient with symptoms of nervous system disorder first gets a general examination.

Examination of the nervous system takes about an hour. It includes tests of brain function, which examine memory of the recent and distant past, the ability to repeat things properly, and the ability to add and subtract. The exam includes an assessment of whether the patient has hallucinations, whether the patient is overactive or underactive, how he dresses, his personal habits, how he relates to other people, and his mood (Is he depressed, elated, or angry, and is the mood appropriate or inappropriate?). These are considered under general headings of behavior and appearance, mood, intellectual capacity, consciousness, and attention span.

Further examination of the nervous system includes examination of speech, reading and writing, vision, hearing, taste, smell, feeling about the face, movement of the eyes and tongue, and swallowing. The examiner then tests the upper and lower limbs for their ability to perceive pain, touch, temperature, and vibration. One of the most important parts of the nervous system examination for coordination and strength is having the patient walk, because walking requires the use of many muscles carefully coordinated so that balance is maintained.

After the neurologist has done the so-called clinical tests, he may, depending upon the complexity of the problem, order special diagnostic procedures. The brain can be examined by computerized cranial tomography, the so-called CT scan (see chapter 32, "X Rays and Radiology"), which combines a computer and X ray to show the anatomy of the brain in thin "slices." The arteries that supply blood to the brain can be examined by ultrasound techniques or by arteriography, in which a catheter is placed in the artery and a radioactive material injected to show circulation and possible blockage. The electricity within the brain cells is measured with the electroencephalograph (EEG). Other tests use radioisotopes, which show the tissues of certain parts of the brain and blood vessels. Electromyography (EMG) and nerve conduction studies use needles to test the condition of the muscles and the speed with which the nerves conduct impulses. Lumbar puncture (spinal tap) samples the fluid that surrounds the brain, measures its pressure, and allows the injection of material for examining the spinal cord and canal. Seldom are all these tests done on one patient. Part of the skill of the neurologist is his selection of tests that will provide the answer with the least pain or potential harm to the patient and at the lowest cost. Skillful neurologists can often make a diagnosis without any special tests.

SYMPTOMS THAT SUGGEST NERVOUS SYSTEM DISEASE

Headache

Probably the most common complaint on earth is that of headache. Almost two-thirds of all people get headaches at one time or another, but only some of these suggest disorder of the nervous system. The head contains many structures that can produce pain, including the sinuses, the eyes, the teeth, and the ears. Contrary to popular belief, injury to the brain itself does not result in headache or pain of any sort because the brain has no pain sensitivity.

The intensity of a headache is not a good clue to the seriousness of its cause. Mild headaches can be early warnings of serious disease, and excruciating ones can have trivial causes. The types of headache that suggest disease of the nervous system are those related to movement (those which occur particularly when a person coughs or bends over), those that are different from one's customary headache, and those that begin out of the blue in a person who has never had headaches before. Even these types of headaches often turn out to be caused by the tensions of life, resulting in contraction of muscles of the face and scalp, rather than a neurological cause.

Doctors usually classify headaches into five groups: vascular, muscle contraction or tension, combined tension and vascular, inflammation, and psychogenic. Vascular and muscle contraction headaches account for 90 percent of all chronic recurrent headaches.

Vascular headache arises when the large blood vessels of the scalp and head are displaced and stretched, pressing on sensitive adjoining tissue and producing pain. Tumors, blood clots, swelling of the brain, hypertension, and diseases of the blood vessels can all cause vascular headache, but the overwhelming majority of vascular headaches are migraine.

Migraine has been defined as "a familial disorder characterized by vasomotor dysfunction and associated with difficulty in adaptation to environmental changes." That means the chronic, recurrent head pain runs in families, stems from a problem with the nerves that control the constriction and dilation of blood vessels, and is usually triggered by outside events. Among the triggering events may be menstruation, diet, fatigue, and exposure to bright lights. About 20 percent of adults, predominantly women in the reproductive years, suffer from migraine. So do five percent of all children. The pain is usually (but not always) located over the temple on one side of the head. It is usually throbbing and severe, with tender distended scalp arteries. Sometimes the artery can be seen pulsating at the temple. The symptoms are worse with sudden head movement or exertion and may last hours or days. They may recur at long intervals or strike several times a week. Some patients have nausea, vomiting, diarrhea, and dizziness. They may be exquisitely sensitive to light, and forced to take refuge in a dark room. In children, headache is often less well-defined and usually does not last as long.

Classical migraine accounts for 20 percent of all cases but gives the condition its name ("migraine" is derived from the Greek "hemicrania," meaning "half the head"). The patient is forewarned of the attack by an aura, caused by constriction of the blood vessels, lasting 10 to 40 minutes. He or she "sees" evanescent light flashes like Roman candles, sparkles, or pinwheels. A common aura is "fortification spectra," geometric patterns like the parapets of a fort. Some patients lose vision in one or both eyes, have tingling in the fingers and tongue, mild confusion, and slurred speech. The aura is followed by a pounding headache that always strikes the same side.

Drawbacks of Pain-killers

One big problem of headache is the use of habituating or narcotic medications to which the patient can become addicted. As a consequence, physicians and patients must be careful not to prescribe or take medicines that can create a dangerous cycle of recurrent headache and addicting medication. Another problem is the use of pain medications (analgesics) such as aspirin or phenacetin. When taken in large doses, they can have side effects that are worse than the headaches. For example, too much aspirin can cause bleeding from the stomach, and phenacetin can lead to chronic kidney disease.

Common migraine involves the entire head. Its victims usually lack the warning aura.

Complicated migraine is characterized by paralysis of eye movement, weakness or paralysis of the limbs, vertigo, tingling, blindness, and even loss of consciousness.

Cluster headache is a variant of migraine that is more common in men over 40 than in women. It gets its name because attacks occur in clusters, sometimes two to three times in 24 hours for days or weeks. The attack can wake the patient from a sound sleep. Pain usually centers on one eye and has been compared to being stabbed in the eye with a red-hot poker. An individual attack lasts 30 to 90 minutes. Often the affected eye streams and the nose runs or is blocked. A man can have a series of attacks, then be free of attacks for years.

Vascular headaches appear to be related to the neurotransmitters serotonin and histamine. At the beginning of the attack accumulations of serotonin cause the capillaries to dilate and the larger vessels to contract. Serotonin is then inactivated and the process is reversed—capillaries constrict and arteries dilate. This explanation is supported by the identification of what is known as dietary migraine. Certain foods whose ingredients mimic the effect of these chemicals have been shown to trigger migraine attacks. Alcohol, red wine, champagne, cheddar cheese, chicken liver, pickled herring, canned figs, monosodium glutamate (MSG, a flavor enhancer used in Chinese dishes), nitrites (in cured meats), chocolate, and fatty and fried foods all can start the cycle. Oral contraceptives have been associated with migraine because falling estradiol levels can provoke an attack.

Treatment for migraine usually begins with an attempt to identify potential "triggers." This may mean changing the diet to eliminate any offending substances such as alcohol, chocolate, cheese, shellfish, and foods containing nitrites or MSG. Women with migraine should not use oral contraceptives. Since low blood sugar can cause headaches, it is important to establish regular meals. Rest and avoidance of stress are important. In migraine-prone children, exercise or vigorous sports can precipitate an attack and should be carefully controlled.

Drugs for migraine fall into two categories: those used for the acute attack and those for prevention of future attacks (prophylaxis).

Acute attack. To stop the pain of migraine, most doctors prescribe aspirin, acetaminophen, or codeine, combined with a mild sedative. If this is not effective, ergotamine tartrate may be used. Ergotamine acts by constricting blood vessels in the scalp and decreasing their pulsation. To be successful it must be taken during the aura of the attack, before the vessel wall begins to dilate. When taken in excess, or when taken by persons with diseased or especially sensitive arteries, there can be unwanted constriction of arteries to the limbs, eyes, or heart. It is used with caution in older persons.

Preventive medications are recommended for patients with more than three severe headaches a month, or when headache is a major problem for more than one week a month. In addition to ergotamine tartrate, there are three major types of preventive (prophylactic) medications, sometimes used in various combinations. All have been shown to affect the serotonin levels. Each has advantages, but each can have serious side effects.

(1) Methysergide is effective in preventing attacks in 60 to 75 percent of cases, but it is not recommended for persons with vascular disease and peptic ulcer. If used for long periods, it may cause "silent" fibroid growths that can interfere with kidney function. These can be avoided by a drug "holiday" of at least one month in six.

(2) Amitriptyline, an antidepressant, inhibits the re-uptake of serotonin. It, too, is given daily. Minor side effects are drowsiness, blurred vision, weight gain, and nervousness. More serious ones are intestinal disorders and retention of urine. It should not be taken by patients with heart disease.

(3) Propranolol, also used for hypertension, is the most recent addition to the preventive-medication arsenal. It appears to have fewer side effects, but is not recommended for patients with cardiac disease and asthma. It can produce nausea and drowsiness.

Minor tranquilizers such as meprobamate and diazepam may be helpful. Biofeedback training also has been used.

Other forms of vascular headache occur in hypoxia, fever, hunger with hypoglycemia, carbon dioxide retention, hangover, and in the early post-concussion state. Excessive use of coffee, tea, or cola drinks may result in caffeine withdrawal, with generalized headache.

Cranial arteritis is an inflammation that commonly affects the temporal artery but can affect any scalp artery, plus the middle cerebral and ophthalmic artery serving the eye. About one-third of patients may lose vision permanently. The diagnosis should be considered in any person over 60 who complains of headache for the first time. Headache may throb at first but soon becomes severe and burning. The affected arteries are tender and firm, but do not pulsate. Sometimes weakness, muscle pain, and low-grade fever are present. Prednisone tends to eliminate the pain and prevent complications.

Tension headache or muscle-contraction headache is the most common form of headache. The pain is usually dull and generalized. It may feel as though someone were tightening a band around the head. There may be a burning sensation and tenderness of the scalp, which may spread to the neck and shoulders. Occasionally the pain may be more concentrated in one part of the head than another.

Symptoms stem from the tightening of scalp muscles, usually in response to tension, fatigue, or emotional stress. The headaches may come and go as episodes of stress recur.

Tension headache should be differentiated from the constant headache that persists for years and is unaffected by any treatment. This uncommon headache is seen in more severe psychological disorders.

Treatment of tension headache usually seeks to uncover underlying conflicts and reduce emotional stress. This may be a long process, because changes in life-style or stressful occupations are not always easily achieved. Mild, nonaddicting analgesics such as aspirin and sedatives are useful. Prolonged tension headache is often associated with depression, so antidepressants may be prescribed, too. Muscle relaxation exercises and biofeedback may help.

Temporo-mandibular joint dysfunction, affecting the joint at the angle of the jaw and spreading through the head, is another source of headache. It is often due to faulty dental work or unconscious jaw clenching during sleep. Dental problems can be corrected (see chapter 18, "The Teeth and Oral Health"), but jaw clenching may be more difficult because it may have an emotional basis.

Trigeminal neuralgia (tic douloureux) is a particularly severe kind of headache, caused by degeneration of or pressure on the trigeminal nerve radiating from the angle of the jaw. The terrible pain is said by some women to be worse than that of a first labor. The attack comes as sudden sharp stabbing pains, always on the same side, the exact location and spread determined by the nerve branch involved. Sometimes the pain can be relieved with tranquilizers, but surgery may be necessary to relieve the pressure.

Intercranial diseases other than vascular disorders cause no more than five percent of headaches. They mainly include tumors, with or without increased intercranial pressure, and irritation of the meninges (brain membranes) caused by hemorrhage or infection (meningitis). They may be signaled by a change in the pattern of headache, by headache accompanied by diminishing vision or difficulty in focusing the eyes, or by headache appearing for the first time in children or after middle age. Tumor can produce intermittent headaches because of pressure of the growth on pain-sensitive structures. It is usually most noticeable in a particular area of the head. The pain may be made worse by coughing or bending, and may wake the person from sleep. Headache caused by hemorrhage under the arachnoid membrane or by meningitis usually occurs suddenly and involves the whole head or the back of the head. There may be loss of consciousness, sometimes blurred vision or loss of sight.

Dizziness, Light-headedness, and Vertigo

A variety of disorders express themselves by what is commonly called light-headedness or dizziness. Although they commonly are lumped together by patients, these two conditions are separated by physicians. Light-headedness refers to a subjective feeling of unsteadiness, possibly associated with a sensation that one is about to faint. There may be some blurred vision and ringing in the ears. Dizziness, or vertigo, makes a person unsteady on his feet because of a feeling that he or everything around him is moving. There is no associated clouding of consciousness, but vision may blur if the surroundings seem to be in motion. The reason for distinguishing between the two sensations is that light-headedness is usually caused by reduced blood supply to the brain, while dizziness results from a defect in function of the balancing apparatus which keeps the body in its correct position in space. There are several causes for each.

Light-headedness. The most common cause of reduced blood supply to the brain is an abnormality in the heart or the blood pressure regulating system (see chapter 3, "The Heart and Circulation," chapter 4, "Hypertension," and chapter 6, "The Blood"). The reduction also may stem from disease of the arteries supplying the brain (see chapter 5, "Blood Vessel Disorders"). Symptoms of light-headedness also may precede stroke, but seldom occur alone. They usually are accompanied by such symptoms as weakness in one side of the body, loss of vision in one eye, or transient ischemic attacks, which are interruptions of blood supply that can cause lapses of consciousness.

Other causes of light-headedness are defects in the blood itself. Anemia, a deficiency of red blood cells, can lower the amount of oxygen reaching the brain. Polycythemia, an excess of red blood cells, can result in thickened blood that does not flow properly through the brain.

Hyperventilation syndrome also is a frequent cause of light-headedness. A person under stress or anxiety begins to breathe deeply and rapidly, which causes him to expel the carbon dioxide in the blood. The blood vessels that supply the brain constrict, lowering the blood supply and inducing a feeling of light-headedness. Often the cause is not recognized. A person with light-headedness should always be asked to breathe deeply in order to assess this possibility.

Vertigo, the medical term for what is commonly called dizziness, describes the feeling that a person's surroundings are moving. In some cases the surroundings seem to be spinning like a top, but more often pitching and heaving, as if one is standing on a boat tossed about by waves. The reason is usually a malfunction of the balancing apparatus, which includes the labyrinth in the inner ear, its nerves, and the brainstem connecting to the cerebellum and cerebrum (see chapter 13, "Ear, Nose, and Throat"). Because the two labyrinths are located in the inner ear adjacent to the organs for hearing, and because their blood supply is from the same source, the two are often affected by the same disease, such as the common ear infection. The labyrinth, three fluid-filled semicircular canals, sense all directions that the head might move in space. Fluid displaced by movement causes discharge of neurons in the labyrinthine nerves, which send messages to the brain. (We have vertigo after riding a merry-go-round because of continued movement of the fluid.) Movements may be unconscious, such as walking, or conscious, as in a person who is tilting his head. Static position in contrast to acceleration is sensed by cells with a bit of sand (otolith) attached. The semicircular canals and their nerves must function equally well. If one is too sensitive or too insensitive, the brain interprets the information as indicating that the surroundings are in motion. It

is similar to an airplane with two engines when one speeds up or slows down and causes the plane to turn.

The diseases that cause this change fall into three major categories: blood vessel disease, nerve disorder, and disease of the semicircular apparatus itself. The most common is Meniere's disease or hydrops. Meniere's disease in its classical form strikes suddenly and is often associated with ringing in the ear or even deafness. The patient often must lie motionless in bed because even the slightest movement such as sitting up or turning incites violent vertigo which may result in nausea and vomiting. The attack may be accompanied by nystagmus, rhythmic jerking of the eyes to one side. Tests are performed by inserting hot and cold water into the ear to find out whether the flow of fluid in the semicircular canals is normal. Attacks are usually short-lived but unfortunately are recurrent. The disease sometimes is hereditary, and the cause is unknown. The treatment is to reduce the sensitivity of the labyrinthine nerves by antimotion sickness pills such as Antivert,® Dramamine,® Bonine,® and Marezine.® The patient is also given diuretics to reduce the amount of fluid in the inner ear.

An especially severe form of vertigo is one which occurs in some persons whenever they change head position. Even the simple act of lying down, sitting up, or turning the head can induce a violent but short-lived attack. The cause is usually in the inner ear, sometimes due to a loss of the otolith, which rolls about loosely within the inner ear. It may result from a head injury or toxicity to certain drugs.

Pain and Numbness

All parts of the body have countless nerve endings. The skin is full of nerve receptors that sense the environment around it. Heat and cold, pain, vibration, pressure, and movement are all "felt" by messages sent to the brain. When this system does not work properly, the patient begins to feel pain, numbness, or peculiarities of sensation—a cold object feels painful or a painful sensation feels hot. Sometimes a patient feels a sensation of pins and needles or tingling. At other times a limb feels as if it has fallen asleep. We have all had the experience of sleeping with an arm in such a position that when we awaken it feels numb and useless, and most of us have had dental anesthesia which makes a part of the tongue or jaw uncomfortably numb.

When a patient complains of pain or numbness in a body part, the physician tests the involved areas with a pin, cotton, tuning fork, and hot and cold objects. The nerves that leave the skin carry the sensations of pain, temperature, pressure, and vibration together so that any abnormality in the nerve will affect all to a degree. When the nerve reaches the spinal cord, the sensations begin to separate and at the brainstem are "felt" in different locations. An abnormality at the spinal cord or beyond may affect only one sensation, a telltale clue.

The brain also puts these sensations into a meaningful relationship, so that not only are the sensations felt, but the shape of the object and its potential use are recognized by the brain. It is possible, for example, to recognize that something is cold, heavy, and sharp but not to be able to recognize that it is a knife except by looking at it. Certain diseases of the brain destroy the ability to integrate this information or to name the object even if one recognizes it. Other diseases destroy our ability to recognize what we see, although touching the object still allows us to identify it.

Peripheral neuropathy is the name given to those disorders affecting the peripheral nerves. A single nerve or many nerves can be involved. Nerves commonly affected are the radial, ulnar, and median nerves of the arm and the sciatic nerve in the lower extremity. Because roots coming from the spinal cord join to form a peripheral nerve, a neurologist tries to determine whether a root or the nerve is affected and whether one or several nerves are involved. Herniated discs and tumors of the spinal cord are common root disorders. Neuropathies result from poisoning by alcohol, drugs, or insecticides, and are a common consequence of diabetes.

Sciatica can be caused by compression of the sciatic nerve as it passes through the muscles of the buttock in its long course from the spinal cord to the foot. Sciatica can cause pain down the leg, areas of numbness, loss of reflexes, and sometimes weakness in the foot. Medication, rest, exercises, instruction in proper use of back muscles, and perhaps surgery to remove a herniated disc are the best treatments.

Shingles (herpes zoster) is caused by an infection of a nerve cell by a virus that is similar if not identical to the chickenpox virus. It causes burning pain in a rash of blebs that usually follows the nerve course. Common sites are the trigeminal nerve of the face and nerves of the torso. Steroid medications bring relief, but there is no cure. The rash tends to subside and disappear in a few weeks, but the pain may remain for months, a condition known as postherpetic neuralgia. In this case several pain relieving medications may be necessary because no one treatment is satisfactory.

Postinfectious polyneuritis (Guillain-Barre syndrome) is a disturbance that affects the nerve roots, sometimes of both arms and legs, along with some of the cranial nerves affecting the face, jaws, tongue, and eyes. Motor as well as sensory nerves are involved, causing weakness, difficulty in breathing, wasting of the muscles, numbness, and loss of reflexes. The disorder may be caused by a postinfectious immune reaction, toxic substances such as insecticides, and serum injections. The onset is sudden, with weakness usually beginning in the legs and sometimes ascending within hours to involve the entire body. The patient may need artificial breathing support (see chapter 8, "The Lungs") because of respiratory paralysis. Symptoms can be relieved by use of steroids.

Compression neuropathy is the direct compression of a nerve as it passes through a narrow canal. In carpal tunnel syndrome the hand is affected, with severe pain in the thumb and fingers, particularly at night. In crossed-leg palsy the nerve to the foot is affected with tingling, numbness, and temporary loss of power in that leg. The condition clears if the person avoids crossing one leg tightly over the other.

Bell's palsy is compression of the swollen facial nerve as it passes through a bony canal in the skull below the ear on its course to the muscles of the face. Pain below the ear is followed by loss of ability to close the eye or smile on the affected side. The paralysis causes the mouth to pull to the other side.

The condition is alarming and embarrassing, but normally clears up within several months, perhaps more rapidly with steroids, electric treatment, and massage. During the time when the eyelid cannot be closed, glasses or a patch must be worn to prevent dust or rough particles from injuring the cornea.

Tremors

Shaking movements have a variety of causes and are classified according to their rhythm, amplitude, and location in the body. One of the most common is the tremulousness that sometimes occurs with aging.

Parkinson's disease, or parkinsonism, stems from loss of dopamine-producing cells in the substantia nigra portion of the basal ganglia. The symptoms are shaking (tremor) of the hands, head, and feet, stiffness (rigidity) of the limbs with slowing of movements (particularly walking), and a stooped posture. The disorder does not affect mental functions and does not lead to paralysis. The earliest manifestations are usually a slight shaking of the hands when trying to perform fine movements such as writing. The disorder usually progresses to more widespread symptoms, but sometimes tremors are not progressive and run in families, in which case they are termed benign essential tremors. True parkinsonism usually progresses to affect other functions such as speech, which becomes tremulous and soft, walking, which becomes slow and shuffling, and posture, which becomes bent forward.

In 1918 a worldwide epidemic of influenza followed by encephalitis, or "sleeping sickness," left enormous numbers of people with postencephalitic parkinsonism. Now most cases are of unknown cause, but the long-delayed aftermath of an earlier virus infection is suspected. In rare instances parkinsonism is caused by hereditary degeneration of the basal ganglia. In these cases mental deterioration also may occur because of cortical involvement. Parkinsonism also can be caused by poisoning, most commonly by certain tranquilizers used for psychiatric disorders.

It is sometimes said that a person with advanced parkinsonism is frozen within his own body because the muscles cannot act fast enough to perform the actions necessary for daily living, such as getting out of bed, dressing, eating, sitting down, and standing up. Fortunately, the handicaps once associated with parkinsonism now can be overcome through the use of levadopa, or L-dopa. This drug, taken by mouth, substitutes for the missing neurotransmitter dopamine, normally secreted by the cells of the substantia nigra. The discovery has made it possible for hundreds of thousands of parkinsonism patients to lead almost normal lives. L-dopa (and its newer modified formulas which include carbidopa), when taken daily in sufficient dosage, can almost totally substitute for the deficiencies of the degenerated cells. Only rarely is it necessary to consider a surgical operation to relieve the tremor as was necessary in the past. The amount of L-dopa necessary to control parkinsonism varies from patient to patient and an individual's tolerance also varies. Too much causes uncontrolled movements of the limbs called choreoathetosis.

Huntington's disease or Huntington's chorea is another movement-producing disorder of the basal ganglia. It is hereditary, affecting men and women in their early 40s and 50s. The disease is dominantly transmitted, meaning that it passes from an affected parent to half the offspring. Tragically, the child may not know whether he or she carries the disease until the first symptoms appear in midlife. By then he or she may have had children.

The first symptoms are usually an involuntary, barely noticeable, movement of fingers, facial muscles, or limbs. The movement occurs both when the person is relaxed and when engaged in activities. As the disorder progresses these involuntary movements begin to interfere with more skilled movements and the person drops objects or stumbles. Speech is interrupted by sudden facial, tongue, and breathing abnormalities that persist despite the person's best attempts to control them. Mental deterioration occurs in many patients as the frontal lobes of the brain are affected.

There may be marked personality change: the formerly neat and meticulous patient becomes slovenly. Sexual and emotional aberrations may develop. Within five to ten years the patient is incapacitated either by uncontrollable movements or by dementia. The disorder can be diagnosed by family history or by the characteristic loss of the caudate nucleus of the basal ganglia (revealed by CT brain scan). The disease cannot be prevented or cured. The drug bromocryptine may modify the tremors.

Other forms of tremor (chorea) are now rare. Sydenham's chorea occurs during active rheumatic fever and persists only as long as the disease is active. Chorea gravidarum has its onset during pregnancy and disappears with delivery.

Dystonia, also a disorder of the basal ganglia, affects the large muscle groups of the limbs, neck, and body, which contract slowly and for a prolonged period of time causing the patient to be contorted into extremely awkward and sometimes painful positions. Dystonia can result from birth injury, can be hereditary, or it can result from unusual reaction to tranquilizers as in torticollis ("wry neck"), an involuntary sustained turning of the head to one side caused by contraction of the sternomastoid muscle in the neck.

Ballism is a rare affliction in which the arm and leg on one side are involuntarily flung about so violently that the joints may be dislocated or the body part injured if it strikes against something. The disorder is caused by a lesion in the corpus Luys area of the midbrain, usually because of a stroke. It usually subsides spontaneously in a few weeks.

Wilson's disease (hepatolenticular degeneration) is a rare but potentially preventable and curable hereditary disorder. The victim is born with an inability to properly use copper obtained in the diet. The metal accumulates in the liver and basal ganglia (see chapter 20, "The Digestive System"), causing hepatitis or parkinson-like symptoms. This potentially fatal disease can be cured with a diet low in copper and medication to remove accumulations of the metal from the body.

Ataxia is the name given to a group of disorders of movement that superficially resemble others classified as tremors but that originate in other parts of the nervous system. Their common characteristic is abnormality of limb placement in response to voluntary movement. The patient is unable to place his feet in desired position rapidly and accurately, and therefore walks with a drunken, rolling gait, similar to the way a person walks on a ship at sea. In advanced ataxia the upper limbs are also affected and the person cannot reach out and touch objects accurately.

The location for this disorder is the cerebellum and its connections. The most common cause is intoxication with alcohol, tranquilizers, street drugs, or toxic substances.

In other instances the disorder is hereditary and develops slowly over many years, often beginning in adolescence. These hereditary ataxias are classified according to the part of the nervous system most affected. Charcot-Marie-Tooth disease results in loss of nerves to the limbs with atrophy of muscles and abnormal sensation. This causes "bird legs" of only skin and bones. There is also a characteristically high arch to the foot and a hammer toe. If the spinal cord is most affected by the disorder it is Friedrich's ataxia. If degeneration of the cerebellum predominates it is Marie's cellebellar ataxia. These disorders are genetically transmitted and are suspected to be caused by enzyme defects in the affected cells, which function normally for years before they begin to die off. There is no known prevention or treatment.

Gilles de la Tourette syndrome affects young people, who develop an uncontrollable grimacing of the face coupled with respiratory movements that cause them to sigh, snort, grunt, and clear their throats. They may utter obscenities in a loud voice for which there is no control or particular underlying motivation. Treatment with the drug haloperidol may be effective. The cause is not known.

Buccolingual dyskinesia is a disorder that can be induced by too many tranquilizers or excessive medication for parkinsonism. It consists of involuntary movements of the jaw, tongue, and face which are particularly disconcerting if the person wears dentures. It may be modified with haloperidol.

Tics are nervous movements such as the repeated shrugging of a shoulder or pulling up of one corner of the mouth. They seldom have a neurological basis, but are related to some inner emotional tension. They occur chiefly among adolescents but may continue through life. Treatment is in the realm of psychiatry.

Forgetfulness

Memory is a term used by physicians and laymen alike, but a physician classifies memory into three categories: immediate, intermediate, and remote. Immediate recall is the ability to repeat accurately information that has just been received. For example, if someone tells you a phone number you can repeat it immediately. Try to recollect it in five minutes; this is intermediate recall. Would you be able to remember the number in two years? Few people could remember it unless they recited it or heard it repeatedly during that time. This is remote recall.

When we are awake, everything we see, hear, or touch is recorded in the brain. Presumably every bit of that information becomes a memory, but most of it is soon forgotten. Have you ever looked at a photograph album and seen pictures of things you did years ago but had completely forgotten? Only stressful, exciting, or perhaps dangerous and anxious experiences can be recollected at will, and even those are often remembered inaccurately. Many memories lost to consciousness remain in the unconscious and can be recalled with appropriate techniques. When a person is born he has his total lifetime supply of nerve cells. Only the circuits that link these neurons together increase. By about age 18 memory prowess is at its best. Subsequently, experience and learning continue to improve our judgment, but the number of cells and their activity begin to decline. With advancing age some people lose enough cells that they cannot function normally. If this occurs before age 65 it is classified as presenile dementia. After 65,

it is called senile dementia. The terms stem from the mistaken notion that the processes differ at different ages.

The young boy can sit at his grandfather's knee for hours and listen to tales of the old days because senile people sometimes have a fabulous memory for the remote past. Ask the old gentleman to dress himself or take a message on the telephone, however, and nothing may be accomplished except confusion. Many senile people are aware of their problem, frustrated and depressed by it, but helpless to do anything about it. Fortunately, the deficiency can be compensated for by understanding and helpful family members who can substitute for the defect in memory just as one would help a person who had lost an arm or leg. Memory loss cannot be corrected, but the family and the physician can do much to reduce the stress that it creates.

The first step is to determine why the brain cannot record new information. There can be many causes. One of the most common and yet most preventable is excessive use of alcohol, which causes death of the cells that record new memories. "Excessive" use of alcohol does not necessarily mean a daily drink or two, but does include the abuse of alcohol to substitute for nutritious foods and the vitamins needed for normal function. Another cause of mental deterioration is endocrine disease, particularly low thyroid function. A third is brain injury with damage to the temporal lobes of the brain. Anyone who has seen a person with a head injury realizes that after regaining consciousness the person is confused and has lost memory of the events that preceded the accident. The common terminology for this condition is "punch drunk," so called because boxers who have had their heads pummeled for many years lose the ability to record memories and live in a confused state. Other diseases that cause memory to change are acute and chronic infections of the nervous system, including syphilis and certain viral diseases. Uncommonly, a stroke can cause a temporary or even a permanent loss of memory.

Communication Abnormalities

Aphasia is the name given to the loss of ability to communicate via speech or to understand the speech of others. It includes the "deaf and dumb" who have never had normal hearing and as a consequence cannot speak words. Another group, however, has normal hearing but sounds are not properly recorded in the brain because of disease. It is as if those around them were speaking an unknown foreign language. A third disorder is the loss of the ability to speak even though one hears and comprehends what is said. This type of aphasia is caused by loss of control over the muscles that guide movements of the mouth, lungs, and chest during speech.

As discussed on page 196, our speech capability is in the brain's dominant hemisphere, usually the side opposite the hand used for writing. Both the representation for hearing and the motor control for speech are located here. They are close together because part of hearing words is the ability to respond quickly with speech.

Stuttering begins in childhood and sometimes persists throughout life, usually during moments of stress. The cause is unknown but in some cases it results from mixed dominance in which the two brain hemispheres compete for control of the neuromuscular apparatus of language.

Reading and writing are a substitute for speech. Reading is the ability to translate symbols into mental images. This occurs in the dominant hemisphere. Writing is symbolic language and requires coordinated control of the arm and hand for making marks. In the growth of normal children speech is acquired some years before reading and writing, a fact commonly attributed to maturation of different areas of the brain. Speech resides in the frontal lobes of the dominant hemisphere. Speech requires hearing, which transmits nerve impulses to the temporal lobes. Connections from the temporal lobe go to the motor area of the dominant frontal lobe and coordinate the impulses that become speech.

Reading and writing require that we see words or symbols. The impulses they create on the retina travel to the visual area of the occipital lobes, then to the parietal regions for interpretation. Writing arises in the parietal region where word symbols are stored, but the movements of the hands are controlled by the dominant frontal lobe. Therefore connections between parietal and frontal regions must function properly for reading and writing to be normal.

Dyslexia is a congenital inability to learn to read, presumably caused by the improper or delayed development of these brain areas or their interconnections. Dyslexia runs in families, affects males predominantly, and has a tendency to occur in families that have several left-handers. Dyslexics write with letter reversals and at times use mirror writing. It is important to recognize that dyslexic children are not intellectually deficient or recalcitrant, but cannot cope with printed symbols. Oral rather than written methods for teaching must be used.

Remedial reading and writing by teaching specialists can produce dramatic improvement in many but not all cases. Treatment often calls for careful support so that children do not develop psychological and behavioral abnormalities resulting from societal and school pressure.

Sleep and Wakefulness

The normal adult sleeps between 25 and 33 percent of his life, infants and children even more. Sleep is vital for refurbishment of the brain, so that it may function normally. Deprivation of sleep, even for only 48 hours, results in abnormalities of behavior which can include paranoia and hallucinations, even convulsions. Precisely what happens during normal sleep is unknown but the reticular activating system of the midbrain, which keeps the two cerebral hemispheres alert, is switched off. Coma is akin to but not synonymous with sleep. Sleep is easily disturbed in some people and sleep disturbance may be one of the early symptoms of psychiatric disorder.

Sleep is of two types, called REM (for rapid eye movement) and non-REM sleep. They alternate at about 90-minute intervals. In REM sleep the eyes move beneath the closed eyelids and dreaming takes place. Muscles of the body stiffen and sometimes twitch. The electroencephalogram (EEG) shows a characteristic alteration in rhythm. There are four progressively deeper stages of non-REM sleep with no eye movement and no dreaming in the usual sense. Each non-REM stage has its characteristic EEG rhythm, too.

When a person falls asleep his stage 1 rapid EEG slows progressively for about 70 minutes until in stage 4 a very slow EEG develops. Then, the rhythms speed up again, eye movement (REM sleep) begins, and dreaming ensues. This cycle is repeated four to six times during eight hours of sleep. The REM periods grow progressively longer. Therefore 20 to 25 percent of sleep is occupied by dreaming.

Disturbances of normal sleep patterns include certain forms of bed-wetting (enuresis), sleepwalking (somnambulism), nightmares, and insomnia.

Insomnia is a major complaint of Americans who have been schooled to believe that eight hours of uninterrupted sleep nightly are essential for good health. Studies have shown, however, that there is an enormous range of "normal" requirements for sleep. Some persons are able to function well on frequent short catnaps, while others require a rigid routine of uninterrupted sleep. Infants and young children require eight to 10 hours of sleep. By age 20 the usual is seven hours and by age 40 it has dropped to six hours. Above age 40 we tend to spend more time in bed but a lesser percentage of that time asleep. After age 60 repeated interruptions of sleep seem to be the norm. Because there is no unanimity of opinion among the public or physicians on how much sleep is needed, the tolerable limits of insomnia are unknown, so enormous quantities of sleeping aids and medications are sold annually. Many are harmless but some create dependency and require increasing use until they are abused. Some persons, particularly if depressed, use them for inducing unnecessarily prolonged sleep to escape their intolerable environment.

Illnesses associated with excessive sleeping are disordered endocrine function, particularly hypothyroidism, narcolepsy, brain neoplasms, metabolic disorders with toxic substances that sedate the brain as in liver, kidney, or respiratory disease, and drugs that sedate the brain.

Insomnia suggests anxiety and hypersomnia (excessive sleep) suggests depression.

Some who complain of continuing fatigue have sleep abnormalities that prevent them from achieving stage 3 or stage 4 sleep, the deepest and most refreshing sleep. In some people this abnormality is so severe that they fall asleep at inappropriate times throughout the day. Respiratory disorders that obstruct breathing may result in recurrent awakening throughout the night. Snoring can be one clue to this abnormality. Sometimes the breathing obstruction results from obesity. The cure is removal of the obstruction, weight reduction for the obese, and in some cases a tracheostomy to bypass the obstruction of the upper air passages.

Narcolepsy is a disorder in which the person may suddenly drop off to sleep without warning and at inappropriate moments, such as while eating, or at dangerous moments, such as while driving a car. In some cases this stems from an abnormality in the reticular activating system, the brain's so-called "sleep center." In other cases it is suspected that the difficulty is emotional. Some persons require brain stimulation through amphetamines to prevent sudden dropping off to sleep. Occasionally, narcoleptic attacks are accompanied by feelings of body paralysis, weakness, or collapse when angry or laughing. The person may drop helplessly to the ground on such occasions. There also may be a compulsion to eat enormous quantities of food, a condition called Kleine-Levine syndrome.

DISORDERS OF THE NERVOUS SYSTEM

Because the nervous system is spread throughout every part of the body and regulates innumerable functions, nervous system disorders can take many forms. Two of the most important are covered in subsequent chapters. Chapter 10, "Epilepsy," deals with electrical disturbances within the brain and the patterns of symptoms those disturbances produce. Chapter 11, "Stroke," describes interruptions of the blood supply to the brain and the consequences.

Other common neurological disorders include demyelinating diseases, infections, tumors, neuromuscular diseases, and nutritional diseases.

Demyelinating Diseases

Axons and dendrites are enwrapped by cells that contain myelin, a fatty substance essential for normal conduction of electrical impulses. Myelin thickness varies along the length of the axons and dendrites and from fiber to fiber. The thicker the myelin the faster the electrical impulse is conducted. Myelin is yellow-white in color while cells are gray. So the white matter of the brain, spinal cord, and peripheral nerves contains myelinated fibers and the gray matter contains concentrations of cell bodies. Certain diseases attack myelin and the special cells that produce it, stripping the cells of myelin or causing scarring (plaque). When this happens the nerve ceases to conduct impulses normally and may even stop conducting completely.

Multiple sclerosis (MS) is the most common of several demyelinating diseases. MS is especially prevalent in the United States but is not equally distributed within the country, nor for that matter around the world. It is concentrated in areas of temperate climate and is rare in the tropics or the Arctic. This suggests to researchers that there may be an environmental or climatic influence. Others suggest that MS is caused by a slow virus that remains in the body for many years until activated by some outside event. Still others think that it is an autoimmune disorder with the patient becoming "allergic" to his own myelin. A third opinion combines the two, suggesting that the virus alters the myelin in such a way that the immune system regards it as a foreign substance. Because the cause of MS is unknown, extensive research is being carried out in areas where the disease is epidemic, such as the Shetland and Orkney Islands off Scotland. There the disease is clustered in families and is especially frequent in women. An increasingly popular theory implicates contagion from dogs that have had distemper.

The disease usually begins during the teens or twenties, rarely after 35. The onset is sudden and can occur in any part of the central nervous system. It may strike in more than one part, hence the name "multiple." Early symptoms may be subtle and fleeting. Visual abnormality, unsteadiness of gait, tremor, sensory impairment, bladder disturbance, paralysis, and slurring of speech can occur alone or in combination. The plaque of demyelination stops normal nerve function for about two weeks and then begins to heal, resulting in improvement or remission. However, healing is seldom complete, so full function may not return to the affected areas. Usually the disorder is quiet, without new symptoms for about two years, whereupon it flares up again. With each exacerbation the patient usually has more loss of neurological function. Some persons, however, never have more than a single attack.

Treatment for MS is nonspecific because the cause is unknown. Many physicians prescribe ACTH or steroids to reduce swelling and inflammation during the acute phase. Physical therapy, low-fat diets, and avoidance of heat are all advocated. Although the disease can progress to severe handicap, it is not fatal. About one-third of MS patients are said to hold regular jobs.

Infections

Infections of the nervous system can involve the brain, spinal cord, or nerves, or the roots that emanate from them (see chapter 28, "Infectious Diseases"). Infection of the brain tissue is called encephalitis, while infection of the membranes covering the brain and spinal cord (meninges) is called meningitis. Infection or inflammation of the nerve roots is called radiculitis, and infection of the nerves is neuritis. The infections may be either bacterial or viral, and may spread from infections elsewhere in the body. At times a brain infection may result in an abscess, a localized pocket of pus in the brain tissue or membranes.

Inflammation of the brain causes headache, fever, nausea, vomiting, and clouding of consciousness, sometimes with coma. There may also be paralysis or numbness in parts of the body, and even temporary blindness or deafness depending on the area of the brain infected. The combination of fever, headache, confusion, delirium, and stupor, especially when accompanied by neck pain, strongly suggests meningitis and is a medical emergency (see chapter 27, "Taking Care of Your Child" and chapter 28, "Infectious Diseases").

Before the advent of antibiotics, any infection in the nervous system was almost invariably fatal. Great epidemics of spinal meningitis, spread by several highly infectious strains of bacteria, would dictate that entire populations be quarantined and that children be kept out of school to contain the spread. Antibiotic treatment can quickly arrest the disease, and also prevents its occurrence by halting bacterial infections elsewhere in the body that might affect the brain. Antibiotics also have reduced the frequency of brain abscess, which frequently resulted from spread of infection from the nasal sinuses or the middle ear. Fortunately, successful treatment of nervous system infections usually leaves no lasting neurological consequences.

Injury

Injuries to the head and brain most commonly result from auto accidents or gunshot wounds, occasionally from falls or sports mishaps. They are most common in the young adult population; auto accidents are the leading cause of disability and death in men and women under 30. These consequences have been reduced by enforcement of a 55 m.p.h. speed limit and the use of seat belts. Helmets for bicyclists and motorcyclists, and safer athletic equipment have also reduced the toll.

Brain injury occurs when the brain impacts against the bony skull, resulting in bruises or lacerations that can have permanent effects. Or there may be bleeding within the brain or over its entire surface. Sometimes the injured brain swells with edema fluid, putting pressure on the cells. There may also be damage if an object penetrates the skull and brain, or from depressed skull fracture which bruises the brain beneath it.

Mild brain injury that merely stuns or dazes is called a concussion. Most head injuries fall into this category. The person may be confused, dizzy, forgetful of the preceding events, and may vomit. He may briefly lose consciousness. Mild injury seldom causes permanent damage, although some patients may experience dizziness, nervousness, restlessness, and headache for weeks or months afterward.

Unconsciousness following a head injury requires prompt medical evaluation by a neurologist or neurosurgeon. So do persistent vomiting, dilation of one pupil, weakness of the limbs, paralysis, and convulsions. In fact, it is wise for anyone who has had a head injury, unless it is trivial, to have a neurological examination, including an X ray and possibly a computerized cranial tomogram (CT scan) to rule out fracture and head off delayed consequences. Some brain injuries, with or without fracture of the skull, can cause lasting damage. When a person is rendered unconscious the brain has been injured. The patient may recover completely, but may develop intercranial bleeding or fluid buildup which requires emergency neurosurgery.

Brain injury is one of the most preventable of neurological conditions, and safety measures to protect the vulnerable brain, such as the use of seat belts and helmets, should be followed by everyone.

Brain Tumor (Neoplasm)

Because the brain nearly fills the rigid skull, any addition or enlargement inside the skull cavity, whether it be a hemorrhage, an infection, swelling from injury, or a new growth in the brain, can cause severe headache until the increase in intracranial pressure is relieved by brain surgery, drugs, or by the natural course of events.

Technically, tumors within the brain, like those that develop elsewhere in the body, fall into two categories, benign and malignant. Because of the confined space within the skull, however, even benign tumors can be life-threatening. The intracranial pressure crowds healthy cells and interferes with their normal functions. Tumors can develop deep within the brain, making removal impossible without destruction of other cells. However, benign growths are often encapsulated. If discovered early and if they are in an accessible area, they often can be removed completely. Malignant tumors, on the other hand, often have roots like a plant and removing them completely is difficult. Additionally, the brain is a frequent target for cancer cells spread from a primary tumor elsewhere. Sometimes it is possible to remove the primary tumor but not the satellite growth in the brain.

Although generations of moviegoers believe that brain tumors announce themselves with sudden, splitting headache or attacks of blindness, early symptoms are seldom so dramatic. In fact, brain tumor may be difficult to diagnose because symptoms are so vague, or resemble those of other conditions. There may be blindness, paralysis of one side of the body, severe headache, seizures, or loss of consciousness. There may be dimmed vision, reduced hearing, bouts of irritation, or loss of emotion or intellect. Some persons experience strange sensations such as auditory hallucinations or strange smells. Obviously, one of these clues alone rarely indicates brain tumor, but a pattern, or symptoms that occur "out of the blue," should receive medical attention.

Treatment depends on the location and the type of tumor involved. There are many types of new growths within the brain. Surgery is the preferred course for those located near the skull, where they may be removed completely. Sometimes the tumor is so deep in the brain that removal can only be accomplished at the risk of causing further damage or death. In these cases a portion may be removed to relieve intracranial pressure and to allow microscopic examination of the cell type, even though the unremoved parts will continue to grow. Deep X-ray treatment may be used afterwards, and is sometimes used alone to retard growth of certain types of tumors. Drugs may be used alone or in conjunction with radiotherapy. An obstacle to drug use has been the blood-brain barrier (see page 194), which presumably filters out harmful substances to the brain, but newer drugs are able to bypass this hurdle.

The use of computerized cranial tomography (see chapter 32, "X Rays and Radiology") has led to earlier and surer diagnosis of brain tumor.

Tumors of the central nervous system can originate within the brain or spinal cord from any of the different cell types contained there, or from the meninges that surround the brain (meningiomas). Furthermore, tumors of the cranial nerves themselves can originate from the optic, trigeminal, or acoustic nerves, or from any of the spinal nerves (neuromas). Neoplasms that arise in other organs of the body can travel to the brain via the bloodstream. There they lodge and grow as metastases. Usually, these metastases arise from the breast, lung, kidney, or thyroid.

Neuromuscular Diseases

Each motor cell in the spinal cord sends instructions via its axon in the peripheral nerve to as many as 100 muscle fibers. When an individual cell is activated, an electrical impulse travels down the axon, causing the fibers to twitch. Impulses from hundreds of motor cells unite these twitches into contraction. Obviously, many thousands of cells must act together to cause contraction of a muscle. In an action as complicated as walking or talking, dozens of muscles must work together. This coordinated activity is synchronized by the brain, which modulates the firing of the spinal cord cells. When the cellular unit is diseased, the result is weakness, rapid fatigue, or wasting of the muscle. Disorders can affect a single muscle or many muscles.

Symptoms. Weakness is the primary symptom of neuromuscular disorder. The distinction between what would be called "normal" fatigue and weakness indicating disease is often difficult. Many people get tired at the end of the day—fatigue is one of the most common symptoms experienced by people. But if the person begins to have double vision, difficulty with swallowing, weakness to the point of collapse, and inability to carry out normal activities, particularly if the weakness affects only one part of the body, then it may signal muscle disease. Weakness of the legs often begins with difficulties with walking, including frequent stumbling, particularly when climbing stairs or walking over carpets. In the hands, the difficulty may be as simple as trying to turn a key in a lock, or as complicated as a coordinated activity such as typing.

Weakness also must be distinguished from fatigue. Fatigue is a symptom everybody experiences. In some cases it is the result of overexertion or exhaustion. In other instances, it is a feeling that one is "out of energy" or tired. It is usually felt throughout the body although it may be confined to muscles that have been overexercised. Weakness, on the other hand, is the loss of ability of a muscle to perform its normal activities when presumably the remaining muscles continue to function normally.

A neurologist is an expert in deciding whether these symptoms are normal, whether they mean disease, or whether they may be psychiatric in origin. Many people who are depressed complain of "weakness" and fatigue as one of the early symptoms. Among the most important clues are the deep tendon or stretch reflexes, electrical tests of the activity of the nerves and the muscles (called electromyograms) and nerve conduction velocities. In addition to the electrical testing, blood studies for the level of the enzymes from the muscles, and at times a muscle biopsy for microscopic examination are necessary. Weakness is a sign of impaired muscle function and its source may be anywhere from the brain area to the pathways that conduct the nerve impulse, even the muscle itself.

Moreover, weakness may be local or general. Certain diseases result in deficiency of function of specific muscle groups. In myasthenia gravis (see page 219), the muscles of the face are often the first affected, so that vision, facial movements, swallowing, and perhaps breathing are impaired, but movement of the arms and legs remains strong. In contrast, a disease of skeletal muscle can result in weakness of the limbs, whereas strength of the muscles about the face and the eyes remains normal.

There are many explanations but one point of importance is that not all muscles are the same either anatomically or chemically. Skeletal muscle is subclassified into red muscle and white muscle. Red muscle is used for sustained contractions as in maintaining posture or holding up a heavy weight. White muscle is used for quick, delicate movement, such as playing the piano. Most muscles have both types of fibers in varying proportions. It is possible for a muscle to have disease of one type of muscle fiber without disease of the other. The white muscle uses more oxygen and fatigues more quickly than red muscle, which has the ability to perform during times when not enough oxygen is available to the body. Red muscle helps to maintain survival in emergency circumstances and is thought to be a more primitive form of muscle, whereas white muscle has evolved for highly coordinated and highly skilled acts.

In classifying diseases of the muscles, it is important for the physician to be able to find out from the patient which circumstances bring on symptoms. Although exercise is the most common precipitating factor, certain diseases produce characteristic disorders. For example, a person who can stand and walk normally may be unable to arise from sitting in a chair. This strongly suggests disease of the muscles that extend around the hips upon the pelvic girdle, so-called proximal muscle-disorder. In another case a patient may be able to sit and rise normally but finds that the foot repeatedly trips against rugs, steps, or small objects when walking. This would suggest weakness of the dorsiflexors of the foot and would imply a distal muscle disorder.

Other disorders affect the extraocular muscles that move the eyes. The symptom is double vision, because one eye "lags behind" the other in its movements and projects an image onto an unusual part of the retina. As a last example, patients with certain muscle disorders find that speech is impaired and swallowing difficult. A distressing result may be regurgitation of fluids back through the nose because of weakness of the muscles of the soft palate.

Most muscle disorders are worse in the evening after the muscles have been used throughout the day. Furthermore, when muscles are cold, they generally perform less well than when they are warmed up through exercise. Continued heating, however, can result in reduced efficiency, and in some instances the muscles will become extraordinarily weak. This may impair the ability to move. For example, the act of reading requires that the eyes shift back and forth across the printed page. In disorders affecting the extraocular muscles, the loss of ability to read is one of the early signs of abnormality. In proximal muscle disorder of the arms, difficulties in brushing one's hair, placing objects on shelves, or washing walls are early symptoms. Impairment of writing ability is a typical symptom of distal muscle disorder.

Pain can be another symptom of muscle disorder. Almost everyone has occasional muscle cramps but repeated cramping in the same muscle group, particularly if not precipitated by exercise, suggests muscle disease. Tender muscles without a particular cause is another symptom of disorder.

Often, symptoms related to muscle are only one manifestation of disease that affects many other organ systems of the body. The muscle symptoms simply may be the first to be evident. The most common example of this is collagen vascular disease, which includes systemic lupus erythematosus, scleroderma, and dermatomyositis (see chapter 15, "Arthritis and Related Diseases"). These diseases produce weakness in various muscle groups, including the smooth muscles of the blood vessels. Vasospasm, with cold, pale fingers and toes or flushed, dusky red fingers and toes, may be the first clue to their existence. The condition leads to intolerance of cold and sometimes to the inability to hold iced drinks or frozen food packages.

It is not always realized that the most important muscle in the body is the heart. The heart is a blood pump which must work properly throughout life beating 60 to 70 times a minute for upward of 70 years for a total of approximately 250 million beats. This contraction, which goes on continuously day and night without our being aware of it, consumes an enormous amount of energy and the force of the contraction is very powerful. Generalized disturbances of muscle also affect the heart muscle, resulting in heart failure.

Some prominent neuromuscular diseases include muscular dystrophy, cerebral palsy, motor neuron disease, and a disorder called myasthenia gravis.

Muscular dystrophy has been identified in several forms, most of which appear to be inherited. The disease is characterized by wasting of the muscles. They enlarge, then begin to separate, with muscular tissue eventually replaced by fat and connective tissue. The disease is usually thought to be relentlessly progressive, although painless, with the victim eventually confined to a wheelchair. The disease may reach the cardiac and respiratory muscles, leading to death. Recent research indicates there are milder forms of dystrophy that go unrecognized or lead to milder consequences.

Duchenne muscular dystrophy is a sex-linked disease, transmitted to boys by their unaffected carrier mothers. It usually strikes early in life, between the ages of 5 and 15. The wasting is usually confined to the muscles of the trunk and legs, so that the boy is clumsy and finds it difficult to rise from a lying position or to stand totally erect. The facial muscles are rarely involved. If they are, it may be difficult for the patient to close his eyes completely while sleeping, or to smile or laugh normally.

Other forms of the disease appear in adolescence or later and may affect either sex. Their progression is slower than in the Duchenne form. The precise cause of the degenerative changes in the muscle is not known. It is believed to be a defect in the enzyme concerned with muscle metabolism. There is no effective treatment for the disease.

Cerebral palsy is not a disease but the name given to a group of conditions affecting muscular control that arise from damage to the developing brain before birth or shortly thereafter. Because brain damage cannot be reversed, there is no cure, but rehabilitation therapy can help minimize its effects. An important development has been public recognition that intelligence is seldom affected, so that palsy victims are able to hold jobs, attend schools, and lead lives more normal than in the past.

Palsy victims are usually classified into three groups according to which part of the brain has suffered damage. The distinction is not clear-cut, however, and some persons have mixed symptoms and characteristics. The majority of cerebral palsy victims are spastic. Their tightly contracted muscles make them walk with a lurching gait, fling their arms, toss their heads, and speak in a guttural voice. Damage in this case is to the motor cortex. Most other patients are athetoid, victims of damage to the basal ganglia. They may have constant, uncontrolled motion of the limbs. Less common is the ataxic form, marked by poor balance and frequent falls, and by tremor of the hands and feet.

The symptoms in all varieties range from mild to severe. Some persons are affected in only one limb, or on one side of the body.

The causes of brain damage leading to cerebral palsy are many. They may result from poor nutrition and poor health in the mother, or from her exposure to diseases in early pregnancy. Those that strike during the last months of pregnancy, when the brain and spinal cord are maturing, may be the most dangerous. Birth complications, drugs, infections, and deprivation of oxygen are also causes. Premature babies are particularly susceptible.

The symptoms usually appear in infancy, when the child is not able to hold the head up, sit erect, crawl, or walk at the expected time. In milder cases, symptoms may not appear for several years. Early rehabilitation therapy is important. Various drugs have been used to relax the contracted muscles, and surgery has been attempted, with success in some cases, to sever the nerves controlling contracted muscles. The heel tendons may also be lengthened to relax tense calf muscles.

Motor neuron disease or amyotrophic lateral sclerosis (not to be confused with multiple sclerosis) is degeneration of cell bodies of the motor cells of the brain and spinal cord, causing a slowly progressive paralysis and wasting of muscles of breathing, swallowing, and of the arms and legs. The hands often show the first signs of wasting and weakness. The legs are affected later. There is no loss of sensation. No specific treatment is available. The cause is unknown although some suspect that it is a slow viral disease.

Myasthenia gravis is a disorder of the synapse between the axon and muscle fibers. The secretion of the neurotransmitter acetylcholine is insufficient to stimulate the muscle fibers to keep contracting. The first few contractions usually are normal, but because the supply of acetylcholine is scant, repeated muscle contractions become weaker and weaker. After a few minutes of rest, the acetylcholine supply builds up again and muscle contraction can be resumed temporarily. This rapid fatigue first involves eye movement, talking, chewing, swallowing, and sometimes breathing and use of the arms or legs. In many cases the disease can be controlled with steroids, or with medications that inactivate cholinesterase, the chemical that inhibits acetylcholine. Removal of the thymus gland is another remedy. The disease may disappear spontaneously but other patients need continued medication. Myasthenia gravis is but one form of myasthenia. Abnormalities of thyroid, certain tumors of the lungs, and toxic substances also may cause similar symptoms or rapid weakness of muscle (see chapter 21, "Allergy and the Immune System").

Cramps often arouse elderly people from sleep, particularly during winter months, with pain in one or both legs. Relaxation, cold, and fatigue cause the attacks. Rising from bed, moving about, and rubbing the legs can relieve them. Other treatments include quinine, procainamide, Benadryl,® and counter-irritation such as acupinch, which is the introduction of pain by pinching the skin. At times muscle cramps signal the onset of neuromuscular disease.

Nutritional Disease

The nervous system is one of the first affected by insufficient or improper quantities of vitamins, minerals, and other substances. Excessive exposure to such substances such as lead, arsenic, and thallium (from organic solvents, polymers, insecticides, herbicides, and certain chemicals used in medications) may cause neurological disorders.

Lack of the vitamin B complex contained in vegetables, grains, and meat can produce nerve problems. Fortunately, these disorders are now uncommon in the United States (although they are prevalent in many less-developed nations), confined primarily to food faddists, people on diets, the impoverished, alcoholics, and those who are alone and depressed. The vitamin deficiency causes painful sensorimotor neuropathy in the feet and legs followed by loss of ability to register new memories, a condition called Wernicke-Korsakoff syndrome. The deficiency is an emergency situation because the lack of thiamine and other components of the vitamin B complex can cause small brain hemorrhages, brain swelling, and death if not immediately treated. Pellegra, due to nicotinic acid deficiency, also can cause dermatitis, neuropathy, and dementia.

Pernicious anemia (subacute combined degeneration of the spinal cord) results from a lack of the ability of the stomach and small intestine to absorb vitamin B_{12} from food (see chapter 20, "The Digestive System" and chapter 6, "The Blood"). Without B_{12} certain cells of the spinal cord and brain die, producing a loss of perception of movement of the extremities and damaging the motor tracts in the spinal cord, again particularly affecting the legs. People with this disorder lose the ability to perceive the position of their feet and toes when moved and as a consequence they stumble and fall easily, particularly in the dark. They have an increasing gait disturbance because their muscles do not move as quickly as they should. Once a serious health problem, especially in the elderly, pernicious anemia can now be diagnosed by determination of the blood level of B_{12}, with the vitamin given by injection periodically for the remainder of the patient's life. Neurological damage, of course, cannot be restored.

Toxic substances ingested or injected by insects or reptiles can be fatal by causing loss of normal neuromuscular function. Botulism is a food-borne disorder resulting from processing and preserving foods in cans or jars in such a way that bacteria can grow and produce their toxin. When eaten it causes paralysis of muscles by inactivating the neuromuscular junction. This is an emergency requiring use of artificial ventilation and other life support systems and chemical antidotes.

CHAPTER 10   **RICHARD L. MASLAND, M.D.**

EPILEPSY

Epilepsy is not a disease but a symptom. It is characterized by recurrent seizures or attacks in which the person experiences a sudden change in sensation or consciousness, or uncontrollable movements, or spasms of the muscles. A number of disorders can bring about this condition, but what the disorders have in common is that they cause the nerves of the brain to become overexcited. The individual cells, which ordinarily function in an orderly, independent fashion, fall into step and begin to beat rapidly and in unison. Because the impulses of the brain are activated by precise and measured amounts of electricity, the condition is one of electrical overload, and the result is overactivity—a seizure. Characteristically, a seizure often comes on suddenly and unpredictably, and lasts from a few seconds to 15 or 20 minutes. Between seizures the person is usually normal. A hard seizure in which there are spasms of the muscles is termed a convulsion.

Epilepsy is one of mankind's oldest recorded disorders and is said to have affected historical figures from Julius Caesar to Leon Trotsky. It also is one of the most familiar disorders. Probably every adult has witnessed a seizure at some time. Nonetheless, many mysteries remain about epilepsy. The precise number of Americans afflicted is not known, but two million is a frequent estimate. The figure means little, in any case, because epilepsy varies widely from person to person. Some persons have one seizure in a lifetime and others have hundreds a day. The attacks vary in severity from a momentary period of confusion to a violent spasm that lasts several minutes.

Depending upon the cause, cases of epilepsy fall into two large groups. One is known by several names: idiopathic, cryptogenic, essential, or *primary* epilepsy. The other is referred to as symptomatic or *secondary*.

In the primary epilepsies, no physical or anatomical abnormality of the brain can be found. Epilepsy is the primary disorder. In these instances, epilepsy results from some constitutional or acquired excitability of the entire brain, and when seizures occur they are generalized, involving the whole brain.

The secondary epilepsies usually result from an injury or an illness that leaves a scar or defect on the surface (cortex) of the brain. The scar irritates the surrounding brain tissues and overexcites them. Seizures originating from such a site or "focus" may start gradually and spread progressively to other parts of the brain. These seizures are spoken of as partial, local, or focal seizures, even though eventually they may involve the whole brain. If there is widespread brain disease or damage, the seizures of secondary epilepsy may originate as generalized ones that involve the entire brain.

THE CAUSES OF EPILEPSY

In the majority of cases of primary epilepsy, the underlying cause is unknown, and a hereditary factor is suspected. But no specific inherited disease is to blame. Instead, many factors seem to be involved, including inborn susceptibility, changes in body chemistry and hormones, and stress, anxiety, and emotional tension, which may precipitate the actual attack.

The secondary epilepsies stem from many forms of brain injury. Cases originating in infancy commonly result from complications of pregnancy, delivery, and the newborn period. In children, meningitis (infections of the membranes around the brain) and accidental head injury can be responsible. Seizures that first begin after the age of 20 suggest the possibility of brain tumor. In the elderly, seizures suggest disorders of the blood vessels of the brain, such as cerebral arteriosclerosis ("hardening of the arteries").

CAUSES OF SECONDARY EPILEPSY

Birth injury and complications of pregnancy	43%
Infection (encephalitis, meningitis)	27%
Head injury	17%
Brain tumor	5%
Other	5%
Unknown	3%

The primary epilepsies usually are first seen between ages 4 and 14. More than 75 percent of all cases of epilepsy start before age 20. Seizures rarely start during middle life or later. When they do, they usually are related to brain tumor or arteriosclerosis.

TYPES OF SEIZURES

Generalized Seizures

The seizures of primary epilepsy are always generalized (involving the entire brain) from the moment they start. The person loses consciousness without warning. The seizure itself takes one of several forms.

Tonic-clonic seizures (grand mal). The grand mal seizure (from the French phrase for "great sickness") is what most persons mean when they speak of a convulsion or "fit." The seizure strikes suddenly. The person loses consciousness and the entire body stiffens and becomes rigid. Breath is expelled with a whistling sound or cry, and the victim drops to the ground. Gradually the rigidity of the body— doctors call it tonus—gives way to jerking of the arms, legs, trunk, and head. The movements are rhythmic and rapid at first, then become intermittent and irregular, the phase called clonus. After five to ten minutes, the jerking ceases. The person remains unconscious for a few minutes. When he regains consciousness, he may be lethargic or confused or drift off again into a heavy sleep. During the spasm he may bite his tongue, and the bowels or bladder may release their contents, causing embarrassment on awakening.

Absence seizures (petit mal). The petit mal ("little sickness") seizure also begins without warning, but is far less startling. It consists of a brief lapse of consciousness, accompanied by loss of awareness and movement. The person develops a blank stare. Eyelids, jaws, and hands may twitch slightly. Unconsciousness usually lasts less than a minute. The person does not fall. As he regains consciousness, he may make a few aimless movements with his hands, but usually recovers rapidly without confusion or loss of memory. He may continue a conversation as if nothing had happened, and the whole episode may not be noticed by onlookers. Sometimes children with petit mal seizures are put down as being inattentive or daydreamers. An electroencephalogram (see page 224), however,

shows the condition clearly. During the attack, persons subject to petit mal seizures have a characteristic pattern of rhythmic electrical disturbances recurring at a rate of two or four per second.

Myoclonic seizures. Myoclonic (muscle jerk) seizures consist of shock-like jerking of the arms and body. They are so brief that loss of consciousness may not be noticeable. The person may be unaware of the jerking movement, and may fling objects or drop them without realizing why he or she has done so. However, in more severe attacks the body suddenly goes limp and the person falls to the floor. These seizures are most common during the first hours after awakening. They sometimes recur repeatedly over a period of minutes, and occasionally fuse into a generalized tonic-clonic attack (what is usually referred to as a convulsion or fit).

Photosensitive seizures can result in either myoclonic or tonic-clonic (convulsion) symptoms. They occur in a small number of persons who react to a bright light or other visual stimulus. The rhythmic flashes of a blinking sign or traffic signal, the repetitive patterns in a checkerboard, flickering TV screen, or moving stairway—any of these can set off a seizure. In an extremely small number of people, loud noises or a particular strain of music may be responsible. The tendency for photosensitive seizures appears to run in families. (Curiously, the seizures also occur in certain breeds of animals.)

Benign epilepsy with Rolandic spikes is an unusual form of primary epilepsy. Its name stems from the distinctive pattern of brain waves seen on the electroencephalogram. The seizures are partial seizures and the electroencephalogram shows a local rather than a general disturbance of brain activity. However, benign epilepsy is not associated with brain disease. It is easily controlled with medicine and tends to disappear after adolescence.

Partial Seizures

Attacks of the secondary epilepsies are even more varied than those of the primary epilepsies. Their characteristics depend upon the area of brain where they start. At the beginning of the attack only a part of the brain is affected, so the person does not necessarily lose consciousness, and even may be aware of the

THE MOST COMMON SEIZURES

Type of Seizure	Percentage of Epileptics Affected
Grand mal only	53
Grand mal plus psychomotor	16
Grand mal plus petit mal	11
Psychomotor only	11
Elementary partial	5
Petit mal only	4
Total	100

Generalized or grand mal seizures (the kind most people mean when they refer to an epileptic convulsion) are the most common type, accounting for more than half of all cases. About 80 percent of all epilepsy cases involve grand mal seizures, either alone or in combination with another kind, such as psychomotor seizures.

impending seizure. There may be a brief premonition or warning sign (called an aura) marking the onset of the attack. This warning usually consists of tingling, numbness or twitching of the face, hand, or foot, or flashing lights or colored balls appearing before the eyes. That may be all there is to the entire attack, or it may spread to become a generalized tonic-clonic seizure with muscle spasms, jerking, and potential loss of consciousness.

Other types of partial seizures (sometimes called "complex" or "psychomotor" seizures) begin with a dreamlike state, peculiar changes in the appearance of the surroundings, sense of strangeness or familiarity, or peculiar taste or smell. Without being aware of it, the person carries out purposeless, automatic, and inappropriate activities, such as plucking at his clothes absently or moving about in an aimless way. A generalized clonic-tonic seizure may follow, but more commonly the automatic unconscious behavior lasts five to ten mintues, then wears off, leaving the subject confused, disoriented, and unaware of the attack and what he or she has done during the interlude.

The premonition (aura) and the limited extent of the local seizure are the distinguishing features of the partial epilepsies that point to a possible brain scar or irritation. This is confirmed by the electroencephalogram, which shows "random spikes"—irregular electrical discharges originating from a local region of the brain rather than the rhythmic disturbances of the entire brain characteristic of the primary epilepsies.

Secondary Epilepsy with Generalized Seizures

When there is generalized brain disease or a generalized disturbance of brain function, the seizures of the secondary epilepsies may be generalized as well. In infants under age one, a condition called "infantile spasms" is characterized by slight but frequent minor episodes. These consist of a sudden cry and sharp jerking of the body, almost as if the infant had been startled. However, the attacks occur many times daily. Older children may have headnodding attacks during which they lose consciousness, then slump forward to the floor. After the age of seven or eight, these attacks may become generalized, with tonic-clonic seizures, attacks of falling, and jerking of the limbs. This form of epilepsy is difficult to arrest, and in 80 percent of the cases leads to mental retardation.

DIAGNOSING EPILEPSY

In diagnosing epilepsy, a doctor first tries to eliminate other possible explanations for seizures. What might appear to be an epileptic attack in fact can result from hysteria, fainting, breath-holding spells in children, or from heart attack, low blood sugar (hypoglycemia), or stroke in an adult.

The primary epilepsies also must be distinguished from the secondary epilepsies, because the two types respond differently to medicines, and because these distinctions help in the search for the underlying cause, which perhaps can be remedied.

Epilepsy is usually diagnosed on the basis of family and personal history, physical and neurological examination, and laboratory tests. The history might disclose injury or disease that occurred before birth or shortly afterward. Of particular importance is the description of the attack, especially its beginning. An epileptic seizure shows unprovoked and unpredictable onset, recurrence, and a stereotyped and consistent pattern of seizure behavior for each individual. The characteristic of the partial epilepsies is the occurrence of the warning sign or premonition.

Physical and neurological exams can uncover a contributing disease or nervous system damage that is involved in the seizures.

Blood chemical studies are used to find abnormalities of blood sugar, calcium, or phosphorus which can be contributing factors, and as a safeguard before starting certain forms of drug therapy.

The electroencephalogram (EEG) is the single most valuable tool for diagnosing epilepsy. The EEG is a harmless procedure for tracing the rhythm and electrical activity of the brain. It amplifies the signals and traces their pattern by activating pens that move across a drum of paper. Brain electrical activity in most persons follows a regular and predictable pattern, changing in a characteristic way during sleep, upon opening the eyes, or when in deep thought.

While the person rests on a bed or in a chair, salt-moistened electrodes are placed on the scalp at various locations. The normal adult's brain wave pattern usually will show a rhythmic fluctuation under resting conditions of 8½ to 12 cycles per second. This is the alpha rhythm. Sometimes the physician wants to obtain both a waking and sleeping record, or asks the person to do an overbreathing exercise or stimulates him with a flashing light. An abnormality of brain activity can be accentuated by these procedures, which also precipitate a seizure occasionally.

A clearly abnormal EEG reading will be found in about 60 percent of persons with epilepsy, even between attacks, and in almost 100 percent of the cases if an attack occurs during the recording. However, such clearcut abnormalities also are observed in up to five percent of the seizure-free population, and in 20 percent of relatives of persons with certain forms of primary epilepsy. Thus they might indicate a predisposition to epilepsy, but not necessarily the disorder itself. Minor irregularities are observed in almost 80 percent of persons diagnosed as epileptic. But these, too, are observed in 20 to 40 percent of the general population. The EEG is known to be more accurate in children than adults.

Computer-assisted tomography, known as the CT scan, is another valuable diagnostic aid (see chapter 32, "X Rays and Radiology"). CT scanners are sophisticated devices that combine X rays and a computer to produce clearer pictures of internal organs than are available from simple X rays. They can record very slight differences in density within the head and can distinguish brain tissue from the water-filled cavities or ventricles within the brain. It produces a shadow picture of the brain that clearly delineates areas of altered density, such as those produced by scar, tumor, or blood vessel disease. About 50 percent of the scans taken of persons with epilepsy reveal some anatomical irregularity. Of persons suffering from primary generalized epilepsy with "absence" seizures, only 10 percent were shown by brain scan to be abnormal.

Two other methods formerly used frequently to diagnose epilepsy have largely been replaced by the CT scan.

Pneumoencephalography is one of those methods. It is a spinal-tap process in which air is injected into a fluid-filled cavity at the lower end of the spine. The air trickles upward and replaces the fluid within the cavities of the

CHARACTERISTICS OF DIFFERENT TYPES OF EPILEPSY

Type	Cause	What Happens
PRIMARY Grand mal and petit mal	Unknown	Generalized attacks without warning. **Grand mal:** Sudden loss of consciousness and stiffening of body; a fall to the ground and jerking of muscles. **Petit mal:** "Absence" seizures—brief lapses of consciousness or "staring spells."
Myoclonic (muscle jerk)	Unknown	Brief jerking of body or sudden fall.
Photosensitive	Strong genetic factor.	Muscle jerk or generalized seizure precipitated by flashing light.
Febrile convulsions	Febrile illness of infancy.	Generalized convulsions during high fever.
Benign Rolandic spikes	Strong genetic factor.	Partial seizures starting in face or arm.
SECONDARY Partial—Elementary	Brain scar or malformation.	Elementary partial seizures preceded by flashes of light, tingling sensation of skin, jerking of face, arm, or leg.
Partial—Complex	Brain scar or malformation	Complex partial seizures preceded by peculiar taste or smell, numbness of lips, face, and throat; or dreamy states; often, automatic, unconscious behavior.
Generalized	Diffuse brain disease.	Diverse, including absences, drop attacks, brief spasms, and generalized convulsions.

brain. Since air is of low density, the empty cavities can then be seen on X ray, and distortion by scar or tumor is disclosed. This test is now used primarily to confirm a diagnosis and before surgery for brain tumor.

Angiography is the other diagnostic method supplanted by CT scanning. It is a procedure in which a liquid that casts an X-ray shadow is injected into the artery supplying the brain. As the liquid courses through the arteries of the brain itself, an X ray is taken. This produces a shadow picture of the blood vessels of the brain. Angiography is useful in diagnosing certain types of tumors and in locating the point where an artery is blocked in victims of stroke. In epilepsy, its primary purpose is to see abnormal constellations of blood vessels which can precipitate seizures.

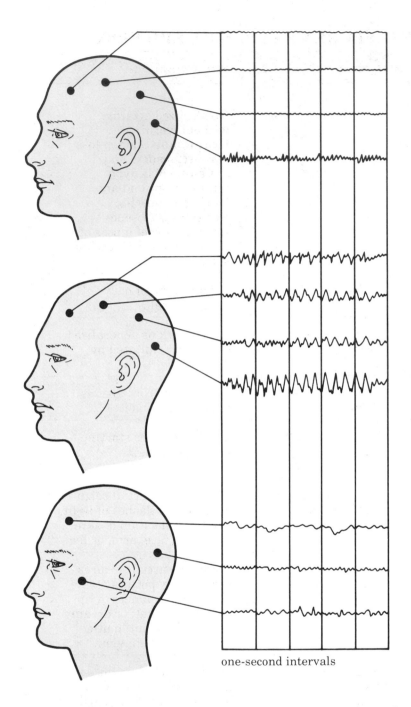

one-second intervals

ELECTROENCEPHALOGRAM

The electroencephalogram (EEG) measures electrical voltages from the brain and is an important diagnostic tool in epilepsy. The top drawing shows the EEG of a normal adult. Electrodes are glued to the scalp in a number of positions with one glued to the ear for reference (not shown). Sensitive voltmeters (channels) record the fluctuating electrical potentials between pairs of electrodes. As many as 30 channels can be recorded, although only four are shown in this diagram. Vertical lines indicate one-second intervals. Most normal EEGs show rhythmic waves at a rate of about seven per second, most evident over the back of the head. This pattern is called the alpha rhythm. The center drawing shows an EEG during petit mal seizure. A momentary lapse of consciousness occurs with each "spike and wave" discharge. These high-voltage discharges appear suddenly and on both sides of the head. The lower EEG is that of a person with partial epilepsy. Sudden spikes arise from that portion of the brain where a scar or other irritation is located. If the spikes become continuous, a focal seizure might occur, appearing first at the site of the spike, then spreading to other parts of the brain.

TREATMENT

Drugs

Unless an underlying cause can be found and treated, epilepsy cannot be cured. Fortunately, however, the majority of seizures can be controlled by anticonvulsant drugs. By taking a few pills a day the overwhelming preponderance of epileptics are completely free of attacks and lead normal lives. A diagnosis of epilepsy no longer must mean a lifetime of seizures.

Reaching the goal of controlling seizures, however, is an exquisitely delicate task.

The type of drug and the dosage must be tailored to the individual and the type of seizure. Considerable adjusting and tinkering may be required before the best regimen is arrived at. People absorb and eliminate drugs differently, so there is no set prescription that fits every case. It may be necessary periodically to measure the level of anticonvulsant drugs in the blood, a procedure known as

EPILEPTICS AND THEIR TREATMENT

Severity	Approximate Number in United States	Percent of Population
Occasional or unrecognized attack—have not sought medical care (estimated)	726,000	.34
Require occasional medical consultation	769,000	.36
Under continuing medical supervision	563,000	.26
In residential facilities	78,000	.04
Total	2,136,000	1.0

More than 2.1 million people–about one percent of the U.S. population–are affected by epilepsy. About one-third of them have attacks so rarely that they do not recognize the condition or have not sought medical help. Another third require only occasional medical help. Only about four percent of all epileptics are in residential facilities for special care.

ACDL, and repeated determinations of the drug level may be required before the optimum dosage is figured. Fortunately, an ACDL measurement today is a simple automated procedure. Even when a patient is taking several forms of medicine only one blood sample is required.

The objective of anticonvulsant drugs is to reduce the sensitivity of the nervous system, and especially to block brain overactivity that triggers the seizure. They do their job by changing the characteristics of the nerve membranes, and possibly by increasing the levels of certain natural substances that help keep brain activity regular. It is important to maintain a constant protection level in the bloodstream, so the drugs must be taken on a regular schedule and exactly as prescribed. To discontinue anticonvulsant drugs suddenly is extremely hazardous. The body apparently adjusts to the medication so that withdrawal can throw the person into an uncontrollable series of convulsions called status epilepticus (see page 230). Changing and discontinuing medication must be carried out over a period of days or weeks to give the body time to adjust.

The commonly used anticonvulsant drugs have been in use for a number of years. They have been taken by millions of people and for long periods of time. Their safety has been thoroughly evaluated, and their use approved only after careful study.

However, there is no drug that does not have undesirable or even dangerous side effects in a few people. The best protection against side effects is for persons taking medicine to be aware of the symptoms of these complications. That will help them recognize problems before they have become serious, and forestall danger.

Descriptions of the commonly used anticonvulsant drugs follow. In each instance the generic name is followed by a brand name.

Barbiturates: phenobarbital (Luminal), primidone (Mysoline), metharbital (Mebaral). These three medicines are especially useful against generalized convulsions and partial seizures. They do not work well against absence seizures.

Barbiturates are sedatives. Although they are not considered habit-forming, they have been subject to abuse, so only a month's supply can be obtained at a time, and a new prescription must be written every six months.

Especially at first, phenobarbital can make people sleepy and sluggish. The effects tend to wear off, but large doses are sometimes required for proper control, so some sluggishness may have to be accepted. In some children, phenobarbital has the reverse effect. They become cranky and overactive, so other drugs have to be substituted.

Phenobarbital is one of the safest drugs for seizure control. Skin rash is the most common sensitivity reaction and may force a change to another drug.

Hydantoins: phenytoin (Dilatin), ethotoin (Peganone), mephenytoin (Mesantoin). The hydantoins were the first drugs widely and successfully used to control seizures. Their introduction in the 1930s ushered in the modern era of epilepsy treatment and permitted persons with epilepsy to lead normal lives. They are particularly effective for various forms of generalized convulsions and for partial seizures. Unlike phenobarbital, they have little sedative effect.

Too great a dosage can cause ataxia, a loss of coordination so that the person cannot control body movements smoothly and walks as if he were drunk. Jerky movements of the eye also may result. When the dosage is reduced, however, these side effects disappear, although continued overdosage can cause permanent unsteadiness.

Some persons taking phenytoin develop overgrowth of the gums. This tendency can be lessened by careful brushing and frequent visits to the dentist. It may be necessary to have the extra tissue cut away periodically.

Rare but dangerous side effects are severe forms of dermatitis, sometimes linked to interference with the blood-forming organs and anemia. Persons taking phenytoin should check with a doctor if they develop serious skin rash, purple spots under the skin, or unusual bleeding from the gums.

Carbamazepine. Although carbamazepine (Tegretol) has been known as an anticonvulsant for over 20 years, its use in the United States has been restricted. However, carbamazepine is widely used in Europe in some forms of childhood and adult epilepsy because it produces neither the sedative effect nor the hyperactive behavior caused by phenobarbital, nor the side effects of phenytoin. Effectiveness is about the same as phenytoin.

Overdose can produce dizziness and double vision, or it can affect the white blood cells. While the dose of carbamazepine is being regulated, frequent blood counts are required so that the dosage can be reduced if the white blood count falls too low.

Valproic acid (Depakene) is the newest addition to the list of anticonvulsant drugs in the United States, although it has been used in Europe since 1965. It is especially effective against absence (petit mal) and myoclonic (muscle jerk) seizures, and can prevent grand mal (convulsion) seizures in some patients. It is least effective against complex partial (psychomotor) attacks.

The great advantage of valproic acid is its lack of sedative effect. Overdoses can produce tremor.

Valproic acid is an oily liquid usually taken in capsule form or as an elixir. Because it can be irritating to the stomach and cause indigestion, it is best taken at mealtimes on a full stomach. Another undesirable side effect is to cause a weight gain. Temporary hair loss occurs in some persons. However, valproic acid's most serious side effect is injury to the liver (hepatitis). Although this occurs only rarely, periodic blood tests are recommended to determine whether the liver is functioning properly.

The suximides: ethosuximide (Zarontin), methsuximide (Celontin), and phensuximide (Milontin). Until the introduction of valproic acid, ethosuximide was the best drug for control of absence (petit mal) attacks. The combination of valproic acid and ethosuximide is still used sometimes. Phensuximide is also employed in absence seizures, but requires large dosages and is less effective. Methsuximide, on the other hand, is more effective for myoclonic seizures and psychomotor attacks.

The suximides have little sedative effect. Overdoses can produce dizziness or unsteadiness. Some patients develop headache or general weakness. Serious side effects such as skin rash or anemia are rare.

The benzodiazepines: clonazepam (Clonapin), diazepam (Valium). Clonazepam and diazepam—the so-called tranquilizers—are powerful anticonvulsants. Clonazepam is especially effective against absence and myoclonic attacks. Unfortunately, the beneficial effects do not always last. Tolerance develops and the seizures recur. Like phenobarbital, the tranquilizers are sedative drugs. Children using them may become irritable and overactive. Serious side effects are extremely rare.

The diones: trimethadione (Tridione), paramethadione (Paradione). Until the development of ethosuximide, valproic acid, and clonazepam, the diones were the only drugs effective against absence attacks. They are rarely used today. Overdoses produce a peculiar visual disturbance and unusual sensitivity to bright light, as though everything were covered by sunlit snow. Even more serious side effects include irreversible injury of the bone marrow and damage to the unborn child of a mother taking the drug. For this reason, the diones are now used only when no other drug is effective.

Phenacemide (Phenurone) is a powerful anticonvulsant, especially effective against psychomotor seizures. It has little sedative effect and is well tolerated by most people. But it, too, has serious side effects—liver injury and mental confusion with hallucinations—and is used only in rare instances where all else fails.

Obviously, a number of drugs are now available to control seizures. Most people become readily and completely seizure-free by using only one or two, such as phenytoin, phenobarbital, or carbamazepine. In more difficult cases, drug regulation may be a long and difficult undertaking, extending over months or even years as dosages are increased or reduced and several drugs are tried and withdrawn.

It is most important to remember that *no* drug cures epilepsy. Drugs only control the seizures. Once begun, drug doses usually must be continued for a number of years. All too often, a person who has had only a few seizures which are then controlled by medication believes himself cured and stops taking medicine. Many persons with seizures can ultimately discontinue medication, but usually only after being free of seizures for several years, and only if they reduce gradually under close medical supervision.

Surgery

In some cases of partial epilepsy, seizures can be eliminated by surgical removal of the brain area where the irritating focus is located. This step is usually taken, however, only when three conditions are met: The seizures cannot be controlled by medication, the point where they originate is in an accessible area, and the removal will not cause intolerable loss of brain function.

LONG-TERM OUTLOOK FOR PERSONS WITH EPILEPSY

Type of Epilepsy	Percent of persons who have been seizure-free for 5 years starting 5 years after diagnosis		Percent of persons who have been seizure-free for 5 years starting 10 years after diagnosis		Percent of persons who have been seizure-free for 5 years starting 15 years after diagnosis	
	All Persons	Without Medication	All Persons	Without Medication	All Persons	Without Medication
Primary all types	62	36	70	42	74	47
Secondary	60	20	61	30	90	54
Having neurologic defect	42	15	45	28	45	30
Type of Seizure						
Grand Mal	70	40	72	51	85	50
Petit Mal	70	40	72	47	80	60
Partial complex	60	30	62	32	65	35
All seizure types	61	30	63	40	70	50

With proper treatment, most persons with epilepsy become free of seizures within five years of diagnosis. The percentage of persons free from seizures increases gradually after that time. The most difficult seizures to control are those with a neurological basis.

Under these conditions, seizure control has been achieved by surgery with very low risk in 60 to 70 percent of cases. The success rate depends upon carefully locating the focus before the operation, which may require long periods of EEG monitoring and even insertion of electrodes into the brain.

Management of a Seizure

A sudden epileptic seizure can be upsetting for an onlooker, but if someone undergoes a seizure in your presence there is no cause for alarm. The seizure will run its course without harm to the person. One sensible step is to prevent the subject from injuring himself by clearing the nearby area of sharp objects.

The head should be placed on a soft surface and clothing loosened around the neck. As the person relaxes, after the rigid portion of the attack, the head should be turned to the side to prevent swallowing of saliva. Open the throat to allow passage of air. This can be done by grasping the angle of the jaw on either side just below the ear and pulling gently forward. Contrary to common belief, nothing should be thrust into the mouth, unless the subject has enough warning to chew on something soft like a handkerchief before the seizure starts. Tongue-biting occurs at the start of an attack. The attempt to protect the tongue later may only result in knocking out teeth. Keep your hands away from the patient's mouth. A person known to have epilepsy can usually return to his usual activities afterwards. He should be left alone and permitted to rest until he has recovered.

In someone not known to have epilepsy, it can be important to observe his or her behavior during the convulsion. This information can be helpful to a physician in establishing the type of seizure.

Status epilepticus. Most seizures end spontaneously after 10 minutes at most. If a seizure continues for more than 15 minutes, or if seizures recur so frequently that the subject does not regain consciousness between them, there is cause for concern. Repeated or continued seizures can develop into a self-perpetuating condition called status epilepticus, in which stopping the seizures becomes increasingly difficult. Emergency medical care is needed, including intravenous medication to stop the attacks, or the condition can be fatal. The most common cause of status epilepticus is sudden discontinuation of medicines.

THE CAUSES OF DEATH OF PERSONS WITH EPILEPSY

Seizure Related Deaths	
Accidental death, drowning, suicide	24%
Sudden death associated with seizure	18%
Status epilepticus (continuous succession of attacks)	9%
Brain disease (tumor)	5%
Non-Neurological Causes	41%
Unknown	3%

More than half of persons with epilepsy die of causes related to their condition. On average persons with epilepsy live 10 fewer years than the general population. However, average figures mean little because the effects of epilepsy vary so widely from individual to individual.

Managing psychomotor seizures. Persons experiencing psychomotor seizures commonly fumble with objects in their surroundings in a semipurposeful way. They may walk or even run without knowing where or why they are going. An observer is often tempted to try to restrain them, but such attempts might provoke anger and cause them to resist. Unless his or her life is endangered, someone having a psychomotor attack should be left alone until the episode ends.

Other precautionary steps. Too much alcohol can set off an epileptic seizure. Persons with epilepsy should avoid drinking, except in moderate amounts. Another cause of seizures is lack of sleep. Violent or exhausting physical exercise causes seizures in some persons, but regular physical activities and participation in sports is recommended. Some epileptics have been prominent athletes. A person with frequent seizures should avoid activities where sudden loss of consciousness could lead to serious injury to himself or others. Obviously, someone who has seizures should not climb ladders or other structures where a fall would cause serious injury. Swimming is permissible under supervised conditions.

Some doctors disagree about whether seizures are triggered by emotional crises, and whether persons with epilepsy can learn to control the attacks by conscious effort. Some subjects have been trained to use biofeedback

RISK TO CHILD WHEN A PARENT HAS EPILEPSY

Type of Epilepsy	Children Affected
Primary generalized seizures	7%
Secondary symptomatic	2%

RISK ACCORDING TO PARENT WITH EPILEPSY

Type of Epilepsy	Children Affected
All types (mother)	5%
All types (father)	2%

RISK IF SISTER OR BROTHER HAS EPILEPSY

Type of Epilepsy	Children Affected
Primary generalized epilepsies	
Generalized convulsion	6%
Absence	7%
Muscle jerk seizures	10%
Photosensitivity	8%
Partial epilepsy	2.5%

The role heredity plays in epilepsy depends on the type of epilepsy involved. For example, a parent with primary generalized seizures is more likely to have a child with epilepsy than a parent who has secondary symptomatic epilepsy. For some unexplained reason, children of epileptic mothers are more likely to have epilepsy than children of epileptic fathers.

to alter their brain rhythm in the belief that it might reduce their susceptibility to seizures. The procedure requires daily training over several months, and benefits appear to diminish when active treatment stops. The procedure is still experimental.

Febrile convulsions. Some young children suffer generalized tonic-clonic convulsions during an illness associated with high fever. Most convulsions stop by themselves within 10 to 15 minutes, but on rare occasions the seizure will not stop and medical treatment is required to bring it to an end. For this reason, an infantile convulsion is considered a medical emergency and help should be sought, even if it proves unnecessary in 99 out of 100 cases. Another reason for seeking medical evaluation is to be certain that the episode represents a simple febrile convulsion, rather than the early symptoms of meningitis or other brain disease.

A single febrile convulsion does not indicate that the child will grow up to have adult seizures, although the chances are slightly higher than for children in the general population. Some children who have experienced febrile convulsion may require anticonvulsant medications to protect against further seizures during fever. The medication is usually discontinued after about age five. Febrile convulsions do not occur after that age.

THE OUTLOOK IN EPILEPSY

The chances that epilepsy will cease spontaneously vary with its cause. Secondary seizures starting in early infancy are often hard to control, even with medication, and frequently have a neurological basis. The partial epilepsies, especially where there is an underlying structural brain defect, also are relatively intractable. On the other hand, the majority of primary epilepsies starting in

INTELLIGENCE LEVELS AMONG EPILEPTIC SCHOOLCHILDREN

IQ	With Brain Disorder	Uncomplicated
Over 130	5%	2%
116–130	5%	29%
101–115	5%	16%
86–100	10%	36%
71–85	5%	14%
51–70	15%	3%
Under 51	55%	—

FREQUENCY OF SEIZURES AT AGE 10 AND 11

Frequency of Attacks in Past Year	Major Attacks	Minor Attacks
None	67%	75%
One only	13%	4%
2–5	10%	5%
6–9	2%	5%
Greater than 9	8%	11%
Total	100%	100%

PSYCHOLOGICAL PROBLEMS OF SCHOOLCHILDREN

Diagnosis	General Population	Epileptic Children
Neurotic	2%	13%
Conduct disorder	2%	10%
Mixed	1%	5%
Total	5%	28%

Top chart shows that schoolchildren with uncomplicated epilepsy have a normal range of intelligence. Subnormal intelligence is common among those with brain disorders. Center chart shows that only 20 percent of epileptic 10- and 11-year-olds have more than one seizure during a school year. Bottom chart indicates that epileptic children have more psychological problems than the general population.

childhood cease during maturity. In one study of a large number of patients with various seizure types monitored for 20 years, 70 percent have been free of seizures for five years.

People who have epilepsy face a greater-than-normal risk of injury and illness. Their mortality rate is more than double that of the entire population. On average, they live 10 fewer years. The causes of death are indicated in the table on page 230. However, averages mean little to an individual because epilepsy varies so widely from person to person.

Insurance companies now recognize individual variations, and both health and life insurance are available for persons with epilepsy, although at higher premiums.

HEREDITY AND EPILEPSY

The role of heredity in epilepsy has been greatly overemphasized. In less than two percent of all cases, epilepsy is one symptom of an inherited disease. But these diseases usually cause physical defects or mental retardation, and epilepsy is a lesser symptom. In cases of symptomatic epilepsy following complications of pregnancy and delivery, head injury, or meningitis, inherited susceptibility plays a role in determining the subsequent occurrence of epilepsy, but that role is so minor that it has little practical significance.

Among the primary generalized epilepsies, inherited susceptibility to seizures can be demonstrated clearly, but whether seizures actually occur depends upon other factors, too.

If a woman is epileptic, the risk that her child will have epilepsy is greater than the risk to a child of an unaffected mother. The risk also is higher than normal for children born into a family where a brother or sister has epilepsy. In both cases the chances range from 2 to 10 percent, depending on the type of epilepsy. When both parents are affected, the chances increase to about 13 percent, which is also the approximate risk when one parent and one child are affected. If both parents and one child are affected, the likelihood of epilepsy occurring in a second child in that family is 33 percent.

It must be emphasized that these figures are averages of large groups of individuals with diverse forms of epilepsy. The risk for any individual or family depends on many factors and can be estimated only on the basis of a complete evaluation by a genetic counselor.

THE SOCIAL CONSEQUENCES OF EPILEPSY

In the days when people were guided by superstition more than by knowledge, persons with epilepsy experienced many forms of discrimination. It can be frightening to witness a seizure, and easy to understand how ignorant people observing the sudden unconsciousness and involuntary movement would believe that the victim was mentally diseased or possessed by an evil spirit. Because no one knew the cause, and because a few families had an abnormal number of epileptics, it was easy to consider the disorder to be inherited or contagious. Even the laws reflected these misconceptions.

Fortunately, these false notions are yielding to scientific knowledge, and our outmoded laws are being repealed. The Epilepsy Foundation of America, a voluntary agency concerned with the welfare of persons with epilepsy, has spearheaded the movement. Here is the epileptic legal status today.

Marriage. Persons with epilepsy can now marry with no legal barriers in every state.

Sterilization. Five states (Arkansas, Delaware, Oklahoma, South Carolina, and Utah) still provide for involuntary sterilization of certain epileptics. Similar laws in nine other states have been repealed.

Adoption. Five states (Arkansas, Florida, Iowa, Missouri, and Utah) have laws allowing annulment of adoption if the child is found to have epilepsy.

Education. Federal law requires that every handicapped child must be educated in the "least restrictive environment" possible. This means most children with epilepsy should be taught in the regular school classroom, especially since those with uncomplicated epilepsy have the normal range of intelligence (see page 232). However, about 25 percent of the children with epilepsy have associated brain damage and require special education. About 18 percent—three times the number in the general population—have problems learning to read (dyslexia). A few have such frequent seizures that they cannot keep up with other children in the regular classroom. In those cases, the state must provide tutoring to supplement classroom instruction, or provide a separate classroom to be shared with other children who have learning problems. Only in rare instances of multiple uncontrolled seizures is home instruction necessary.

Improper treatment. The recent increase in drug abuse among the general population has caused added problems for persons with epilepsy, especially those who experience complex partial (psychomotor) seizures. These persons may be confused for a few minutes after their attack. If someone tries to restrain them or force them into a car or ambulance, they may become frightened or begin to fight. Unfortunately, authorities sometimes think they are drunk or drugged. It may be some time before their condition is recognized. Even then, an emergency-room physician unfamiliar with the case might be uncertain about what treatment, if any, is needed. For this reason, the Epilepsy Foundation of America issues an identification badge with the diagnosis, the epileptic's name, and an emergency telephone number. Police and emergency personnel are under instructions to look for such identification.

ACCIDENT RATES OF EPILEPTICS, DIABETICS, AND STROKE VICTIMS

Condition	Accidents Per Million Miles
Epilepsy	16
Diabetes	15
Stroke victims	14
General population	8

The accident rate among drivers who have epilepsy is not much more frequent than among those with other medical problems, but is about twice the rate of the general population.

Driving. The automobile kills 50,000 people every year, and causes severe head injury to more than 200,000 others, of whom 2,000 to 4,000 will later develop epilepsy. To operate a car requires constant alertness, and it is obvious that people subject to frequent lapses of consciousness should not drive.

Yet, to lack a driver's license in our society is a serious handicap. Some jobs require driving. In many communities driving is the only way to reach work. For this reason, even though there are increased risks involved, society permits persons with epilepsy to drive if seizures have been controlled for a reasonable period of time. The accident rate for known epileptic drivers is higher than the national average (see the table above), but not significantly higher than that of certain other groups, such as teenage males. Epileptic drivers account for less than one percent of all accidents. Compared to the accident toll from speeding or drunken driving, that is insignificant.

To maintain his driving privilege, however, any person who has experienced a lapse of consciousness, from whatever cause, is required to report it on his license application, or to report it afterwards if he already has a driver's license. Seven states require a physician who treats a person with epilepsy to report the patient to a state authority. However, the primary responsibility to report belongs to the patient.

The individual who remains under medical supervision and is consistent in taking medicine will be granted a license after freedom from seizures for one to two years. Some states will grant limited license privileges after shorter periods of time.

Employment. The most serious problem for many epileptics is finding a job. Many employers consider their work places unsafe for persons with epilepsy. In truth, few jobs are that hazardous. Indeed, a work place that is not safe for the person with epilepsy is not entirely safe for anyone. One study showed that more employees were injured by sneezing than by convulsions. Anyone can trip, fall, sneeze, or faint. Increasingly, employers are under pressure to make their work places safe for everyone.

Many states now have laws forbidding an employer to discriminate against a person with a handicap. In addition, the Federal Rehabilitation Act of 1973 prohibits federal grant recipients and contractors from discriminating in employment against handicapped persons. The act requires any such organization to make "reasonable accommodation" to the "known physical or mental limitation of an otherwise qualified handicapped applicant or employee unless (it) can demonstrate that the accommodation would impose an undue hardship on the operation of its program." "Accommodation" implies not only changes in the physical environment of the work place, but also such things as flexibility of work hours, including time off for illness.

Still, some persons with extremely frequent uncontrolled seizures or related disabilities remain unable to work. The Social Security Administration considers a person totally disabled if he or she has a major convulsion more than once a month or a minor attack more than once a week.

In employment, too, epilepsy is so individual in its effects that no rules apply to everyone. Some persons have seizures only at night. For them, the risk of injury at work is minimal. Others have a prolonged warning or premonition (aura) before a seizure. They have time to lie down or go to a safe place. Persons suffering from absence seizures (petit mal) do not fall or move about. There is no hazard to them or others unless they are in control of dangerous equipment. Persons with complex partial seizures present a problem because they may walk into dangerous situations during their unconsciousness and automatic behavior.

STATE LAWS REGULATING DRIVING BY EPILEPTICS

Doctors are required to report names of their epilepsy patients to a state agency in seven states:

California, Connecticut, Delaware, Georgia, Montana, New Jersey, Oregon.

License granted after *2 years* freedom from seizure:

Connecticut, District of Columbia, Florida, New Jersey, West Virginia, Wisconsin (varies).

License granted after *18 months* freedom from seizure:

Massachusetts, New Hampshire, Vermont.

License granted after *1 year* freedom from seizure:

California, Colorado, Iowa, Kansas, Kentucky, Louisiana, Maine, Michigan, Minnesota, Nevada, New York, North Carolina, Ohio, Oregon, Pennsylvania, Utah.

License granted after *6 months* freedom from seizure:

Wisconsin (limited license), Washington (limited license).

License procedure uncertain, depending upon doctor's recommendation and other information:

Alabama, Alaska, Arizona, Arkansas, Delaware, Georgia, Hawaii, Idaho, Indiana, Maryland, Mississippi, Missouri, Montana, Nebraska, New Mexico, North Dakota, Oklahoma, Rhode Island, South Carolina, South Dakota, Tennessee, Texas, Virginia, Wyoming.

Hospitalization. Years ago, people with severe, uncontrollable epilepsy were cared for in epileptic colonies where they could live and work within a protected environment. At present, the only persons with epilepsy living in institutions are those who also are mentally retarded or ill. Even for them, the trend is to develop living arrangements within their community, such as cooperative apartments or supervised group homes with associated sheltered workshops. These arrangements allow persons with epilepsy to remain in the community and still receive social and physical protection and medical care.

Psychological problems. In view of the stresses in their lives, it is not surprising that many persons with epilepsy suffer from psychological problems. Anxiety, lack of self-assurance, and restless or irritable behavior are common among schoolchildren. Adults have problems, too. Although the epileptic seizure might not be frightening to the person who has it, the experience of public loss of consciousness plus the frightened reaction of parents, friends, and others can be upsetting. Add

to this the potential social rejection at home and school, or loss of employment, and the stage is set for anxiety and depression. An added burden is the effect of medicine. Phenobarbital in particular slows the thought processes and produces sleepiness and irritability. In children it produces restlessness, hyperactive behavior, and misbehavior. Fortunately, newer drugs are less likely to have this effect.

Epilepsy and violent behavior. There is a false belief that people with epilepsy often commit crimes during an attack. This misunderstanding probably arises because some people become confused during a psychomotor seizure, and if efforts are made to control their aimless behavior, they may become frightened and violent. But this is a matter far different from the conduct of a deliberate criminal act or unprovoked attack. Studies of prison populations, including prisoners with epilepsy, have failed to demonstrate that the crimes committed by epileptics differed significantly from those of others in similar walks of life.

CHAPTER 11   JOHN STIRLING MEYER, M.D.

STROKE (VASCULAR DISEASE OF THE BRAIN)

Stroke (called apoplexy or cerebral vascular accident in old terminology) means a sudden brain disturbance caused by an interruption of the blood supply. It results from disease of the blood vessels supplying the brain (cerebrum). This condition is usually termed "cerebrovascular disease." The arteries carrying blood to the brain are most commonly involved, but in rare cases the disease occurs in the veins that remove blood from the brain.

TYPES AND SYMPTOMS
OF STROKE

There are three general types of stroke: cerebral hemorrhage, cerebral thrombosis, and cerebral embolism.

Cerebral hemorrhage is caused by rupture of a cerebral blood vessel with bleeding into the brain (intracerebral hemorrhage) or under its covering membranes. Depending on which membrane, this bleeding is called subarachnoid hemorrhage or subdural hematoma.

Cerebral thrombosis stems from obstruction of a cerebral blood vessel when a blood clot forms within its walls. The clot may be caused by abnormal thickening of the blood, damage to the vessel wall from arteriosclerosis (hardening of the arteries), atherosclerosis (fatty deposits in the vessel walls), inflammation of the arteries (arteritis), or inflammation of the veins (phlebitis). If the blood supply is completely stopped or reduced below one-fourth of its normal level, softening of the brain (called cerebral infarction) results. Infarction causes permanent brain damage.

Cerebral embolism is obstruction of a cerebral artery by a blood clot or a foreign body which usually has migrated from another part of the body's circulation. An example is a blood clot breaking off from a damaged heart and being transported to a main artery of the brain. Another example is when a clot that has formed on the inside wall of one of the two carotid or two vertebral arteries in the neck travels up to the brain and blocks a major artery branch that brings blood to the brain. The clots commonly fragment and lodge in the left middle cerebral artery, which in right-handers supplies the speech areas of the brain. This artery also supplies the nerve cells controlling movement of the right side of the body, particularly the right arm and leg.

Common symptoms. When the blood supply to part of the brain is suddenly interrupted, there will be a corresponding loss of the functions controlled by that part of the brain. Depending on location, this may include loss of speech (aphasia) or slurred speech, confusion, paralysis of one side of the body (hemiplegia), paralysis of one side of the face, paralysis of movement of the eyes with squint, unequal pupils, staggering and loss of coordination (ataxia), loss of sensation to parts of the body, headache, nausea, vomiting, and loss of consciousness.

Frequency. In the United States stroke is the third most common cause of death after heart disease and cancer, and it is the most common disabler. Two million Americans are disabled by stroke. Fortunately, thanks to control of hypertension and other risk factors, the incidence is decreasing.

Aging and stroke. Chronological age and physical age are not the same because some people age more rapidly than others. Nor is age a disease, although diseases increase with advancing age. Some 80-year-olds are strikingly free of arteriosclerosis. However, the peak incidence of stroke is reached after age 50 and continues through the 70s. Men have a higher incidence in the earlier decades than women, possibly because of some protective effect of female hormones. Women tend to catch up with men in stroke incidence after the menopause.

Severity and Consequences

Besides being classified by cause, strokes also are classified by their severity and consequences.

Transient ischemic attacks or "TIAs" are brief episodes of symptoms caused by temporary interruptions of the blood supply to the brain. They last from a few minutes to less than 24 hours, with complete recovery.

Reversible ischemic neurological deficits (RINDs) are small cerebral infarctions from which almost complete recovery results after three weeks to three months.

Recognizing TIAs and RINDs is important because if proper treatment is begun, major strokes can be prevented. For example, at least 11 percent of cerebral thromboses are preceded by warning TIAs, and 41 percent of patients with TIAs will proceed to the permanent damage of cerebral infarction if the condition is not treated properly.

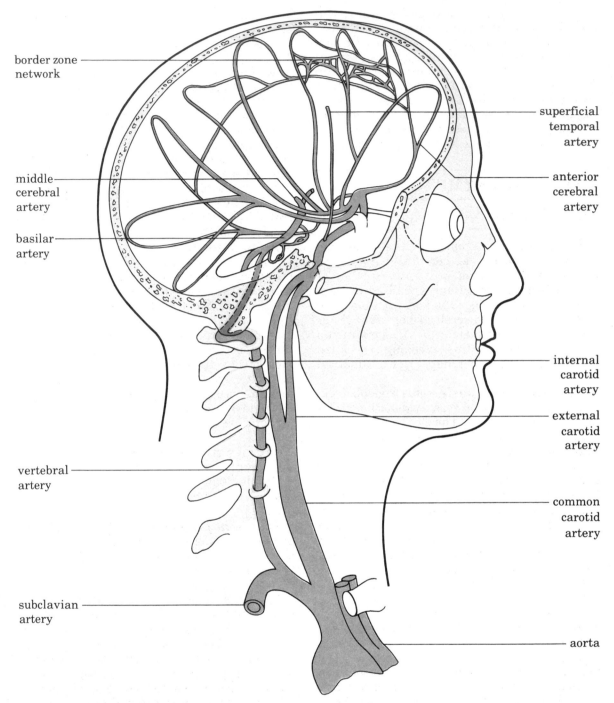

border zone
network

superficial
temporal
artery

middle
cerebral
artery

anterior
cerebral
artery

basilar
artery

internal
carotid
artery

external
carotid
artery

vertebral
artery

common
carotid
artery

subclavian
artery

aorta

ARTERIES AND THE BRAIN

The two major arteries carrying blood to the brain are the internal carotid artery and the vertebral artery. Stroke can occur when either of these major arteries is blocked. The collateral blood supply is usually shunted via *the anterior cerebral artery, the blood vessels of the eye, the border zone network, and branches of the basilar artery. The collateral vessels are shown in black.*

A progressing stroke is caused by infarction of the brain, which usually worsens for five days, and then improves to become a completed or stable stroke with permanent loss of some central nervous system function. Because it is sometimes difficult to distinguish cerebral infarctions caused by thrombosis from those caused by embolism, they are sometimes listed together under the term atherothrombotic brain infarction (ABI).

Multiple cerebral infarction can lead to permanent confusion and memory loss, termed multi-infarct dementia. The mortality rate from cerebral infarction is 30 to 40 percent.

Patients with cerebral hemorrhage usually have high blood pressure (hypertension). The course is characterized by the sudden onset of headache, severe loss of brain function, nausea, vomiting often progressing to coma, and death within a few days. The death rate for strokes due to cerebral hemorrhage is 80 to 90 percent. Fortunately, they are far less common than strokes caused by ABI.

Transient ischemic attacks (TIAs) also may be classified into two major groups according to the part of the brain served by the affected vessels. They are vertebrobasilar arterial insufficiency (VBI) and carotid arterial insufficiency. As shown on page 238, the carotid system supplies the front and middle portion of each brain hemisphere and the vertebral arteries join to form the basilar and posterior cerebral arteries, which supply the brain stem, cerebellum, and rearmost occipital lobes.

As shown on page 240, temporary interruption of the blood supply to the brain stem, cerebellum, and occipital lobes can cause attacks of dizziness, unsteady gait, clumsiness, thick speech, cortical blindness, double vision, and falling spells without loss of consciousness. Temporary interruption of the carotid blood supply can cause weakness of the opposite side of the body, trouble with speech formation (expressive aphasia), memory and personality changes, difficulty writing (agraphia), loss of sensation on the opposite side of the body (contralateral hemianesthesia), difficulty calculating (acalculia), inability to comprehend music (amusia), difficulty in initiating movement of the limbs (ideomotor apraxia), difficulty understanding speech (receptive aphasia), and confusing of the left and right sides.

VBI also can cause temporary amnesia for up to 24 hours. These episodes are characterized by complete loss of recent memory, with disorientation to time, place, and identity of others. The person may have complete confusion and loss of memory about the entire event when he or she recovers the next day.

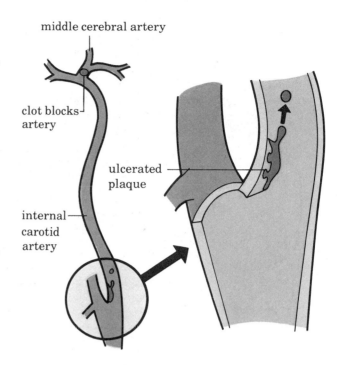

middle cerebral artery

clot blocks artery

ulcerated plaque

internal carotid artery

HOW STROKES OCCUR

Strokes frequently are caused by atherosclerosis of the internal carotid artery of the neck, which supplies blood to the brain, as shown in the left portion of the diagram. Plaque develops on the inner surface of the artery (enlarged view, right), narrowing the channel and roughening the arterial walls. Turbulent blood flow through the narrowed area dislodges the material and carries it to the brain, where it may form a plug in an artery (top left). The result can be a brief interruption in blood supply, called a transient ischemic attack (TIA), or a stroke. The narrowed blood vessel can be reamed out surgically, a procedure called carotid endarterectomy.

Apart from TIAs caused by emboli, symptoms also can arise when a carotid artery, middle cerebral artery, or vertebral artery is completely blocked and the blood supply to the brain's "anemic territory" is supplied by other vessels shunting it around the blockage (collateral circulation). When there is a fall in blood pressure or irregular heart action, the collateral circulation may fail and stroke symptoms result.

The harmful deposits of atherosclerosis (hardening of the arteries) occur commonly in certain portions of the blood vessels that supply the brain. These vessels include the aorta, subclavian, and innominate arteries in the

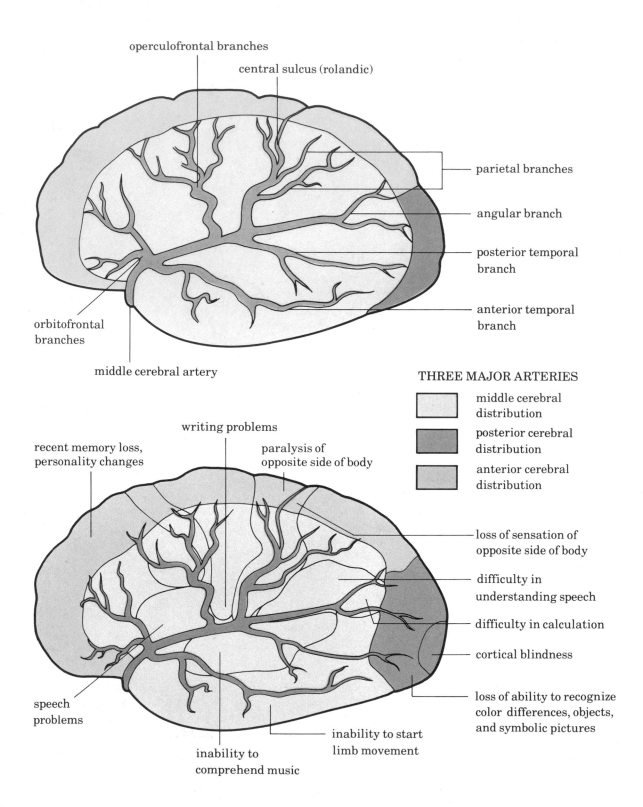

operculofrontal branches

central sulcus (rolandic)

parietal branches

angular branch

posterior temporal
branch

anterior temporal
branch

orbitofrontal
branches

middle cerebral artery

THREE MAJOR ARTERIES

middle cerebral
distribution

posterior cerebral
distribution

anterior cerebral
distribution

writing problems

recent memory loss,
personality changes

paralysis of
opposite side of body

loss of sensation of
opposite side of body

difficulty in
understanding speech

difficulty in calculation

cortical blindness

speech
problems

loss of ability to recognize
color differences, objects,
and symbolic pictures

inability to start
limb movement

inability to
comprehend music

CONSEQUENCES OF STROKE

*An interruption of blood supply to
the brain can cause a variety of
neurological problems, depending on
the location of the blockage and the
part of the brain supplied by the
blocked artery. Top drawing shows the*
*brain's three major cerebral arteries
and the portions of the brain supplied
by each. The lower diagram shows the
location of several brain functions and
the neurological problem that results
when blood supply is halted to each.*

chest, the carotid and vertebral arteries in the neck, and the basilar, middle cerebral, posterior cerebral, and anterior cerebral arteries in the brain. The most common blockage sites stemming from atherosclerosis are shown on page 242.

INTRACRANIAL BLEEDING

Bleeding within the brain or under its membranes, called intracranial bleeding, is a common form of stroke. There are five general types of these hemorrhages.

Cerebral hemorrhage. Thanks to control of hypertension, the incidence of all types of cerebral hemorrhage is declining. Severe hypertension damages the walls of the cerebral vessels, with thickening of the smooth muscle and loss of elastic tissue. This is followed by scarring and deposit of fats within the lining of the vessels. This degenerative process can result in rupture of the vessel with bleeding into the substance of the brain, called hypertensive intracerebral hemorrhage. This is the most serious form of stroke and carries a high mortality rate.

Subarachnoid hemorrhage and aneurysm. Intracranial bleeding also may arise from a defect present at birth in the walls of the cerebral arteries. The arterial wall lacks a segment of normal smooth muscle and elastic tissue layers, which weakens the wall. The weak segment stretches and gradually enlarges to cause a ballooning or "blowout" in the wall, called an aneurysm. The thin-walled aneurysm eventually may burst or rupture, bleeding into and through the thin arachnoid membrane that covers the brain. This is called a subarachnoid or meningeal hemorrhage. The result is sudden excruciating head pain, stiff neck, nausea, vomiting, and collapse. If the hemorrhage also extends into the brain substance and damages major nerve pathways, it is called a meningo-cerebral hemorrhage. Paralysis on one side of the body, dilated pupils, double vision, and paralysis of eye movements may result, followed by loss of consciousness. The condition can occur at any age, but is most common in the 40s and 50s. The outlook is better if the person remains conscious and if paralysis is minimal. Patients who go into deep coma usually die.

Subdural hemorrhage or hematoma. Hemorrhage under the outer hard covering (dura) of the brain most commonly arises from head injury but occasionally results from a ruptured aneurysm. The clot must be removed surgically by drilling a hole in the skull or turning a flap of bone to gain access to it (see chapter 31, "Understanding Your Operation").

Malformed blood vessels. An arteriovenous malformation (AVM) is a tangle of thin-walled vessels. After birth these vessels did not differentiate properly into thick-walled arteries, well-supported capillaries, and tissue-reinforced veins. These abnormal vessels shunt blood directly from arteries to veins in the cerebral circulation, returning blood to the heart without nourishing the area of brain they were intended to supply. Because these thin-walled veins carry blood under arterial pressure, they are liable to rupture and cause bleeding into the brain. They also are a common cause of epilepsy or convulsive seizures.

Other causes. Disorders of the clotting properties of the blood can cause brain hemorrhage. These disorders include hemophilia, leukemia, Hodgkin's disease, and sickle-cell anemia. The excessive use of anticoagulants or blood thinning drugs can cause hemorrhage (see chapter 6, "The Blood"). Head injury, infections, and brain tumors also are potential causes of bleeding in the brain.

THE BRAIN AND
ITS BLOOD SUPPLY

The brain has the highest demand for energy of any organ. One-fifth of the blood pumped from the heart goes to the brain. If the blood supply is suddenly cut off, loss of consciousness occurs in 10 to 12 seconds. Oxygen and glucose are brought to the brain by the arterial blood. Ninety-nine percent becomes carbon dioxide and water, but a small amount of lactic acid is produced. These are normally carried away promptly by the veins. If the blood supply is reduced, less oxygen is provided and more lactic acid is produced. Removal is slowed down, and these acid waste products accumulate. Lactic acid and carbon dioxide stimulate the brain vessels to dilate so that blood flow is increased, thereby providing more oxygen and glucose to the brain and improving the washout of these accumulations. When the brain does work such as thinking, more energy is consumed and more acid products are formed, so blood flow is increased. This response fails in patients after a stroke.

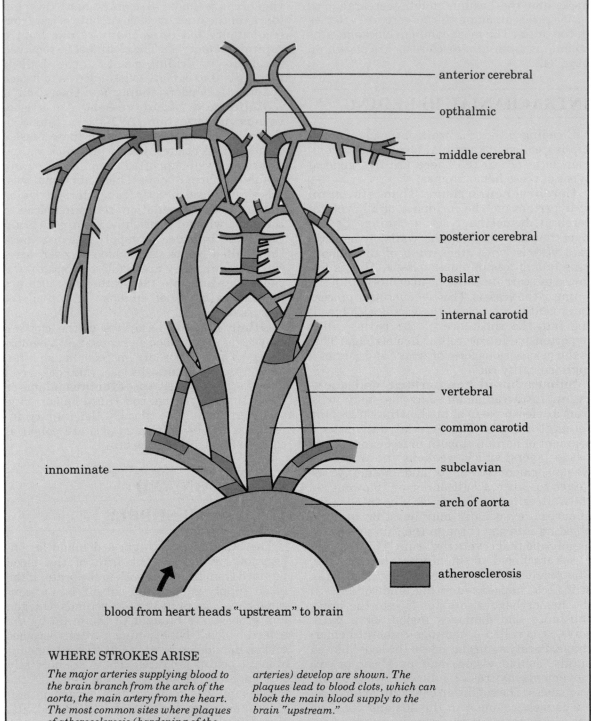

anterior cerebral

opthalmic

middle cerebral

posterior cerebral

basilar

internal carotid

vertebral

common carotid

innominate

subclavian

arch of aorta

atherosclerosis

blood from heart heads "upstream" to brain

WHERE STROKES ARISE

The major arteries supplying blood to the brain branch from the arch of the aorta, the main artery from the heart. The most common sites where plaques of atherosclerosis (hardening of the arteries) develop are shown. The plaques lead to blood clots, which can block the main blood supply to the brain "upstream."

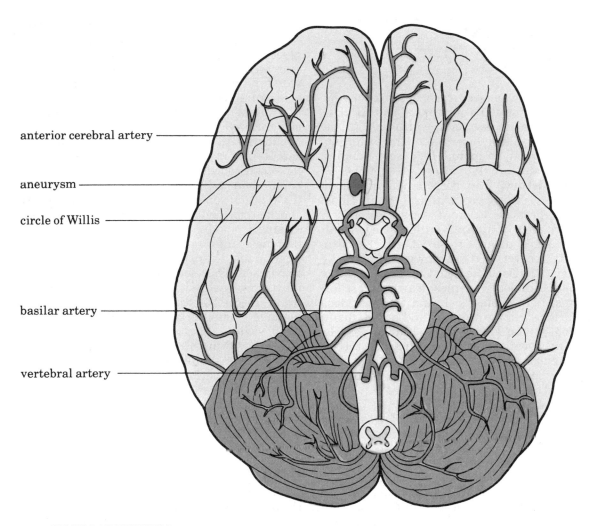

anterior cerebral artery

aneurysm

circle of Willis

basilar artery

vertebral artery

BRAIN ANEURYSM

A weak-walled, distended area of an artery is called an aneurysm. The balloon-like enlargement is susceptible to rupture and causes hemorrhage under the brain's arachnoid membrane. In this illustration the brain, viewed from below, has an aneurysm of the anterior cerebral artery, a common site. In most cases an aneurysm can be corrected surgically with a clip so it will not rupture again.

The blood flow to the brain normally remains constant despite changes in blood pressure. The brain arteries dilate when the blood pressure falls and constrict when it rises. This mechanism fails if there is marked arteriosclerosis, particularly if the blood pressure falls too low. Very low blood pressure will cause normal people to faint or lose consciousness due to anemia of the brain, but it may precipitate a stroke in patients with arteriosclerosis or hypertension. This normal regulatory mechanism also fails when the blood pressure becomes exceedingly high. Headache and confusion usually result and cerebral hemorrhage may occur.

STROKE RISK FACTORS

We know that many cases of stroke can be prevented or lessened by treatment of risk factors that tend to cause cerebral arteriosclerosis and stroke. These include high blood pressure, diabetes mellitus, elevated fats in the blood (hyperlipemia), heart disease, obesity, and smoking. Most physicians believe that early diagnosis and treatment of hypertension, diabetes, excessive blood fats, and heart disease are important in preventing strokes. They also recommend keeping weight down and avoiding the smoking habit.

DIAGNOSIS AND PREVENTION

The patient who faces a risk of stroke or who has had warning signs of stroke (TIAs, RINDs) should make an early appointment to be examined by his or her doctor. The examination will probably include a case history, a physical exam, and laboratory tests.

Case history. The person will be asked about the risk factors in himself or in blood relatives, because stroke and risk factors for stroke frequently run in families. The patient will be asked about any brief attacks with complete recovery (TIAs) or with incomplete recovery (RINDs). The blood pressure will be recorded and blood samples drawn to test for diabetes, high cholesterol, and triglycerides. The patient will be weighed and asked about smoking habits. The heart and major vessels in the neck will be examined with a stethoscope. Arteriosclerotic plaques in the major arteries of the neck frequently cause abnormal noises and may decrease the pulse of the artery when felt with the fingers.

Physical examination. Neurological tests will attempt to define any temporary or permanent damage to the nervous system. This includes evaluation of the state of consciousness, which is usually impaired in severe strokes. Changes in consciousness can be simply classified as coma (without response to pain), semicoma (responds to pain but otherwise unresponsive), drowsy, confused, or mentally clear. Speech, memory, and the patient's orientation to time, place, and person are evaluated. The neck is tested for stiffness, which occurs in subarachnoid hemorrhage.

Examination of the eyes is important. The ophthalmoscope is used to inspect the optic nerve at the back of the eye. In intracranial hemorrhage or massive infarction, pressure on the nerve or hemorrhages around it may be seen. Paralysis of eye movements, paralysis of one side of the face and body (hemiplegia), or loss of sensation (hemisensory loss) may occur. The tendon reflexes, checked by tapping the tendons with a rubber hammer, may show increased or decreased response because of brain damage.

Laboratory tests. The urine should be examined for evidence of kidney disease. Blood samples are tested for the following: red blood cell count (high counts thicken the blood and predispose to stroke), white blood cell count (elevated in leukemia and infection), blood sugar (up in diabetes), cholesterol, triglycerides (up in hyperlipemia), urea content (elevated in kidney failure), and enzymes (elevated in liver failure, some heart attacks, and brain infarction).

A spinal tap or lumbar puncture may be carried out under local anesthetic by inserting a needle into the lower spine to draw off a small sample of spinal fluid. The sample is examined for fresh blood, found in subarachnoid and brain hemorrhage. The electrocardiogram (ECG) and often the echocardiogram are checked for evidence of cerebral embolism arising from the heart, and the chest X ray provides information about complicating pneumonia, heart failure, and enlargement of the heart. The electroencephalogram (EEG) may show localized slowing or reduction of the brain electrical activity because of stroke damage. Computerized axial tomography scan (CAT scan) helps to locate hemorrhages and infarcts within the brain. The vessels in the neck can be examined by ultrasound, which may reveal arteriosclerotic narrowing. All the above tests are harmless (noninvasive) and carry no risk for the patient.

Finally, cerebral arteriography is recommended if surgical treatment is contemplated or diagnosis is in doubt. This is accomplished by passing a catheter through the femoral artery in the groin, through the aorta to the carotid and vertebral arteries (which supply the brain), and then injecting a radiopaque dye containing iodine. X-ray pictures of the head and neck trace the passage of the dye through the arteries of the brain so that any blockage, narrowing, or other problem will be noted with precision.

TREATMENT

The first step in treatment of stroke is prevention. There is now considerable evidence that the risk of stroke can be reduced by public education concerning early detection and treatment of hypertension, diabetes mellitus, hyperlipemia, obesity, heart disease, and avoidance of smoking.

When transient ischemic attacks (TIAs) begin to occur, the patient should report them immediately to his or her physician so that an evaluation can be carried out and a program of secondary prevention can begin. Risk factors should be treated. If disease of the heart is the cause of cerebral embolism, some irregularities can be corrected with medication, others can be corrected with surgery.

Surgery

If examination of a patient with carotid transient ischemic attacks discloses large arteriosclerotic or atherosclerotic plaques, the plaques can be removed under general anesthesia. The surgery is accomplished by making an incision in the artery, reaming out the plaque lining and its wall, and sewing the artery together again. A graft of sterile knitted dacron plastic or vein taken from the leg can be used to restore the artery to its normal width. This operation is called a carotid endarterectomy and the complication rate is usually less than 1 in 20. If the carotid or middle cerebral artery is completely blocked, a scalp artery, usually the superficial temporal artery (STA), can be carried through the skull after removing a window of bone, then joined to the middle cerebral artery (MCA) beyond the blockage to shunt blood around it and to supply the brain. This shunt operation is called an STA-MCA bypass.

Medical Management

The majority of cases of stroke and TIA do not require surgery and can be treated by medical means. The chief objective is to prevent the formation of blood clots on the atherosclerotic plaques within the vessel wall by use of medication.

When an arteriosclerotic plaque or roughening forms within a vessel wall, small sticky elements in the blood called platelets collect on the roughened surface. This is followed by the accumulation of a protein meshwork called fibrin, which forms the beginning of the white clot (fibrino-platelet deposition). When mixed with red cells it enlarges and becomes the firm and familiar red clot that is seen on the surface of most wounds as they cease to bleed. Certain medicines inhibit the formation of platelet deposits. These include aspirin, dipyridamole, and sulfinpyrazone.

Many patients with TIAs thus are treated with one aspirin twice a day. Controlled clinical trials have shown that patients receiving aspirin had fewer TIAs and strokes than those who did not receive aspirin. Or patients may be given anti-blood-clotting drugs of the warfarin type, which prevent the fibrin deposition phase of clotting. These carry a far greater risk of hemorrhage than aspirin, however, and controlled clinical trials have shown less satisfactory results.

Treatment of subarachnoid hemorrhage begins with complete bed rest to minimize the risk of further bleeding. Pain-relieving drugs and sedation are usually required because head pain is severe. Fluids are restricted in the early stages to minimize brain edema or swelling. Supplementary potassium may be required if there has been depletion of this important mineral because of vomiting.

Certain drugs can enhance clotting of the blood in patients with subarachnoid hemorrhage. The most widely used in the United States is epsilon-amino-caproic acid. It may be given during the first two weeks after rupture and active bleeding from an intracranial aneurysm to cause clotting within the aneurysm and to stop the bleeding.

After arteriography has shown the cause of bleeding, intracranial surgery is usually recommended to clip or remove the aneurysm or AVM (see chapter 31, "Understanding Your Operation"). All intracranial operations carry considerable risk but untreated aneurysm or AVM carries a much greater risk of death or repeated ruptures. Occasionally, if the aneurysm arises directly from the carotid artery, the surgeon elects to close the carotid artery in the neck gradually in order to reduce blood pressure within the aneurysm.

Treatment of progressive stroke. In general, the recommended treatment of acute, progressive stroke is conservative medical care. Certain exceptions are when the CAT scan shows a hemorrhage on the surface of the cerebral hemispheres or in the cerebellum, where it can be removed surgically.

Medical treatment is begun by nursing the patient on complete bed rest lying flat on the back or on the side, with frequent turning to prevent bedsores. The paralyzed limbs are regularly exercised through a full range of motion at least once or twice per day to prevent frozen joints (contractures). This requires expert and dedicated nursing care. Blood pressure, pulse rate, and body temperature are charted daily. Pneumonia and urinary tract infections are common complications of stroke that the doctor must watch for diligently. A semiconscious or lethargic patient usually requires a catheter to drain the bladder and must be fed intravenously or via a tube through the nose to the stomach. Patients with breathing problems may require a plastic airway or tube or operation to open the windpipe.

Brain swelling (cerebral edema) commonly accompanies brain infarction or hemorrhage. No entirely satisfactory treatment has been found but medication can be given to draw water out of the brain tissue and back into the bloodstream.

After the acute stroke has subsided (usually in four to five days), feeding with a stomach tube may replace intravenous feeding. The patient should be encouraged to eat again as soon as possible.

Heart Disease and Treatment of Stroke

About 20 percent of the strokes that do not involve bleeding are caused by embolism from the heart, where either fibrinoplatelet emboli or red clots break off and lodge in the brain. The former cause TIAs or brief neurological symptoms. The red clots cause more serious neurological damage. The emboli from the heart may arise from diseased heart valves. The mitral valve and the aortic valve (see chapter 3, "The Heart and Circulation") most commonly are affected, by rheumatic fever or infections in the bloodstream called subacute bacterial endocarditis. Or they may arise from disturbances of normal heart rhythm, most commonly atrial fibrillation, where the upper chambers of the heart are beating faster than the lower chambers. As a result, blood clots form in the atria and break off to form emboli. Blood clots also can result after a "heart attack," which is coronary artery disease or thrombosis of the main arteries supplying the heart muscle. Rarely in young adults, the mitral valve may periodically prolapse (invert like an umbrella blowing out in the wind) and emboli may arise from clots forming on the prolapsed valve. Surgical replacement of diseased valves during open heart surgery sometimes produces emboli.

Emboli are usually treated with aspirin or other platelet-inhibiting drugs. Anticoagulant drugs are sometimes used to prevent red clot formation, but unless carefully supervised by the physician, an overdose can result in accidental hemorrhage within the body.

If atrial fibrillation is the cause of blood clot emboli, normal rhythm of the heart can be restored with medications or by external application of electrical shock to the heart.

If the blood clots arise from coronary thrombosis or diseased heart valves, open heart surgery often repairs the problem.

Stroke Caused by Thrombosis of a Cerebral Vein

Stroke caused by blockage of veins is very rare. Sometimes it occurs in women immediately after childbirth, and in rare instances it occurs in both men and women as a complication of cancer and dehydrated or emaciated states. It is a rare complication of the use of oral contraceptive pills. Diagnosis is made based on history, neurological examination, EEG showing slowing of brain waves, CAT scan abnormalities, and abnormal filling of the veins during arteriography. Treatment is medical. Intravenous infusion to restore fluids or clot-dissolving and anticoagulant drugs are used. The outlook is better than when the stroke is caused by a blocked artery.

REHABILITATION

For booklets on care of the stroke patient contact your local American Heart Association chapter and the National Institute of Neurological Communicative Disorders and Stroke, Bethesda, Maryland.

As indicated, physical therapy should begin the day after the stroke, with full range of passive motion exercises once or twice daily.

At home, the patient should be encouraged to raise himself to a sitting position with assistance and to maintain this position without help. A sling may be helpful in supporting the paralyzed arm and a short leg brace in supporting the paralyzed lower leg. When sitting, the patient should be taught to lift the paralyzed arm and flex it across the lower chest. The weak leg and foot may also be assisted by the normal limbs in learning to sit and stand once again. Next the patient learns to walk with help, first in the parallel bars, later with a walker or with a cane. The patient is then ready to learn to care for himself, and to handle utensils with one hand. A wheelchair may be used until the patient can walk unaided.

Most communities have rehabilitation facilities, including physical therapy and occupational therapy programs, for the patient who has recovered from the acute stroke. If loss of speech persists, retraining is needed.

What can you do to minimize your risk of a stroke? Have your heart and blood pressure and your blood sugar and blood lipid levels checked regularly (at least once a year) by your physician. Watch your diet and weight, exercise regularly, and avoid smoking. If you should have any TIAs as described earlier in this chapter, tell your doctor immediately.

REHABILITATION EXERCISE AFTER A STROKE

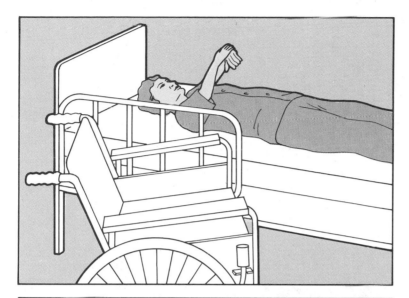

Learning to move from bed to wheelchair, the stroke patient with a paralyzed left side uses the nonparalyzed limbs to move the paralyzed ones. In a lying position, he or she first lifts the left arm across the chest.

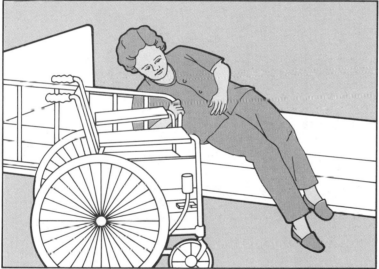

In the second step, the patient grasps the bed rail with the nonparalyzed right hand. The nonparalyzed right leg is tucked under the left, so that the legs may be rolled and swung off the bed.

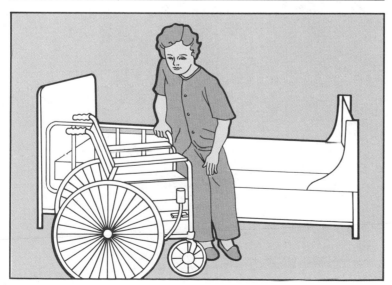

In the third step, the patient uses the bed rail to push into a sitting position, then leans on the nonparalyzed right leg to move into the wheelchair. The chair is kept in a locked position so that it does not move during the shift.

CHAPTER 12   BRUCE E. SPIVEY, M.D.

THE EYES

Vision—seeing and interpreting what we see—has always been one of the most precious and guarded of human gifts. It is intricately woven into the texture of our culture and the complexity of our civilization. Our religions elevate vision to a power of the gods: "Your eyes shall be open and ye shall be as gods..." are the words from Genesis 3:5. Our legal system is, in large part, based on bearing witness. Cults throughout all cultures produce "seers." Artists and poets place beauty in the eye of the beholder.

Of the five human senses, sight is probably the most important, yet we often take it for granted. We glance at a bus schedule, focus quickly on the television screen, catch hues of the rainbow in soap bubbles, and recognize fine lines of worry on the face of a friend, yet give no thought to the miraculous way these images are produced, or to how much we depend on them. But when our sight is threatened, it is a different story. A public-opinion survey by Research to Prevent Blindness Inc. shows that Americans rank loss of vision second among afflictions they fear most, behind cancer but ahead of life-threatening heart disease or stroke. Blindness is the chief cause of disability in the United States.

There is, for the most part, good reason for this fear, even though children who are born without sight or who lose vision at an early age develop and mature far more normally than children born without hearing. Most of our activities and occupations today are based on the ability to see and interpret what we see. Skills as diverse as reading and driving are basic to getting along in society. Entertainment and much of art are basically visual, and we all know the family down the street that absolutely could not survive without TV.

What, then, is vision? How do we see? How do we learn to make meaning of what we see? What can go wrong in the process of vision? Most importantly, how can we maintain good vision? And if, at any age, something does go wrong with our vision, how can we treat it?

As with many parts of the body, modern medicine does not have all the answers to these questions. We do not know how the brain works to integrate vision. We do not know what causes most cataracts in aging, why children are born cross-eyed, or why the part of the retina we must have to read disintegrates in some older people and not in others. On the other hand, because the front of the eye is transparent, we can see more of its abnormalities than any other organ of the body except the skin. Thus, we can quickly detect problems of the eye and treat them precisely. Ophthalmology, the medical study dedicated to maintaining good vision and preventing or treating eye disease, is the oldest medical specialty in which physicians concentrate exclusively on one organ system. Whereas medicine and surgery are general medical studies, ophthalmology became a distinct specialty more than 100 years ago.

Although eye care has been a human concern for centuries, in recent years it has progressed dramatically. New ways have been devised to restore or improve the sight of many who otherwise might have been sentenced to a lifetime of darkness. New drugs and nonsurgical techniques are used to treat diseases that otherwise could lead to blindness, and surgeons routinely probe the interior of the eye. The operating microscope, other miniaturized and highly specialized instruments, and innovative procedures can accomplish delicate repairs to restore useful vision. Some serious eye problems still remain beyond the reach of even the most advanced medical and surgical methods, but hope remains that even those can someday be conquered.

THE NATURE OF VISION

Before we can answer the questions, "What is vision?" and "How do we see?" we must understand the eye as an organ of the body and the structures that surround, protect, and expand its visual capabilities.

The eye, as so many others have said, is like a camera. Although that analogy is a useful one, it hardly describes the sensitive, versatile, flexible, and enduring structure of the human eye. The eye can automatically control the amount of light that enters it. It can focus on precise detail or perceive objects, light, and movement at the outer edge of the visual range. It has its own lubrication system. With proper care, eyes last a lifetime for most people, needing little more than external readjustment in the form of prescription lenses once we get past the age of 45 or so. Moreover, to the physician, the eye is a window into the patient's internal world, a peephole through which blood vessels and nerve endings of the eye can be viewed to reveal representative characteristics of health or disease in the rest of the body.

To understand this sensitive and complex organ and the diseases or disorders that affect it, we should extend the oversimplified camera comparison and take a brief lesson in the anatomy of the eye.

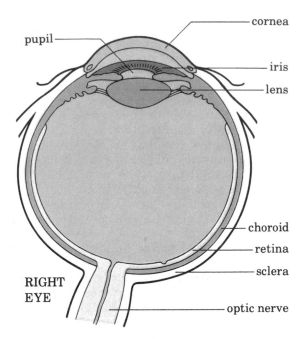

pupil
cornea
iris
lens
choroid
retina
sclera
optic nerve
RIGHT
EYE

ANATOMY OF THE EYE

This horizontal cross section shows the arrangement of the major parts of the eye. Light enters through the cornea, passes through the pupil, which is an opening in the iris, then through the crystalline lens, and is focused on the retina. The choroid is a layer important to the eye's nutrition. The sclera is visible at the front as the "white of the eye." Light is converted by the retina to nerve impulses that travel through the optic nerve to the brain.

Structure and Function of the Eyes

The eyeball, or globe, is about the size of a table tennis ball and fits into a skeletal pocket of protection in the skull called the orbit, or socket. The eye itself is made up of intricate layers, all of which serve a particular function.

The outer coat consists of two parts, the cornea and sclera, that are tough but sensitive. The sclera is the white of the eye and protects it from injury and irritation. The cornea, an extension of the sclera at the front of the eye, is not white but perfectly clear so that light can pass through. It protects the iris and pupil. Because it has a concentration of nerve endings, the cornea is one of the structures in the body most sensitive to pain, as anyone who has suffered a bit of sand or even an eyelash scratching its surface can confirm. This sensitivity is an alarm system, a protective mechanism that triggers other reflexes such as blinking and tearing, which guard the eye against injury.

Another layer, the conjunctiva, covers the white sclera of the eye and the inside of the eyelids. By manufacturing oily secretions, it prevents friction when the eye moves. When people suffer from hay fever or other allergies, it is the conjunctiva that becomes red and irritated. It is also the membrane infected in cases of "red eye" (see page 274).

Behind these outer layers in the interior of the eye lies the pupil, the small black-looking aperture that allows light to enter. The size of the pupil and the amount of light that enters the eye are controlled by the surrounding iris, the colored part of the eye. It contains two small muscles plus pigment and blood vessels, and contracts or expands with exposure to light. In darkness, the iris muscles allow the pupil to become larger, so that more light can enter the eye. In bright light, the pupil becomes smaller to keep out an excess.

The color of your iris, like the color of your skin, depends upon hereditary factors that dictate the amount of pigment it contains. People with fair hair and skin usually have less pigment so that their eyes are usually gray, green, or blue. People with dark hair and dark skin usually have brown or nearly black eyes.

Behind the pupil sits the lens, a flexible, transparent structure about the size of a lentil that focuses light by changing its shape, a process termed accommodation. The lens is made of a clear protein substance that can, just like the white of an egg, become less flexible and less clear as we age. It is held in place behind the pupil by fine fibers called zonules, thin thread-like strands that pull to stretch the lens, change its shape, and connect in turn to a circular muscle structure called the ciliary body. The contractions and relaxations of the ciliary body plus the elasticity of the lens control focusing.

The structures of the eye in front of the lens are collectively termed the anterior chamber. This portion of the eye is filled with a watery fluid called the aqueous humor. It is a substance manufactured by the cells that cover a part of the ciliary body called ciliary processes. This fluid helps the anterior chamber keep its shape by maintaining just the right amount of pressure, much like a basketball or football keeps its shape by being filled with just the right amount of air.

Between the outer protective layer of the eye, the sclera, and the inner lining, the retina, is the choroid, a sheet of capillaries that nourish half of the retina and thereby contribute profoundly to the energy necessary for the sensation of sight.

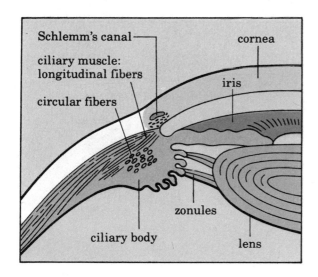

Schlemm's canal
ciliary muscle:
longitudinal fibers
circular fibers
cornea
iris
zonules
ciliary body
lens

THE ANTERIOR CHAMBER

An enlarged view of the anterior chamber of the eye shows the relationship of its structures. The iris rests on the lens, which, with the cornea, encloses the anterior chamber. The anterior chamber is filled with aqueous fluid. The lens is delicately suspended by fine ligaments called zonules attached to the ciliary body. The ciliary muscles, with both longitudinal and circular fibers, change the shape of the lens for focusing. Aqueous fluid drains from the eye via Schlemm's canal. Function of the canal is important in the eye diesase glaucoma.

The retina is the innermost lining of the eyeball, which, like film in a camera, lines the back of the eye and receives the image that the lens focuses on it. Unlike film, we do not roll it up and send it in for processing. Rather, it continuously functions by regenerating itself. Most important, and most miraculous, it transmits that image via cells called rods and cones through the optic nerve to the brain. Rods, scattered across the retina, pick up the impulses that are especially important in peripheral vision and in seeing light, shape, and movement. They also help us to see in dim light. By contrast, cones function to give us precise or central vision, the kind we need to thread a needle or read fine print. Although spread throughout the retina like the rods, the cones are especially concentrated, really packed like sardines, in one particular tiny area no larger than the head of a hat pin, at the macula, the center of the retina.

In addition to providing central vision, the cones are responsible for our perception of color. The process by which color is perceived is not fully understood. Basically, there appear to be three types of color receptors in the cones that respond to various wavelengths of light reflected by a colored object. These are changed into electrical impulses that result in color vision in the brain. Although color blindness, or, more accurately, a color vision deficiency, is relatively common (see page 256), no gross physical differences can be detected in the eyes of people who are color deficient.

The retina and its rods and cones, all located behind the lens, are collectively called the posterior segment of the eye. This segment is filled with a gelatinous fluid called the vitreous humor.

Ultimately, the nerve fibers that are spread densely throughout the retina collect at the optic disc or nervehead and form the optic nerve, a cord of more than one million individual nerve fibers that transmits the light patterns formed on the retinal screen to the visual centers of the brain. The eye is, in fact, connected to the brain in a relationship that no other part of the body enjoys.

Related Structures of the Eye

The eye is one of the most sensitive and delicate human organs, so it must be well protected against injury. A number of related structures help keep it in good operating order. The first line of defense is the bony orbit in which the eye rests. These tough surrounding skull bones enclose the eye completely except for the frontal openings. They also protrude somewhat at the eyebrow and cheek to deflect blows. In addition, a fatty layer of tissue within the socket cushions the eye and acts as a shock absorber.

Eyelids and eyelashes protect the eye, too. By closing, the eyelid covers the eye, protecting it from foreign bodies or exposure. This usually happens so quickly that we cannot control it. This instantaneous reaction is called the blink reflex. Eyelashes function as protective devices, too, blocking out larger intrusions such as raindrops or snowflakes. Long, lustrous lashes are not nature's devices for flirtation. They're actually a line of defense instead of attack.

The blink reflex protects the eye in another regular, automatic manner. It washes the eye every two to ten seconds by spreading tears across its sensitive surface. Lacrimal glands in the upper eyelid produce this salty, lubricating, and bacteria-killing substance which is vital to the eyeball. Without tears, the cornea

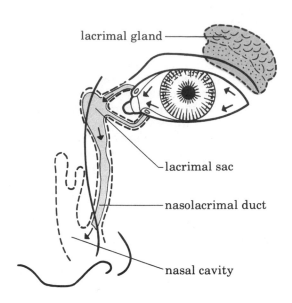

THE LACRIMAL SYSTEM

Tears produced constantly by the lacrimal and other glands in the upper part of the eye socket flow over the front of the eye to lubricate it. They collect in the lacrimal sac at the inner corner of the eye and drain through the nasolacrimal duct into the nose. That is why the nose runs when a person cries.

would dry, become irritated and inflamed, and the eye would be destroyed. We get a dripping nose when we cry because excess tears are fed into the nose via the usual drainage mechanism from the inner corner of each eye through tiny tubes called lacrimal ducts, and the rest are discharged over the lids as tears.

Movement of each eye is controlled by three pairs of muscles that shift the eye vertically, horizontally, and diagonally in a coordinated fashion. It is because our eye muscles function in tandem that the eyes can focus on the same object at the same time—one of the critical factors in developing depth perception. Because there is a distance between the two eyes, the images we see fall on two very slightly different corresponding points in the two retinas. This slight difference—within a small tolerance—produces an important stimulus throughout the entire nerve connection from the eye to the occipital lobe in the brain. When those images are integrated by the brain, we are able to interpret depth perception, or stereopsis. People who have lost vision in one eye or whose eye muscles do not function in tandem lack this perception.

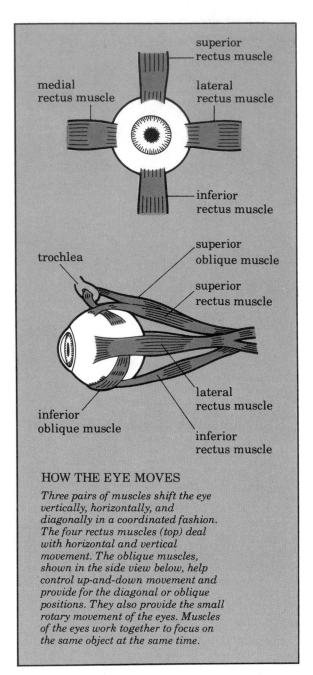

HOW THE EYE MOVES

Three pairs of muscles shift the eye vertically, horizontally, and diagonally in a coordinated fashion. The four rectus muscles (top) deal with horizontal and vertical movement. The oblique muscles, shown in the side view below, help control up-and-down movement and provide for the diagonal or oblique positions. They also provide the small rotary movement of the eyes. Muscles of the eyes work together to focus on the same object at the same time.

The Physiology of Vision

How we see—the physiology of vision—is something science cannot fully explain. We do not know exactly how light impulses are changed into a visual image in the brain. We do know, however, that the eye structures bring an image into focus on the retina, convert the energy of light into nerve impulses, and transmit these electric currents over the optic nerve to the back of the brain, then forward to other parts of the brain. It is with the brain, not the eyes, that we "see."

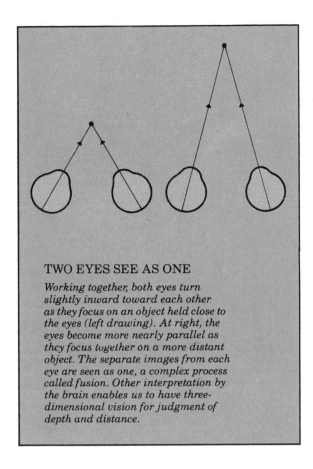

TWO EYES SEE AS ONE

Working together, both eyes turn slightly inward toward each other as they focus on an object held close to the eyes (left drawing). At right, the eyes become more nearly parallel as they focus together on a more distant object. The separate images from each eye are seen as one, a complex process called fusion. Other interpretation by the brain enables us to have three-dimensional vision for judgment of depth and distance.

The process of seeing begins the moment light strikes the outer surface of the eye, because the curved cornea, a convex lens, starts the focusing process by bending light rays inward. The lens does the fine focusing work, becoming thicker to bring objects near us in focus and stretching thinner when we need to focus on objects farther away. Simultaneously but independently, the iris adjusts the size of the pupil and admits as much light as is appropriate for optimal vision. This light-admitting and focusing machinery directs light impulses to the retina's light-sensitive nerve endings, the rods and cones. These cells connect with others, the final connection in the eye becoming the visual fiber layer which coalesces into the optic nerve.

We do not know what happens in the visual cortex of the brain to change what was light and is now electrical impulse to the visual imagery we call sight. We do know how the nerve connections are established. The visual image in the eye is converted by the optical mechanism to one which is initially upside down. The optic nerve from each eye meets in the optic chiasm where about half of the fibers from one eye cross to the other side allowing representation from the inner half of each retina to cross to the opposite side of the brain.

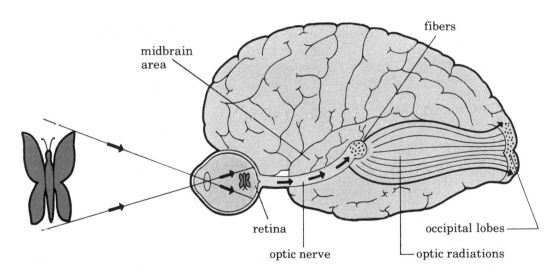

HOW THE BRAIN "SEES"

The nerve pathways of vision in the brain are shown in cross section. Rays of light falling as the inverted image of a butterfly on the retina excite nerve impulses in the rods and cones of the retina. Nerve impulses follow the *pathways of arrows in the optic nerve to the midbrain area and in fibers called optic radiations that make intricate connections in the occipital lobes in the back of the brain.*

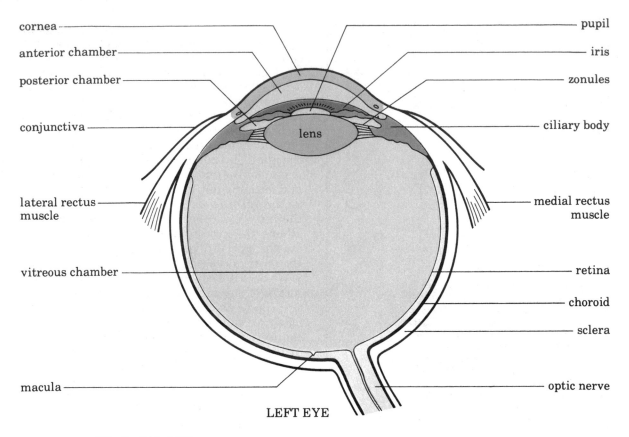

cornea

anterior chamber

posterior chamber

conjunctiva

lateral rectus muscle

vitreous chamber

macula

pupil

iris

zonules

ciliary body

lens

medial rectus muscle

retina

choroid

sclera

optic nerve

LEFT EYE

THE TOTAL EYE

The eye and some related structures are shown in this cutaway diagram. The organ itself rests in a protective socket in the skull called the orbit and its movement is controlled by three pairs of muscles.

THE EYE AND THE BRAIN

This drawing of the underside of the brain shows how nerve impulses from either eye travel along the optic nerve and partially "cross over" at the optic chiasm. Impulses from the inner half of each retina cross over to the opposite side of the brain, as traced by the arrows, while impulses from the other half of the retina do not. Collective impulses arrive at the midbrain junctions on either side of the brain and travel over fibers that collect in the occipital lobe.

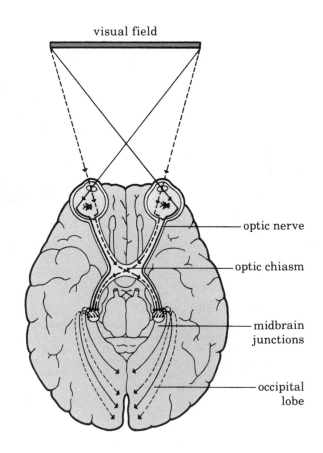

visual field

optic nerve

optic chiasm

midbrain junctions

occipital lobe

CARE OF THE EYES

Several different specialists provide eye care in the United States, and many of us frequently are confused by their titles as well as whose services we need at a particular time.

The Eye Care Professionals

An ophthalmologist is a physician who specializes in medical and surgical care of the eye and the structures surrounding it. As a rule of thumb, he or she is the professional most qualified by training to advise you on most eye problems. (If you need eye care and do not know an ophthalmologist, you usually can obtain a name from your local medical society or from the American Academy of Ophthalmology, Box 7424, San Francisco, CA 94120.)

A board-certified ophthalmologist is the product of a college or a university undergraduate program plus four years of medical school. After a year of broad medical training as an intern, he or she obtains an additional three to five years of specific training in an ophthalmology residency program and often has one or more years of additional subspecialty training. These eight to twelve years of medical education after college prepare him or her to handle the evaluation, diagnosis, and treatment of eye problems and disorders related to the surrounding structures of the eye as well as their central connections to the brain.

Subspecialists have additional, highly specialized years of training. Pediatric ophthalmology, the cornea, the retina, neuro-ophthalmology, and plastic and reconstructive surgery of the eye are some of the ophthalmic subspecialty areas.

An ophthalmologist determines whether a person needs glasses. Beyond that, he or she can treat both medical and surgical problems relating to the eye. Being both a medical and surgical physician is an unusual quality in these days of technical medicine. An ophthalmologist is the only eye care provider who holds an M.D. degree.

An optometrist, after two to four years in college, adds four years of specialized education before practicing. The degree is an O.D., doctor of optometry. Optometrists are primarily prepared to examine the eyes, prescribe glasses, and screen for eye disease. They also are trained to perform other diagnostic techniques such as testing visual fields, color vision, and the movement of the eye. Optometrists possess some of the same skills as ophthalmologists, but they are not trained to diagnose or medically treat eye disease, nor can they perform surgery.

Opticians are trained to make eyeglasses from a prescription written by an ophthalmologist or an optometrist. In addition to understanding optics, they can translate the prescription into spectacles or contact lenses for the patient. In many states, opticians are licensed to fit contact lenses.

An ocularist has two years of supervised education and up to five years of additional training in learning to fabricate and manufacture false eyes (prostheses). These "glass eyes" (a misnomer today, because most are made of plastic) are needed when a person loses an eye and substitutes an artificial one for cosmetic purposes.

Other care providers include a variety of ophthalmic and optometric technicians or technologists with specific training who help the ophthalmologist or optometrist. They may test visual acuity, perform the initial tests for refraction and ocular motility, and execute diagnostic tests such as visual fields, ultrasonography, or electrophysiology. In a few instances, they assist in fabricating or fitting contact lenses.

Eye Examinations

Contrary to common opinion, most people *do not* need an eye examination once a year. No annual checkup prevents ocular disease, although timely visits to an ophthalmologist or optometrist will usually detect eye problems before they become severe.

A child should be given a routine screening examination at the age of six months and again by the time he or she is three or four. Screening exams are important, because it can be difficult for a parent to recognize that a child has visual problems. Your child's eyes should be tested again around the age of 10 unless school screening tests reveal a special difficulty or specific problems appear earlier, such as crossed eyes, pupils that appear white, or eyes that are unequal in size.

Because the eyes, like the rest of the body, often have a growth spurt during puberty, teenagers should have their eyes tested every two to four years. Then, unless a person experiences unusual or recurring difficulty, he or she probably does not need another eye examination until about age 40, when most of us develop the need for reading glasses. After the age of 55, we all should seek eye examinations every two to three years unless we experience eye problems. Obviously, a person will require more frequent visits if he has a history of ocular disease, a family history of glaucoma, difficulty seeing from one or both eyes, or a general systemic disease such as diabetes, which can result in eye problems.

Here is what is usually included in an initial comprehensive eye examination:

In the first phase, the eye specialist asks your "eye history"—family problems, general medical problems, medications, history of eye problems, eye injuries, glasses. This is highly important in any medical evaluation, for your eyes or for your health in general, and you can improve the quality of your exam by providing as much information as possible.

Then, the eye specialist will test your vision with and without glasses, test each eye separately, and test both together. The test is usually done at a distance of 20 feet or with mirrors to create the effect of a 20-foot examination. It is a distance that, for technical purposes, has been chosen arbitrarily to record visual function. The distance of 20 feet helps define a vision rating. "Normal" vision is 20/20, which means that a person can see at 20 feet what other "normal" people with "normal" vision can see at 20 feet. However, many people see better than 20/20.

The most common method of measuring vision is the familiar Snellen chart, which tests the ability to distinguish letters of the alphabet in different sizes or numbers or the capital letter E. The chart that uses only the letter E allows testing of preschool children or others who are not able to identify accurately all alphabetical letters or numbers. They can simply indicate which direction the prongs of each "E" face to have their visual acuity measured.

The eye specialist will then look at the external appearance of your eyes, including the eyelids and their linings, the tear ducts, the color and structure of the iris, the number and location of blood vessels in the white part of the eye. He or she also will check movement.

A refraction, which is testing the eyes for glasses, is done either by putting special frames on your nose or by using a phoropter. The patient sits behind this large machine, which allows the examiner to test vision with a variety of glass lenses. These determine which modifications will help you see best.

Next, the eye specialist or a technician will test for muscle balance to make certain that the eyes work together. In this test you must look at targets. By covering and uncovering your eyes as well as using a polarized lens, the doctor determines how well your eyes can fix on the same target and the accuracy of your depth perception, or stereopsis.

A test for color vision might be part of the examination. In this test, you probably will look through a binocular sighting device or directly at a series of pseudo-isochromatic color plates. Here dots of primary colors are printed on a background of similar dots in a confusion of colors. A person who cannot readily recognize a simple pattern, such as a number, in these dots is usually judged to have a color deficiency, or congenital inability to distinguish certain shades of green from shades of red. About eight percent of American males and one-half percent of females are "color-blind" in mild to moderate degree. This deficiency, however, is seldom a handicap.

Next may come a test for clarity of cornea and lens. This test uses a slit lamp, or biomicroscope, that magnifies the front portions of your eye up to 20 times or more. Using the slit lamp, the examiner can observe variations in these structures, which can indicate the presence of eye disorders.

An applanation tonometer attached to the slit lamp allows pressure within the eyes to be measured. Other devices, such as the air puff tonometer or a plunger mechanism called the Schiotz tonometer, are used for screening tests, but the applanation tonometer is the most accurate. Measuring intraocular pressure, a most important test, is relatively simple and painless. It is the most common and reliable means to check for the presence of glaucoma (see page 264), a leading cause of blindness in the United States and a disease that can be prevented if caught in early stages.

The eye specialist then dilates the pupils by using drops in order to see the back of the eye (the retina). This examination is performed with an instrument called an ophthalmoscope. The examination includes the area of highest resolution directly in the back of the eye, and the retinal periphery, the sides where infections and tumors occur.

At the end of a routine examination your doctor might prescribe eyeglasses. This is usually done to correct the four most common vi-

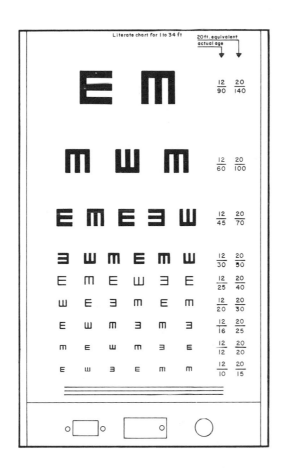

Literate chart for 1 to 34 ft

20 ft. equivalent
actual age

$\frac{12}{90}$	$\frac{20}{140}$
$\frac{12}{60}$	$\frac{20}{100}$
$\frac{12}{45}$	$\frac{20}{70}$
$\frac{12}{30}$	$\frac{20}{50}$
$\frac{12}{25}$	$\frac{20}{40}$
$\frac{12}{20}$	$\frac{20}{30}$
$\frac{12}{16}$	$\frac{20}{25}$
$\frac{12}{12}$	$\frac{20}{20}$
$\frac{12}{10}$	$\frac{20}{15}$

THE BIG E

The Snellen eye chart is the most common method of measuring vision. This version, using only the capital letter E, allows the eye specialist to test preschool children or others who are not able to recognize all letters of the alphabet. Variations of this chart use all letters or numbers. The figures at the right represent distances based on a 20-foot scale.

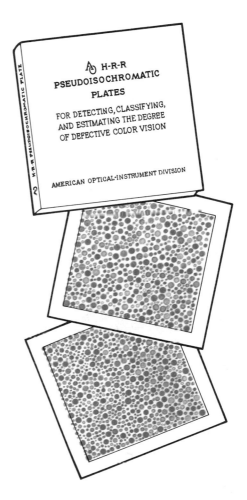

sual problems: nearsightedness (myopia), farsightedness (hyperopia), astigmatism, and presbyopia.

If you are nearsighted, you probably have an eye somewhat longer than normal from front to back (lens to retina). You can see to read very well but objects in the distance are blurred without glasses. Nearsightedness is common and readily corrected by wearing glasses or contact lenses.

If you are farsighted, your eyes are shorter than normal. You generally can see things well at a distance and nearby until you approach age 40, when you may need glasses to read.

A third common condition, astigmatism, occurs when the front part of the eye, the cornea, is not perfectly round as a basketball might be, but more curved in one direction than the other as a football might be. The eye bends the light rays as they enter and that distorts the images. To help someone with astigmatism see properly, opticians will grind cylinders into the lenses of glasses according to the prescription written by an ophthalmologist or optometrist. It is not uncommon to be both nearsighted or farsighted and astigmatic.

TESTING COLOR VISION

Colored plates like these help determine a person's ability to perceive color. Persons with normal color vision will see the geometric shapes. Those with a color deficiency will see a different shape or none at all. Mild to moderate color deficiency is seldom a handicap.

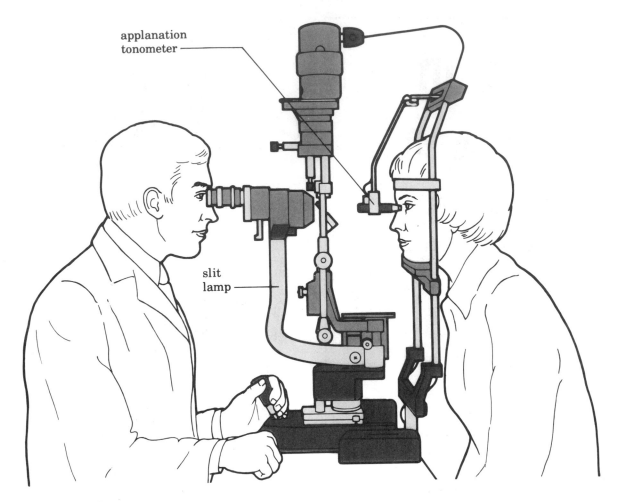

applanation tonometer

slit lamp

EYE EXAMINATION

Among the sophisticated instruments used during eye examinations is the applanation tonometer, which measures the pressure inside the eye. It is attached to the slit lamp, which enables the doctor to look into the front and back of the eye, and, with special attachments, to examine the retina. Measuring eye pressure is important in the detection of glaucoma, a leading cause of blindness.

Glasses and Contact Lenses

Most people wear spectacles to correct vision problems, but contact lenses are becoming increasingly popular. This is partly because many people who need visual correction believe they are more attractive without glasses. But the reasons are not only cosmetic. In cases of profound myopia, contact lenses correct vision better than standard lenses.

There are two types of contact lenses. Hard contact lenses are made of a hard plastic and are, in a sense, a miniature pair of glasses except that they rest directly on the cornea of the eye rather than on the bridge of the nose. Soft contact lenses are made of a slightly different plastic material that has a high water content, which allows them to conform closely to the shape of the eye. Soft contact lenses were developed because some persons found hard lenses irritating. Soft lenses are larger and more malleable than hard lenses, and in some cases can be worn for longer periods. Many athletes wear contact lenses that are larger than the usual cosmetic lens, covering enough of the eye's surface to fit under the eyelid. The lid then acts as a harness, holding the contact in place.

Low vision aids are a third type of optical device used by those with substantially lower than normal vision. These are magnifiers or specially constructed high-power lenses and telescopes. They help in cases of macular degeneration in older persons or in pathologic conditions that reduce vision markedly.

NEARSIGHTEDNESS

In myopia (nearsightedness) the image of an object, unless it is held close to the eyes, falls in front of the retina instead of upon it (top drawing), and the object is seen indistinctly. A concave lens of proper curvature corrects the condition by bringing the object into focus on the retina, as shown in bottom drawing.

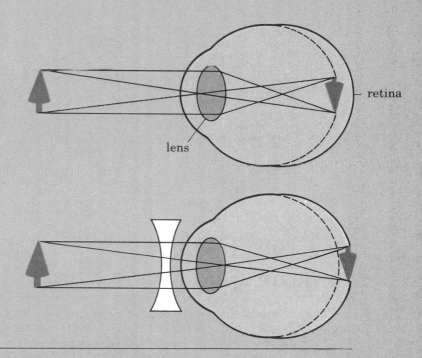

FARSIGHTEDNESS

In hyperopia (farsightedness) the image of an object is focused behind the retina of an eyeball that is too short for the focusing mechanism (top drawing). A convex lens brings the light rays into focus on the retina, as shown at bottom. Farsighted persons may be able to see things sharply by thickening the lens of the eye, a process called accommodation. However, this involuntary effort involves inner muscles of the eye and causes eye fatigue if the hyperopia is of sufficient magnitude.

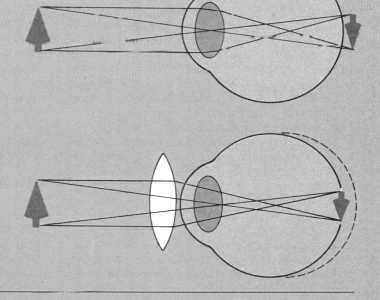

ASTIGMATISM

The result of irregular curvature of the cornea, astigmatism is comparable to the distortion produced by a wavy pane of glass. The drawing shows light rays 3 and 4 in sharp focus on the retina, with light rays 1 and 2 focused in front of the retina. The result is a blurred image, where the horizontal line is in focus and the vertical line out of focus. A cylindrical lens in the proper axis brings the light rays into even focus and corrects astigmatism.

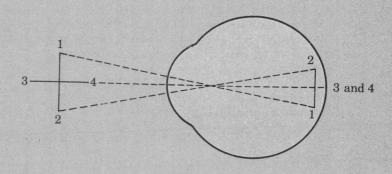

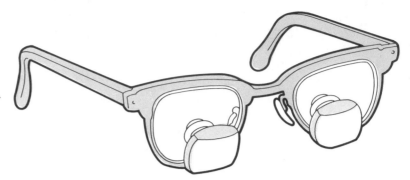

Special visual aids are useful for persons with low-vision handicaps or for the working comfort of people with normal vision. The drawing shows a type of magnifying binocular spectacles that permit convenient magnification in such occupations as dentistry, surgery, and on assembly lines where minute pieces are used.

HOW THE EYES GROW, DEVELOP, AND AGE

The eyes are probably a baby's most mature organ at birth. They are approximately five-sixths the size of an adult eye and will develop faster than any other part of the body. Although it is obviously impossible to test an infant's vision in the way we test adults, pediatric ophthalmologists using special tests estimate that the normal visual resolution ability of a newborn is somewhere between 20/30 and 20/70. Not a bad starting skill for a beginner! Of course, the baby has not learned to interpret what is "seen."

By the age of three months a baby can see light and shadow, distinguish color, focus on objects near and far away, even put together the sophisticated visual signals that distinguish Mother from any other woman in the room. The child usually develops normal visual acuity between the ages of three and five. By the time he or she reaches school age, a child with normal vision has nearly reached full visual potential.

Like the rest of the body, the eyes change during puberty, reaching maturity before the rest of the body. Just as they experience a spurt in the growth of their bones, many adolescents experience a growth of their eyes as well. The eyes of a young person who previously had no visual problems may grow too large and thus too long—longer, that is, than the lens can accommodate to focus properly. Then, for the first time, a young person needs glasses to correct nearsightedness.

But just as they are one of the first organs to mature, our eyes are one of the first to age. We can measure objectively the effects of aging. As the eyes and their owner grow older, the lens begins to lose its elasticity. Our ability to see nearby and distant objects clearly requires that the lens, the focusing mechanism at the front of the eye, make adjustments. These adjustments are made automatically and are a focusing process that many automatic focusing cameras imitate incredibly well. The circular muscle called the ciliary body contracts and relaxes to help the lens change shape. Unfortunately, however, as the protein of the lens progressively hardens, by about age 40, ciliary muscles working through the zonules (see page 250) can no longer compress or stretch the lens enough to change focus from distance to near. The condition progresses throughout life, although it reaches a functional maximum at about age 55. The need for progressively stronger bifocals reaches its maximum about that time.

EYE PROBLEMS DECADE BY DECADE

Because the eyes develop in a chronological fashion, problems of the eye tend to follow a chronological pattern, too. Occasionally, for instance, a baby is born with cataracts, but cataracts are primarily a problem of later years. Similarly, the need for bifocals usually becomes apparent in middle age. Eye problems usually can be categorized according to the decades in which they commonly occur.

Problems of Childhood

Most babies are born with normal eye function, but it is important for a pediatrician to evaluate the infant's eyes at birth. The examination should check the clarity of the cornea, inspect the vascular structure (blood supply) of the optic nerve head, and test for muscular paralysis. The doctor should check for a variety of other problems that are either congenital (present at birth) or inherited (passed down genetically from one or both parents, but not always immediately apparent). These conditions can include cataract (clouding of the lens), glaucoma (abnormal fluid pressure within the eye), ptosis (droopy eyelid), and strabismus.

Strabismus is by far the most common problem of the early years. It affects 3 to 5 percent of newborn children. In strabismus, the eyes fail to work together to focus on a single object. Just as two horses hitched to a wagon must learn to pull in the same direction, a baby's eyes and brain must develop the ability to work as a team.

In strabismus, one eye deviates in or out from the line of focus while the other looks directly at the object. Dissimilar information thus comes from the two eyes. A baby looking out from his or her crib may see parents in one eye and a rattle in the other— a confusing and disturbing message for the brain to sort out.

The brain is an amazingly resilient organ, but when it receives separate and confusing images it is forced to make a choice. It must decide to see either the parents or the rattle, selecting one and ignoring the other. In time, a "preferred" eye is established because the brain tends to disregard information transmitted by the deviated one. Sometimes the eyes alternate, so that first one is used, then the other. If the eyes cross, one usually becomes preferred. If the condition is allowed to persist, the visual potential, the brain's ability to process information coming from the "weak" eye, is lost, and that eye may never become a completely functional organ. Untreated strabismus frequently results in amblyopia, or reduced vision.

There are two types of strabismus that lead to reduced vision. The most common is esotropia, or crossed eyes. A hereditary factor is involved, but it is not the usual hereditary pat-

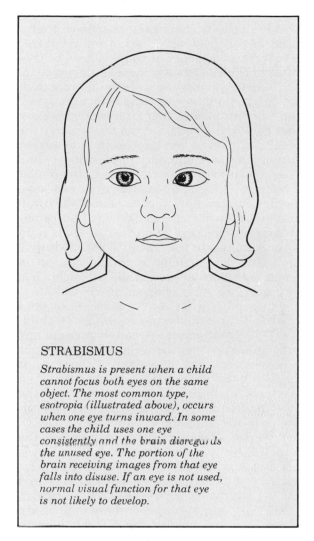

STRABISMUS

Strabismus is present when a child cannot focus both eyes on the same object. The most common type, esotropia (illustrated above), occurs when one eye turns inward. In some cases the child uses one eye consistently and the brain disregards the unused eye. The portion of the brain receiving images from that eye falls into disuse. If an eye is not used, normal visual function for that eye is not likely to develop.

tern and therefore not absolutely predictable. Esotropia is usually noticeable to parents during the early months of life.

Exotropia, the outward deviation of one eye, might not be noticed until a child is six or seven. Surgery will then be necessary to readjust the eye muscles. Good vision usually is retained in each eye in exotropia.

Ptosis, or droopy eyelid, also causes reduced vision if it droops completely, because the information from one eye is suppressed in the brain and visual potential does not develop.

Many pediatricians used to believe that a child would "grow out of" strabismus, but this is an erroneous belief. If you seriously believe that your child shows the eye deviation of strabismus, you should have an ophthalmologist examine your child before the age of three or four months. Some physicians believe that the earlier the treatment, the better the results. Glasses (even bifocals in some cases), surgery, or a combination of surgery and glasses can help align the eyes in the proper direction. Once aligned, the eyes can send similar information to each side of the brain and binocular vision can develop. Laboratory studies on monkeys and other animals indicate that if early treatment is not instituted, binocular development is unlikely to occur. Some say binocular vision must be established by one or two years of age or it will be lost.

Retinoblastoma is a far more serious but relatively uncommon eye disorder of childhood. This malignant eye cancer appears any time from a few months of age to seven or eight years. In one-third to one-half of the cases, it appears to be inherited. Symptoms are often minimal. A white pupil or a crossed eye are the most noticeable early signs. Generally, children will not complain of pain.

When this disease occurs in only one eye, the afflicted eye is usually removed. If both eyes are attacked, the most seriously affected is removed and its mate is treated by radiation and chemotherapy. As with other types of cancer, the disease may spread elsewhere in the body. However, if retinoblastoma is caught early, treatment may be successful.

Tearing is a common and disturbing disorder in infants, although not generally a sight-threatening problem. Tear ducts drain through a connection into the nose, the nasolacrimal duct, which in an infant is a very small passageway. Not infrequently, the duct does not function properly for weeks or even months after birth, so that the eyes stream steadily. Usually the duct will open spontaneously, but if tearing in one or both eyes persists, and it is obvious that the tear drainage mechanism is faulty, an ophthalmologist should be consulted. By a simple and relatively pain-free probe of the duct, he can open the faulty membrane, which permanently solves the problem in almost every case.

Although most eye problems of childhood are apparent to fathers and mothers, it is important for a child to have an ophthalmological examination before he or she begins school.

This will help disclose whether the eyes can perform the visual tasks critical to reading and other schoolwork. Young eyes cannot always be successfully tested much before that time because many subjective tests require the child to be able to recognize and identify letters of the alphabet. However, any parent with questions about a child's vision should not wait for this examination. Abnormal vision usually can be treated successfully if it is recognized promptly.

The need for visual correction often shows up at this time. It is not always possible for a parent to recognize that a child has seeing problems until schoolwork begins. A school screening examination and an ophthalmologist's examination will disclose nearsightedness, farsightedness, or astigmatism. Glasses should then be prescribed as soon as possible and the parent should see that the child wears them.

Problems of the Teens

Eye injury is the major problem between the ages of 10 and 20. Historically, boys have suffered more eye injuries than girls, but that may change as girls join Little League baseball, soccer, and other athletic activities and expose themselves to other accident risks of childhood. Major penetrating injuries from darts, pencils, air rifles, or sharp sticks require immediate and sophisticated surgical repair. It is amazing what severe injuries can be treated successfully with modern techniques. Yet, because of the delicate nature of the eye, even minimal injuries sometimes have disastrous outcomes. The result depends primarily on the severity and location of the injury.

The bulk of eye injuries, fortunately, can be treated successfully. Treatments cover a spectrum of medical and surgical techniques. A cut can often be stitched with tiny sutures and the eye covered with a patch until it heals. Antibiotic drops prevent infection and damage. Modern developments in instrumentation save many injured eyes that formerly would have been lost.

In rare cases an eye cannot be saved and must be removed. The procedure sounds horrible, but surgically it is not difficult. A ball of plastic or similar material is placed where the eye was and the patient is fitted with a prosthesis by a well-trained ocularist. The surgeon may affix the plastic globe or ball to the muscles of the eye, or may simply place it in the orbit. The plastic eye, which is like a large and thick contact lens, then moves much as the normal eye does, pushed and pulled by the eye muscles and the surrounding tissue. Because a good ocularist usually can duplicate a patient's natural eye, the cosmetic outcome is generally excellent, and most people learn to function almost normally with one eye.

Adults who have lost an eye complain at first of their "blind" side or are annoyed by loss of depth perception. One patient complained that the most difficult problem was to relearn how to pour coffee accurately. But with time and patience, most people adapt and lead relatively normal lives. Instead of binocular or normal depth perception, they learn to function with monocular (one eye) cues to judge the relative distance of objects.

"Pink eye" or conjunctivitis (inflammation of the conjunctiva) is a common though minor problem of the teen years (as well as before and after). Pink eye occurs when blood vessels in the eye become congested or engorged, giving the white of the eye a pinkish hue. The condition can result from an injury, or because the eye is rubbed too vigorously, but most commonly the cause is an upper respiratory infection that spreads to the eye. It is most often caused by a virus. Virus pink eye usually resolves itself within several weeks and does not necessarily require medical treatment. On the other hand, bacterial infections are usually accompanied by more purulent pus-like discharge and crusting and should be medically treated. They respond rapidly to an antibiotic, while a viral conjunctivitis does not. And a viral conjunctivitis, in contrast to one of bacterial origin, has an associated swelling and tenderness of the lymph node in front of the ear on the affected side.

Styes, a frequent and annoying disorder, are localized red spots or swellings that develop near the lid margin of the eye. They are analogous to boils of the skin. Styes are little abscesses of bacteria (usually a staphylococcus infection) in the glands of the lid margins. They sometimes drain spontaneously, as other abscesses do, but may require an ophthalmologist to open them.

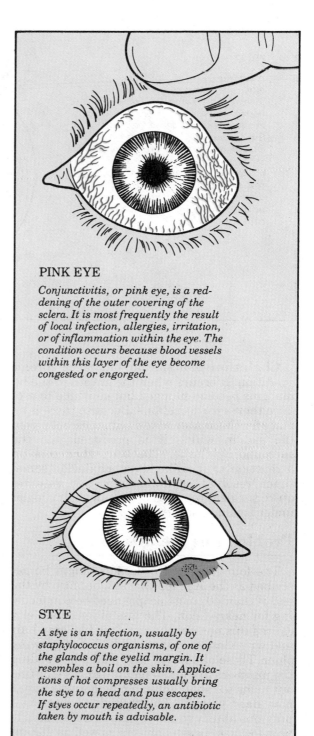

PINK EYE

Conjunctivitis, or pink eye, is a reddening of the outer covering of the sclera. It is most frequently the result of local infection, allergies, irritation, or of inflammation within the eye. The condition occurs because blood vessels within this layer of the eye become congested or engorged.

STYE

A stye is an infection, usually by staphylococcus organisms, of one of the glands of the eyelid margin. It resembles a boil on the skin. Applications of hot compresses usually bring the stye to a head and pus escapes. If styes occur repeatedly, an antibiotic taken by mouth is advisable.

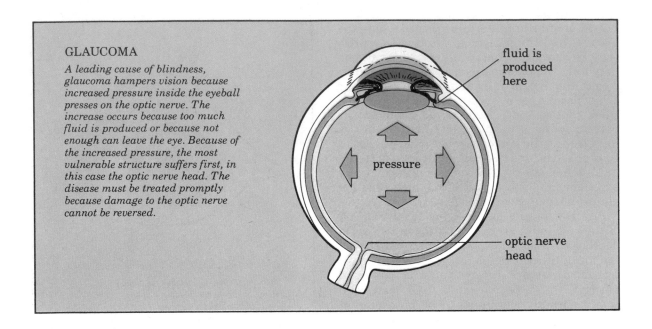

GLAUCOMA

A leading cause of blindness, glaucoma hampers vision because increased pressure inside the eyeball presses on the optic nerve. The increase occurs because too much fluid is produced or because not enough can leave the eye. Because of the increased pressure, the most vulnerable structure suffers first, in this case the optic nerve head. The disease must be treated promptly because damage to the optic nerve cannot be reversed.

fluid is produced here

pressure

optic nerve head

Chalazion is a similar but more chronic condition. It occurs when the glands in the lid margins become plugged but continue to produce their own secretions. Because there is no place for this material to drain, it escapes from the sac in which it is produced into the surrounding tissue. The body then sets up a reaction to it. Like styes, chalazion sometimes resolves spontaneously, but may require surgical removal by an ophthalmologist under local anesthetic.

Problems of the 30s and 40s

The fourth and fifth decades might be described as the Age for Glasses, because by the end of their 40s most people need help in focusing for near vision. The loss of lens elasticity causes this normal change. It is like grey hair and wrinkles, an unavoidable fact of growing older. Those of us who have difficulty reading the numbers in the telephone directory, or find our arms too short to scan the morning paper, now need glasses. The farsighted lose their previous ability to see objects at a distance. To help focus on nearby objects as well as distant ones, some need bifocals, which are glasses divided into focal lengths for both close and dis-

tant vision. Some are fortunate and need only minimal correction for distance or simply require reading glasses which they can purchase at a drug or department store. (It is advisable to have an eye exam before seeking such help.) Finally, there are those who see life with a slight to severe blur, apparently preferring vanity to clarity. For them, we can only hope that what they don't see won't hurt them.

Glaucoma also becomes more common during the 30s and 40s, although it can occur at any age. Glaucoma is the result of increased fluid pressure inside the eye that presses on and damages the optic nerve, causing a loss of vision. The increased pressure may be caused by an abnormal production of fluid, by an inability of a normal amount of fluid to leave the eye (the result of a blocked or faulty drainage system), or by secondary reactions to other eye problems or injuries.

Chronic glaucoma, also known as simple or open-angle glaucoma, is the most common and vexing form of the disease. Usually, it is a painless, progressive disease that can result in blindness if not treated. Many persons notice no symptoms until some vision has been lost. To treat it, an ophthalmologist must reduce the pressure. The doctor can prescribe a variety of eye drops, including Pilocarpine,® which improves the outflow of fluid from the eye, epinephrine compounds, which decrease the production of eye fluid, and Timolol,® which appears to do both. Certain pills also may be prescribed to reduce the production of fluid.

CORNEAL ULCERS

There are several types of corneal ulcers, but by far the most common is dendritic ulcer, shown in the top drawing. It results from infection by the herpes simplex virus, which also causes cold sores. The lower drawings show different stages of bacterial ulcer erosion. Top to bottom: Invasion of the superficial layer of the cornea; then of deeper layers of the cornea, and finally perforation. Corneal transplant, the most successful of transplant operations, is necessary to restore useful vision in severe cases of corneal scarring.

DENDRITIC ULCER

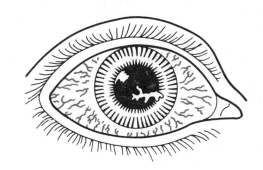

BACTERIAL ULCER

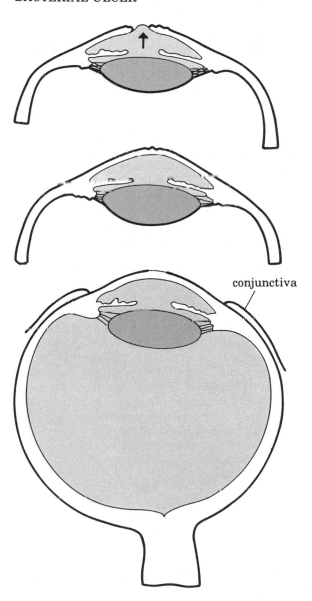

conjunctiva

Sometimes the combination of drops and pills is unsuccessful in controlling the pressure and surgery is required. Surgery is generally successful in lowering the pressure and stopping the disease. It is important to note, however, that when loss of visual field occurs as a result of glaucoma, it is a permanent loss and cannot be improved. That is why early screening for glaucoma is important.

Fortunately, chronic glaucoma can be treated if it is detected early. Prevention means simply taking a screening test to measure the intraocular pressure in the course of a regular eye exam. Because glaucoma appears to be hereditary, people with a family history should have the intraocular pressure and sometimes even their peripheral visual field measured regularly and routinely. Measuring the peripheral field (how well we see objects to the side of the main line of vision) is a critical way to check the presence of the disorder. Elevated pressure inside the eye appears to disrupt the normal flow of blood to peripheral areas of the retina and optic nerve. If this pressure remains high, the peripheral visual field is affected first, but because we generally notice only what we look at directly, we seldom are aware of peripheral visual loss.

Closed-angle glaucoma, also known as acute glaucoma, a less common form, is often an episodic event producing halos in the vision and causing eye pain. It is thus more readily noticed. It can be cured with an operation called an iridectomy. The ophthalmologist removes a small piece of the iris, and that allows the aqueous humor, the fluid trapped in the front part of the eye, to drain. This usually restores normal eye pressure.

Secondary glaucoma occurs with inflammations, infections, or injury within the eyeball. Treatment of the underlying disorder generally improves the "secondary" glaucoma.

An ophthalmologist will diagnose glaucoma if he finds pressure, optic nerve damage, and visual field loss. All are considered necessary to make the diagnosis. Doctors used to believe that high pressure alone in the eye was an indication of the disorder, but we know now that certain people can have relatively high pressures in their eye and not have glaucoma or visual field loss.

Corneal diseases also appear in the 30s and 40s, although sometimes they do not occur until the 50s or later. Deteriorating or degenerating corneal tissue is the cause.

Herpes simplex keratitis is the most common corneal disease. Although there are a multitude of other infections, it accounts for 90 percent of corneal diseases. The cause is the same virus that produces cold sores and, like cold sores, corneal infections tend to recur once the virus has become established. Herpes simplex keratitis is not painful. In fact, the sensation of pain on the normally sensitive cornea is greatly reduced. The infection's particular danger is that it can erode the cornea and produce dense scars that impair vision. Ophthalmologists usually prescribe eye drops to treat the disease, or they may scrape the cornea and patch the eye. Severe corneal disease may require corneal transplant surgery.

The cornea is a clear structure that has no blood vessels of its own. When it becomes cloudy, light cannot transfer images to the retina as it does in normal vision. In performing a transplant, the surgeon removes part of the diseased cornea and replaces it with a segment of cornea from a donor, usually a person who has bequeathed his eyes for this purpose. The new section is then sutured into place with strands much finer than human hair. Although this procedure is technically difficult, it has become the most successful of all transplant operations. The outcome in most cases is excellent, with sight often restored to normal or near normal.

Retinitis pigmentosa may show itself during the teens, but is more common in the middle years. A layer of the eye, the retinal pigment epithelium containing the rods and cones, begins to degenerate. The process starts at the periphery of the retina and gradually moves toward the macula in the center. People with this condition suffer from marked loss of night vision and narrowing of the visual field, so they are sometimes said to have "gun-barrel vision." Retinitis pigmentosa, like many eye disorders, is frequently hereditary. It is painless, generally progressive, and can result in near blindness, or at least marked narrowing of the visual field, similar to that of advanced glaucoma. But despite its severity, we know little about how to halt or cure it.

Malignant melanoma, usually thought of as a skin cancer, is the most common cancerous eye tumor of adult life. It attacks the pigmented layers of the eye, the choroid and iris. Depending on its location, a melanoma may grow to fairly large size without affecting vision. If the cancer is in the choroid, the eye is often removed, but the outlook is much more favorable than with melanomas of the skin.

Clouding of the vitreous, the semi-liquid, gel-like substance in the central portion of the eye, also can damage vision, especially in later life. The darkening or clouding usually is caused by blood leaking into the eye from hemorrhages on the retina. The hemorrhages result from diabetes or from a direct blow or puncture would to the eye. The blood or tissue blocks vision by preventing light from passing unobstructed to the retina.

A remarkable new procedure, vitrectomy, is now used to clear the patient's vision. Using extremely fine instruments, the ophthalmologist makes an incision through the sclera, the tough outer covering of the eyeball, and removes the vitreous humor from the eye, replacing it with liquid, such as a saline solution. Many persons whose vision was severely limited have had significant improvement after such an operation. In a similarly delicate operation, the ophthalmologist may also sever pre-retinal membranes that grow spontaneously, grind them with a precise instrument, and remove them from the eye by suction.

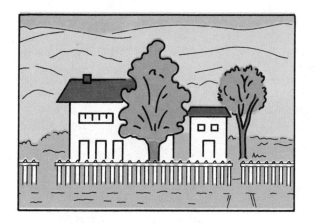 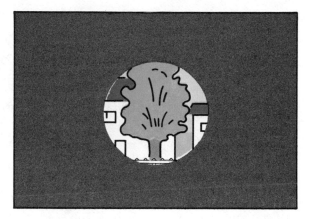

GUN-BARREL VISION

Persons whose vision is impaired by retinitis pigmentosa suffer from a narrowing of the visual field, as if they were looking through a gun barrel. A person with normal vision would perceive the scene on the left. One with retinitis pigmentosa eventually loses *peripheral vision and sees only a small portion of the scene, as shown at right. Similar impairment of the visual field may occur in advanced stages of glaucoma, although in each case it is unlikely that the remaining visual field would be perfectly round.*

The Later Decades

Cataract is the most common eye problem that strikes men and women in their 50s, 60s, 70s, and 80s. Cataracts occur when the normally clear lens becomes cloudy. This is a perfectly natural biochemical phenomenon, as our analogy to the egg white (page 250) shows. Both the egg white and the lens are made primarily of protein, which hardens and yellows with age. The aging lens not only cannot stretch as well to focus light waves, but it also begins to block light on its way to the retina, obstructing vision.

An estimated nine out of ten 65-year-olds show some sign of cataract or changes that lead to cataract, but that does not mean their vision is impaired. Some cataracts are minor and do not require surgery because they do not impair vision. A cataract is simply cloudiness of a normally clear lens and if it is in the edge of the lens, no visual loss is apparent. Moreover, a cataract often develops at such a gradual pace that it does not advance to the point of destroying or impairing eyesight during the person's lifetime.

Thus you might have a cataract but not need to have it removed. Only when a person is unable to drive, read, or perform the visual tasks necessary in daily life should cataract surgery be considered. Medicine no longer believes it is necessary for a cataract to "ripen" before it can be surgically treated, nor is it necessary for cataracts to develop to any predetermined point. In many cases the rate of development and visual loss is unequal in the two eyes. Sometimes a dense cataract can develop in one eye, while little or no problem occurs in the other.

It is important to seek medical help, however, because neglected cataracts remain a leading cause of loss of vision. The early warning signs of the condition are hazy vision or poor night vision. When the cataract victim drives in bright sunlight or at night, the clouded lens will "scatter" light, causing a dazzling effect.

Tremendous advances in cataract surgery have occurred in the past 30 years. More than 98 percent of the 400,000 operations performed annually are successful.

Today, ophthalmologists use two basic techniques: They remove the entire lens, or they remove the cataract but leave the posterior capsule of the lens intact. Sometimes a miniature cryogenic probe is used, which instantly freezes the lens and capsule to the probe. A newer procedure, phacoemulsification, makes use of an ultrasonic device that breaks the lens into minute particles that are gently sucked from the eye. The patient and physician together must discuss the various types of

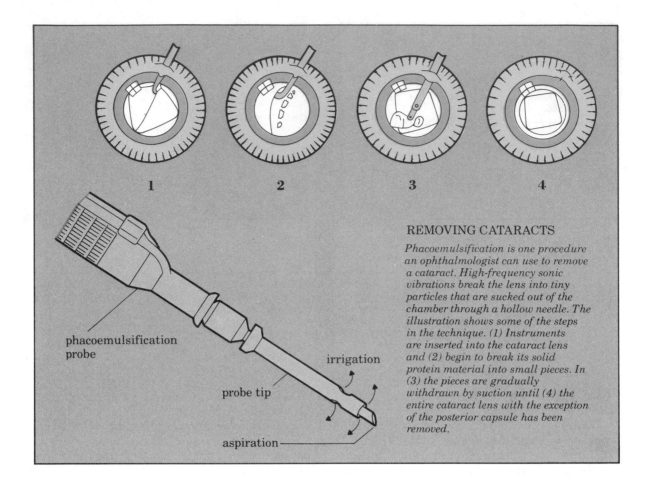

1   2   3   4

phacoemulsification probe

irrigation

probe tip

aspiration

REMOVING CATARACTS

Phacoemulsification is one procedure an ophthalmologist can use to remove a cataract. High-frequency sonic vibrations break the lens into tiny particles that are sucked out of the chamber through a hollow needle. The illustration shows some of the steps in the technique. (1) Instruments are inserted into the cataract lens and (2) begin to break its solid protein material into small pieces. In (3) the pieces are gradually withdrawn by suction until (4) the entire cataract lens with the exception of the posterior capsule has been removed.

cataract procedures and make a decision on which is best for that particular patient. No one procedure is applicable to all cases.

These days, recuperation from cataract surgery is rapid and relatively painless. A cataract patient in the 1960s was hospitalized seven to ten days, but today he or she usually stays two or three days. Rarely do hospital stays extend beyond four days unless there are complications. After recovery, the cataract will not return, although it is common for cataract to develop in the other eye. Sometimes a thin membrane must be removed at a later date if phacoemulsification is used.

Vision aids after cataract removal. If the cataract lens is removed from the eye, so is the eye's natural focusing mechanism. A patient who has had a lens removed is described as aphakic. Many people assume it takes a long time to adjust to vision without a focusing mechanism, but most patients return to useful vision within days, and often "normal" vision returns within several months. Today, an aphakic's ability to focus can be artificially or technically replaced in one of three ways: with glasses, contact lenses, or intraocular lenses.

Eyeglasses are the most traditional and probably still the most common way of helping the aphakic patient. Unfortunately, they are also the most difficult to adjust to. The aphakic patient does not see as normally as he used to, for aphakic glasses magnify his vision up to 30 percent. Therefore, a person cannot wear a cataract eyeglass lens in one eye and a normal lens in the other because his brain becomes confused by the difference in image size.

Contact lenses have provided one solution to this problem. Although contacts magnify the visual image nearly 10 percent, this is a magnification our brain seems to tolerate. At one time, contacts were not recommended because of the difficulty in insertion and removal, particularly for the elderly. But continuous or prolonged contact lens wear has proven highly successful for many. Soft lenses have been developed that can be worn for a month or longer

glasses contact lenses lens implant

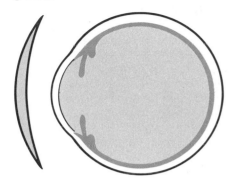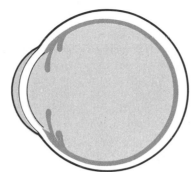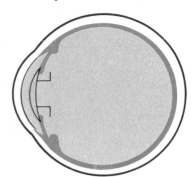

REPLACING THE LENS

There are three ways to substitute for a missing natural lens that has been removed in a cataract operation. The most common way is to use strong eyeglasses. A second method uses a contact lens. The third technique is *surgical insertion of an intraocular lens into the eye itself. The most appropriate method must be determined by the patient and the ophthalmologist.*

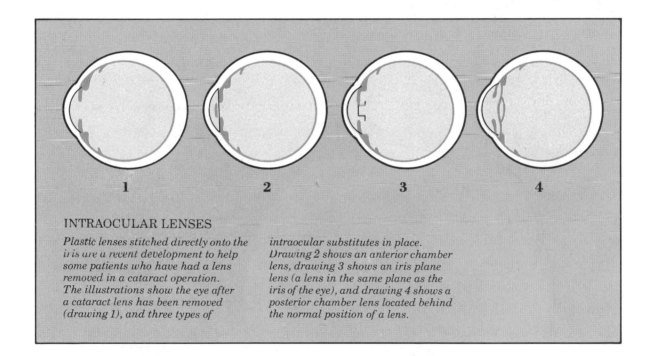

INTRAOCULAR LENSES

Plastic lenses stitched directly onto the iris are a recent development to help some patients who have had a lens removed in a cataract operation. The illustrations show the eye after a cataract lens has been removed (drawing 1), and three types of *intraocular substitutes in place. Drawing 2 shows an anterior chamber lens, drawing 3 shows an iris plane lens (a lens in the same plane as the iris of the eye), and drawing 4 shows a posterior chamber lens located behind the normal position of a lens.*

without removal, and improvements continue to be made. In fact, the industry hopes to perfect a lens that can be worn continuously at least up to six months.

Intraocular lenses are recommended for some aphakic patients. An intraocular lens is a plastic substitute for the natural lens that has been removed. It is placed and sometimes stitched into place inside the eye in approximately the position of the lens at the time of cataract surgery. A successful intraocular lens provides the most normal vision for aphakics. But because of technical difficulties and uncertainty about inserting plastic material inside the eye—or anywhere in the body for that matter—its use has been limited. The procedure is increasingly popular, although the effects 30 or 40 years after surgery are unknown.

Thus, intraocular lenses have been reserved for older persons, or for those who would have difficulty inserting contact lenses.

Retinal disorders are the second most common problem, after cataracts, of the later decades. There are three main types: macular degeneration, peripheral retinal degeneration, and retinal detachment.

Macular degeneration is an increasingly common disorder but its cause is not fully known. It affects the macula, the high-resolution or "fine-tuning" part of the retina, which we need for close work such as reading and threading a needle. It is an orange-yellow area in the center of the retina.

Macular degeneration appears to run in families. It occurs when the blood supply to the macula hemorrhages or when other fluid collects in the vicinity of the macula, reducing central visual sharpness. A person with macular degeneration retains vision to the side but has difficulty reading or fine-focusing on any object directly in front of him. Sometimes this reduction is marked, sometimes it is minimal.

Certain types of macular degeneration can be stabilized by coagulating the hemorrhaging vessels with laser burn. Other types are untreatable.

Peripheral retinal degeneration is simply the change or destruction of tissue in the retina's periphery. Around the eyeball toward the front of the eye various developmental retinal structures are found. Many are normal variations and cause no visual problems. In some people, however, for reasons unknown, degenerative changes develop in this peripheral area. The changes go by a variety of names such as "lattice degeneration," "snail tracks," "paving stones," "cystoid degeneration," all describing what the eye specialist sees when he or she examines this part of the eye. There are virtually no visual symptoms because we do not notice the use of this portion of our eye. The problems are generally discovered during a thorough eye examination. The important point, however, is that retinal detachments, a more serious condition, can develop from certain peripheral retinal degenerations. It is also important to note that retinal degeneration occurs somewhat more frequently in people who are nearsighted.

Retinal detachment occurs when a hole in the retina allows liquid vitreous in the center of the eye to seep behind the retina and push it away from the back of the eyeball. The process is much the same as when moisture collects

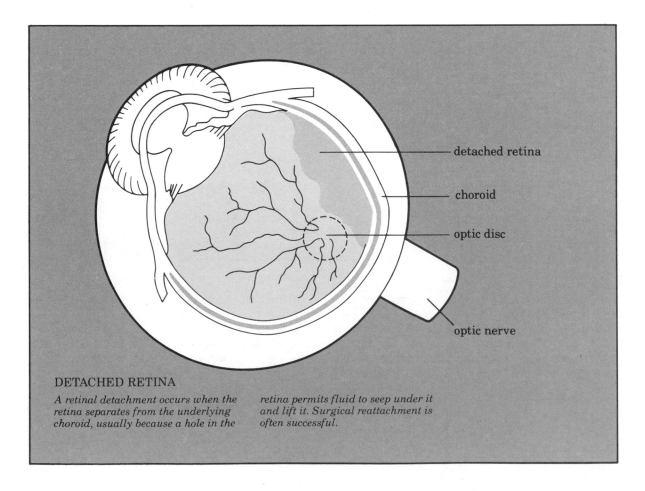

DETACHED RETINA

A retinal detachment occurs when the retina separates from the underlying choroid, usually because a hole in the retina permits fluid to seep under it and lift it. Surgical reattachment is often successful.

detached retina

choroid

optic disc

optic nerve

behind wallpaper, producing a fluid bubble. Loss of vision occurs because the retina is pulled away from part of its blood supply. Symptoms include black "floating spots" or a constant dark spot in the field of vision. Sometimes the victim feels as if a curtain has been pulled in front of his eyes. Generally, ophthalmologists can successfully treat this condition through surgery. If the hole is very small and the fluid behind it very minimal, they can freeze or burn the area surrounding the hole so that a scar seals it. The techniques are called cryotherapy and photocoagulation, respectively. A laser beam is one method used for the burning process.

If the hole is large and the amount of fluid great, or if other conditions exist, an ophthalmologist will place a silicone pillow over the sclera at the site of the hole or an encircling band around the eyeball to force the separated layers together and help seal the hole. If the retinal detachment can be treated before it reaches the macula, there is an excellent chance for good vision. A high percentage of the operations for retinal detachment are successful.

Low vision aids. Some old people tend not to complain of poor vision because they accept the myth that vision naturally dims with age. Others are unduly pessimistic, falsely believing that it is only a matter of time before they become blind. Persons with macular degeneration do *not* go blind. Their ability to read, to recognize friends at a distance, or to perform other tasks that require close visual attention is markedly impaired, but they retain peripheral vision, which allows them to move around freely. Many still enjoy television. They can perceive the general movement on the screen but not facial expressions. For these individuals, low vision aids and appliances can help.

The needs of the individual with low vision are the detection, prevention of further progression and, if possible, treatment of the disease; expert advice on optical aids such as strong reading lenses, magnifiers, and telescopic lenses; and psychosocial services, instruction, and rehabilitation. Spectacles are the best form of aid for prolonged reading. Other aids are hand-held or stand magnifiers and monocular telescopes small enough to fit into a pocket. There are devices other than magnifying lenses that are helpful. Examples are colored filters to enhance contrast, large print books and magazines, large print checks and playing cards, large print telephone dials, and special fixtures for stove and refrigerator dials. The decision to license a driver is the responsibility of each state. The decision involves general driving ability as well as vision.

For some people, advice in managing their everyday lives (shopping, cooking, and taking care of themselves and their homes) will be more important than an optical aid. The person who cannot travel safely, efficiently, and alone needs the training offered by schools and agencies for the visually handicapped. Some may want to consider learning Braille in cases where sight will one day disappear completely.

When a person has a corrected visual acuity of 20/200 or less and a visual field of 20 degrees or less, he or she can be classified as "legally blind." That means the person becomes eligible for an extra income tax deduction and can get educational benefits from the state. "Legal blindness" is a legal, not a medical, term. It does not necessarily mean that the person is totally blind or will go blind.

BLINDNESS

Blindness is confined to no particular age group. It respects neither the very young nor the very old. Generally, it results from disease or injury, although a small percentage of people are born blind each year.

Research to Prevent Blindness, Inc., a nonprofit foundation dedicated to preventing and curing blindness, estimates that in the United States alone four million new cases of eye disease occur each year and 500,000 are considered "legally blind." According to the National Society to Prevent Blindness, another national nonprofit organization, more than 25 percent of those who lose their sight are blinded by retinal disorders, nearly 14 percent by cataracts, and 12 percent by glaucoma. For more than 11 percent of the diseases that lead to blindness, the causes are unknown. Most major cities in the United States support a local chapter of the National Society to Prevent Blindness. Most also support Lions Clubs. The Lions Eye Foundation is one of the leading international organizations dedicated to helping the visually impaired. The yellow pages of your telephone directory may list sources of aid under "Blind Institutions."

SYSTEMIC DISEASES
THAT AFFECT THE EYE

Generalized diseases that originate elsewhere in the body can affect the eyes, but because physicians can look through the eye to see its internal tissues, it becomes a marvelous diagnostic structure. Without having to cut through a layer of skin, a doctor can examine the blood vessels of the retina with an ophthalmoscope or directly photograph a condition that is simultaneously occurring in less accessible parts of your body. This is especially important in diseases of the blood.

Atherosclerosis produces deposits called plaques which can be found in the larger blood vessels such as the aorta, which is the body's main artery, or its major branches. Plaques normally do not develop inside the eye because the blood vessels are too small. Frequently, however, small pieces of plaque break off from the walls of the major blood vessels and lodge in smaller vessels of the eyes. By observing these plaques or by recording the history of occasional visual loss, your ophthalmologist often detects symptoms or sees the evidence of vascular disease.

Arteriosclerosis (see chapter 5, "Blood Vessel Disorders") also can be detected by looking inside your eye. Thickening blood vessel walls or changes that occur when artery and vein cross one another are pieces of evidence that show your blood vessels are aging throughout the rest of your body. For reasons like these, general eye exams can be of help to any patient who seeks a general health evaluation.

Diabetes (see chapter 17) is sometimes detected and monitored by observing its effects on the blood vessels of the eye. Indeed, diabetic damage to the blood vessels often occurs most prominently in the eyes.

Diabetic retinopathy, damage to the retina caused by diabetes, is a leading cause of blindness. It occurs when blood vessels of the retina disintegrate, causing blood to collect or to seep between the retinal layers. Sometimes, because of diabetes-caused blockage in normal capillaries, new blood vessels form, and they also hemorrhage and spill their contents into the vitreous.

A wide spectrum of visual changes can occur in a person suffering from diabetic retinopathy, and any diabetic should consult an ophthalmologist if he or she begins to experience changes in vision. In fact, any individual who has had diabetes for seven to ten years should have regular eye examinations.

Photocoagulation is the primary treatment for certain types of diabetic retinopathy. A xenon or argon laser is used to burn certain portions of the retina to reduce the need for oxygen in the retina and to coagulate new blood vessels that form in the center. These new blood vessels are extremely fragile and tend to bleed easily.

Toxoplasmosis, an infection which can be transmitted by the mother to her child before birth, causes a scar on the baby's retina. The child may be born with visual damage, or this scar, containing toxoplasmosis organisms in cyst form, can be reactivated throughout the child's life. It can be associated with further bouts of active inflammation or infection, particularly in the retina. Close association with cats seems to be common but not the only cause of this condition.

Histoplasmosis, a fungus disease particularly common in the Midwest (see chapter 8, "The Lungs"), produces a condition in the eyes of younger people which resembles macular degeneration. The treatment is directed at the disease itself. It is very difficult to prevent visual loss, however, if the infection centers in the macular area.

Arthritis, particularly the rheumatoid variety and a condition called Sjogren's syndrome (see chapter 15, "Arthritis and Related Diseases"), is another generalized disease that manifests itself in your eyes. The relationship is unclear, but it frequently causes "dry eyes," that are painfully dry and scratchy because the eyes cannot produce enough tears. Juvenile arthritis, particularly that affecting the spine, can inflame the front of the eye and cloud vision. Infrequently it causes loss of an eye due to secondary glaucoma, cataracts, or degeneration of the eye because of the inflammation.

Worms common to dogs and cats, particularly the dog tapeworm, *Toxocara canis,* can affect children who play with puppies and result in an infection of the eye which creates destructive eye abnormalities.

Congenital malformations of the blood vessels, such as hemangiomas and angiomas affecting the brain, also frequently result in damage to the eye.

Trachoma, rarely seen in the United States now except among certain American Indian tribes, is one of the leading causes of

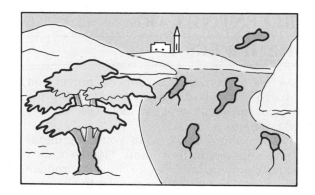 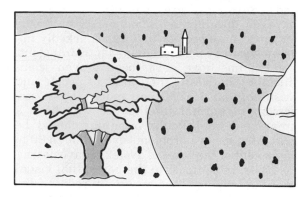

SPOTS BEFORE THE EYES

Transparent "floating" spots across your vision (left drawing), a common occurrence, are normal and should cause no concern. Sudden showers of black spots that affect your vision, as in the right drawing, may represent a more serious eye problem and you should see an ophthalmologist immediately.

blindness in the rest of the world. Caused by a virus-like organism, this disease particularly affects the cornea, as well as the lining of the lids, the conjunctiva. It can be treated with antibiotics, but until recently treatment has been sporadic because the disease occurs in under-developed cultures.

Allergies (see chapter 21) are a frequent but less serious cause of eye problems. In the spring, summer, and fall hay fever sufferers allergic to weeds and pollens often suffer from inflammation of the conjunctiva as well as irritation of the generalized mucous membrane. Allergies to dust, animals, or cosmetics also produce severe itching, redness, and weeping in the eyes. The proper treatment for these irritations is to alleviate the offending allergen, but symptomatic relief can be obtained with medications applied directly to the eye such as antihistamines and, in extreme cases, cortisone administered under medical supervision.

COMMON SYMPTOMS
AND THEIR SIGNIFICANCE

There are many misconceptions about eye problems and treatments. They include:

Spots before your eyes. One of the most common complaints an eye specialist hears is that the patient sees small, web-like floating spots. If the spots are very small and constant, they almost invariably are caused by the aging process of the vitreous as it changes from a gel into liquid and strand-like components. These strands, which develop patterns like cobwebs or spots, can be annoying but are not serious.

They are particularly obvious if an individual looks at a clear wall, moves his eyes, looks at the sky or "looks for" the spots. In contrast, however, sudden showers of spots that look like multiple black dots frequently represent a much more serious condition. They result from a break in a small blood vessel and commonly are associated with retinal detachments. If you see hundreds of black spots, you should seek immediate attention from an ophthalmologist.

Headaches. People often blame their headaches on their eyes but rarely are they right. A person who does not have properly prescribed glasses or who is beginning to need glasses often complains of headaches and tired eyes. Once he or she is fitted with the proper prescription, the ocular cause of the headaches is alleviated. Headaches in the back of the head generally have nothing to do with the eyes. They are usually caused by tension.

Tired eyes. Middle-aged persons who complain that they can read for only a short time won't increase their reading time with eye exercises but can improve it by changing their prescription. In children these complaints may indicate that their ability to focus on near objects is inadequate. This so-called "convergence insufficiency"—we all must "converge" in order to read—can often be handled with proper diagnosis and simple exercises. However, "perceptual visual training and eye exercises" are generally of no help and have no documented scientific basis. Some "experts" may profess they can markedly improve vision by perceptual visual training, but their claims have never been proven scientifically. They dupe thousands of people and waste a great deal of their money. Dyslexics, persons of normal intelligence who have a great deal of difficulty reading, should be evaluated for eye problems even though 90 to 95 percent of the cases of dyslexia have no ocular basis. In contrast to the perceptual visual training "experts," the experts in reading disorders or learning disability specialists are trained professionals who can make a significant difference in a child's reading ability.

Bulging eyes. Certain people complain that their eyes appear to be bulging. This is most likely a hereditary trait, dependent upon the shape of the orbit which is usually similar to those of one or both parents. A small prominence of the eyes should be no functional concern. However, if you notice that one eye protrudes more than the other or that your eyes are developing a rather marked stare or an upper lid retraction, you should see a doctor. The most frequent cause for this condition is hyperthyroidism (see chapter 16, "The Hormones and Endocrine Glands"). Unilateral bulging, or proptosis, when one eye becomes far more prominent than the other, is definitely abnormal and requires prompt attention.

Eye strain. Many people question how long they can read or watch television without straining the eyes. Others ask how closely they should hold a book or how close to the television screen they should sit. Like any other part of the body, eyes will present problems if you overwork them, but these are not usually persistent or severe. If the athlete training for a weightlifting competition lifts weight for 12 hours a day, it is likely that his body will complain. Similarly, if you read for 12 or more hours a day or watch television for prolonged periods, you may have transient headaches, irritations, or discomfort with your eyes. Reading is easiest in proper light, but even reading in dim light will not cause permanent damage to your eyes.

PREVENTIVE CARE
OF THE EYES

As in most instances, an ounce of prevention is worth a pound of cure in eye care. Simple common sense can prevent most eye injuries and problems.

Eye injuries. Individuals pounding metal on metal are asking for trouble. Metal pounded on another metal surface can chip and produce a sliver which can easily penetrate the eye. Goggles may be troublesome, time-consuming, or uncomfortable, but they are still the best way to prevent unnecessary eye injury. If an injury of this nature does occur, immediate treatment by an ophthalmologist is needed.

Trauma. A severe direct blow to the eye sometimes results in a small break of blood vessels inside the eye. The eruption may clear without problems, but it is extremely important that it be examined by an ophthalmologist. In this condition, vision may be reduced. The person may require hospitalization and certainly should have pressure inside the eye measured. If the blood does not absorb within a reasonable time, the injury requires ophthalmic treatment, sometimes surgery.

Red eye. After coughing, choking, or straining in some other manner, you may note a bright red spot in the white part of your eye. Even rubbing your eye can cause this type of bleeding. This spot is called a subconjunctival hemorrhage and is not dangerous, nor is it associated with decreased vision. The blood, contained entirely on the outside surface of the eye, does not penetrate inside and should disappear in seven to ten days. But if you notice frequent or recurrent red spots occurring spontaneously, you should consult a doctor. These hemorrhages could be the result of abnormal blood vessels or of a bleeding tendency that has not made itself apparent in another way.

Another type of "red eye" is cosmetic, the result of smog, smoky rooms, dust, allergies, or other irritants. Routinely using eyedrops to "get the red out" is unrewarding, except to the manufacturer of the eyedrops. The only exception is some cases where prolonged allergenic irritants make drops necessary or helpful on a regular basis. On the other hand, using eyedrops to whiten your eyes produces only the most temporary relief. Depending upon the drop you use, you can even irritate or damage your eye by using drops too frequently.

Chemical burns. Lyes and commercial or home-cleaning ammonias and fertilizers can cause loss of vision or even blindness (see chapter 35, "First Aid"). Lye burns are many times

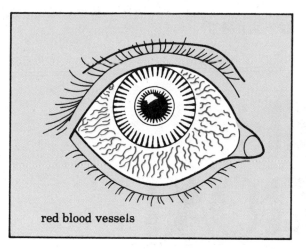

red blood vessels

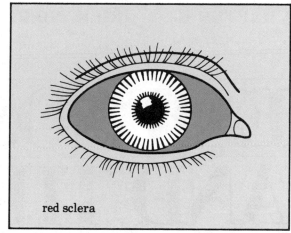

red sclera

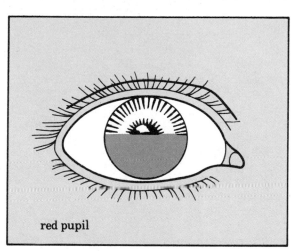

red pupil

RED EYES

Red eyes can be caused by many problems and vary in severity. The top left drawing illustrates a common condition in which blood vessels become enlarged because of a minor infection or irritation. The condition in the top right drawing, although serious in appearance, is usually not dangerous because the blood remains in the outer layers of the eyeball. The lower right drawing represents a serious problem that must be treated by an ophthalmologist immediately because bleeding has occurred inside the eye.

more dangerous to your eye than acid burns. Acid denatures the protein of your eye immediately but does not continue to cause problems because it neutralizes quickly. Lye will continue to burn for a long time. Wash your eyes with water immediately. This is the best home treatment for any such injury. Individuals working with acid or alkali materials should wear glasses and make extensive efforts to prevent the potential for spilling or splashing such material into their eyes. Immediate irrigation and rapid ophthalmic care produce the best outcome if a chemical burn occurs, although severe lye burns carry high probability for loss of vision or loss of the eye.

A chapter on the eyes can only begin to describe the marvelous gift of sight and list only a few of the more common problems and eye diseases. There are, however, two important messages. First, our eyes are precious, flexible, sensitive, and enduring. They are not only amazing mechanisms in themselves, but work intricately with other organs to perform the tasks involved in seeing. The realists may argue with romantics, but if our eyes are not windows to the soul, they are windows through which a physician can look to see the health of the rest of the body as well as the health of the eyes. They deserve our respect and care.

That is the second message. Eye care providers agree that many causes of blindness are still unknown. They agree that some diseases causing blindness cannot successfully be treated. They also agree that eye health care in the United States is the best in the world. By using good judgment and taking simple precautionary measures, most eye injuries can be prevented. By consulting an ophthalmologist when early signs of eye problems or diseases occur, many of them can be cured or treated. Windows to the soul? Possibly. Windows to the external world? Certainly. A precious gift that deserves the best of care.

CHAPTER 13   RICHARD R. GACEK, M.D.

EAR, NOSE, AND THROAT

When we speak of something as unnecessary, we sometimes say we "need it like a hole in the head." We have several holes in the head and they are, in fact, quite important to our well-being. The passageways of the ears, nose, and throat, and their internal mechanisms deal with such essential matters as hearing and understanding speech, communicating with others, filtering and warming the air we breathe, balance, smell, tasting and enjoying food, and preparing it for digestion. These passageways enter the head from different directions, but within the bony recesses of the skull they connect. Therefore, the ears, nose, and throat are often regarded as a unit and thought of as a single medical specialty.

THE EARS

Structure and Function

The function of the ears is not only to collect sound, but to give it meaning. It is no coincidence that Shakespeare's character Mark Antony urges friends, Romans, and countrymen to "lend me your ears," or that the Bible says "he who hath ears to hear, let him hear." These are pleas for understanding, not mere audition. Sounds are simply air vibrations that have no meaning until they are collected by the external ear, transmitted across the eardrum through the internal parts of the ear, then converted to nerve impulses that travel along the auditory nerve to the brain. As the brain sorts out visual impulses and tells us what we "see," so it unscrambles auditory impulses and interprets what we "hear."

The auditory system is one of the most sensitive and discriminating of all the senses, able to distinguish faint puffs of air issued by a human voice or the particular notes of a musical instrument. Hearing is basic to communication, pleasure, protection, and safety.

Structurally, the ear is divided into three parts, the external, middle ear, and inner ear.

The external ear is the part we can see. The pinkish, bendable, question-mark shaped appendage on either side of the head plays only a minor part in sound reception, although its curving channels do help to funnel sound to less visible parts of the ear. The ear canal (the hole in the head), of which we see only the opening and a bit of the tube, is also part of the external ear. It is a passageway about 1¼ inches long, ending at the eardrum, or tympanic membrane.

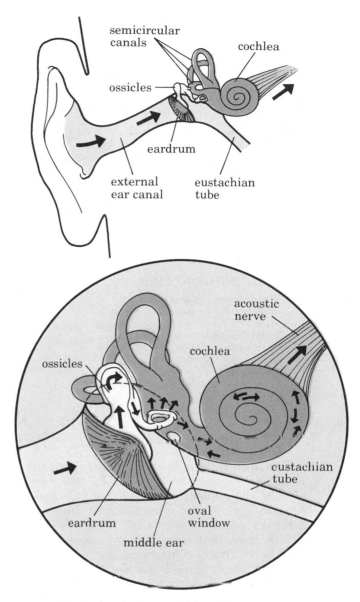

TRANSMISSION OF SOUND

Arrows show how sound waves are converted to nerve impulses. Entering the external ear canal (at left in the top drawing), the sound waves cause the eardrum to vibrate. The vibrations are transmitted across the middle ear space by three small bones called ossicles. The movement of each bone increases the amplification of the sound. The movements excite the fluids in the inner ear, which excite the nerve endings in the acoustic nerve, which in turn carries the impulses to the brain for interpretation.

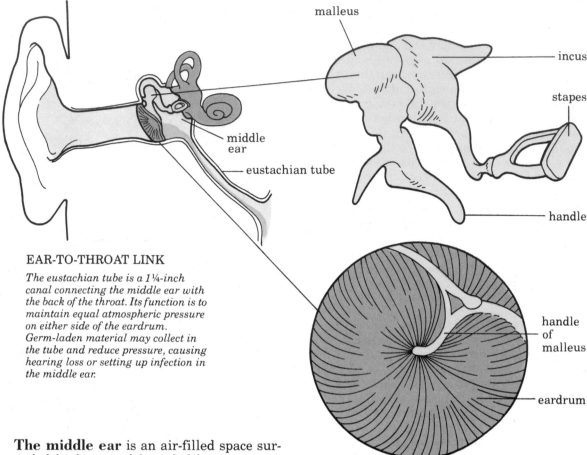

malleus

incus

stapes

handle

middle ear

eustachian tube

EAR-TO-THROAT LINK

The eustachian tube is a 1¼-inch canal connecting the middle ear with the back of the throat. Its function is to maintain equal atmospheric pressure on either side of the eardrum. Germ-laden material may collect in the tube and reduce pressure, causing hearing loss or setting up infection in the middle ear.

handle of malleus

eardrum

THE MIDDLE EAR BONES

The conducting system of the middle ear is based on three bones, the tiniest in the human body. Named for their presumed resemblance to everyday objects, they are the malleus (hammer), the incus (anvil), and the stapes (stirrup). The malleus handle, connected to the eardrum, receives its vibrations and transmits them across the bone chain to the stapes, which is connected to the oval window of the inner ear.

The middle ear is an air-filled space surrounded by bone and bounded by two membranes, the eardrum on the outer side and a flexible membrane separating it from the inner ear on the inner side. A narrow tube slants downward from this air space to the back of the throat. This passageway, about 1½ inches long, is called the eustachian tube. Hourglass-shaped, it is about the diameter of a pencil at either end, narrowing at the isthmus in the center to about one millimeter. The tube's function is to allow air to enter the middle ear space and maintain equal atmospheric pressure on either side of the eardrum. Balanced pressure is necessary to keep the eardrum working properly. A partial vacuum in the middle ear space pulls the eardrum inward and prevents it from vibrating normally. This often happens when the eustachian tube is blocked by infection, congestion, or tumor, and fluid collects in the middle ear.

Just about everyone who has flown in an airplane or traveled in a high-speed elevator knows about the equalization of pressure in the middle ear. The atmospheric pressure at the top of a skyscraper is less than that at the ground floor, and when the elevator drops swiftly, the low-pressure air is trapped inside the middle ear by the quick descent. It pushes

its way out through the eustachian tube, and we may hear or feel a distinct pop. Sometimes congestion keeps the air trapped even after we have reached ground level, reducing hearing or even causing pain.

The main job of the middle ear is amplification. When a person speaks or a tree falls, sound waves radiate in all directions from the source of the noise. The sound waves travel until they meet resistance. In the case of the listener's ear, that resistance is the eardrum. This tough but delicate membrane is jarred into movement just as any other drumhead vibrates when struck. But in the case of the eardrum, the movements are very slight. A high frequency sound moves the eardrum less than a billionth of a centimeter, but that is enough to set off the process of hearing. The vibrations activate the three bones of the middle ear, the ossicles, connected in a chain across the middle ear space.

The middle ear bones are named for their real or imagined resemblance to everyday objects: the malleus (hammer), the incus (anvil), and the stapes (stirrup). The malleus, the outermost of the trio, is in contact with the eardrum. When sound strikes the eardrum, its vibrations are transmitted to the malleus. These vibrations of the malleus, in turn, stimulate the incus, which passes them along to the stapes, the innermost bone. The amplitude of the vibration increases with each step. The footplate of the stirrup bone is attached to a flexible membrane covering an opening into the inner ear called the oval window. Moving back and forth like a piston, the stapes sets in motion the fluids of the inner ear. In the short but intricate journey from eardrum to inner ear, the sound wave is amplified as much as 20 times.

As your stereo amplifier must be well protected against damage, so must the delicate mechanism of the middle ear. Tiny muscles and ligaments secure the structures of the middle ear so they can vibrate properly. The largest muscle, the tensor tympani, pulls the hammer bone inward and increases the tension of the eardrum, like tightening a drumhead. The stapedius muscle tightens the stapes, particularly in the case of loud noise, to restrict the tiny bone's movement and protect against excessive stimulation, which can lead to nerve deafness.

The inner ear is the area where the sound vibrations are converted into electrical impulses that eventually reach the brain. It is a delicate structure of membranes, hair cells, and nerve fibers, bathed in fluid called perilymph and protected by the hard temporal bone of the skull. When the footplate of the stapes bone moves to and fro in the oval window, it sets off corresponding movements in the fluid of the inner ear. A second membrane-covered opening, the round window, allows for release of the pressure exerted on the fluid and permits waves to form within the inner ear.

The rhythmic waves stirred up in the inner ear fluid excite a highly delicate organ that is at the heart of sound reception. This is a tubular, bony structure lined with a membrane containing more than 20,000 hair cells tuned to vibrate to sounds of different frequencies. Coiled like a snail shell—hence its name, cochlea, from the Latin word for snail—the structure is sometimes described as a spiral piano keyboard. If the spiral were stretched out, it would measure about an inch and a half in length, but in its coiled configuration it occupies no more space than a pea. The hair cells at one end of the keyboard respond to sounds at high frequencies, up to 20,000 cycles per second; those at the opposite end respond to low ones, down to 16 cycles per second, just as the 88 keys of a piano are graduated from treble to bass. The receptors for the bass are at the innermost turn of the spiral. Nerve endings are contained in a complex, slightly elevated structure over the floor of the tube contained by the cochlea. This area is known as the organ of Corti.

As the sensitive hair cells arranged along the cochlea are shaken by the oscillations of the fluid around them, they initiate an electrical impulse that is transmitted to the individual nerve fibers, which then merge into the auditory nerve. These impulses are carried into the central auditory pathways of the brain and ultimately to the cerebral cortex, where their pattern is interpreted as a sound. This remarkably effective and complex arrangement allows us to distinguish sounds from the deep boom of the kettledrum to the highest shrill of the piccolo.

Balance and Equilibrium

The inner ear also contains two other types of sense organs, which help us to maintain equilibrium. Near the cochlea are three semicircular canals that occupy the three planes in space. They perceive changes in angular movement. The second set of organs, the flat position receptors or otolith sense organs (individually known as the utricle and saccule), oriented in horizontal and vertical planes respectively, detect changes in position or forward and backward movement. The sense organs of equilibrium, collectively known as the labyrinth because of their serpentine course within the vestibule of the inner ear, are composed of hair cells and nerve fibers much like those of the organ of hearing. When the hair cells are stimulated by a covering membrane set in motion by movements of another inner-ear fluid, the endolymph, an electrical impulse is transmitted to the vestibular or balance nerve which connects to the cerebellum and to the brainstem area that controls muscles of the eye, trunk, and limbs. When a person moves his head, this complex system of canals, sacs, membranes, fluid, and nerves brings about reflex muscle contractions of the eyes and limbs that tend to maintain the body in an erect position.

As might be expected, since the balance and hearing organs are housed within the same compartment of the temporal bone, they are often affected by the same disorders. For example, infection of the labyrinth (labyrinthitis) will cause hearing loss, dizziness, and vomiting. The symptoms usually last for several days, and can leave both permanent nerve deafness and disequilibrium, which is eventually compensated for.

Bone and Air Conduction

Any vibrations that stimulate the acoustic nerve are audible, but they do not always reach the nerve in the same way. Vibrations can reach the hearing nerve directly over the bony structures of the head or by sound waves that strike the eardrum and are transmitted across the middle ear space. The first is called bone conduction, the second air conduction.

We hear by bone and air conduction all the time, although air conduction predominates in general hearing or listening. Bone conduction is especially related to speaking, and is a kind of feedback control in hearing your own voice. Think of the first time you heard your own voice on a tape recording. It probably sounded unfamiliar, probably higher-pitched, almost the voice of a stranger. The primary reason for the difference is that when you speak, the sound is reaching you by both air and bone conduction. The resonance of the bones gives the sound its deeper pitch. When you hear it via an outside source, such as a tape recording, only air conduction is used. The resonance is eliminated.

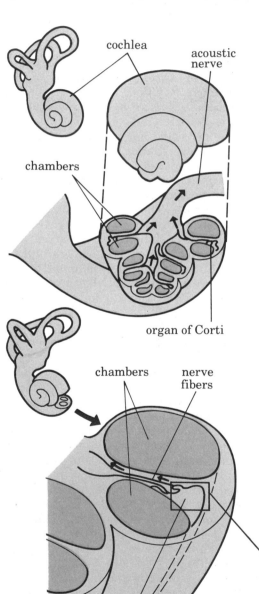

CENTERS OF HEARING

Inside the inner ear, the cochlea (top drawing) contains chambers that bring fluids in contact with the organ of Corti, from which nerve impulses are carried to the cochlear branch of the acoustic nerve. The center drawing shows the organ of Corti in relationship to the chambers, nerve fibers, and cochlear duct. The microscopic inset (lower right) shows the hair cells that excite the nerve fibers going to the brain.

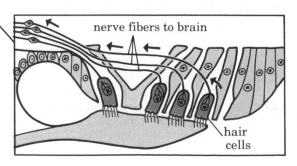

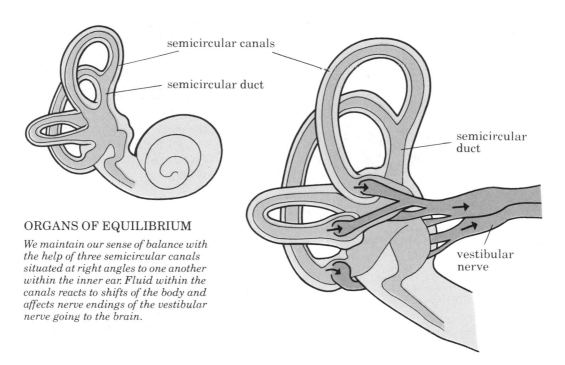

semicircular canals

semicircular duct

semicircular
duct

vestibular
nerve

ORGANS OF EQUILIBRIUM

We maintain our sense of balance with the help of three semicircular canals situated at right angles to one another within the inner ear. Fluid within the canals reacts to shifts of the body and affects nerve endings of the vestibular nerve going to the brain.

Air and bone conduction differences are important in tests of hearing. If a person hears air conduction sounds poorly but bone conduction sounds quite well, the site of hearing trouble is probably in the middle ear. If he cannot hear bone conduction vibrations, he probably suffers from nerve deafness as a result of impaired structures in the inner ear.

Impaired Hearing

Relatively few persons are totally deaf, completely unable to receive sounds. But a large number—more than seven million Americans—have some degree of hearing loss. Many, perhaps most, have a deficiency that stems from growing older. The young ear normally can hear tones in a range of 16 cycles per second up to 20,000 cycles per second, and possibly more. A person older than 60 usually is not able to hear sounds above 8,000 or 10,000 cycles per second.

The loss in the high frequency range that occurs with aging happens to almost everyone. It usually comes on gradually and is probably related to a number of factors: heredity, exposure to noise over many years, or as a result of nerve damage caused by such conditions as diabetes and hypothyroidism. The degenerative process may involve hair cells, nerve fibers, or other mechanical structures of the inner ear.

Although a slight loss of ability to hear high tones is seldom severely disabling, significant involvement of the entire frequency range will make even ordinary conversation difficult or impossible to understand. The frequency range from 500 to 2,000 cycles per second is crucial for hearing and understanding speech. Inability to hear well within this range can be a serious personal and social handicap. Hard-of-hearing persons are often blamed unfairly for being rude and inattentive if they do not answer questions asked in conversational tones.

Although aging is perhaps the most common cause of hearing loss, it is not the only one. A variety of hearing impairments affect young and old. Hearing loss may be divided into two types: conductive deafness and nerve (sensorineural) deafness. Often a mixture of the two occurs. Occasionally, a person cannot hear even though the hearing apparatus and system are intact. The cause of the deafness is a psychological one.

The two types of hearing impairments have different causes. Conduction deafness results from a failure of airborne sound waves to be conducted efficiently through the ear canal and tympanic membrane over the middle ear and auditory ossicles to the inner ear. Any obstruction along this route results in a conductive hearing loss because the sound messages never get a chance to stimulate the nerves in the inner ear. In perceptive or nerve deafness, the transmission of sound is normal, but the inner ear or its nerves fail to perceive the sound.

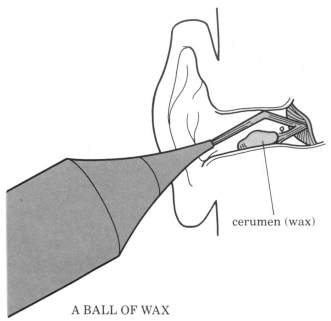

A BALL OF WAX

cerumen (wax)

Impaired hearing can result from something as simple as accumulated wax, which hinders sound waves from reaching the eardrum. The wax (cerumen) can be removed by a doctor who injects warm fluid (above) which is reflected off the eardrum and forces the wax loose. Matches, toothpicks, and cotton-tipped swabs should not be used to loosen wax because of possible damage to the eardrum.

The obstruction that causes conductive hearing loss may occur in the external ear or the middle ear. The ear canal may be closed by accumulated wax or bony tumors (exostoses) resulting from swimming in cold water. A less common cause is failure of the ear canal to develop normally. In the middle ear space, fluid accumulation, defects of the eardrum, or fixation of the auditory bones may be the culprit.

Nerve or perceptive deafness implies damage in the inner ear or its nerve supply. Commonly, the high frequencies are affected more than the middle or lower ranges. Nerve deafness can be sudden or gradual. Since it is irreversible and untreatable, nerve deafness is the most frustrating type of hearing loss. The most common reasons for nerve deafness are aging, acoustic injury resulting from exposure to high-intensity noise, reaction to drugs (such as certain antibiotics or aspirin), infection of the labyrinth, temporal bone fracture, prenatal infection with rubella (German measles) or other viruses, and meningitis.

Tests of Hearing

The standard unit of loudness of sound is called the decibel. It is not an absolute measurement of a sound's power, but compares its strength to that of other sounds. For example, a whisper is rated at 20 decibels, conversation at 50 or 60 decibels. Injurious noise, such as train wheels shrieking in the subway, rates 100 decibels, the whine of a jet airplane 140 decibels. Most hearing tests measure loss in terms of loss of decibels.

The most simple and practical test of hearing is simply to detect whether a person can hear a whisper or normal conversation at a given distance, or to have him or her listen to the ticking of a watch. Professional testing may include both speech perception and the perception of tones. In a speech test, the person is tested for ability to understand the complex sound of a word. Tone perception uses a tuning fork with a specific vibrating frequency. The tuning fork is particularly useful in distinguishing conductive deafness from nerve deafness. Normally, the sound of a tuning fork heard via the ear canal (air conduction) is louder than when the fork is applied to the bone behind the ear (bone conduction). In a person with normal hearing or one with nerve deafness, sounds traveling through the air are heard louder than those transmitted through bone. This is called a positive tuning-fork test (the Rinne test). When bone conduction is heard louder than air, the test is said to be abnormal or negative.

A physician can get a general idea of the type and severity of hearing loss with these methods of testing, but more precise evaluation requires an instrument called an audiometer. This instrument emits pure tones that can be graded in decibels. The physician can chart the patient's response to pure tones at different intensities; this chart is called an audiogram. The doctor can also test the patient's ability to respond to speech and get an evaluation of speech perception.

A tympanometer is an instrument used by a physician or technician to test whether a person (often a child) has fluid in the middle ear or a conductive or perceptive hearing loss. The test shows whether the eardrum and the middle-ear ossicles move normally, or whether their movement is limited by accumulated fluid. It is often used to screen school children to identify those who should then be evaluated by an ear specialist (otologist).

The audiometer requires the tested person to respond to what he thinks he hears, and therefore is subjective. A modern objective

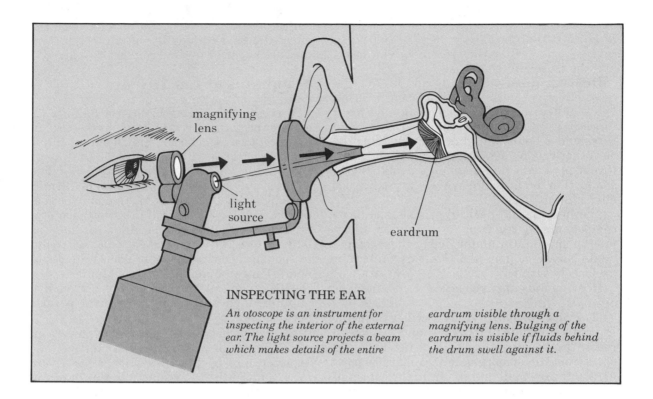

INSPECTING THE EAR

An otoscope is an instrument for inspecting the interior of the external ear. The light source projects a beam which makes details of the entire eardrum visible through a magnifying lens. Bulging of the eardrum is visible if fluids behind the drum swell against it.

form of testing relies on the recording of electrical waves in the hearing nerve or auditory pathway of the brain in response to a signal. This more precise form of hearing test, called brainstem-evoked response audiometry, requires specialized equipment usually present only in large medical centers. It is advantageous in measuring hearing in patients who are otherwise unable to respond, such as infants, patients who have had strokes, and patients with psychophysiological forms of hearing loss.

Deaf Infants and Children

Some infants are born deaf or with a serious hearing loss, and early recognition of their condition is extremely important. Certain signs can alert a parent to the presence of significant hearing loss. One warning signal is a child's failure to respond to a loud noise like a bang or a clang. If a six-month-old does not cry or appear startled under those circumstances, it may suggest hearing impairment. By the age of nine or ten months a normal infant can locate a sound quite well and will turn the head in that direction. The deaf infant does not respond.

Another important sign of significant hearing loss in infants is failure to develop speech at normal age. A deaf infant may go through the babbling stage like other babies, but soon gives it up if he or she cannot hear his or her own voice. The child is shut off from the world of sound and as he or she grows older, communicates only with grunts or gestures. As soon as a parent notices such signs, the child should be brought to an audiologist or otologist for special hearing tests.

In a few nurseries, a new method is being used to evaluate or screen newborn infants for hearing loss. In this method, sounds are delivered that should produce a physical response from the baby. Extremely delicate sensors connected to the crib record the infant's movements, however fine. The test cannot evaluate level of hearing, but can identify newborns at high risk for hearing loss. Later tests can assess the loss more precisely.

Treatment

In a child, conductive hearing loss is usually managed with a hearing aid early in life. Corrective surgery is carried out when the child is 10 years or older. Sensorineural or nerve hearing loss also dictates a hearing aid at first. Other rehabilitative measures, such as courses in lip-reading, take a long time, require the assistance of trained personnel, and at times require special schools. The rule, however, is that the earlier the handicap is discovered, the earlier the treatment can begin and the more effective it is.

Hearing aids. For many adults, too, the most effective method of combating hearing loss is a hearing aid. The hearing aid's main function is to amplify sound, raising the threshold of hearing higher than the impaired ear otherwise possesses. Amplification is useful for persons who have nerve deafness or a conduction deafness for which surgery is not advisable.

The hearing aid basically consists of three components: a receiver, an amplifier, and a microphone or stimulator. Today, these components can be compressed into tiny units that are barely visible.

Hearing aids may be classified in a number of ways.

(1) Power or gain. This describes the hearing aid's ability to amplify a sound in order to reach the hearing threshold of the impaired ear. Generally speaking, low gain or low powered aids are small and can fit in the ear canal or around the ear. These are called ear level aids. Hearing aids that require greater power or amplification need a large power source, usually attached around the body or chest with a cord leading to the stimulator in the ear. These are called body aids.

(2) Monaural or binaural. Monaural aids are fitted in one ear, binaural aids in both ears. A monaural hearing aid can be quite effective for a person who requires amplification in only one ear or, in the case of a bilateral nerve loss, has one ear with a better inner ear function. Binaural hearing aids allow the user to locate sound more effectively and increase the sensitivity to hearing by several decibels. One type of monaural aid allows the patient to perceive sounds received on the side of a profoundly deafened ear by carrying them across the head to the normal ear.

(3) Air conduction or bone conduction aids. An air conduction hearing aid fits into the ear canal and presents the amplified sound to the eardrum, which then transmits the sound across the ossicular chain to the inner ear at increased sound pressure levels. A bone conduction aid employs a vibrator or stimulator on the bone of the skull, preferably behind the ear on the bulge called the mastoid process. The bone-conducted sound is then perceived directly by the inner ear and hearing nerve. The bone conduction aid is used in persons who do not have a normal ear canal or in persons who suffer a fungal infection of the ear canal that causes irritation. However, the effectiveness and fidelity of air conduction aids are superior to bone conduction aids.

Symptoms of Ear Disease

Vertigo, the feeling of loss of balance, is another prominent symptom of ear disease. In its worst form, the victim may feel that his or her surroundings are spinning, or that he or she is falling down or falling to the side. The sufferer may also feel nauseated, may vomit, or be lightheaded or dizzy. Vertigo may be sustained, lasting for several days because of a prolonged affliction of the inner ear such as labyrinthitis, or it may be episodic, occurring in spells that last anywhere from minutes to hours. For example, the spells of Meniere's disease (see page 291) have a duration of from five minutes to several hours, with clear periods between.

A third variety of vertigo occurs in certain positions, and is called positional vertigo. The experience of positional vertigo is as severe as in labyrinthitis except that the duration of positional vertigo is much shorter, lasting only seconds.

The presence of a disorder in the balance, or vestibular, system may be indicated by a condition called nystagmus, in which the eyes oscillate during the episode of vertigo or disequilibrium. This is produced by an imbalance in the eye reflexes, which are normally used to help maintain the body's position in space. The imbalance is caused by an abnormal train of impulses from the diseased inner ear compared to the normal opposite ear. The standard method of evaluating the ear for a disturbance in the vestibular system is the caloric test, in which a stimulus to the lateral semicircular canal is produced by injecting cold or warm water into the ear canal. The cold or warmth is transmitted across the middle ear space to the inner ear where the fluids in the semicircular canals are caused to move, much as one sees the water level rise in a pot of boiling water. As the fluids circulate, the balancing organs are stimulated, activating their connection to the eye muscles. In a normal patient, stimulation of one ear will result in eye movement equal in duration and intensity to that when the opposite ear is stimulated. A test that reveals a diminished response in one ear indicates a disturbance in the vestibular system of that inner ear and suggests that more specialized tests are required to determine whether infection, tumor, or other causes are responsible.

Tinnitus, or noise heard in the ear, is a common inner ear symptom. It occurs in almost any condition where some form of inner ear degeneration has occurred, including those of aging or where nerve damage is produced. Thumping like a heartbeat in the ear may indicate a blood vessel tumor in the middle ear. Any episode of tinnitus should be investigated and an evaluation of inner ear function and examination performed.

Facial paralysis also may stem from ear problems. The most common form is Bell's palsy, the cause of which is unknown. It is thought that the facial nerve becomes swollen in its course through the temporal bone surrounding the ear. Other forms of facial paralysis may signal serious disease in the inner, middle, or outer ear. The causes include malignant or benign tumors of the temporal bone, and chronic or acute infection of the middle ear space. Tumors of the internal auditory canal, the canal through which the nerves travel from the brain to reach the temporal bone, occasionally produce facial weakness, nerve hearing loss, and loss of equilibrium.

DISORDERS AFFECTING

THE EAR

Infections of the outer, middle, and inner ear occur in either acute or chronic forms and produce different symptoms.

Outer Ear Infections

Infection of the external or outer ear is commonly referred to as "swimmer's ear" because of its frequency during the summer months or swimming season. Essentially, swimmer's ear is an infection of ear canal skin and is more properly termed a dermatitis. It causes a feeling of fullness and extreme discomfort in the ear after swimming in contaminated water or after an irritation in the ear canal. Hearing is not usually affected unless the ear canal is completely closed by the swelling. Pressure on the ear or movement of the jaw joint during speaking or chewing can cause pain. A slight fever may accompany the infection. The usual treatment consists of antibiotic ear drops, local heat, aspirin, and in rare cases, antibiotics by

mouth. The infection is usually over quickly and it rarely recurs. In persons with chronic or recurring infection of the ear canal because of skin allergy, hearing loss may result because scar tissue narrows the ear canal opening. In this case, surgery may be necessary to remove the infected skin of the ear canal and eardrum and replace it with healthy skin from another part of the body.

Malignant otitis. A particularly dangerous form of external ear infection occurs in elderly diabetics. This severe infection is usually called malignant otitis or necrotizing external otitis. It can result in death from progressive involvement in the bone of the skull and its major blood vessels and nervous structures. External ear infection in an elderly diabetic requires immediate attention by a specialist (otolaryngologist).

Infections of the Middle Ear and Mastoid

Serous otitis media. A common condition, all too familiar to many parents, is serous otitis media, fluid in the middle ear space. This problem, which in its acute form can produce excruciating earache in children, can cause temporary hearing loss that can become permanent if not treated properly. The fluid accumulation results from obstruction in the eustachian tube, apparently because the tube has not yet developed fully. The muscles and cartilage of the tube are believed to be floppy, leading to improper ventilation and chronic obstruction. The condition appears to run in families, supporting the belief that it is developmental.

The customary symptoms are poor hearing and recurrent ear infections. Fluid usually can be found in the middle ear by an otologist's examination or during a hearing test. Decongestants usually do not help clear the tube, lending support to the theory of developmental lag. Treatment is directed at relieving the hearing loss and halting the parade of infections. An incision is made in the eardrum (myringotomy) to drain the fluid behind it, and a tiny ventilating tube is placed in the incision. Healing seals the tube in place and forms a conduit to ventilate the middle ear space. The tubes as a rule are rejected by the eardrum after a few months. If the condition returns, the tubes may have to be replaced.

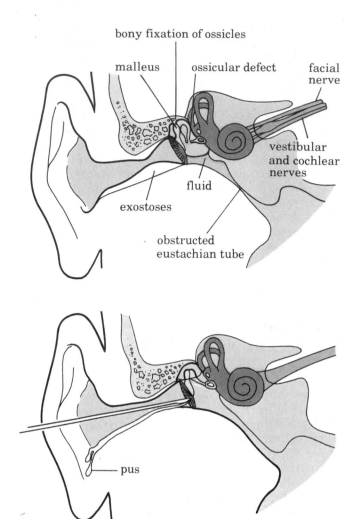

bony fixation of ossicles

malleus   ossicular defect   facial nerve

vestibular and cochlear nerves

fluid

exostoses

obstructed eustachian tube

pus

EAR INFECTIONS

Infection can occur in the external or middle ear. Exostoses (top drawing) are a form of bone overgrowth that narrows or obstructs the external ear canal. Middle ear infection is common in children and can have serious consequences if not treated properly. When the eustachian tube is obstructed, fluid accumulates behind the eardrum, preventing the drum from moving normally and providing a site for infection. An untreated infection can cause a bony fixation of the ossicles. To remove fluid, a myringotomy (lower drawing) is performed to make a tiny hole in the eardrum, equalizing pressure and promoting drainage.

Middle ear infections usually follow an upper respiratory infection of the nose and throat. Although it is possible that bacteria move up through the eustachian tube to the middle ear space, the speed with which the infection occurs suggests that it is probably blood-borne. The symptoms are pain around the ear, high fever, and diminished hearing, caused by the collection of bacteria and pus in the middle ear space and adjoining mastoid-cell compartment. The infection is usually treated first with antibiotics, but if the treatment is not successful, a myringotomy may be necessary to drain the pus. The condition usually clears completely with early treatment, but if treatment is delayed or inadequate, the infection may invade the bone around the mastoid cells. The result, acute mastoiditis, causes swelling behind the ear, high fever, and other signs of serious illness. Before antibiotics, it was often necessary to drain infected bone particles and pus from the mastoid cells via an incision behind the ear, a procedure called simple mastoidectomy. Thanks to antibiotics and early treatment, acute mastoiditis and mastoidectomy are rare today.

Chronic middle ear and mastoid infection may result from an inadequately treated acute ear infection where the drum has ruptured and drained but infection lingers within the membranes. Or it may occur when skin grows into the middle ear and the mastoid through a perforation in the eardrum. The skin may then form a sac or a cyst with a skin lining. The outer layer of cells of the membrane, as they are discarded, accumulate in the sac, liquefy, and produce a foul-smelling ear drainage. This cyst, or cholesteatoma, is able to erode bone. Because of this property and the favorable environment for infection, a chronic inflammatory process is set up. Eventually it may involve such important structures as the labyrinth, facial nerve, and the dural covering of the brain. Although local antibiotic therapy can help to diminish drainage and chronic middle ear and mastoid infections, the only consistent way to restore the hearing mechanism is surgical removal of all infected tissue and repair of the eardrum and middle ear ossicles. In recurrent acute and chronic infections of the middle ear, part or all of the eardrum and various middle ear bones may be destroyed. The destruction can be repaired surgically. The repair, called tympanoplasty, can be undertaken in one of two ways. The first involves repositioning of the middle ear bones so that

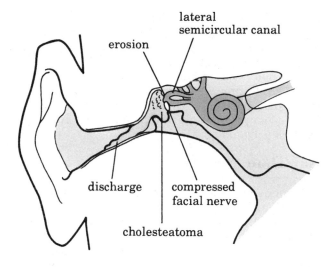

CHOLESTEATOMA

A middle ear cyst, or cholesteatoma, arises when skin grows through an eardrum perforation. Discarded cells from the membrane collect in the cyst and begin to erode the bone. Consequences may be erosion of the semicircular canals, which causes vertigo, or compression of the facial nerve, which causes facial paralysis. The infected area must be removed surgically and the bones and eardrum repaired if necessary.

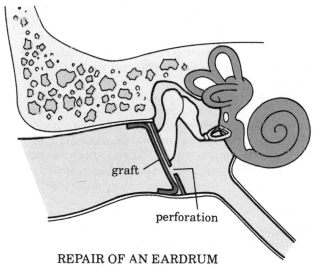

REPAIR OF AN EARDRUM

Tympanoplasty can repair damage to the eardrum caused by infection, cholesteatoma, or a perforating instrument. Tissue is grafted from the temporalis muscle on the side of the head to close the perforation. If the structures in the inner ear work freely, hearing is likely to improve.

contact is made from the eardrum to the stapes bone. The second involves insertion of an artificial strut between the bones still present. The eardrum perforation is closed with a graft from the temporalis muscle on the side of the head. This muscle has a thin but tough fibrous covering and closely resembles the texture of the eardrum. The chances for successful repair of an eardrum are better than 90 percent. If the structures in the middle ear work freely, improvement in hearing may be gained, too.

Inner Ear Infection

Infection of the inner ear is called labyrinthitis and may be caused by bacteria or virus. Symptoms of bacterial labyrinthitis are perceptive hearing loss and sustained vertigo. It usually results from an extension of infection in the middle ear and mastoid compartment, sometimes from an acute middle ear infection. The infectious process usually enters the labyrinth through the oval or round windows or through an opening in the bony labyrinth. Total nerve deafness and loss of balance usually result. However, the important aspect of managing bacterial labyrinthitis is the prevention of the dangerous complication of meningitis by the proper use of antibiotics and drainage of the inner ear.

Viral labyrinthitis usually affects only hearing, not the sense of balance. Commonly, the patient wakes up with a sudden hearing loss. Less commonly, the patient is unaware of the loss until hearing is tested. A few persons have mild disequilibrium, but usually only hearing symptoms are present. Mumps also can affect the ear in this manner. There is no known effective treatment for viral labyrinthitis.

Trauma

Temporal bone trauma may result from a head injury that produces a fracture of the skull. The two types of temporal bone fracture are called longitudinal and transverse. Longitudinal fracture is more common and involves the middle ear and the ear canal. The usual symptoms are bleeding from the ear and hearing loss because of blood in the middle ear space. About one in four persons also suffers facial paralysis. Treatment is usually nonsurgical unless complete facial paralysis has occurred. Surgery is usually recommended if there is conductive hearing loss caused by a tear in the tympanic membrane or dislocation of the middle ear ossicles.

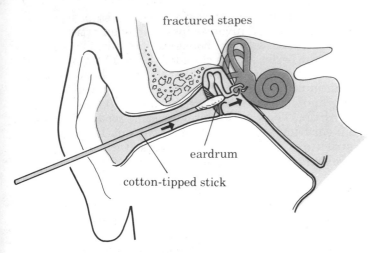

fractured stapes

eardrum

cotton-tipped stick

PERILS OF EAR-PICKING

Using a sharp object to remove wax from the ears can have serious consequences. Even a cotton-tipped swab can penetrate the eardrum and dislocate or fracture the stapes bone. The injury can cause severe pain and bleeding. If it also causes disequilibrium and a staggering gait, emergency treatment is needed.

Transverse fracture of the temporal bone occurs through the inner ear and the internal auditory canal, producing nerve deafness and sustained dizziness. Again, no treatment can preserve inner ear function in this form of fracture. Surgery is reserved for only those cases in which facial paralysis has also occurred.

Direct damage to the eardrum can be produced by a penetrating injury from a toothpick, hairpin, or a cotton-tipped stick inserted into the ear canal and then accidentally pushed toward the eardrum. The usual result is severe pain and bleeding from a laceration of the ear canal skin. Sometimes the tympanic membrane is perforated. If the victim also loses the sense of balance, emergency surgical attention by an otologist is required. This is because the injury has probably dislocated the stapes bone, causing an opening to develop in the inner ear. If this opening is not repaired early, the patient may lose hearing.

Acoustic trauma occurs when high-energy sound waves damage the hair cells of the inner ear. If this happens repeatedly, permanent nerve deafness can occur. Usually the first exposure leads to a temporary loss of hearing which gradually returns over a period of hours. This is referred to as a "temporary threshold shift" and indicates that the noise is harmful to the sensitive inner ear. Repeated exposure to the same noise level can bring

irreversible hearing loss caused by hair cell degeneration. Once that happens, no treatment can restore hearing. Prolonged high-intensity noise (registering 85 to 90 decibels or above) should be avoided in occupational or social environments. Electronically amplified music has been shown to damage the inner ear in this way, and some rock musicians have become permanently deaf.

Ear Damaging Drugs

Various antibiotics belonging to the family of aminoglyocides are considered ototoxic, meaning they can damage the structures and function of the ear. The common offenders are neomycin, kanamycin, dihydrostreptomycin, vancomycin, streptomycin, and gentomycin. Neomycin, kanamycin, dihydrostreptomycin, and vancomycin primarily damage hearing, attacking the hair cells of the cochlea and causing a loss of ability to discriminate high tones. Once it occurs, the loss worsens with prolonged use of the drug and is irreversible. Decreased kidney function allowing buildup of the damaging drug in the bloodstream can accelerate the process.

Streptomycin and gentomycin are different. They affect balance before they affect hearing. The symptoms of streptomycin and gentomycin damage initially are loss of coordination and balance caused by destruction of the hair cells of the balancing organs. Once the drug is stopped and the vertigo has disappeared, the patient can regain a sense of equilibrium with the aid of vision and sensors in joints. If the drug is continued, nerve deafness may occur, too, as the auditory labyrinth becomes involved. Nevertheless, streptomycin has been useful in the management of disorders of disequilibrium when it is felt that both inner ears are abnormal and it is desirable to destroy the balancing organs to preserve hearing in both ears.

Other commonly used drugs with ear damaging potential are aspirin and quinine. Aspirin is toxic in prolonged high doses, greater than 15 to 20 tablets per day. Only the auditory system is affected, and hearing can be restored even after several years. Quinine produces a nerve hearing loss which is irreversible and which may be transmitted from a pregnant woman to her fetus.

Birth Defects

The birth defects that are treatable affect the auricle and external auditory canal of the outer ear. The most common are failure of the outer ear to develop (agenesis) or development of a very small outer ear (microtia). These are usually accompanied by a closed or absent external-ear canal (atresia). An abnormally small outer ear can be reconstructed by a series of plastic operations. But these multiple procedures are time-consuming and frequently the results are less than satisfactory. Lack of an external auditory canal when the inner ear is normal presents a conductive hearing loss, but this can be treated surgically or by use of a hearing aid. Surgery is usually reserved for cases where both ears are involved. When the opposite ear is functioning normally, surgical treatment is not required because it adds little to overall hearing ability and carries the risks of facial nerve and inner ear damage. When a child is born with both external ear canals closed, a hearing aid is used early in life to help language development and sound perception until the child is older. Even the most successful surgery, however, produces less than normal hearing and surgical repair of middle and outer ear malformations depends on the presence of a normal inner ear. Defects of the inner ear are not treatable. They range the entire spectrum from severe, with total loss of hearing, to mild, with hearing virtually normal.

Tumors of the Temporal Bone

The most common benign tumor of the external auditory canal is a bony growth that results from swimming in very cold water. Repeated formation of bone produces mounds that narrow the diameter of the ear canal. At first the mounds produce only a feeling of blockage or a tendency toward recurrent external ear inflammations but ultimately they may fuse, producing a conductive hearing loss. Surgical removal is usually successful.

The most frequent malignant tumor of the external auditory canal and the middle ear occurs primarily in the elderly—skin cancer arising from lining of the ear canal. This form of malignancy may result from chronic infection, another especially good reason for the early and complete eradication of ear infection. The indications of malignancy are pain and bleeding from the ear canal. Early diagnosis and treatment either by surgery or radiation is essential to eradicate the malignancy.

The most common tumor of the temporal bone surrounding the ear, however, is a benign growth called a glomus jugular tumor which arises in the middle ear space. The initial symptom is usually a pulsating ear noise (tinnitus) accompanied by hearing loss. Careful examination of the eardrum and structures behind it along with X rays of the temporal bone confirm the diagnosis. The tumor is usually removed surgically unless it is so large that an operation might endanger the patient's life. In that case radiation therapy may be used to slow tumor growth.

An unusual tumor in the temporal bone arises from the eighth hearing and balance nerve in the internal auditory canal. These benign tumors are called acoustic neurinomas and begin in the cells surrounding the nerve

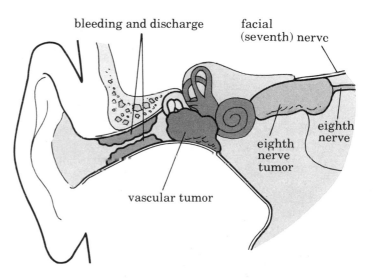

bleeding and discharge

facial (seventh) nerve

eighth nerve

eighth nerve tumor

vascular tumor

TUMORS OF THE EAR

Tumors may arise in the external, middle, or inner ear. Benign or malignant growths may occur in the bone or the skin of the external ear canal, producing blood and discharge. They may be treated with surgery or radiation. A benign vascular tumor which develops in the middle ear space can cause hearing loss or pulsating noises in the ear. An acoustic neurinoma, a tumor of the eighth cranial nerve, begins in the cells surrounding the nerve fibers. It can cause both hearing loss and imbalance. If not removed, it may grow toward the brainstem, causing serious complications.

fibers. The first symptoms are usually nerve deafness with noise in one ear. A few persons have minor episodes of disequilibrium over a period of years. When the tumor is small, it occupies only the internal auditory canal, producing hearing and imbalance symptoms. As the tumor grows larger, it expands toward the brainstem and neurosurgery becomes necessary to prevent serious complications.

Degeneration of the Inner Ear

Degeneration of the hearing and balance organs of the inner ear is a common consequence of the aging process. Everyone knows someone aged 50 or 60 who has lost some hearing, particularly in the high frequencies. As the degeneration of the inner ear hair cells and nerve fibers continues, a greater portion of the hearing spectrum is involved. As more nerve fibers are lost, the ability to understand speech is lost, too. Unfortunately, the only effective way to restore hearing is by use of a hearing aid.

When and how much hearing we lose is largely determined by how much our parents and grandparents lost. But other traumatic events during life—exposure to noise or injurious drugs, for instance—are also involved.

Dizzy spells and loss of coordination may also result from degeneration of the various vestibular sense organs. The condition cannot be treated. The elderly victim must avoid situations where sudden loss of equilibrium could cause injury.

Conditions of Unknown Cause

Otosclerosis is a formation of a bone overgrowth for unknown reasons in the region of the oval window, thus limiting movement of the stapes bone (stirrup). Since the stapes bone transmits sound pressure waves from the tympanic membrane across the ear to the inner ear fluids, impairment of its piston-like movement produces a gradual conductive hearing loss. This hearing loss usually begins in the 20s and 30s, is more common in women than men, and frequently shows a hereditary pattern. Loss is gradual and progressive. Both ears are usually affected. Victims are otherwise normal, with few ear infections, and can usually hear well

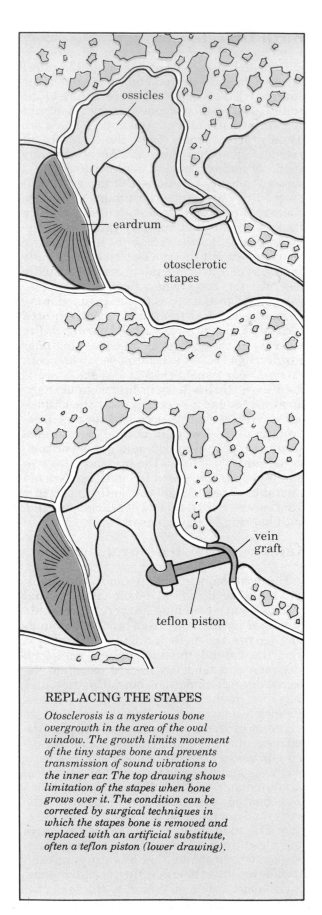

ossicles

eardrum

otosclerotic stapes

vein graft

teflon piston

REPLACING THE STAPES

Otosclerosis is a mysterious bone overgrowth in the area of the oval window. The growth limits movement of the tiny stapes bone and prevents transmission of sound vibrations to the inner ear. The top drawing shows limitation of the stapes when bone grows over it. The condition can be corrected by surgical techniques in which the stapes bone is removed and replaced with an artificial substitute, often a teflon piston (lower drawing).

over the telephone if the sound has been amplified. A hearing aid can help, but surgery is preferable because it is usually successful. An operation called a stapedectomy is carried out under local anesthesia through the ear canal. After the tympanic membrane is elevated, the stapes bone is removed and an artificial substitute—a piston or a tiny bit of wire—is inserted into the oval window. Hearing returns immediately. The sudden restoration of hearing is dramatic and rewarding. The chances of success are better than 90 percent.

Meniere's disease, another mysterious condition, involves both the hearing and balance organs. In this disorder, a patient has both a hearing loss and episodes of vertigo, usually a feeling that the world is spinning. The episodes last from one to several hours. The severe vertigo usually is accompanied by nausea and vomiting. The person is usually completely well between attacks, and many say hearing also improves between attacks. Hearing is often worst during or soon after an attack of dizziness.

Meniere's disease occurs usually in only one ear, and has its onset in middle or later life. Its most dangerous consequence is that the dizzy, spinning feeling may strike without warning, potentially endangering the person's life. Not surprisingly, many Meniere's patients lead extremely anxious, tense lives, fearful of the sudden attacks of vertigo.

Although the cause of Meniere's disease is uncertain, it is known that a buildup of fluid occurs in one of the compartments in the inner ear. When the membranes containing the accumulated fluid reach a breaking point, they rupture and release a substance that poisons the balancing and hearing nerve fibers, which causes the symptoms. Repeated healing and rupturing of the membranes lead to the recurring vertigo and the fluctuating hearing loss. Although many medications have been recommended, no drug has a proven effect on either the hearing loss or the vertigo of Meniere's disease. However, symptoms may be somewhat controlled with sedatives. Most surgical forms of treatment are designed to relieve the vertigo by eliminating either the sense organs or the nerve fibers to the balancing sense organs.

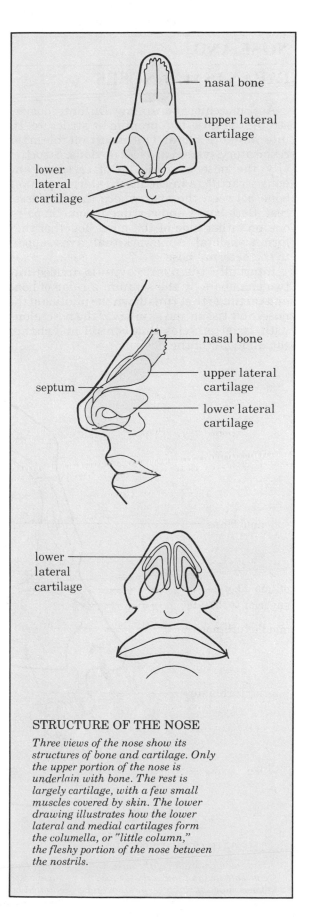

STRUCTURE OF THE NOSE

Three views of the nose show its structures of bone and cartilage. Only the upper portion of the nose is underlain with bone. The rest is largely cartilage, with a few small muscles covered by skin. The lower drawing illustrates how the lower lateral and medial cartilages form the columella, or "little column," the fleshy portion of the nose between the nostrils.

NOSE AND

PARANASAL SINUSES

As Pinocchio and Jimmy Durante demonstrate, the nose is a prominent structure. Its internal workings and its important role in the respiratory system are less obvious. Structurally, the nose is made up of cartilage and bone—cartilage in the most external portion, bone between the eyes where the eyeglasses rest. Both bones and cartilages come in pairs, one on either side of the nose. Together they form a skeletal framework that gives support to the external nose.

Internally, the nasal cavity is divided into two chambers by the septum, a ridge of bone and cartilage that runs down the midline of the nose. Soft tissue and skin cover the nose, along with facial muscles that control and change the diameter of the nostrils.

The respiratory function takes place in the nasal cavity. It is literally the place where the respiratory system begins, and its job is to prepare inhaled air for entry into the lungs. The inside of the nose is made up of extensive areas of mucous membrane. Most are concentrated in three scroll-like structures called turbinates at the back of the nose. These projections from the nasal cavity are rich in blood vessels and mucous glands. As the air passes their membranes, it is moistened by the glandular secretions and warmed by the circulating blood. This air conditioning system is the reason the lungs are not chilled even by the coldest air of winter, and may explain why Europeans have longer noses than the broad, flat ones of many Asians and Africans. The European needs more membrane area to warm the chill air than does a resident of the tropical zone.

The nasal cavity also houses a filtering and cleansing system. Hairs in the nostrils and

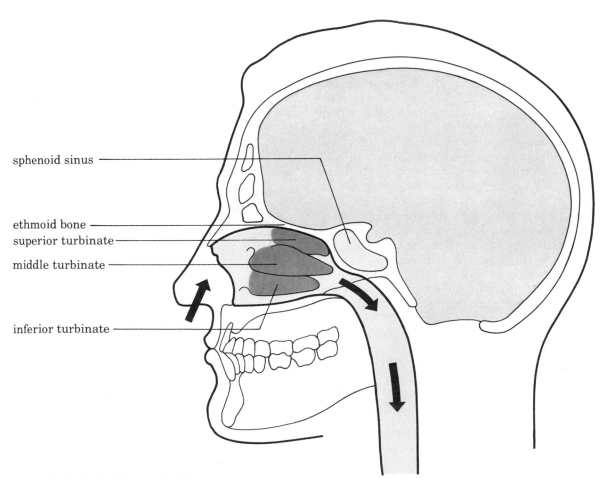

sphenoid sinus

ethmoid bone
superior turbinate

middle turbinate

inferior turbinate

THE "AIR CONDITIONER"

Mucous membranes of the nose, concentrated in three scroll-shaped bones called turbinates, moisten and warm inhaled air on its way to the lungs. These spongy tissues are rich in blood vessels and mucous glands. The ethmoid bone forms the floor of the brain and the roof of the nasal cavity.

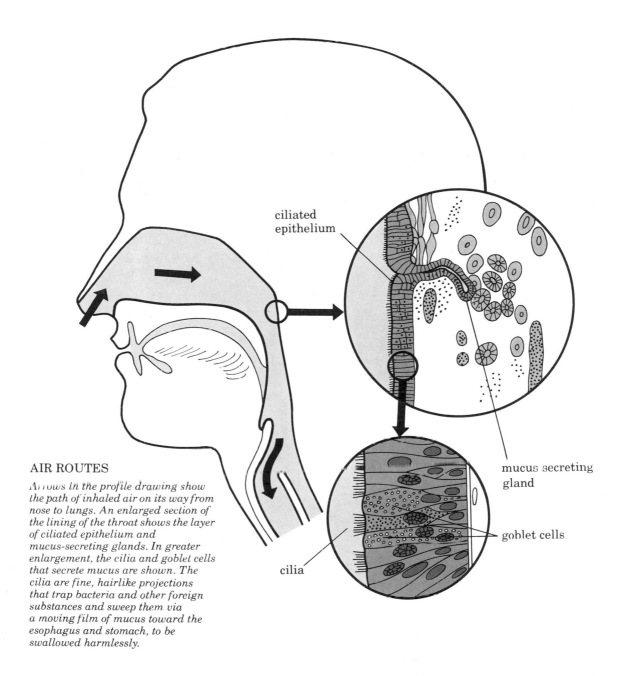

ciliated epithelium

mucus secreting gland

goblet cells

cilia

AIR ROUTES

Arrows in the profile drawing show the path of inhaled air on its way from nose to lungs. An enlarged section of the lining of the throat shows the layer of ciliated epithelium and mucus-secreting glands. In greater enlargement, the cilia and goblet cells that secrete mucus are shown. The cilia are fine, hairlike projections that trap bacteria and other foreign substances and sweep them via a moving film of mucus toward the esophagus and stomach, to be swallowed harmlessly.

finer ones within the cavity catch particles in the air before they can reach the lungs (as your soiled handkerchief discloses after a few hours in a smoky, dirty atmosphere). They also remove bacteria from the inhaled air. The nasal secretions contain substances called lysozymes which destroy the trapped bacteria. The particles, the dead bacteria, and more resistant species are then carried to the back throat by sweeping motions of feathery projections called cilia, where they are swallowed harmlessly and pass into the stomach.

In addition to respiration, a vital function of the nose is smell, or olfaction. The smell receptors are located in the top portion of the nasal cavities. They are approximately one-half inch square and have a yellowish tinge, in contrast to the surrounding pink tissues. The millions of tiny nerve endings of the olfactory nerve pass through the cribiform plate and form the first cranial nerve to the brain.

In order to be detected by the olfactory nerve, odors must be airborne and soluble enough to be dissolved in the mucous secretions of the nose. The air currents of the nose are designed to carry volatile odors toward the

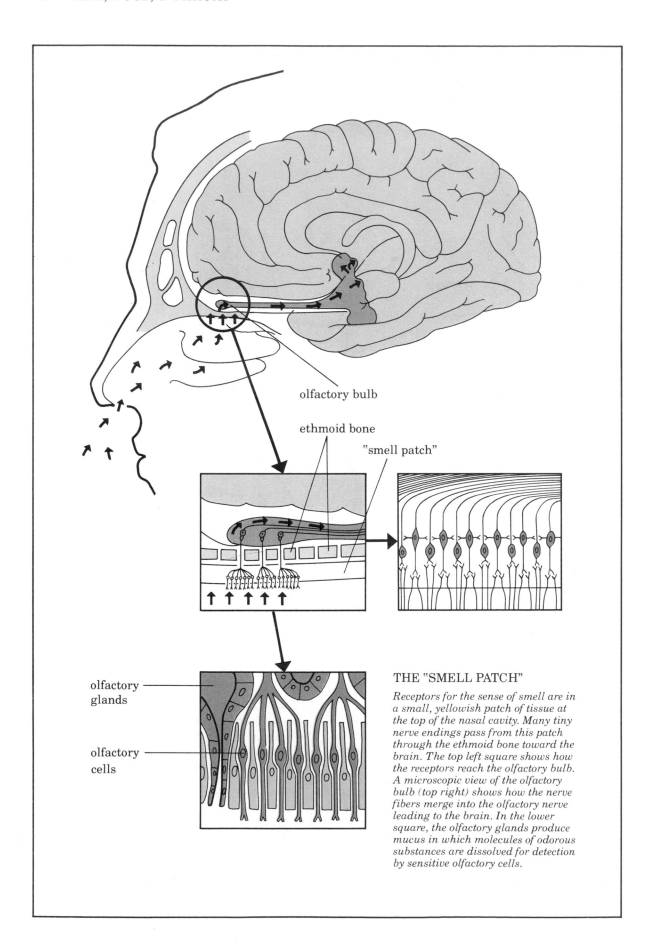

olfactory bulb

ethmoid bone

"smell patch"

olfactory
glands

olfactory
cells

THE "SMELL PATCH"

*Receptors for the sense of smell are in
a small, yellowish patch of tissue at
the top of the nasal cavity. Many tiny
nerve endings pass from this patch
through the ethmoid bone toward the
brain. The top left square shows how
the receptors reach the olfactory bulb.
A microscopic view of the olfactory
bulb (top right) shows how the nerve
fibers merge into the olfactory nerve
leading to the brain. In the lower
square, the olfactory glands produce
mucus in which molecules of odorous
substances are dissolved for detection
by sensitive olfactory cells.*

top of the nose (where the smell receptors are located) in an arc-like fashion before passing into the nasopharynx. We may lose the sense of smell (a condition called anosmia) because of a simple obstruction in the nose, such as when congestion from a cold swells the membranes of the nose, or when viruses attack the olfactory nerve and destroy the nerve endings.

The sense of taste is closely related to smell, although the sense organs of taste are located in a far removed area, the tongue. Taste buds are not the minute protuberances or papillae that we see on the surface of the tongue, but are microscopic cellular structures located within the tissue of those papillae. There are about 250 taste buds per papilla, but the number gradually diminishes with age to about 90 per papilla. The sense of smell has no way of classifying different types of odors, but taste can be broken down into four sensations: bitter, salt, sweet, and sour. They are distinguished by taste buds in particular surface areas of the tongue. For example, salt is perceived along the tip and front sides of the tongue. Sweet is detected further back on the sides, sour along the sides in the rear. Bitter is sensed farthest back, across the base of the tongue.

Although the functions of taste and smell are separate at the level of their sense organs, the central pathways mix, so one is dependent on the other. When an abnormality in taste occurs, smell is also affected, and when an abnormality of smell occurs, taste is affected. This explains why a cold in the nose interferes with our ability to taste food.

The senses of smell and taste enhance our enjoyment of the delicate odors and subtle flavors around us, but their proper function is far less important (and far less developed) than in other animals. Nevertheless, they have a protective function, alerting us to possible danger, such as leaking gas or contaminated food. It is best to keep them in good repair.

The Paranasal Sinuses

The paranasal sinuses are a series of air spaces filling the bones of the face. They are extensions of the nasal cavities. Their exact function is not known, but it is thought that by forming air spaces within the bones of the skull, they lighten and perhaps strengthen the skull. The sinuses also add a source of mucus to humidify the inhaled air.

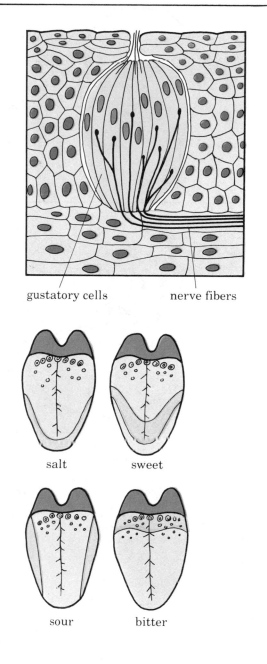

gustatory cells   nerve fibers

salt   sweet

sour   bitter

THE SENSE OF TASTE

A single taste bud is sensitive to only one of the four primary sensations of taste. The taste buds of the tongue are not uniformly distributed. The lower drawing shows the location of buds sensitive to salt, sweet, sour, and bitter tastes. The top drawing, a cross section through a taste bud, depicts how dissolved substances on the surface make contact with spindle-shaped cells, producing impulses that travel over nerve fibers to the brain.

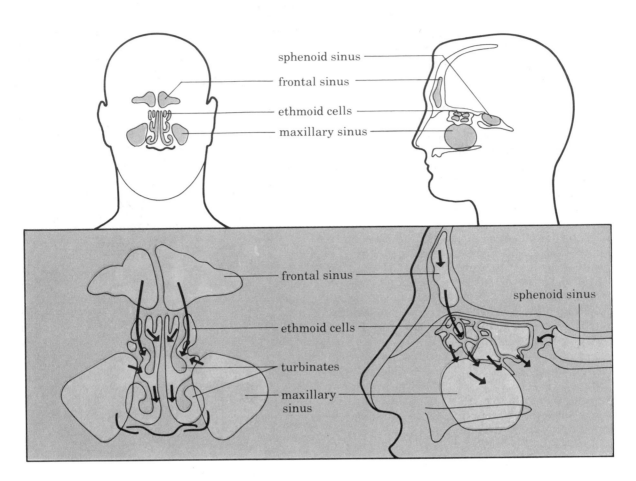

sphenoid sinus

frontal sinus

ethmoid cells

maxillary sinus

frontal sinus

sphenoid sinus

ethmoid cells

turbinates

maxillary sinus

PARANASAL SINUSES

The four major sinuses and their locations are: The frontal sinuses above the eyes and behind the root of the nose, the ethmoid sinuses at the root of the nose between the eyes, the sphenoid sinus in the center of the

skull, and the maxillary sinuses in the cheekbones. The lower drawing shows the direction of drainage from the sinuses, all of which normally drain into the nasal cavity.

There are four major pairs of sinuses, one-half of each pair lying on either side of the midline of the face. Their mucous membranes are a continuation of the nasal mucous membrane, and they open into the nasal cavity by means of tiny openings called ostia.

The frontal sinuses lie in the bone above the eyes and behind the root of the nose. They vary greatly in size and sometimes are completely absent. (Their absence seldom seems to be noticed.)

The ethmoid sinuses form a labyrinth of five to 15 small areas separated by thin bony partitions at the root of the nose between the eyes. They surround the opening into the frontal sinus and extend to the rear to the sphenoid sinus.

The sphenoid sinus is in the center of the head and surrounds the pituitary gland.

The maxillary sinuses develop separately from the ethmoid and sphenoid sinuses and are located in the cheekbone under the eye. Each one has roughly the shape of a pyramid although considerable variations occur. This sinus, because it is close to the roots of the teeth, can cause dental symptoms when it becomes infected. Conversely, infection of the roots of the upper teeth can produce an infection in the sinus.

Disorders of the Nose and Paranasal Sinuses

Injury. Because of its prominence on the face, the nose is particularly subject to injuries. Most involve only the cartilage, but injury to the nasal and facial bones is not uncommon. Fracture of the nasal bones or dislocation or fracture of the septum calls for the prompt attention of a physician, because failure of these injuries to heal properly can lead not only to a misshapen nose but to malfunction of the nasal airway. A broken nose is usually reset by simply elevating the bones into place, but sometimes it is necessary to wire the fractured segments together to maintain position.

Nosebleed (epistaxis) is the nasal injury most of us are most familiar with. Bleeding may result from a direct blow to the nose, from nosepicking, drying of the mucous membranes, or violent sneezing or nose-blowing. Most nosebleeds involve damage to the small blood vessels in the lower septum, so bleeding is forward, out of the nostrils. These anterior nosebleeds usually can be controlled by pinching the nostrils together, as if clamping them with a clothespin. Five to ten minutes of pressure will usually halt most minor nosebleeds. However, if bleeding cannot be controlled by pressure or if blood flows backward into the throat, packing by an otolaryngologist may be needed to control the flow. This may require three or four days of hospitalization until the blood vessel has clotted. If bleeding still does not stop, it may be necessary to tie off the artery.

Some people, especially children, have recurrent minor nosebleeds. These should be brought to the attention of a specialist. In rare cases, repeated nasal bleeding may indicate the presence of a tumor. More commonly, simple measures are required to prevent the recurrence. The usual treatment is to cauterize the offending vessels of the septum. Less commonly, the artery is tied off.

Infection. Breathes there an American man, woman, or child who is not familiar with nasal infection? The common cold, with its streaming nose, watery eyes, and (often) hacking cough, is the most ubiquitous of ailments. Its technical name (or rather the name for the symptoms it produces) is rhinitis, inflammation of the nasal mucous membranes. If the infection obstructs the sinus openings or spreads into the sinuses, it is called sinusitis.

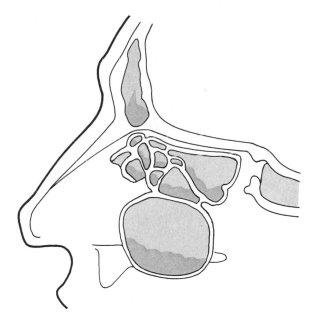

CLOGGED SINUS

Thick, infected secretions may collect in any of the sinus cavities if drainage is obstructed, producing pain. The first aim of treatment is to provide free drainage. The infection frequently develops from a nasal infection and may be acute or chronic.

Acute rhinitis or sinusitis may be caused by a viral infection, a bacterial infection, or both. Besides the running nose, the person may also develop a fever. The nasal discharge may be thick and yellow, rather than clear. In sinusitis, there may be pain in the area of the face over the sinuses. Often the collected fluid or pus and thickened mucous membranes may be visible in the sinuses by X ray.

Rhinitis and sinusitis are treated primarily with antibiotics (mainly to prevent secondary bacterial infection in cases of viral rhinitis) and decongestants to shrink the mucous membranes and allow better drainage of the sinuses. Viral rhinitis is usually self-limiting.

If a sinus infection is not treated, is treated inadequately, or recurs, changes may occur in the mucous membranes, producing a chronic sinusitis. The result is intermittent pain and

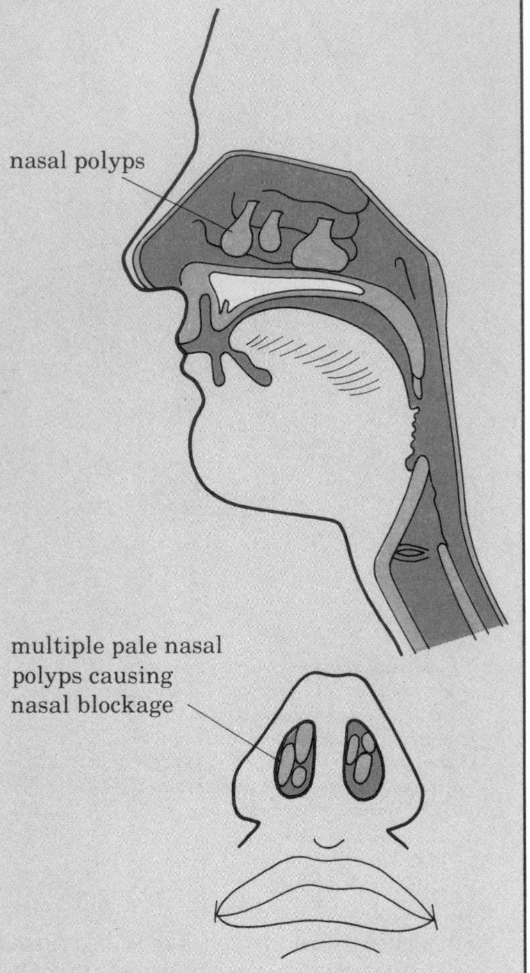

nasal polyps

multiple pale nasal
polyps causing
nasal blockage

NASAL POLYPS

*Nasal polyps, a common nasal
outgrowth, are soft, pendulous
growths from lining membranes of the
nose. Polyps are often associated with
allergies. If they become extensive
enough to block passage between the
nose and paranasal sinus, they must
be removed surgically.*

Tumors. Most tumors of the nose are benign. The most common are nasal polyps, which are extensions of swollen sinus mucous membranes caused by a nasal allergy such as hay fever. These enlarge gradually over a long period of time and produce varying degrees of nasal obstruction. If they become extensive, they may block the passage between nose and paranasal sinuses and produce a secondary paranasal sinusitis. When this happens, the polyps must be removed surgically. Since they largely arise from the ethmoid sinus, cleaning it out (ethmoidectomy) is necessary to achieve lasting control of the polyps. Medical control of the allergic process which produced the polyps in the first place is also necessary to prevent their recurrence.

A second benign tumor of the nose is called inverted papilloma and arises from the lining of the nose and ethmoid sinus. It may well be the result of a virus infection. This tumor, although benign, should be removed promptly to relieve obstruction and avoid the possibility of malignant change.

Malignant tumors may involve the sinuses, most commonly the maxillary sinus, but also the ethmoid and the frontal sinuses. The first indication is usually a painless enlarging deformity of the bone over the involved sinus and obstruction of nearby structures such as the tear duct (causing tearing), compression of eye muscles (causing double vision), or compression of nerves (causing numbness). Bleeding from the nose is also a cardinal sign. If the malignancy is confirmed by biopsy, it is usually treated by a combination of radiation therapy and surgery.

PHARYNX AND LARYNX

The throat portion of the ear-nose-throat is also known as the pharynx. Usually, the mouth to which it adjoins is included in that term, too. The pharynx is a long muscular tube that extends from the back of the nose into the swallowing tube (esophagus). It is generally divided into the nasopharynx, oropharynx, and hypopharynx. Each level has its own important function.

headaches over the sinuses, plus a persistent drainage from the nose. X rays show thickened mucous membranes and sometimes bone damage. Surgery may be necessary to remove the inflamed and infected mucous membrane. Prompt treatment is important, because meningitis and brain abscess can result, particularly from infections in the frontal, sphenoid, and ethmoid sinuses.

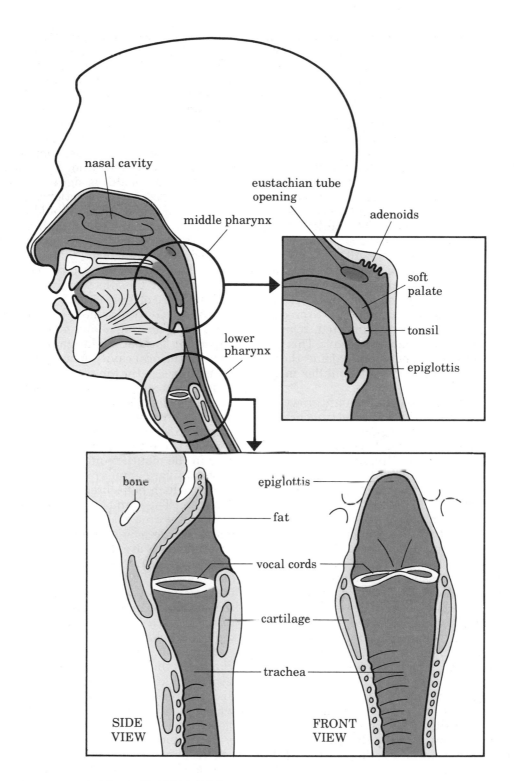

NOSE AND THROAT

Important features of the nose and throat and their interrelationship are shown above. The enlargement at upper right shows the middle pharynx, also known as the tonsillar area. Below, two views of the lower pharynx show how speech and breathing are controlled. The vocal cords are two muscular bands that contract when we swallow to prevent liquids or solids from entering the lungs. They also rhythmically control the expulsion of air from the lungs into the mouth and throat, where it is formed into words or sounds.

The nasopharynx, located above the soft palate and behind the nose, connects the nasal cavity and the oropharynx. It therefore has a function in the breathing process. The eustachian tubes that ventilate the middle ears connect to the nasopharynx on both sides. Thus, a blockage in the nasopharynx may obstruct the airway, the eustachian tube, and middle ear.

Adenoid. The most common tissue mass to block the nasopharynx is the adenoid. It is a normal mass of lymphoid tissue which during childhood infections may greatly enlarge and obstruct the nasopharynx. The child usually compensates by breathing through the mouth. Snoring is a common result of enlarged adenoids and the obstruction also can cause fluid to collect in the middle ear space, producing a conductive hearing loss. If the adenoid mass becomes large enough to produce such symptoms or becomes infected, removal (adenoidectomy) becomes necessary. This procedure is performed under general anesthesia. The adenoids usually become smaller in the teen years.

Angiofibroma. A second benign growth of the nasopharynx is a blood-vessel tumor called an angiofibroma. This tumor is unusual because it occurs only in adolescent boys. The usual symptoms are difficulty in breathing through the nose, recurrent nosebleeds, and a bulging deformity of the cheek if the tumor has extended into the sinuses. Although these tumors are benign, they should be removed because they destroy the surrounding tissue. Removal is accomplished through the nose or through the back of the throat. Because of the potential for excessive loss of blood, the operation must be carried out by an experienced surgeon in a major hospital center.

The oropharynx forms the rear portion of the oral cavity. Its main purpose is swallowing. The major problem here arises from the tonsils, masses of lymphoid tissue that occur at the junction of the oropharynx and the oral cavity.

Children's tonsils normally enlarge and become inflamed during periods of infection. The enlargement may partially obstruct the throat and interfere with swallowing or breathing.

Sometimes a secondary infection arises in the inflamed tissue, and persists after the original infection has subsided. This condition, called tonsillitis, often includes severe sore throat, high fever, earache, difficulty swallowing, and swollen lymph nodes in the neck.

Tonsil infections decrease as the child grows older, but tonsillectomy during early childhood has become one of the most common surgical procedures. It is usually not recommended unless the child's health is significantly affected by severe, recurrent infections. Doctors disagree about when tonsils should be removed. However, most ear, nose, and throat surgeons consider the occurrence of four to five documented cases of bacterial tonsillitis a year for more than three successive years sufficient indication for tonsillectomy (see chapter 27, "Taking Care of Your Child").

The oral cavity also has roles in chewing and speaking. The tongue and mouth muscles are important for both. Malignant tumors may occur in the oral cavity, usually on the floor of the mouth or in the tongue. The first indication is usually a sore or irritation, sometimes accompanied by bleeding. A sore area, especially in a person who smokes and drinks heavily, should be examined carefully if the soreness persists three to four weeks. Any suspicious area in the mouth requires a biopsy.

The salivary glands provide the saliva in the mouth, which helps break down food and aids digestion. The glands are located primarily in the parotid area near the ear and in the submaxillary area at the angle of the jaw. The parotid glands are the largest salivary glands, and being near the surface, show swelling quite readily. The most common problems are benign tumors, painless masses, or lumps in the cheek or in the front of the ear. They usually are removed surgically to prevent malignant change.

Mumps is a viral infection of the salivary glands. In the past, it was a common and often serious illness of childhood, but it has nearly disappeared in the United States because of widespread immunization. Bacterial infections of the salivary glands usually are treated with antibiotics.

The submaxillary glands sometimes develop stones which obstruct the flow of saliva. The gland swells, particularly during eating. Repeated obstructions are often accompanied by infection and pain, in which case the gland probably should be removed surgically.

The hypopharynx is the lower part of the pharynx and also contains the larynx. Its functions are primarily in swallowing and speaking. Malignant tumors sometimes develop in the swallowing area, or a sac (diverticulum) may collect food. Either can cause difficulty in swallowing. Anyone who has a swallowing problem that persists for more than four weeks should be examined by a specialist.

The larynx is the cartilaginous box felt in the front of the neck as the Adam's apple. It is the entrance into the trachea and the lungs. Its main functions are speech, respiration, and protection of the airway during swallowing.

The vocal cords of the larynx are two muscular bands that contract during swallowing to prevent solids or liquids from entering the lungs. This is the primary function for which the larynx was designed. In higher forms of life, including man, these vocal cords are trained to control the expulsion of air from the lungs into the mouth and throat. These puffs of air are formed into sounds or words by the tongue, lips, and cheek muscles.

The larynx also has a respiratory role. It separates the vocal cords to allow inhaled air to enter the trachea and lungs.

The main problems that affect the larynx relate to hoarseness or breathing difficulty. The specialist examines the larynx by inserting a small mirror into the patient's mouth to look at the vocal cords while the patient breathes and speaks. In this way the doctor can determine whether a tumor or infection is present.

The most common problem with the larynx is infection (laryngitis). Laryngitis refers to an inflammation of tissues around the larynx which produces spasm of laryngeal muscles. The result is hoarseness and discomfort or pain in the throat. Laryngitis of bacterial origin can be treated with antibiotics, by inhaling steam, or simply by resting the voice.

A special form of laryngitis, laryngotracheitis, occurs in infants and is called croup. It results from a virus infection that causes the cords to swell and narrows the space between them. This condition usually occurs in children one year old or younger, when the diameters of the larynx and trachea are still very small. Even a slight swelling will produce significant airway obstruction, called stridor. The child will have a blocked nose, breathe noisily, have a "croupy" cough and a low grade temperature. Croup is potentially life threatening and medical attention should be sought immediately (see chapter 27, "Taking Care of Your Child"). Cortisone and antibiotics may be given to reduce the swelling. A tracheotomy or intubation become necessary if the swelling does not recede.

Another form of infection in the child larynx is epiglottitis, an infection of the upper part of the larynx over the vocal cords. Loose membranes in this part of the larynx may swell and completely obstruct the larynx above the vocal cords. A bacterial infection is usually responsible. Epiglottitis occurs primarily in children aged two to four and almost always requires a tracheotomy or intubation because of a threat to the airway.

In adults, a common condition is polyps of the vocal cords, representing accumulations of mucous membrane and fluid producing hoarseness. They may result from prolonged shouting, such as at a football game, talking too much, or from inhaling cigarette smoke. These polyps should be removed surgically.

Cancer of the vocal cord is also associated with cigarette smoking, particularly heavy smoking accompanied by heavy drinking. This form of cancer strikes about 9,000 Americans a year, the overwhelming majority of them white men in their 50s and 60s, and most of them city-dwellers. The rate has been rising gradually for several decades, although not as rapidly as lung cancer.

Persistent hoarseness is the primary symptom of vocal cord cancer. Any hoarseness that lasts longer than four weeks should be investigated by a specialist to search for a growth on the vocal cord margin. When the cancer is small and limited to the vocal cord, chances for cure are more than 90 percent and may be achieved by radiation therapy alone. Sometimes removal of the vocal cord (partial laryngectomy) also may be effective in treating the cancer and preserving a fairly normal voice.

If the tumor or the cancer has been neglected for many months and involves not only the vocal cord but other regions of the larynx, complete removal of the larynx (total laryngectomy) is necessary. After such an operation, the trachea is brought out to the skin as a permanent opening into the windpipe, and the swallowing tube is sutured closed so that the person may eat normally. The swallowing tube is used to develop a substitute form of speech called esophageal speech. The person is trained to swallow air into the stomach, then belch it up into the mouth to be formed into words by the tongue and mouth muscles. At least two-thirds of those whose larynxes have been removed can learn esophageal speech.

The lymph nodes of the neck are glandular structures that drain the mouth, throat, and the larynx and provide a mechanism for the body to limit the spread of infection or tumor from these areas. Enlarged lymph nodes in the neck not associated with infection should be viewed suspiciously as reflecting a primary tumor somewhere in the pharynx, larynx, or nasopharynx. Such a lymph node or lump in the neck, if persistent, should be seen as soon as possible by an otolaryngologist.

PLASTIC SURGERY

OF THE FACE

Plastic or cosmetic surgery is performed primarily for appearance, not to improve function. The most common plastic surgical procedure is rhinoplasty, or surgery to change the shape of the nose. Most deformities of the nose, even conspicuous ones, do not interfere seriously with the health of the owner. And many deformities are so slight that the nose can be considered normal-looking for all practical purposes. Nevertheless, even a deformity that appears minor to others may justify correction on the basis of improving the owner's psychological well-being, or because a new nose may advance his or her career. Entertainers in particular may feel that they fare considerably better professionally with a more attractive nose.

A competent ear, nose, and throat surgeon or plastic surgeon can correct large and small deformities of the nose. A bony hump, a large nose, a wide nose, or irregularities of the nasal tip may be corrected by surgery to remove the bone and cartilage forming the deformity. Incisions are made within the nostril so that scars are not visible later. By separating the skin from the nasal bone and cartilage, the surgeon saws or chips away at the bone and reshapes it by fracturing and remolding the structures.

In deformities such as a saddle nose, where a loss of tissue exists, bone grafts or cartilage grafts from other parts of the body may be inserted. This surgery is performed under local or general anesthesia and requires hospitalization for three to five days. A protective splint or cast is placed over the nose until scar tissue can begin to anchor the grafts. The patient may have a swollen nose and blackened eyes for a week to 10 days. Patients usually are able to return to work two weeks after surgery.

The nasal septum divides the nose into two cavities and is almost always tilted to one side or the other to varying degrees. Most nasal septal deviations do not interfere with breathing enough to require correction. However, the nasal septum must be altered routinely during plastic surgery of the nose, so any deviation is corrected at that time, both to improve the airway and to remake the septum to accommodate the newly shaped nose. The bone and cartilage are removed and replaced in a straightened position.

An uncommon but obvious deformity of the nose that can be surgically corrected quite successfully is rhinophyma, the huge, reddish, bulbous nose made famous by comedian W. C. Fields. This condition is caused by an overgrowth of the sebaceous glands under the skin of the nose (see chapter 7, "The Skin"). Surgery consists of shaving down the excess tissue and allowing new skin to grow over the shaved area.

OTOPLASTY

Many persons are born with one or both ears protruding because of failure of the ear cartilage to form curvatures or to form them adequately. These "dumbo" ears often are the target of ridicule, especially in childhood. Protruding ears can be successfully "pinned back," with significant psychological gains. It is generally agreed that surgery should be carried out before the child enters school. The most common age is about four or five.

The surgery consists of removing excess skin in the groove behind the ear, then exposing the cartilage of the ear by elevating the skin on the back surface of the ear so that the cartilage may be handled. The surgeon then breaks the spring of the cartilage in the area where a fold is to be formed, and the cartilage is sewn into the desired position. This procedure is done under general anesthesia and requires hospitalization for only a few days. However, a protective dressing is usually worn for a week until the sutures are removed. The operation is rarely performed on an adult, although there is no age limitation.

Congenital absence or gross malformation of the outer ear can be corrected surgically, but a large number of surgical procedures are needed. They involve imbedding cartilage under the skin step by step to build a structure resembling an ear. The finished product is not a perfectly normal ear, but it supports glasses and takes away the stigma of a completely absent ear.

A number of surgical procedures are effective in dealing with the effects of aging on facial skin. The skin loses elasticity with age, and parts of the face droop. Excessive wrinkles about the eyes and forehead, sagging cheeks and chin, and formation of excess skin, sometimes with bags of fluid under the eyes, are common in the older face. Two common and effective surgical procedures are blepharoplasty (removal of bags under the eyes) and face-lift.

Blepharoplasty consists of removing the excess skin and carefully suturing the remaining defect in a horizontal fashion to minimize the scar. This operation can often be carried out in the surgeon's office under local anesthesia. Face-lift consists of undermining the facial skin through an incision strategically located in the hairline or around the ear so it will not be noticed. The surgeon separates the skin from the underlying tissues and draws it up tight like a lampshade, removing the excess skin and suturing the incision. A total face-lift can be carried out under local or general anesthesia and requires hospitalization for a few days. A partial lift can be done under local anesthesia in an office. No face-lift is permanent, because the aging process continues, but repeat lifts can be done with success.

CLEFT LIP AND CLEFT PALATE

A cleft in the lip or the palate results from stunted development of the bones and soft tissues of the mouth sometime before birth, probably in the sixth to eighth week of prenatal life. The exact cause is unknown, and may vary from case to case. It is probable that a hereditary factor, however distant, may play a role, or that a maternal infection or illness during the sixth to eighth week of pregnancy is instrumental.

The usual cleft is limited to one side of the palate midline and extends into one nostril. In addition to the speech defect that may occur later, feeding difficulties usually occur in infancy because milk backs up into the nose.

Cleft palate can be corrected in one or several stages, depending on the age of the child and the magnitude of the defect. Surgery consists of bringing the tissues together by means of carefully planned incisions and flaps. It is preferable to repair the cleft quite early, when the baby is healthy and gaining weight. Surgery not only corrects an obvious functional defect, but boosts parental morale by eliminating the deformity.

The end results of cleft-palate surgery are so good that there is no excuse for such a defect to go uncorrected in a young patient healthy enough to tolerate the operation. Speech therapy is usually necessary afterwards to help the child form sounds through the coordination of muscles of the palate and mouth. The follow-up treatment usually involves a team of plastic surgeons, ear, nose and throat surgeons, plus dental, speech, and hearing specialists. Afterwards the cleft-palate patient may develop problems of fluid accumulation in the middle ears because of the involvement of muscles that open the eustachian tube. These problems are usually corrected by draining fluid and inserting a ventilating tube.

CHAPTER 14   DONALD B. LUCAS, M.D.

THE
BONES
AND
MUSCLES

Anyone who watches a ballerina glide effortlessly across a stage or an athlete perform a seemingly impossible feat of skill is witnessing the human body performing at the peak of perfection. It is the musculoskeletal system that allows these highly trained individuals to perform, just as it enables all of us to carry out the multitude of tasks associated with daily living.

Bodily movements depend upon the coordinated use of bones, ligaments, muscles, tendons, fascia and bursae, and their associated nerves and blood vessels, all of which constitute the musculoskeletal system. These tissues are subject to wear and tear, injury, and diseases that make themselves known to us as pain, weakness, and deformity. While doctors talk in scientific terms, patients think in terms of "sore elbows," "aching backs," and "feet that are killing me."

THE SKELETON

The bones of the body form the basis of the musculoskeletal system. They house and protect the soft parts of the body, and enable the body to maintain posture. Their joints, or articulations, allow for mobility.

The muscles that attach to the bones are the motors which furnish the power for all bodily movements. Electrical impulses sent out from the spinal cord cause the muscles to contract in an organized fashion. As the muscles shorten during contraction they pull on the lever-like bones through leaders called tendons, causing the bones to move against one another at the joints. For each set of muscles that produces motion in one direction, there is another set to reverse the motion. For example, one group makes a fist and another set extends the fingers. Another example is the biceps and triceps combination of the upper arm. The biceps flexes the forearm and the triceps extends it. Precision movements usually require both sets of muscles acting in unison, one shortening and the other lengthening, to provide the utmost control.

The bones have other jobs. They contain blood-forming elements in their marrow cavities constantly at work turning out red blood cells. Other cells are busy forming new bone or repairing defects.

The skeletal framework has a central or axial component consisting of the skull, backbone, ribs, and pelvis. These house the vital organs essential to life. Attached to the axial skeleton are the extremities, the arms and legs, which make up the appendicular skeleton.

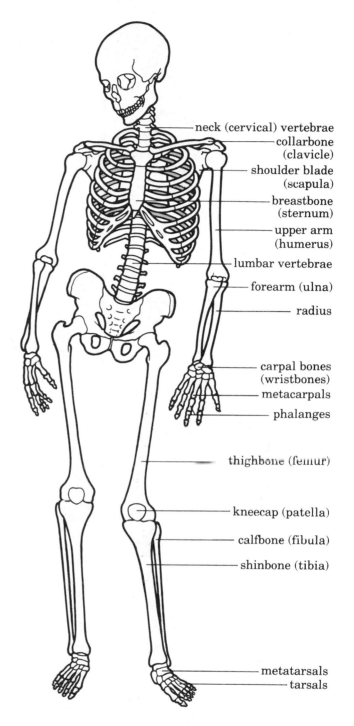

neck (cervical) vertebrae
collarbone (clavicle)
shoulder blade (scapula)
breastbone (sternum)
upper arm (humerus)
lumbar vertebrae
forearm (ulna)
radius
carpal bones (wristbones)
metacarpals
phalanges
thighbone (femur)
kneecap (patella)
calfbone (fibula)
shinbone (tibia)
metatarsals
tarsals

THE HUMAN SKELETON

The human skeleton consists of 206 bones, the most prominent of which are designated above. Names given to groups of bones include the spine, pelvic girdle, shoulder girdle, rib cage, and skull. The spine rests on the pelvic girdle and supports the shoulder girdle, rib cage, and skull. Some bones are separate at birth but fuse as we grow older.

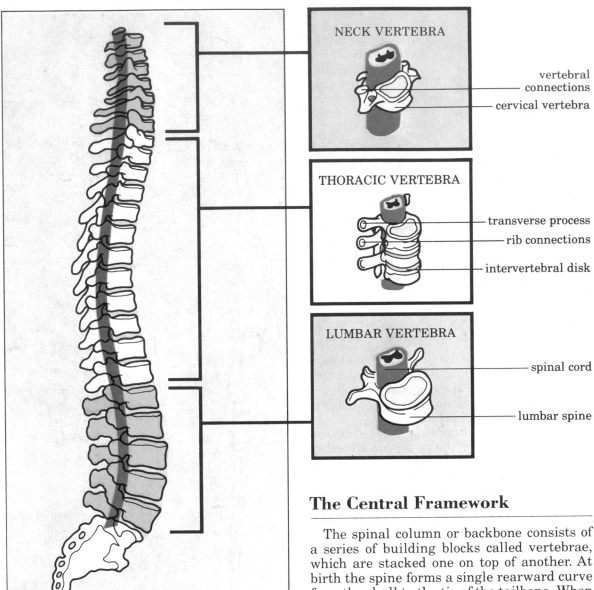

NECK VERTEBRA

vertebral connections

cervical vertebra

THORACIC VERTEBRA

transverse process

rib connections

intervertebral disk

LUMBAR VERTEBRA

spinal cord

lumbar spine

THE SPINE

The spine has four curves that give it stability. The seven topmost vertebrae constitute the cervical or neck section, which supports the head. A representative vertebra at upper right illustrates the vertebral body and connections to adjoining vertebrae. The middle or thoracic vertebrae anchor the rib cage. The transverse process, rib connections, and intervertebral disk are shown in the representative section. Heavier vertebrae make up the lumbar spine. They rest on the fixed sacrum, five vertebrae that have fused early in life. The vertebral cross section at lower right shows the placement of protection for the spinal cord.

The Central Framework

The spinal column or backbone consists of a series of building blocks called vertebrae, which are stacked one on top of another. At birth the spine forms a single rearward curve from the skull to the tip of the tailbone. When the infant gains enough strength to hold up the head, a reverse curve develops in the neck region. When the infant can stand erect, a similar curve forms in the lower back. The resultant four curves add stability to the spine and enable it to accommodate adjacent soft tissues.

A single vertebra is roughly circular with a flat top and bottom. Bony projections called processes provide attachment for muscles. Accommodation is made for the spinal cord by two processes that project rearward around the cord before uniting to form the familiar spinous process readily felt when the finger is run up the middle of the back. Each vertebra has two small articulations projecting downward and upward called intervertebral facets. They guide and limit intervertebral (between the vertebrae) motion.

Between the vertebrae, pads of elastic and stiff cartilage act as shock absorbers and permit motion in all directions. These pads are called intervertebral disks. A healthy disk is about the size and shape of a cookie, with an outer ring of dense elastic covering a center of gelatinous material. The disk sucks in fluid from the surrounding tissue. While we are upright during the day, the fluid is partially squeezed out, causing a slight decrease in height. It is regained while we sleep and we are restored to normal height in the morning. It is this structure that often gives way to aging and stress so that it presses against spinal nerves and causes varying degrees of pain, weakness, and numbness.

Special terms are applied to the areas included in the curves of the spine. The cervical or neck region has seven vertebrae. The topmost and tiniest of these is the atlas, which carries the head. Below the cervical region is the thoracic segment of 12 vertebrae to which 12 pairs of ribs are attached. The topmost 10 pairs end in cartilage at the front and are attached to the sternum or breastbone. The lowest two pairs do not attach in front and are called floating ribs. It is not unusual to have 11 or 13 pairs of ribs. Extra ribs attached to the bottom cervical vertebra are called cervical ribs. These may press on spinal nerves and cause tingling, numbness, or weakness in the arms and hands.

The five lowest movable vertebrae complete the backbone and comprise the lumbar area. The lowermost vertebra rests on the sacrum, which is composed of five vertebrae that fuse into one solid bone early in life. The junction between the movable lumbar spine and the fixed sacrum (lumbosacral joint) is the site of great strain and wear and tear. Pain here is

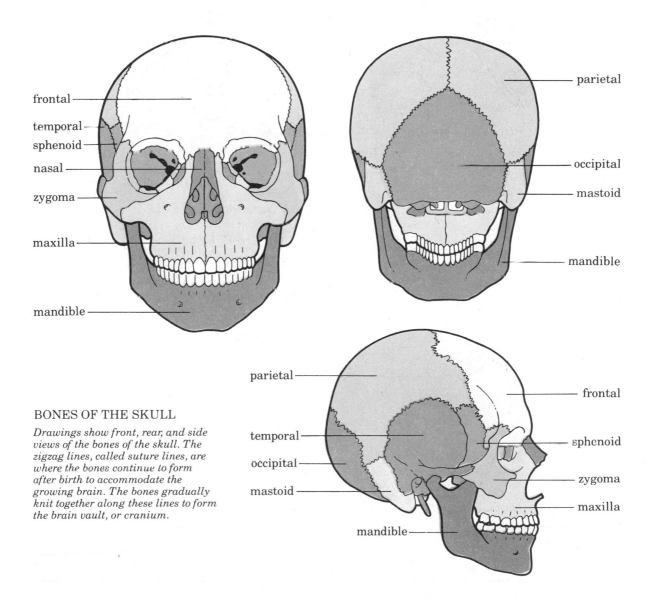

BONES OF THE SKULL

Drawings show front, rear, and side views of the bones of the skull. The zigzag lines, called suture lines, are where the bones continue to form after birth to accommodate the growing brain. The bones gradually knit together along these lines to form the brain vault, or cranium.

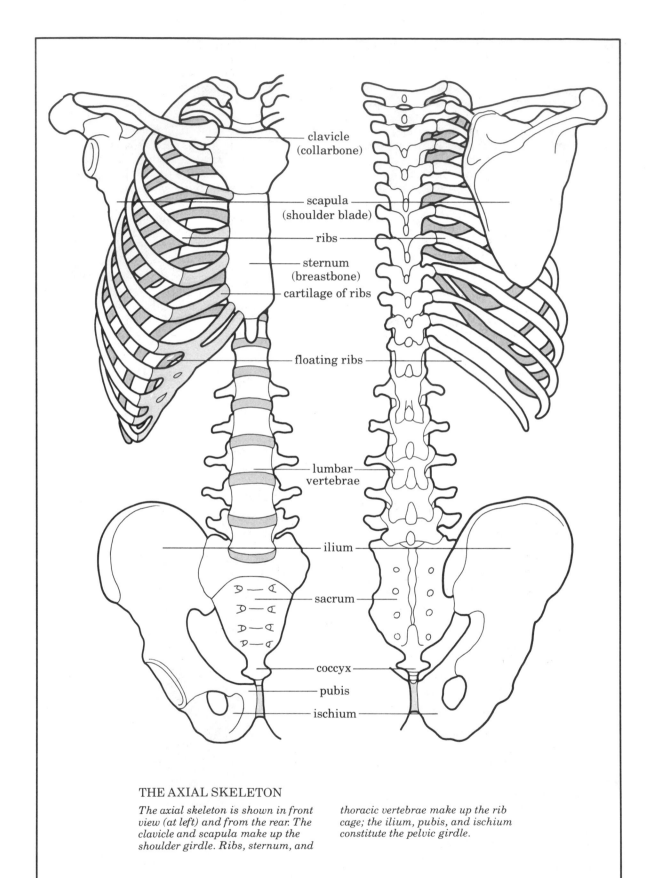

clavicle
(collarbone)

scapula
(shoulder blade)

ribs

sternum
(breastbone)

cartilage of ribs

floating ribs

lumbar
vertebrae

ilium

sacrum

coccyx

pubis

ischium

THE AXIAL SKELETON

The axial skeleton is shown in front view (at left) and from the rear. The clavicle and scapula make up the shoulder girdle. Ribs, sternum, and thoracic vertebrae make up the rib cage; the ilium, pubis, and ischium constitute the pelvic girdle.

common, giving rise to the terms "lumbago" and "acute and chronic low back strain." Below the sacrum is the tiny tailbone or coccyx, which curves forward. It, too, is made up of small fused segments, but slight motion does occur between the sacrum and the coccyx so that the joint sometimes becomes sprained.

The skull perched on top of the spinal column contains 22 bones (plus six more if the tiny ossicles of the middle ear are included). The brain vault or cranium is composed of eight flat bones knitted together in irregular suture lines. A newborn infant's skull is quite pliable and the familiar "soft spots" or fontanels are cranial areas where bone has not yet formed. Suture lines are points at which bone continues to grow as the cranium develops to accommodate the enlarging brain.

In all, the adult complement of bones numbers 206. We "lose" approximately 60 bones by fusion as the skeleton matures. We have so many bones, each with its medical name, that it is hardly possible or even useful to try to remember them. It is more practical to refer to the drawings on page 305 if you want to locate certain bones in your body or remind yourself that the tibia is the shinbone.

The Appendages

The appendicular skeleton is concerned with locomotion and manipulation—moving about and handling things. The joining of the bones in the extremities (the arms and legs) is for the most part quite different from that in the axial skeleton. Capping the ends of the bones is a smooth, glistening, rubber-like cartilage that enables the bones to move easily on each other. These synovial joints are lubricated by a few drops of slippery fluid secreted by the synovial membrane surrounding the joint. Outside the synovium are stout bands of elastic tissue (ligaments) that bind the bones together to prevent dislocation and limit motion. Muscles attach to bones by means of tendons placed at intervals to take advantage of the leverage provided by the bones. Broad bands of fibrous tissue called fascia frequently reinforce joints, act as muscle attachments, or otherwise separate the extremities into compartments. Bursae are thin-walled sacs containing a few drops of fluid that are located between soft tissue and bony parts to prevent wear. The various joints are designed so that by their shape and bindings they act as hinges, balls and sockets, slides, or pivots.

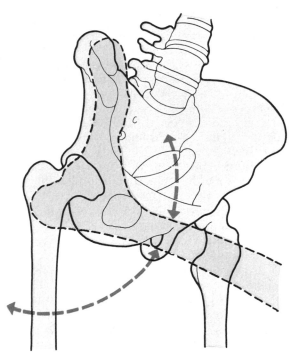

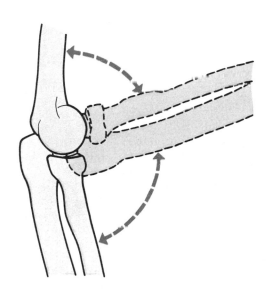

TWO TYPES OF JOINTS

Two types of joints are the ball-and-socket of the hip (top) and the hinge of the elbow. Arrows show the range of motion permitted by each joint. In the ball-and-socket joint, the rounded head of the thighbone, called the femur, fits into a cup-shaped cavity, the acetabulum, in the pelvis. As the femur moves, the head of the thighbone rotates in its socket. The hinge of the elbow permits the forearm to be raised or lowered. It also allows the forearm to be rotated, as in turning the palm up or down.

The upper extremity is suspended from the axial skeleton by muscles. This arrangement provides maximum mobility. The shoulder blades (scapulae), which provide shallow sockets (glenoids) for the upper arm bones (humeri), "float" freely on the upper chest wall under muscle control. The collarbones (clavicles) also lend support through their muscle attachments, but they hinder motion by holding the arms away from the body. Animals of the cat family have no collarbones and can bring their shoulders together, allowing them to squeeze through narrow spaces.

Each lower extremity is attached to the body by means of a deep socket (acetabulum) in the pelvis which provides maximum stability, in contrast to the mobile upper extremity. The pelvis is composed of three pairs of fused bones. The easiest to recognize is the ilium, which has a crest that bulges outward and which is often called the hip, although the true hip joint is several inches lower. Uniting the two ilia behind is the sacrum. The union forms the two sacroiliac joints, which are tightly bound and seldom cause pain in spite of the cry, "my aching sacroiliac." We sit on the ischia, and the two pubic bones complete the circle in front.

THE STRUCTURE
OF BONE

A pillar of long bone is much stronger than reinforced concrete, much lighter, and more flexible. Two types of bone work together—compact or hard bone, and spongy or cancellous bone. Bones are commonly classified as flat, such as those in the skull; or as long and hollow, such as those in the legs.

A long bone like the femur, between the hip and knee, has a hard, tubular outside and an internal cavity filled with marrow. Flat bones have two layers of compact bone enclosing a spongy middle. The bulging ends of long bones are honeycombed with spongy bone. There appears to be no rhyme or reason to the helter-skelter arrangement of tiny pockets, but the thin walls are arranged along stress lines to give the greatest weight-bearing strength.

Disregarding water, bone is about two-thirds mineral and one-third organic matter—chiefly the protein collagen. Elements are so intimately mixed that if minerals are dissolved out by acids, leaving the organic material, the bone retains its shape but is much too soft to support stresses. Similarly, if the organic matter is removed by heating, the remaining minerals preserve the original shape but the bone crumbles to ashes at a touch.

Whole bone is a community of living cells that are impregnated with mineral salts.

Nearly all bone surfaces are covered by a tough membrane called the periosteum. Bone cells receive nourishment from blood vessels that weave through the periosteum and reach the spongy interior directly or through an intricate network of tiny canals. Nerve fibers follow similar routes. The periosteum is where we feel sensations when the bone is subjected to pain or pressure.

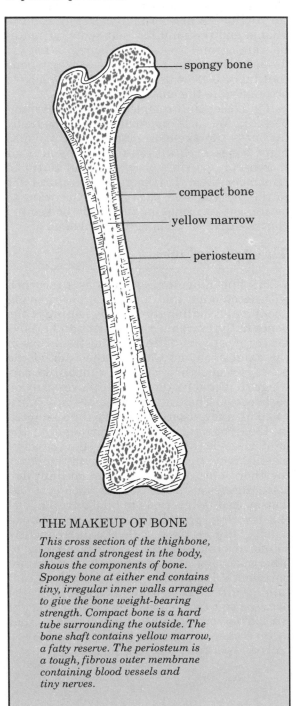

spongy bone

compact bone

yellow marrow

periosteum

THE MAKEUP OF BONE

This cross section of the thighbone, longest and strongest in the body, shows the components of bone. Spongy bone at either end contains tiny, irregular inner walls arranged to give the bone weight-bearing strength. Compact bone is a hard tube surrounding the outside. The bone shaft contains yellow marrow, a fatty reserve. The periosteum is a tough, fibrous outer membrane containing blood vessels and tiny nerves.

Growth and Repair

Bone grows and repairs itself in complicated ways. In essence, certain cells secrete the bony matter and many become imprisoned in it. At the same time, other cells dissolve away bits of bone and help to sculpture materials to the proper shape. This simultaneous bone-building and bone-destroying process goes on within the bone itself. The ends of long bones of children, sites of active growth, are separated from the main bone by a layer of cartilage. Cartilage does not turn into bone, but is replaced by bone. At about age 20, the cartilaginous growth plate becomes a part of the larger bone. Then the bone grows no longer and the subject no taller.

When a bone is broken, lacerated tissues pour out sticky secretions which stiffen into a bulgy deposit. Little by little, bone-making cells from the periosteum and fractured bone ends penetrate the deposit of secretions and replace it with spongy bone (callous) which holds the injured parts more firmly in place. This in turn is removed gradually by bone-dissolving cells, with the spongy bone slowly replaced by hard bone.

Red Cells and Minerals

In small children, the hollow central shafts and the ends of the long bones contain red marrow. As the bones mature, the red marrow in the shaft is gradually replaced with yellow marrow, which is composed mostly of fatty material. Red marrow is where red blood cells are manufactured in prodigious numbers, not at a rate of thousands per minute, but millions. These stupendous factories are located in spongy bone, such as in the ends of long bones and spongy parts of flat bones of the skull, ribs, pelvis, breastbone, and spine. Yellow marrow does not have immediate cell making duties. It serves an important part of the body's fatty reserve.

We need a certain amount of calcium to keep the heart beating, contract muscles, and help blood to clot. Most of our calcium is stored in the skeleton in complex combinations with phosphorus and tiny amounts of a few other minerals. But the skeletal warehouse is not a mere repository. Its salts are constantly seeking an equilibrium with the rest of the body, an equilibrium that is never attained for long. Consequently, there is a continuous scurrying of traffic into and out of the skeleton—first a deposit of calcium is received, later a with-drawal order arrives for calcium to be delivered to the blood supply, perhaps to spark the heartbeat or help muscles do their work.

In short, the concept of bones as dull, inert girders and pillars, as unchanging and uninteresting as concrete, is far from the truth. Bone is living tissue that is constantly undergoing changes and being reabsorbed and reconstructed. It may seem rigid, but is remarkably plastic, and any continued pressure can cause bone to change its shape. The bones of children are especially pliable and to a limited degree usually respond to measures necessary to correct defects.

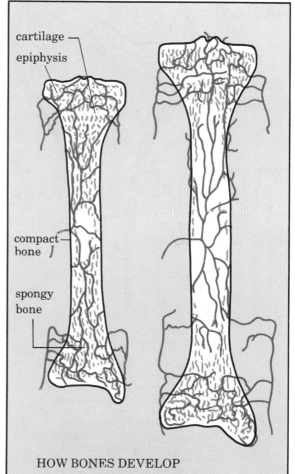

cartilage
epiphysis
compact bone
spongy bone

HOW BONES DEVELOP

The young developing bone at left shows epiphysis, bone separated in early life from the long bone by cartilage. It also shows spongy bone being replaced by cartilage, and compact bone taking form on the exterior. In the drawing at right, the epiphysis has united with the main bone, the marrow cavity has enlarged, and the deposit of compact bone has thickened. Blood vessels traverse the covering membrane and the bone matrix.

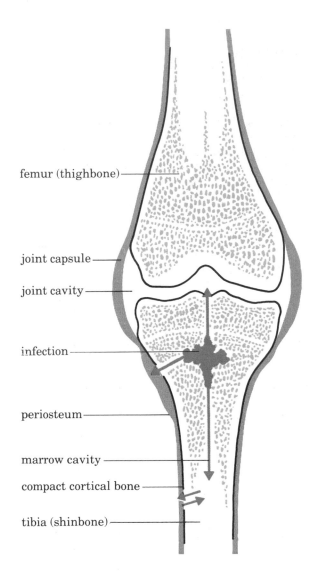

femur (thighbone)

joint capsule

joint cavity

infection

periosteum

marrow cavity

compact cortical bone

tibia (shinbone)

BONE INFECTION

*Infection within a bone (osteo-
myelitis) is far less common than
in the past, thanks to antibiotics, but
it still can be a dangerous disease
if not detected and treated. Commonly
caused by bacteria carried in the
bloodstream, osteomyelitis usually
occurs in the long bones of children,
such as in the knee joint shown
above. The arrows show how the infection, once lodged, spreads from the
spongy bone of the tibia into the joint
cavity, compact bone, periosteum, or
marrow cavity. From the marrow
cavity the infection can spread
throughout the body.*

DISEASES OF THE BONE

Osteomyelitis

Osteomyelitis is an infection resulting from the growth of germs within the bone. The long bones are most often affected in children, and the short, flat bones of the spine and pelvis are most often affected in adults.

In children the infection usually is caused by staphylococci and less commonly by strep-tococci. The germs may reach the bone through the bloodstream (hematogenous), from an infection elsewhere in the body, by direct spread from infected tissues near the bone, or as the result of a wound or open fracture.

The first symptoms of hematogenous osteo-myelitis are usually pain and tenderness near a joint. The pain increases rapidly in intensity so that children may refuse to move the af-fected limb. Fever follows; illness is evident. The signs and symptoms are usually sufficient for a doctor to make the diagnosis. Changes may not appear on X ray for eight to ten days. To wait for X-ray signs to confirm the diag-nosis is to wait too long.

Treatment. Before the introduction of an-tibiotics, acute hematogenous osteomyelitis was a dangerous and crippling disease. Today, antibiotics have revolutionized treatment, and mortality has been reduced to less than one percent. However, unless osteomyelitis is treated promptly with antibiotics, the symp-toms may be masked, the signs suppressed, and the infection may become chronic. If local signs do not begin to subside within a day after starting antibiotic treatment, the site of in-flammation must be opened for drainage.

Cases of acute hematogenous osteomyelitis that are diagnosed late show extensive local destruction of bone and associated soft tissue abscesses. Unfortunately, extensive infection is difficult to control, and chronic osteomyeli-tis with draining pus may be present for years.

A complication of acute osteomyelitis is spread of the infection into one or more joints (septic arthritis). Fluid from the joint must be sampled by aspiration and the bacteria iden-tified. Antibiotics are administered intrave-nously or directly into the affected joint. Surgical drainage of the joint is necessary in some instances.

Another possible complication of acute or chronic osteomyelitis in children is retarda-tion of growth because of damage to the car-tilage of long bones.

Osteoporosis

Osteoporosis is abnormal porousness or "thinning" of bone caused by insufficient production of the protein in which calcium salts are deposited. The most common type is "post-menopausal osteoporosis," occurring in a large proportion of women after natural or artificial menopause. There may be no symptoms until some area of fragile bone fractures with only slight provocation, such as a crushed vertebra resulting from bending or a relatively minor jolt. "Senile osteoporosis" occurs to some degree in all aging persons. In advanced stages, deformities of the spine resulting from collapsed vertebrae are not uncommon.

Hormone deficiencies are primarily involved, but there are many contributing causes. They include poor nutrition for many years, or poor assimilation at the bone-forming site even though the diet is good, menopause and aging, prolonged bed rest, immobilization, inactivity, impaired blood supply to bone, or various diseases such as forms of rheumatoid arthritis.

Treatment depends upon the stage and nature of the osteoporosis, and upon remedy of underlying factors if possible. Sex hormones are commonly prescribed, and a substantial protein diet, sometimes with minerals to assist calcification, although this requires careful supervision by a physician because excessive mineral intake can harm the kidneys, especially of an immobilized patient. Activity to the extent that it is tolerated is encouraged, but precautions must be taken to prevent further fractures. In osteoporosis of the aged, the patient should be regarded as being marked "fragile, handle with care."

Osteomalacia

Osteomalacia is also called "adult rickets." Bone changes are similar to those of childhood rickets, except that they are more diffuse because there are no special areas of growth in adults. In its simplest form, osteomalacia is a deficiency disease, rare in the United States, but it may also result from impaired assimilation of nutrients when the older person's body, for reasons unknown, can no longer properly use certain substances from food. Treatment with a high calcium, high phosphorus diet and vitamin D usually gives prompt and often dramatic relief from the disease.

Paget's Disease

(osteitis deformans)

This is a relatively common bone disease among persons over 40 years of age. It is a chronic process of bone overgrowth, destruction, and new bone formation. In the course of the disease, bone becomes deformed and its internal cellular architecture disordered. The patients often have arteriosclerosis and impaired blood supply to the bones. The disease is not diffuse but "spotty," with a predilection for bones of the spine, skull, and lower leg. The onset is insidious so some patients do not seek medical help for years. The disease might become arrested or progress slowly. Spontaneous fractures may occur but heal normally. A hearing aid frequently becomes necessary because of damage to ear bones. There is no specific treatment, but some measures can relieve pain.

THE SPINE

Posture. Because the joints of the spine and appendages are flexible, posture is an ever-changing state rather than a static condition. It is partly a matter of choice, as demonstrated by a soldier at attention versus one at ease. If the body is held in a rather fixed position over a period of months and years, ligaments and muscles tend to contract so that a relatively fixed posture develops. The rigidity usually can be overcome but only with persistent exercises. The best posture is one that satisfies the emotional and intellectual needs of the individual and leaves the body feeling as relaxed as possible.

Changes in posture are controlled by the abdominal muscles. Weak and flabby abdominal muscles allow the pelvis to tilt downward, which results in a swayback in the lumbar region and a round back in the thoracic region. When the abdominal muscles tighten or contract, the lumbar curve flattens and the thoracic spine extends, giving the body an alert attitude.

The erect spine is under stress at all levels, but the stress increases progressively from top to bottom. The greatest stress is between the lowermost lumbar vertebra and the sacrum. A swayback or sagging spine is often a source of chronic postural pain because the ligaments are stretched and more weight is borne on the small facet joints than was intended. Decreasing the lumbar curve by strengthening the abdominal muscles usually will correct the painful condition. Persistent swayback deserves an examination by a physician.

Low back pain can be caused by a variety of mechanisms. The most common are acute injury or degeneration of the joints, ligaments, muscles, or intervertebral disks.

Referred pain, which is pain that hurts where it does not originate, can be felt in the back as a result of nerve root irritation. Muscles that are in spasm because of attempts to protect some local injury can also become painful. Sometimes the entire back hurts as the victim hunches and stiffens to guard against painful movement.

Acute back sprain is usually produced by a sudden bending of the spine, as in a fall or a "snatch lifting" motion. The force tears ligaments or compresses disks, producing pain and protective muscle spasm. These injuries usually heal in three weeks if protected against further sprains. It is necessary for some patients to wear a corset-like support during the healing period.

Chronic back strain, also called postural fatigue, is a condition in which there is no violent, sudden, precipitating incident, but the structures are subjected to prolonged tension greater than they can withstand. Symptoms usually come on gradually and progressively get worse. The symptoms usually are aggravated if the person is fatigued, but they can be improved by lying down or by physiotherapy.

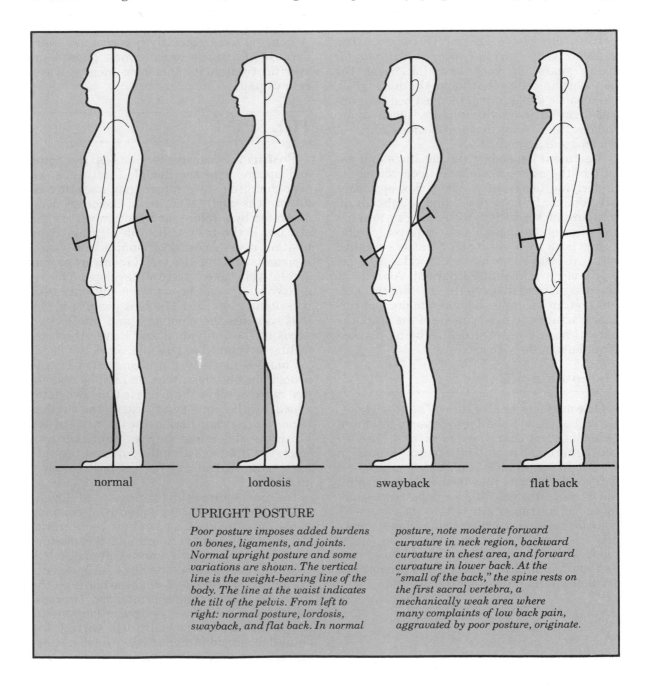

normal   lordosis   swayback   flat back

UPRIGHT POSTURE

Poor posture imposes added burdens on bones, ligaments, and joints. Normal upright posture and some variations are shown. The vertical line is the weight-bearing line of the body. The line at the waist indicates the tilt of the pelvis. From left to right: normal posture, lordosis, swayback, and flat back. In normal posture, note moderate forward curvature in neck region, backward curvature in chest area, and forward curvature in lower back. At the "small of the back," the spine rests on the first sacral vertebra, a mechanically weak area where many complaints of low back pain, aggravated by poor posture, originate.

Treatment is difficult because the main cause for chronic strain is postural fatigue. The outlook is not always good, particularly if it is not possible to change an occupation associated with the strain or if the fatigue results from obesity or severe depression.

Disk trouble. The intervertebral disks are buffers or "shock absorbers" between the bony vertebrae. After age 20 it is normal for disks gradually to degenerate. Less weight is borne on the pulpy central portion and added strain is placed on the sensitive outer casing, giving rise to aching pain. Because the greatest strain occurs in the lower back, the pain usually is confined to that region. As degeneration progresses, the pain is likely to change slightly in location and severity, and may be felt in the legs.

Early degeneration of the disk usually does not cause pain unless strain is added. The strain can be slight but prolonged, such as the strain brought on by sitting during a long automobile trip without getting out frequently to stretch. There is usually only mild local tenderness in the back, and X rays may show nothing abnormal. Treatment should include rest, followed by muscle-strengthening exercises and avoidance of strains.

Ruptured disk or slipped disk. This refers to a specific condition in which the pulpy body at the center of an intervertebral disk ruptures or protrudes through a break in the surrounding casing. When the herniated fragment presses on an adjacent nerve root, severe pain (sciatica) is felt in the buttock, the back of the thigh, and even into the foot. Numbness and weakness may follow. The victim often tilts the body to one side (sciatic scoliosis) to lessen the pain. The sciatic nerve pain is made worse by coughing, straining, sneezing, or jarring movements. The victim finds that it is difficult to make leg movements that stretch the sciatic nerve. Routine X-ray films seldom disclose the level and extent of the slippage. A myelogram (X ray of the spinal canal after injection of a special dye) may be necessary.

Treatment usually consists of simple bed rest. Often symptoms will subside, indicating that a herniation did not occur or that the fragment was small and became walled off. If conservative treatment fails, it usually is necessary to remove the free fragment and the remaining degenerated portion of the disk.

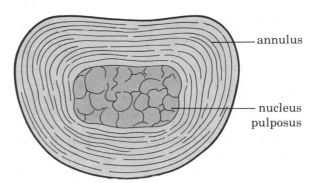

NORMAL DISK BETWEEN VERTEBRAE

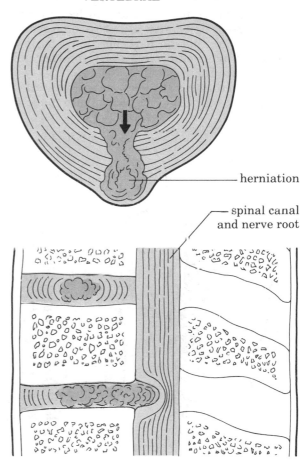

SLIPPED DISK

A "slipped disk" occurs when the intervertebral disk, which acts as a shock absorber between vertebrae, breaks out of its capsule and presses on an adjoining nerve. The top drawing shows a cross section of a normal disk viewed from above. Its nucleus pulposus is contained within its casing. In the center illustration, the casing has ruptured, allowing the nucleus to protrude into a bulge. The side view shows how the bulge impinges on a nearby nerve.

Spondylolisthesis refers to spontaneous forward displacement of a lumbar vertebra caused by a bony defect between the vertebra and the arch that encloses the spinal canal. The defect may be congenital or may have developed in early life. The slippage results from disk degeneration. Spondylolisthesis can exist without any sign of backache and is often discovered accidentally during a routine physical examination.

When symptoms do occur, they usually appear as low lumbar backache with or without accompanying sciatica. Treatment is the same as for disk degeneration. In young, growing children, the spine may have to be fused to prevent gross deformity. If there are no symptoms, a young person need not be restricted. Many teenagers and young adults lead normal lives despite their spondylolisthesis.

Scheuermann's disease, sometimes called "adolescent round back," is a common cause of backache among teenagers. For unknown reasons, growth changes in the thoracic vertebrae give them a wedge-shaped formation which increases the usual thoracic curve. In the active stage of the disorder, which lasts from two to five years, there may be some pain.

This self-limiting disorder is not serious, but may result in an undesirable deformity. Treatment usually involves little more than restriction of activity and back muscle exercises. In severe cases, bed rest followed by the wearing of a spinal brace, or even a surgical fusion, may be necessary.

Scoliosis is a term used to describe a lateral curvature of the spine. It may be associated with a variety of disorders but, basically, it is caused by either faulty bone structure or inadequate supporting muscles. The deformity usually appears in childhood and increases in varying degrees because of uneven growth of the vertebrae. The deformity is usually most noticeable in the thoracic region because the ribs on one side protrude backward and accentuate the normal curve. When normal growth ceases, the deformity stops progressing except for a very small amount attributable to the disk degeneration of aging.

Idiopathic scoliosis is by far the most common type, and is usually first recognized in the prepuberty period. It occurs predominantly in girls. The curve is usually to the right in the chest region and to the left in the lumbar region. Its cause is unknown. A doctor should be consulted as soon as the deformity is recognized because close observation and treatment are necessary to prevent a potentially severe deformity.

Treatment for all types of scoliosis is a combination of exercise, bracing, and surgical fusion, depending on the type, the rate of increase, and the severity of the deformity. At all costs, a severe deformity of the chest is to be avoided because it may encroach on the lungs and increase the workload of the heart, even resulting in eventual heart failure.

Minor deformities can be detected on physical examination. Some schools have screening programs to detect early cases and bring them to the attention of the parents.

Scoliosis sometimes occurs when a person compensates for a sideward tilt of the pelvis produced by a short leg or by an apparent shortening of the leg caused by hip or knee contraction. The scoliosis disappears if the pelvic tilt is corrected before growth alterations occur in the spine.

SCOLIOSIS

Lateral curvature of the spine, called scoliosis, is compared with the normal spine (right). There are several forms of scoliosis, some of which can be corrected with exercise. Other types cause deformity of the bony parts of the spine and require braces or surgical repair.

Torticollis or wry-neck. This deformity of the seven vertebrae of the neck causes a person to carry the head tilted to one side, with the chin thrust forward and pointed toward the opposite side. The muscles on the affected side are contracted. The most common form is found in newborns and is associated with a swelling of the neck muscles that is incorrectly called a tumor. The child's muscles can often be manipulated gently to correct the deformity. If not corrected, it may be necessary later to divide the contracted muscle surgically.

Adult wry-neck is less common. It occurs spasmodically, for reasons not known. This malady, known technically as spasmodic torticollis, does not respond to ordinary therapeutic measures and may be associated with emotional strain. The condition is different from the well-known "stiff neck," in which muscle pain running up one or both sides of the neck may cause the sufferer to hold the neck in a rigid position. The pain of stiff neck may result from tooth pain or from hunching the shoulders to protect against a cold draft. It usually responds well to heat, rest, and aspirin.

Whiplash injuries. "Whiplash injury" is a term that has fallen into disrepute among physicians because it does not describe any specific abnormality or anatomical disorder. It is a general descriptive term such as "dyspepsia" or "lumbago," but it is still used in courts as if it had a specific medical meaning.

The injury usually is sustained in an automobile accident that causes the head to be thrown forward suddenly and then jerked backward, or vice versa, like the cracking of a whip. The brunt of the injury is borne at the level of the fifth neck vertebra where muscles and ligaments can be torn and strained. Occasionally, there is associated bone or nerve damage, but this is not common.

The injury is similar to a badly sprained ankle, and treatment is similar. The neck should be protected by a soft felt or sponge rubber collar for two or three weeks. Anti-inflammatory medications, heat, and massage are helpful in relieving symptoms. Occasionally victims have persistent headaches afterwards.

All the symptoms appear to be aggravated by emotional factors, and a nervous, tense person generally takes longer to recover than a calm person.

Degenerative arthritis of the spine. Inflammation of joints (arthritis) may stem from a variety of problems. The most common is wear and tear associated with growing older. An earlier injury, infection, or faulty development of the joints may hasten the onset of this condition, which is called degenerative arthritis. Degenerative changes occur commonly in the intervertebral joints of the upper and lower back, and are particularly common among persons who do heavy work. Marked degrees of arthritis can exist without causing any symptoms, but if symptoms are triggered by some relatively minor stress, they are likely to be persistent. Even without aggravation, symptoms eventually arise in the affected area. Usually there are periodic attacks of discomfort lasting a few weeks, followed by periods of freedom from pain. In mild cases treatment is unnecessary, but more severe cases require physiotherapy, braces or corsets, or anti-inflammatory medications.

THE SHOULDER

Pain in the shoulder can be caused by many conditions not originating in the joint itself. For instance, the pain's source may be in the lungs, the diaphragm, or the heart. Shingles, disturbances in the neck, and muscular dystrophies can also produce shoulder pain.

Impingement syndrome (bursitis). Most shoulder pain, however, is caused by degenerative changes in the small tendons that make up the rotator cuff. The muscles attached to those tendons turn the arm inward and outward and work with the deltoid muscle in raising the arm over the head. Between the rotator cuff and the overlying deltoid muscle is the subdeltoid or subacromial bursa. The two layers of the bursa are lubricated and permit the humerus, or upper arm bone, with its rotator cuff, to glide smoothly beneath the soft deltoid muscle and the acromion, which is the hard, overhanging projection of the shoulder blade. The deep layer of the bursa becomes locally inflamed when degeneration begins in any of the rotator cuff tendons to which it is attached. As the tendon passes beneath the acromion when the arm is elevated between 60 and 120 degrees, the inflamed bursa is pinched, causing the sharp pain that we know as bursitis. There is usually little or no pain during motion on either side of this middle arc of movement.

Calcium deposits may build up in the degenerating tendons, thereby increasing the inflammation, impingement, and pain. The calcium may liquefy and rupture into the bursal sac. This produces a generalized bursitis and a shoulder immobilized by severe pain.

Treatment. Often unnecessary in mild cases, treatment may involve exercises and short-wave diathermy, a form of deep-heat treatment. Aspirin or injections of cortisone derivatives and exercises are also used. Rarely is it necessary to remove calcium deposits surgically. In cases of acute bursitis, a period of rest in a sling may be required before starting an exercise program. In older persons who suffer chronically recurring pain and who do not respond well to conservative treatment, it may be necessary to remove part of the acromion surgically.

Tendon and muscle tears. Tears in tendons and muscles are common causes of pain around shoulder joints. An incomplete tear of the rotator cuff where muscles are attached to bone is one of the causes of the impingement syndrome described earlier. A complete tear greatly hinders the raising of the arm throughout its range of movement. Complete tears are often produced by minor accidents, such as falling on the outstretched hand. There is immediate pain in the shoulder that worsens during the next few hours and may be so great that drugs are necessary to control it. The victim, who is usually over 45 years of age, is unable to raise the arm. The point of the shoulder may be tender to the touch.

The outlook is good if the tear is repaired surgically within a few days of its occurrence. If an operation is delayed it is unlikely that full shoulder movement will return. After the operation the arm usually is held away from the side in a plaster cast for several weeks.

Frozen shoulder. Also known as pericapsulitis or adhesive capsulitis (inflammation of a membranous sac enclosing a part), frozen shoulder is an ill-understood condition. Patients with this condition complain of moderate pain and marked limitation of movement. The pain, a dull ache, comes on gradually in the shoulder and upper arm. Movement is restricted in all directions.

Usually the stiffness gradually disappears, but it may take six months to a year. The pain disappears sooner, but in early stages the arm needs rest in sling.

Recurrent shoulder dislocation. This is a condition in which repeated dislocations of the glenohumeral joint occur. The dislocations usually occur when raising or extending the arm without any great violence, even while stretching, swimming, putting on a coat, or brushing the hair. Dislocations are rare in some cases, but in others they are so frequent that they interfere with daily activities. Often the patient is able to relocate the shoulder himself or with the help of a friend.

The reasons some primary dislocations of the shoulder heal without further trouble while others go on to repeated dislocations are not fully understood. However, there is no doubt that if a primary dislocation is not properly reduced (replaced in normal position) and immobilized, the risk of recurrent dislocation increases.

No abnormalities will be found if the shoulder is examined when not dislocated. Even X rays show nothing abnormal unless a special

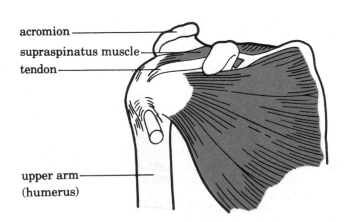

acromion
supraspinatus muscle
tendon

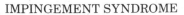

upper arm
(humerus)

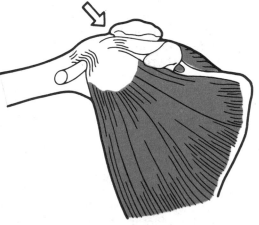

IMPINGEMENT SYNDROME

Impingement syndrome is the name frequently given to shoulder pain that occurs when the arm is raised toward a horizontal position. In drawing at left the arm hangs normally at the side and there is no pain. As the arm is raised, the supraspinatus muscle and its tendon are pinched pain- *fully between the upper arm bone and the acromion, which is the point of the shoulder. The condition often occurs if these tissues are swollen or inflamed, and can no longer glide smoothly between the bones. Calcium deposits in the tendons aggravate the problem.*

view, called a medial rotation view, is taken. This view usually will show a bony defect on the head of the arm bone, thought to be produced by "denting" with a sharp margin of the shoulder blade. This dent allows the head to dislocate completely when the arm is moved to a susceptible position.

There is no simple, effective treatment. If the dislocations occur frequently and are troublesome, an operation should be performed. There are several procedures, but all try to strengthen the capsule of the joint and slightly limit its range of outward rotation. When successful, the operation yields a shoulder that can be used for hard work. Many athletes who suffered repeated shoulder dislocations in college have been able to withstand the violent contact of professional football after a successful repair operation.

Joint replacement. In recent years arthroplasty, or joint replacement, is being performed more frequently to salvage motion and relieve pain about the glenohumeral joint. Replacement of the head of the humerus with a metallic implant following painful malunion, septic arthritis, tumor excision, and rheumatoid disease is quite successful in relieving pain, but less so in restoring motion. Nevertheless, a useful shoulder can be expected.

The acromioclavicular joint. This joint connects the outer end of the collarbone and the acromion process of the shoulder blade. Degenerative changes in this joint produce pain that usually is confined to the joint. The pain is made worse when the joint is used extensively, particularly for overhead work such as painting a ceiling.

Examination of the joint does not show any soft tissue thickening, but bony outgrowth can be felt at the edges of the joint. The arm can be raised to a horizontal level without discomfort, but raising it above this level causes pain. X rays show that the joint has been narrowed and show the presence of bony outgrowth at the edges.

Heat, rest, a sling, and aspirin are usually satisfactory. Occasionally, operation is necessary if symptoms are severe and do not respond to treatment. The most satisfactory operation is "decompression" of the joint by removing the outer end of the collarbone.

This joint also is prone to persistent dislocation (shoulder separation) brought about by injury. In most cases the displacement is minimal and the symptoms slight. The outer end of the collarbone sticks up beneath the skin. The rest of the shoulder girdle and arm hang lower than the collarbone. Usually little or no treatment is needed except a sling for rest. An operation is rarely necessary, but if performed, the most effective procedure is removal of the outer end of the collarbone.

Sternoclavicular joint. The inner end of the collarbone occasionally dislocates, either permanently or when the shoulders are braced back. This in-and-out displacement can be troublesome, but there is no effective conservative treatment. If the pain and disability are severe, removal of the inner end of the collarbone may help.

THE ELBOW

When the arm is held straight by the side, the elbow is bent slightly outward at an angle of about 10 degrees in men and 15 degrees in women. This is known as the "carrying angle," and if it is greatly increased the resulting deformity is known as "cubitus valgus."

Cubitus valgus usually occurs because of poor union of a fracture of the lower end of the has been affected by disease or injury. The deformity is harmless and usually not readily noticeable. Function of the arm is not disturbed, but a possible complication is ulnar nerve neuritis.

The ulnar nerve, which supplies most of the muscles of the hand, passes around the back of the elbow joint and is exposed to direct injury at the point of the elbow known as the "crazy bone." When the carrying angle is greatly increased, the nerve is bent sharply around the angle and repeated injury may damage it. Scarring around and within the nerve may produce numbness, tingling in the hand, and weakness and wasting of small hand muscles supplied by the nerve. When symptoms of nerve damage occur, it may be advisable to have the nerve transposed by an operation that removes it from danger by placing it at the front of the elbow.

Cubitus varus is the opposite deformity in which the normal carrying angle is reduced or even reversed. The causes of the deformity are the same as those of cubitus valgus. There is usually no disability from this deformity, although cosmetic appearance varies from what is considered normal.

Tennis elbow. A name commonly applied to any disorder causing pain on the outer side of the elbow joint is tennis elbow. Only in a few people is it caused by playing tennis. Any activity that requires rotary movements of the forearm and a firm grip of the hand (using a screwdriver, for instance) can cause the symptoms. There is pain and tenderness at the rear of the elbow where extensor muscles originate. The pain often radiates down the back of the forearm, and can change into widespread aching in all the forearm muscles, particularly if extensive gripping is involved. A similar condition occurs on the inner side of the elbow at the point of origin of the flexor muscles of the wrist and fingers, but is much less common.

Many mild cases require no treatment. When treatment is necessary a variety of conservative measures are available. The most common are rest, diathermy, and injection of local anesthetics combined with cortisone derivatives. Immobilization in a sling or even a plaster cast is often helpful in early cases. Operation is occasionally necessary in severely disabled patients who have not responded to conservative treatment. Results are not always predictable, but usually the pain disappears after healing has taken place.

The elbow is second only to the knee as a site of osteochondritis dissecans (see page 328). This is a condition in which a fragment of cartilage and bone becomes detached, occurring most often in teenagers. Pain is moderate and movements usually are limited somewhat, but "locking" of the elbow does not occur until the fragment is completely detached. X rays first show an area of irregularity. Later a cavity and the bony fragment lying free within the joint—a "joint mouse"—may be seen.

Several months of immobilization may be necessary in these early cases. If the fragment has separated or is ripe for separation, it must be removed by incision.

Degenerative arthritis. This is less common in the elbow than elsewhere because the elbow is not a weight-bearing joint. When arthritis does occur it generally results from injury or disease of the joint surfaces. Relatively minor stresses repeated over several years can be as damaging as a major fracture. For example, workers who regularly use compressed air drills sometimes develop severe degenerative changes in the elbow joint.

Symptoms are pain and limitation of movement. The joint aches for a considerable time after heavy use. In some patients the first abnormal sign is locking of the joint by a loose fragment of cartilage or bone.

Massage and diathermy or other forms of local heat are useful, particularly if the joint can be rested. Often, restriction of activity combined with anti-inflammatory medicines is sufficient treatment. Operation is rarely needed. When an operation is performed, loose bodies usually are removed, and in exceptional circumstances the joint stiffened in the most useful position. Another alternative is an operation in which the destroyed surfaces are removed (excisional arthroplasty) and the joint left movable. Total elbow joint replacement with implants has been less successful than in other joints.

Ruptures of the biceps. This muscle of the upper arm can rupture at either end, but rupture is extremely uncommon at the "elbow end." It usually occurs in a middle-aged person during lifting or pulling, and is only slightly painful. There is little loss of power and little interference with customary work. When the arm is used, a portion of the muscle fails to harden causing a soft bulge lower in the arm. Repair of the rupture is seldom necessary.

THE WRIST AND HAND

"Sprained wrist" is a common lay diagnosis but it is often wrong. The true sprained wrist is rare. Symptoms are more frequently caused by a fracture, a dislocation, or arthritis.

Persistent pain in the wrist following an accident is a serious symptom that needs thorough investigation. X rays are essential. Fracture of the navicular bone above the thumb is common, and if left untreated can produce crippling arthritis of the wrist. Falls on the back of the hand can chip small flakes of bone that cause troublesome symptoms for weeks.

If these causes of symptoms can be excluded, then "sprained wrist" can safely be diagnosed and successfully treated by strapping or temporary immobilization in a plaster cast.

DeQuervain's disease. A common cause of pain in the thumb side of the wrist is a thickening of the sheaths covering two of the tendons which pass to the thumb. This stenosing tenovaginitis, or DeQuervain's disease, is more common among women than men. In general, repetitive actions such as typing, or strenuous actions such as prolonged gripping, produce the symptoms, which come on gradually. There is pain at the base of the thumb radiating to the nail and up into the forearm, and tenderness is present on pressure over the thumb side of the wrist.

Sometimes the condition cures itself if the wrist can be immobilized and if the actions that cause it can be avoided. Cortisone derivatives injected into the sheath usually bring prompt relief. In more stubborn cases, surgical incision of the tendon sheath is necessary.

Ganglion of the wrist. A ganglion is a cystic swelling which occurs in association with a joint or tendon sheath. The cyst is generally thought to be a degenerative lesion. Ganglia occur most commonly on the back of the wrist, but also can arise around the knee or ankle.

Usually there are no symptoms except occasional slight discomfort. Since they are harmless, ganglia can safely be left untreated and many disappear spontaneously. Aspiration of the ganglion to remove fluid followed by injection of a cortisone derivative often will eliminate the cyst. Large ganglia or those which cause pain or pressure symptoms may require surgical removal. This is not always easy, because the whole cyst and its root or pedicle must be dissected. Recurrence is uncommon, however, if the cyst is completely removed.

Median nerve compression. Pressure on the median nerve where it enters the wrist (the carpal tunnel) is a common cause of discomfort of the hand, especially in persons over 40 or in patients who have sustained a Colles' fracture (see page 332). This big nerve passes along the middle of the arm and forearm and enters the hand at the wrist joint along with all the flexor tendons to the fingers. Thickening of the tendon sheaths and arthritic changes at the wrist tend to reduce the size of the tunnel through which the nerve passes.

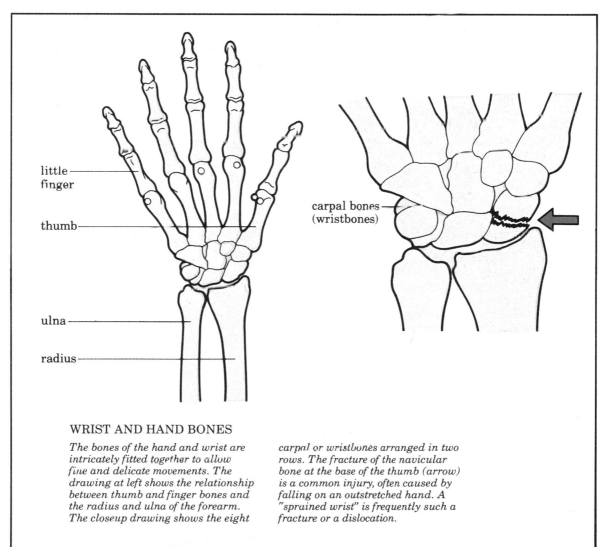

little
finger

thumb

ulna

radius

carpal bones
(wristbones)

WRIST AND HAND BONES

The bones of the hand and wrist are intricately fitted together to allow fine and delicate movements. The drawing at left shows the relationship between thumb and finger bones and the radius and ulna of the forearm. The closeup drawing shows the eight carpal or wristbones arranged in two rows. The fracture of the navicular bone at the base of the thumb (arrow) is a common injury, often caused by falling on an outstretched hand. A "sprained wrist" is frequently such a fracture or a dislocation.

Because the nerve is softer than the tendons, it is subjected to considerable pressure with accompanying discomfort.

Symptoms are tingling, vague or sharp pain, and perhaps numbness in the thumb, index, and long fingers. If pressure has been present for some time there will be clumsiness in fine movements. The victim may drop dishes, and wasting of the thumb muscles may be apparent. The pain is often worst at night. Shortly after falling asleep the victim is awakened by intense discomfort in the hand which does not go away until the hand is exercised. Only a few men suffer from this condition. It is common among expectant mothers during late pregnancy. The symptoms usually disappear after delivery.

Rest occasionally helps. A cortisone derivative injected into the carpal tunnel often relieves the symptoms. When conservative treatment fails, the volar carpal ligament may be partly or completely removed to relieve pressure on the nerve.

Degenerative changes. Such changes at the wrist are common because of the frequency with which the joint surfaces are damaged. Symptoms are tenderness around the joint, pain, and limitation of movement. Mild cases can be relieved by resting the wrist with a molded leather or plastic splint. Some persons will not wear splints indefinitely and request surgery, but the only reliable method involves complete stiffening of the wrist.

Degenerative changes of the finger joints are quite common in elderly people and in most cases no treatment is required except aspirin to relieve pain. The joint at the base of the thumb may be seriously affected. Movement is painful, the joint is prominent and thickened, and range of motion is reduced. If the symptoms are severe, operation will be necessary. Occasionally, replacement of the finger joint is attempted.

Dupuytren's contracture. This is a thickening of tissue (fascia) of the palm which causes fingers to be pulled down into the palm. It also can occur in the sole of the foot. It appears to run in families, but the exact cause is unknown. Changes are most common in the little finger side of the palm. The condition strikes men more often than women and usually starts as a small nodule at the base of the ring finger. As the condition progresses, other nodules appear and firm bands may spread into the fingers. Conservative treatment is in-

effective. When the deformity is disabling, it is necessary to sever the constricting band.

Trigger finger. This disorder results from constriction that prevents free movement of tendons in the sheath. Despite its name, it can occur in any finger. The tendons develop a "waist" opposite the constriction, tend to swell, and the swollen segment often develops into a nodule that has difficulty entering the sheath when the finger is extended. Usually a snap is felt and a click heard as the finger bends or extends. Cortisone injections can relieve the problem. If the injection fails, the constriction in the sheath may have to be divided surgically.

Boutonniere deformity. Also known as "buttonhole" deformity, this results when the central extensor tendon on the base of the middle joint of a finger is cut or ruptured. In the fully developed deformity, the middle joint is bent at a right angle. An immediate operation is needed to reattach the tendon to the bone. Satisfactory treatment is extremely difficult if the deformity is neglected for many weeks after the original injury. Then it may be necessary to stiffen the joint in a better position.

Mallet or baseball finger. This deformity, in which the tip of the finger bends as much as 45 degrees, is caused by rupture or tearing of the attachment of the extensor tendon. The force to do this is a sudden violent blow on the tip of the finger, as in "miscatching" a baseball.

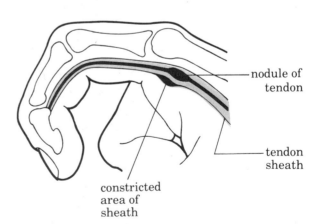

nodule of tendon

tendon sheath

constricted area of sheath

TRIGGER FINGER

Any of the fingers can be affected by the malady known as trigger finger. It occurs when a constricted area develops in the tendon sheath, preventing free tendon movement. The tendons swell opposite the constricted area and form a nodule which has difficulty entering the sheath when the finger is extended. When it does enter the sheath, a snap is often heard.

Immobilizing the joint for about six weeks immediately following injury usually realigns the joint. Old injuries or those which have not responded to immobilization treatment should have surgery to reattach the ruptured tendon.

THE HIP

The hip is a major weight-bearing joint and is subject to many conditions directly connected with the thrust of body weight. It is a ball-and-socket joint with very strong ligaments surrounding and strengthening it.

Many children with hip troubles are brought to a doctor when parents note some abnormality after the child starts to walk. A hip limp in a very young child usually is a congenital dislocation if it is painless, or caused by acute suppurative arthritis (see right) if it is painful.

Congenital dislocation. This spontaneous dislocation occurs before or shortly after birth as a result of an abnormality of development, usually a flattening of the acetabulum (the cup-shaped cavity in the pelvis) in which the end (head) of the thighbone rests. Girls are affected at least five times more often than boys. Heredity plays a part. A woman with this condition has an increased chance of giving birth to a child with the same condition. The congenital dislocation occurs more often in one hip than in both.

Warning signs in a newborn are limited outward motion from the hip, particularly when the infant is lying on the back with the knees bent to 90 degrees, and asymmetrical "folds" of the fat tissue of the leg. The buttock, groin, and thigh folds on the affected side are usually deeper and higher up on the leg than on the normal side. Thigh folds can be asymmetrical in infants who are normal, but asymmetry of the groin and buttock folds as well is rare except in congenital dislocation of the hip.

When the affected hip is moved, a "click" can be heard. X-ray examination shows that the socket is shallow and the bony roof slopes upward and outward so that the thighbone can easily slide upward out of the socket.

Fortunately the condition generally is recognized soon after birth in babies examined regularly by a pediatrician or followed in well-baby clinics.

Treatment. The basic aim is to place the head of the thighbone in the socket and to retain it there until the socket has had time to develop. Several different methods are used. Probably the most satisfactory is to stretch tight muscles gradually, then replace the thighbone under general anesthesia, followed by immobilization of the leg and hip joint in a plaster cast. After removal of the cast, a bar may be attached to the baby's shoes to hold the legs apart and to limit hip movement. In infants with slight dislocations, splinting may be sufficient. An operation may be necessary if the hip cannot be returned to its proper place or if the socket fails to develop satisfactorily.

If the condition is discovered early and treatment is started within the first six months of life, the results will be excellent in nearly every case. If treatment is delayed because it is not recognized until the child starts walking, the prospects for a satisfactory result decrease. In late cases, a reconstructive operation may help at first, but after age 35 increasing amounts of pain are common.

Acute suppurative arthritis. Pyogenic (pus-producing) arthritis of the hip occurs relatively frequently in infants and young children. In infants it usually results from infection elsewhere, such as pneumonia, impetigo, or middle ear infection. The baby is obviously sick, has a sudden onset of high fever, holds the hip joint bent, and resists examination.

Fortunately, the infecting organism is sensitive to antibiotics. Sometimes the doctor must surgically drain the hip joint to prevent destruction of bone. When treatment is started

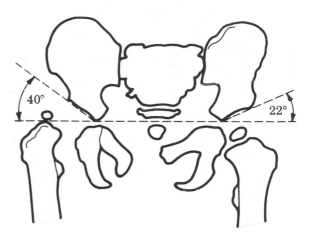

HIP DISLOCATION

Congenital hip dislocation results from abnormal development of the acetabulum, the cup-shaped socket in which the thighbone fits. Normally, the angle between the horizontal and the upper half of the acetabulum is 22 degrees, as on the right side above. In abnormal cases, the angle may be 40 degrees, allowing the thighbone to slip from its socket.

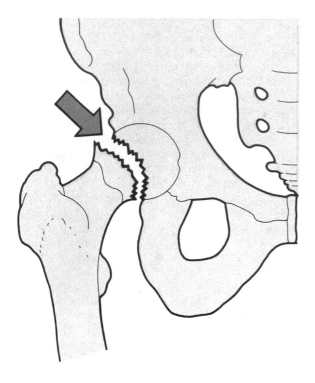

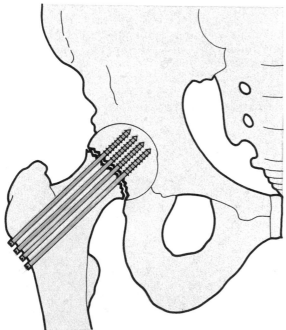

SLIPPED EPIPHYSIS

Slipped epiphysis, which happens in late childhood, can occur at any growth center but is most common at the hip joint, where the rounded head of the thighbone slips from its normal cartilage connection with the rest of the bone (top drawing), causing an unstable joint, limping, and pain. A cluster of fine-diameter, threaded nails can be inserted through the bone (lower drawing) to hold the slipped parts in position.

late, the joint cartilage already has been destroyed in many cases.

Perthes' disease is now one of the common hip diseases of children between three and eight. It is three times more common among boys than among girls.

The specific cause is not known, but a local reduction of blood supply leads to collapse of the head of the thighbone (femoral head). The condition goes through three stages—onset, activity, and healing—that may cover three years. The onset is marked by pain in the thigh or groin associated with a limp. During the active stage the head of the thighbone softens and deforms. Healing is gradual, but the head may be permanently deformed, increasing the probability of degenerative arthritis of the hip later in life.

The diagnosis of Perthes' disease is made principally from X-ray examination. The objective of treatment is to prevent the soft femoral head from being deformed into a grossly distorted shape. Immobilization with braces or in a cast, with the legs held widely apart, seats the ball in the round socket and avoids distortion. Limited weight is also important. Sometimes an operation must be performed to realign the pelvic bone and limit stress on the femoral head. No medicine or other known treatment will accelerate healing, nor is there any way to restore the femoral head to normal after it has become grossly deformed.

Slipped femoral epiphysis, also known as coxa vara, is a condition which occurs in late childhood. The rounded top of the thighbone slips from its cartilaginous connection with the rest of the bone and is displaced downward and backward. Usually this is a gradual development, but a fall or injury can cause sudden displacement.

Symptoms usually begin with gradually increasing pain in the hip plus a limp. Movement of the hip joint is limited. The displacement can be seen on X ray.

Because the condition worsens until growth has ceased or the epiphyseal cap has united with the shaft, an operation is usually necessary. If there is minimal slipping, several small screws are inserted across the cartilage plate to prevent further displacement. In acute severe slipping, manipulation and screws are required. In late severe slipping, it may be necessary to sever and realign the bone.

Degenerative arthritis of the hip generally is not common until after age 60, but can occur at any age in adults. Earlier cases usually result from congenital abnormalities or injury. The basic cause is wear and tear.

The first symptom is pain about the hip. It usually can be relieved by "taking it easy" at work and play. As the pain gradually increases, anti-inflammatory medications are helpful. As the hip becomes stiffer and more painful, it may be necessary to use a cane.

Various forms of surgery can be performed on the arthritic hip. Stiffening the hip (fusion) to minimize movement eliminates the hip pain permanently but may cause low back pain because of the added strain on the back during walking and sitting. Changing the thrust of the body weight through the pelvis by realigning the thighbone (osteotomy) retains limited hip motion but does not always relieve pain. Remodeling the hip joint (arthroplasty) is the most popular, because it restores motion and usually relieves pain. None of the operations is suitable for everyone. Choice depends on state of the tissue in the affected hip and the condition of the other hip and the spine.

Arthroplasty of the hip has been undergoing constant change over the past 50 years as doctors study the long-term results, and as new materials and improved care allow for better technology. Doctors now speak of "total hip replacement," but there are many variations designed to treat any type of hip problem. Some replace only the ball on the end of the thighbone. Others replace the ball and resurface the socket. Generally speaking, the ball is replaced by a metallic knob secured with methylmethacrylate and the socket is lined with high density polyethylene also secured with the same "acrylic cement."

Total hip replacement in older patients, since the procedure was developed in 1960 by Dr. John Charnley, an English orthopedist, has produced outstanding results in most instances. Generally pain is gone immediately after surgery, and the patient can walk as soon as the wound heals. Severely handicapped patients have been restored to near normal activity, comfort, and gait by the operation. Complications can occur as with any operation in this age group, but it appears Dr. Charnley's operation is here to stay. The procedure is being adapted to younger people as the technology improves. In general, however, the longer one can put off this type of operation, the more assurance that the new hip will last for a lifetime.

Bursitis of the hip. This bursitis may occur following surgery but also happens spontaneously in older people, especially those suffering from gout. Pain and tenderness over the point of the hip joint mark the site of the bursa that has become inflamed. When the condition is acute, sufferers find it difficult to lie on the affected side or to walk without a limp.

Heat, rest, and anti-inflammatory medications are used to treat the condition. Injection into the bursa of a local anesthetic combined with a cortisone derivative usually brings immediate pain relief.

THE KNEE

It is often said that the knee is the joint least likely to succeed. Situated midway between the hip and the foot, it is subject to enormous stresses that must be withstood by four relatively small ligaments—one on either side and two inside the joint. Those on the sides prevent sideward displacement and those on the inside prevent backward and forward displacement. Because of the leverage applied through the thigh and leg bones, ligament injuries to the knee are common among athletes as well as others who sustain falls or direct blows to the knees.

Loosely attached to the surface of the leg bone (tibia) are two half-moon-shaped cartilages (menisci) that cradle the knuckles of the thighbone (femur), and serve to lubricate the surface of the femur as well as to bear some of the weight transmitted across the joint. These cartilages frequently are torn during twisting injuries to the knee.

Knee movements are controlled by the hamstring muscles of the thigh which bend the knee, and by the powerful four part quadriceps muscle which straightens the joint. It is this thigh muscle which plays an important role in assisting the ligaments to withstand stresses when weight is borne on a partly bent knee. Situated in the tendon of the quadriceps muscle just before it attaches to the leg bone is the familiar kneecap (patella). This small bone glides over the end of the thighbone, preventing wear to the quadriceps tendon and at the same time providing leverage to increase the strength of the quadriceps muscle.

Patella-femoral syndrome. Technically referred to as chondromalacia patellae, this occurs in young men and women, and involves the junction of the kneecap and thighbone. Victims complain of pain under or around the kneecap, catching of the joint, and stiffness. The condition is aggravated by pro-

KNEE INJURIES

Athlete's knee injuries usually result from a severe impact or twist on a bent, weight-bearing knee. A side tackle on a football player can drive in the knee and cause strain on the four principal ligaments supporting the joint, as shown in the close-up. The medial ligament on the inner side of the knee is the one most commonly stretched (strained) or torn, as in the illustration at top. Frequently the cartilage in the joint (meniscus) is also torn. The tear interferes with joint function, causing swelling and collection of fluid.

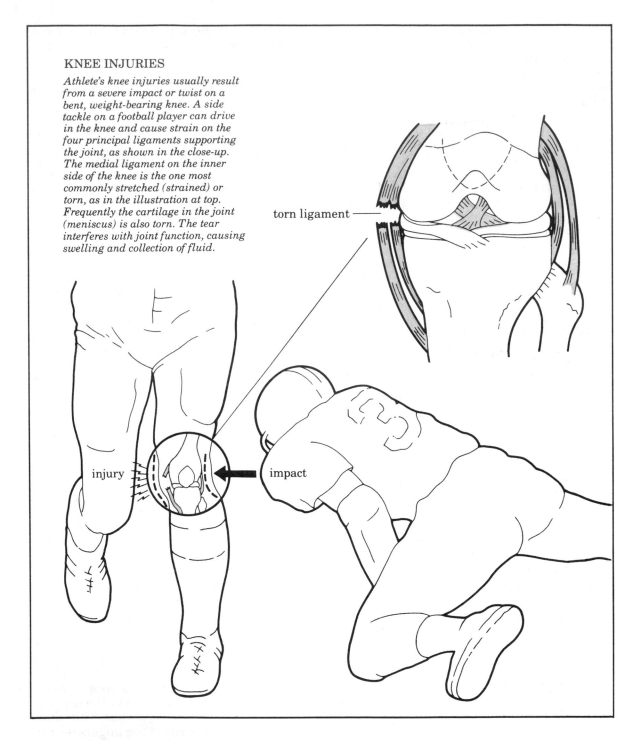

torn ligament

injury   impact

longed sitting with the knees bent, stair climbing, deep-knee bending, and negotiating hills. The kneecap feels tender and there is swelling because of fluid in the joint.

The cause is not clear, but appears to be associated with overactivity, slight malalignment of the patella, minor softening of the cartilaginous surface of the patella, and weakness of the quadriceps muscle.

Treatment consists of quadriceps strengthening exercises with the knee in extension and anti-inflammatory medications. It may be necessary to avoid positions that aggravate the condition. The kneecap is only rarely removed surgically. The best prescription is patience. The problem usually is resolved with conservative treatment.

Recurrent dislocation of the patella usually is a developmental condition affecting both knees and most commonly occurring in teenage girls. Injury is occasionally the cause. The dislocation is to the outer side, the kneecap slipping over the edge of the femur as the knee is bent. It can occur spontaneously while walking, running, or turning suddenly. The pain is acute and the girl is unable to straighten her knee. Another person can easily extend the joint by straightening the knee and the patella slips back into position.

After the first dislocation, the inner border of the kneecap usually feels tender, indicating the point where the quadriceps tendon has pulled away. The joint is filled with fluid. The torn tendon must be repaired surgically, followed by four to six weeks with the knee immobilized. A vigorous exercise program to restore strength to the quadriceps muscle is necessary afterwards. Following this treatment dislocation probably will not recur.

In persons whose tissues tend to stretch easily, recurrent dislocation becomes a chronic problem. Repeated dislocations predispose to early degenerative arthritis. Additional surgery may be necessary to realign the kneecap in an effort to prevent dislocation.

Torn ligaments. The four principal ligaments of the knee joint frequently are strained or torn in sports and accidents. These injuries can be serious and must be treated promptly if disability is to be avoided. If the ligament is completely torn, the best treatment is early surgical repair. Moderate sprains can be treated by immobilizing the knee in a plaster cylinder or brace. Minor injuries are treated by wrapping the knee and avoiding strains during healing.

All ligament injuries cause wasting of the quadriceps muscle, and intensive exercises are necessary to strengthen the muscle and provide future protection for the joint.

Torn cartilage. An acute tear of one of the knee cartilages is common in young people with an athletic bent. A tear occurs when a substantial twisting force passes through a bent knee. The initial pain is sharp; it is difficult to straighten the knee. The knee is said to be "locked." Swelling soon follows. Fluid (effusion) can be felt and the knee is tender over the joint line, usually on the inner side.

Because the cartilage does not show on film, routine X ray will not disclose the tear. Instead a radiopaque dye must be injected to the knee joint. The dye passes along the torn surface and can be seen on X ray film.

Another technique allows the torn cartilage to be observed directly. A lighted fiberoptic device with a small eyepiece is passed through a tiny surgical opening. With the aid of this arthroscope, the physician can see the extent of the tear.

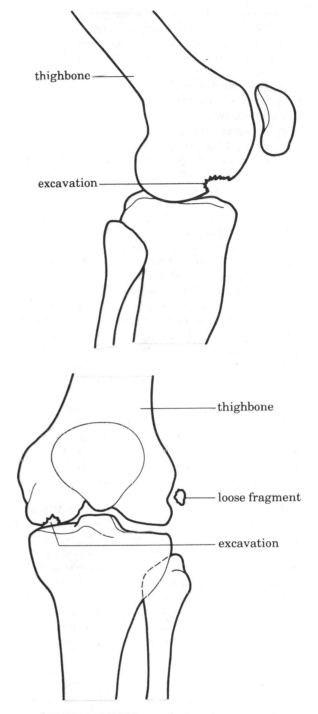

"JOINT MOUSE"

A "joint mouse" is a loose bit of bone and cartilage in the joint cavity, most commonly found in the knee. It may occur because a local reduction of blood supply causes the death of a small area of bone and its overlying cartilage. The dead fragment separates from the rest of the bone and floats in the cavity. Side and front views show a loose fragment that has separated from the rounded end of the thighbone, leaving an excavation that is visible on X ray.

Treatment is based on the amount of damage and the fact that cartilage does not heal itself. Immediate therapy is to keep weight off the leg, usually by resting in bed with the joint elevated.

If the tear is small and does not interfere with knee movement, symptoms usually will subside in two to six weeks. If not, surgery may be necessary. The torn portion of the cartilage may need to be removed, or the edges of the tear rounded off. Most surgeons leave the undamaged portion because it can continue to serve a useful purpose.

In some cases, cartilage is removed via the arthroscope, which can be fitted with miniature surgical blades. Because only a tiny incision is necessary, the patient may be walking again within a few days. Otherwise the rehabilitation period is six to eight weeks.

Degenerative tears of the knee cartilage also occur in older persons even without injury. The cartilage tears when the person simply squats or kneels. The diagnosis and treatment are the same as for the acute tear.

Degenerative arthritis may occur years later as a complication of this injury even if the cartilage is removed.

Bowlegs represent an outward bending of the knee joint. A mild degree of bowing, followed by a period of straightening and even slight overcorrection which may produce knock-knees, is common in children. No treatment is necessary unless the condition persists.

Knock-knees are produced by inward bending of the knee joint. The condition is common in children between the ages of three and five. It occasionally is associated with a deformity of the hip. In the absence of bone disease the condition usually corrects itself spontaneously in a few years.

A severe knock-knee case that continues to the age of 10 definitely requires surgery, either to remove a wedge from the femur to correct the angle, or to retard bone growth so that it eventually straightens the legs.

Osteochondritis dissecans. This is a fairly common condition, usually occurring in late adolescence. A section of the joint surface of a bone dies, along with its overlying cartilage. Eventually the fragment may separate and form a loose body in the joint. The knee joint is affected most often. Injury is probably a predisposing factor.

At first the knee feels weak and aches vaguely. Symptoms are worsened by exercise and may persist when the knee is at rest. The doctor may discover wasted muscles and slight fluid in the joint. X rays show a well-defined, crescent-shaped excavation in the bone substance.

Treatment consists of surgical removal of the fragment if it has separated and is loose in the joint. If it has not separated, the fragment often can be encouraged to "grow back" by an operation that drills small holes in the fragment to allow new blood vessels to enter from the depths of the bone. In some cases the fragment requires a metallic pin to hold it in place.

In young people, the knee can be immobilized in a plaster cast and an operation avoided. The cast may have to be worn for several months.

Degenerative arthritis is probably more common in the knee than in any other joint because the knee is so vulnerable to repeated injury and stress. Obesity, previous fracture or disease, and malalignment between bones of the joint also contribute to its wear and tear.

The principal symptoms are limited movement and gradually increasing pain, often made worse by relatively trivial strains or twists.

When significant overweight is a factor, losing weight may reduce the pain and stiffness. An exercise program and anti-inflammatory medications enable many persons to carry on for many months in moderate confort, although they should avoid climbing stairs and walking over uneven ground.

Surgical realignment of the tibia (leg bone) by sectioning (osteotomy) alters the weight distribution across the knee and generally reduces the pain. The femur and tibia can be resurfaced with metal or plastic (total knee arthroplasty), but pain relief is less predictable than when performed in hip replacement. In some instances, stiffening the knee joint by fusion is the only feasible method of pain control, but results in stiff knee gait.

THE ANKLE

The ankle is the joint between the foot and the leg bones. The weight-bearing leg bone (tibia) has a downward projection along its inner side (medial malleolus) that pairs with the projection of the fibula (lateral malleolus) on the outer side, forming a yoke to house the upper foot bone (talus). The surface of the talus is curved and allows the foot to tip forward and backward as it does in walking. As the calf muscles tighten, the foot is tipped downward and the body is lifted and propelled forward by the force transmitted upward across the ankle joint. The joint is stabilized by ligaments on both sides.

Beneath the talus is the heel bone (calcaneus). This joint permits motion at right angles to the ankle joint and allows the foot to tip from side to side and to accommodate itself to uneven surfaces. Thus, the ankle and heel joints comprise a "universal joint."

Sprained ankle. The most common disability to affect the ankle joint is the all too familiar "turned ankle" (sprain). A misstep on uneven ground can result in a partial tear on the outer (fibulo-talar) ligament. Small blood vessels are ruptured, causing a large collection of blood to form beneath the skin, followed in 24 hours by swelling of the ankle and foot. When the injury is first seen by a doctor, an X ray should be obtained to determine whether a break in the fibula also has occurred.

Treatment includes rest with the foot elevated. An ice pack applied to the ankle mass may prevent hemorrhage and swelling during the first few hours. An elastic bandage, adhesive strapping, or a walking plaster cast then may be required to support the ankle, depending on the severity of the sprain. It is usually possible to walk as soon as pain permits. A sprain generally is slow to heal and pain is out of proportion to the severity of the injury. If the lateral ligaments are torn completely, surgical repair may be necessary. An associated broken bone will require additional treatment.

Degenerative arthritis frequently affects the ankle joint and usually results from fractures. Pain and stiffness are the signs. Restricted activity and anti-inflammatory medications help in the early stages. Later it may be necessary to immobilize the joint with a brace. An operation to stiffen the joint (fusion) is a last resort. Early attempts at total ankle arthroplasty have been disappointing, but with improvement in material and technique, this procedure could become an alternative.

THE FOOT

A painless normal functioning foot is taken for granted by most of us most of the time. Yet everyone at some time has experienced "aching feet" for one reason or another and has felt utterly miserable.

The foot contains 26 bones and 33 articulations, joined together by more than 100 ligaments. Nineteen muscles provide control of the foot. The bones are arranged in two arches—a lengthwise arch and a crosswise arch. The arches are determined by the shape of the bones and the supporting ligaments of the joints.

The feet support the weight of the body, and act as levers to raise the body and move it forward in walking or running. In normal, rapid walking, body weight meets the ground at the heel, moves along the outer border to the ball of the foot, then across the line of metatarsal heads (the long bones connecting to each toe), and is transferred into the big toe. This rolling, progressive shift of body weight cannot occur in a foot that is rigid. A foot that is functioning normally changes its shape with every step to accommodate the forces passing through it.

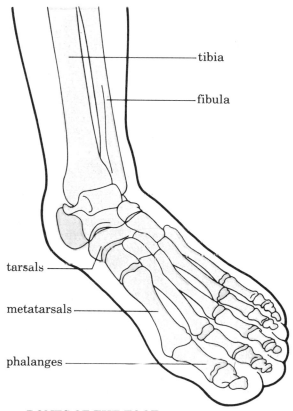

BONES OF THE FOOT

The bones of the foot and their ligaments provide remarkable flexibility and easy, rolling shift of body weight. Despite variations in size and numerous articulations, the bones work smoothly together to support the weight of the body and move it forward. Most people have aching feet at times, but it is not normal for feet to hurt.

Foot strain. The arches and supporting structures in the foot can be affected by acute or chronic strain. Acute strain usually is caused by an isolated incident that grossly overtaxes the foot. Symptoms usually respond to rest. Chronic strain of the foot can be caused by excess weight, excessive fatigue, occupational demands, abnormal gait, and faults or diseases within the foot. Most of the symptoms occur in the midtarsal area between the hindfoot and forefoot.

Treatment, which usually is helpful immediately, requires support for the longitudinal arch sufficiently high to relieve strain on the ligaments. Every effort should be made to remove the primary cause because it is not good for the foot to become permanently reliant on arch supports.

Metatarsalgia. This refers to pain in the ball of the foot. Usually the primary cause is weakness in the foot muscles. Wearing high-heeled shoes aggravates the symptoms.

Pain can be relieved by wearing low-heeled shoes in which small, domed supports (metatarsal pads) are placed. When correctly placed, these pads distribute the weight over a larger area and relieve the pressure on the metatarsal heads. A metatarsal pain associated with numbness between the third and fourth toes may be caused by a small tumor on one of the nerves. This condition can be relieved by surgical removal of the tumor.

Children's Foot Problems

Flat feet. Babies' feet are always flat and it is senseless to worry about "flat feet" in infants and toddlers before the arch of the foot has had time to develop. Even when a child first begins to stand, the foot is very mobile and flattens when it bears weight. All that is required in footwear is a soft, pliable protective shoe. True flat feet are so uncommon that the diagnosis should be made by a qualified orthopedist.

Pigeon toe. Also called toe inturning, this is common in the early stages of walking. At this stage of walking there are often signs of bowlegs, knock-knees, or inward twisting of the leg. In the vast majority of cases, all these abnormalities correct themselves spontaneously as the child grows.

Clubfoot. There are two usual forms of clubfoot, congenital talipes equinovarus and calcaneovalgus. Both deformities, which are present at birth, respond well to treatment provided it is started quickly. A series of corrective plaster casts usually will restore a normal contour to the foot, although sometimes minor operations also are necessary to relieve tightness in tendons and ligaments.

It is vital that children who have the deformity be examined at regular intervals to be sure that the correction is maintained. It is often found that so-called "relapsed" clubfeet have not been checked often enough. If a relapse is detected early, recasting will restore the correction.

Webbed toes. Webbing (a connecting membrane between digits) is not uncommon. When it occurs between the fingers, correction is necessary, but not in webbed toes. There is usually no difficulty in fitting shoes, normal function of the foot is rarely if ever affected, and surgical treatment is usually unnecessary.

Elevated little toe. Occasionally there is a hereditary disposition for the fifth (little) toe to be elevated above the others. Symptoms develop when attempts are made to force the foot into ordinary shoes. Treatment is unnecessary unless pain persists. An operation designed to lengthen the shortened tissues will relieve the pain.

Children's shoes. Except for fashion, the only reason for wearing shoes is to protect the feet from weather and injury. A shoe does nothing to help the development of the muscles or arches of a normal foot. Barefoot walking is the best possible treatment for growing feet.

Loose-fitting cloth booties are all that is necessary for infants before they start to walk. When the time comes to fit shoes to a baby's foot, the shoes must conform to the shape of the foot and must be large enough to allow normal movement of the foot within the shoes. The soles and uppers should be of supple leather. Neither arches nor heels are necessary.

A child's shoes should be inspected regularly to be sure that they are large enough. There should be a space of one-half to three-fourths of an inch between the end of the big toe and the end of the shoe when the child is standing.

The widest portion of the shoe should correspond with the widest portion of the foot. Shoes that are too short gradually will cause the toes to flex, and persistence of this position may lead to weakness of muscles of the foot and further deformity of the toes. Stockings that are too short also can constrict the feet. When a growing child needs larger shoes, he or she usually needs larger stockings.

Adult Foot Problems

Women have much more foot trouble than men, principally because of the shoes they wear. Pointed shoes cram the toes together and produce pressure symptoms such as corns and calluses and hammer toe. Shoes of this shape force the foot into an abnormal posture that leads to poor distribution of body weight, not infrequently felt as backache. Constant wearing of such shoes can cause bunion formation.

In young people these deformities are reversible. For example, when pregnant women wear low-heeled shoes their foot symptoms invariably improve and they lose their calluses and corns. Women who consistently wear high heels may suffer shortening of the calf muscles to such an extent that walking barefoot or in low heels is extremely uncomfortable.

Bunion. Also called hallux valgus, bunions are a common deformity of the adult female foot. They also can occur in men. The defect is an obvious thickening and swelling of the big joint of the big toe which forces the big toe toward the little toe. There is a protuberance on the inner side of the foot where the "hinge" bends when walking, and instead of being straight, the big toe develops an inward angle.

Once the deformity is established, it is self-perpetuating and will get progressively worse if untreated. In elderly people with bunions, surgery is not warranted and shoes should be made to fit the deformed foot. In younger persons there is no real alternative to surgical correction.

Hallux rigidus (stiff toe). Pain and stiffness in the big joint of the big toe is quite common. It is usually produced by repeated minor injuries or a single major accident that overextends the toe with great force. Degenerative joint disease follows. If pain and limitation of toe movement are sufficiently troublesome, relief can be obtained by surgery.

Hammer toe. Hammer toe usually is caused by cramping the toes into shoes that are too small, although it can be produced by muscle imbalance in the foot even if shoes fit properly. Most often the clawlike deformity affects the second toe. Symptoms usually are produced by pressure, and may be alleviated by padding. If not, surgery gives excellent relief from the deformity.

Ingrown toenail. Ingrown toenail usually affects the big toe. Commonly, the edge of the nail is driven into soft tissues by the pressure of tight shoes, or a crushing blow may initiate local injury. The forward edge of the nail as well as the side may cut into soft tissue if the nail is trimmed too short. If the area is not infected, the victim may be able to draw the overgrown tissue away from the nail after hot soaks of the foot. Thus the cutting edge of the nail can be freed, and a wisp of cotton placed to cushion the contact area. This should be done daily after the bath until the "corner" of the nail has grown beyond the point where it cuts into flesh. However, if the condition was caused by tight shoes, it will recur unless roomier shoes are worn. When infection is present, removal of a portion of the nail by simple surgery usually is necessary and successful. To prevent ingrown toenail, the nail should be trimmed squarely, with enough projection at the corners to prevent gouging and possible infection of underlying tissues.

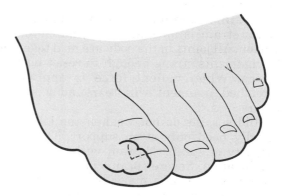

INGROWN TOENAIL

Ingrown toenail commonly results from trimming the nail too short, especially at its corners. This permits the edge of the nail to gouge into soft tissue, causing painful inflammation. Trimming the nail squarely so that the corners project slightly beyond soft tissues helps to prevent ingrown toenail.

SPRAINS, DISLOCATIONS, FRACTURES, CONTUSIONS

The increased emphasis on physical fitness for both sexes and for young and old has led to greatly expanded participation in all types of physical activity ranging from individual and group exercise programs to amateur and professional athletic competition and softball games at picnics. Obviously, an increase in musculoskeletal injuries accompanies the increased exposure of the body to physical forces.

Lack of conditioning greatly increases the risk of injury. Neophyte joggers who extend themselves too rapidly experience swollen, painful knees and ankles (synovitis), sore muscles (strains), painful tendons (tenosynovitis), and occasionally broken bones in the foot and leg (stress fractures).

Inexperienced roller skaters in the park frequently sustain broken wrist bones (Colles' fractures), dislocated elbows, broken arm bones, and sprained and broken ankles. Hang glider participants are subject to massive injuries such as a broken back, hip, leg, or pelvis when the winds fail.

A well-planned conditioning program does much to prevent injury. A knowledge of the risks involved in any activity forewarns and helps avoid injury. Familiarity with equipment and terrain also lessens the risk of injury. In spite of the best laid plans, however, accidents do happen.

Sprain. A sprain is an injury to a ligament, and a strain is an injury to a muscle or its tendon. All joints in the body are held together by ligaments strong enough to resist normal forces. When violent force is applied, a stretched ligament will tear and a sprain occurs.

Mild sprains do not weaken the joint and usually need only strap support. The great majority of sprains do well with plaster immobilization. Severe sprains usually produce a complete tear of a major ligament and are best treated by surgical repair of the torn tissues. Sometimes the ligament remains intact and tears away from its bony attachment, perhaps carrying a small piece of bone with it. X rays will show whether the bony fragment is near its original site or whether the ligament is curled upon itself. If it is curled it cannot heal satisfactorily and must be repositioned surgically.

Dislocation. A dislocation occurs when the force applied to a joint is greater than that necessary to produce a strain, resulting in displacement of the bone from its normal position in the joint. Dislocations must be reduced (returned to proper position) as soon as possible, and usually an anesthetic is necessary to relax the spasm in surrounding muscles. Occasionally, manipulation does not succeed, usually because some torn tissue or an adjacent tendon is interposed between the joining surfaces. In such cases an operation may be necessary. Once the bone is returned to its proper position, the torn tissues must be given time to heal before allowing movement in the joint. Three weeks is usually the minimum.

Fracture. A fracture is a break in a bone. When the skin is broken the fracture is open or compound. When the skin is not broken the fracture is closed or simple. The strength of bones varies from person to person and depends on age. In elderly people the bones are relatively weak; in children they are more flexible.

A common fracture among older persons is the Colles' fracture of the wrist, caused by a fall on an outstretched hand. The force crushes the radius bone of the forearm just above the wrist, so that the hand can be displaced backward. Because of the crushing, the fracture frequently heals with a characteristic deformity called the "silver fork" deformity. When the hand and forearm are placed palm down on a table, the alignment resembles the reverse-curve shape of a fork's tines and its bent handle.

Among young active adults, ankle fractures are the most common. A spiral break of the fibula, the outer, smaller bone of the leg, is often the result of a twisting fall, as in skiing. A tendon frequently tears loose with the smaller bit of broken bone.

Young children frequently suffer an incomplete or "greenstick" fracture of the long bones, in which the break occurs only on one side, as in a half-broken green branch.

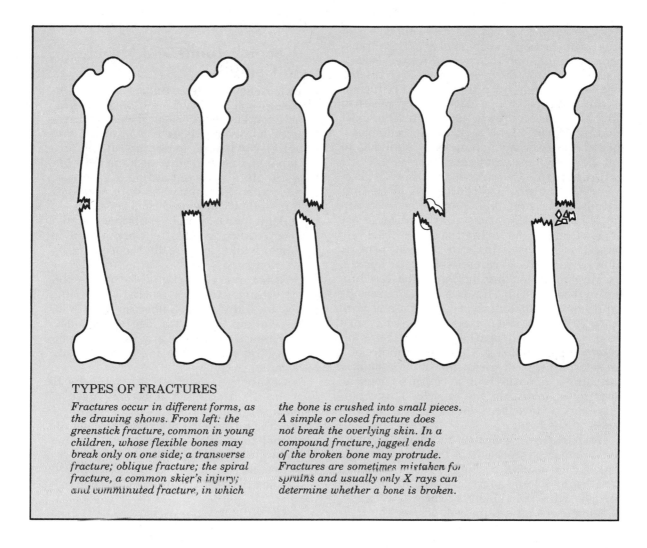

TYPES OF FRACTURES

Fractures occur in different forms, as the drawing shows. From left: the greenstick fracture, common in young children, whose flexible bones may break only on one side; a transverse fracture; oblique fracture; the spiral fracture, a common skier's injury; and comminuted fracture, in which the bone is crushed into small pieces. A simple or closed fracture does not break the overlying skin. In a compound fracture, jagged ends of the broken bone may protrude. Fractures are sometimes mistaken for sprains and usually only X rays can determine whether a bone is broken.

The physician who treats fractures is concerned with obtaining the best functional result for the fractured bone. This does not require perfect anatomical positioning. Bone is a living tissue and is capable of uniting fractured parts that have not been exactly replaced in their original positions. Because of this capacity for repair, it is possible to treat most fractures by manipulations that place the broken ends close enough to each other for good union to occur. A good blood supply at the fracture site is necessary for repair to occur. Healing is usually more rapid in children than in the elderly.

During healing the fracture area must be protected from excessive movement. Several methods of immobilization are used. The most common is a plaster cast which is easily applied and removed. Some fractures may be treated in the early days after injury by various methods of traction on the limb. A pull can be applied to a limb by adhesive tape stuck to the skin or a metallic pin placed through an unbroken part of the bone or an adjacent bone. By such means the fracture can be controlled through the healing process and minor adjustments can be made in the position of the broken bones.

Some closed fractures are so grossly unstable that they constantly shift and need to be immobilized internally by fixing with screws or pins. However, any operation contains risk. Most physicians are conservative in their care of fractures because of the risk of complications and because few fractures need an operation.

Names are given to the different types of breaks in the bone, such as greenstick, transverse, oblique, spiral, or comminuted (see illustration). But all types of breaks are treated by the same general principles: (1) reduction of the fracture into a satisfactory position; (2) maintenance of fracture reduction until healing is sufficient to prevent redisplacement; (3) restoration of normal function to muscles, tendons, and joints.

Contusion. Often associated with fractures and sprains are contusions of the soft tissues. The usual "black and blue" spots are caused by blows that crush the fatty tissue just beneath the skin, tearing the small blood vessels. These require little or no treatment. A blow with more force can contuse a muscle, causing some tearing of fibers and bleeding within the muscle. This is a far more serious injury in terms of length of disability and pain. However, unless the muscle is completely torn apart, it will heal together by scar tissue following a period of rest. Complete rupture of a muscle requires surgical repair. Occasionally calcium is deposited in a contused muscle, forming bone within the muscle. This condition, called myositis ossificans, may require surgical removal.

Restoration of function. A vital part of treatment is restoration of function after the fracture has united. When the cast is removed, it is usual to find joint stiffness and muscle atrophy, which is a shrinkage or wasting away of the muscle caused by lack of use. The stiffness and atrophy are directly proportional to the age of the patient and the period of immobilization. It is often hard to decide how soon a cast can be removed from an elderly patient in order to prevent gross stiffness and yet allow the fracture to heal.

Physiotherapy is of great help in the mobilization of a stiffened limb, but movement and muscle contractions by the patient are the key to success. Most restoration of function occurs during the first three or four months. After this period, recovery slows and may not be complete for a year or more.

Keeping Joints and Muscles in Condition

Experienced athletes understand the importance of conditioning in any physical activity. The inexperienced weekend athlete, however, frequently plunges into activity without loosening up beforehand, and fails to stay in shape between workouts. To prevent stiffness, soreness, and potential injury—and to feel better—follow these conditioning steps:
- Begin with simple calisthenics and short walks, gradually working up to longer walks, jogging, and more lengthy workouts.
- Start every workout with muscle-stretching exercises (such as touching the toes) and joint-limbering calisthenics. Follow them with jogging in place.
- Increase the pace of any workout gradually. Do not plunge immediately into vigorous activity.
- Choose sports and activities suitable to your conditioning. Limit the length of each workout at first.
- After any period of exercise, schedule a cool-down period. Follow with a hot shower and rubdown, if possible.
- Rest any injury or soreness. Do not be heroic or try to "come back" too soon.

MAJOR MUSCLES

The muscles of the human body are almost too numerous to name. Those concerned with movement are illustrated. The topmost layer of muscles is shown on the left side of the figure. Underlying muscles (deep musculature) are named on the right side. Some bones are included as points of reference.

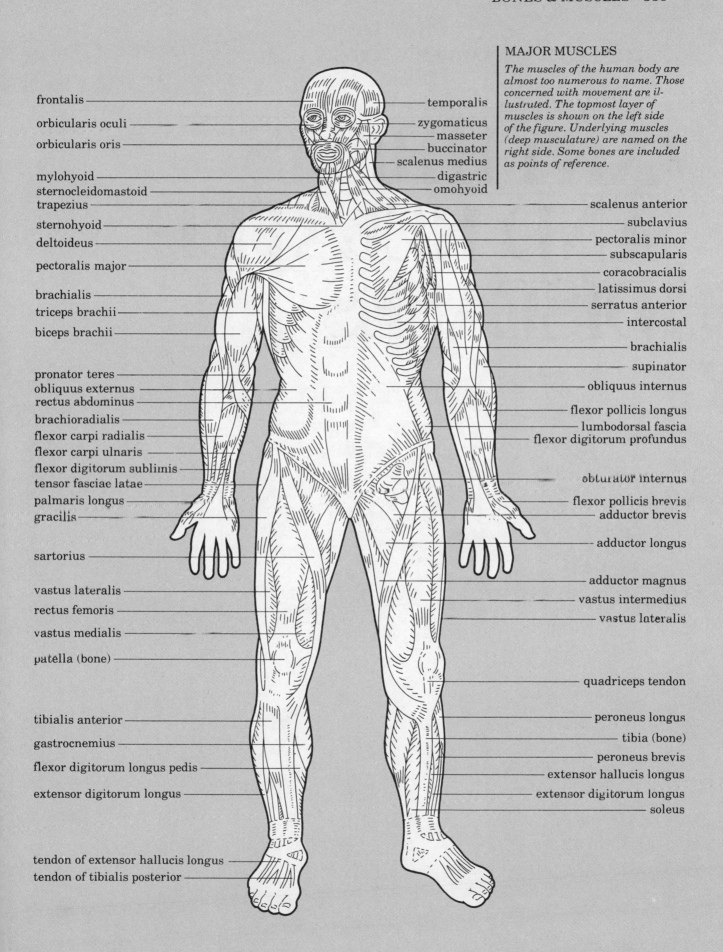

frontalis

orbicularis oculi

orbicularis oris

mylohyoid
sternocleidomastoid
trapezius

sternohyoid

deltoideus

pectoralis major

brachialis
triceps brachii
biceps brachii

pronator teres
obliquus externus
rectus abdominus
brachioradialis
flexor carpi radialis
flexor carpi ulnaris
flexor digitorum sublimis
tensor fasciae latae
palmaris longus
gracilis

sartorius

vastus lateralis
rectus femoris

vastus medialis

patella (bone)

tibialis anterior
gastrocnemius
flexor digitorum longus pedis
extensor digitorum longus

tendon of extensor hallucis longus
tendon of tibialis posterior

temporalis
zygomaticus
masseter
buccinator
scalenus medius
digastric
omohyoid

scalenus anterior
subclavius
pectoralis minor
subscapularis
coracobracialis
latissimus dorsi
serratus anterior
intercostal
brachialis
supinator
obliquus internus
flexor pollicis longus
lumbodorsal fascia
flexor digitorum profundus

obturator internus

flexor pollicis brevis
adductor brevis

adductor longus

adductor magnus
vastus intermedius
vastus lateralis

quadriceps tendon

peroneus longus
tibia (bone)
peroneus brevis
extensor hallucis longus
extensor digitorum longus
soleus

CHAPTER 15   WARREN A. KATZ, M.D., F.A.C.P.

ARTHRITIS AND RELATED DISEASES

Almost everyone at some time will develop arthritis. The disease has been known throughout history, traces of it having been found in skeletons of dinosaurs. Our prehistoric ancestors had arthritis of the spine, and arthritis can be detected in Egyptian mummies through their wrappings by modern X-ray techniques. Arthritis strikes people of all ages in all parts of the world. Along with its variants, it is responsible for more disability and time lost from work than any other illness. Few diseases cause more suffering for more Americans—not cancer, not heart disease, not diabetes.

It seems astounding at first, then, that many people lack a clear understanding of what arthritis is and how serious it can be. But the misunderstanding is less surprising on second thought, because the term arthritis has so many different meanings. There is no single definition for arthritis. Several terms may be applied to the same condition, and there are more than 100 types of arthritic diseases.

What Is Arthritis?

The ancient Greeks described "rheumatism" as an evil humor (mucus) that flowed from the brain and other organs and inflicted pain. Today, "rheumatic" or "rheumatologic" is a broad term embracing all conditions that produce pain and stiffness in joints or other parts of the musculoskeletal system, usually excepting fractures or congenital abnormalities. Arthritis is one type of rheumatism. In its narrowest sense it means inflammation ("itis") of the joint ("arthros"). In reality, arthritis is interpreted in different ways. For example, when a young mother with painfully stiff and swollen joints complains of "arthritis," she most likely refers to her rheumatoid arthritis. Her grandfather's "arthritis" that causes him some stiffness in the back and knees might be caused by osteoarthritis. Her harried, stressed executive husband rubs his neck and agonizes that his "arthritis" is killing him. He means that fibrositis and muscle spasms are causing him discomfort. Technically, his joints aren't even involved.

Connective tissue disorders, also referred to as collagen diseases, affect not only the joints but the skin and internal organs as well. They tend to be more severe than arthritis, and may even be fatal, but they are usually classified as a rheumatic disease, and are treated by rheumatologists. A rheumatologist is a physician, usually an internist, who has undergone extensive training in rheumatology, which is the study of all rheumatic diseases, including arthritis, bursitis, tendinitis, fibrositis, myositis, certain types of neuralgia, gout, and connective tissue diseases.

Who Gets Arthritis?

There are many types of arthritis. Some are acute, others chronic. Some are common, others rare. Some affect a single joint, others all joints. Arthritis may be associated with generalized illness, but more often it is an entity unto itself. The more than 100 types of rheumatic disease are caused by injuries, infections, metabolic disturbances, or tumors. In many cases, the cause is not known.

The Arthritis Foundation estimates that more than 32 million Americans suffer from one form of arthritis or another. Some types of arthritis are peculiar to certain age groups. For example, rheumatic fever is basically a disease of children. Gonococcal arthritis, a venereal disease, afflicts mostly young people in their teens and twenties. Persons with rheumatoid arthritis are most often young to middle-aged adults, whereas gout occurs in those middle-aged and older. A disorder called polymyalgia rheumatica strikes only the aged. Some forms of rheumatism such as lupus erythematosus are more prevalent in women, yet men are more likely to develop a disorder known as ankylosing spondylitis. Men and women are equally prone to most rheumatic diseases. No one is immune from arthritis.

JOINTS AND THE MUSCULOSKELETAL SYSTEM

A total of 206 bones form the supporting skeleton of the body. Bones are found in all shapes and sizes depending upon location and function. They may be long, short, flat, tubular, straight, or curved. Some bones such as those in the skull are firmly fixed to adjacent bones with minimal movement possible at the point where they join. Most joints, however, are capable of a wide range of motion. Can you imagine what we would be like if the bones of the body were fused to one another? We would not be able to sit, stand, or walk. For that matter, we would not be able to move at all. Each

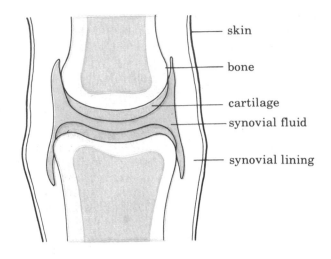

skin

bone

cartilage

synovial fluid

synovial lining

ANATOMY OF A JOINT

Where two movable bones meet, a joint is formed. A membrane called the synovial lining forms a capsule between the bones. The lining secretes synovial fluid, which lubricates and makes joint movement easier. Cartilage caps the end of each bone to cushion impact and prevent damage. Tight bands of ligament (not shown here for clarity) link the bones across the joint. Ligaments allow motion and at the same time limit it. Tendons cross the joint to provide stability, and it is protected by muscle, fat, and skin.

joint moves billions of times in a lifetime and, although joints can deteriorate as a result of wear and tear, most hold up well considering the abuse they take.

A joint is defined as a connection of two movable bones covered by a membrane that secretes joint fluid. The joint itself is covered with ligaments, fascia, tendons, muscles, fat, and skin. The cap of cartilage at the end of each bone provides a relatively low friction surface between the bones. Cartilage is composed of cells that produce a mucus-like substance and collagen fibers. Both provide considerable strength and elasticity so that the cartilage can act as a shock absorber and combat shearing forces. The joint fluid or synovial fluid is a viscous, light yellow liquid secreted by the membranes that line the joint. It facilitates joint motion, lubricates, and aids in exchange of nutrients the tissues need.

Ligaments are tight bands that link one bone to another across the joint. A ligament's flexibility varies from one joint to another depending upon how much motion that joint is intended to have. Without ligaments the entire skeleton would collapse. Tendons are tough, spindled ends of muscle composed of densely packed collagen fibers. They, too, attach to bones to impart both stability and motion to the joints. The brain sends messages to the muscles to contract or relax. In response the joints move.

DIAGNOSIS OF
RHEUMATIC DISEASES

Many rheumatic diseases are readily diagnosed because their symptoms are so characteristic. Symptoms are still the main way to identify rheumatic disorders, but a battery of simple and sophisticated tests also helps to pinpoint the problems.

Symptoms and Physical Signs

There are six major categories of symptoms that may occur in rheumatic disorders:

Pain is the major symptom of almost all rheumatic disease. It may arise from the joint or the surrounding structures. It may be mild, severe, constant, or intermittent. Individual response to pain is so variable that no two people react the same way to the same painful stimulus. Melzak in *"The Puzzle of Pain"* wrote, "pain...is a highly personal, variable experience which is influenced by cultural learning, the meaning of the situation, intention and other cognitive activities." René Leriche wrote, "There is only one pain that is easy to bear, and that is the pain of others." When a physician evaluates pain for diagnostic purposes, he considers the location, onset, frequency, duration, and severity, among other factors.

Stiffness is the feeling, independent of pain, that the joints are tight and do not move as well as we would like them to. Some people describe it as resistance, a lack of get-up-and-go, or difficulty in limbering up. All of us feel stiff for short periods once in a while, especially the morning after a day of vigorous activity. Many rheumatic diseases, notably rheumatoid arthritis, are characterized by prolonged morning stiffness that sometimes lasts several hours.

Weakness and disability accompany some rheumatic conditions, especially when the joints are inflamed or when the illness has been prolonged. In some disorders local weakness is the predominant symptom. For instance, a patient with polymyositis (see page 350) has great difficulty arising from a chair. Disability depends on many factors, including the type of arthritis, number of joints involved, severity of the illness, presence of deformities, and quite importantly, motivation. A positively motivated patient can minimize his disability. His or her own needs often can influence the degree of disability.

Swelling of the joint may result from fluid within the joint, engorged synovial tissues, bony enlargement, or a combination of these factors. Severe swelling is easy to detect, but mild degrees of swelling are less noticeable. Sometimes the first symptom of a rheumatic disease is swelling of one or more joints, not necessarily accompanied by pain.

Tenderness characterizes most painful joints, but not always. The physician may be able to diagnose a condition by the location of tenderness. For example, patients with subdeltoid bursitis complain of pain in the upper arm, yet the tenderness usually is limited to the outer portion of the shoulder. Heat and redness are additional clues to inflammation. A red-hot, swollen, exquisitely tender big toe is a tipoff to gout.

Deformities, single or multiple, are so characteristic in certain rheumatic diseases that a doctor usually can diagnose the problem solely by examining the deformity. Deformities may be caused by a combination of changes in the joints, muscles, ligaments, tendons, or skin. Deformities do not necessarily imply disability or crippling, but the primary goal of any treatment program is to prevent any deformity from developing.

Each rheumatic disease has its own constellation of symptoms and signs that enable the physician to make the diagnosis accurately in most cases. However, if the clinical features are mild, atypical, or few in number, considerable diagnostic skill is required. The nature of the illness, its severity and duration, as well as the training and ability of the physician, determine how readily a diagnosis can be established.

Special Tests

A physician who suspects arthritis can perform a variety of blood, urine, synovial fluid, and X-ray tests. But only in rare instances are any of these tests by themselves critical. Instead, they usually serve as guides to support the doctor's suspicions.

X rays are important for the full assessment of many types of arthritis because they frequently disclose the destructive process going on within the body, and help to confirm a clinical diagnosis. For example, if a few joints in the hand are inflamed, the physician may not be able to tell whether the patient has rheumatoid arthritis, psoriatic arthritis, infectious arthritis, or gout. The X-ray examination often will easily differentiate among them.

Radioisotopic scanning. The principle of bone and joint scanning is based upon the concentration of previously administered radionucleotide tracers (see chapter 32, "X Rays and Radiology") in areas of inflammation and new bone formation. Technetium 99m is the most commonly used isotope. A scan may "light up" an area that the physical and X-ray examinations fail to disclose as abnormal. These studies are helpful in detecting inflammation of the joint, bone tumors, Paget's disease, osteomyelitis, and avascular necrosis (concentrated areas of bone death).

Electromyography. Skeletal muscles and nerves emit electrical impulses that may be detected just as the impulses emitted from the heart are detected by an electrocardiogram. Electromyographic and nerve conduction studies give vital information about the state of muscles and nerves. As a result, the site of the disease can be precisely located. These tests are particularly helpful in finding nerve entrapments and muscle inflammation.

Arthroscopy is a relatively safe, simple procedure that permits inspection inside the joint, using a large needle, bright light, and magnifying lens. The procedure eliminates the need for major surgery in order to search for tumors, foreign bodies, inflammation, or changes in the joint. Remarkably, even small pieces of tissue may be removed for analysis, but the procedure can be used only in large joints.

Laboratory tests. The red blood cell sedimentation rate is a relatively inexpensive laboratory indicator of inflammation in the body regardless of cause. The test screens out noninflammatory disorders and tells the

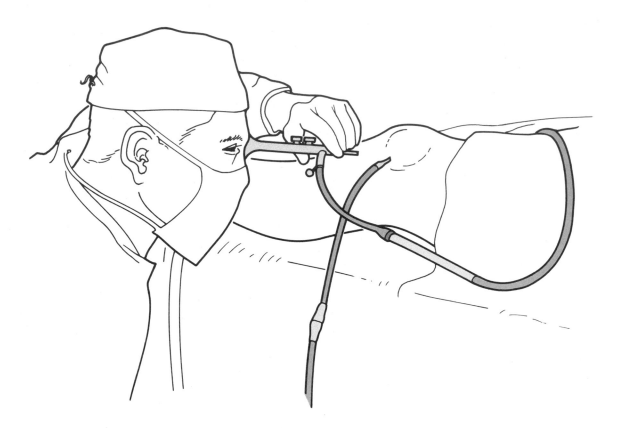

LOOKING INSIDE A JOINT

The arthroscope permits inspection
of the knee or other large joints with-
out surgery. With a large needle
and lighted magnifying eyepiece, the

doctor can look directly inside for joint
injuries, tumors, or foreign objects. He
also can remove bits of cartilage or
tissue for laboratory tests.

physician when to investigate further. It measures how quickly red cells separate when a blood sample is allowed to stand in a tube for one hour. The test result tends to be normal in noninflammatory rheumatic diseases such as osteoarthritis and fibrositis, but it is higher in rheumatoid arthritis, other connective tissue diseases, infectious arthritis, gout, and poly-myalgia rheumatica.

The latex fixation test for rheumatoid factor is a measure of certain protein antibodies in the blood. These so-called rheumatoid factors are higher than normal in 70 to 80 percent of patients with rheumatoid arthritis. Factors may also be found in certain other rheumatic and nonrheumatic diseases, so their value in diagnosis is limited. However, the higher the level of rheumatoid factor, the more likely the diagnosis of rheumatoid arthritis.

The antinuclear antibody and LE cell phenomenon (LE prep) help make a more precise and earlier diagnosis of systemic lupus erythematosus and other connective tissue diseases. The test consists of labeling known cellular (nuclear) antigens with a fluorescent material. If antibodies to any of the antigens are present in a blood sample, distinct patterns can be seen with a fluorescent microscope.

Synovial fluid analysis. Normal synovial fluid, the lubricating substance of the joint, consists of extremely large, heavy molecules and is highly viscous. When the joint is diseased, the fluid may increase in quantity, become inflamed, and contain abnormal elements such as white cells, crystals, strands of collagen, and bacteria. Analysis of the fluid may help to identify the condition.

Biopsy. The removal of a bit of tissue for examination usually implies a search for malignancy. But in rheumatic diseases biopsy of the joints, muscles, skin, blood vessels, and other structures is done to allow precise assessment of these tissues.

RHEUMATIC DISEASES

Nonarticular Rheumatism

Not all rheumatic diseases affect the joints directly. Nonarticular rheumatism encompasses rheumatic conditions of tissues around the joint—muscles, ligaments, tendons, fascia, bursa—rather than inside the joint. It also includes certain conditions in which pain is felt in joints far from the immediate cause. There are many forms of nonarticular rheumatism, including some of the most common disorders seen by rheumatic disease specialists. These disorders affect patients of all ages but a preponderance are seen in middle-aged patients.

Bursitis is an inflammation of a small lubricating sac, or bursa, located between muscle layers or between a muscle and bone. Bursae, located throughout the body, reduce friction. One or multiple bursae may become inflamed, a condition called bursitis. Subdeltoid or shoulder bursitis is the best known, but any bursa can be affected. Symptoms include pain while lying on or moving the involved joint. Joint motion is often limited. Sometimes the bursal area is swollen, red, and tender.

Tendinitis is the inflammation of one or more tendons. It is often precipitated by injury. Persons in certain occupations are more likely to develop shoulder bursitis or tendinitis as a result of overuse or misuse of the joint. Symptoms of tendinitis are identical to those of bursitis.

Ligament problems result from strain or a tear. Ligaments also may become painful and tender as a result of chronic irritation. Tennis elbow (epicondylitis) is an example. In this condition, the tendons of the forearm become painful and tender where they attach to the ligaments in the elbow. An incorrect swing of a tennis racquet can cause tennis elbow, but the disorder also may occur in those who do not play tennis. Bursitis, tendinitis, and tennis elbow are treated with anti-inflammatory drugs, cortisone injections, exercises, protective devices, and surgery in rare cases.

Nerve entrapments occur when certain nerves become compressed by distortions or inflammations.

• **Thoracic outlet syndrome** occurs when poor posture, local injury, or congenital abnormalities narrow the upper rib cage opening

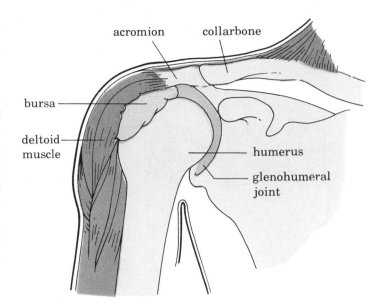

BURSITIS

Inflammation of a bursa, a lubricating sac between muscles or between muscle and bone, can cause excruciating pain. The most common form occurs in the shoulder. When the arm is moved, the swollen bursa may become pinched between the upper arm bone (humerus) and the point of the shoulder (acromion). Sometimes the shoulder is tender, swollen, and red.

where the nerves and major blood vessels pass from the chest cavity into the arm. The result is arm pain, numbness, and occasionally swelling, especially when sleeping, reaching, or carrying.

• **Carpal tunnel syndrome** occurs when the nerve passing from the arm through the wrist into the hand is compressed by inflamed and swollen tendons or narrowing of the tunnel by systemic disease. Carpal tunnel syndrome during pregnancy is common. Sometimes fractures distort the canal and compress the nerve. Regardless of cause, the patient experiences numbness, tingling, or pain in the thumb or second, third, and fourth fingers.

Symptoms often strike at night and awaken the sufferer. Momentary relief may be obtained by shaking the hand or running it under warm water. Carpal tunnel syndrome is common but the cause usually cannot be detected. Heat, wrist splints, and local injections of cortisone tend to relieve symptoms, but sometimes surgery is necessary to relieve the pressure in the wrist.

Fibromyositis, also known as fibrositis, is not a disease in the usual sense of the word because neither pathologic nor physiologic

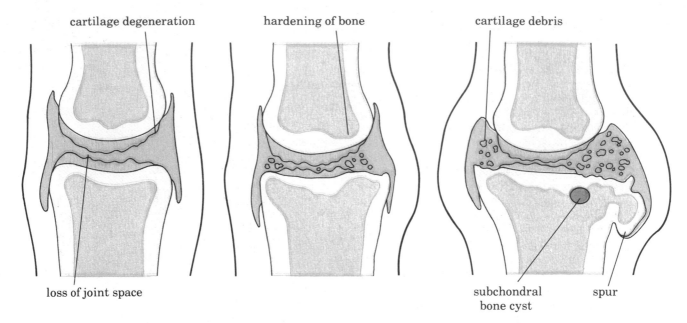

cartilage degeneration   hardening of bone   cartilage debris

loss of joint space   subchondral bone cyst   spur

STAGES OF ARTHRITIS

The changes of degenerative arthritis begin gradually and may cover many years. In the early stage (left drawing) cartilage softens and develops cracks and fissures, forming an uneven surface and narrowing the joint space. Later (center drawing) the underlying bone attempts to repair the damage by new growth. Crumbled bits of cartilage and bone float in the synovial fluid, interfering with joint motion. In advanced arthritis, cysts may develop in the bone, joint space is greatly narrowed, and the synovial capsule is distorted by bone spurs.

changes have been clearly demonstrated. However, the pattern of symptoms and, in many instances, the response to therapy is so characteristic that it is recognized as a disease. Patients with fibromyositis complain of pain in several areas arising from muscles and ligaments and tendons around the joints. The neck, shoulders, back, elbows, and outside of the thighs are common sites. On examination, the doctor finds tender areas that show no swelling, heat, or redness. These are often referred to as "trigger points" because pressure on one may cause pain in many places.

Patients with fibrositis are young or middle-aged and may be under a great deal of emotional or physical stress or may be depressed. Some experts believe that emotional tension is converted to painful muscle spasm. Laboratory and X-ray studies are normal. Treatment varies but generally consists of heat or ice applications, muscle relaxing and analgesic drugs, and injections of a combination of a local anesthetic and cortisone into the trigger points. Many patients seem to respond well to antidepressant drugs even though they are not necessarily depressed.

Osteoarthritis

Osteoarthritis is a degenerative disorder of one or more joints. It is sometimes referred to as wear-and-tear arthritis or degenerative arthritis. Most experts agree that the breakdown process begins in cartilage or in bone under the cartilage. In otherwise healthy people cartilage gradually deteriorates over a span of many years as part of aging, but in osteoarthritis the process seems to be accelerated. Sometimes a single traumatic event appears to be responsible, sometimes multiple minor injuries appear to be. In some cases the cause of injury is obvious, such as falling off a truck and twisting or fracturing an ankle. It should come as no surprise that former professional football players fall victim to osteoarthritis more often than people who have led more sedentary lives. Yet, most of us probably injure the joints frequently during our lifetime, often without being aware of it. Obviously there are other causes of osteoarthritis besides trauma.

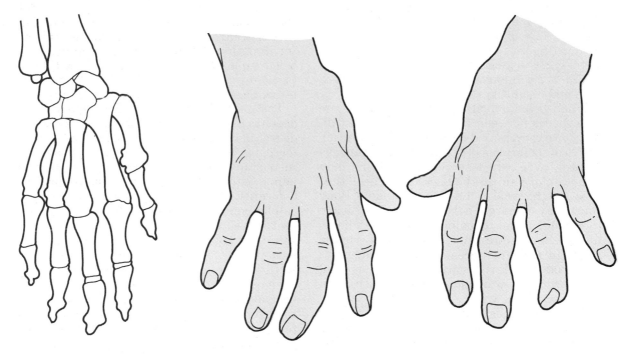

ARTHRITIS OF THE HAND

Small joints of the fingers are a common site of arthritis. Degenerative changes in the joint, joint space narrowing, and spur formation give the fingers a snakelike configuration

and a squared appearance at the base of the thumb. The changes are seen on X ray. Arthritis confined to the finger joints appears to run in families.

Some persons appear to be predisposed to develop osteoarthritis in many relatively inactive joints. Doctors suspect, based on experimental evidence, that increased amounts of certain enzymes cause a premature breakdown of cartilage in these persons' joints. Also, certain metabolic diseases are associated with osteoarthritis (it is more common in diabetes, for example). Other types of arthritis, infection, and congenital abnormalities are causes of secondary types of arthritis. Heredity plays a role in some cases; osteoarthritis confined to the small joints of the hands tends to run in families. Some closely bred laboratory animals predictably develop osteoarthritis.

Osteoarthritis is the most common type of arthritis. It is the type we mean when we say that all of us will develop arthritis sooner or later. Almost everyone over age 70 has osteoarthritis of the neck, although some are not bothered by it. Because deterioration is gradual, most cases of osteoarthritis are not diagnosed before age 40. Both sexes are affected. Women may notice that it appears abruptly after menopause.

Early symptoms are dull pain and stiffness in a few joints. At first, discomfort is most noticeable in mornings, but soon the patient may become aware of aches that come and go during the day. Mild activity or limbering up may lessen the symptoms, but extensive activity tends to worsen them. The housekeeper with osteoarthritis of the knees may have difficulty descending stairs, climbing onto a stool, or standing for long periods, while the secretary with small finger involvement may find typing, buttoning, or other fine finger movements difficult.

As the disease becomes more advanced, pain is persistent and certain activities become laborious, even impossible. The physician's first examination may show little more than tenderness and mild swelling, or there may be bony protuberances (spurs), growths that interfere with joint motion. Redness and warmth are unusual, and rarely is joint motion severely painful until later in the course of the disease.

In advanced cases, the joint may actually crunch when moved, a phenomenon called crepitus. Range of motion is limited. Still later, certain joints may become loose or deformed.

The hands may take on a snakelike appearance because of deviations in the small joints. If your fingers are knobby or bumpy, you may have early osteoarthritis. The base of the thumb is a common site and may cause severe pain and disability.

When osteoarthritis strikes the neck, the disc spaces between the vertebrae almost always are compressed because of degeneration (cervical spondylosis). The process is not always painful, even when advanced. Patients may complain of pain in the back of the neck that shoots to the head or top of the shoulders. Bony spurs may compress nerve roots as they leave the spinal canal, causing pain that radiates into the hand and even muscle weakness in the arms. In rare instances spurs may compress the blood vessels that carry blood to the brain, and bizarre neurologic symptoms and even stroke may follow.

Few people escape back pain during a lifetime. In the older age group osteoarthritis seems the most common cause, although physicians cannot always be sure because osteoarthritic changes are commonly found in the lumbar spine even in X rays of people who have no symptoms. The hips cannot be straightened and the knees are bowed. Osteoarthritis of the ankle is usually a consequence of previous injury.

Osteoarthritis is painful and may limit function, but fortunately it rarely confines the sufferer to a wheelchair or bed. Only the joints are affected; there are no other manifestations. Joint pain that worsens with activity in a middle-aged or older person is highly suggestive of osteoarthritis. A physician's physical examination usually confirms it. X rays may be recommended to support the diagnosis and give an indication of how far the disease has progressed. In early cases, there will be only a few spurs and increased density of bone next to the joint (sclerosis). Advanced disease may show holes in the bone (cysts), irregularity of the bone surfaces, and narrowed joint space. Blood tests are useful because they can rule out diseases that mimic osteoarthritis. Arthroscopy and bone scan may indicate osteoarthritic changes before the routine X ray.

There are several variations of osteoarthritis. Primary generalized osteoarthritis is a slowly progressive form characterized by involvement of more than one joint, especially in the hands. Modest inflammatory changes take place in the joints. In certain neurologic conditions such as those caused by syphilis or diabetes, the sensation of pain is diminished so that some joints cannot receive the body's message to ease up on an overstressed joint. The excess wear and tear causes a destructive "neuropathic arthritis." In a vascular necrosis, blood supply to the joint is diminished. Bony tissue dies, and the ease of joint motion is altered. Secondary osteoarthritis sets in.

The method used to manage osteoarthritis depends on the number of joints involved, the degree of disability, and the person's tolerance for pain. A program of joint conservation—instructing the patient how to use the affected joints with minimum strain—helps prevent deformity. Certain occupations, for example, call for continued use of the hands and persistent stress. Protecting the joints with proper splints enables their continued use and impedes the osteoarthritic process. With arthritis of the lower extremities, prolonged weight-bearing and continued stair climbing should be avoided. Canes, crutches, and walkers help remove weight from the joints, help relieve pain, and may even stem further damage. Heat and range of motion exercises are invaluable in most cases. Intermittent cervical or pelvic traction is useful in osteoarthritis of the upper and lower back.

Medications can reduce pain and inflammation. Most rheumatologists have found nonsteroid anti-inflammatory drugs beneficial even though inflammation may not be apparent. Injections of cortisone into a few affected joints can alleviate pain, stiffness, and to an extent, disability. However, these drugs cannot be administered too often.

Surgery is helpful when there is intractable pain and need for improved function of the joint. Operative procedures include debridement (removal of destroyed tissues), arthroplasty (joint reconstruction), and joint replacement. Hips and knees are replaced frequently. Small finger joints are inserted less often. Osteotomy is an operation in which a wedge of bone is removed for better joint realignment. Most surgical procedures for osteoarthritis require two to six weeks of hospitalization.

Rheumatoid Arthritis

Rheumatoid arthritis is a chronic inflammatory condition not only of the joints, but of some internal organs as well. Anyone at any age can be afflicted with this disease, but it strikes most commonly between 20 and 45, and

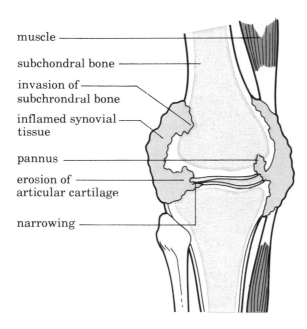

muscle

subchondral bone

invasion of subchrondral bone

inflamed synovial tissue

pannus

erosion of articular cartilage

narrowing

RHEUMATOID ARTHRITIS

The changes of rheumatoid arthritis are extensive and involve all parts of the joint. Cartilage erodes, narrowing the joint space. Underlying bone is invaded and destroyed. The capsule and ligaments are thickened and become contracted or overstretched. New areas of tough fibrous tissue are formed. The joint usually becomes deformed and movement is difficult, painful, and fatiguing.

onset is rare after 60. It is characterized by persistent pain, progressive deformity, and at its worst, profound disability. Rheumatoid arthritis usually starts insidiously. In early stages, the hands, feet, and other joints ache and are stiff. The patient has difficulty with fine finger movements such as buttoning. He is clumsy and tends to walk stiff-legged because full weight-bearing causes pain in the hips, knees, and toes. He has morning stiffness that lasts several hours. The joints gradually swell and become difficult to move. Forming a fist, for example, is nearly impossible. At first, symptoms may be intermittent, but gradually they become persistent and involve almost all the joints in the body. Most patients are so tired that even a minimal chore is exhausting.

The inflammatory process eventually invades cartilage and the surrounding structures. The joint capsule, tendons, and ligaments may become contracted or overstretched, and joint deformities result. Nodules may develop beneath the surface of

the skin in areas of friction. The heart, lungs, spleen, eye, and blood vessels may become involved. Sjogren's or sicca syndrome is a complication that causes malfunction and dryness of the lubricating glands of the mouth, eyes, respiratory tract, vagina, and rectum (see chapter 12, "The Eyes").

The inflammatory changes and deformities of advanced rheumatoid arthritis are so characteristic that the diagnosis is not difficult. However, until significant changes are seen, diagnosis may be difficult. Nonspecific measures of inflammation such as the sedimentation rate are abnormal. Rheumatoid factor (see page 340) is found in the serum of most patients, sometimes in concentrated amounts. Many patients with active arthritis are anemic. X rays may show loss of bone density, cysts or erosions, and even complete destruction of the joint.

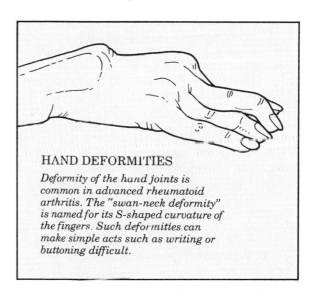

HAND DEFORMITIES

Deformity of the hand joints is common in advanced rheumatoid arthritis. The "swan-neck deformity" is named for its S-shaped curvature of the fingers. Such deformities can make simple acts such as writing or buttoning difficult.

The cause of rheumatoid arthritis, despite thousands of experimental investigations, is not known. The most prevalent theory is that a virus, small bacteria, or other microorganism is harbored in the joint. Local tissues form antibodies against the foreign invader, but in the process of interacting with the microorganisms the antibodies become altered and are no longer recognized by the body itself. The body forms new antibodies to fight the altered old ones (rheumatoid factor). This immune reaction triggers a flood of inflammatory substances that increase the surrounding circulation with swelling, heat, and sometimes redness. Somehow, the process becomes self-perpetuating.

Management of rheumatoid arthritis is complex. The most important consideration is for patients and their families to become familiar with the nature of the disease, the usual courses, tendencies for ups and downs, and the consequences of failing to adhere to a regimen of therapy.

Drugs play a major role. Analgesics, nonsteroidal anti-inflammatory drugs, systemic cortisone, cortisone injections into the joints, and a group of drugs called remittive agents, including gold salts, penicillamine, and antimalarial drugs, used singly or in combination, are helpful for most patients. The remittive group is most likely to sustain improvement but must be administered for months or even years, and they have more side effects. However, in most instances the benefits outweigh the adverse reactions.

But drugs used without other supporting methods are likely to fail. Physical and occupational therapies play valuable roles. Heat, cold, exercises, splints, braces, and supportive devices not only prevent and correct deformity but relieve pain. Most patients fail to realize that a single warm towel over an inflamed joint will usually provide as much relief as a potent analgesic.

Almost all patients with rheumatoid arthritis can benefit from some form of physical or occupational therapy. Patients who are bedridden may learn to move to a chair independently. Those in a wheelchair can be made to walk. Many who cannot carry on manual activities of daily living can have those abilities restored, while those with pain can be given at least symptomatic relief. One of the most important phases of the management of rheumatoid arthritis is joint conservation, because it minimizes stress and prevents further damage.

Twenty years ago, joint surgery in rheumatoid arthritis was virtually unheard of. Today, inflamed joint linings are successfully removed to alleviate pain and impede destructive changes. Joints can be realigned. Numerous surgical restorative procedures are available for most joints, including partial or total replacement. Older patients with rheumatoid arthritis are often concerned about whether they can tolerate the surgery. Generally, age is no barrier.

The psychological problems of rheumatoid arthritis are vast. Rheumatoid arthritis, because of its potential for pain and disability, affects not only the patient but family, friends, and any person close to the patient. Relatives and friends may be a great help in a rehabilitation program. They can remind the patient to take medication, help in home exercise programs, and, most importantly, can be encouraging and motivating.

It is a disastrous experience at any age to be struck down by a chronic painful illness such as rheumatoid arthritis. A patient is bound to meet frustrations and from time to time express anger at those around him, including his physician. Logic, patience, equanimity, and an air of confidence will eventually be rewarded. Most of the problems of rheumatoid arthritis can be overcome so that the patient will become an independent, productive person who is an asset rather than a burden to society.

Juvenile Rheumatoid Arthritis

The Arthritis Foundation reports that 250,000 children in the United States bear the diagnosis of juvenile rheumatoid arthritis. Three forms are recognized, but in reality they may turn out to be separate diseases. The cause of rheumatoid arthritis in children is not understood any better than is the adult form.

About 50 percent of patients with juvenile rheumatoid arthritis have what is termed the polyarticular form, which means more than one joint is affected. These children tend to have less morning stiffness and greater involvement of the neck, sacroiliac, and temporo-mandibular jaw joints. They also have more flexion contractures, in which the joints tense and contract and fail to maintain normal alignment. The jaw may be recessed (micrognathia) and the child may stop growing before reaching normal height. There is a greater tendency for fever and a transient, orange-tinted rash on the torso. Nodules under the skin like those seen in adults are rare.

A second type, pauciarticular rheumatoid arthritis, involves fewer joints and affects about one-third of child victims. Knees, ankles, hips, elbows, and wrists are most commonly involved. Fortunately, this type tends to disappear by the teens, although some cases go on to the polyarticular phase. While the joint manifestations of pauciarticular arthritis are more benign than other types, inflammation of the anterior chamber of the eye (iritis) can lead to blindness without much warning.

A few children have the acute systemic form of juvenile rheumatoid arthritis called Still's disease. They may become suddenly and seriously ill with high temperatures, a generalized rash, lymph node enlargement, and even involvement of the heart, lung, and spleen. The joints may appear not to be involved, in which case diagnosis is often difficult.

Rheumatoid arthritis in children is managed as it is in adults but with great emphasis on educational programs, physical therapy, recreational programs, and emotional support. Drugs and surgery are used to a lesser degree. Aspirin is a mainstay because most other nonsteroid anti-inflammatory drugs have not been tested in children under 14. Cortisone helps to reduce inflammation but has numerous side effects including stunted growth. Corticosteroids are needed for iritis when blindness is impending. Gold salts have been found to be safe but not as effective as in adults. Penicillamine and antimalarials are not yet advised for young children because they have not been fully tested. However, they may be tried in older children and young adults who develop the juvenile form of rheumatoid arthritis.

The treatment goals in children are to reduce pain, prevent deformity, maintain function, and prevent blindness by periodic eye examinations. The child should not be overly sheltered but encouraged to lead as normal a life as possible. Hospitalizations should be minimized, and children should attend regular schools and play with their peers.

Ankylosing Spondylitis

Imagine what it is like to go through life unable to bend forward or sit in a chair because the spine is poker straight. Some patients with advanced ankylosing spondylitis, an inflammation of the spinal and sacroiliac joints, must live this way. Young and middle-aged men are the most frequent victims. Initial symptoms are low back pain on either or both sides. Stiffness is profound, particularly in the morning. Gradually, pain ascends along the spine. The neck tightens, until after several years it may be difficult or impossible to turn the head. Sometimes shoulders, hips, knees, and other joints may be painful and restricted.

Almost all persons with ankylosing spondylitis have HLA (human leukocytic antigen) B27, a specific type of genetic marker detected on white blood cells (see chapter 6, "The Blood"). HLA B27 may be likened to the blood cell types A, B, or O, but only four to eight percent of the population bear this genetic marker, thus simplifying diagnosis. Patients with early ankylosing spondylitis resemble those with structural abnormalities of the back or generalized inflammatory arthritis. X rays of advanced cases show fusion of the entire spine with calcified ligaments ("bamboo spine").

Management programs for ankylosing spondylitis emphasize physical therapy to maintain good posture and drugs to reduce inflammation. Aspirin and other nonsteroid anti-inflammatory drugs play a valuable role. Cortisone, gold, and other remittive agents are used less. Surgery is restricted to realigning badly deformed spines, but fortunately the procedure rarely has to be performed. Psychological problems in this group are similar to those in rheumatoid arthritis. Most persons continue to work despite severe disease.

Psoriatic Arthritis and Reiter's Syndrome

Most patients are surprised to learn that psoriasis, a chronic scaling disease of the skin, is associated with arthritis. In some cases arthritis symptoms precede the skin rash. Young and middle-aged adults are the most frequent sufferers. In this condition, which closely resembles rheumatoid arthritis, several joints become acutely or chronically inflamed with pain, redness, heat, and swelling. Involvement in the hand joints and diffuse swelling of the fingers or toes (sausage digit) are striking. It is not clear how psoriasis relates to arthritis.

Reiter's syndrome is a peculiar combination of arthritis, conjunctivitis (pink eye), urethritis (redness and discharge at the opening of the penis), balanitis (inflammation of the penis), keratodermia blennorrhagicum (rash on the palms and soles with nail changes), and painless mouth ulcers.

In both psoriatic arthritis and Reiter's syndrome, anti-inflammatory drugs and local injections of cortisone relieve pain and disability. The course of both diseases is unpredictable. Attacks are briefer and lead to less damage than in rheumatoid arthritis.

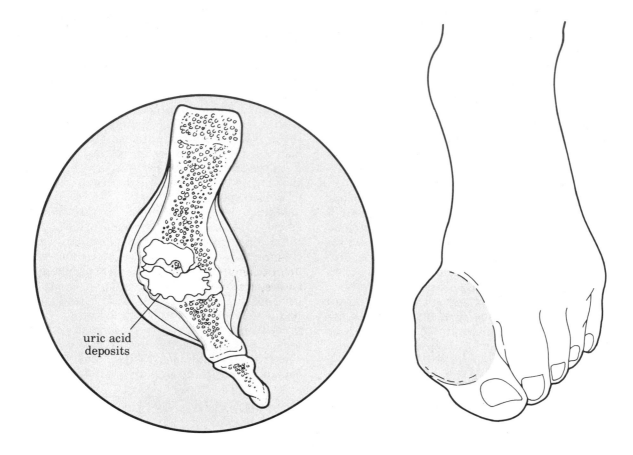

uric acid
deposits

A GOUT ATTACK

An acute attack of gout usually strikes the joint of the big toe, causing swelling and extreme pain. It occurs when crystals of uric acid (urate) are deposited in the joint (enlarged drawing). Gout frequently appears suddenly, often striking while the person is asleep. Pain and swelling may subside within a few days without treatment, but may recur later.

Infectious Arthritis

Infectious arthritis is uncommon. Its beginning is dramatic, with the appearance of the cardinal signs of inflammation—pain, swelling, redness, and profound disability. Infants, elderly adults, and the chronically ill are most prone to develop it. Staphylococcus, streptococcus, diplococcus, influenza bacteria, and other germs are responsible. Young adults are susceptible to gonorrheal arthritis of one or two joints.

Most patients with infectious arthritis appear sick, as with a "flu" or other illness. Fever is usually present. Tuberculosis may cause a more sustained low-grade destructive arthritis in the joints. The infection is usually recognized by isolating the infecting organism from joint fluid, blood, or other specimens.

Treatment consists of intravenous antibiotics, joint drainage, and physical therapy to prevent permanent joint deformities.

Gout and Pseudogout

Gout is an ancient disease, descriptions being found in the Bible. It has been known as the "rich man's disease" and the disease of kings because it notoriously affects high-livers and overindulgers of wine and food. Benjamin Franklin, Michelangelo, and Martin Luther are famous victims. However, anyone may develop gout. Middle-aged and older men are most prone, while women almost never have gout before menopause.

Gout usually appears suddenly. One or two joints, often adjoining each other, become inflamed. The typical patient reports going to bed feeling well but awakening during the night with excruciating pain, usually in the big toe. The other joints of the feet, ankles, knees, elbows, and wrists are subject to gouty attacks, too. Untreated, the attacks usually subside in a few days, but may recur periodically.

Gout strikes people who have excessive amounts of uric acid in the body. Crystals of the acid collect in the connective tissues, notably the joints. It is not known why the crystals are found in some people who have elevated amounts of uric acid and not in others. Over the years the crystals coalesce to form larger collections known as tophi. These are often visible as nodules just below the surface of the skin, particularly in the elbows and hands.

Most attacks of gout occur without explanation, but some are precipitated by stress, injury, increased alcoholic intake, and dietary excesses, hence the presumed association with high living.

Treatment of gout is designed to reduce acute inflammation and prevent recurrences. With potent anti-inflammatory drugs or colchicine, an old drug produced from the roots of the meadow saffron, a properly treated attack will subside in 24 to 48 hours. Colchicine may also be prescribed daily for several years to prevent further attacks. If the amount of uric acid in the body is excessively high, or if there are large deposits of crystals, then drugs may be used to reduce the level of uric acid. Probenecid (Benemid®) and sulfinpyrazone (Anturane®) reduce blood uric acid by promoting excretion through the kidneys. Allopurinol (Xyloprim®) is another effective drug that controls uric acid by preventing its formation. Large crystal deposits may be removed surgically.

Pseudogout gets its name from its resemblance to gout. But instead of the uric acid crystal, the culprit is a calcium pyrophosphate particle. As in gout, one or several joints are acutely inflamed, but there are no tophi. Pseudogout affects the elderly of both sexes. Many patients also have diabetes mellitus or other metabolic diseases. Blood calcium levels are rarely high. The disease is diagnosed by analyzing synovial fluid for crystals and X-ray detection of calcium deposits in cartilage. Treatment includes nonsteroid anti-inflammatory drugs and aspiration of joint fluid. Colchicine is of less value than in gout.

Systemic Lupus Erythematosus (SLE)

SLE is the prototype of connective tissue diseases, a group of disorders caused by nonspecific, noninfectious inflammation of the supporting systems of the body and internal organs. The diseases apparently stem from autoimmunity, the phenomenon by which the body forms antibodies against some of its own tissues. The process may strike the joints, skin, blood vessels, nervous system, muscles, kidneys, or the lining of the heart, lungs, and other internal organs. Tissue destruction can result.

Full-blown SLE most often strikes women, mostly young to middle-aged; it is rare after menopause. SLE causes fever, arthritis, mouth ulcers, loss of hair, kidney disease, pleurisy, pericarditis (inflammation of the heart lining), seizures, and other nervous system problems. A sun-sensitive rash may appear over any part of the body, but a blush over the nose and cheeks most commonly characterizes the disease. Anemia, low white cell count, and a reduced number of blood platelets result in serious complications. All organs may suddenly be affected simultaneously or they may be affected in turn. Blood studies usually show evidence of the body reacting against itself. The extent of illness in SLE is variable. Some patients are desperately ill while others have recurrent, mild manifestations for years.

Treatment, of course, depends upon the nature and severity of illness. Aspirin and other nonsteroid anti-inflammatory drugs help reduce fever and joint pain but usually are not a match for the more severe internal problems caused by SLE. Cortisone is the mainstay of therapy. Sometimes high doses by mouth or injection are needed. Other drugs that suppress the immune system also may be tried. Plasmapheresis, a method of removing blood and treating red cells (see chapter 6, "The Blood"), is used in severe cases. Attention is given to the prompt detection and treatment of other infections that may prove fatal if missed. Many patients with SLE must avoid the sun or they suffer a flare. Sunscreen lotions and broad-brimmed hats help those who must go outdoors. Cortisone ointments reduce the lupus rash.

SLE places a great deal of stress on the patient and family. Marital conflicts are not unusual. Anxiety and depression are common. The stresses must be dealt with. Most patients can be assured that they will do well with proper follow-up and treatment. Fatigue and systemic illness may adversely affect sexual relationships. Infertility can be a problem but once conception takes place, most patients, contrary to customary belief, do well during pregnancy. Careful observation is needed in the period after childbirth.

Systemic Sclerosis

(Scleroderma)

Systemic sclerosis is an uncommon connective tissue disease in which the skin is the major target. It results from excessive deposits of collagen, the main structural protein of the body. Initially, the skin over the extremities becomes swollen and then taut, giving a "hidebound" appearance. Skin may turn color and be punctuated by small ulcers at the fingertips. As the skin tightens, joints contract in flexion, particularly the elbows and fingers. The mouth opening narrows, the nose beaks, and breathing may be restricted because drum-tight skin over the chest limits expansion. Internal organs may be affected, notably the esophagus, lower gastrointestinal tract, kidneys, lungs, and heart. Swallowing may become difficult, and diarrhea may ensue. If the kidneys or lungs are attacked, the disease can be fatal.

Scleroderma is usually heralded by Raynaud's syndrome, characterized by purplish discoloration of the fingers and toes or painful blanching upon exposure to cold. However, not all cases of Raynaud's result in scleroderma.

Treatment of scleroderma is disappointing. To a degree the flexion contractures can be prevented by physical and occupational therapies. Swallowing difficulty and Raynaud's phenomenon can be eased by medication, but the skin cannot be predictably softened. The internal organs in particular fail to respond to treatment. Several experimental drugs are being investigated, including immunosuppressive drugs, penicillamine, colchicine, and dimethysulfoxide (DMSO).

Vasculitis

Vasculitis is characterized by inflammation and blockage of arteries and their branches. There are many different types, each having its own complex of symptoms. The best known is polyarteritis nodosa, in which the blocked vessels prevent blood from flowing to vital organs, damaging them. The heart, lungs, kidneys, gastrointestinal tract, and nervous system may be sources of pain and other signs of tissue destruction. Fever, joint pain, and skin rashes of various types also occur.

A peculiar type of vasculitis is referred to as giant cell arteritis or temporal arteritis. It involves the blood vessels of the head, almost always in the elderly. On one side of the head, headaches, visual disturbance, and pain on chewing may develop, depending upon which blood vessels are inflamed. Much less frequently, strokes may occur. Temporal arteritis is sometimes associated with polymyalgia rheumatica, a type of rheumatism that affects the elderly and is easily confused with rheumatoid arthritis. In this disorder the entire body aches, especially the neck, shoulders, back, thighs, and groin. Stiffness may be profound, particularly in the morning. Patients are apt to feel depressed or fatigued, and may appear to be chronically ill. Yet there is little for the physician to find on physical examination. Sufferers are often dismissed as old people who complain a lot. However, the sedimentation rate is almost always markedly elevated, a sign of inflammation. Fortunately cortisone in varying doses is highly effective treatment for temporal arteritis and polymyalgia rheumatica. Patients with polymyalgia rheumatica note the abrupt disappearance of their symptoms. Other types of vasculitis also respond to cortisone if tissue damage is not extensive.

Polymyositis

In polymyositis the muscles become inflamed, causing weakness and a limited degree of pain. Sometimes disability is so profound that the patient finds it difficult to rise from a chair, put on a coat, or lift. Polymyositis may be accompanied by a prominent rash on the face, chest, extremities, and knuckles (dermatomyositis). Diagnosis is made by finding elevated enzymes from muscle in the blood, by special tests to measure muscle electrical activity (electromyogram), and by muscle biopsy. Treatment with high doses of cortisone is usually effective.

MANAGEMENT OF ARTHRITIS
AND RELATED DISEASES

"Nothing can be done for arthritis" is a pessimistic aphorism that is heard not only among patients and their families but physicians as well. Dramatic cures are not likely in arthritis and similar diseases, but as a result of a comprehensive approach to most arthritis patients, marked improvements in pain relief and lessened disability can be achieved. Drugs alone, physical and occupational therapy alone, surgery alone, or tender loving care alone will not bring about desired results, but a combined approach usually will be effective.

Drugs

There are many different types of drugs for arthritis, each used in a different way. Analgesics such as aspirin relieve pain but do not alter the basic disease in any way. Anti-inflammatory drugs reduce pain, redness, heat, and swelling. Remittive drugs are capable of inducing complete although not always permanent disappearance of some maladies, notably rheumatoid arthritis and the connective tissue diseases. Some drugs are used specifically for certain forms of arthritis—colchicine for gout, antibiotics for infection.

Anti-inflammatory drugs. Inflammation is basic in almost all rheumatic diseases. A primary aim, therefore, is usually to reduce inflammation. Aspirin and related compounds have been in widespread use to reduce inflammation since the beginning of the century. Most people are familiar with aspirin as a pain killer and headache remedy, but for reasons that are not understood it also reduces inflammation significantly. Inexpensive and available in many forms, aspirin is the standard against which other nonsteroid anti-inflammatory drugs are measured.

To be most effective, aspirin must be given in proper doses. For the average person, this means 10 to 14 five-grain tablets daily. Most patients can tolerate even higher doses. It is important to take the medication with food to prevent gastrointestinal irritation. However, some forms are buffered to make gastrointestinal upset less likely. Furthermore, some aspirin preparations are coated to dissolve in the lower gastrointestinal tract, where undue gastric acidity is less likely, rather than in the upper tract. Other side effects of aspirin include ringing of the ears, temporary deafness, and small amounts of bleeding through the gastrointestinal tract. In more serious cases, there may be gastric and small bowel ulcers, abdominal cramps, and more extensive hemorrhage. The side effects of aspirin in most instances are related to the size of the dose. Both young children and the elderly are more sensitive to moderately large doses. Fortunately, true aspirin allergy, resulting in a rash and wheezing, is rare.

In 1952, phenylbutazone and subsequently a closely related compound, oxyphenbutazone, were introduced as potent anti-inflammatory drugs (grouped with aspirin in the "nonsteroid" category to distinguish them from the steroid cortisone and its derivatives, described below). They are highly effective in reducing rheumatic inflammation, but are associated with a relatively high rate of toxic reactions, some of which are quite serious, so their use is limited. Since 1965, several new nonsteroid anti-inflammatory drugs have been approved by the U.S. Food and Drug Administration and dozens more are being investigated. These drugs do not contain aspirin, but have about the same effectiveness. Side effects vary. Each can cause gastrointestinal upset but less often than aspirin. Ringing in the ears, deafness, and metabolic disturbances do not develop as with aspirin. However, skin rash and fluid retention are not uncommon. These drugs must be administered cautiously to persons with high blood pressure and congestive heart failure.

Unquestionably, the most potent anti-inflammatory agent is cortisone, classed as a steroid hormone. The adrenal glands under the influence of the pituitary hormone ACTH (adrenocorticotropic hormone) normally produce cortisone, especially at times of emotional and physical stress. The natural hormone can now be duplicated synthetically. Synthetic cortisone can effectively reduce joint inflammation, and inflammation of the internal organs can be brought under control with the administration of relatively large doses.

The response of a sick person to cortisone and its derivatives may be dramatic. Some patients are symptom-free only two days after being extremely sick with a life-threatening illness. But high doses bring numerous side effects. Indeed, all patients who take enough

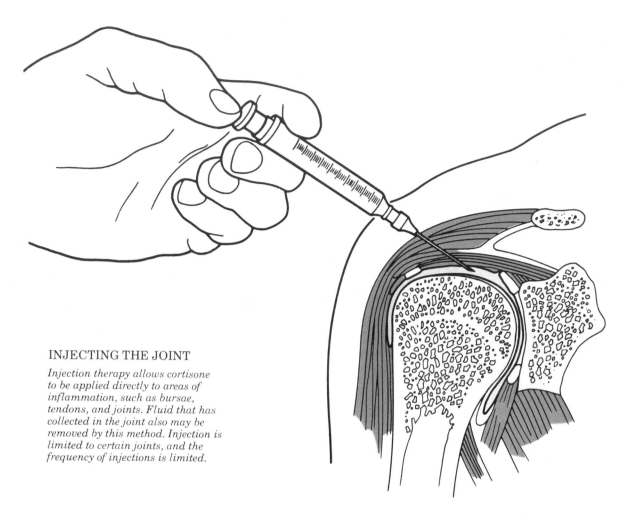

INJECTING THE JOINT

Injection therapy allows cortisone to be applied directly to areas of inflammation, such as bursae, tendons, and joints. Fluid that has collected in the joint also may be removed by this method. Injection is limited to certain joints, and the frequency of injections is limited.

cortisone in high enough doses will suffer some unwanted reaction. Therefore, cortisone must be used judiciously. It may be the patient's best friend or worst enemy.

Injection therapy. Cortisone can be injected safely into joints, bursae, tendon sheaths, and other areas to reduce inflammation. Cortisone administered this way does not enter the general circulation and thus is less likely to cause the multiple toxic effects that occur when it is given by other routes. One or more inflamed joints may be injected, especially if they are impeding a rehabilitation program. If fluid is present in the joint, it may be removed by aspiration before injection of cortisone. Sometimes aspiration itself will relieve pain and stiffness. Physicians vary in their opinions on how often joints can be injected. As a general rule, more than once a month is too often.

Remittive agents. Gold salts, penicillamine, and antimalarial drugs are classed as remittive agents because they are capable of bringing about a complete or partial remission, the state in which all symptoms and signs of arthritis have disappeared. Gold salts are used almost exclusively in the treatment of rheumatoid and psoriatic arthritis. Penicillamine, for many years used for certain nonrheumatic conditions, recently has been approved for treatment of rheumatoid arthritis. Antimalarial drugs are employed against rheumatoid arthritis and for some types of systemic lupus erythematosus (SLE).

Gold salts. Many persons ask whether gold salts really contain gold. The answer is yes, but in water-soluble compounds, not in the solid, expensive form. Gold has been used for more than 50 years to treat rheumatoid arthritis, although the way it works is not understood. It usually has been reserved for severe cases, but there is a trend toward using it earlier in the disease. Gold is effective; more than half the patients experience good or excellent results. It usually takes at least six weeks to see benefits.

Gold is injected into the muscle on a weekly basis at first, but gradually the frequency is reduced to monthly maintenance doses. Doctors now believe that gold can be administered indefinitely if the patient does not experience adverse reactions. Although gold causes side effects, primarily in the skin, kidneys, and blood, these reactions have been exaggerated. Almost everyone can tolerate gold, and if problems develop, the drug can be discontinued temporarily and resumed later. An oral form of gold is being studied.

Antimalarial compounds like chloroquine and hydroxychloroquine accidentally were found to be helpful in treatment of rheumatoid arthritis as well as malaria. The drugs are administered by mouth once or twice daily and, like gold, take more than six weeks to produce a response. Adverse reactions are different from gold. They include nausea and damage to the cornea and retina of the eye. That damage can diminish vision if the drug is taken in high doses for many years. Therefore, periodic eye examinations are necessary when using antimalarial compounds.

Penicillamine, used in rheumatoid arthritis, is chemically related to penicillin but is not an antibiotic. It is administered orally in increasing doses until a satisfactory response is achieved. Complete remission with loss of joint inflammation has been seen in many cases. The drug has side effects, the most common being skin rash. A serious blood and kidney problem can occur. For these reasons, penicillamine is usually reserved for patients with severe rheumatoid arthritis who fail to respond to other forms of therapy.

Physical and Occupational Therapy

Physical and occupational therapy programs are exceedingly important in the management of almost all types of arthritis. When properly used, they relieve pain, improve function, and may impede the progress of the disease or at least stem significant disability. Rest, exercise, manipulation, traction, heat or cold, and numerous self-help devices all can help patients with musculoskeletal problems.

Rest. Rest may be interpreted in different ways. Complete confinement to bed is not necessary or desirable. Although adequate sleep at night and periodic rest during the day will probably enable the arthritic patient to regain stamina, prolonged bed rest deconditions the body and can cause significant shrinkage and weakening of the muscles. However, both physical and emotional stress often aggravate the arthritic process, so arthritics should not push themselves to the point of fatigue.

Resting the involved joints is also important in order to relieve pain, to prevent deformity caused by overstretched ligaments or tendons, and to allow inflammation to subside. The arms and legs can be rested by use of pillows, splints, casts, and braces. A simple, inexpensive canvas splint for the wrist is desirable for maintaining normal use and alleviating pain.

Exercise. Daily exercise of both arthritic and nonarthritic joints is important in order to maintain functional range of motion, to prevent further deforming changes, and to strengthen weakened muscles. Exercise can prevent pain by gently stretching contracted tendons or by eliminating small degrees of instability. Exercise can be prescribed even if the person is confined to bed. A therapist's help is needed for a few exercises, but most can be performed by the patient independently.

Heat and cold. Heat or cold can help the arthritic joints and the surrounding muscles. Cold appears to be preferred by most patients to relieve pain of injuries, while heat is preferred for more chronic, persistent types of arthritis. It makes little difference how heat is delivered, although some patients prefer one method to another. Hydrotherapy—whirlpools or swimming pools—allow the patient to exercise while receiving heat. Paraffin dips are useful for the hands or feet. Many patients feel more comfortable with moist heat packs than with dry forms such as a heating pad, infrared therapy, diathermy, and ultrasound. Hydrocollator packs filled with heat-retaining resin and moisturizing heating pads can be bought commercially. One way to apply moist heat at home is to wrap a hot, damp towel in plastic and then place a heating pad on top. Of course, it is necessary to avoid wetting the appliance. A towel must be placed between the hot pack and the skin in all cases to avoid severe burns. There is no support for the colloquialism "the hotter the better." The proper temperature is the one that feels comfortable and relieves pain.

EXERCISES FOR ARTHRITIS

Daily exercise is important in combating all forms of arthritis. Exercises shown here cover both the joints that are involved in arthritis and those that are not. These exercises help to maintain range of motion, prevent deformity, strengthen weakened muscles, and reduce pain. Most of them can be performed by the patient without help, and can be done even if the person is confined to bed or a wheelchair. A few more advanced exercises require the assistance of a trained therapist who can gently limber stiff joints.

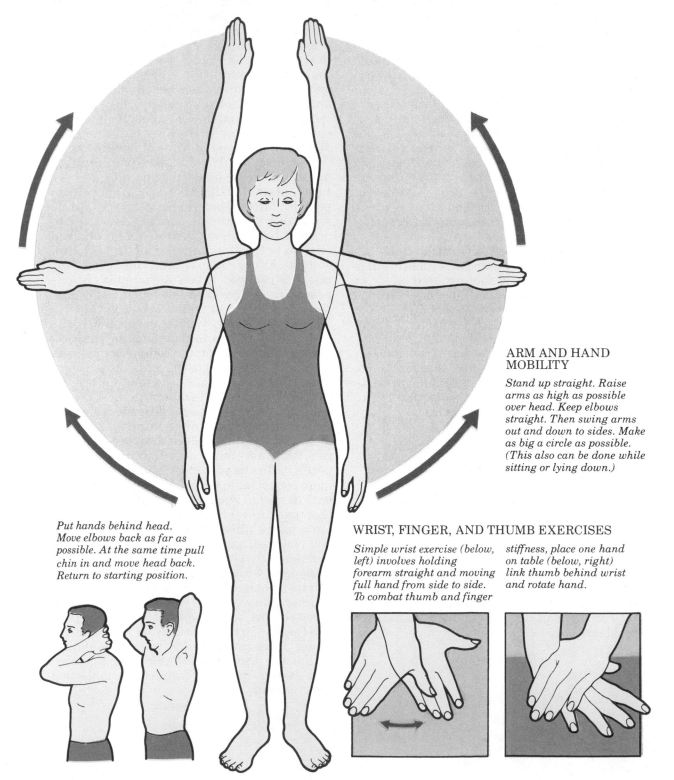

ARM AND HAND MOBILITY

Stand up straight. Raise arms as high as possible over head. Keep elbows straight. Then swing arms out and down to sides. Make as big a circle as possible. (This also can be done while sitting or lying down.)

Put hands behind head. Move elbows back as far as possible. At the same time pull chin in and move head back. Return to starting position.

WRIST, FINGER, AND THUMB EXERCISES

Simple wrist exercise (below, left) involves holding forearm straight and moving full hand from side to side. To combat thumb and finger stiffness, place one hand on table (below, right) link thumb behind wrist and rotate hand.

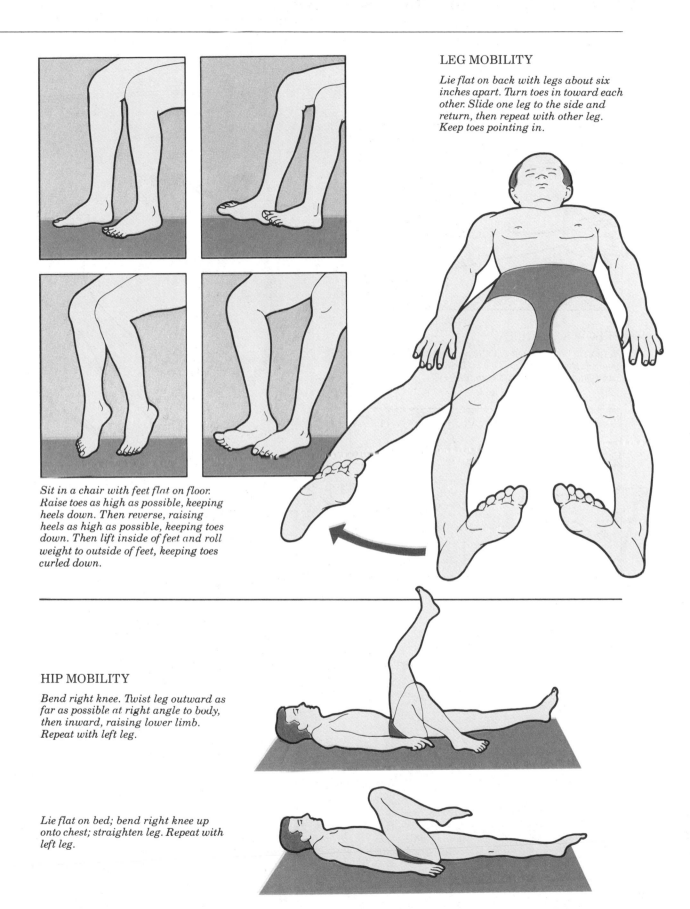

LEG MOBILITY

Lie flat on back with legs about six inches apart. Turn toes in toward each other. Slide one leg to the side and return, then repeat with other leg. Keep toes pointing in.

Sit in a chair with feet flat on floor. Raise toes as high as possible, keeping heels down. Then reverse, raising heels as high as possible, keeping toes down. Then lift inside of feet and roll weight to outside of feet, keeping toes curled down.

HIP MOBILITY

Bend right knee. Twist leg outward as far as possible at right angle to body, then inward, raising lower limb. Repeat with left leg.

Lie flat on bed; bend right knee up onto chest; straighten leg. Repeat with left leg.

EXERCISES FOR ARTHRITIS, continued

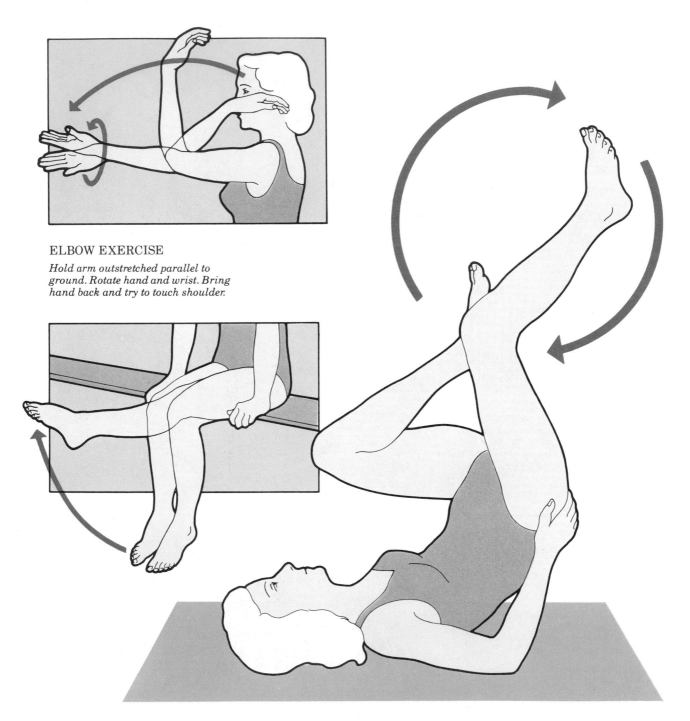

ELBOW EXERCISE

Hold arm outstretched parallel to ground. Rotate hand and wrist. Bring hand back and try to touch shoulder.

KNEE EXERCISES

Sit on bench or high chair (above, left) with legs dangling. Raise one leg parallel to ground. Repeat with other leg. Lie on back with legs elevated (above). Rotate the feet as if you were pedaling a bicycle.

SHOULDER EXERCISE

Lie on back with hands over head. Slowly bring arm along floor until it touches your side. Then raise arm through the air to overhead position. Repeat with other arm.

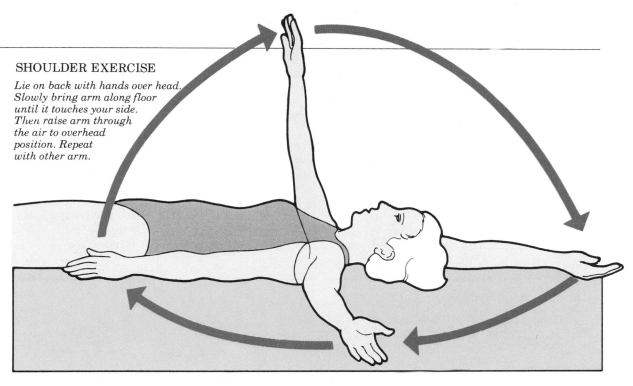

ANKLE EXERCISE

With leg dangling, rotate ankle, first in one direction, then in reverse. Repeat with the other ankle.

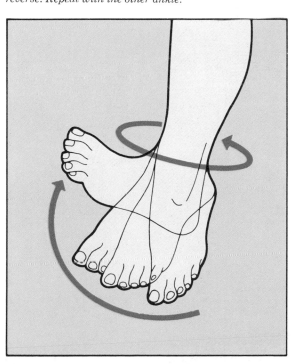

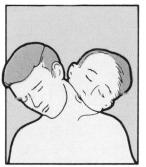

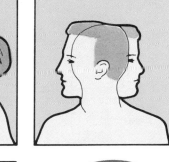

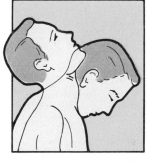

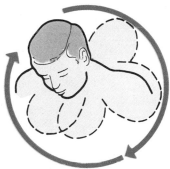

NECK EXERCISES

Bend head forward to rest chin on chest, then arch neck backward as far as possible. Next tilt head to bring right ear as near shoulder as possible. Repeat for left side. Hold head erect; turn to bring chin even with right shoulder, then to left. Drop chin to chest. Rotate head clockwise in complete circle.

Massage and manipulation. Massage is a comforting form of physical therapy that warms the skin. When combined with manipulation of the joints, it may reduce muscle spasm and improve range of motion. Traction is also used to stretch contracted or improperly aligned joints. In the case of cervical or lumbar disc disease, intermittent traction appears to reduce pain and muscle spasm. Whether massage, manipulation, or traction is used, it is extremely important that it be administered by someone competent. It should be avoided if joints are dislocated.

Assistive and self-help devices. Canes, crutches, wheelchairs, braces, and certain shoes are examples of assistive devices that aid movement by relieving pain and reducing stress loads. These devices require instruction by trained personnel.

When, despite all therapeutic attempts, no way can be found to improve function of individual joints so that a person can operate independently, self-help devices may be useful. Many of these are available commercially, although some must be fabricated by the physician or by a therapist. Examples include utensils, tools, and toothbrushes with enlarged handles to permit easy gripping. Clothing can be altered to make dressing, buttoning, and lacing shoes easier. There are several

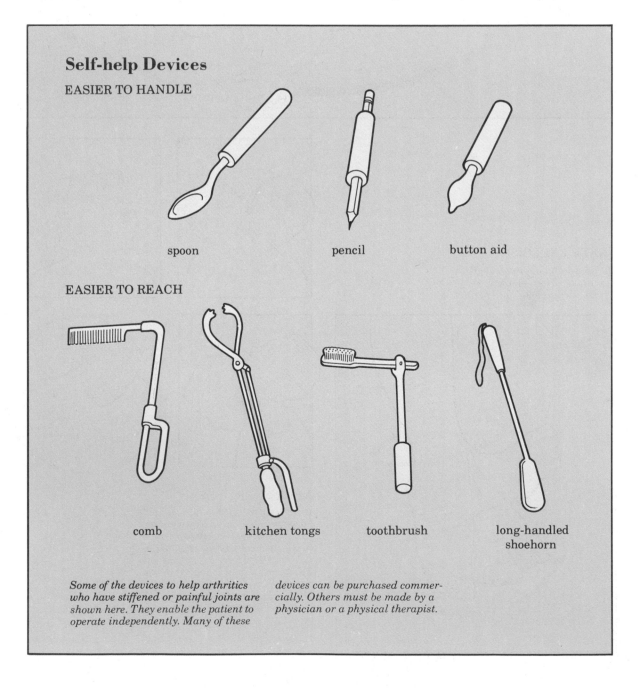

Self-help Devices

EASIER TO HANDLE

spoon   pencil   button aid

EASIER TO REACH

comb   kitchen tongs   toothbrush   long-handled shoehorn

Some of the devices to help arthritics who have stiffened or painful joints are shown here. They enable the patient to operate independently. Many of these devices can be purchased commercially. Others must be made by a physician or a physical therapist.

books available on self-help devices, and information is readily available from the Arthritis Foundation.

Joint conservation. With or without self-help devices, patients can be instructed in the proper use of their joints in daily living. For example, isn't it easier for a person with arthritic hands to hold a pot between two extended palms rather than stressing the wrist by holding it with the handle in one hand? Similar physical and occupational therapy can be self-taught or instructed by the physician or physician's assistant. More sophisticated therapy programs are best administered by occupational or physical therapists.

Arthritis Surgery

We often hear a person with arthritis lament, "Oh, if only I could have new joints!" As a result of some exciting developments in orthopedic surgery, it is now possible for new joints to replace the old. Artificial hip joints, knees, and small joints of the finger can be easily inserted. Elbow, shoulder, and wrist replacements are still being investigated.

Total joint replacement surpasses the advantages of medication in cases of advanced disease. Relief of pain and significant gains in range of motion can be obtained in all patients. Complications of surgery are not common.

Artificial joints of the hands are made of a silicone rubber compound, Silastic, that is extremely flexible but durable. The larger hip joint usually consists of three components: a high-density polyethylene or plastic cup that serves as the socket of the hip, a smooth stainless steel ball that serves as the head of the thighbone, and a methyl methacrylate cement that holds the two in place. Similar combinations of plastic and stainless steel are found in knee replacements. Total joint replacements have become so successful that other forms of joint surgery including arthroplasty (remodeling of the joint) and synovectomy (removal of the inflamed joint lining) have become much less common. Other surgical procedures include tendon transplants, osteotomy, in which a wedge of bone is removed so that the limb may be straightened, and joint fusion, which sacrifices joint mobility to provide stability and relief of pain. In addition, impinged nerves may be released by cutting surrounding soft tissues. In some instances arthritis surgery can be preventive, such as removing a jagged end of a wrist bone that could rupture the hand tendons.

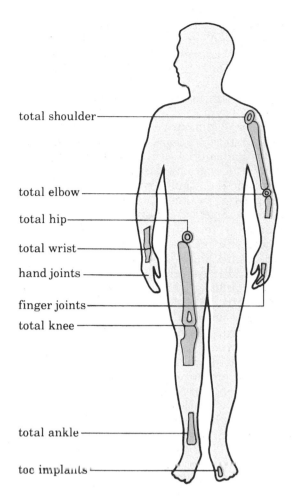

total shoulder

total elbow

total hip

total wrist

hand joints

finger joints

total knee

total ankle

toe implants

REPLACEABLE JOINTS

Artificial joints can often restore motion and eliminate pain and stiffness for many arthritics. The diagram above shows which joints can be replaced. Artificial hip, knee, and finger joints are most successful. Others are still in development stage.

Psychosocial and Sexual Problems of Arthritis

It is little wonder that arthritis, the prototype of chronic disease, can cause significant psychological problems. Persistent pain, limitations of movement, physical disabilities, generalized weakness, fatigue, and visible crippling place a great emotional burden on arthritics. A quick temper, anxiety about the future, and depression are common reactions. Some patients suffer from poor body image, feelings of lost masculinity or femininity, concerns about dependency on others, altered sexual libido, and job problems.

Arthritis may actually arise out of stressful situations, and almost all types of arthritis tend to be aggravated by environmental stress. On the other hand, some patients find secondary gains in being sick, perhaps because of the attention or sympathy they receive.

Sexual problems are a common result of arthritis. Systemic illness such as rheumatoid arthritis can cause loss of sexuality. The pain, limitation of motion, fatigue, and weakness may impede the act of sexual intercourse. Distracting pain, fatigue, and drugs may cause impotence. Fear of failure, fear of causing joint damage, fear of pregnancy, and in many instances fear on the partner's side of harming the mate, may make either participant avoid sexual relationships. If orgasm is achieved, sudden muscle cramping of a joint might result.

Diseases such as systemic lupus erythematosus strain many relationships. Patients may shy from social activities, and may find it difficult to make new friends. They may feel a burden to friends, and even relinquish leadership or participatory roles in community activities. Arthritis patients may find it difficult to carry on with their job, or may be reluctant to take on a job change. Indeed an employer may refuse to alter the job qualifications for the individual. Some arthritis sufferers must stop working because of permanent or temporary disability.

Despite the great personal, social, sexual, and job difficulties, there are many ways for the patient to normalize his life. Individual, group, sexual, and vocational counseling prove beneficial in the overwhelming majority of the cases.

Hospitalization

Most patients with arthritis-related diseases do well while living at home. However, hospitalization may be needed for those who fail to respond to outpatient treatment. This is particularly true in patients who require certain treatments not available outside the hospital. Hospitalization may make it easier to provide medication and physical therapy, and is required for most types of surgery. The hospital provides a setting in which the patient can be treated not only by the attending physician but the orthopedic surgeon, physiatrists (specialists in physical medicine), psychiatrists, psychologists, social workers, vocational rehabilitation counselors, occupational and physical therapists, and arthritis rehabilitation nurses.

Weather, Spas, Acupuncture and Diet

Weather. It is not an old wives' tale that patients with arthritis become achy before a storm. Controlled scientific studies have proven that most patients worsen within a few hours after the start of a drop in barometric pressure and a rise in humidity. Indeed, some patients claim to be greatly improved in the southwestern part of the United States where the climate is dry and the atmospheric pressure stable. However, patients who are contemplating a move solely for relief should be warned that changes in job, removal from precipitating stresses, relaxation, and different patterns of exercise also might be responsible for improvement. The decision to move to a different climate must be based on medical, psychological, and economic factors.

Spas throughout the world, particularly in Europe, promise relief and even cures for arthritis. These warm baths, most of them alkaline, frequently do make the patient feel better, at least temporarily. But cures are not to be had for most types of arthritis as a result of spa therapy. Although some spas have been operating for centuries, the effects of mineralized waters are still not proven.

Acupuncture has been used effectively in certain types of musculoskeletal conditions, but in the systemic forms of arthritis with multiple joint involvement, results have been disappointing. In the few investigative studies completed, objective signs of inflammation have not been altered by acupuncture.

Special diets for rheumatoid and other types of arthritis are sometimes recommended in publications. Under certain circumstances a low purine diet may help patients with gout. A weight reduction diet may ease the pressure on the joints in an obese person. Otherwise, the role of diet in causing or relieving arthritic symptoms is not clear.

UNPROVEN REMEDIES

AND QUACKERY

Arthritis quackery is big business, according to the Arthritis Foundation. More than $950 million is spent each year on worthless nostrums, devices, and other alleged forms of therapy, some of which are downright dangerous. It is hard to pick up a weekly tabloid without finding articles on arthritis vaccines or miracle treatments with bee venom, cobra venom, or alfalfa tea. Some promote electrical devices, uranium dust, or radioactive mitts. Of course, there is the well-known copper bracelet for which some individuals have paid hundreds of dollars.

In most instances the public is intentionally bilked because the quack is well aware that the remedy is worthless. Sometimes the promoter has good intentions but has failed to prove scientifically that the treatment works.

There is a scientific way to study most drugs and treatment methods. This consists of treating half of a group of patients with the method under investigation. The other half, which serves as the control group, receives placebo treatment (inactive ingredient). As many as one-third of the patients in a placebo group are likely to respond favorably. This is why some worthless methods might cause improvement, at least temporarily. The risk and high cost of those treatments is considerable. Be wary if a remedy is advertised as exclusive, if it is dispensed as a secret medication without a label, or if it is promised as a *cure* for arthritis.

THE WAR AGAINST ARTHRITIS

Arthritics have the same needs, worries, hopes, and aspirations as their unafflicted neighbors. They may or may not have pain. They may or may not be handicapped. However, they are people, entitled to the same legal and social rights as everyone. They deserve the best care available. The war against arthritis begins with educating the public about the frequency and dangers of arthritis, and about the encouraging progress made in managing this group of potentially crippling diseases. The public must be made aware of the warning signs of arthritis and where to obtain help. It is critical that the patient and family be informed of the comprehensive approach to arthritis and of the treatments available to combat it. Of great importance, too, is the education of physicians, nurses, and allied health professionals in the early diagnosis and treatment of rheumatic diseases.

Research. Many of the approximately 3,000 rheumatologists in the United States

perform research projects to discover the cause and new treatments for many forms of arthritis. Some type of clinical or laboratory experimentation is being done at almost every medical school in this country. Research is sponsored by the federal government under National Institutes of Health programs. The Arthritis Foundation and other private foundations also provide research support.

The Arthritis Foundation is the national voluntary health association in the United States devoted to seeking the causes and cures of arthritis and its related disorders, as well as improved care for those who have the disease. The Arthritis Foundation carries out a nationwide research program and supports training programs to increase the number of qualified physicians and health professionals to undertake arthritis research and treatment. It sponsors arthritis centers devoted to research, teaching, and treatment. Furthermore, the Arthritis Foundation promotes medical education for all professionals engaged in patient care. A major goal of the organization is to increase public awareness of arthritis and the social and human cost imposed by this group of diseases. Most of the Arthritis Foundation's programs are managed through chapters distributed throughout the United States.

National Arthritis Act. On January 4, 1975, the National Arthritis Act was signed by President Gerald Ford. The act established an 18-member National Committee on Arthritis and Related Musculoskeletal Diseases to study the problem and develop a plan with recommendations for action. The act also provided for an Arthritis Coordinating Committee of the Federal Government, plans for community demonstration projects, comprehensive arthritis centers, an arthritis data bank, and programs for epidemiology, research, arthritis screening, and education.

Local government. Municipal governments are becoming more concerned with the plight of all who suffer chronic disabling diseases such as arthritis. In some cities there are offices for the handicapped. Several states have programs for research, public education, and professional education.

The war against arthritis can be fought most effectively by patients and their families. No one should accept the concept that nothing can be done about arthritis. Treatment is available, but it is up to the patients and those around them to seek it.

CHAPTER 16   CLARK T. SAWIN, M.D.

THE HORMONES AND ENDOCRINE GLANDS

Why do boys become men? Or girls women? Why does someone with an overactive thyroid become nervous, jittery, and intolerant of hot weather? All these events and many other changes that take place in our bodies are caused by hormones.

The idea that something in the blood affects the various tissues of the body is thousands of years old. So is the observation that certain organs—the testes, for example—manufacture some substance that causes changes such as hair and muscle growth in distant parts of the body. But only in the last 80 years or so have we finally obtained trustworthy evidence that blood contains active substances, realized what they are, and determined where they come from. We now know that hormones (the word comes from a Greek word meaning to excite or stimulate) are chemicals secreted into the bloodstream by special cells. Carried by the blood, hormones reach other cells in the body and stimulate those cells. Not every cell in the body is stimulated, of course, because hormones do not do their work at random. They act only on cells able to respond to the hormone. A cell must have a specific receptor for a particular hormone before that hormone can work.

The exact number of hormones produced and secreted within the human body is not known, and perhaps never will be. There may be a hundred (a partial list is on page 364). All together, the hormones make up one of the major control systems for regulating the body's activities, the other being the nervous system.

"Even our destiny is determined by the endocrine glands."

—ALBERT EINSTEIN

But while the nervous system causes changes rapidly, from a matter of seconds to a maximum of a few minutes, the hormone actions are more gradual, taking place in several minutes to hours, lending stability to the change. The quick-acting nerve impulses and the slower-acting hormones thus maintain homeostasis, the body's ability to operate normally despite internal change and external stress. They also help perpetuate the species by coordinating reproduction. In many cases, the hormonal and nervous control systems are so closely coordinated that it is hard to separate their functions.

If hormones are to exert control over the body, their actions cannot be continuous. If they were, the body's responses would go off in all directions. So hormone secretion itself is under control, regulated so that just the proper amount of a hormone is secreted. Usually, when the effect of a hormone reaches a certain level, that effect itself shuts off secretion. This is called negative feedback.

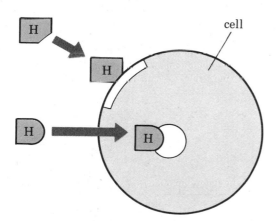

A HORMONE IN ACTION

In order to act, a hormone (labeled H in the drawing above) must attach to a specific receptor on the cell surface or inside the cell. Like a key and lock, only certain hormones fit certain receptors, allowing them to act on the cell body.

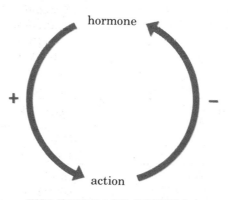

THE FEEDBACK SYSTEM

Secretion of a hormone stimulates a cell's action, indicated by the plus symbol in the drawing. When action reaches a certain level, secretion is shut off by the action itself, indicated by the minus symbol. The system is called negative feedback and helps the body to maintain homeostasis, its state of normal balance.

THE PRINCIPAL HORMONES AND GLANDS

Gland	Hormone
Hypothalamus and brain	Thyrotropin-releasing hormone (TRH) LH-releasing hormone (LRH) Growth hormone-releasing factor (GHRF) ACTH-releasing factor (CRF) Prolactin-releasing factor (PRF) Somatostatin Neurotensin Substance P Endorphins/enkephalins Catecholamines: norepinephrine, epinephrine, dopamine
Pineal	Melatonin
Anterior pituitary	Thyrotropin (TSH) Follicle-stimulating hormone (FSH) Luteinizing hormone (LH) Corticotropin (ACTH) Growth hormone (GH) Prolactin (PRL)
Posterior pituitary	Vasopressin (ADH) Oxytocin
Thyroid	Thyroxine (T_4) Triiodothyronine (T_3) Calcitonin
Parathyroid	Parathyroid hormone (PTH)
Adrenal cortex	Hydrocortisone (cortisol) Aldosterone
Adrenal medulla	Epinephrine Norepinephrine
Ovary	Estradiol Progesterone Relaxin Inhibin
Testis	Testosterone Inhibin
Placenta	Estradiol Progesterone Chorionic gonadotropin Placental lactogen
Pancreatic islet	Insulin Glucagon Somatostatin
Kidney	Renin (leads to angiotensin II) Erythrogenin (leads to erythropoietin) Activated vitamin D (from skin)
Thymus	Thymosin Thymopoietin

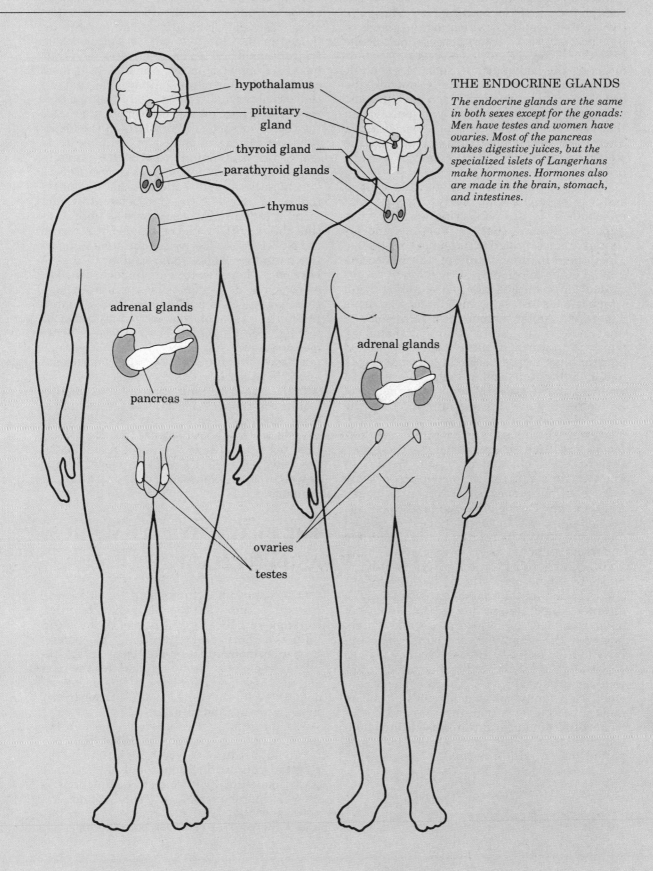

hypothalamus
pituitary gland
thyroid gland
parathyroid glands
thymus
adrenal glands
adrenal glands
pancreas
ovaries
testes

THE ENDOCRINE GLANDS

The endocrine glands are the same in both sexes except for the gonads: Men have testes and women have ovaries. Most of the pancreas makes digestive juices, but the specialized islets of Langerhans make hormones. Hormones also are made in the brain, stomach, and intestines.

Most hormones are secreted by special tissues that do little or nothing else. These are the endocrine glands, which means glands of internal secretion. "Internal secretion" means into the blood. "External secretion" means either to the body surface, such as sweat, or into the gut (which is technically "outside" the body), such as saliva or stomach acid. In some cases a hormone comes from a specialized cell that is not a gland, but part of another organ. There are hormone-producing cells in the stomach, intestinal wall, kidney, even the brain.

Although we often refer to this control system for regulating body activity and metabolism as the "endocrine system," it is important to note that its functions and activities are not limited to the endocrine glands. Thus the functional unit of the endocrine system is the hormone, not the gland.

Medical scientists are reasonably certain which tissues are endocrine glands. The list is generally taken to include the pituitary on the underside of the brain, the hypothalamus, which is above the pituitary, the thyroid and parathyroids in the neck, the adrenal cortex and medulla atop each kidney, the ovaries in women, the testes in men, the islets of Langerhans, which are specialized cells in the pancreas, and the pineal gland in the brain. However, we are still discovering new hormones produced in areas such as the brain, thymus, stomach, and intestine. We do not know much about the actions of these newly discovered hormones so it is hard to say whether they can be abnormal and cause disease. As a result, most of what is considered endocrine disease is related to the recognized endocrine glands.

How do we tell if an endocrine disorder is present? Sometimes there is an obvious change, such as the coarse-featured face in a disorder called acromegaly or the absence of menstrual bleeding in several diseases. Often, however, the symptoms are subtle, particularly in mild or early disease. Or they may be vague and not at all specific, such as fatigue or weakness. So suspicion is the key. The person who "feels funny" or that person's physician must suspect an endocrine disorder and test for it. Fortunately, endocrine disease is fairly uncommon. Most of the time the test for a suspected disease will be normal.

What do we test for? In general, there can be either too much or too little secretion of a hormone. The endocrine glands can become inflamed or develop a tumor or cancer which triggers abnormal hormone secretion and thus has effects apart from the tumor itself. In most cases we can measure the hormone that we think is abnormal. Ten or fifteen years ago it was difficult to measure hormones because they occur in such tiny amounts in the blood. However, the development of hormone tests using the radioimmunoassay has revolutionized the diagnosis of endocrine diseases (among others) and made possible diagnoses that could only be guessed at before. Development of radioimmunoassay was so important that the scientists who originated it received the Nobel Prize. The technique uses radioactive hormones (hence *radio*) and antibodies to hormones (hence *immuno*) to measure hormone levels in blood. Most assays are so sensitive that less than one-hundredth of an ounce (0.3 milliliters) of blood is all that is needed for testing. Being able to make these delicate measurements has allowed us to intervene much earlier and more successfully in cases of endocrine disorder.

In the case of inflammation or tumor, merely feeling the gland (palpation) may be enough to raise suspicion. This is the case with the thyroid, testis, and sometimes the ovary. After that, tests can clearly define the problem. Often, however, special X rays are needed for the less accessible glands, such as the pituitary or adrenals.

THE BRAIN, HYPOTHALAMUS, AND PITUITARY

One remarkable thing about the endocrine system is the way the hormones interact. Hormones produced in one part of the body can influence hormonal secretions elsewhere. Proper hormone function is often an interlocking series of steps, each necessary for the next one to take place. Nowhere is this more evident than in the relationship of the brain, hypothalamus, and pituitary.

The pituitary gland, located almost in the center of the skull, used to be called "the master gland" because its secretions stimulate the secretions of certain other glands and because its hormones deal with such basic functions as growth, metabolism, and reproduction. We now know that the "master gland" is in fact under the control of the hypothalamus, that

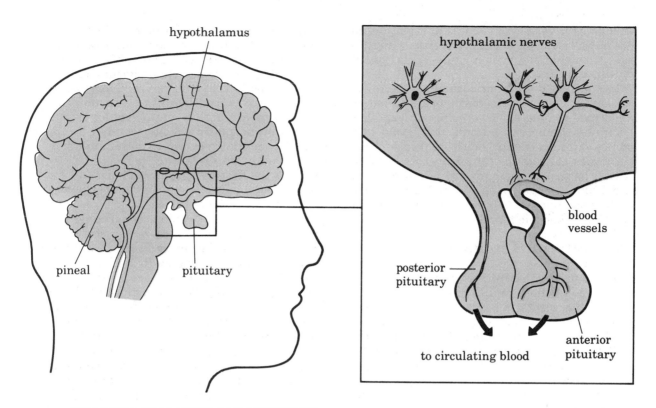

hypothalamus

pineal

pituitary

hypothalamic nerves

blood vessels

posterior pituitary

to circulating blood

anterior pituitary

THE HYPOTHALAMUS AND PITUITARY

The hypothalamus in the brain connects to and controls the pituitary gland. Hypothalamic nerves run into the posterior pituitary and secrete posterior pituitary hormones directly into the blood. Other portions of the hypothalamus secrete hormones into blood vessels that carry them into the anterior pituitary and stimulate secretions of hormones directly from there into the circulating blood. Still other hypothalamic nerves appear to act on other parts of the brain. The pineal gland's function is not clear but it may have some effect on reproduction.

area of the brain situated directly above it. The hypothalamus controls the front part (anterior) of the pituitary by secreting its own hormones, which then flow into the pituitary via tiny connecting blood vessels. The posterior or rear portion of the pituitary is an extension of the hypothalamus, which secretes its own hormones and is not really a separate gland at all.

Thus the hypothalamus, although technically a part of the brain concerned with such matters as sleeping and waking, body temperature, and appetite, is also very much an endocrine gland. The nerves that make up the hypothalamus, including those going to the posterior pituitary, themselves secrete hormones. This phenomenon, called neurosecretion, is a prime example of how closely the endocrine and nervous systems are linked.

The hypothalamic hormones have a major role in exerting control over the pituitary. But we know now that these hormones and many hormonelike substances occur not only in the hypothalamus but in many other parts of the brain and structures attached to it, such as the pineal gland. Besides controlling the hormones of the pituitary, these brain hormones probably act to regulate mood, alertness, sensitivity to pain, and such behaviors as eating, drinking, and sexual activity. For example, the endorphins, so-called because they act like morphine, are peptides, small proteins that decrease the sensation of pain and regulate secretion of some of the pituitary hormones.

The pineal, named for its resemblance to a small pine cone, is a gland-like structure attached to the upper edge of the inner portion of the brain. It makes melatonin, so-called because it lightens the color of frog skin, and contains some hormonelike peptides. While melatonin is affected by light—secretion increases in darkness—and may regulate the hormones involved in sexual function, we do not have a clear picture of what it does. In rare cases a pineal tumor can cause early sexual maturation in boys.

In addition to making hormones, the brain responds to many of the hormones secreted by endocrine glands elsewhere in the body. For example, changes in adrenal or thyroid hormones can cause depression or mania, and sex hormones can act on the brain to stimulate sexual behavior. So the brain is not only an endocrine organ, although admittedly a poorly understood one, but an organ highly affected by other endocrine glands.

The Anterior Pituitary

The anterior pituitary secretes six hormones, all of them small proteins.

Follicle-stimulating hormone (FSH) and luteinizing hormone (LH) are related to reproduction. FSH stimulates the growth of the follicle in the female ovary in preparation for ovulation and fertilization. Luteinizing hormone causes ovulation, the process in which the egg cell is expelled from the follicle and moves down the fallopian tube toward a possible rendezvous with a male sperm (see chapter 26, "Pregnancy and Childbirth"). LH also helps form the corpus luteum ("yellow body," named for its color) from the ovarian follicle after ovulation, which is why it is called "luteinizing."

Both FSH and LH also directly stimulate the ovary to secrete its own hormones, estradiol and progesterone. (Any substance that behaves like estradiol is called an estrogen, and one that behaves like progesterone is called a progestin.) These ovarian hormones cause breast development and feminization in women and are the type of hormones used in oral contraceptive pills. Although the names follicle-stimulating hormone and luteinizing hormone describe actions on the ovary, both hormones are found in men as well, where they stimulate the testes. FSH causes spermatozoa to develop, and LH stimulates secretion of the male hormone testosterone, which causes men to develop muscles and beards, and also supports development of spermatozoa.

Since the ovary and the testis are the gonads, or organs of reproduction, FSH and LH are also called gonadotropins ("affecting or changing the gonads"). Both FSH and LH are themselves controlled by a hypothalamic hormone called LH-releasing hormone (LRH). The name is something of a misnomer because LRH stimulates the secretion of both FSH and LH, so it is sometimes called gonadotropin-releasing hormone (which is too hard to say easily).

Thyroid-stimulating hormone (TSH), also called thyrotropin, is another anterior pituitary hormone. TSH stimulates the thyroid gland in the neck to secrete its hormones. The principal action of the thyroid hormones, thyroxine and triiodothyronine, is to maintain metabolism at a high enough level for tissues to function normally. TSH is secreted by the pituitary on cue from the hypothalamic hormone, thyrotropin-releasing hormone (TRH). TRH was the first hypothalamic hormone discovered, a major advance in endocrinology that also won a Nobel Prize.

A fourth pituitary hormone is adrenal cortical tropic hormone (ACTH), or corticotropin, which stimulates the adrenal cortex, an endocrine organ atop the kidney, to secrete its hormones. The two main hormones of the adrenal cortex (the outside portion of the gland) are hydrocortisone, also called cortisol, and aldosterone. Hydrocortisone plays a major role in the regulation of blood sugar and aldosterone in maintaining salt and water balance.

These four anterior pituitary hormones all act on other endocrine glands to cause secretion of other hormones. The remaining two anterior pituitary hormones do not. They are growth hormone (GH), also called somatotropin, which stimulates growth, at least up to a maximum, and prolactin (PRL) which stimulates the production of milk in the nursing mother. The hypothalamus controls growth-hormone secretion by secreting a releasing factor not yet chemically identified, and an inhibiting peptide called somatostatin. The hypothalamus also exerts this double control over prolactin. It makes a prolactin-releasing factor, which stimulates, and dopamine, which inhibits.

The Posterior Pituitary

The posterior pituitary secretes two hormones: antidiuretic hormone (ADH), which acts to prevent the flow of urine, and oxytocin, which stimulates the uterus and the breast to contract. Antidiuretic hormone is also called vasopressin because large amounts can raise the blood pressure. Like aldosterone, ADH is important in fluid balance. Its major action is to cause the kidney to retain water. The only known functions of oxytocin are to enhance the contractions of the uterus during childbirth and to stimulate milk flow during nursing. But oxytocin is secreted at other times, too, and exists in men as well. We do not know what it does in nonpregnant women or in men.

Pituitary Hormone Deficiency

What can go wrong with the pituitary hormones? If one or more of them is not being produced, or is being secreted in insufficient amounts to carry out its function, or if secretion is so great that the target organ is overstimulated, characteristic symptoms will be seen. If thyroid-stimulating hormone is missing, for example, the thyroid will be underactive or hypothyroid. Symptoms include fatigue, lethargy, puffiness, and occasionally weight gain. If the gonadotropins, FSH and LH, are missing, the ovaries or testes will not make their hormones. The patient is hypogonad and sexual function will not be normal. If ACTH is missing, the adrenal cortex will not secrete its hormones properly, leading to weakness, fatigue, lack of stamina, and sometimes difficulty in maintaining the blood sugar. The lack of growth hormone (GH) causes no difficulty in a fully grown adult but in a child it will lead to a form of dwarfism. Prolactin deficiency is rare but can result in poor lactation in the mother after giving birth. Sometimes only one pituitary hormone is missing but more often two or more are deficient. When all are lacking, the patient has panhypopituitarism, a word derived from Greek which means a complete absence of pituitary function.

The two principal causes of pituitary hormone deficiency are pituitary tumors and hypothalamic disease. Sometimes the hypothalamic disease stems from a kind of tumor known as craniopharyngioma, but sometimes we do not know the reason for the disease. Careful testing for each of the pituitary hormones will define which ones are missing so the treatment can be designed specifically for that patient.

A child who lacks growth hormone can be given injections of the substance and will grow to a relatively normal height. But human growth hormone is scarce and expensive, because the only source has been extraction from the pituitaries of dead persons. Recently, human growth hormone has been made in the laboratory using techniques of recombinant DNA. The hope is that this scarce hormone will soon be available for more widespread use.

Replacing the other missing pituitary hormones is less difficult because in most cases a different hormone can be substituted. For example, thyroid hormone will compensate for a lack of TSH. Similarly, the treatment for ACTH deficiency is hydrocortisone, an adrenal cortical hormone. For a deficiency of FSH or LH, testosterone is usually the treatment in men and an estrogen in women. Treatment with sex hormones, however, does not correct the inability to ovulate or to make sperm. It only stimulates the secondary effects such as hair growth and muscular development. So, if fertility is important, the gonadotropins themselves (FSH and LH or a similar preparation) must be injected. This is a practical approach in women but often is not successful in men. A deficiency of prolactin cannot be treated but is quite rare.

Correcting pituitary hormonal deficiency, of course, does nothing for the disease that caused it. Since the cause is often a tumor in the pituitary, the usual approach is either surgery or radiation. In the past, pituitary surgery was difficult and somewhat hazardous, because the gland lies deep within the skull. In recent years, a new surgical technique, transsphenoidal hypophysectomy, which enables the surgeon to go back under the nose to the pituitary, has made the operation much safer.

Deficiency of the hormones of the posterior pituitary is less common. Oxytocin deficiency conceivably could lead to poor uterine contractions during childbirth, but few cases are recorded. On the other hand, lack of antidiuretic hormone (ADH) leads to a profuse watery urine. A person may produce as much as 10 to 15 quarts of urine a day. ADH deficiency is called diabetes insipidus and should not be confused with diabetes mellitus, the diabetes most of us have heard about in which the urine contains large amounts of sugar. Anything that damages the hypothalamus, such as a hypothalamic tumor or a head injury, can cause diabetes insipidus but often there is no known cause. The treatment is to replace ADH. For many years, persons needing ADH had to be injected with an extract of cow pituitary. Now the patient simply sniffs a synthetic form of ADH one to three times a day, which reduces the excessive urine outflow.

Excessive Pituitary Hormones

Too much pituitary hormone production is usually limited to only a single pituitary hormone in each case and is almost always caused by a pituitary tumor. Furthermore, only a few of the pituitary hormones seem to be involved: growth hormone, prolactin, or ACTH. Excessive secretion of the others is so rare that such a case would be published in a medical journal.

Excessive growth hormone secretion causes acromegaly in a fully grown person or giantism in a person who has not yet reached adulthood. Acromegaly literally means an increase in the size of the hands and feet, but there is also enlargement of the nose, jaw, tissues over the eyes, and many of the internal organs such as the liver and heart. The facial features become coarse with thickened skin and a large tongue. There may be high blood pressure (hypertension) and increased sweating because of enlargement of the sweat glands. Acromegaly usually is slowly progressive over 10 to 20 years and is hard to detect in its early stages. Family and friends of an acromegalic may not even notice the changes because they occur so gradually. Looking at old photographs may suddenly disclose what has happened over the years.

Giantism is acromegaly that begins before the bones have stopped growing. Excess growth hormone causes not only the changes in hands, feet, and internal organs, but a marked increase in height as well. Some of the tallest people listed in *Guinness' Book of World Records* were victims of giantism. The ultimate height can reach eight to nine feet. Note, however, that the overwhelming number of basketball players and other tall persons are naturally tall, the product of genes and nutrition, not disease.

Excessive growth hormone secretion frequently can be suspected simply by looking at the person. Measurement of blood levels of growth hormone will then confirm whether the condition exists. Both acromegaly and giantism decrease life expectancy and should be treated. Because the cause is almost always a pituitary tumor, the treatment is radiation, surgery, or a combination. In some cases, drug therapy may be useful. A drug called bromocriptine directly inhibits secretion of growth hormone. With treatment, many of the changes in the soft tissues will return toward normal. Changes in bones such as the jaw, however, are permanent but will not worsen if treatment is successful.

Sometimes a child, usually a girl, grows far sooner and more rapidly than her peers. Her parents become worried and remain so even though growth hormone measurements are normal. The problem is cultural, not physical. In our society it is easy to be a tall man but difficult to be a tall woman, and very difficult to be a 10-year-old who towers over her classmates.

The ultimate height of a rapidly growing girl can be limited, although most physicians would advise against it. The easiest method is to induce early puberty by giving the girl estrogens. During normal puberty the long bones in the legs, which largely determine final height, first undergo a growth spurt, then stop growing altogether. By giving estrogen well before puberty occurs, one can stop bone growth at a younger age and produce a shorter person. Whether this should be done requires a careful assessment of all considerations, physical and emotional, involving the child, parents, and physician.

Excessive prolactin secretion can cause galactorrhea, which is secretion of breast milk anytime except after giving birth. The condition is more common in women, probably because the breasts are more developed, but occurs in men, too. Men may have no accompanying symptoms except impotence, probably caused by prolactin's interference with FSH and LH secretion from the pituitary. Women often have disrupted menstrual periods or the periods stop entirely, also probably caused by interruption of FSH and LH.

When excessive prolactin is suspected, measurement of prolactin confirms the diagnosis. The cause is usually a pituitary tumor. In many cases the tumor is small and requires special techniques to locate and treat. The usual treatment is surgical removal of the tumor. Sometimes, however, no tumor is found and the medication bromocriptine is used, as it is in an excess of human growth hormone. Bromocriptine blocks the secretion of prolactin (it acts like the hypothalamic hormone dopamine) effectively in most patients and in some cases decreases the size of the tumor.

Excessive ACTH secretion causes a similarly excessive secretion of hydrocortisone from the adrenal cortex and leads to Cushing's disease (see page 378).

The treatment of a pituitary tumor, whether by radiation or surgery, can stop growth of the tumor or excessive hormone secretion but can also cause hormonal deficiencies not present before the treatment. Periodic testing for hormonal deficiency is important after surgery or radiation so that appropriate treatment can be started.

THE THYROID GLAND

The thyroid gland is in the front of the neck and weighs about an ounce. It has two lobes, lying on either side of the midline and joined just below the larynx. If the neck muscles are thin, you can see the thyroid gland move upward during swallowing. An enlarged thyroid or a lump on the gland thus can be felt or seen on examination.

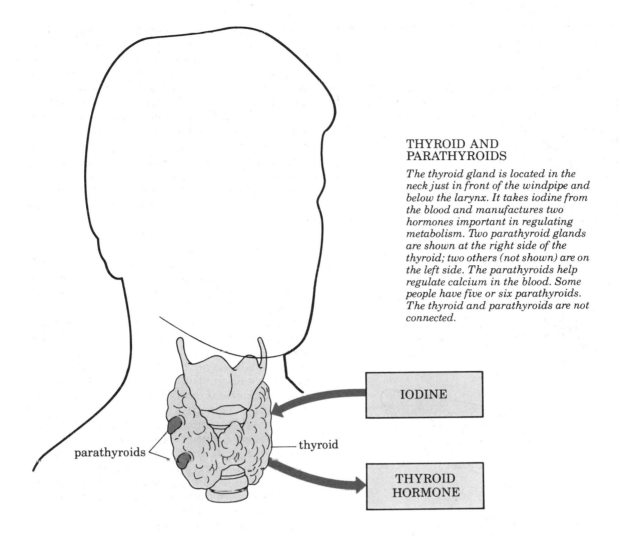

THYROID AND PARATHYROIDS

The thyroid gland is located in the neck just in front of the windpipe and below the larynx. It takes iodine from the blood and manufactures two hormones important in regulating metabolism. Two parathyroid glands are shown at the right side of the thyroid; two others (not shown) are on the left side. The parathyroids help regulate calcium in the blood. Some people have five or six parathyroids. The thyroid and parathyroids are not connected.

parathyroids

thyroid

IODINE

THYROID HORMONE

The thyroid takes iodine from the blood and makes it into the two thyroid hormones, thyroxine and triiodothyronine, which it then secretes on signal from the pituitary hormone thyrotropin, or TSH. Thyroxine is abbreviated T_4 because it contains four iodine atoms and triiodothyronine is abbreviated T_3 because it contains three iodine atoms. T_3 is the more potent of the two. Much of the T_3 in the blood is not secreted by the thyroid, however, but is made from T_4 by other tissues such as the liver, which remove one of the iodine atoms.

The thyroid hormones together act to maintain the metabolism of the entire body. They enhance oxygen consumption, speed up chemical reactions, and help the brain develop and function properly. They help determine whether we are hungry or full, energetic or tired, nervous or calm. With too little thyroid hormone we become mentally sluggish and physically lethargic. With too much, we become jumpy, irritable, and ravenous.

Thyroid secretion is an excellent example of how hormones are controlled by negative feedback. Secretion of the thyroid hormones depends on the secretion of thyrotropin (TSH), which in turn is controlled by TRH, the thyrotropin-releasing hormone from the hypothalamus. When T_4 and T_3 reach the proper levels, negative feedback inhibits further secretion of thyrotropin. An interruption anywhere in the chain can thus disturb normal thyroid function. Thyroid hormone deficiency, or hypothyroidism, occurs if either TRH or TSH is missing, or if the thyroid itself is defective, which is by far the most common cause. An overactive thyroid (hyperthyroidism) produces too much thyroid secretion and is almost always caused by a thyroid problem, rarely by an excess of thyrotropin.

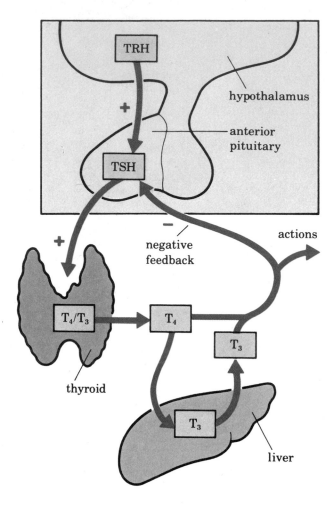

THYROID SECRETION

The two thyroid hormones, T_4 and T_3, bring about many actions in the body, but these can occur only after T_4 has been converted to T_3 in the liver or other organ. The pituitary controls the thyroid via the thyroid-stimulating hormone called thyrotropin (TSH), which in turn is regulated by thyrotropin-releasing hormone (TRH) produced by the hypothalamus. When proper levels of T_4 and T_3 have been reached, negative feedback halts the flow of TSH from the pituitary.

Thyroid Tests

Because of the several hormones involved, there are many ways of testing thyroid function when a disorder is suspected. No one method is best, and the test should be tailored to the suspected disorder. The easiest test is to measure the level of T_4, which will diagnose clear-cut excess or deficiency of thyroid hormone. Often, however, things are not clear-cut and other tests must be used.

Sometimes, when thyroid deficiency is suspected, the level of T_4 will not be clearly in the low range, even though it may be too low for that person. If so, the pituitary will sense the deficiency of T_4 and secrete more thyrotropin, a normal response of negative feedback control. So thyrotropin levels sometimes must be measured, too, to determine whether thyroid hormone secretion is adequate.

Similarly, in suspected hyperthyroidism, T_4 may be only slightly elevated or in the "high normal" range. But the output of thyroid hormone may be still too great for that person's needs. The person's pituitary will sense the excess and shut off secretion of thyrotropin, even when it is stimulated with TRH, the hypothalamic hormone that normally turns it on. Thus, an injection of TRH that does not increase secretion of thyrotropin may unmask hyperthyroidism.

Other tests can examine both thyroid function and thyroid anatomy. Radioactive iodine and sometimes other radioactive elements such as radioactive technetium are often used and are safe in the small amounts needed. After the patient drinks or is injected with the radioactive element, the amount taken up by the thyroid is counted with a modern version of the Geiger counter. An overactive thyroid takes up a lot of radioactivity and an underactive thyroid only a little. At the same time, a thyroid scan, which is a "picture" of the pattern of radioactivity taken up by the thyroid, shows whether one part of the thyroid takes up more or less radioactivity than the rest.

Hypothyroidism

Severe, overt hypothyroidism is a serious disease. Fatigue, sleepiness, lack of energy, a dull and sluggish mental state, decreased metabolism, and a puffy, thickened skin (myxedema) are all common symptoms. The condition comes on over a long period of time. The patient and his relatives or friends may be unaware of what is happening. Milder degrees of hypothyroidism are more common, but they are difficult to detect. The primary symptoms, fatigue and lethargy, are nonspecific because many persons feel tired and lack pep, yet they are not hypothyroid.

Identifying the hypothyroid is most difficult at the extremes of age. The newborn and the elderly show almost no outward symptoms. Yet an untreated hypothyroid infant will develop into a cretin, a mentally and physically retarded dwarf, probably requiring lifetime care.

Although only one in 4,000 newborns is hypothyroid, it is less expensive to screen all babies for hypothyroidism than to care for the few unfortunate victims. Testing for thyroid function is therefore routine at most hospitals. Treatment begun shortly after birth can reverse the condition.

In the case of the elderly some form of screening might be useful, although the consequences of poor thyroid function are less clear-cut than in newborns. Mild hypothyroidism occurs in four to seven percent of persons over age 60, especially in women. But the symptoms are nonspecific and resemble those occurring in many older persons such as tiredness or changes in memory. Treatment with thyroid hormone may help but should be individualized, depending on the patient's overall health. In sum, any time hypothyroidism is suspected it is probably wise to test for it.

Most hypothyroidism is caused by damage to the thyroid gland itself, and is called primary hypothyroidism. In the newborn the likely cause is abnormal development of the thyroid. In adults it is usually caused by either chronic inflammatory destruction of the gland or by previous treatment of hyperthyroidism, which has tilted the balance in the other direction. In the rare cases where hypothyroidism is due to deficiency of pituitary or hypothalamic hormones, it is called secondary hypothyroidism.

Primary hypothyroidism caused by chronic inflammation of the thyroid usually occurs because of a faulty immune system, the system the body uses to fight off harmful invaders. In this case, the body mistakenly generates antibodies against its own thyroid. These antibodies attack the gland and will slowly destroy it if not treated. This immunologic defect often runs in families, and if one member is hypothyroid, others probably should be checked. The defect also may be part of a pattern in which other glands, especially the adrenals and parathyroid, are affected. They should be checked as well.

The treatment of hypothyroidism, whatever the cause, is to replace or supplement the missing hormone. In the past the most common way was to use a preparation called desiccated thyroid, made from the dried thyroids of cattle and pigs. This treatment, the first hormone therapy ever used successfully, is still widely employed, but most patients now take tablets of synthetic thyroxine (T_4), eliminating the need for animal material. The pills usually are taken on a daily basis, but the proper interval and amount of thyroxine is not the same for everyone. In primary hypothyroidism with an elevated thyrotropin level, the correct amount is the dose that brings the thyrotropin down into the normal range. Thyrotropin must be carefully measured during treatment to ensure that the patient takes neither too much nor too little thyroxine.

Because a sluggish thyroid is blamed for "that tired feeling" and a general lack of energy, many persons take thyroid hormone as a kind of nonspecific tonic. Taking thyroid as a pep pill is a definite mistake, one that can have serious consequences. No one should take thyroid hormone without a well-defined diagnosis of thyroid insufficiency.

Hyperthyroidism

Almost everyone has known someone with an overactive thyroid. The hyperthyroid person is jumpy, irritable, sweats a lot, often loses weight, and may have protruding eyes. Most have a large thyroid or goiter (goiter simply means a large thyroid). Most cases of hyperthyroidism are caused by Graves' disease, named after Robert Graves, the 19th century Irish physician who was one of the first to describe its characteristics. Like many cases of primary hypothyroidism, Graves' disease is the result of a faulty immune system, but in this case antibodies overstimulate the thyroid instead of destroying it. In fact it is not unusual for both hyperthyroidism and hypothyroidism caused by immune defects to occur in different members of the same family.

Less commonly, hyperthyroidism may result from overactive areas within the thyroid gland or because a person takes too much thyroid hormone.

Many people are nervous and anxious but do not have hyperthyroidism. A clearly elevated thyroxine (T_4) level makes the diagnosis, but if the thyroxine is only slightly elevated, measurement of T_3 or injection of TRH is needed to define the problem.

There are several treatments for hyperthyroidism, which means that none of them is perfect. In some persons the disease is spontaneously reversible. Someone taking too much thyroid hormone should simply stop, for instance. But the usual hyperthyroid person with Graves' disease requires active treatment. Although the disease will disappear with time, it may take many years to do so.

Possible treatments include antithyroid drugs to block the synthesis of thyroid hormone, radioactive iodine, or surgery. The latter two destroy most but not all of the thyroid gland. Note that none of the treatments clearly affects the immune defect. Because radioactive iodine and surgery frequently lead to the opposite extreme, hypothyroidism, several years later, they generally are not used in younger patients. An antithyroid drug controls hyperthyroidism in all cases if the dose is large enough but the hyperthyroidism may return when the drug is stopped, so therapy must go on for months or even years. The best approach is open discussion of the available treatments between the patient and the physician with careful consideration of the pros and cons before using any of them. Because hyperthyroidism can recur after any treatment and hypothyroidism can occur after surgery or radioiodine (and less commonly after antithyroid drugs), careful follow-up of all hyperthyroid persons is necessary for many years.

Subacute Thyroiditis

Sometimes a person will get a "sore throat" that never seems to go away and lasts for several weeks or even longer. The problem may actually be an inflamed thyroid. The thyroid is tender, the overlying skin is often red and warm and there may be a fever. If this happens suddenly it is called acute thyroiditis. More often it develops over several days or weeks and is called subacute thyroiditis. Many doctors think the inflammation is caused by a virus although this is difficult to prove. It is not caused by an immune defect. When the gland is acutely inflamed, large amounts of thyroid hormone may be released into the bloodstream, causing a temporary form of hyperthyroidism. Once the inflammation subsides the hyperthyroidism disappears. Later, because the thyroid takes time to heal, temporary (rarely permanent) hypothyroidism can occur. Not all patients have all of these phases. In the usual patient, the disease lasts several weeks to months, and a few patients may have recurrent episodes.

If the thyroiditis is mild, simple measures such as aspirin to quell the symptoms may suffice. If it is more severe, treatment may include thyroid hormone, which appears to suppress the gland's activity, or other anti-inflammatory drugs such as prednisone or indomethacin.

Goiter, Thyroid Nodules, and Thyroid Cancer

Goiter means an enlarged thyroid and is not a specific disease. Sometimes the enlargement feels bumpy and so is called a nodular goiter. Nodular thyroids are fairly common in the United States. One study showed that four percent of the population is affected. Most of these patients are euthyroid, neither hypothyroid nor hyperthyroid, with normal hormone levels. Euthyroid goiter is thought to be caused by some minor abnormality in the thyroid leading to a slight increase in thyrotropin (the hormone that controls the thyroid), which in turn causes a modest growth of the gland. In the past iodine deficiency was probably the cause of many euthyroid goiters but this is unlikely in the United States today because the American diet contains sufficient iodine. In other parts of the world, however, iodine deficiency still occurs, and, especially if combined with an intrinsic thyroid defect, can lead to strikingly enlarged thyroid glands and a greatly swollen neck.

Diffuse or nodular goiter can be left untreated if it does not seem to be growing and if the person's hormone levels are normal. More often, the patient is treated with modest doses of thyroid hormone on the assumption that a slight degree of thyroid deficiency exists. Therapy, of course, is necessary if the patient with goiter turns out to be hypothyroid. Treating nodular goiter with thyroid hormone may make the nodule shrink or disappear.

Thyroid cancer is a major concern of many patients and physicians when there is a thyroid nodule. If several nodules can be felt, the likelihood of cancer is quite small, so concern centers on patients who appear to have only a single nodule. In reality, even these usually have several nodules which are found only after removing the thyroid surgically. The evidence indicates that five to ten percent of these nodules contain tissue that looks like cancer (carcinoma). However, this kind of carcinoma does not seem to kill many persons because the overall mortality from thyroid carcinoma is quite low. Thus what is carcinoma under the microscope (the five to ten percent of single nodules just mentioned) is often not biologically malignant. Interestingly, some of the nodules containing carcinoma shrink or disappear after treatment with thyroid hormone.

Findings that increase the suspicion of biologically malignant carcinoma in a thyroid nodule are: a nodule that is extremely hard to the touch, does not move on swallowing, is associated with hoarseness, or gets larger rather than smaller after taking thyroid hormone. Another important clue is radiation treatment to the head, neck or upper chest years before. The previous radiation increases the chance that a thyroid nodule contains cancer. Sometimes a radioactive scan or "picture" (see page 372) shows little or no radioactivity in the nodule. When it is "cold," the likelihood of carcinoma is higher.

In any case, even if the nodule contains a cancer, it is slow growing and there is usually ample time for the patient and doctor to assess the effect of giving thyroid hormone. In most cases a reasonable first step is to give T_4 by mouth for several months to a year, while the nodule or lump is being observed. If the nodule shrinks, no further treatment is necessary and the patient can continue to take T_4. If the nodule continues to grow, surgery may be done. If the nodule does not change much during T_4 treatment, or if other findings suggest a higher likelihood of carcinoma, many physicians would advise surgery. Many others, however, reserve surgery for the nodule that grows despite thyroid hormone.

THE ADRENAL GLAND

In the mid-19th century, Thomas Addison, a British physician, saw several patients who felt weak and lethargic, and had a peculiar darkening of the skin. He did not know what caused the illness, and the patients died. He later found that all had diseased adrenal glands. Dr. Addison knew nothing of hormones but he was the first to connect a clinical disease with a disorder of the adrenal glands. Adrenal insufficiency caused by adrenal damage is now called Addison's disease.

There are two adrenal glands, one on top of each kidney ("adrenal" is a Latin word meaning "next to the kidney"). Each adrenal gland is in fact two separate glands. The outer portion, the adrenal cortex, makes two principal hormones, hydrocortisone (also known as cortisol) and aldosterone. The adrenal cortex also secretes small amounts of male and female hormones (androgens and estrogens). The inner portion of the gland, the adrenal medulla, makes its own two hormones, norepinephrine (noradrenalin) and epinephrine (adrenalin).

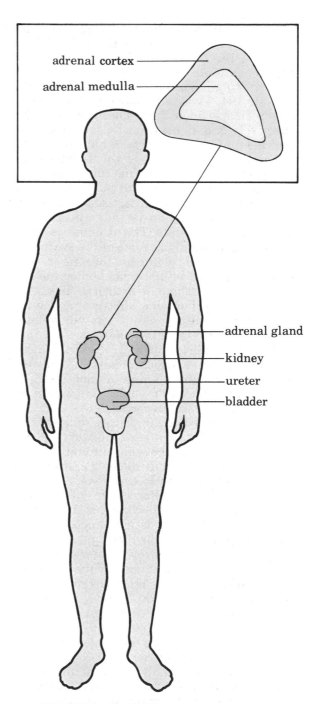

ADRENAL GLANDS

The adrenal glands are located atop the kidneys but have no direct connection to them. The cortex, or outer part, makes the two steroid hormones hydrocortisone and aldosterone. The medulla, or inner part, is an entirely separate gland and makes epinephrine (adrenalin) and norepinephrine.

After its discovery in the late 19th century epinephrine was considered the only adrenal hormone. But treatment with epinephrine did not cure patients with Addison's disease, so the search for other hormones continued. Not until the late 1940s was a hormone of the adrenal cortex clearly identified. The first one used effectively in patients was cortisone. Later we realized that hydrocortisone, which has a similar chemical structure, is the hormone actually secreted by the adrenal cortex. Both are now useful treatments. Still later, many synthetic derivatives of hydrocortisone were made in an attempt to avoid its side effects when used in large amounts. The attempt was only partially successful but some of the synthetics such as prednisone or dexamethasone are now widely employed in many non-endocrine diseases such as asthma or arthritis. The other adrenal cortical hormone, aldosterone, was the most recently discovered; it was not isolated and synthesized until the 1950s.

Both hydrocortisone and aldosterone are steroid hormones, which means they have a chemical structure similar to cholesterol. In fact, both are made from cholesterol within the adrenal gland. Hydrocortisone is called a glucocorticoid because it is a corticoid (adrenal cortical steroid) that affects glucose (sugar or carbohydrate) metabolism throughout the body. It tends to keep the blood sugar normal. In large amounts hydrocortisone can cause diabetes mellitus. "Glucocorticoid" is, however, somewhat of a misnomer. It has several other actions that may be more important than those on glucose metabolism but are not as well understood. Hydrocortisone enhances the heart's ability to contract, helps maintain normal blood pressure, and has a role in brain function. When hydrocortisone is lacking, patients do not think clearly and can become depressed.

Aldosterone is called a mineralocorticoid because its major effects are on mineral metabolism, principally sodium and potassium. Sodium, dissolved as sodium chloride or common salt, is the main constituent in the blood. Without sodium the volume of blood would shrink, the vascular system would collapse, and in a short time we would become dehydrated and die. When animals evolved from living in water to living on land, a mechanism was needed to prevent loss of salt and water from the body. Aldosterone is primarily responsible for retaining critical sodium, a task it performs by acting on the kidney. Antidiuretic hormone (ADH), secreted by the pituitary, works with it to retain water.

Even though hydrocortisone and aldosterone are both made by the adrenal cortex,

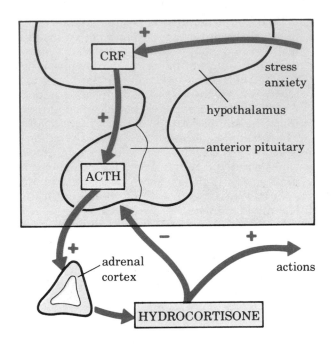

HYDROCORTISONE

Hydrocortisone from the adrenal cortex influences many body functions, including sugar metabolism, heart contractions, and blood pressure. It also acts to control its own secretion through negative feedback. The pituitary hormone ACTH stimulates secretion of hydrocortisone, then negative feedback partially shuts off ACTH to keep the system in balance. The brain hormone CRF regulates both hormone levels. In times of stress or anxiety, increased secretion of CRF steps up the amounts of hydrocortisone, with effects on sugar, heart, blood pressure, and other functions to help handle the stress.

they are controlled by entirely different mechanisms. This is not surprising considering their different functions. Hydrocortisone (cortisol) is completely under the control of ACTH (corticotropin) from the pituitary gland, which in turn is controlled by the hypothalamus. The amount of ACTH secreted depends on three things. One is the usual negative feedback effect, where a rise in cortisol inhibits ACTH secretion. The other two controls are related to the brain and hypothalamus. ACTH and cortisol secretion are higher in the morning than in the evening. This daily (or diurnal or circadian) cycle is set by the sleep-waking cycle and by the light-dark cycle acting through the brain. Further, any kind of stress, whether physical or psychological, increases the ACTH level, again a brain-mediated effect. Since ACTH determines cortisol secretion, the level of cortisol in the blood is affected both by the time of day and by the physical and mental state of the individual.

The pituitary has relatively little control over aldosterone secretion. Instead, the circulating blood volume is the major influence because the blood volume is largely determined by the amount of salt in the body, and aldosterone's main action is to retain salt. When blood volume drops, the kidney senses the decline and secretes a substance called renin. Renin is a kind of hormone of the kidney. More precisely, it is an enzyme that acts on a protein called renin substrate to make angiotensin I, a small peptide. Almost immediately another enzyme converts angiotensin I to a slightly smaller peptide, angiotensin II. Angiotensin II is the principal stimulator of aldosterone secretion. With the rise in aldosterone, more salt is retained by the kidney. The salt winds up in the bloodstream and increases the blood volume. Angiotensin II also acts to narrow blood vessels and helps to maintain the blood pressure directly (blood pressure falls if blood volume is too low). When everything is back to normal, the whole mechanism that triggered the increased aldosterone will slow down and return to its normal steady state.

The hormones made and secreted by the inner part of the adrenal (the adrenal medulla) are epinephrine (adrenalin) and norepinephrine (noradrenalin), and are called catecholamines. The adrenal medulla is actually an extension of the so-called sympathetic nervous system, which makes norepinephrine, too—another example of the close interlocking of nervous and hormonal function. The catecholamines—the "fight or flight" hormones—help the body respond quickly to various types of stress. For example, standing up suddenly tends to decrease blood flow to the brain. A sudden drop in blood sugar can also be dangerous to the brain. Epinephrine from the adrenal medulla and norepinephrine from the sympathetic nerves help keep the blood pressure and blood sugar from falling too low. Anxiety, fear, injury, and excitement also activate the sympathetic nervous system and the release of catecholamines. We say they "get the adrenalin flowing." This activation also causes a heightened sense of awareness, a feeling of tension, a rapid pulse, and sweating. The effects are familiar to almost everyone.

What can go wrong with the adrenal gland? The main problems are too little or too much hormone production or a tumor.

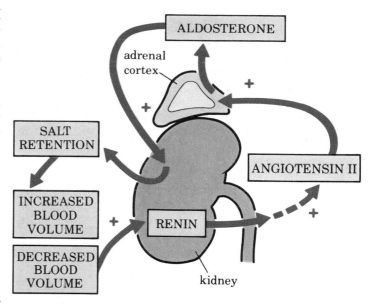

HORMONES AND BLOOD VOLUME

When the blood volume falls because of dehydration, lack of salt, or massive bleeding, a complex process takes place. The kidney (center) senses the loss and secretes into the blood a hormonelike substance called renin. Renin causes the formation of angiotensin, which in turn stimulates the adrenal cortex to secrete aldosterone. The circuit is complete when aldosterone acts on the kidney to prevent it from excreting salt in the urine, thereby helping it to retain salt in the body. The blood volume increases and tends to return to normal because most of the blood is simply a weak solution of salt water.

Adrenal Insufficiency

Lack of adrenal cortical hormones can be caused by direct damage to the adrenal cortex (primary adrenal insufficiency or Addison's disease) or to a deficiency of ACTH from the pituitary (secondary adrenal insufficiency). The symptoms meticulously described by Addison more than 100 years ago are still typical.

Severe Addison's disease causes weakness, lethargy, lack of energy, mental depression, light-headedness, and an inability to think clearly. The skin darkens, and is sometimes mottled, with black freckles and milky patches. There may be both loss of salt into the urine, causing the person to eat extra salt, and a tendency toward low blood sugar (hypoglycemia). Sometimes, particularly under a stress such as infection, surgery, or injury, the symptoms are catastrophic, including shock and complete cardiovascular collapse. This is known as acute adrenal insufficiency.

Deficiency of both cortisol and aldosterone is more likely with primary adrenal insufficiency. Here the negative feedback effect of the low cortisol causes increased secretion of ACTH from the pituitary. The large amount of ACTH (and similar peptides) usually darkens the skin. In secondary adrenal insufficiency, the lack of ACTH causes mostly cortisol deficiency because ACTH has little effect on normal aldosterone secretion. Another form of secondary insufficiency is lack of aldosterone alone because of low renin secretion by the kidney. In this form the symptoms are mainly loss of salt into the urine and a high level of potassium in the blood.

Measurement of blood levels of cortisol and sometimes aldosterone may make the diagnosis. Often, however, the results are equivocal and an adrenal stimulation test is needed. An injection of ACTH in a normal person causes a brisk rise in both cortisol and aldosterone. If this rise does not happen there is adrenal insufficiency. Other tests distinguish whether the poorly functioning adrenal is of the primary (adrenal destruction) or secondary (ACTH deficiency) type.

Treatment of adrenal insufficiency is now fairly straightforward, but before the 1940s the condition was often fatal because the hormones—and therefore the cause—were unknown. When cortisol is deficient, the treatment is to give cortisol (hydrocortisone) or cortisone. When aldosterone is lacking, aldosterone itself taken by mouth does not work well and a synthetic mineralocorticoid, called 9-alpha-fluorohydrocortisone (Florinef®), is used instead. Many patients with primary adrenal insufficiency must take both cortisol and Florinef.® Still, the usual daily medication alone is not complete treatment because any severe stress increases the body's need and can cause acute adrenal insufficiency. The person must be careful to carry an extra supply of cortisone or hydrocortisone and take it in the event of moderate or serious injury. He should also be equipped with a bracelet, necklace, or wallet card informing others of his condition in case an accident renders him unconscious.

Congenital adrenal hyperplasia (CAH) is a special kind of insufficiency which is present at birth and usually shows up at birth or later in childhood. It is uncommon.

The problem is not destruction of the adrenal cortex but a defect in the enzyme machinery that makes the hormones. Cortisol is not produced, leading to a high ACTH level, and, since the adrenal tissue is still intact, the ACTH causes it to grow. One result can be excessive secretion of male hormones, the so-called adrenogenital syndrome. A young girl may become masculinized and a boy will have what looks like early puberty. Severe cases bring cardiovascular collapse in the first few days after birth.

Treatment of congenital adrenal hyperplasia is the same as for other forms of adrenal deficiency, using both cortisol and a mineralocorticoid as needed. If treatment is started early enough, the high ACTH will be lowered to normal while the child is still quite young and the abnormal sex hormone production will stop. Because the adrenal defect begins before birth, masculinizing of a girl can occur while still in the mother's uterus. The medical treatment after birth is the same but genital abnormalities must be corrected by surgery.

Excessive Adrenal Function

When there is an overactive adrenal cortex, the extra hormone is either cortisol or aldosterone but not both.

Cushing's syndrome. Too much cortisol causes Cushing's syndrome, named after Harvey Cushing, the neurosurgeon who first defined it in 1932. The person is obese, sometimes only in the body without fat arms or legs, usually has a red face and thin skin, and may have high blood pressure. The thin skin stretches easily which leads to stretch marks (striae). Women may have extra hair on the face or chest and the menstrual cycle may be disrupted or stop. There can be metabolic effects such as a higher blood sugar, thin bones that can lead to fractures, and poor protein synthesis in muscles and other tissues, which can cause weakness and poor healing. Most patients do not have all of these symptoms and may have only one or two.

A common cause of Cushing's syndrome is simply taking too much glucocorticoid, such as the synthetics prednisone or dexamethasone. They are often prescribed for other diseases such as asthma and arthritis. If Cushing's disease happens spontaneously without taking any medication to cause it, the diagnosis is often only suspected and needs specific testing for confirmation. The basic test is the measurement of blood cortisol. A clear elevation is a definite sign, but many patients do not have this. Instead they have an abnormal cortisol pattern. For example, the cortisol level might not fall in the evening as it normally should. A good test for the disease is the suppression test. A synthetic glucocorticoid, usually dexamethasone, suppresses the cortisol level in a normal person by the usual negative feedback mechanism. However, in the person with Cushing's disease the cortisol level fails to decline normally.

Spontaneous Cushing's syndrome is usually caused by a small pituitary tumor secreting too much ACTH, which in turn raises the cortisol level. Sometimes the extra ACTH does not come from the pituitary but from a malignant tumor elsewhere in the body, such as a lung cancer (ectopic ACTH secretion). Less often Cushing's syndrome is caused by excessive secretion of ACTH-releasing factor from the hypothalamus or by an adrenal tumor, either benign or malignant, directly secreting too much cortisol. Another unusual cause is drinking too much alcohol, in which case the answer is to stop the alcohol. Because treatment of Cushing's syndrome depends on whether the type is pituitary, adrenal, or ectopic, tests must be done to identify the type.

The treatment of spontaneous Cushing's syndrome is basically surgical. A pituitary tumor usually can be removed by the procedure known as transsphenoidal hypophysectomy (see page 369). An alternate treatment is to remove both adrenal glands. Sometimes conditions are not right for surgery so radiation or drugs are used instead. Surgery is also the therapy for an adrenal tumor.

Cushing's syndrome is an expected side effect of using large amounts of glucocorticoids to treat asthma or arthritis. Often it can be avoided by careful attention to the timing of the dose and the amount taken, and, of course, it will disappear when the medication is stopped. Afterwards, however, the asthma, arthritis, or other illness may flare up again. Moreover, while taking corticoids, the patient's own ACTH secretion is shut down, and when corticoid treatment stops, it takes some time for ACTH secretion to start up again. Until it does there will be modest but temporary adrenal insufficiency.

Too much aldosterone causes high blood pressure and low blood potassium. When an excess is suspected because of the low potassium in a patient with hypertension, both aldosterone and renin are measured. Too much aldosterone would be expected to suppress renin through its negative feedback effect. If aldosterone is in fact too high, the renin level will be quite low. Most persons with primary aldosteronism have a single adrenal tumor that can be removed surgically. However, sometimes both adrenals secrete excessive aldosterone and no tumor can be found. An aldosterone-blocking drug, spironolactone, is then used.

The Adrenal Medulla and Disease

Destruction of the adrenal medulla rarely causes deficiency of epinephrine or norepinephrine because the sympathetic nerves throughout the body make up for the shortage. Sometimes, however, a large part of the sympathetic nervous system, including the adrenal medulla, is damaged. This can lead to low blood pressure, with light-headedness and fainting, and a tendency toward low blood sugar. Treatment is difficult, mainly involving drugs similar to norepinephrine but which last longer. Treatment can also involve giving medication to retain salt, which increases the blood volume, making fainting less likely to occur.

Excessive secretion of epinephrine and norepinephrine is almost always caused by a pheochromocytoma, a tumor in one or both adrenals named because its cells take on a gray color after staining. This tumor may cause high blood pressure, headache, palpitations, and sweating. If suspected, the diagnosis usually can be made by measuring the hormones or their by-products in the urine. Treatment is surgical, following special X rays; it is important to know which adrenal is involved. Occasionally the tumor is found outside the glands, not in either one.

Nonfunctioning Adrenal Tumors

An occasional adrenal tumor has no effect on hormone production. Since there are no hormonal effects, the tumor usually grows to a large size and is finally detected simply by its size or perhaps by the pressure it exerts on the kidney. Surgery is the treatment, but if the tumor is malignant, drugs also may be used.

CALCIUM, BONES, AND HORMONES

When thyroid surgery was perfected in the late 19th century, some patients afterwards developed a peculiar tingling, particularly in the hands and face. Some became irritable, sometimes had sudden spastic contractions of the muscles, or even underwent epilepsy-like seizures. The surgeons were puzzled at first, but later realized that the symptoms were caused by a low level of calcium in the blood, a condition known as hypocalcemia. We now know that the thyroid surgery damaged the nearby parathyroid glands, which are responsible for keeping the blood calcium normal.

Calcium is important for every tissue in the body. The amount of calcium in the blood stays within a narrow range. Whenever there is too much (hypercalcemia) or too little (hypocalcemia), tissue function deteriorates and characteristic symptoms occur.

Calcium salts are also the main component of bone and are mainly responsible for its strength. Bone is an active, living tissue, with new bone constantly being formed and old bone resorbed. However, changes in bone calcium are relatively slow compared to the rapid, fine control of blood calcium.

Blood and bone calcium are closely interrelated. Bone contains more than two pounds of calcium and acts as a storage site to be drawn upon whenever the blood calcium falls too low. The other main source of calcium for the blood is the diet. Most comes from milk or a milk product such as cheese. A quart of milk contains about one gram (1/30th of an ounce) of calcium.

If the blood calcium is to stay constant there must be careful regulation of absorption of dietary calcium, of resorption from bone, and of urinary losses. The hormones that regulate calcium are parathyroid hormone (PTH), calcitonin, and vitamin D. Vitamin D, although called a vitamin because it seemed a necessary part of the diet, is actually a hormone made by the skin under the influence of sunlight. In fact, even though vitamin D is now added to milk by law, most of the vitamin D in the blood is made by the skin.

Parathyroid hormone is secreted by the parathyroid glands, so-called because each pair is located near the lobes of the thyroid gland. There are normally four, but some people have as many as seven. Despite the location, there is no connection between the parathyroid and thyroid gland and their hormones have different actions. Parathyroid hormone causes the blood calcium to rise by stimulating bone cells to break down bone mineral and by stimulating the kidney to resorb calcium that otherwise might be excreted in the urine. Parathyroid hormone secretion is controlled by the level of blood calcium in a simple negative feedback fashion. When calcium goes up, secretion goes down.

The vitamin D released from the skin into the blood is rather inactive. It becomes potent after passing through the liver and the kidney (see chapter 22, "The Kidneys and Urinary System"). The kidney product, called 1,25-dihydroxycholecalciferol or "1,25-D," stimulates calcium absorption from the intestine. It also acts on bone to enhance both the formation and resorption of bone calcium. Since parathyroid hormone enhances the formation of "1,25-D" from vitamin D, both act together to help maintain blood calcium and the structure of bone.

A third calcium hormone, calcitonin, lowers the blood calcium, the opposite of the effect of parathyroid hormone. It comes from parafollicular cells in the thyroid gland but these cells have nothing to do with the secretion of T_4 or T_3. How calcitonin functions to help control the blood calcium is not clear. It may act only when the blood calcium goes too high in an attempt to bring the levels back to normal.

Hypocalcemia, a severely low level of blood calcium, usually produces the symptoms recognized by the 19th century surgeons. These include irritability, muddled thinking, spastic muscle contractions, and even seizures. The condition most often results from a deficiency of parathyroid hormone (hypoparathyroidism). This may be a defect present from birth or may be caused by immune destruction of the parathyroid glands (as happens with the thyroid or the adrenals), or result from previous neck surgery that has damaged the parathyroids. The ideal treatment would be to substitute parathyroid hormone but it is not available. So doctors use large doses of vitamin D, or perhaps the more potent "1,25-D" form, and give extra calcium by mouth. The combination is usually enough to keep the blood calcium reasonably close to normal.

Vitamin D deficiency produces a modest degree of low blood calcium levels, but the main effect is on the bones. When the deficiency occurs in children because of both a poor diet and poor exposure to the sun, the disease is called rickets. With insufficient calcium, the growing bones become structurally weak and bend. Rickets is now rare but used to be fairly common in large cities of the early 1900s where tall buildings and coal smoke cut off the sun-

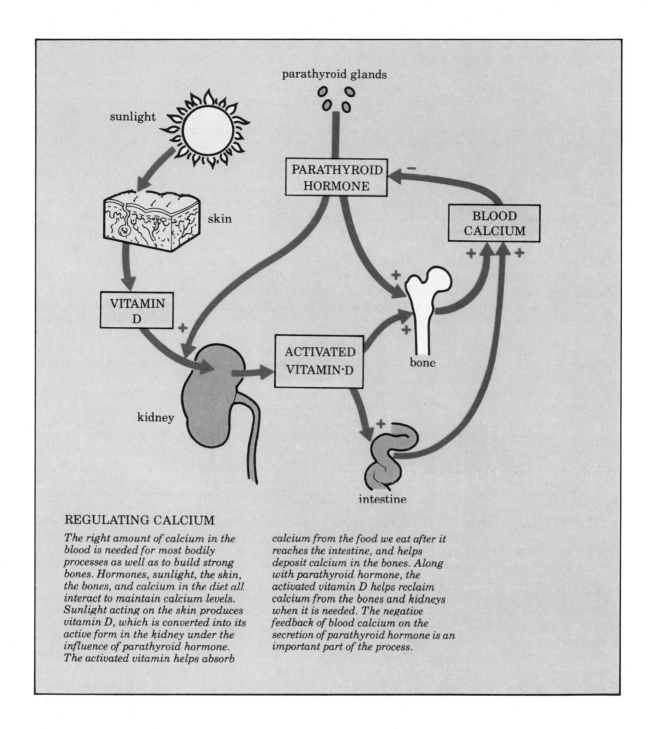

REGULATING CALCIUM

The right amount of calcium in the blood is needed for most bodily processes as well as to build strong bones. Hormones, sunlight, the skin, the bones, and calcium in the diet all interact to maintain calcium levels. Sunlight acting on the skin produces vitamin D, which is converted into its active form in the kidney under the influence of parathyroid hormone. The activated vitamin helps absorb

calcium from the food we eat after it reaches the intestine, and helps deposit calcium in the bones. Along with parathyroid hormone, the activated vitamin D helps reclaim calcium from the bones and kidneys when it is needed. The negative feedback of blood calcium on the secretion of parathyroid hormone is an important part of the process.

light. In adults, vitamin D deficiency may be more common than suspected, particularly in the elderly. Besides a somewhat low blood calcium, the bones may be thin and somewhat soft, a condition called osteomalacia (see chapter 14, "The Bones and Muscles"). In both children and adults the treatment is vitamin D by mouth and calcium added to the diet. The doses of vitamin D needed, however, are much lower than those required in hypoparathyroidism.

Hypercalcemia, excessive calcium in the blood, causes vague and nonspecific complaints such as lethargy, constipation, "not feeling well," or, if severe enough, coma. Some of the causes are rather rare, such as taking too much vitamin D or a generalized disease called sarcoidosis (see chapter 8, "The Lungs"). Usually, excessive blood calcium is caused by excessive secretion of parathyroid hormone or by a malignant tumor elsewhere in the body, such as a lung cancer. Sometimes it is caused by drugs, particularly the thiazide drugs used in treating hypertension. If discontinuing the drugs does not return the blood calcium to normal, measuring parathyroid hormone or looking for a tumor in organs such as the lungs or kidneys will help in the diagnosis.

A high level of parathyroid hormone along with high blood calcium indicates hyperparathyroidism. Usually this is caused by a benign tumor of one of the parathyroid glands, which can be removed surgically. Sometimes more than one parathyroid gland is involved, perhaps all, or the offending gland is an "extra" gland located in an odd place such as the chest. If the hypercalcemia persists after the operation, X rays and measurement of parathyroid hormones in many veins at once will help pinpoint the abnormal glandular tissue before doing a second operation. When the degree of hypercalcemia is slight, phosphate salts by mouth can be used without surgery but there must be careful follow-up with periodic measurements of the blood calcium.

When a malignant tumor causes the high blood calcium, treatment should be aimed at the tumor. But if the problem is severe, the situation is life-threatening and the calcium must be lowered quickly. Large amounts of intravenous sodium and various drugs must be used. Even these measures have only temporary benefit unless the malignant tumor can be controlled.

THE HORMONES
AND REPRODUCTION

An individual need not reproduce but the species must or it perishes. In fact, a person who lacks the hormones needed for reproduction lives a fairly normal life in most ways.

For successful reproduction there must be a precise sequence of events leading to the birth of the child (see chapter 26, "Pregnancy and Childbirth"). At almost every step of the way one hormone or another is important. Not only are hormones needed for the development of the spermatozoa in men and the eggs (ova) in women, but they are also necessary for the normal sexual behavior that leads to fertilization, for carrying a normal pregnancy to a successful conclusion, and for ensuring the production of milk after birth.

The knowledge that sexual behavior in men is related to some substance from the testes has been known for centuries. The first endocrine experiment, performed in 1849, was a testis transplant to a castrated rooster, which then strutted about and behaved like a normal rooster. Unfortunately, this sort of experiment led to much quackery in the late 19th and early 20th centuries, including transplanting monkey testes into men who complained of impotence. Scientists gradually were able to isolate and identify the hormones of the gonads in both men and women. By the 1930s we knew that the principal male hormone was testosterone and the female hormones of the ovary were estradiol and progesterone. All of these are steroid hormones like hydrocortisone and have a structure similar to cholesterol.

In men, testosterone is responsible for masculinizing the body, both when a male fetus is developing in the uterus and at puberty when boy becomes man. Testosterone is secreted by the interstitial cells (Leydig cells) of the testis. Before birth, testosterone secreted by the testis of a male fetus causes the development of the male genitalia including the scrotum and penis. Fetal testosterone also acts on the brain to "prime" it for normal male sexual behavior after birth. During childhood, testosterone secretion is actually lower than before birth, but it rises again during puberty. Then it causes hair growth on the face, pubic area, and other parts of the body, increased size of the penis, a major increase in muscle size and strength, and a growth spurt. The growth spurt is caused by testosterone's action directly on bone, especially the long bones of the legs. Some teenaged boys may grow half a foot in a year. The growth spurt is only temporary, however, because after two or three years of stimulating bone growth testosterone eventually stops the long bones from growing at all. Once testosterone acts on bone, the final length of the bone, and the ultimate height of the man, are already determined.

At puberty, too, the rising level of testosterone acts on the brain to develop the libido, or sexual desire, generally directed toward the opposite sex. Testosterone acts on the testis itself to stimulate development of active and fertile spermatozoa. Testosterone also develops the prostate gland and seminal vesicles which contribute fluid to the semen (see chapter 23, "The Male Reproductive System"). The spermatozoa and this carrying fluid are ejaculated together during sexual intercourse. If intercourse is timed properly and an egg has been ovulated in the woman, fertilization occurs.

The actions of testosterone are sometimes due to the hormone itself, as in muscle. But in other tissues, such as the prostate gland, the testosterone is converted to dihydrotestosterone, an active product of testosterone. Any compound that masculinizes is an androgen. Both testosterone and dihydrotestosterone are androgens. A testosterone-like steroid that

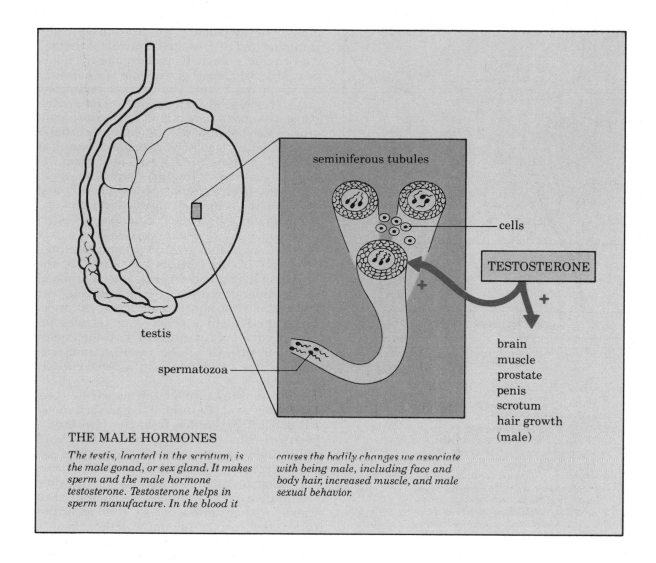

seminiferous tubules

cells

TESTOSTERONE

testis

spermatozoa

brain
muscle
prostate
penis
scrotum
hair growth
(male)

THE MALE HORMONES

The testis, located in the scrotum, is the male gonad, or sex gland. It makes sperm and the male hormone testosterone. Testosterone helps in sperm manufacture. In the blood it causes the bodily changes we associate with being male, including face and body hair, increased muscle, and male sexual behavior.

has more action on muscle than on the penis or hair growth is called an anabolic steroid. Anabolic steroids are sometimes used by athletes to increase muscle strength, but the evidence of their success is weak and prolonged use may lead to infertility.

Testosterone secretion is directly under the control of the pituitary and hypothalamus. The hypothalamic hormone known as LRH stimulates the secretion of luteinizing hormone (LH) from the pituitary, which in turn acts on the Leydig cells to increase testosterone secretion. Puberty in boys is probably a result of changes in the hypothalamus that lead to increased LRH secretion and activation of this entire system. As with other pituitary hormones, there is negative feedback control under which a rise in testosterone shuts off the secretion of LH.

Besides secreting testosterone the other principal function of the testis is spermatogenesis, making new spermatozoa. Here, too, the right hormones are needed. Both FSH and LH from the pituitary and testosterone from the Leydig cells contribute. Sperm formation occurs in the seminiferous tubules which make up the bulk of the testis. Inside each tubule are cells that develop into the spermatozoa. Next to them are supporting cells called Sertoli cells. FSH acts on the Sertoli cells while LH stimulates testosterone secretion from the nearby Leydig cells. Together testosterone and the Sertoli cells support the formation of new spermatozoa. There is probably a negative feedback effect here as well. Something in the sequence of spermatogenesis seems to feed back on the pituitary to inhibit the secretion of FSH. That unknown substance has been named "inhibin."

The female hypothalamic and pituitary hormones are the same as the male and the

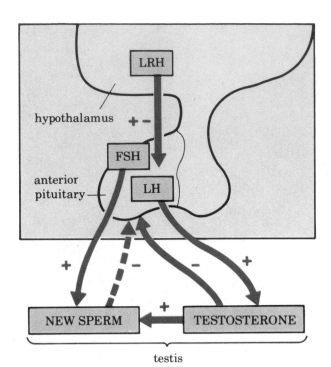

MALE HORMONE CONTROL

The hypothalamus and pituitary play an important role in the male sex function. Follicle-stimulating hormone (FSH) from the pituitary controls new sperm formation and luteinizing hormone (LH) controls testosterone. Both are controlled by the hypothalamic secretion known as luteinizing hormone releasing hormone (LRH). Testosterone and possibly the sperm themselves have a negative feedback effect on both FSH and LH.

breast development, maturation of the genitalia, and the redistribution of fat that occurs in adult women. It also develops the libido (sexual desire), another example of a hormone acting on the brain. The adrenal androgens may be responsible for the growth of hair in the pubic area and in the armpits. Girls also have a growth spurt at puberty although it is usually not as great as in boys. Growth is due mostly to estradiol, perhaps with some effect from the small amount of androgens. As in boys, these hormones first stimulate bone growth and then stop the bone from growing further.

After puberty the menstrual cycle is often irregular, but eventually settles into a regular pattern. After each menstrual bleeding, FSH and LH act together to stimulate the growth of a single ovarian follicle, a group of cells surrounding the egg. The follicle grows during the first half of the menstrual cycle, called the follicular phase, and secretes increasing amounts of estradiol. Estradiol helps stimulate growth of the endometrium, the lining of the uterine cavity, to receive a fertilized egg.

About midway through the menstrual cycle the higher level of estradiol triggers a burst of LH and FSH secretion from the pituitary, a positive feedback effect. The sudden high level of LH causes the enlarged follicle to erupt, releasing the egg, which begins its travels down the fallopian tube (oviduct) toward possible fertilization. The follicle collapses, then rapidly changes into a denser, solid structure called the corpus luteum ("yellow body"), which lasts until the next menstrual bleeding. The second half of the menstrual cycle is thus called the luteal phase. The corpus luteum continues to secrete estradiol and also secretes progesterone.

The combination of estradiol and progesterone from the corpus luteum makes the endometrium develop into a suitable place for the implantation of a fertilized egg. If fertilization occurs (in the fallopian tube), the egg begins to divide and forms a small cell mass called the blastocyst. It takes about one week for the blastocyst to travel down the fallopian tube into the uterus. By then the endometrium is properly developed to receive it. The blastocyst implants into the endometrium and begins to develop into the placenta and the fetus.

If no fertilization takes place, the corpus luteum begins to fail. It makes less and less estradiol and progesterone. Without them the developed endometrium deteriorates and is carried away in the menstrual flow about two weeks after ovulation. The reason pregnancy

general pattern of reproductive hormones is similar. LRH from the hypothalamus increases the pituitary secretion of follicle-stimulating hormone and luteinizing hormone, which in turn stimulate the ovary. The important difference is that the ovary secretes different steroid hormones, estradiol and progesterone, and does so cyclically, at intervals about four weeks apart. While the male secretion of luteinizing hormone and testosterone and the production of spermatozoa are reasonably constant, in women the egg and the ovarian hormones are released in a monthly pattern which causes menstrual (which means monthly) bleeding (see chapter 26, "Pregnancy and Childbirth").

When puberty occurs in girls the hypothalamus-pituitary-gonad axis is activated, as in boys, with increased secretion of estradiol from the ovary. The adrenal glands secrete weak androgens, too. Estradiol brings about

stops menstrual bleeding is that part of the implanted blastocyst begins to form the placenta and make hormones that keep the corpus luteum alive. In a sense menstrual bleeding is a failed pregnancy.

During pregnancy the placenta secretes several hormones of its own. Human chorionic gonadotropin (HCG) acts exactly like LH. Its main function seems to be the maintenance of the corpus luteum for a few weeks. (Its presence is the basis for pregnancy tests.) After a while the placenta also makes estradiol and progesterone, and the hormonal output of the corpus luteum is no longer needed. HCG also stimulates testosterone secretion by the testis of a male fetus. The large amounts of progesterone and estradiol contribute to the growth of the uterus and to the breast development needed for lactation after the child is born. Progesterone also keeps down uterine contractions and prevents premature birth.

We do not know why pregnancy ends and birth occurs when it does, but it may be because of a fall in progesterone and a rise in estradiol. Estradiol tends to increase uterine contractions. Apparently, the combination of more estradiol, lowered progesterone, and secretion of oxytocin from the posterior pituitary causes progressive contractions that eventually bring on birth.

Lactation, or milk secretion, begins shortly after birth. During pregnancy the breasts develop in preparation for lactation largely because of placental estradiol and progesterone, and because of increased secretion of prolactin (PRL) from the mother's pituitary. Lactation does not usually occur during pregnancy because estradiol and progesterone, while they develop the breasts, block lactation itself. After birth, placental estradiol and progesterone disappear, relieving the blockage. The high prolactin persists because it comes from the mother's pituitary. The breasts then engorge and milk secretion begins. When the infant suckles at the breast, oxytocin secretion from the posterior pituitary is stimulated; oxytocin causes the small milk glands in the breast to contract and the milk squirts out. Suckling also tends to maintain prolactin secretion. Thus, both prolactin and oxytocin are important hormones for effective nursing. If the mother does not nurse the child or if the child stops nursing later, milk secretion stops, too, in part because prolactin and oxytocin secretion cease when there is no suckling.

While the mother is nursing, ovulation usually does not occur. But this is at best an unreliable contraceptive because the inhibition of ovulation is not always complete. Why nursing inhibits ovulation is not clear but the high pro-

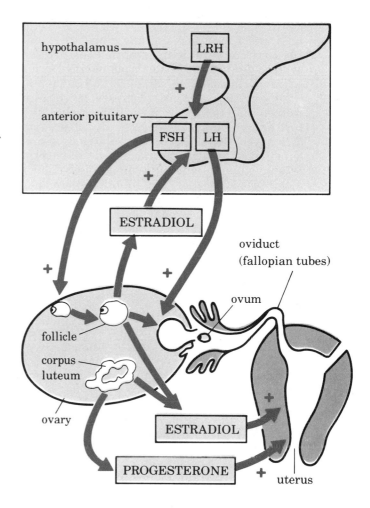

SEX HORMONES IN WOMEN

A chain of hormones secreted cyclically is responsible for menstruation and pregnancy. It begins with the release of luteinizing hormone releasing hormone (LRH) from the hypothalamus. Influenced by LRH, the pituitary secretes follicle-stimulating hormone (FSH) and luteinizing hormone (LH), which together stimulate the growth of the egg-containing follicle in the ovary. As the follicle develops it makes the hormone estradiol. Estradiol prepares the lining of the uterus for a possible conception and also causes a burst of secretion of FSH and LH. The large amounts of FSH and LH propel the ovum from the follicle into the oviduct to await fertilization. The empty follicle becomes the corpus luteum and secretes yet another hormone, progesterone. Estradiol and progesterone further develop the uterine lining for the possible implantation of a fertilized egg. If there is no fertilization, the lining is sloughed off in menstrual bleeding and the cycle begins again.

lactin probably interferes with secretion of FSH and LH. When nursing stops, FSH and LH secretion resume in a few months, and the pituitary-ovarian-uterine cycle begins anew.

The hormones involved in reproduction and their control are clearly complex, more so in women than in men because of the cyclical nature and the major changes during pregnancy. Whenever anything is complicated, many things can go wrong, and at any of several levels: hypothalamus, pituitary, testis, or ovary. Disorders of reproductive hormones rarely cause death but the psychological and emotional effects can be devastating. Disturbances of sexual function and inability to have children are not matters most men and women take lightly. Neither are such problems as excessive body hair or menstrual difficulties, including absence of menses. Hormonal defects are not always the cause of these disorders, but generally a careful study of the appropriate hormones in the man or woman is still needed before a hormone defect can be ruled out.

In men, common problems include impotence (inability to get and maintain erection for successful sexual intercourse), decreased libido (lack of interest in sexual activity), and infertility (inability to father children despite apparently normal sexual function).

Impotence increases with age. It may be a normal part of the aging process in some men, although certainly not in all. Most impotent men do not have defective testosterone (the most common cause of impotence is psychological) but blood testosterone should be checked. A low testosterone level is probably more common than many doctors think. Such a deficiency is easily treated, preferably by testosterone injections every two to four weeks, if the man is otherwise healthy.

Diabetes mellitus is another common cause of impotence but in those cases the testosterone level is usually normal. The cause is usually diabetes-related damage to the nerves involved in erection and it is generally not reversible. Other hormone changes that can uncommonly cause impotence are hypothyroidism, easily tested for and treated, and excessive prolactin, which is also easily detected and usually means a pituitary tumor.

Poor libido is most often caused by psychological problems or by some chronic illness, but also may result from testosterone deficiency. Infertility usually does not stem from a hormonal defect but sometimes can be caused by poor FSH or LH secretion from the pituitary.

Finally, if there is a low testosterone level, more tests should be administered to identify the cause. Primary hypogonadism gets its name because the gonad, in this case the testis, functions poorly because of some intrinsic defect. Sometimes a boy is born with the defect but makes just enough testosterone to get through a relatively normal puberty. Or the damage may occur later in life. In either case, the low testosterone level of primary hypogonadism causes a high blood LH level because of the negative feedback. Thus a low (or low normal) testosterone and a high LH make the diagnosis. If blood testosterone is low and LH is normal, the defect is probably in the pituitary or hypothalamus, which is secondary hypogonadism. Here X rays are needed to look for a pituitary tumor, along with measurement of other pituitary hormones.

Gynecomastia, which means female-like breasts, commonly occurs in boys at puberty. It is of no concern then, because it usually goes away. But gynecomastia at other times of life is worrisome. It may be related to hypogonadism and low testosterone, but it may also indicate excessive production of an estrogen as a result of a tumor of the testis, or in rare cases the result of a tumor of the adrenal or some other organ. Often the cause is evident, such as certain drugs or other endocrine or non-endocrine disease, such as cirrhosis of the liver. If not, careful testing must be done.

Rarely a boy may start to masculinize and begin the changes of puberty several years early. This is called sexual precocity and means he is producing too much testosterone, at least for his age. Sometimes caused by a testis, adrenal, or pineal tumor, sometimes by a metabolic defect in the adrenal cortex, sexual precocity also may reflect early maturation of the whole hypothalamic-pituitary mechanism for puberty. It is important to identify the cause, not only to get rid of a possible tumor or to correct a defect but because if the condition is left untreated, bone growth will stop too soon and the boy will become a short man.

Amenorrhea, the absence of menstrual flow, occurs when the ovary does not secrete estrogen so that the endometrium does not develop.

This is the female form of primary hypogonadism. There can be causes other than the lack of estrogen. If menstruation has never occurred, the girl may have some structural abnormality in or near the uterus or no ovaries at all. Sometimes pituitary or hypothalamic damage is responsible. If menses have stopped in a woman who formerly menstruated regularly, it may indicate pregnancy or menopause. If neither seems likely, it may be that psychological strain and unusual diets are acting through the hypothalamus to disrupt FSH and LH secretion, without which menses would not occur. Other causes of amenorrhea in an adult woman are pituitary tumors, excessive testosterone or other androgens, too much (sometimes too little) thyroid hormone, and some drugs. A woman who has been using oral contraceptives may have amenorrhea after she stops. The treatment of amenorrhea depends on the cause, but if estrogen is missing, oral estrogen is usually given.

Sometimes a woman will have reasonably normal menstrual cycles but not be able to become pregnant. She is called infertile. There are many causes for infertility; sometimes the cause is never found. As with amenorrhea, there are several possible hormone defects. She is obviously producing some FSH, LH, and estrogen because menstrual cycling does occur, but secretion may be too slight to stimulate ovulation. If ovulation is normal and followed by the formation of a corpus luteum, the corpus luteum should secrete progesterone. Measuring blood progesterone about a week before the next expected menstrual period is usually the doctor's first step. If it is too low, something is wrong with ovulation or with the corpus luteum, and both are needed to become pregnant. There may be a problem with androgens or thyroid hormones as well.

Some women have too much facial and body hair, or at least think they do. This is called hirsutism. Often, the "extra" hair is normal, particularly if it is light in amount and limited to the upper lip, face and chest, and if other women in the family show a similar pattern. If the hair growth seems greater in amount or extent or if it has recently increased, there may be an endocrine cause, especially if accompanied by infertility, irregular periods, or even amenorrhea. A possible explanation is excessive testosterone (or some other androgen) from either the ovaries or adrenals, perhaps caused by a tumor in either gland. More often there seems to be a functional defect. In the ovaries defective function can lead to large, cystic ovaries that make abnormal amounts of testosterone. The condition is called the polycystic ovary or Stein-Leventhal syndrome. Measurement of blood testosterone may not be much above normal, and it is often not easy to tell if the excess is coming from the ovaries or the adrenals. Careful physical examination may be more informative. If there are clear-cut polycystic ovaries, medical or surgical treatment to cause ovulation will certainly help infertility and may correct the hirsutism. If not clear-cut, oral contraceptives or adrenal corticoids may suppress testosterone secretion enough so that the hirsutism improves. Only occasionally, however, does the excess hair disappear altogether.

HORMONES AND AGING

In the past the aging process was believed by some to be caused by a decrease in one or more hormones. The idea probably arose because sexual function decreases in both sexes, and ovarian hormone secretion obviously decreases in women with age. The menopause, or the cessation of menstrual bleeding, is in fact due to failure of the ovaries to continue to secrete estradiol, and this lack does cause some decrease in sexual function in women. However, the tissues of the body seem to age independently of most hormones. Thus aging itself does not seem to be caused by a generalized deficiency of hormones.

Still, there are changes in hormone secretion with advancing age. The female menopause is one. Whether there is a male menopause has been argued for decades. Certainly sexual function decreases as men get older but only in some does testosterone secretion fall significantly. Thyroid, parathyroid, and adrenal function remain reasonably intact in the elderly although there may be more mild primary hypothyroidism in older persons than we currently suspect. The secretion of pituitary hormones also seems intact except for some blunting of growth hormone secretion which may not mean much at this stage of life. Of course, FSH and LH secretions from the pituitary rise when the gonads fail. This happens in all women after the menopause and in those men with poor testosterone secretion. TSH also will be high if there is primary hypothyroidism.

CHAPTER 17   ALDO A. ROSSINI, M.D.

DIABETES MELLITUS

Diabetes is a disease that affects at least five percent of the American population. It is the third leading cause of death in the United States. Also known as diabetes mellitus or "sugar diabetes," it has been described by medical writers for nearly 4,000 years, but not until this century was it treated effectively. Diabetes affects many organs of the body, and is an incurable, lifelong condition. What we now call diabetes includes several different diseases, all of which can produce the same derangement of the body's use of fuel. But, whatever its causes, the major characteristic of diabetes is the body's inability to regulate the level of "sugar," or glucose, in the blood.

Although its symptoms were first described in an Egyptian papyrus about 1,500 B.C., diabetes received its modern name from the Greeks, who called it by their word for "siphon" because, as Aretaeus wrote in the second century A.D., "The fluid does not remain in the body, but uses the man's body as a ladder to leave it." This "melting down of the flesh and limbs into urine," as he described it, often began without warning in children and young people. Besides frequent urination, it brought terrible thirst that nonetheless was powerless to prevent water loss, coma, and death. Physicians watched the process helplessly, not even knowing which organ was responsible, although the sweetness of the patients' urine prompted the Romans to append the name "mellitus" or "honeylike," and led some to suspect that sugar was involved.

Indeed, it is now known that people with diabetes tend to build up a higher than normal level of sugar, or glucose, in the blood because they lack a hormone called insulin, the chemical messenger responsible for moving glucose out of the blood to other parts of the body.

THE TYPES OF DIABETES

Doctors recognize two types of diabetes. One type is called juvenile diabetes, ketosis-prone diabetes, or insulin-dependent diabetes. Only 15 percent of all diabetics have this type. They usually develop it when they are children or young adults—under age 40—and they are usually thin. These persons have a total or almost total lack of the hormone insulin, which is necessary to maintain normal sugar levels in the blood. They usually need daily injections of insulin or they may develop a dangerous condition called ketosis, in which glucose and acids in the body reach harmful levels.

The more common type of diabetes, which 85 percent of diabetics have, is called mature-onset or adult-onset diabetes, ketosis-resistant diabetes, or non-insulin-dependent diabetes. Patients usually develop it after age 40, and they are usually overweight. Indeed, reducing weight may make the diabetes improve or disappear. These persons are able to make some insulin, often enough to avoid needing injections but not enough to keep their blood glucose level normal all the time. Although, like insulin-dependent diabetics, they are at risk of developing long-term complications, they usually have enough insulin of their own to avoid ketosis.

THE NORMAL ROLE

OF INSULIN

To understand diabetes, one must understand the hormone insulin and its role.

Insulin is produced by the pancreas, an organ that lies below and behind the stomach and weighs about one-half pound. Much of the pancreas is made up of glands that produce enzymes, chemicals that digest food. But lying among these digestive glands are tiny islands of cells called islets of Langerhans (named for the German doctor who discovered them in 1869). The islets contain four kinds of cells: alpha cells, beta cells, somatostatin cells, and polypeptide cells. Although the functions of the last two types are uncertain, it is known that the beta cells produce insulin and the alpha cells produce another hormone, glucagon.

The beta cells are the most numerous in the islets. They are the body's only insulin source, and in a normal person they release insulin constantly in whatever amount is needed to keep the level of glucose in the blood within narrow limits. Beta cells release insulin in response to the arrival in the bloodstream of fuel obtained from food.

If the body is thought of as a machine, the food "fuels" it can use are of three kinds: carbohydrates, fats, and proteins. Carbohydrates (cakes, candy, fruits, and starchy foods such as bread and potatoes) are broken down by digestion into glucose. Proteins (steak, cheese, fish) are broken down to amino acids. Fats (butter, cream, bacon) are broken down to fatty acids. Glucose, amino acids, and fatty acids are all basic fuels of the body, and when any of them enter the bloodstream after a meal, they stimulate the beta cells to release insulin.

COMPARING THE TYPES OF DIABETES		Juvenile	Adult
	Other names	Insulin-dependent Ketosis-prone	Insulin-independent Ketosis-resistant
	Percentage of all diabetics	15%	85%
	Age of onset	Usually before 25	Over 40
	Body type	Thin	Overweight
	Insulin	Absolute deficiency	Relative deficiency
	Onset	Very rapid	Gradual

Insulin can be likened to a hose that funnels these fuels into the machine—that is, into the muscle cells, fat cells, liver cells, and other body tissues that need them. Insulin allows the liver to remove glucose and amino acids from the blood and transform them. The glucose is converted to glycogen, a storage fuel, and the amino acids are converted to body proteins. Some amino acids are trapped in the liver and converted to glucose by means of the hormone glucagon, which is also released from the pancreatic islet at the time amino acids are ingested. Insulin also facilitates movement of glucose and amino acids into other tissues, such as muscles that can use glucose or amino acids for fuel or convert amino acids into muscle protein. Finally, insulin expedites the movement of fatty acids into fat cells, where they become storage fuel. Insulin also stimulates the liver to turn extra glucose or amino acids into fat for storage. In the end, any of the three kinds of fuel can end up as fat, because insulin efficiently prevents excess fuel from being wasted. That's why a person who takes in more fuel than the body needs for immediate activities becomes obese.

After a full meal a large amount of insulin is produced, and by transporting glucose out of the bloodstream, it keeps the glucose level from rising too high. Then, if the person eats nothing more for six or eight hours, the glucose level gradually falls. As it does, the amount of insulin in the blood also falls.

When the blood glucose and insulin levels become low, the body tissues—liver, muscle, and especially fat—respond by breaking down storage fuels to produce more glucose. These storage fuels are glycogen, protein, and the glycerol portion of stored fats. As it enters the bloodstream, this glucose stimulates the beta cells to release a little more insulin, which halts the storage fuel breakdown. In this way, the glucose level in the blood is kept within a narrow range, even in the fasting state.

INSULIN'S ROLE
IN DIABETES

What happens in the body of a diabetic? In someone with juvenile diabetes who produces no insulin, the machine breaks down from lack of fuel. When the diabetic eats, the three basic fuels appear in the bloodstream, but the beta cells release no insulin in response. Without insulin, the body tissues—liver, muscle, fat, and others—have no way to remove fuel from the blood and convert it into protein or storage fuels. Glucose and other fuels remain in the bloodstream.

But the body tissues do not "know" that glucose is already in the blood. Just as in a normal person who has been fasting, the diabetic has little or no insulin in the bloodstream, and the body tissues respond by trying to produce glucose and other fuels. Muscle protein is broken down into amino acids, fat stores into fatty acids, and liver glycogen into glucose. Amino acids and fatty acids traverse the bloodstream to the liver, which converts the amino acids into more glucose and the fatty acids into a new fuel, ketone acids. The final result is that blood glucose levels rise higher and higher, and the ketone acids begin to accumulate.

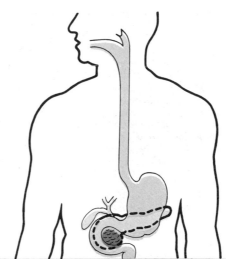

PHYSIOLOGY OF DIABETES

Diabetes centers on a malfunction of the pancreas, a large organ lying behind the stomach (top drawing). The pancreas contains small islands of tissue known as islets of Langerhans (center drawing). The islets are made up of four types of cells (bottom drawing). Beta cells, the most numerous, are the body's only source of insulin, a hormone that regulates the amount of glucose in the blood. Alpha cells produce another hormone, glucagon, also involved in glucose regulation. The role of the somatostatin and polypeptide cells is uncertain.

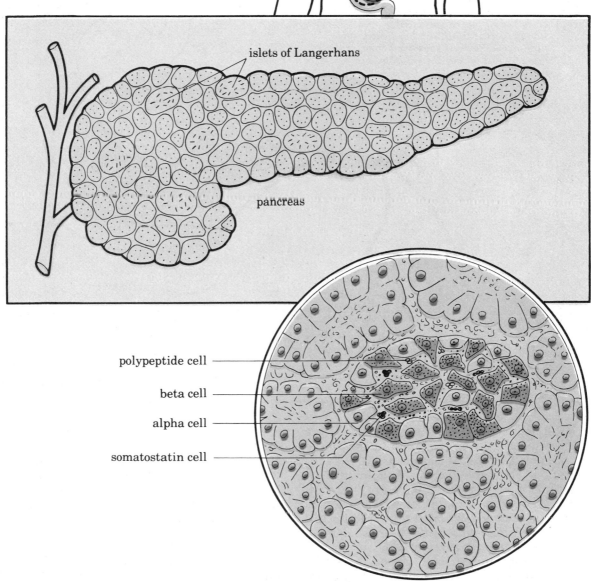

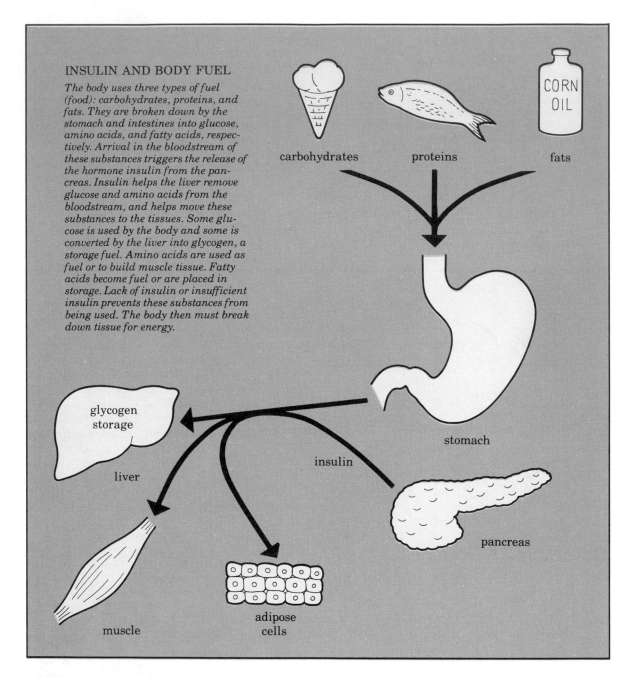

INSULIN AND BODY FUEL

The body uses three types of fuel (food): carbohydrates, proteins, and fats. They are broken down by the stomach and intestines into glucose, amino acids, and fatty acids, respectively. Arrival in the bloodstream of these substances triggers the release of the hormone insulin from the pancreas. Insulin helps the liver remove glucose and amino acids from the bloodstream, and helps move these substances to the tissues. Some glucose is used by the body and some is converted by the liver into glycogen, a storage fuel. Amino acids are used as fuel or to build muscle tissue. Fatty acids become fuel or are placed in storage. Lack of insulin or insufficient insulin prevents these substances from being used. The body then must break down tissue for energy.

carbohydrates

proteins

fats

CORN OIL

stomach

glycogen storage

liver

insulin

pancreas

muscle

adipose cells

With no insulin, the tissues of the diabetic's body respond as if he were starving—and he is, because the tissues cannot use the available fuel. Thus, the diabetic feels hungry all the time, eats enormous quantities, but cannot gain weight. His muscles waste away (as protein is broken down) and may cramp painfully. He is constantly tired, because none of the body tissues get enough fuel. Finally, the high level of glucose in his blood forces the kidneys to excrete large amounts of glucose via the urine, and the glucose draws excess water with it. So the diabetic urinates excessively, loses water from the body, and is constantly thirsty as a result. If glucose and ketone acids reach extremely high levels, the diabetic enters the dangerous state called ketosis or ketoacidosis, which leads to coma and death if not treated quickly.

These are the consequences of having no insulin at all—the absolute insulin deficiency of severe juvenile diabetes. But adult-onset diabetics do not completely lack insulin. Some insulin is still manufactured by the beta cells and released as fuels arrive, but not enough insulin is produced to keep the blood glucose down to normal levels at all times. Reasons for the insulin deficiency vary, but whatever the cause, the adult-onset diabetic cannot use body fuels as well as a normal person. He or she usually has enough insulin to move *some* of the fuel into cells and prevent ketosis. In fact, the adult-onset diabetic is often overweight rather than thin like the juvenile-onset diabetic. But because of the high glucose level in his blood, the adult-onset diabetic frequently loses glucose in the urine, leading again to the classic diabetic symptoms of excessive urination and excessive thirst.

How does a person know whether he or she has diabetes? When should a physician suspect the disease? In a person with adult-onset diabetes, the onset may be gradual and very subtle, with almost no noticeable change in habits or apparent health. In a child, the disease often begins dramatically.

Juvenile diabetes sometimes appears during a period of stress such as illness or pregnancy. However, in most cases no precipitating condition can be identified before it begins. Juvenile diabetes usually starts in childhood, including the teens, or less commonly during young adulthood. It can be heralded by fatigue and weakness. The young victim may notice that he or she urinates frequently and is compelled to get up during the night to do so. Thirst may be constant, accompanied by an increase in appetite. But despite "eating like a horse," the new diabetic steadily loses weight. He or she may notice muscle cramps or blurred vision, and may suffer from lingering infections or slow healing wounds.

Mature-onset diabetes has the symptoms of frequent urination, excessive thirst, and increased appetite, but they are less common than in juvenile diabetes. Instead, the mature-onset diabetic may suffer urinary or skin infections, especially yeast infections in the vagina (causing itching and a whitish discharge) or red, itchy irritation in the groins, armpits, and under the breasts. Sometimes small, raised reddish-yellow spots appear on the skin because of increased fat in the blood. Some persons develop numbness and burning or tingling of the hands, feet, or legs. A few suffer blurry vision or frequently have their eyeglass prescription changed. And, like juvenile diabetics, many adult-onset diabetics feel tired and run-down.

These symptoms, especially in combination, should lead one to consult a doctor. Diabetes is common, easy to test for, and easy to treat. There is evidence that prompt treatment minimizes complications and reduces risk of associated diseases of the eye, kidney, and nervous system.

THE CAUSES OF DIABETES

Although the causes of diabetes are still not understood, much has been learned in recent years about who is at highest risk of becoming diabetic. Both juvenile and mature-onset diabetes tend to run in families, and the two types behave as if they were separate diseases, seldom occurring in the same family.

But heredity is not the only factor, and diabetes is not passed from parent to child in an easily predictable way, like a trait carried on a single gene. A person's environment and lifestyle interact with heredity to determine whether he or she will become diabetic.

In mature-onset diabetes, being overweight is the major risk factor. The mature-onset diabetic has an insulin deficiency partly because he or she has large fat cells, so large that they create a greater demand for insulin than the beta cells can keep up with. Overweight people often have large fat cells, so they risk becoming diabetic. Obesity is a problem that fat parents tend to pass on to their children, probably both through genes and life-style, so they also pass on their increased risk of diabetes. In the United States, the increasing incidence of diabetes may be explained by our tendency to overeat (40 percent of the American population is obese). The connection between diabetes and obesity has been studied among Yemenite Jews, a group of people who formerly lived in the desert, usually were thin, and had a low incidence of diabetes. As they moved to the city, the frequency of obesity increased and so did diabetes.

Juvenile diabetes is a problem of beta cell absence rather than an increased demand by fat cells, and its causes are being aggressively studied. Heredity plays a role. For instance, the children of two juvenile diabetic parents have about a 30 percent chance of becoming diabetic. In research on cells and organ transplants, scientists have studied many protein antigens, or "markers," that occur on all human cells. Each of us has our own set of antigens, but certain groups of people have antigens in common. Researchers have found two particular antigens that occur frequently in juvenile diabetics, making them wonder whether the "genes" for diabetes are passed on in association with the genes for those particular markers.

Viruses also have been implicated in diabetes. As early as 1864, a Norwegian scientist noticed that diabetes increased after a mumps epidemic. Since then, about 20 viruses or virus particles have been connected with diabetes, so it seems likely that no single virus sets off the disease. Diabetes occurs in children more often at ages when they are likely to be exposed to certain virus strains for the first time. Some researchers have suggested a possible explanation that the body, in fighting off a virus infection by making protein antibodies and special cells to attack the invading virus, inadvertently makes antibodies that attack some of the antigens (protein markers) on its own cells. This backfiring of the normal immune mechanism has been shown to occur in other diseases such as lupus erythematosus, rheumatic fever, and glomerulonephritis (see chapter 21, "Allergy and the Immune System"). Another possible mechanism is that an altered protein is produced by the beta cells or an altered cell surface occurs that is perceived by the body as foreign. Thus, a person with the cell antigens (markers) associated with diabetes develops the disease because when he or she produces antibodies to fight off a routine virus infection, the antibodies attack not only the virus, but the person's own beta cells. This autoimmune response destroys the beta cells and produces diabetes.

Other factors can set off diabetes or aggravate it. Normal aging may cause higher levels of blood glucose, as the pancreas "wears out" or the body tissues become less sensitive to insulin's effect. Certain drugs may elevate blood glucose levels. The thiazide diuretics, commonly used to treat high blood pressure, may do so by lowering potassium levels in the blood, and birth control pills apparently sometimes interfere with insulin. Thyroid hormones and cortisone may raise the blood glucose through complicated actions on the body's metabolism. These and other hormones are affected by illness and stress, such as a heart attack or a severe injury. Consequently, glucose levels may rise during such episodes (or even during pregnancy) only to return to normal when the stress is removed.

DIAGNOSING DIABETES

Besides the common symptoms, other factors may influence a doctor to test a patient for diabetes: a family history of the disease, an early heart attack, an unusually high blood sugar level during a hospital stay, a tendency for a woman to have unusually large babies, or a propensity to develop skin sores that heal slowly. Several tests are available.

The most common screening test measures the fasting blood sugar level. This test determines the amount of glucose in a small sample of blood obtained first thing in the morning, when the patient has eaten nothing since the night before. If glucose levels are normal, it indicates that the person is making enough insulin to keep glucose within the proper range. If glucose is higher than normal, it may mean that the body is not producing enough insulin, and that storage fuels are breaking down and raising the blood sugar in response. Although the "normal" numbers vary at different laboratories, a fasting blood sugar level more than 20 percent above a laboratory's normal limit suggests diabetes.

If the first test shows a high fasting blood sugar, the doctor usually does a second, the two-hour postprandial blood sugar test, to confirm the presence of diabetes. For this test, the patient eats a large meal and has his or her blood sugar measured two hours later. The meal puts stress on the beta cells by creating a demand for insulin, and their ability to produce insulin is measured by whether the blood glucose level has returned to a normal level two hours after eating. A two-hour blood glucose level of more than 20 percent above the laboratory's normal limit is considered an indication of diabetes. (The normal level two hours after a meal is 120 mg%, meaning 120 milligrams of glucose in 100 milliliters of blood.) Most doctors repeat these tests when they obtain a high reading to be certain there is no laboratory error before deciding that a patient has diabetes. They also take into account that blood sugar levels normally are slightly higher in older people.

Testing the urine for glucose is another way to look for diabetes, and is important for insulin-taking diabetics to do at home (see page 398). It is of little value, however, in diagnosing the disease, because glucose levels in the blood may rise to two or three times normal before the kidneys begin to spill glucose in the urine. Part of the job of the normal kidney is to conserve glucose, not excrete it, and a diabetic's blood glucose may rise dangerously high before this conservation mechanism is overwhelmed and the urine test becomes positive. (The normal kidney threshold is approximately 180 mg% of glucose, which means that 100 milliliters of blood contain 180 milligrams of glucose.)

Other tests sometimes used to diagnose diabetes are the glucose tolerance test, the tolbutamide tolerance test, the leucine tolerance test, and the cortisone priming test. All challenge the beta cells to produce insulin, but most diabetes specialists now feel they are no better than the two-hour postprandial blood sugar repeated two or three times.

Low Blood Sugar (Hypoglycemia)

The problem of low blood sugar is the opposite of diabetes. Hypoglycemia refers to all the symptoms that occur in a diabetic during an insulin reaction: nervousness, sweating, trembling, drowsiness, and others. Low blood sugar in normal people can indeed produce these symptoms, and recent publicity has touted hypoglycemia as the long-overlooked explanation for the vague feelings of malaise most people experience at times. In reality, the symptoms of hypoglycemia do occur repeatedly in certain people when their blood sugar falls too low, but the disease is not common. Patients with reactive functional hypoglycemia develop a low blood glucose level two to four hours after eating because of an overactive insulin release, primarily in response to carbohydrates. If the symptoms and the low blood sugar level can be demonstrated by an oral glucose tolerance test, in which the patient's blood glucose is measured repeatedly up to five hours after a glucose meal, then the patient may show improvement by turning to a diet low in carbohydrates and high in protein.

Although persons with reactive hypoglycemia do not appear to have an increased risk of diabetes, similar symptoms and low blood sugar may occur three to five hours after eating in a few patients with early diabetes. Rarer causes of hypoglycemia, such as excess insulin release after stomach surgery or excess insulin caused by a pancreatic islet tumor, require more specialized tests and treatment.

COMPLICATIONS OF DIABETES

Beyond the obvious need to prevent acute problems like ketosis, it is important to find and treat diabetes in order to minimize its long-term complications. The long-term effects of the disease are serious and involve every organ of the body. Although specialists disagree on whether all complications can be prevented by keeping the blood glucose at a normal level, research indicates that some complications are related to high blood glucose levels, and are reduced by control of blood sugar. Almost all agree that the length of time a person has had diabetes also has a great bearing on the complications.

Compared to the normal population, diabetics are 25 times more prone to blindness, 17 times more prone to kidney disease, five times more prone to gangrene, and twice as prone to heart disease. Although heart disease is the leading cause of death among diabetics as a whole, juvenile diabetics are particularly vulnerable to kidney failure. In fact, half of juvenile diabetics die of kidney failure by the time they have been diabetic for 25 years.

Given these figures, it is understandable that research efforts to find the causes of diabetes' complications and to understand their relation to high blood sugar have been intense. There is mounting evidence that controlling blood sugar helps prevent damage to the eyes, kidneys, and nerves. Normal blood glucose levels also improve the function of blood cells and the body's metabolism. But doctors are less optimistic that control of blood sugar lowers the diabetic's high risk of heart disease and damage to large blood vessels.

The major complications of diabetes affect the eyes, nerves, kidneys, and blood vessels. The disease does damage in a number of ways. In the eye, abnormal shifts of water and chemicals can impair vision by causing swelling of the lens (which may improve when blood glucose is brought back to normal). The patient may experience blurry vision. If the blood sugar level is elevated for a prolonged time, cataracts may develop in the lens and eventually require surgery. Glaucoma is common in diabetics, and can impair vision if not treated.

But the most dangerous visual complication is diabetic proliferative retinopathy, the process of damage and abnormal growth of small blood vessels in the retina of the eye. Less than five percent of diabetics become blind, but that is enough to make diabetes a leading cause of blindness. Early retinopathy can be helped by blood glucose control, but more advanced retinopathy may require laser treatment (see chapter 12, "The Eyes," and chapter 31, "Understanding Your Operation"). Photocoagulation through the laser beam is a procedure by which areas of the retina are burned and scarred by a highly concentrated beam of light. This seals off the leaking blood vessels and often improves vision, avoiding blindness or hemorrhage and detachment of the retina. Vitrectomy is a procedure in which fluid and blood in the vitreous chamber of the eye are removed and replaced with a salt solution. This technique has provided vision to patients who have lost vision in one or both eyes. Less severe changes called background retinopathy may produce small red dots on the retina (microaneurysms) which occasionally bleed and scar.

Like the eyes, the nerves of diabetics can malfunction because of chemical abnormalities associated with high glucose levels or because of damage to the tiny blood vessels that feed the nerves. The results include tingling or burning of the skin, weakness, dizziness, diarrhea, bladder problems, and impotence. Nerve damage can decrease pain sensation in the hands and feet, which is dangerous for diabetics because foot injuries may occur without the person sensing normal pain. This is further aggravated by poor healing because of inadequate blood supply. The pain is usually worse at night, while resting, or on cold, wet days.

Kidney failure, as noted, is a particularly severe problem in juvenile diabetics, but mature-onset diabetics also are vulnerable. Diabetic kidney damage appears to be related to both impaired blood supply and abnormal glucose levels, and can make the diabetic's kidneys more vulnerable to infection and to destruction by high blood pressure. Kidney failure may require dialysis—use of an "artificial kidney"—or transplantation. All diabetics should have a yearly urinalysis and blood test to check kidney function.

Because of diabetes' damage to blood vessels (by mechanisms that are still not understood), diabetics run a higher risk of heart disease, and have heart attacks at younger ages and with fewer warning signs of pain than nondiabetics. After age 40, vessels supplying the limbs and skin are affected. In addition, the function of white blood cells diminishes and the combination makes diabetics prone to infection and slow wound-healing. Blood supply to the feet can become so poor that the tissues break down, and an apparently minor cut can fail to heal, become infected, and even lead to gangrene and amputation. For this reason, diabetics are instructed in foot care and warned against going barefoot and against wearing tight shoes and stockings. Special attention to other parts of the body, such as the mouth and genital areas, is necessary. Diabetics also are warned against smoking, high cholesterol, and obesity.

Even though control of blood sugar clearly does not *cure* diabetes, it improves so many aspects of the disease that doctors agree every effort should be made to bring high glucose levels down to normal and keep them there. The treatment of diabetes and prevention of its complications is a lifelong project for doctor and patient. The patient must understand the disease and cooperate with the doctor in planning control through diet, exercise, and medication, if necessary. He or she also must know what worsens diabetes, and the side effects of medicines.

TREATMENT OF DIABETES

The two types of diabetes are treated somewhat differently, even though the goal of lowering blood glucose is the same. In mature-onset diabetes, some insulin is usually present, so treatment concentrates on increasing the natural supply and its effectiveness in the body. Often mature-onset diabetics are overweight, with large fat cells that create a high demand for insulin. A reducing diet not only decreases fat cell size, but apparently makes the diabetic more sensitive to his own insulin and increases the amount available.

Whether the diabetic is insulin-dependent or not, the diet is based on five factors: total calories, percentage and type of carbohydrates, percentage and type of fats, meal spacing, and adjustments for exercise or complicating disorders.

For most patients who are taking insulin, the total calorie intake should be between 1,400 and 2,700 a day, with the exact amount depending on daily activity and desired weight of the patient. (Growing, active young people need more calories.) The usual distribution is 160 to 230 grams of carbohydrates, 65 to 125 grams of protein, and 60 to 40 grams of fat. Fats are usually kept low in proportion to protein in the diabetic's diet.

It is important, too, that meals be eaten regularly and on time. The usual schedule is three meals and two snacks. Usually one-fifth of the daily calories are given for breakfast, and two-fifths each for lunch and dinner. The mid-afternoon and bedtime snacks are subtracted from the noon and evening meals.

For the diabetic who is not insulin-dependent, three divided meals of approximately equal calories are recommended. The calorie total is normally kept low.

The optimum diet usually is worked out by a doctor and a dietitian. It may have a high fiber content, which has been found to be beneficial in diabetes. Regular exercise is encouraged because it helps the patient lose weight and because it lowers blood glucose. When a patient is very obese or has great difficulty losing weight, doctors may employ a diet high in protein and low in carbohydrates, and also may use behavioral modification techniques. The diabetic diet centers on well-balanced meals that are tailored to individual needs, likes, dislikes, and life-style.

Most Americans have a sweet tooth, and diabetics are no exception. The most frequently asked questions about diabetic diets concern artificial sweeteners. Chemical sweeteners such as cyclamates and saccharin, as well as slower metabolized non-glucose carbohydrates such as fructose, sorbitol, and xylitol, are often used. The long-term effects of fructose and sorbitol have not been evaluated, but some researchers suspect that xylitol has cancer-causing properties.

The chemical sweeteners have been controversial. The U.S. Food and Drug Administration has banned the use of cyclamates because laboratory tests on animals strongly suggest that they cause cancer. Saccharin has been implicated as a cause of bladder cancer in animals, but most scientists consider the data inconclusive, and this sweetener has not been banned.

A walk through the supermarket shows a variety of canned foods labeled "dietetic." They are generally more expensive than other canned foods and the diabetic receives no nutritional benefit for the added cost. Only a few diabetics would benefit from using them.

Often diet and exercise are adequate treatment for mature-onset diabetes. If blood glucose levels remain too high, most doctors consider insulin injections the best measure. If a patient is unable or unwilling to learn insulin self-injection, or if diet alone cannot control glucose, a doctor may prescribe an oral hypoglycemic agent, a pill to lower blood glucose levels. The pills are not a form of insulin.

There are two classes of oral medications but only one, sulfonylurea, is available in the United States. Oral hypoglycemics work by increasing insulin manufacture and release by the beta cells and by affecting glucose metabolism elsewhere. Although the medication lowers blood sugar, its long term success rate in keeping glucose levels normal is estimated at 20 to 30 percent. A controversial research project, the UGDP (University Group Diabetes Project) study, has raised the question of whether patients taking oral hypoglycemic pills had a higher death rate, especially from heart disease, than other diabetics. The study results were inconclusive, and other studies are being conducted. The pills occasionally lower blood glucose and sodium levels too far, causing lethargy, nervousness, confusion, and other symptoms. Other side effects include skin rash, nausea, vomiting, diarrhea, and flushing, especially after drinking an alcoholic beverage.

For the juvenile diabetic, diet and exercise are also essential, but the approach is different. Because juvenile diabetics are so often children, they must eat frequently in order to grow. And because they take insulin daily, diet

ORAL HYPOGLYCEMIC MEDICATIONS (sulfonylurea)

Type	Length of Action
Dymelor® (Acetohexamide) 250 mg (white) 500 mg (yellow)	12–18 hours
Diabinese® (Chlorpropamide) 100 mg (blue) 250 mg (blue)	36 hours
Orinase® (Tolbutamide) 500 mg (white)	6–8 hours
Tolinase® (Tolazamide) 100 mg (white) 250 mg (white) 500 mg (white)	12–18 hours

Instead of injecting insulin, a few diabetics can use drugs that lower the blood sugar level when taken orally. The chart shows trade names of four, the dosages available, and how long each is effective.

INSULIN PREPARATIONS

	Onset of action (hours)	Peak of action (hours)	Length of action (hours)
Short			
Regular	1	2–4	6–8
Semi-lente	1½–2	5–7	12–18
Intermediate			
NPH	1–2	8–12	20–32
Lente	1–2	8–12	26–30

The injectable insulin diabetics use is available in several preparations that vary in how quickly they act and how long they last. Those most com- *monly used are regular insulin, which takes effect in about an hour, and the intermediate forms, which some diabetics need only once a day.*

must be carefully regulated to correspond with the insulin dose, keep the blood glucose level as constant as possible, and avoid an insulin reaction from a blood sugar level that is too low. Calorie requirements change as children gain height and weight, and food intake must be spaced throughout the day to avoid rapid zigzags in glucose levels. Juvenile diabetics also must learn to increase food intake on days when they exercise vigorously because exercise lowers glucose levels and decreases insulin requirements. Urine must be tested for glucose frequently to decide whether the insulin dose is adequate. Although juvenile diabetic diets usually limit sugar consumption, diabetics must always keep sugar available—candy, juice, soft drinks—to eat in case of an insulin reaction. It is also recommended that high cholesterol and saturated fats be avoided.

Injectable insulin is one of the landmark success stories in medical research. Its development dates only from the 1920s but the groundwork was laid a hundred years earlier. Nineteenth century doctors observed that diabetes appeared to stem from a malfunction of the pancreas. In 1869, a German pathologist, Paul Langerhans, narrowed it to the tiny islets of tissue that bear his name (see page 389). Other investigators established that keeping these islets healthy prevented laboratory animals from becoming diabetic. Then in 1922,

two Canadians, Dr. Frederick G. Banting and Charles H. Best, a young student, succeeded in extracting from the islets a hormone with which they could control blood sugar levels in laboratory animals. The hormone was insulin. Shortly afterward they treated their first diabetic patient and the results were dramatic. Although injectable insulin was not then and is not now a cure for diabetes, it quickly revolutionized treatment and kept alive millions of diabetics who otherwise would have wasted away in a diabetic coma.

Today injectable insulin is manufactured from pork and beef pancreases, and comes in several preparations with different durations of effect. The most commonly used types are regular insulin, whose peak activity comes two to four hours after injection, and NPH and Lente intermediate insulin, which peak in eight to 12 hours. Many diabetics take only a single injection of intermediate insulin in the morning. Others take a mixture of intermediate and regular insulin, or more than one injection per day. The amount of the dose is determined by a doctor, who first prescribes a low dose and then tests the diabetic's blood and urine, slowly increasing the daily dose until blood glucose levels are nearly normal. The diabetic learns how to give himself or herself injections and how to decide whether to raise or lower the dose slightly depending on the presence of glucose in the urine.

Even young children can administer insulin to themselves. Injection is performed under the skin, the site rotated among such areas as thigh, abdomen, hip, and arms.

WARNING SIGNS OF INSULIN REACTIONS

Pallor	Nervousness	Tingling around the mouth
Headache	Perspiration	Inability to concentrate
Dizziness	Blurred vision	Drowsiness or fatigue
Confusion	Irritability	

At the first sign of any of the above warning signs, give sugar immediately in one of the following forms:

- Sugar—5 small cubes, 2 packets, or 2 teaspoons
- Fruit juice—½ to ⅔ cup
- Carbonated beverage—6 ounces (not diet or sugarless soda pop)
- Candy—Three candy mints or ⅓ candy bar

Although insulin treatment becomes more complicated during pregnancy, illness, or surgery, and although some diabetics develop resistance to animal insulin and produce "antibodies" to it, most insulin-dependent diabetics can become expert at treating their own illness.

A number of self-administered tests are now available to help diabetics. Glucose monitoring techniques are the most recent. A blood sample is obtained by pricking the finger with a small sterile needle and a drop of blood is placed on a strip impregnated with a chemical reagent. After about a minute, the excess blood is washed off the strip and the color change that occurs can be compared to an established scale to determine glucose content. By taking several samples during the day, a diabetic can continuously monitor blood glucose levels, but time, effort, and cost make the test productive for only some persons.

Other tests measure urine sugar levels by dipping a chemically treated strip into a morning urine sample. There are a variety of these tests, and all involve a color change in the strip in reaction to the concentration of sugar in the urine. The tests vary in expense, accuracy, and difficulty of administration. The exact test used by the patient should be determined by both the patient and the physician. The urine-testing technique is the mainstay of determining outpatient control of diabetes.

The diabetic patient, his friends, and family should know the symptoms of and treatment for an insulin reaction, which occurs when the body has an excess of the hormone compared to the amount of glucose. Most reactions are perceived by the diabetic and can be readily checked with a quick acting sugar (two teaspoons of sugar, a half cup of fruit juice, six ounces of a regular (non-dietetic) soft drink, two candy mints). The symptoms vary. They include hunger, nervousness and irritability, trembling, pallor, perspiration, headache, blurry vision, confusion or abnormal behavior, crying, drowsiness, and abdominal pain. Occasionally, a reaction is more severe, and the diabetic passes out and is unable to eat. A one-milligram injection of glucagon may be life-saving. If unconscious, the diabetic should be taken to a hospital emergency room. The symptoms of low insulin and a very high blood sugar level (ketosis)—a particular danger in juvenile diabetics—also include hunger, weakness, dizziness, confusion, headache, abdominal pain, and passing out. A positive urine test for glucose can help distinguish between the two, but when symptoms occur it is always best for the diabetic to take sugar at once and call the doctor or go to the emergency room because both conditions are dangerous. It should be remembered that all the symptoms of low blood sugar can be caused by oral hypoglycemic pills as well as by insulin, although this rarely happens.

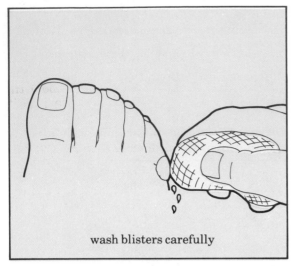

wash blisters carefully

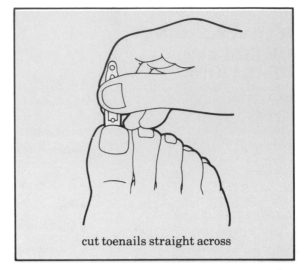

cut toenails straight across

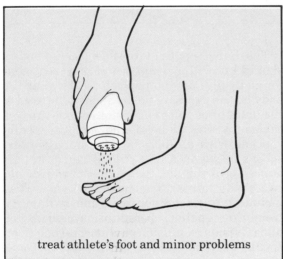

treat athlete's foot and minor problems

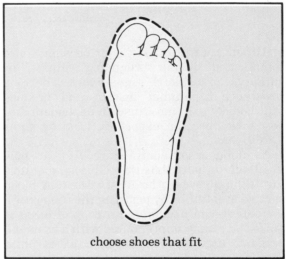

choose shoes that fit

FOOT CARE AND DIABETES

Care of the feet is especially important for diabetics because long-standing disease can damage the nerves so that pain and temperature change are not felt, and because blood vessel damage can impair circulation so that minor wounds do not heal properly. The steps shown above should be part of a diabetic's regular foot care. In addition, a diabetic should examine the feet daily for red spots, bruises, cuts, blisters, or cracks, and should wash them daily with mild soap and dry them well. He or she should never go barefoot and should keep feet warm on cold days, but not with a hot-water bottle or heating pad, which can cause unnoticed burns.

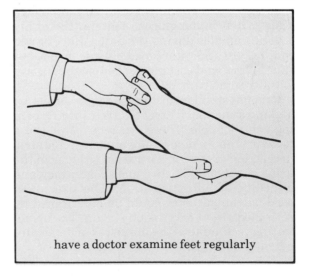

have a doctor examine feet regularly

Special Problems of the Diabetic

Besides the daily control of blood sugar, the treatment of diabetes demands that a doctor or nurse provide regular counseling and support. The diabetic must assume responsibility for control of the disease. He or she must consider what to eat, what to do, and how to care for the body more carefully than most people. A youthful diabetic may rebel against limits on diet or alcohol intake. In the middle years, the diabetic must work harder than other adults to reduce the risk factors for heart disease such as smoking, high blood pressure, and high cholesterol consumption. Parents of diabetic children learn to live with the frightening risks of ketosis, insulin reactions, and decreased life expectancy, while children of diabetic parents might have to live with a parent's blindness, heart problems, or kidney failure.

At first, parents often experience shock, disbelief, grief, and guilt when they learn that a child has diabetes. Adjustments by the whole family are needed. The parents must understand that how they accept the disease and deal with it affects how the child deals with it. Parents must protect, but not demand. If the child is under age seven, parents generally must assume total responsibility for treatment, but beyond that age the child must begin to assume responsibility for care of the disease. Overanxious parents create an overanxious child, lacking self-confidence and unprepared for future independence. The parent should learn to "give a little" about dietary restrictions but not become overindulgent. On the other hand, the diabetic child should get no preferential treatment, and discipline meted out to other family members should be shared by the diabetic. Adolescent diabetics often deny their disease and dependence on others. Encouragement, reenforcement, and allowing them to make their own decisions may help them learn that diabetics can lead a full life with some restrictions. Pamphlets and assistance can be obtained from groups active in education and care of the diabetic. Workshops and group meetings can be helpful. The more parents and young diabetics know about the disease, the better they are able to care for it.

Finally, the diabetic undergoing surgery needs careful monitoring to prevent wide swings in glucose levels, and the pregnant diabetic faces a much higher risk than other women of losing her baby or having a premature or low birth weight infant. Recent evidence suggests that well-controlled pregnant diabetics are capable of having babies with no higher risk of problems than the nondiabetic. This can be accomplished by frequent visits to the obstetrician and the aid of a specialist to help control the blood sugar during pregnancy.

General Hygiene

A special consideration for diabetics is general hygiene. Proper care of teeth and gums is strongly recommended. There is ample evidence that diabetics have an increased incidence of both gum and tooth problems. Uncontrolled diabetics appear to have more cavities as well as a higher incidence of gum disease, apparently because of the elevated levels of blood sugar. Some of these problems can be prevented by frequent brushing and flossing to prevent plaque formation. Diabetics are encouraged to have frequent dental checkups. A diabetic's skin may be dry and itchy, and may require the use of lanolin creams after a bath or shower to trap water in the skin and prevent cracking. The diabetic should examine the feet daily, checking for infection, bruises, cuts, and blisters. Shoes that fit properly are imperative, and new shoes should be broken in slowly. The diabetic should always wear shoes or slippers and never walk barefoot. Pumice stones should be used to buff calluses. Toenails should be kept short and cut straight across. Because they may lack pain sensation, diabetics should never use hot water bottles or heating pads on their feet, and must avoid prolonged soaking of the feet. At the earliest sign of infection, a podiatrist or physician should be consulted, because small problems become magnified in diabetics.

THE FUTURE FOR DIABETICS

The future treatment of diabetes lies in the research laboratories, and some exciting innovations may soon be available for patients. Transplantation of pancreatic islet tissue has been attempted, and specialists are working on ways to overcome the problem of tissue rejection. Other researchers are developing implantable insulin pumps that would work like the pancreas to deliver small, constant doses of insulin. Drug researchers are seeking inhibitors of glucagon and other hormones that work against insulin, and still others are seeking to identify chemicals that would prevent development of diabetic cataracts and

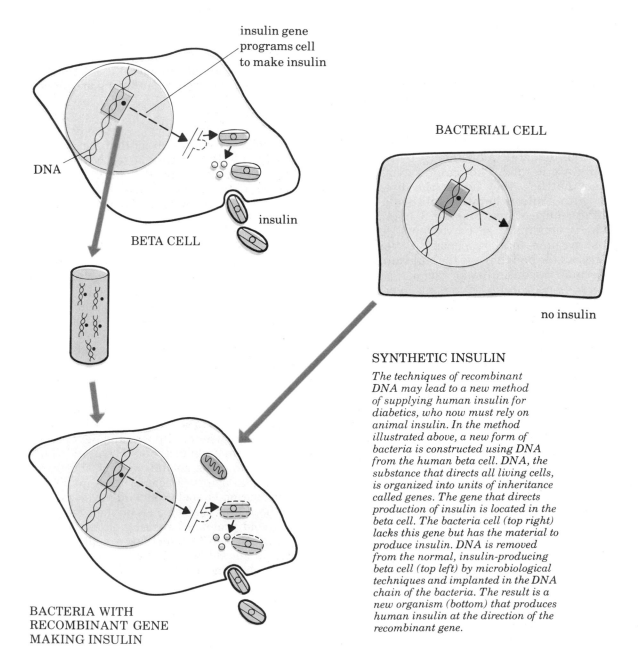

insulin gene programs cell to make insulin

DNA

BETA CELL

insulin

BACTERIAL CELL

no insulin

BACTERIA WITH RECOMBINANT GENE MAKING INSULIN

SYNTHETIC INSULIN

The techniques of recombinant DNA may lead to a new method of supplying human insulin for diabetics, who now must rely on animal insulin. In the method illustrated above, a new form of bacteria is constructed using DNA from the human beta cell. DNA, the substance that directs all living cells, is organized into units of inheritance called genes. The gene that directs production of insulin is located in the beta cell. The bacteria cell (top right) lacks this gene but has the material to produce insulin. DNA is removed from the normal, insulin-producing beta cell (top left) by microbiological techniques and implanted in the DNA chain of the bacteria. The result is a new organism (bottom) that produces human insulin at the direction of the recombinant gene.

blood vessel damage. Finally, the causes of diabetes are being investigated in animals as specialists look for ways to prevent genetic tendencies toward the disease, and for ways to develop a vaccine to short-circuit the immune system's attack on beta cells.

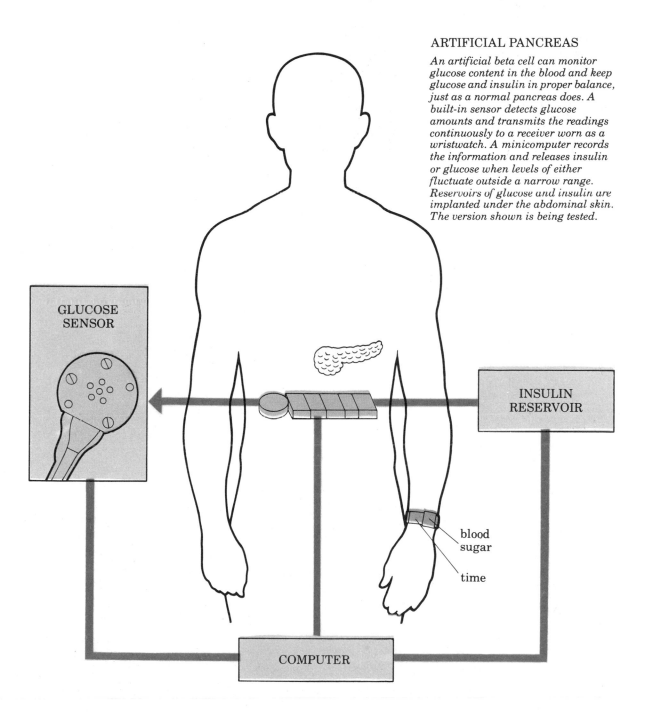

ARTIFICIAL PANCREAS

An artificial beta cell can monitor glucose content in the blood and keep glucose and insulin in proper balance, just as a normal pancreas does. A built-in sensor detects glucose amounts and transmits the readings continuously to a receiver worn as a wristwatch. A minicomputer records the information and releases insulin or glucose when levels of either fluctuate outside a narrow range. Reservoirs of glucose and insulin are implanted under the abdominal skin. The version shown is being tested.

GLUCOSE SENSOR

INSULIN RESERVOIR

blood sugar

time

COMPUTER

CHAPTER 18   ROBERT A. BAGRAMIAN, D.D.S., Dr. P.H.

TEETH AND ORAL HEALTH

In the 1960s and '70s, a series of television advertisements for toothpaste depicted delighted youngsters returning from a visit to the dentist shouting, "Look, Mom! No cavities!" Not many Americans can make that boast, at least not for long. Periodontal disease and dental caries, the technical name for the decay that produces cavities, are two of the most prevalent chronic diseases in our society. Hardly an American exists whose mouth does not testify to their ravages and their repair.

A few figures indicate the scope of American dental problems. In a typical year more than 100 million of us—about half the U.S. population—pay at least one visit to the dentist. The total bill for dental care exceeds $10 billion annually. One American in four over the age of 29 wears one complete upper or lower denture. Half of the adult population has periodontal disease. Nine of ten Americans are victims of tooth decay, and the average six-year-old already has 3.7 decayed teeth.

Not all the consequences are so easily measured. Untreated dental diseases and disorders can lead to toothache, tooth loss, impairment of the victim's general health, and costly replacement services. They affect our enjoyment of food, the kind of appearance we present to the world, and how we feel about ourselves. Even when properly treated, dental diseases leave a permanent "scar" in the form of a filling, a bridge, a missing tooth, loss of gum tissue, or an artificial denture.

Fortunately, modern dental practice stresses prevention as much as it stresses the treatment of dental disease—saving teeth as well as doctoring them. Dentists in the 1980s generally try to help patients understand the basis of oral health. A visit to a dentist's office now encompasses lessons in oral hygiene, diet, and fluoride treatments to help prevent tooth loss. And when it does come time to deal with dental problems, they can be handled with minimal pain and discomfort.

TEETH: THEIR FUNCTION AND STRUCTURE

What are the functions of teeth? There are several important and obvious ones:

Preparation of food for digestion is their main purpose. The 32 teeth of the adult human are designed to bite, tear, and grind morsels of food into a semi-liquid that can pass down the gullet and into the digestive system. A full complement of healthy teeth permits a wide selection of food and encourages a well balanced diet. A poor set of teeth or less than

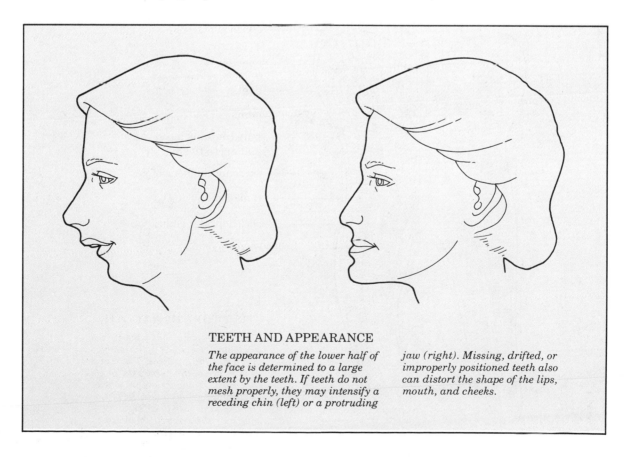

TEETH AND APPEARANCE
The appearance of the lower half of the face is determined to a large extent by the teeth. If teeth do not mesh properly, they may intensify a receding chin (left) or a protruding jaw (right). Missing, drifted, or improperly positioned teeth also can distort the shape of the lips, mouth, and cheeks.

a full set of teeth may limit us to soft, mushy foods and semi-liquids that need little or no chewing, provide limited nutrition, and constitute a monotonous diet.

Personal appearance, not surprisingly, relies on healthy teeth and gums, as advertising incessantly reminds us. Many persons become socially withdrawn because of poorly arranged, unsightly, or diseased teeth. Inflamed and swollen gums not only are unattractive, but can cause bad breath. The appearance of the lower half of the face is determined to a large extent by the teeth. The receding (retrognathic) jaw and the protruding (prognathic) jaw are two examples of dental abnormalities involving improper "meshing" or contact of upper and lower teeth. Teeth that are missing, drifted, or improperly positioned also may distort the shape of the lips, mouth, and cheeks.

Good speech also depends on good teeth. Many sounds are formed by the position of the tongue or lips against the teeth. People who lack upper front teeth may have difficulty speaking distinctly. Misaligned teeth, overbite, and other irregularities can contribute to problems of articulation and communication.

Structure of the Teeth

Each tooth is composed of a crown and a root. The crown is the visible part. The root, usually two or three times longer than the crown, fits into the bony socket in the jaw. It is attached to the bone beneath the gum by a tough membrane or ligament. A constriction in the contour of the tooth where the crown and root join is called the neck.

A tooth is composed of four types of tissue: enamel, cementum, dentin, and pulp. Dental enamel, the hardest tissue in the human body, coats the crown. The root is covered with a bone-like substance called cementum. The ends of the fibers in the ligament attaching the tooth to the jaw are embedded in the cementum. This tough fibrous attachment is called the periodontal membrane.

Most of the tooth beneath the enamel and cementum is made of an ivory-like material called dentin. Dentin contains minute tubules arranged in a nearly parallel radial fashion. The tubules extend to the enamel and cementum from the center chamber of the tooth. This construction provides elasticity that the harder and more brittle enamel lacks.

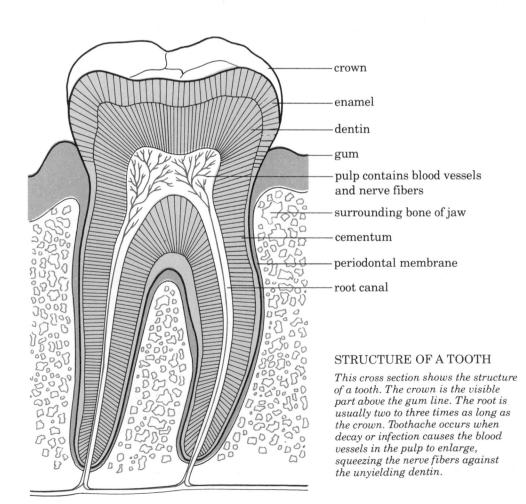

crown

enamel

dentin

gum

pulp contains blood vessels and nerve fibers

surrounding bone of jaw

cementum

periodontal membrane

root canal

STRUCTURE OF A TOOTH

This cross section shows the structure of a tooth. The crown is the visible part above the gum line. The root is usually two to three times as long as the crown. Toothache occurs when decay or infection causes the blood vessels in the pulp to enlarge, squeezing the nerve fibers against the unyielding dentin.

The small channel that runs through the center of the tooth from the crown to the root tip contains the dental pulp. In the crown this channel widens to form the pulp chamber. In the root it is called the root canal.

The pulp is composed of soft tissue containing small blood vessels and nerve fibers and provides moisture to the dentin through the dentinal tubules. If the pulp is destroyed by disease or accident, the dentin becomes more brittle. The soft tissue that constitutes the pulp serves as a cushion that allows slight changes in the circulation of the blood into the pulp without noticeable pressure on the nerve fibers. The blood flow, however, can be altered by the irritation caused by very hot or cold food or by infection accompanying tooth decay. If the irritation is severe or prolonged, the vessels enlarge and pressure develops. Because of the unyielding dentin surrounding the pulp, this pressure squeezes the nerve fibers. This pressure is interpreted as pulsating or throbbing pain—in short, a toothache.

TOOTH DEVELOPMENT

A human being develops two sets of teeth during a lifetime. The first set, the primary teeth—also known as deciduous, "baby," or "milk" teeth—are 20 in number. Eight of them, the four above and four below in the front of the mouth, are called incisors. They are equipped with cutting edges to shear or bite off food. Next to them on either side, upper and lower, are the canines, also called cuspids

or "eye teeth." There are four, each equipped with a pointed tip for tearing food. Behind each canine are two molars, making a total of eight. Molars have the largest crowns and are arranged so that when the jaws close, their surfaces mesh to produce grinding action.

Eruption

Although teeth normally are not visible when a baby is born, the buds that develop into teeth have been in place since about six weeks after conception. Mineral salts, mainly calcium phosphate and carbonate, are deposited in these buds to form the teeth starting about the sixteenth week of prenatal life.

The crowns of the incisors are fairly well developed at birth, but the teeth usually do not push through the gum for several months. The first to appear are usually the lower central incisors, one on either side of the midline of the lower jaw. The average age of eruption is between six and nine months after birth, but eruption time and sequence varies for each child. Some teeth may begin to appear as early as three months, which can create nursing problems. Conversely, a child's first tooth may not appear until after nine months. However, if tooth eruption is markedly delayed, a dentist or pediatrician should be consulted.

Teething

A baby usually fusses while cutting primary teeth. The sharp edges pushing their way through the gum tissue can be uncomfortable,

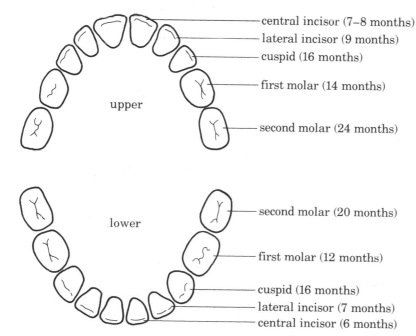

central incisor (7–8 months)

lateral incisor (9 months)

cuspid (16 months)

first molar (14 months)

upper

second molar (24 months)

second molar (20 months)

lower

first molar (12 months)

cuspid (16 months)

lateral incisor (7 months)

central incisor (6 months)

BABY TEETH

The first baby tooth usually arrives at about six months, but may appear as early as three months or as late as nine months. Teeth continue to arrive through the first two years of life. Babies commonly fuss while teething, but teething itself does not cause illness.

to say the least, and some infants react vigorously. Teething itself does not make children ill, but it is important for parents to be sure that the child's irritability is not the sign of real illness mistakenly thought to be symptoms of teething.

A baby may drool during teething, or bite, chew, or gnaw any object he or she can place in the mouth. The baby may work the lower jaw forward or from side to side in an attempt to rub the gum pads together over the erupting tooth. Teething rings and other objects of suitable size and firmness may help to satisfy the urge to push the teeth through the overlying gum tissue. At first the baby may need help learning to handle these objects. To soothe the irritated gums, teething rings can be chilled. Cool foods or ice may help.

Primary teeth cause more discomfort during eruption than do permanent teeth. Most of the permanent teeth replace primaries that have been shed recently, so they have a path to follow. The 12 permanent molars do not have any primary teeth to succeed, but when they erupt (around the ages of 6, 12, and 17), the discomfort is less annoying. Most youngsters at those ages find a slightly sore gum only mildly incapacitating.

Some parents assume that primary teeth can be neglected because they eventually will be replaced by a second set. But diseased primary teeth can cause infection and pain, and the premature loss of primary teeth can prevent proper growth and development of the jaw. The resulting collapse in the size of the jaw can cause crowding and irregularities in the position of permanent teeth. This irregular positioning, in turn, may make permanent teeth more susceptible to the diseases and disorders of adolescent and adult life.

Shedding the Primary Teeth

Increasing pressure on the roots of the primary teeth from the permanent teeth growing beneath them causes their roots to be absorbed little by little. The attachments remain sturdy enough for the primaries to function properly until just before the permanent teeth replace them. If for some reason a permanent tooth does not form, the primary tooth may remain in place throughout adult life.

A child usually loses the lower front teeth first, normally at six to seven years. The upper front teeth loosen and drop out not long afterwards. The "second-grade smile" caused by two to four missing front teeth may make it difficult for the child to pronounce sounds such as "s," "z," and "sh" (commonly known as lisping), or eat particular foods that require biting,

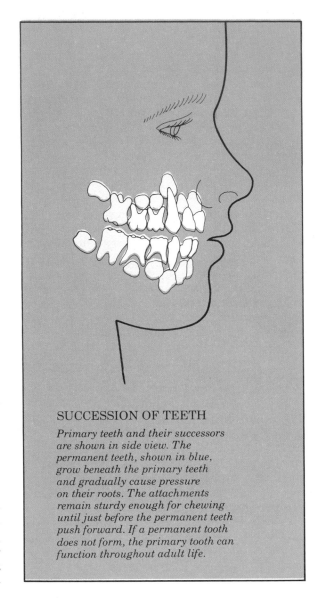

SUCCESSION OF TEETH

Primary teeth and their successors are shown in side view. The permanent teeth, shown in blue, grow beneath the primary teeth and gradually cause pressure on their roots. The attachments remain sturdy enough for chewing until just before the permanent teeth push forward. If a permanent tooth does not form, the primary tooth can function throughout adult life.

such as corn. Normal speech and eating usually return with the replacement teeth.

The chart on page 409 gives approximate ages when permanent teeth appear. If baby teeth remain in the mouth considerably beyond these ages, a dentist should be consulted. The dentist probably will want an X-ray examination to determine whether a permanent tooth is developing and to locate its position in the jaw.

Normally there are 32 permanent teeth. The increase from 20 to 32 is produced by the addition of eight bicuspid teeth and four third molars, the so-called "wisdom teeth." The eight bicuspids replace the eight primary molars, usually between the ages of 10 and 12.

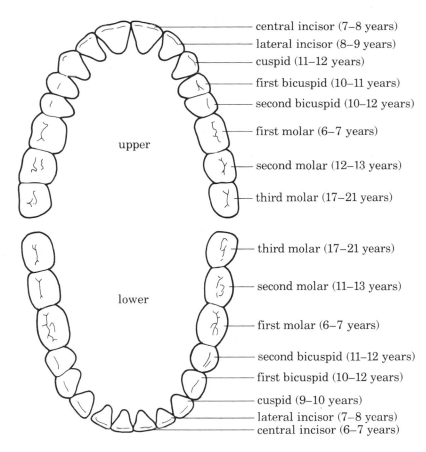

central incisor (7–8 years)
lateral incisor (8–9 years)
cuspid (11–12 years)
first bicuspid (10–11 years)
second bicuspid (10–12 years)
first molar (6–7 years)

upper

second molar (12–13 years)
third molar (17–21 years)

third molar (17–21 years)
second molar (11–13 years)
first molar (6–7 years)

lower

second bicuspid (11–12 years)
first bicuspid (10–12 years)
cuspid (9–10 years)
lateral incisor (7–8 years)
central incisor (6–7 years)

THE PERMANENT TEETH

Permanent teeth begin arriving at age six, when the lower front teeth and the first molar appear. Primaries drop out and new permanent teeth are added over the next 10 to 15 years. If the arrival of permanent teeth is delayed substantially, a dentist should be consulted.

The first permanent molar already is forming at the time of birth. It pokes through the gums to the rear of the last "baby" molar at about six years of age, without a tooth being lost. This tooth is often called the "six-year molar." Almost all children acquire it before the seventh birthday, regardless of whether previous eruptions have been early or late.

Although the new addition is considerably larger than the primary molars, many parents do not realize that it is a permanent tooth destined to last a lifetime. The six-year molars are usually the most decay-prone of all the permanent teeth. Dental caries frequently is found first in the pits and grooves of their chewing surfaces. More than one child in four has a beginning cavity in one of these molars by the age of seven. Some show spots of decay when the teeth are barely through the gum. If the decay is not found and corrected with a filling, this important tooth may be lost.

The first permanent molar is the "keystone" of the dental arch. If loss occurs while the jaw is still developing, other teeth may shift into improper positions. That can impair jaw development and facial appearance, and set up a chain reaction detrimental to dental and general health. The first permanent molar should receive attention as soon as it appears.

The second permanent molars usually make their appearance between the ages of 11 and 13, and the third molar between 17 and 21. The third molars, called wisdom teeth, often cause difficulties if the jaws are too small to allow one or all of them to emerge. That forces the teeth to remain completely embedded (impacted). Wisdom teeth also may become a source of trouble because they press on adjacent teeth, or because infection develops under the gum flap. Surgical removal is sometimes necessary.

ORAL DISEASES, ACCIDENTS AND ABNORMALITIES

Tooth Decay *(dental caries)*

Tooth decay affects about 97 percent of the U.S. population. A person who has never had a single dental cavity resulting from the inroads of decay is rare indeed. The problem is most prevalent during childhood and adolescence, and it begins early. Fifty percent of normal two-year-olds have at least one spot of decay. The average 11- to 15-year-old gets 1.5

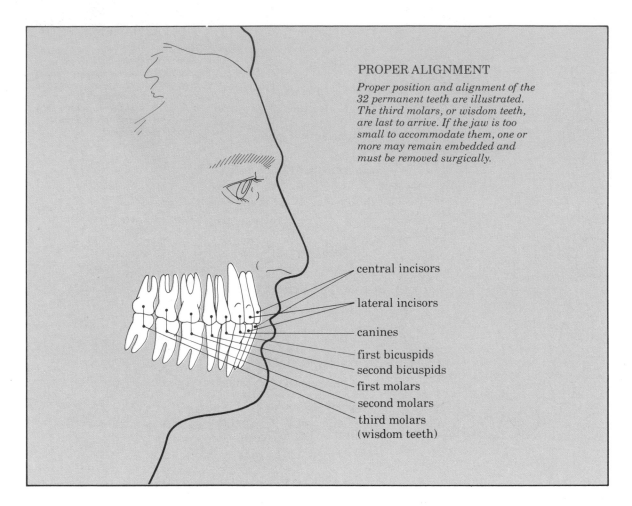

PROPER ALIGNMENT

Proper position and alignment of the 32 permanent teeth are illustrated. The third molars, or wisdom teeth, are last to arrive. If the jaw is too small to accommodate them, one or more may remain embedded and must be removed surgically.

central incisors
lateral incisors
canines
first bicuspids
second bicuspids
first molars
second molars
third molars
(wisdom teeth)

new cavities a year, and the average 17-year-old has nine decayed, missing, or filled teeth out of a complement of 28. Some dentists believe that adults have fewer cavities only because most of the vulnerable teeth have been attacked and repaired already.

Decay occurs in areas of the mouth where bacteria and food debris accumulate and remain undisturbed. The bacteria react with the carbohydrates of the foods to produce an acid that dissolves tooth enamel. There are three types of decay, categorized by location:

• Pit and fissure decay develops on the biting and chewing surface of the rear teeth.
• Smooth-surface decay occurs in areas between teeth where they adjoin.
• Root-surface decay attacks the dentin on the lower portion of the tooth crown where the gum tissue has receded (usually in later life).

What the three have in common is that they develop in areas not readily cleansed by saliva or toothbrushing.

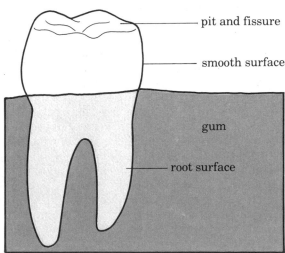

pit and fissure
smooth surface
gum
root surface

COMMON DECAY SITES

Three common areas of decay are the pits and fissures of chewing surfaces of the rear teeth, smooth surfaces between the teeth, and the root surfaces below the gum line. Root surface decay usually occurs in later life after the gum has receded. Decay occurs because all three areas are poorly cleansed by saliva or toothbrushing.

No precise cause and effect has ever been established for tooth decay. It appears that many elements must interact in order for decay to develop. Some of these relate to the tooth and mouth structure itself, inherited resistance or susceptibility, contour of the teeth, composition and arrangement of the teeth, character and amount of saliva, and the presence or absence of tooth-strengthening fluorides in the drinking water from birth. Variations in diet and the presence or absence of certain strains of bacteria also play a part. All must fit together in exactly the right combination for decay to begin.

Decay usually starts with a single microscopic spot, then gradually widens and deepens until a noticeable and sometimes painful cavity is seen. Once decay has occurred, the destroyed part of the tooth must be treated and restored. This involves removing the decay completely to stop the process from advancing, then shaping the cavity to receive a filling. The purpose of the filling is to restore the original shape and contour of the natural tooth so it can maintain its function. Filling materials are usually made of silver and gold for strength when used in back teeth, while tooth-colored materials of porcelain and plastic are used in the front teeth to look natural.

Prevention and Control of Tooth Decay

Because four elements must be present to promote decay, the destructive process can be broken by intervening in these ways:
• Modifying the diet.
• Controlling the bacteria by keeping the mouth clean.
• Increasing the resistance of the teeth to decay by using fluorides or sealants.
• Periodic dental examinations.

Diet. The average American eats between 90 and 100 pounds of refined sugar a year. Twenty-five to 40 pounds would be more than enough to supply all the calories needed from carbohydrate sources for good nutrition.

Too much sugar is detrimental to health for several reasons. It appeases appetite, lessens the desire and capacity for more nutritious foods, and it contributes to poor nutrition, especially in children, who are big sugar consumers. Most important from a dental point of view is that the sucrose of refined sugar provides a special attraction for the bacteria involved in tooth decay. More than any other foodstuff, it promotes tooth decay.

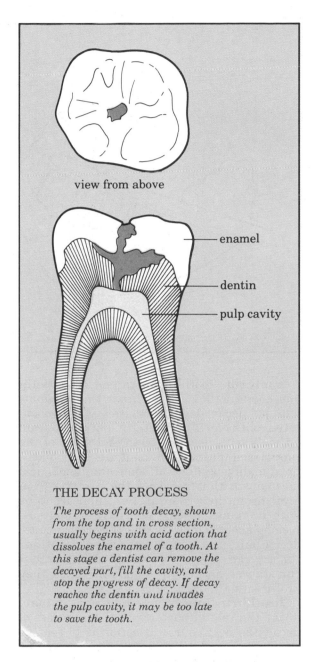

view from above

enamel

dentin

pulp cavity

THE DECAY PROCESS

The process of tooth decay, shown from the top and in cross section, usually begins with acid action that dissolves the enamel of a tooth. At this stage a dentist can remove the decayed part, fill the cavity, and stop the progress of decay. If decay reaches the dentin and invades the pulp cavity, it may be too late to save the tooth.

Sucrose turns up in some surprising foods, as a glance at the labels will tell you. They include such unlikely candidates as ketchup and mayonnaise, not to mention "unsweetened" cereals and white bread. But the biggest source of concentrated sugar is in candy, pastries, jams, and soft drinks. Children in particular eat these sweets between meals several times a day. Their teeth are repeatedly exposed to substances that can be the basis for harmful acid formation.

Changing the diet to less fermentable foods means substituting fresh fruit, nuts, and cheese for highly concentrated sugars.

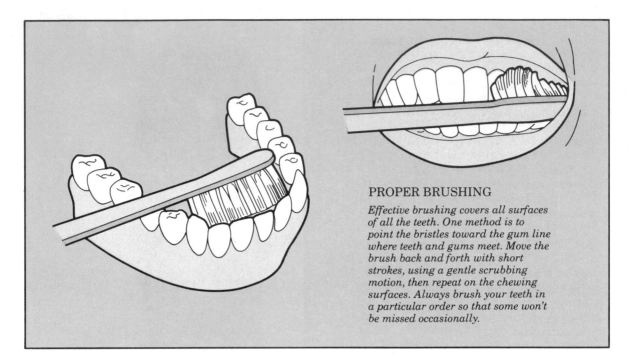

PROPER BRUSHING

Effective brushing covers all surfaces of all the teeth. One method is to point the bristles toward the gum line where teeth and gums meet. Move the brush back and forth with short strokes, using a gentle scrubbing motion, then repeat on the chewing surfaces. Always brush your teeth in a particular order so that some won't be missed occasionally.

Bacteria. Tooth decay cannot occur without bacteria. Research shows that animals without decay develop cavities when inoculated with certain bacteria obtained from animals with decayed teeth. Yet some of the inoculated animals do not develop decay, presumably because of some immunological mechanism that prevents the bacteria from growing in their mouths. So it appears to be with humans. Researchers have strong suspicions about which strains of bacteria cause decay, but investigation has not yet identified them positively or discovered the exact circumstances and environment in which they proliferate.

Toothbrushing. Since questions remain about the role of bacteria and the process of decay, the best course of action is to remove the bacteria and the sugars on which they feed as quickly as possible. Acid begins to form minutes after sugar has entered the secluded areas of the mouth and formation reaches its peak 15 to 30 minutes later. Thus teeth should be brushed immediately after eating for greatest effectiveness. Brushing first thing in the morning or before going to bed makes the teeth look better, stimulates the gum tissue, and may make the mouth feel fresher, but it is not much help in controlling tooth decay.

How you brush is important, too. Brushing only the prominent surfaces will allow bacteria and food debris to accumulate in hard to reach areas.

A toothbrush should have a flat brushing surface with soft bristles. The brush should be of such a size that it can reach every tooth.

One effective method of brushing is to point the bristles toward the gum line where the teeth and gums meet. Move the brush with short back-and-forth strokes using a gentle scrubbing motion. Be sure to brush both inside and outside surfaces of all teeth. Do the same gentle scrubbing motion on the chewing surfaces. Develop a habit of brushing the teeth in a definite order so that some surfaces won't be missed. Store the toothbrush where it will dry quickly. Get a new toothbrush when the bristles become frayed and worn.

Fluoride. Fluoride (which is a chemical compound of the element fluorine and some other element, usually a metal) occurs naturally in some water supplies, and has been found extremely beneficial in reducing tooth decay. Up to 65 percent fewer cavities have been found among residents of areas with a fluoridated water supply. Those who benefit most are children conceived, born, and raised where the waterborne fluoride is at the optimum amount.

The remarkable benefits of fluoride in combatting tooth decay were discovered almost accidentally. The story began in the early 1900s when a young Colorado dentist, Dr. Fred McKay, began to investigate a distinctive brown stain that commonly discolored the teeth of his patients. Further investigation showed similar stains on the teeth of residents of other Rocky Mountain areas, as well as those of residents of Texas and Arizona.

Curiously, although the stains were geographically widespread, they were not found everywhere in those areas, but only in certain communities.

First theories blamed "something in the water." Iron, calcium, and lime were suspected. But studies found no unusual amounts of those substances. Not until the early 1930s, when analytic methods had advanced to allow tests for trace elements, was it discovered that differences in fluoride content in the water were responsible for the stains.

The United States Public Health Service then joined the investigation, assigning a full-time dental officer, Dr. Trendley Dean, to work with Dr. McKay and others in investigating the phenomenon. Thousands of schoolchildren were examined, and hundreds of water supplies tested for fluoride throughout the country. A definite link was established between the amount of fluoride in the water and the intensity of the brown stain. Equally important, and to their delight, researchers unexpectedly found a similar link between the fluoride content and the community's level of tooth decay. Results showed levels of decay lower than those of the general population when the water supply contained fluoride concentrations of about one part per million. And there was little or no staining of teeth. Areas where the brown stain had been prevalent were found to have from 2 to 14 parts per million. But, where the water contained from 0.8 to 1.2 parts per million of fluoride, the residents showed fewer caries with no accompanying brown staining.

The next step was to add natural fluoride artificially to water supplies to test whether the association was one of cause and effect. During the late 1940s and early 1950s, controlled studies were undertaken by different investigators in Michigan, Illinois, New York, and Ontario. The results were clearly positive in all four areas. When fluoride was added to water in proper amounts, there was a significant reduction of decay (about 65 percent), with no signs of brown stain, and no adverse health effects. Meanwhile, health studies of persons who had used water supplies with excessive amounts of fluoride all their lives disclosed no adverse health effects. The conclusion was that fluoride, when used at the recommended level of one part per million, is a safe and effective oral health measure. Water fluoridation has continued to be studied and the verdict of safety and effectiveness reconfirmed.

How fluorides work. Chemically, fluoride has a strong propensity to react with calcium, a major building block of teeth. The calcium forms a new substance in the tooth that is less soluble in the acids associated with tooth decay. Moreover, fluoride in the tooth substance and in saliva has a bacteria-killing (bacteriocidal) effect, and thus does not allow the bacteria to grow. If the protective fluorides are present in the body fluids during the prenatal period of tooth formation, they are built into the tooth substance. This is why children conceived in a fluoridated area derive great benefit.

Topical fluorides. Fluorides also can provide a significant amount of protection when applied periodically to the surfaces of the teeth. This treatment also takes advantage of the affinity of fluoride and tooth structure. When fluoride is painted on the surface enamel of the tooth, the tooth takes it up and thus becomes more resistant to acid. Residents of non-fluoridated water areas can have fluoride solutions applied to their teeth by a dentist, usually in the forms of a gel-like substance, a liquid, or a mouth rinse.

Studies have shown that topical fluoride applications can reduce children's tooth decay by as much as 40 percent. The major drawbacks are time and expense. And the treatment must be repeated regularly because the benefits are not sustained. Most dentists recommend that it be done annually.

A new method of receiving fluorides is via mouthwash. Mouthwash containing fluoride is an effective means of combatting decay if it is used daily as prescribed. The least effective means of receiving fluoride is by daily use of a fluoridated dentifrice. But although this is not as effective as other methods, daily brushing with fluoridated toothpaste is still recommended.

Sealants. Another method of improving resistance to decay is to use a group of materials called sealants. The biting surfaces of the back teeth are usually the first to decay. A plastic coating can be applied to the fissures and grooves of these teeth to protect against decay. The material is applied by trained dental personnel, requires no drilling, and is painless. The coating provides strong protection for the biting surfaces, but should be used with fluoride therapy for other areas of the teeth.

Periodic examinations. Another means of controlling tooth decay is regular examination by a dentist to detect small cavities early and correct them promptly with proper fillings. Examinations should begin about the time of a child's third birthday, about one year

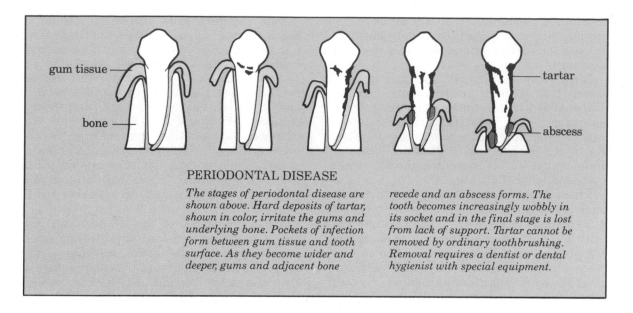

PERIODONTAL DISEASE

The stages of periodontal disease are shown above. Hard deposits of tartar, shown in color, irritate the gums and underlying bone. Pockets of infection form between gum tissue and tooth surface. As they become wider and deeper, gums and adjacent bone recede and an abscess forms. The tooth becomes increasingly wobbly in its socket and in the final stage is lost from lack of support. Tartar cannot be removed by ordinary toothbrushing. Removal requires a dentist or dental hygienist with special equipment.

after all the primary teeth have erupted. Even at that early age, almost half of all children already will have one cavity.

Parental fears and anxiety about dental visits can easily be conveyed to young children. Conversely, parents can do much to prepare the child by explaining procedures or arranging a "get acquainted" visit to the dentist before treatment.

Visits should then take place routinely, about every six months. Some may need more frequent treatment, others only an annual checkup. The interval can be determined by experience and the judgment of the dentist. The main purpose, of course, is to detect problems early and treat them before extensive and expensive damage occurs.

Periodontal Disease

Periodontal disease is an inflammation that results in destruction of the tissues supporting the teeth. It is a major dental problem and is the primary cause of tooth extraction in persons 35 or older. Many victims are unaware of the problem because it usually develops painlessly and progresses slowly.

Gingivitis. The simplest and most common form of periodontal disease is an inflammation of the gums known as gingivitis. It begins with a slight swelling along the gum margin of one or more teeth. The gum tissue in the area may have a slightly reddish tinge. As the condition grows worse, the puffiness and color change become more pronounced, the "collar" of gum tissue loses its tight adaptation to the tooth surface, and the tissue bleeds on slight pressure. Usually there is no pain, and often the person is not aware of anything unusual.

During pregnancy, gums may become inflamed and bleed. This form of gingivitis can be lessened with oral hygiene and usually disappears after the birth of the baby.

Periodontitis. If the inflammation of the gums is not treated, the gum tissue gradually may separate from the tooth and a pocket may form between the soft gum tissue and the hard tooth surface. When that happens the gingivitis, which is limited to gum surface, has developed into a more deep-seated condition called periodontitis. Now bacteria, saliva, and food debris begin to collect in the pockets and intensify the destructive process. The adjacent bone is destroyed, more attaching tissue is lost, and the pocket deepens and widens. Eventually the tooth loosens and begins to move during chewing. This causes additional irritation. The effect is comparable to rocking a post back and forth in the ground. The tooth becomes more and more movable in its socket. By the time teeth become noticeably loose or begin to shift so the gaps open between them, considerable damage has been done. Many people do not become aware of their periodontal problem until this stage is reached.

Treatment. Unless periodontal disease is treated early, the task becomes more difficult because the destroyed tissue cannot be replaced. Thus the dentist attempts to arrest the destruction as soon as possible to preserve the remaining support tissue. These measures include calculus removal and gum surgery (gingivectomy).

Calculus removal. One of the most important ways to check periodontal disease is meticulous cleaning and polishing of the tooth surfaces, particularly the surfaces adjacent to or beneath the gum tissue. In most people there is a tendency for calcium and other mineral salts contained in saliva to combine with bacteria, food particles, and salivary sediment. This debris is called plaque. In its soft form it can promote tooth decay. It can also harden into a substance called dental calculus or tartar.

Plaque attaches itself to the teeth in areas along the gum line and between the teeth. Good brushing and other means of tooth cleaning can remove most of the deposits while they are soft, but if they are left undisturbed because of poor oral hygiene, or remain in place 24 hours or more, ordinary methods of hygiene may not remove them, and they solidify.

These solidified mineral deposits irritate the gums and underlying bone. They intensify the destructive process in the adjacent gum and bone tissues and act as a center for further collection of debris.

The hard and soft accumulations must be removed by a dentist or a dental hygienist. They use small instruments to scrape off the hard coating and polishing devices to clean and brush the surface.

After the hardened deposits have been removed, the patient can prevent or slow their recurrence by faithfully following a cleaning program prescribed by the dentist or dental hygienist. No single routine can be prescribed for everyone because of the differences in mouths and in the accumulation of debris. Your dentist can best decide the proper method for you. Conscientious and sustained home care by the patient is critical to prevent or control periodontal disease.

Gum surgery. If tooth cleaning does not prevent or cure periodontal disease, it may be necessary to remove the gum tissue that has been separated from the tooth, a procedure called gingivectomy. This eliminates areas of stagnation and irritation. It produces greater areas of tooth surface to be kept clean by the patient and dentist, but also makes these surfaces more accessible to good cleaning and prevention of disease.

Preventing periodontal disease. Good oral hygiene is most important. That includes frequent and thorough scaling of the teeth above and below the gum line, followed by regular brushing. Both must be carried out faithfully and completely. The teaching and practice of oral hygiene should begin early.

Vincent's Infection

(trench mouth)

An acute infection of the gums is known as necrotizing gingivitis, trench mouth, or Vincent's infection. The gums become painful, swollen, and inflamed. The inside of the mouth may show blisters and ulcerations. A greyish-yellow membrane usually covers the inflamed areas, and the breath has an unpleasant odor. This disease requires treatment by a dentist as soon as possible. Proper care, especially a thorough cleaning, usually brings relief in 24 to 48 hours. Painting the gums or mouthwashes are not effective. Further treatment will be necessary to clear the condition and to prevent recurrence.

A condition called aphthous stomatitis is frequently confused with Vincent's infection, especially in children. It is extremely painful and has a somewhat similar appearance. However, the inflammations may appear in other areas of the mouth besides the gums. The lips and exterior portions of the mouth may also be infected. Stomatitis is believed to be a viral infection. It is stubborn to treat, but usually cures itself in a week to ten days. The aphthous ulcer or troublesome "canker sore" is a form of this condition. This lesion usually occurs on the inside of the cheek or lips or where the cheek and gum join.

Tumors

It has been estimated that two to five percent of all cancers occur in or around the mouth. Oral cancer is detected in 20,000 people each year. The cure rate is poor because cancer around the mouth usually invades rapidly and spreads to deeper structures. About 7,000 persons die each year from oral cancer.

Malignancies in the mouth begin painlessly and seldom interfere with oral functions at first. The victim may be unaware of the cancer for some time, and the delay in recognition and treatment permits the cancer to spread. As with other cancers, the earlier that malignancies in the lip, tongue, cheek, palate, or gums are detected and removed, the more favorable the outcome is likely to be.

The need for early recognition of growths or non-healing sores in the mouth is an important reason for regular dental examinations. The dentist's examination should include not only inspection of the teeth but a careful appraisal of all the tissues lining and adjoining the oral cavity.

Irritation appears to be associated with cancer development. That is why rough edges on teeth or fillings should be smoothed as soon as possible. Bridges or dentures that are loose or do not fit properly should be adjusted promptly. Repeatedly assaulting the mouth with extremely hot drinks or highly spiced foods can be hazardous. Oral cancer also is more prevalent among those who smoke or chew tobacco. Overexposure of the sensitive areas of the lips to sunlight is another possible cause.

Any unusual lesion should be watched for. One of these is called leukoplakia. It appears as a leathery white patch or patches anywhere on the mucous membrane lining the mouth or covering the tongue. The surface may be smooth and thin, raised and thick, roughened and fissured, or ulcerated. Leukoplakia results from irritation and may become malignant if not treated.

Benign growths, called polyps and papillomas, also can be found in the oral cavity. These outgrowths of soft tissue are often subjected to irritation during chewing or toothbrushing. Although these tumors are not malignant, they can become so and should be kept under strict observation. If they are in a position to be repeatedly irritated, they should be removed.

Cleft Lip and Palate

Cleft lip and palate occur because certain tissues of the lip and palate fail to unite while the fetus is developing in the womb. The condition is discovered at birth. Cleft palate occurs in approximately one in 700 newborns in the United States. Clefts vary widely in severity and location. They may involve the lip, the hard palate (roof of the mouth), the soft palate, or any combination of these structures. In some instances, the upper jaw and lip may be affected. Clefts can occur on one side only (unilateral) or on both sides (bilateral).

The causes of cleft palate are unknown but may involve a combination of factors including genetics, hormones, drugs used by the mother during pregnancy, environment, and disease. Recent advances in treatment have greatly helped cleft palate patients. The treatment is a long process and involves an entire team of specialists. Among those involved are medical personnel (pediatrician, plastic surgeon, ear, nose, and throat specialist), dental (general dentist, orthodontist, and oral surgeon), and speech therapy specialists. Surgical repair of the cleft, usually done in stages, not only greatly improves appearance, but increases ability to eat, drink, and speak normally. Prosthetic speech aids that fit in the mouth not only improve speech, but can help with eating and drinking. Because children with cleft palate seem more prone to tooth decay and gum disease than others, oral hygiene is particularly important. As for all children, proper care of primary (baby) teeth is extremely important.

Occlusion

Occlusion refers to the way the upper and lower teeth mesh when the jaws close. A few teeth may strike each other early and thus be subjected to excessive pressure. Or teeth may be positioned so that the force of tooth contact is not directed vertically toward the end of the root, but instead tends to wedge the teeth sideways. Such movement may put abnormal stress on the bony attachment.

A dentist may adjust the occlusion by carefully grinding certain tooth surfaces to obtain a more equal distribution of the biting pressures. The dentist may even make changes in the alignment of the teeth, or construct a splint to hold two or more adjacent teeth together, providing them with mutual support against the biting strains. Splints usually are employed only when teeth already have become loose. They help preserve some teeth for further service.

Bruxism

Some people have a habit of clenching or grinding their teeth, particularly during sleep. This habit is known as bruxism. The extra stress it places on the supporting tissues of the teeth can be damaging. It is sometimes necessary for the person to wear a mouth guard, particularly at night, to relieve this strain and eliminate the habit.

Tooth Loss

If a tooth or several teeth are lost, there is a tendency for the neighboring teeth to shift toward the empty space created by the loss. These teeth may then be in such a position that they are less able to tolerate the stress of chewing. Such tooth "migration" also may open spaces between the remaining teeth. This allows food fibers and particles to pass between the teeth and pack against the gum, setting up an irritation that can cause destruction of tissue or even bone. This is why it usually is important to insert a bridge to substitute for the missing tooth or teeth as soon as possible.

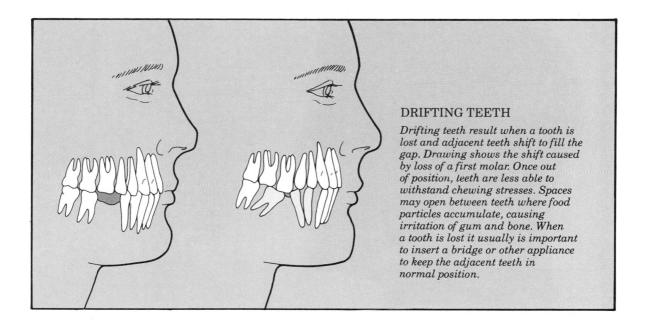

DRIFTING TEETH

Drifting teeth result when a tooth is lost and adjacent teeth shift to fill the gap. Drawing shows the shift caused by loss of a first molar. Once out of position, teeth are less able to withstand chewing stresses. Spaces may open between teeth where food particles accumulate, causing irritation of gum and bone. When a tooth is lost it usually is important to insert a bridge or other appliance to keep the adjacent teeth in normal position.

The rough edges of cavities along the gum line cause irritation that can lead to the destruction of deeper tissues. The edges of poorly fitting crowns or fillings can have the same effect. These defects must be corrected promptly to maintain good dental health.

Temporo-mandibular Joint Disturbances

The lower and upper jaws are connected by two joints, one on the right side and one on the left, called temporo-mandibular joints. They are in front of the external opening of the ears and consist of an extension upward of the lower jaw (mandible), which has a rounded end fitting into a socket in the base of the skull. The bony parts are held together by ligaments and muscles. The arrangement of the temporo-mandibular joints is responsible for the variety of movements that the lower jaw can make, including chewing, swallowing, and talking.

Like other joints in the body, these joints are susceptible to diseases such as arthritis and cancer. Their close relationship to the teeth, however, often brings about changes not common in other body joints.

The symptoms of temporo-mandibular joint disturbances include a clicking noise upon opening the mouth or while chewing, an inability to open the mouth fully, a deviation of the lower jaw to one side upon opening the mouth, pain when opening the mouth, soreness in the side of the face, pain in the region of one or both joints when chewing, and recurrent headaches in some instances. The lower jaw may be susceptible to recurrent dislocation of the joints when the mouth is opened wide because of a weakness in the joint structure.

Dental conditions that may contribute to or cause these disturbances are malocclusion of the teeth or uneven bite. (Bite is the relation between the upper and lower teeth when the mouth is closed and the teeth are brought into contact.) Other causes are: over-closure of the bite, over-opening of the bite, poorly fitting dental restorations, and habits such as grinding or clenching of teeth.

In examining anyone with the above complaints, the dentist usually takes X rays of the joint and carefully studies the patient's bite, any dentures, tooth care, and general health.

Treatment may involve grinding the teeth to adjust an uneven bite, replacement of the improper restorations, special appliances to correct habits, corrections of malocclusion, use of physical therapy such as massage and special exercises, and in some severe cases a complete reconstruction of the patient's occlusion.

Malocclusion

Straightening teeth. Orthodontics is the branch of dental science that treats the misalignment of teeth and jaws, the so-called "crooked teeth." A dentist who specializes in such treatment is known as an orthodontist. He is primarily concerned with the detection, prevention, and correction of irregularities in

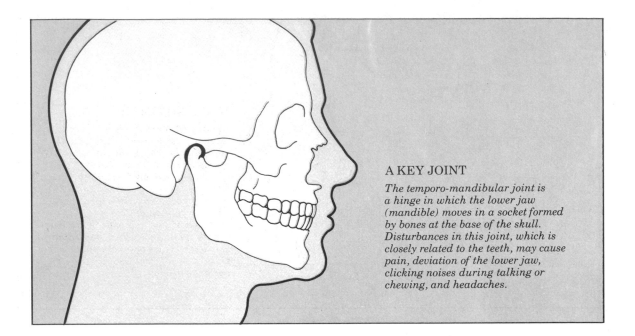

A KEY JOINT

The temporo-mandibular joint is a hinge in which the lower jaw (mandible) moves in a socket formed by bones at the base of the skull. Disturbances in this joint, which is closely related to the teeth, may cause pain, deviation of the lower jaw, clicking noises during talking or chewing, and headaches.

the position of the teeth, any improper relationship of the jaws, and the associated facial deformities and speech imperfections.

Heredity is one of the most important factors producing the crowding or spacing of teeth and the way in which the upper and lower teeth mesh when the jaws are closed. Other factors that influence the development of these irregularities (known as malocclusion) may be the early loss of the primary teeth, dietary and growth disorders, and undesirable habits such as prolonged thumb-sucking.

Poorly positioned teeth can interfere with the proper chewing of food, impair appearance, and may lead to psychological problems. They also are more vulnerable to decay or periodontal disease. Usually the irregularities are not outgrown but can be corrected.

A number of devices have been developed for applying gentle pressure to move the teeth. They usually include bands around the teeth with wires attached, and are used with other means to reposition the teeth and to influence the growth and contour of the jaws. The treatment also may require removal of several teeth so that sufficient space exists for the teeth to come into proper alignment. The proper time for starting treatment, the time required, and the type of treatment depend on the extent of the malocclusion.

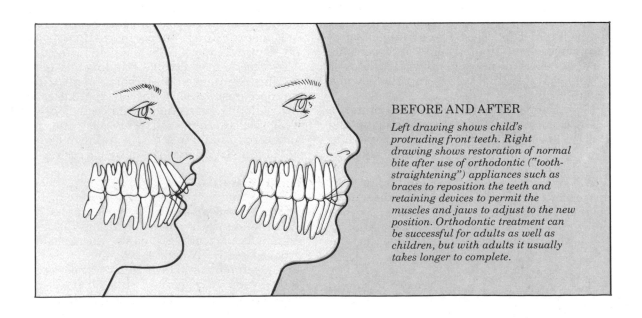

BEFORE AND AFTER

Left drawing shows child's protruding front teeth. Right drawing shows restoration of normal bite after use of orthodontic ("tooth-straightening") appliances such as braces to reposition the teeth and retaining devices to permit the muscles and jaws to adjust to the new position. Orthodontic treatment can be successful for adults as well as children, but with adults it usually takes longer to complete.

Thumb-sucking. Infants are born with a natural instinct to suck. Thumbs and fingers are readily available to satisfy this need. Thumb-sucking produces no lasting effect on the arrangement of the permanent teeth and the development of the jaws unless the habit continues after age four. Even then, potential damage depends on the frequency and intensity of the habit. Persistent thumb-sucking over a period of years, however, may result in unsightly spacing and protrusion of the child's upper front teeth.

Tongue-thrusting may occur when a child has enlarged tonsils and adenoids or has a mouth too small to accommodate the tongue. Other children develop a habit of biting the lips or thrusting the tongue between the teeth during times of tension. Although these habits usually do not noticeably irritate the tongue or lips, sufficient pressure can be exerted over a period of time to alter the position of the teeth and cause malformation of the jaws. Such habits usually develop in older children after a number of their permanent teeth have erupted. As soon as the habit is recognized, a dentist should be consulted. The dentist may need to construct an appliance to protect the teeth or to help break the habit.

Space maintenance. Early loss of baby teeth can result in a lack of space that will prevent the permanent tooth from coming into the mouth properly. When a baby tooth is lost early, there is a tendency for the surrounding teeth to attempt to fill the void. Here, too, it may be necessary for a dentist to insert an appliance to maintain the empty space. These space maintainers are usually simple bits of plastic and wire, and can be permanent or removable.

Accidents. A significant number of teeth are lost due to accidents and injuries, but recent advances in safety and prevention plus government regulation have helped reduce those losses. Automobile seat belt systems and padded automobile interiors have helped lower the number of facial injuries. The regulations in contact sports for protective equipment have significantly reduced other forms of injury. Hard helmets, face protectors, and mouth guards are now required in many sports. Other preventive measures include replacement of hard swing seats with canvas seats for youngsters, plus careful playground supervision. Teeter-totters and drinking fountains, however, remain particularly dangerous.

It is important to know that a tooth which has been completely "knocked out" can be replanted by a dentist if treatment begins within an hour or two. Success is largely dependent upon how quickly treatment can take place.

TOOTH LOSS
AND REPLACEMENT

An X-ray examination may reveal an abscessed tooth, frequently to the amazement of the patient. This pocket of infection represents the loss or destruction of tissue. It may have occurred because the pulp or "nerve" within the tooth has died from an irritation, from infection caused by deep decay, or from a hard bump on the tooth that the individual may not remember. Death of the pulp can occur painlessly or it can cause excruciating pain. As a result of the dead and usually infected pulp tissue within the root canal, the bone around the end of the root may dissolve. This area appears as a dark shadow in the X-ray picture. Affected teeth require treatment or extraction, the sooner the better.

Generally, pulp irritation causes pain. This means some form of treatment is required. Years ago it usually meant extraction of the tooth, but now these teeth can be saved by the branch of dentistry known as endodontics. The pulp is removed while the patient is under local anesthesia, followed by the preparation and filling of the root canal. The cause of the irritated pulp and subsequent toothache most often is a deep cavity.

Sometimes, particularly in children before the root has fully developed, it is possible to clean out the decayed material and cover the pulp area with a medicated cement. This procedure is known as pulp capping. In other circumstances, the portion of the pulp near the cavity may be removed and the medicated cement carefully placed over the amputated pulp stump. This treatment is known as pulpotomy or pulp amputation. These techniques may keep the pulp alive until the root is fully formed, allowing the conventional root filling to be done later. In some cases capped pulps remain alive and require no further treatment.

Saving a "Dying" Tooth

Pulp irritation may be so severe that the pulp tissue dies or will die if left in the tooth. If the tooth is to be saved, the pulp tissue must be removed, the canal prepared medically, and then sealed with a root filling.

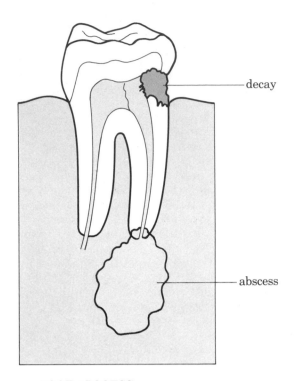

decay

abscess

ROOT ABSCESS

An abscess at the root of a tooth may result from infection caused by deep decay, as shown above, or from irritation or a hard bump. If the pulp is dead as a result, no pain will be felt and the abscess may be discovered on routine X-ray examination. To prevent damage to surrounding bone, the tooth must be extracted or treated by endodontics, in which the pulp is removed and the root canal filled and capped.

When the pulp has been dead for some time and has not been removed, changes take place in the bone around the root. When a considerable amount of bone has been destroyed, and the end of the root also shows signs of shrinkage and roughening, an operation known as periapical surgery (root resection, root amputation, or apicoectomy) may be performed to save the tooth.

This operation requires the exposure of the root end by making an opening through the overlying gum and bone. The small mass of inflamed tissue is scraped out of the bony cavity at the root end, the root end is sealed, and then the window in the gum is closed with sutures. Periapical surgery is usually done on the easily accessible and single-rooted front teeth. It has been highly successful in saving teeth that otherwise would have had to be extracted.

Fractured Teeth

When a tooth is broken off, its dental pulp chamber often is exposed. If it is, and if enough of the tooth remains to permit the missing crown portion to be replaced with an artificial substitute, the pulp must be removed and the root canal filled. If the pulp is not exposed, a protective cement may be applied to the fractured dentin surface and the repair observed to see whether the pulp will survive the injury. The observation period may vary from a few days to several months.

Discolorations

Occasionally the crowns of teeth darken after the root has been filled. The discoloration is caused by blood that seeped into the dentin before treatment, or by oral secretions invading the dentin beneath a crown filling that does not seal the cavity tightly. The discolorations can be corrected through a process known as bleaching. The technique is fairly simple. Bleaching agents are applied within the tooth to remove stains that are in the dentin. However, bleaching is not used for the removal of superficial stains that may be polished off the enamel.

Sometimes the discoloration reappears after a few years and another bleaching is required.

Tooth Extraction

Although it is possible today to keep teeth for a lifetime, there are instances in which extraction may become necessary. If diseased teeth are not treated in time, decay can destroy so much tooth structure that restoration becomes impossible. Gum disease, if allowed to advance, also can destroy so much bone and supporting structure that the tooth becomes too loose to be maintained. In both cases, to leave the tooth is to leave a source of oral infection. And a patient may feel unable to afford the large expense necessary to restore and maintain the teeth. Extraction may be necessary along with construction of complete dentures to restore dental function and appearance.

Thanks to pain medication and advances in equipment, extraction methods are much improved. Following extraction of a tooth, the wound in the jaw usually heals in a few days without complications. It is desirable for the patient to limit activity for several hours following an extraction. This helps to slow blood circulation, thereby reducing bleeding and helping a firm blood clot to form in the socket.

Care After Extraction

Swelling often develops in the face after an extraction. The reaction usually is not serious and can be minimized or prevented by the application of an ice bag or a moist, cold cloth. It should be kept in place for 15 minutes each hour and repeated for several hours.

The mouth should not be rinsed until the day after the extraction. This allows the blood clot to remain undisturbed. After the first day the mouth can be rinsed gently with warm salt water, made by dissolving one-half teaspoon of salt in eight ounces of warm water. Routine but careful brushing of the remaining teeth should be resumed the day after the extraction to keep the mouth clean and lessen the possibility of infection.

Bleeding usually stops shortly after tooth removal. Some oozing or actual bleeding may continue for several hours or even persist into the next day. Continued bleeding may be controlled by gently using a clean piece of gauze to wipe away the blood that has collected in the area of the wound, then folding clean gauze into a pad of proper size so that when placed over the wound, the teeth can be tightly closed and firm pressure made by pressing the gauze with the teeth against the bleeding area. The pressure should be maintained for half an hour, and the procedure can be repeated, if necessary. If bleeding persists or occurs in considerable amount, the dentist should be consulted.

Continue eating without interruption after tooth extraction, making an effort not to miss a meal. Choose soft foods to avoid disturbing the blood clot. Soft boiled eggs, soups, custards, and ground meat are recommended. Solid foods can be added as soon as they can be chewed comfortably and without dislodging the clot.

Most extraction wounds heal without complications. If considerable swelling, continued bleeding, severe or prolonged pain should develop, instructions for relief should be obtained from the dentist.

Dry Socket

Dry socket is a complication that sometimes develops following the extraction of a tooth. As the name implies, the blood clot that normally forms in the socket shortly after tooth removal fails to develop or is lost. This leaves the bony wall of the socket bare and unprotected, exposing the bone to bacteria, saliva, and food debris. The lining of the socket contains many sensory nerve endings and when these are open to such an irritating environment, severe pain can develop.

A sedative medication may be prescribed to reduce the pain of dry socket. The area must be kept as clean as possible, and an anesthetic dressing placed in the open socket until nature develops a protective covering for the exposed bone. Healing usually is delayed and several days pass before the pain disappears.

The reasons a dry socket forms are not fully known. Some believe it results from a rapid bacterial action. Others suspect a fault in the blood clotting mechanism. Rinsing the mouth too vigorously following extraction, sucking on the area, and manipulations by the tongue also tend to dislodge the clot.

Crown and Bridge

In some instances it is necessary to restore or cover the entire crown of a tooth. This is usually done if the tooth has been broken down because of decay or injury. The crown is reduced and smoothed with a dental drill and then a cover or crown is made from a model of the patient's tooth. The materials are usually gold with plastic or porcelain similar in color to natural teeth. A crown can be made to look very much like the missing tooth.

When missing teeth are to be replaced, it is possible to fix the new (replacement) teeth permanently by means of a bridge. Teeth adjacent to the space are prepared for crowns, and the entire unit is soldered together and permanently cemented into the mouth. These replacements usually are very durable.

Partial Denture

This is a removable appliance that replaces one or more missing natural teeth. The "partial plate" is held in the mouth by clasps that grip the adjacent natural teeth. "Partials" must be cleaned after each meal, because food particles can be trapped under them and cause harm to the natural teeth. The partial denture should not be left out of the mouth because the natural teeth may shift position, making the denture fit poorly or not at all. This is not as satisfactory as a fixed bridge in terms of comfort, appearance, or function.

Complete Dentures

A full set of "false teeth," upper and lower, is necessary much less frequently than in past years. False teeth are considered a last resort, and are seldom prescribed for young people, as they previously were.

Dentures made today are much superior to those of years ago. Materials have been developed which make dentures more lifelike and durable, less bulky or porous. Modern techniques have improved their fit and function. Individuals can be less concerned with the cosmetic aspects of dentures because they look more natural and are more likely to mesh properly for eating and speaking than in the past. Dentures should be checked and the mouth periodically examined by the dentist to eliminate soreness or tender areas, to assure that the dentures fit properly, and to see that supporting tissue is healthy.

ORAL HEALTH FOR SPECIAL GROUPS

The dental needs of some segments of our society are not met in ordinary dental practice. In recent times, society has begun to take more responsibility for these special groups such as senior citizens, the chronically ill, and the physically or mentally handicapped. Barrier-free designs for public buildings and senior citizen discounts for restaurants, theaters, and public transportation are indicative of this concern and interest. Heightened awareness of these groups and the development of specialized dental equipment have allowed dental care to be brought to patients in settings such as nursing homes, hospitals, training centers, and schools. Treatment programs have been established in a variety of locations throughout the nation by hospitals, dental schools, public health departments, private agencies, and federal agencies.

Oral Health During Pregnancy

A misconception still persists that a developing fetus can withdraw calcium from the mother's teeth and thus cause cavities. The old wives' tale, "For every child, a tooth," has not been proven in scientific study. The fetus does require calcium, but the fetal supply does not come from the dental enamel of the mother. If the mother's diet does not provide an adequate supply, the fetus can "steal" calcium from the mother's bones. However, calcium cannot be withdrawn from tooth enamel into the bloodstream and circulated to another tissue, to an organ, or to a growing fetus. It is fixed and can be removed only by external action, such as acid forming on the tooth surface (as in dental caries) or by cutting with dental instruments.

If a woman seems to have more tooth decay during pregnancy, the cause is more likely to be a letdown in oral hygiene or an increase in between-meal snacks. If she has had bouts of nausea and acid regurgitation, the natural acid-neutralizing agents in the mouth may be used up or less able to combat the acids formed by fermenting food. That is why the pregnant woman should practice meticulous oral hygiene.

Some pregnant women experience inflammation of the gums (see page 414). As with all gingivitis patients, keeping the teeth clean and removing calculus (tartar) deposits, rough cavity margins, and other sources of irritation will reduce the amount of swelling and inflammation. When the teeth are in good condition, gum tissue usually returns to normal soon after delivery of the baby.

HOW TO BE A WISE DENTAL CARE CONSUMER

Choosing a Dentist

It is prudent to select a family dentist before a dental emergency occurs. A dentist who maintains a general practice can provide routine dental care and is qualified to refer patients requiring specialized treatment to a specialist. Some of these specialists include endodontist (root canal treatment), orthodontist (straightening of teeth), periodontist (gum treatment), and exodontist (tooth extraction). A pedodontist is a dentist who treats only children.

There are several ways to find qualified dentists: Ask knowledgeable friends, neighbors, and co-workers; contact faculty members of area dental schools or hospitals that maintain a dental service; make inquiry to local dental societies; consult the American Dental Association Directory found in public libraries and dental school libraries; and ask your family physician or pharmacist for recommendations.

The Initial Visit

An initial visit will allow you to evaluate the dentist in several areas. Consider the efficiency and general appearance of the office as well as the dentist and the staff. Note whether the office location is convenient, and whether appointments are easy to schedule. The informed person will want a dentist who stresses prevention and uses the latest techniques for treatment and prevention.

Since X rays are a valuable diagnostic tool, it is routine for a dentist to request a full set of mouth X rays for a new patient. If recent X rays are available from a previous dentist, these can be used instead. The radiation exposure during mouth X rays is minimal.

Fees should be discussed during the initial visit. Fees vary with the procedure or treatment needed. The dentist should be willing to discuss fees and payment plans before initiation of any services. Many dentists employ office managers who can discuss financial arrangements with the patient.

If you are not able to reach your dentist in an emergency, other dentists usually provide emergency treatment, telephone consultations, or referrals.

Insurance

Unlike medical insurance, which can be purchased on an individual basis, dental insurance usually can be obtained only through group plans (such as those of labor unions). In 1977, about 48 million Americans, or one in five, were covered by dental insurance. Most plans do not cover all dental health expenses. The plans usually are designed to encourage regular check-ups for preventive care. When dental disease is discovered and treated while still in a minor stage, it is less costly to the patient and the insurance company.

Financial Aid

Many communities offer low-cost or no-cost dental care through dental school clinics, public health clinics, and dental health care centers. Information regarding these programs can be obtained by contacting area dental schools, the local dental society, or the local health department.

Problem Solving

If a patient is displeased with dental services or feels that the fees are unreasonable, he or she should discuss the matter with the dentist. Most dentists want to know if the treatment has not achieved the expected results. An alternative treatment or a consultation with another dentist may be in order. If, however, the problem cannot be satisfactorily remedied in this manner, the patient may ask for help from the local dental society. The case will be reviewed by a panel of dentists called a peer review committee. Often one member of the peer review committee may resolve the dispute by meeting with the patient and dentist. Or the complaint may be reviewed by the entire committee. The treatment record is studied and an oral examination of the patient conducted.

Although this procedure is voluntary (no laws require the dental societies to perform this service), many cases have been resolved through it. However, dental practice laws in each state and a state board of dentistry regulate the practice of dentistry and protect the public from dentists who do not perform within the law or who are not licensed to practice.

To contact local dental societies for information, consult the yellow pages of the phone directory under the listing of "associations" or "dentists," or call a local dentist for the phone number. Or you may contact your county health department or the American Dental Association, 211 East Chicago Avenue, Chicago, Illinois 60611.

Oral Health Products

The American Dental Association, although not a governmental agency, traditionally has evaluated dental products. Those proven to be both safe and effective carry the association's approval. With so many products available, it is best to consult with your dentist, who may recommend a particular type or brand based on personal need.

Toothpaste (dentifrice), the toothbrush, and dental floss remove plaque. While plaque should be removed at least once a day, the dentist may recommend brushing more frequently for certain oral health conditions.

To remove stains and plaque, the toothpaste must have some degree of abrasiveness, but toothpaste containing too many abrasive elements can affect restorations (fillings) and injure surrounding gum tissue. The dentist can help select a toothpaste that removes plaque but is not too abrasive to cause harm.

Toothpastes containing fluoride provide the greatest benefits. Fluoride dentifrices and a fluoridated water supply can help reduce decay, dental experts agree.

Toothbrushes come in two types, manual or electric. Neither has been proven more effective than the other. The choice depends on individual preference, although some children find a powered toothbrush more interesting and therefore use it more consistently and thoroughly. Powered toothbrushes may be beneficial to persons with certain physical handicaps. When considering a manual toothbrush, be sure that the brush head can reach all areas of the mouth. Many persons prefer a soft-bristled brush. However, your dentist may have specific recommendations for you about bristles.

Dental floss. Two types of dental floss can be purchased, waxed and unwaxed. Although unwaxed dental floss may be more acceptable for plaque removal, waxed floss may be easier to use, especially if the teeth are close together. Floss daily, following the procedure recommended by the dentist. Removal of plaque by floss can be important in maintaining good oral hygiene.

Oral irrigating devices. These devices spray water onto gums and teeth to remove loose food particles and debris. They should not be used *instead* of a toothbrush or dental floss. They can be used as an additional aid in maintaining cleanliness, especially by persons wearing dentures or orthodontic bands.

A dentist should be consulted before you use this device, because incorrect pressure can injure tissues in some people.

Mouthwash. While mouthwash may make your mouth feel or taste better, mouthwash without fluoride has not been proven beneficial in removing plaque, and cannot prevent tooth decay or periodontal disease. Mouthwashes that do not contain fluoride should be considered primarily cosmetic and should not be substituted for the toothbrush, toothpaste, and dental floss.

Halitosis. Americans spend a quarter of a billion dollars annually on mouthwashes, fluoride toothpastes, and breath mints in an effort to cure bad breath (halitosis). Halitosis means a condition in which a chemical compound or series of compounds produced within the body result in an unpleasant odor on the breath. The condition can be caused by decaying material deep within the tooth or surrounding tissue, such as food particles that provide nutrients for *Streptococcus mutans,* a strain of bacteria. Decayed teeth also can cause bad breath, as can periodontal disease and gum infection. Infections in the nasal cavity, sinuses, or upper respiratory tract, a deviated septum, or infected tonsils and adenoids are other possible causes. So are gallbladder disease, ulcers, and some blood conditions such as anemia and hemophilia.

Breath odors may originate in the intestines rather than the mouth or respiratory tract. Garlic or onion odors return to the mouth after being absorbed in the bloodstream, then are exhaled through the lungs. The liver and intestines can be irritated by lack of vitamin C and D. Low carbohydrate diets which contain high levels of proteins and fats may also cause bad breath. Individuals exposed to certain chemicals such as mercury, lead, and nickel may be subject to bad breath when these materials are inhaled and then absorbed into the bloodstream.

During sleep, the normal flow of saliva is reduced, so that the cleansing action that functions when we are awake and when we chew food is not present. This condition is aggravated by food particles left in the mouth overnight which are quickly acted upon by bacteria and cause strong odors.

Good oral hygiene is the best preventive method for halitosis. This includes flossing, brushing (even gentle brushing of the tongue), and regular cleaning by a dentist once or twice a year. Diet control is also important. Avoiding highly spiced foods such as onions and garlic, and avoiding alcohol and tobacco, will help reduce halitosis. Cutting consumption of fatty foods such as cheese, butter, and whole milk may help. If the condition is due to a medical problem such as a sore throat, antibiotics will help reduce the infection and hence the related odor. A medical doctor should be consulted if such a condition is suspected. Mouthwashes and similar products will mask breath odors temporarily, but they do nothing to alleviate the cause and have no long-lasting effects.

MODERN DENTAL PRACTICE

Personnel

During recent years the numbers of trained auxiliary personnel who assist dentists have greatly expanded. More and more functions in a dental office are being delegated to relieve the dentist of simple and routine procedures so he or she can concentrate on the more complex aspects of care. The emphasis in most offices is on patient education and the sharing of responsibility for oral health.

Here are some of the personnel in modern dental offices.

• Dental hygienists can directly treat patients. With two to four years of formal training, they are licensed to clean and scale teeth and tissue, provide patient education, and help the dentist with other procedures.

• Dental assistants usually have two years of formal training. Certification is required in some states. They assist the dentist at chairside, but are not legally permitted to treat patients independently, although some states allow treatment under supervision.

• Laboratory technicians follow the prescriptions for construction and repair of oral appliances, dentures, and the like. They work in a commercial laboratory or in the dental office.

Equipment

Dental equipment has undergone a dramatic transformation since about 1970. The equipment has become modernized, and bright, warm colors have replaced the traditional pale tones. The dental chair is now a modular reclining lounge chair. Much of the dental equipment is now recessed or built into cabinets. The dental light is now small and unobtrusive rather than the large, bright fixture patients have stared at for years.

Dental service has changed, too. An example is the equipment used to prepare teeth for fillings and crowns. For years dentists have used rotary tools (drills). These cutting instruments rotated at a top speed of 5,000 revolutions per minute. Vibration, pressure, and heat made the patient uncomfortable. Today, drills are powered by air turbines and rotate at speeds as fast as 300,000 revolutions per minute. Only a light touch is required to cut enamel and dentin at those high speeds. And because the rotations are so rapid, the sense of vibration is eliminated. A spray of water and air is directed at the area being cut to keep the temperature at a comfortable level.

Procedures

Perhaps the most important improvement and modernization has taken place in dental treatment. The orientation of modern practice is prevention. Procedures performed in the dental office are aimed at preventing future problems. The recent advances in endodontics have made it possible for patients to retain most teeth. The present-day practice of treating the root canal of teeth has been of great benefit. Orthodontics (tooth straightening) has also helped prevent problems.

Dental X rays. Good X-ray pictures can reveal the early development of disturbances in the teeth and jaws that the dentist cannot detect simply by looking in the mouth. Decay in hidden surfaces between the teeth, or beneath a filling, or at the bottom of a narrow pit or groove in the chewing surface may be disclosed by X rays long before it might be otherwise detectable. The height of the bone surrounding and supporting the teeth, the amount of bone destroyed by periodontal disease, the development of root abscesses and cysts, the presence of unerupted teeth or broken root fragments embedded in the bone also can be determined by X rays.

It is usually desirable to have an X-ray examination at periodic intervals to give the dentist a continuing record of any change in the teeth and the bone around them. Comparing the series of pictures may lead to earlier detection of disease and permit the dentist to check on the effectiveness of previous treatments.

With modern shielded apparatus and high-speed X-ray film, only a small amount of radiation is required for a complete set of dental pictures. The small fraction that could possibly reach the more sensitive cells of the body is less than everyone receives routinely from cosmic rays from space.

Dental materials. Materials used to fill and replace teeth are constantly being improved. These materials must meet exacting requirements. They must be strong enough to

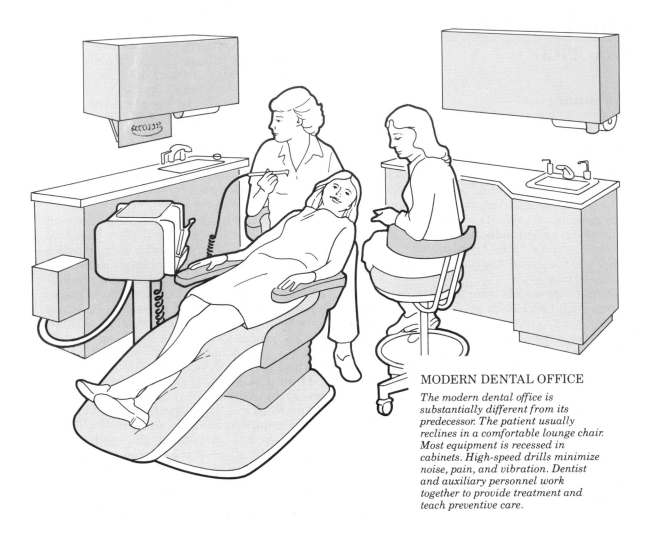

MODERN DENTAL OFFICE

The modern dental office is substantially different from its predecessor. The patient usually reclines in a comfortable lounge chair. Most equipment is recessed in cabinets. High-speed drills minimize noise, pain, and vibration. Dentist and auxiliary personnel work together to provide treatment and teach preventive care.

withstand the stress placed on them in the process of chewing. The restorative material must not be dissolved, discolored, or permeated by the fluids in the mouth, and must not expand or shrink appreciably after being placed in a cavity. And these materials must be nonpoisonous, of course. If possible, they should resemble the color and appearance of natural teeth or gums. Several materials meet these requirements and are widely used. They include gold, silver, porcelain, synthetic porcelain, and acrylic resins.

Gold has had extensive use. Originally very thin strips of pure gold foil were malleted into a cavity. The purity and malleability of the gold under pressure allowed the bits to fuse together into one solid mass, filling the cavity. Gold foil restorations make excellent and durable fillings, but many patients object to the malleting procedure and to the appearance of the filling.

The gold inlay was introduced as a cavity filling in the early 1900s. It is based on the development of a precision casting process. The prepared cavity is filled with softened wax, which is then carved to the proper shape for the tooth. A mold is made of the wax pattern, the wax is eliminated, and molten gold cast into the empty mold. The materials and techniques for making this type of restoration have been greatly refined, and today the cast inlay made of a hard gold alloy is in wide use. Although the inlay is made to fit the cavity precisely, it must be sealed into the tooth with dental cement.

The silver filling is really an alloy (amalgam) of several metals including silver, tin, and mercury. It is produced by mixing a combination of powdered tin and silver with mercury to form a soft mass. Small bits are carried into a cavity and packed against each other until the cavity is filled and the excess mercury squeezed out. The amalgam hardens in a short time, and while it is hardening it can be carved to the desired contour. Silver or amalgam fillings are more brittle than gold and if not mixed properly they tend to shrink or expand.

Porcelain is used as a cavity filling material and in construction of porcelain crowns. The porcelain is a mixture of clay-like materials blended together in powder form to resemble a natural tooth. The blended powders are converted to a plastic state by moistening, and the mass is contoured into the desired form. It is then solidified by baking at high temperature. The porcelain restoration is natural in appearance, but has the disadvantage of being more fragile than one made from a metallic mixture. A "jacket crown," as the name implies, requires the removal of the natural enamel and replacement with a cover of baked porcelain that restores the surface of the crown back to its original contour.

Synthetic porcelain (silicate cement). These fillings are usually placed in the front part of the mouth because of their natural appearance. They are made from porcelain-like powders that are mixed with a liquid, usually phosphoric acid. The mixture is packed into a cavity and sets into a solid crystalline mass in a few minutes. It makes a pleasing restoration because it is hard to distinguish from natural enamel, but it is not as durable as most other filling materials because it has a tendency to wash away.

Acrylic resins were first developed in the early 1940s, and have undergone constant improvement and acceptance in their suitability for dental applications. Various forms of acrylics are used in denture construction, in filling materials, as decay preventives in sealants, and as a means of fixing orthodontic appliances to the teeth. Acrylic resins provide many of the properties of an ideal dental material. They can be molded to any shape or form, they are durable, and they can be easily shaded to match gums or teeth.

Drugs. Research has improved the medications used in dental treatments. Antibiotics are now available to prevent or quickly eliminate dental infections that were exceedingly painful and dangerous to manage a few years ago.

Like their patients, dentists have long been interested in lessening the pain associated with dental operations. It was a dentist, H.G. Wells, who first demonstrated the possibility of overcoming pain during a surgical operation by using nitrous oxide (laughing gas) as a general anesthetic. The local anesthetics widely used in dental practice are continually being improved. Modern local anesthetics are relatively painless and work quickly. Tranquilizers and sedatives before and after treatments have done much to remove apprehension, discomfort, and pain from dental visits.

When Toothache Strikes

Unfortunately, many toothaches seem to strike when a dentist is not available, usually at night. Here are emergency steps to be taken until a dentist can be consulted:

Gently rinse the mouth and affected area with warm water. Remove any debris or food from the tooth cavity and mouth. A small wad of cotton can be used to fill the cavity and protect it from the air and fluids in the mouth. If available, a few drops of oil of cloves can be placed on the ball of cotton. Under no circumstances should any medications or drugs such as aspirin be placed in the mouth, on the tooth, or near the affected area. Aspirin can damage tissue and cause a serious "aspirin burn" if left in contact with the gums.

If swelling is present, a cold compress should be placed on the cheek in the area of the swelling for 15 minutes and then removed for 15 minutes. This can be done for several hours to control the swelling. If pain persists, aspirin can be taken.

Even if pain subsides, a dentist should be consulted promptly. Dental problems never heal by themselves.

CHAPTER 19   HOWARD N. JACOBSON, M.D.
J. TIMOTHY HESLA

NUTRITION

We eat three (or more) meals a day, often without paying a great deal of attention to what we consume. But what we eat and how our bodies use it are basic to the maintenance of health. The dinner plate is not only a meal but a prescription.

Man has long understood that good food is essential for strong bodies, but only recently have the complexities of that relationship been understood.

The study of human nutrition, compared to the study of chemistry or physics, is a young science. In fact, the first vitamin was not isolated until 1912. A Polish scientist, Casimir Funk, observed that people who ate unpolished brown rice did not suffer from beriberi, while those who ate polished white rice were subject to the disease. His subsequent research enabled him to isolate a substance in the rice bran which he named "beriberi vitamine."

Since 1912, great strides have been made in our knowledge of food and its effects on human health, although many mysteries remain to be solved. It is still true, for instance, that if the nation's top nutrition scientists created their best synthetic diet which reflected all of our nutrition knowledge, such a diet would not sustain life.

THE COMPOSITION OF FOOD

Natural foods come in an astounding variety of "packages." The orange "package" that is the pumpkin bears little resemblance to the yellow banana, yet both are foods. Nor would anyone likely confuse grain with a grape. Despite this amazing and colorful array of packages, all foods have one characteristic in common: They are composed of chemical compounds. The early task of nutrition scientists was to classify this great variety of foods according to a meaningful system. Thus, foods are classified according to the substances they contain in the greatest amount—carbohydrates, fats, or proteins. Of course, this does not mean that carbohydrate foods such as cereal grains do not contain some protein, or that a high-protein food such as beef does not contain certain amounts of carbohydrates and fats.

The chemical compounds that make up foods are termed nutrients, so called because they provide the nourishment the body needs for normal growth, development, and activity.

The nutrients can be divided into two basic categories: organic matter, which means living things such as plants and animals, and inorganic matter such as zinc, copper, and iron. About 50 nutrients have been identified. All are essential to our physical and mental health, although the precise amount we need of each nutrient has not been determined.

Energy: The Chain of Life

The sun is a source of virtually unlimited energy. In the chain of life all living things depend on it, because without sunlight, plants could not grow, and plants provide the basic food source for all animals, including man.

In a complex chemical process, plants take carbon and oxygen (carbon dioxide) from the air and combine it with nitrogen from the soil and hydrogen from water. These elements are acted upon by the plant enzymes. Then, in the phenomenon called photosynthesis, the radiant energy of the sun acts on chlorophyll cells containing these elements. The resulting chemical reaction is the most significant process in the world.

In that reaction, the inorganic compounds hydrogen, nitrogen, and carbon dioxide are converted to organic compounds in the form of sugar and related substances. This is the first and most vital link in our food chain. Photosynthesis creates the primary food of the biological world, glucose (sugar). All other energy-containing molecules, such as starches, fats, and proteins, are derived from glucose either directly or indirectly. Glucose is also a basic building block of cellulose, a main component of the walls of plant cells and the wood of trees.

Man needs only three things to survive: food, water, and oxygen. In photosynthesis, two of the three are produced, because not only does photosynthesis manufacture food, but it also gives off oxygen as a by-product. Without this simple yet mysterious process, man could not survive.

CLASSIFYING FOODS

Foods are classified as carbohydrates, fats, or proteins based on which of the three they contain in greatest amount. These charts show the range of nutrients in four common foods. The bars show what percentage the food contributes to the U.S. Recommended Daily Allowance of each nutrient. A healthy adult needs 100 percent of each nutrient.

MILK
8 FLUID OUNCES (244 GRAMS)
FORTIFIED WITH VITAMIN D
150 CALORIES

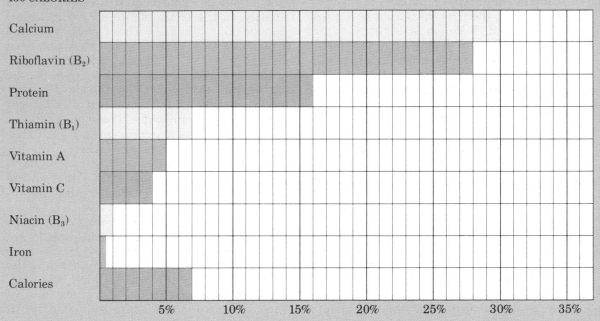

CHEESE PIZZA
ONE-FOURTH OF A MEDIUM PIZZA
WITH ENRICHED CRUST
350 CALORIES

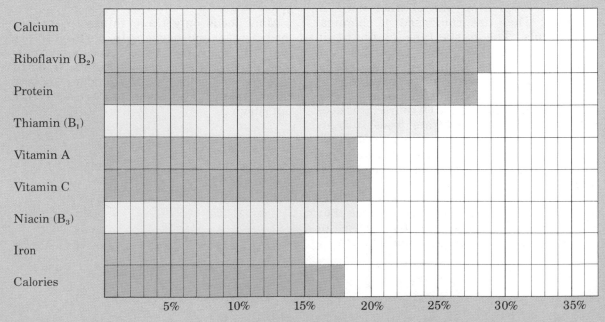

BANANA
MEDIUM SIZE
101 CALORIES

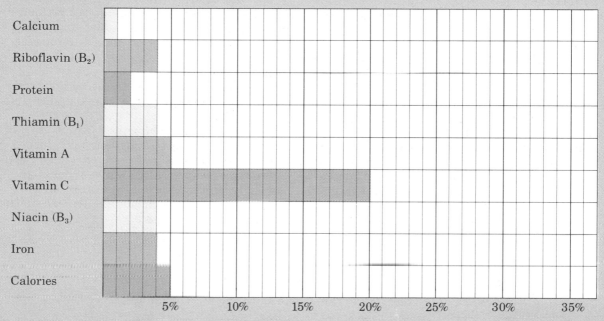

BEEF LIVER
3 OUNCES (85 GRAMS) FRIED
198 CALORIES

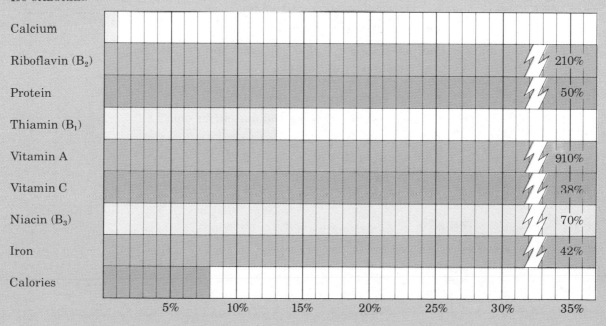

Energy: How It's Measured

In nutrition, the energy needed for all life processes, such as digestion, the heartbeat, and maintaining body temperature, is measured in calories. The "calories" that weight watchers pay so much attention to is the amount of heat required to raise the temperature of one kilogram of water from 15 to 16 degrees centigrade. (Nutrition scientists, to be more precise, might refer to the food calorie as a kilo calorie or "large" calorie, becaue it contains more energy than the "small calorie" chemists and physicists often use.) Applying this measurement to food, we find that one gram of fat contains nine calories, more than twice the number contained in carbohydrates or proteins, which contain four calories per gram.

Not all human beings have the same calorie requirements for normal growth, development, and health maintenance. The number of calories (or the amount of energy) needed varies with age, height, weight, and recreational or work activities. While total calorie needs differ from individual to individual, every diet must contain a variety of foods.

CARBOHYDRATES: THE FIRST LINK IN THE FOOD CHAIN

Carbohydrate food substances are derived mainly from plants, and therefore are among the most common food sources. They are composed largely of sugars and starches. Carbohydrates in the form of the simple sugar called glucose can be found in such foods as corn syrup, vegetables, grape sugar, and honey. Fructose, another simple sugar, can be found in fruits as well as in vegetables and honey. Simple sugars are called monosaccharides. There are three double sugars, known as disaccharides:

Sucrose, a combination of glucose and fructose, is found in sugar cane, beets, and fruits and vegetables.

Lactose combines galactose, which is the product of lactose after digestion, and glucose. It is found in milk.

Maltose is a combination of two types of glucose. It is found in sprouting grains, and is a chief ingredient in such commonly used malt beverages as beer and ale.

CARBOHYDRATES

Simple Sugars (monosaccharides)	Glucose: corn syrup, grape sugar, honey, vegetables
	Fructose: vegetables, honey, fruits
	Galactose: produced from lactose in digestive process
Double Sugars (disaccharides)	Sucrose (glucose + fructose): maple, cane, beet, and sorghum sugars; fruits and vegetables
	Lactose (galactose + glucose): milk
	Maltose (glucose + glucose): grain sprouts and grain products such as beer
Chains of Simple Sugars (polysaccharides)	Starch: legumes, grains, vegetables
	Glycogen: stored in liver and muscle for energy
	Cellulose: found in plants (a fibrous, undigestible structural material)
	Pectins: ripe fruits (seen commonly as the gel in fruit jellies)

Carbohydrates, our chief form of energy, come in simple, double, and chain forms. Starch is a chain of simple sugars. Carbohydrates are derived primarily from plants, and are a common food source.

Polysaccharides are chains of simple sugars. Pectin, for example, is the gel formed from ripe fruit in combination with water. Starch, a simple-sugar chain contained in such foods as grains, vegetables and legumes (peas, peanuts, beans, and alfalfa), is an excellent source of carbohydrates.

Carbohydrates are our chief form of energy. Compared to foods high in protein, carbohydrate foods such as fruits, vegetables, and cereal grains are readily available and affordable. Recent research also indicates that complex starchy carbohydrates, often containing fiber or bran, require more time to digest, which allows for greater absorption of the nutrients.

Energy from carbohydrates. The process of extracting energy from carbohydrates begins as soon as food is placed in the mouth. Here, starches and other polysaccharides are chewed and mixed with saliva, which contains a powerful enzyme that breaks them down. The breakdown continues in the stomach and small intestine. All carbohydrate foods are broken down into the sugar glucose, and the glucose molecules are absorbed into the bloodstream through the intestinal wall. The glucose is then transported to the liver where some of it is converted to glycogen. This complex carbohydrate is the body's form of readily available stored energy. When the body is saturated with glycogen, the remaining glucose is converted into fat and stored for future energy needs.

FATS: FRIEND OR FOE?

Fat is necessary in the diet. Problems arise, however, when too great a proportion of the diet consists of fats. According to the U.S. Senate Subcommittee on Nutrition in the publication, "Revised Dietary Goals," about 40 percent of the average American diet is fat. The committee recommended that this amount be reduced. By reducing the amount of dietary fats, the incidence of cardiovascular diseases such as stroke and heart attack could be lowered, the subcommittee said. Of course, other factors may contribute to heart disease, such as cigarette smoking, lack of exercise, and heredity. Yet intake of fats is considered one of the significant risk factors.

Why are fats necessary? Fats have some properties that other foods do not. First, no other food substance can provide an essential nutrient called polyunsaturated linoleic acid. The body can synthesize other fatty acids from foods, but only in the presence of linoleic acid. Linoleic acid itself must be consumed in the form of fat.

Next, fats are the most concentrated form of food energy. As previously noted, fats contain more than twice as many calories as carbohydrates or protein.

Fats from food also carry the important fat-soluble vitamins A, D, E, and K.

Fats appear in many foods. Chief sources include butter, margarine, cream, salad dressings, cooking oils, lard, bacon and other meats, fish, and poultry. Fats also are present in natural foods such as nuts, avocados, and chocolate, and they are found in dairy products of all kinds. Salad oils and cooking oils are 100 percent fat while butter and margarine are about 80 percent fat.

Cholesterol is a naturally occurring material that the body itself produces. It is also found in various foods of animal origin. Cholesterol is necessary for the proper function of the brain and nervous system, and is found in almost all cell tissues. Cholesterol also plays a role in the digestion of fats and is needed in the synthesis of certain hormones.

The body produces about two grams of cholesterol each day. This amount should serve the body's daily needs. Therefore, eating foods high in cholesterol can raise the level of cholesterol in the blood.

Americans appear to have higher levels of cholesterol than certain other populations. Why this is so is not known. Some researchers assert that high cholesterol figures prominently in heart disease, while others think that its role has been overstated (see chapter 3, "The Heart and Circulation," and chapter 16, "The Hormones and Endocrine Glands"). Until the relationship is proven or disproven, it would be well to follow recommendations of the U.S. Senate Subcommittee on Nutrition and reduce consumption of fats below 40 percent of the diet.

A SAMPLE LISTING OF PROTEIN SOURCES

	Energy				Nutrients				
	Calories	Percentage of Calories from Protein	Percentage of Calories from Carbohydrates	Percentage of Calories from Fats	Protein gm	Thiamin (B₁) mg	Riboflavin (B₂) mg	Niacin (B₃) mg	Iron mg
Frankfurter 2 oz (57 gm)	172	17	2	81	7.0	0.09	0.11	1.4	0.9
Ham, baked 3 oz (85 gm)	179	61	0	39	25.7	0.56	0.26	4.9	3.2
Meat loaf 3 oz (85 gm)	230	28	23	48	15.3	0.27	0.24	3.4	2.4
Tuna 3 oz (85 gm)	168	62	0	38	24.5	0.04	0.10	10.1	1.6
Egg, fried, large (50 gm)	108	28	0.7	71	6.9	0.05	0.15	0.1	1.2
Egg, hard-cooked, large (50 gm)	82	35	2	64	6.5	0.05	0.14	0.1	1.2
Peanut butter 2 tbsp (32 gm)	186	17	12	71	8.9	0.04	0.04	5.0	0.5
Peanuts, salted ¼ cup (36 gm)	211	15	13	71	9.4	0.12	0.05	6.2	0.8
Peas, blackeye ½ cup (124 gm)	94	23	74	4	6.3	0.20	0.05	0.5	1.6
Corn 5″ ear (125 gm)	114	9	82	10	4.1	0.15	0.13	1.8	0.8

PROTEIN: LINKING THE FOOD CHAIN

As we have seen, we depend on food for energy, and the best sources of energy are fats and carbohydrates. Much of this energy is used in activities such as work and recreation. However, a good deal of it is expended without conscious effort. Our hearts pump blood with powerful muscular contractions 60 or 70 times a minute without our asking. Damaged cells and tissues are continuously being repaired and replaced. In our early years, teeth, bones, and muscle are being formed. All of this takes energy, yet it happens without our conscious control.

In a sense, all of this growth, development, and maintenance of our bodies is done through the "guidance" of protein. If fats and carbohydrates provide the energy, protein might be said to provide the organization of that energy.

Proteins are large molecules constructed of hundreds, even thousands, of smaller molecules. These smaller molecules are called amino acids. Nutrition scientists have identified 22 amino acids. Nine of them are categorized as "essential" amino acids because they must be furnished by the diet. The body can manufacture the others, but it cannot produce the nine basic amino acids. From these 22 substances, the body synthesizes the hundreds of proteins that it requires for its highly specialized functions. Protein within the cell of a fingernail, for instance, can be used only for the growth and repair of that material, and a surplus of it cannot be transferred to help the growth of a tooth.

Although protein is vital for growth, maintenance, and repair of bodily tissue, it has other equally important functions. Proteins are present in the structure of enzymes, and thus help break down other foods for digestion. Many hormones that regulate our metabolic processes are proteins. And nucleoproteins are carriers of our genetic potential, or inherited characteristics, in the living cell. Our muscles are made up of proteins that need continual repair and replenishment.

Protein for Energy: A Myth?

It was once widely believed that protein was an abundant source of energy. Many athletes trained under the assumption that a diet high in protein would enhance physical performance. Now we know that protein can indeed be a source of energy, but only under the following circumstances: (1) If the diet contains an excessive amount of protein and the amino acid "pool" is full, the remaining amino acids will be chemically reconstituted and stored as fat for energy reserves; (2) If the diet is insufficient in carbohydrates and fat, protein will be broken down into compounds that can be used for energy. Of course if protein must be used for the basic requirement of energy, it cannot be used for its primary functions. Clearly then, protein *can* be used for energy, but only when the fundamental sources (carbohydrates and fats) are in short supply or when there is an excess of protein in the system.

Protein Sources

Protein is found in ample supply in a variety of foods, both plant and animal. Meats and fish are excellent sources, as are eggs, milk, and cheese. Vegetable sources include beans, such as navy beans, soybeans, and kidney beans; a variety of lentils and peas; grain cereals, including rye, oats, wheat, millet, and corn; and nuts such as peanuts and cashews.

For those who eat the typical American diet, which includes foods from animal sources, daily replenishment of the amino acid store is not difficult. In fact, most adult Americans consume more than 40 to 60 grams of protein per day, the level recommended by the Food and Nutrition Board of the National Research Council. For those who prefer a meatless diet, however, it is more difficult to select foods that give the proper balance of amino acids. Here's why:

Because of the similarity in the biochemical makeup between man and other animals, a portion of beef, for instance, supplies all nine of the essential amino acids in the proper amounts. (One essential amino acid is histidine, which is necessary for children to reach their full growth potential. Research is inconclusive, but it may be an essential amino acid in the adult years as well.)

Vegetables, however, do not offer complete protein in which all nine essential amino acids are present, with a few notable exceptions such as soybeans. Therefore, combinations of vegetables must be eaten to achieve the proper balance of essential amino acids.

THE ESSENTIAL AMINO ACIDS

Requirements in milligrams per gram of protein

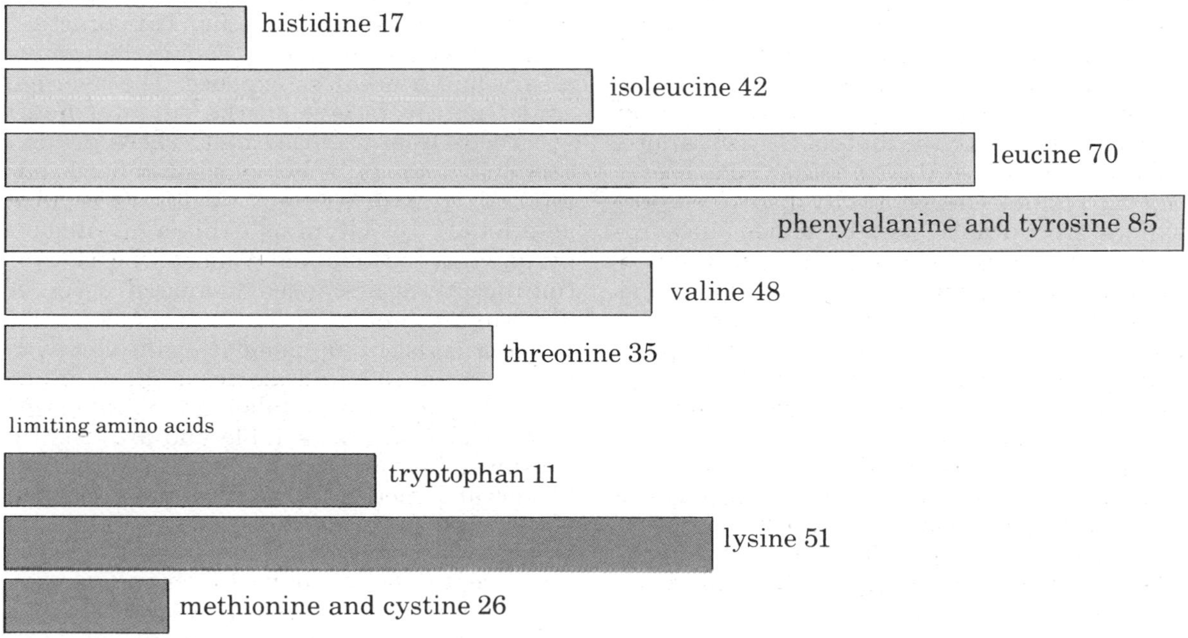

histidine 17

isoleucine 42

leucine 70

phenylalanine and tyrosine 85

valine 48

threonine 35

limiting amino acids

tryptophan 11

lysine 51

methionine and cystine 26

Nine of the amino acids are essential because the body cannot synthesize them. They must be provided by food. Three of the nine are called "limiting" amino acids because they must be consumed in proper quantities and proportions or they restrict the value of the other six. All essential amino acids are present in animal protein such as beef, but in a meatless diet combinations of vegetables must be eaten to get all nine.

Three of the amino acids have been called "limiting amino acids." If a person consumes 100 percent of the daily requirement of six amino acids, yet consumes only 30 percent of the daily requirement of any of the limiting amino acids, the value of the consumed amino acids is limited to 30 percent.

Thus, in a meatless diet, one vegetable must provide the amino acids that the other is missing. But what could be a complicated protein theory is quickly uncomplicated by milk. A glass of milk with each meal will supply any amino acid missing from the vegetables.

VITAMINS: AGENTS

OF CHANGE

Traditionally, vitamins have been defined as organic substances required by the body in small amounts for the processes of life. Generally, these substances must be derived from the foods we eat because the body cannot produce its own vitamins. (Vitamin D may be regarded as an exception because this "sunshine vitamin" is produced in the skin in combination with the ultraviolet rays of the sun.)

Thirteen vitamins have been identified, and the body requires each of them in certain amounts to sustain life. Until the late 18th century, for example, most long sea voyages were plagued by disease and death. Many ships lost up to 50 percent of the crew members to an illness called scurvy caused by a lack of vitamin C. Then, in 1753, a Scottish physician experimented with the diets of British sailors, substituting one food for another and observing the results. He eventually discovered that sailors who drank lime or lemon juice remained free from the ravages of scurvy. When Captain James Cook made his voyage around the world in 1772–1775, he took on fresh supplies of fruits and vegetables at every port, and not one seaman died of scurvy. The practice quickly spread, and as a result, British seamen are nicknamed "limeys" to this day.

Vitamins act as catalysts, or agents of change, causing chemical reactions among the other nutrients to assure the smooth operation of the bodily functions. (The chart on the opposite page lists the vitamins, their functions, and the deficiency symptoms.)

Yet, despite all that has been learned about vitamins, there remains a good deal of uncertainty among consumers and nutrition scientists alike. Most prominent, of course, is the continuing debate over the role of large doses of vitamin C in preventing the common cold.

The U.S. Recommended Daily Allowances for vitamins, set by the Food and Drug Administration, are determined by the amount needed each day to maintain health in healthy people. A safety margin is built in to allow for individual differences in diet and metabolism (see page 438).

This conservative procedure is safer than trying to determine the maximum amount that can be taken before one's health is jeopardized.

Most nutrition scientists agree that the role of vitamins is preventive. That is, if vitamins are consumed in the amounts recommended, one will not be susceptible to any of the deficiency diseases. It has yet to be demonstrated that any vitamin *cures* any disease (other than the deficiency diseases). Vitamins, then, are not medicine. They are part of the body's sophisticated preventive maintenance system.

Vitamin Supplements: Not Without Risk

Millions of Americans supplement their diets with multivitamin pills. This practice, although generally harmless, may be unnecessary and a needless expense. The average American can receive all the vitamins he or she needs from a varied diet. There are exceptions, however. A heavy smoker needs additional vitamin C. Heavy drinkers require additional B vitamins—thiamin, niacin, pyridoxine, and folic acid. Women who use oral contraceptives also need increased doses of vitamin B-complex.

The true risk of supplementing the diet with large amounts of vitamins lies in the different ways vitamins are metabolized. Vitamins A, D, K, and E are fat soluble and are usually consumed in foods containing fat such as liver, butter, and cheese. The fat soluble vitamins, if not used up in life process functions, are stored in the body, mainly in the liver. For instance, two ounces of beef liver will provide all the vitamin A one needs for a week.

The remaining nine vitamins are water soluble. Once the body absorbs the necessary amount of vitamin C, for example, the body will excrete the excess. There is little danger of "overdosing" on the water soluble vitamins.

VITAMINS

	Vitamin	Why it's needed	Symptoms of deficiency	Sources
FAT SOLUBLE	**A**	Needed for growth of bones and teeth; for healthy skin and mucous membranes; for normal vision (it is part of visual pigments of the retina).	Night blindness; rough skin and mucous membranes; no bone growth; cracked, decayed teeth; drying of eyes.	Liver, eggs, cheese, butter, fortified margarine, milk; yellow, orange, and dark green vegetables (carrots, broccoli, squash, spinach).
	D	Essential for normal bone growth and maintenance of strong bones.	Rickets (in children), retarded growth, bowed legs, malformed teeth, protruding abdomen. Osteomalacia (in adults).	Milk, egg yolk, liver, tuna, salmon. Made on skin in sunlight.
	E	Necessary for normal red blood cells, muscles, and tissues; prevents oxidation of vitamin A and fats.	Breakdown of red blood cells. Symptoms in animals but not in man.	Vegetable oils, margarine, whole grain cereal and bread, wheat germ, liver, dried beans, green leafy vegetables.
	K	Essential for normal blood clotting.	Hemorrhage (especially in newborns).	Green leafy vegetables and milk, vegetables in cabbage family.
WATER SOLUBLE	**Thiamin (B$_1$)**	Needed to release energy from carbohydrates and for synthesis of nerve-regulating substance.	Beriberi; mental confusion, muscular weakness; swelling of heart; leg cramps.	Pork (especially ham), liver, oysters, whole grain and enriched cereals, pasta, and bread.
	Riboflavin (B$_2$)	Needed for release of energy to cells from carbohydrates, proteins, and fats; maintenance of mucous membranes.	Skin disorders, especially around nose and lips; cracks at mouth corners, eyes very sensitive to light.	Liver, milk, meat, dark green vegetables, whole grain and enriched cereals, pasta, and bread, mushrooms.
	Niacin (B$_3$)	Works with thiamin and riboflavin in energy-producing reactions in cells.	Pellagra skin disorders, especially parts exposed to sun, smooth tongue; diarrhea; mental confusion; irritability.	Liver, poultry, meat, tuna, whole grain and enriched cereals, pasta, and bread, nuts, dried beans and peas. Made in body from amino acid tryptophan.
	Pyridoxine (B$_6$)	Participates in absorption and metabolism of proteins; use of fats; formation of red blood cells.	Skin disorders; cracks at mouth corners; smooth tongue; convulsions; dizziness; nausea; anemia; kidney stones.	Whole grain (but not enriched) cereals and bread, liver, avocados, spinach, green beans, bananas.
	Cobalamin (B$_{12}$)	Necessary for building of genetic material, formation of red blood cells, functioning of nervous system.	Pernicious anemia, anemia; degeneration of peripheral nerves.	Liver, kidneys, meat, fish, eggs, milk, oysters.
	Folic acid (Folacin)	Helps form body proteins and genetic material; formation of hemoglobin.	Anemia with large red blood cells; smooth tongue; diarrhea.	Liver, kidneys, dark green leafy vegetables, wheat germ, brewers yeast.
	Pantothenic acid	Needed for metabolism of carbohydrates, proteins, and fats; formation of hormones and nerve-regulating substances.	Not known except experimentally in man; vomiting; abdominal pain; fatigue; sleep problems.	Liver, kidneys, whole grain bread and cereal, nuts, eggs, dark green vegetables, yeast.
	Biotin	Formation of fatty acids, release of energy from carbohydrates.	Not known except experimentally in man; fatigue, depression, nausea, pains, loss of appetite.	Egg yolk, liver, kidneys, dark green vegetables, green beans. Made in intestinal tract.
	C (Ascorbic acid)	Helps the maintenance of bones, teeth, blood vessels, formation of collagen, which supports structure; anti-oxidant.	Scurvy, gums bleed, muscles degenerate, wounds don't heal; skin rough, brown and dry; teeth loosen.	Many fruits and vegetables, including citrus, tomato, strawberries, melon, green pepper, potato.

United States Recommended Daily Allowances For Vitamins

Vitamin	Infants	Children 1 to 4 years	Children over 4 and adults	Pregnant or lactating women
A IU	1500	2500	5000	8000
D IU	400	400	400	400
E IU	5	10	30	30
C mg	35	40	60	60
Folic acid mcg.	100	200	400	800
Thiamin (B_1) mg.	0.5	0.7	1.5	1.7
Riboflavin (B_2) mg.	0.6	0.8	1.7	2
Niacin (B_3) mg.	8	9	20	20
Pyridoxine (B_6) mg.	0.4	0.7	2	2.5
Cobalamin (B_{12}) mcg.	2	3	6	8
Biotin mcg.	50	150	300	300
Pantothenic acid mg.	3	5	10	10

IU = International unit   mg. = milligrams   mcg. = micrograms

Recommended Daily Allowances for vitamins are established by the U.S. Food and Drug Administration. With exceptions for differences in metabolism and special circumstances, vitamin supplements generally are not necessary, and massive intake of some vitamins can have serious consequences. No allowances have been determined for vitamin K.

It also would be difficult to consume overdoses of the fat soluble vitamins as they naturally occur in food. Yet, there are those who feel that if a small amount of a vitamin is good for you, large amounts are even better. This kind of thinking can lead to serious consequences in the case of vitamins A and D. Infants need only 400 International Units (IU) of these vitamins daily. If this amount is increased to 40,000 IU (or 75,000 to 100,000 for adults), serious, even life-threatening symptoms can develop. These include sudden loss of appetite, nausea, vomiting, and intense thirst. Fatalities have been recorded in which arteries, heart, and lungs have become calcified, rendering the tissue inflexible and bonelike.

The average American who eats good quality food in variety and abundance has no need for supplementary vitamins. Vitamins do indeed work wonders by acting on the other nutrients and guaranteeing the smooth operation of the life processes, but they are by no means "wonder drugs" and should not be regarded as such.

MINERALS AND WATER

Thus far we have talked about organic nutrients, which are nutrients derived from living sources such as plants and animals. There is another class of nutrients that are inorganic in composition and vital for a normal, healthy life. These are the minerals. Some of them are identical to the material that is mined from the earth: zinc, copper, magnesium, potassium, and iron, for example.

Like vitamins, minerals are required in minute amounts and are found in a variety of food sources. Unlike vitamins, which do not become a part of the bodily composition but fulfill their function by causing change, minerals do become part of our body structure. Our skeletons and teeth are made largely of calcium. Iron is a chief component of red blood cells. Magnesium and phosphorus are found in our bone structure.

Although a normal, varied diet will meet all of the body's essential requirements for minerals, there are circumstances under which supplementation is recommended.

MINERALS

Mineral	Functions	Symptoms of Deficiency	Food Sources
Calcium	Necessary for hard bones and teeth; muscle contraction, especially normal heart rhythm; transmission of nerve impulses; proper blood clotting; and to activate a number of enzymes.	In children: stunted growth, retarded bone mineralization; poor bones and teeth, skeletal malformation (rickets). In adults: osteoporosis (brittle, porous bones resulting from demineralization).	Milk and hard cheeses, dark green leafy vegetables, small fish eaten with bones, soft cheeses, dried beans and peas, broccoli, artichokes, sesame seeds.
Phosphorus	Necessary (with calcium) to form and strengthen bones, as part of the nucleic acids, and for metabolism of fats and carbohydrates.	Deficiency is seldom seen in humans eating a normal diet. Weakness, bone pain, loss of minerals, especially calcium, from bones, poor growth.	Organ meats, meats, fish, poultry, eggs, milk and cheese, nuts, beans, and peas, whole grains.
Magnesium	Activates enzymes in carbohydrate metabolism and release of energy. Helps regulate body temperature, nerve and muscle contraction, and protein synthesis.	Deficiency is seen only in alcoholism or in people on a diet limited to a few highly processed foods. Weakness, tremors, dizziness, spasms and convulsions, delirium, and depression.	Whole grains, nuts, beans, green leafy vegetables. Processing may result in high losses of magnesium.
Sulfur	Part of proteins, especially in hair, nails, and cartilage; part of the B vitamins thiamin and biotin; takes part in detoxification reactions.	Deficiency not found. A diet adequate in protein (several amino acids contain sulfur) will provide sulfur.	Eggs, meat, milk and cheese, nuts, legumes.
Sodium	Is the major component of fluid outside cells. It regulates water balance, muscle contractions, and nerve irritability.	Deficiency is rare. Nausea, diarrhea, abdominal and muscle cramps. Excess: probably a factor in inducing high blood pressure; certainly a low-sodium diet is essential to reduce blood pressure.	Salt, salted foods, monosodium glutamate, soy sauce, baking powder, cheese, milk, shellfish, meat, fish, poultry, eggs.
Potassium	Major constituent of fluid inside cells. With sodium, needed to regulate water balance, nerve irritability, muscle contraction, and heart rhythm. Necessary for protein synthesis and glucose formation.	Muscle weakness, nausea, depletion of glycogen, rapid heart beat, heart failure. Excess: not known.	Widely distributed in foods. Fruits, like dates, bananas, oranges, cantaloupe, tomatoes, vegetables, especially dark green leafy vegetables, liver, meat, fish, poultry, milk.
Chlorine	Part of the fluid outside the cells. Takes part in the formation of gastric juice, absorption of vitamin B_{12} and iron. In stomach, suppresses growth of microorganisms in foods.	Vomiting, diarrhea.	One-half of table salt (with sodium).

TRACE MINERALS (those needed in minute amounts)

Mineral	Functions	Symptoms of Deficiency	Food Sources
Iron	Transports and transfers oxygen in blood and tissues. Part of hemoglobin in blood, myoglobin in muscles, protoplasm of cells, cell nuclei, and many enzymes in tissues.	Faulty digestion, changes in body levels of enzymes containing iron, cell damage, low iron stores, microcytic anemia (red cells smaller, level of hemoglobin in them is lower).	Liver, eggs, lean meats, dried beans and peas, nuts, dried fruits, whole grains, and green leafy vegetables.
Iodine	Vital constituent of the thyroid hormones thyroxine and triiodothyronine, which regulate basal metabolism and influence growth, mental development, and deposition of protein and fat in the body.	Goiter, and, if the mother has a severe iodine deficiency in the first three months of pregnancy or before conception, cretinism in infants.	Iodized salt is the sure source, plus seafood, vegetables grown near the sea where soil is rich in iodine, and butter, milk, cheese, and eggs if the animal's ration has been rich in iodine.
Manganese	Part of many enzymes. Necessary to synthesize complex carbohydrates, fat, and cholesterol, to use glucose and fats, for muscle contraction and proper development of bones.	Deficiency so far seen only in animals, with symptoms including sterility and abnormal fetuses, bone deformation, and muscle deformities.	Abundant in most foods, both plant and animal. Whole grains, legumes, and nuts are good sources.
Copper	Acts with iron to synthesize hemoglobin in red blood cells; necessary for glucose metabolism, formation of nerve walls and connective tissue.	In some infants fed cow's milk, a deficiency inhibits hemoglobin formation, causing anemia. Deficiencies in adults are unknown. Excess: in Wilson's disease, a rare metabolic-defect, there is abnormal storage in liver and other tissues. Can result in uremia, heart defects, hypertension, death.	In most foods. Organ meats, shellfish, nuts, dried beans and peas, and cocoa are good sources. (Like iron, it is absent from dairy products.)
Zinc	A component of insulin and enzymes important to digestion, protein metabolism, and synthesis of nucleic acids.	Deficiency is rare in the U.S.; retarded growth, even "dwarfism," retarded sexual development, anemia, poor wound healing. Excess: nausea, vomiting, diarrhea, fever.	Wheat germ and bran, whole grains, dried beans and peas, nuts, lean meats, fish, and poultry.
Fluorine	Normal component of teeth; prevents dental decay. May also be necessary with calcium and vitamin D to maintain strong bones and prevent demineralization in later life.	Deficiency results in tooth decay in young children, possibly osteoporosis in adults. Excess causes mottling of tooth enamel, deformed teeth and bones.	Water, either naturally or artificially fluoridated at a concentration of one part per million.
Chromium	Metabolism of glucose and protein, synthesis of fatty acids and cholesterol, insulin metabolism.	Poor use of glucose, perhaps caused by impaired insulin metabolism.	Corn oil, meats, whole grains.

Iron-deficiency anemia is the most common of the deficiency problems. It occurs primarily in women of childbearing age who lose iron during the menstrual cycle, and pregnant women or nursing mothers whose needs for increased iron are not met even with a special diet.

While the dietary needs for minerals, including the trace minerals, are well known, researchers continue to discover that additional substances play an essential role in our diets. One day, arsenic may be added to the list of essential trace elements. It may be said with authority, however, that the rule that applies to vitamins also applies to minerals: Consume good quality foods in appropriate amounts with plenty of variety, and your dietary needs will be met.

Water. The human body is 50 to 70 percent water. This calorie-free fluid makes possible all of life's processes. It transports blood, passes nutrients through membranes, and is the vehicle by which bodily wastes are excreted.

Individuals have been known to survive for weeks with no appreciable intake of food. However, losing one-fifth of the body's water without replacing it can be fatal.

Our bodies require about 1½ quarts of water per day. Most of it comes from foods with a high water content such as soup, milk, or other beverages.

DIETARY GOALS FOR
AMERICANS

Increasing concern about the role of nutrition in chronic diseases such as diabetes, stroke, and cancer has led to attempts to formulate national dietary goals aimed at disease prevention. Greatest attention has been given to overconsumption of such substances as fat, refined sugar, cholesterol, and salt. It has been suggested that Americans increase their consumption of fruits, vegetables, whole grains, poultry, fish, skim milk, and vegetable oils, while cutting back on foods high in fat, salt, and sugar.

This approach is now being studied in attempts to manage and prevent diseases such as diabetes and heart attack. Research may indicate more precisely the best food choices for alleviating these conditions.

For the normal, healthy person, some understanding of the nutritive value of foods is essential to plan proper meals and develop good dietary habits. But it is not necessary to remember in minute detail the amount of nutrients in individual foods or groups. It is sufficient to know that foods of certain groups are similar in their content of major nutrients, and to recognize the group to which a food belongs.

One might classify foods into many groups. But as a practical matter of diet planning and education, a convenient guide to the composition of an adequate diet is that prepared by the U.S. Department of Agriculture, in which common foods are divided into five basic groups. Foods in a group have similar nutritive values. Selection of foods as indicated in the table on page 442 provides adequate amounts of important nutrients automatically.

NUTRITION'S ROLE
IN THE LIFE CYCLE

The essential role of nutrition in growth and in the maintenance of health, and the effects of inadequate diet at all ages have been amply demonstrated.

Since life is a continuum from generation to generation, a convenient starting place for a discussion of nutrition in the life cycle is with pregnancy, because here the nutritional needs are shown with greatest clarity.

Maternal Nutrition

The pregnant woman and her developing fetus or the lactating mother require a nutritionally sound diet plus additional amounts of certain nutrient-rich foods.

History records a long list of theories regarding the dietary needs of pregnant women. These recommendations and restrictions become popular for varying periods of time and then are superseded by new ones. Lately, as our knowledge about nutrition, reproduction, and the human cycle of growth has increased, recommendations for healthy pregnancies have been refined.

THE BASIC 5 FOOD GROUPS FOR ENSURING ADEQUATE DIETS

Milk Group
(two or more cups daily)

Children	3 to 4 cups	Pregnant women	4 or more cups
Teenagers	4 or more cups	Nursing mothers	6 or more cups
Adults	2 or more cups		

Milk alternates that have equivalent calcium content:
Cheddar-type cheese: 1-inch cube = ½ cup milk
Cream cheese: 2 tablespoons = 1 tablespoon milk
Cottage cheese: ½ cup = ⅓ cup milk
Ice cream: ½ cup = ⅓ cup milk
Ice milk: ½ cup = ⅓ cup milk

Meat Group
(two or more servings daily)

Beef, veal, pork, lamb, poultry, fish, shellfish, and organ meats (liver, kidney, heart)

Meat substitutes:
Dry beans, dry peas, lentils, eggs, and peanut butter

A serving consists of:
2 to 3 ounces (no bone) of cooked meat, poultry, or fish; 2 eggs;
1 cup cooked beans, dry peas, or lentils; 4 tablespoons peanut butter

Vegetable-Fruit Group
(four or more servings daily)

A good source of vitamin A should be eaten at least every other day. Sources include broccoli, carrots, sweet potatoes, winter squash, pumpkin, and dark green leaves. Good fruit sources of vitamin A include apricots and cantaloupe.

A good source of vitamin C should be eaten daily. Sources include citrus fruits and juices, melons, fresh berries, broccoli, brussels sprouts, leafy greens, potatoes cooked in jackets, cabbage, cauliflower, spinach, peppers, tomatoes, and tomato juice.

A serving consists of:
½ cup of fruits or vegetables; ½ grapefruit or cantaloupe; 1 medium apple, banana, orange, or potato

Bread-Cereal Group
(four or more servings daily)

All whole grain, enriched, or restored breads and cereals. Ready-to-eat or cooked cereals Cornmeal, crackers, flour, macaroni, spaghetti, noodles, rice, rolled oats, baked goods made with whole grain or enriched flour

A serving consists of:
1 slice of bread; 1 ounce of ready-to-eat cereal; ½ to ¾ cup of cooked cereal, macaroni, noodles, rice, or spaghetti

Fats, Sweets, and Alcohol

Foods that provide low levels of nutrition compared with the number of calories are classified in a fifth group, the fats, sweets, and alcohol group. They include butter, margarine, mayonnaise, salad dressings, candy, sugar, jams and jellies, soft drinks, alcoholic beverages, and unenriched breads and pastries. A minimum number of servings is not suggested because these foods are "extras," providing mainly calories.

Studies of large numbers of women in various parts of the world have shown that a woman's weight before pregnancy and her gain during pregnancy are the predominant influence on the weight of the baby at birth. We now know that birth weight is the best indicator of the degree to which the newborn has achieved its growth potential. Other studies demonstrate that providing supplementary food to low-income mothers increases the birth weight of the infant, reduces the incidence of low birth weight, and assures that the baby can achieve its natural potential. In brief, all these studies call attention to the special groups of women who are at greatest risk of nutritional deficiency and who can benefit the most from nutritional guidance and support.

The high-risk pregnancy. Women at the highest risk of nutritional problems during pregnancy are: (1) adolescents; (2) women who have had three or more pregnancies during the past two years; (3) women with a history of poor outcome of previous pregnancies; (4) women with an inadequate food budget; (5) food faddists following bizarre or nutritionally restricted diets; (6) heavy smokers, drug addicts, or alcoholics; (7) women who require a therapeutic diet for chronic disease; (8) women who are seriously underweight or overweight. Women likely to face nutritional risk during prenatal care include those who have a low hemoglobin level. "Low" is defined as a hemoglobin count of 11 grams and "deficient" is below 10 grams. (Average is 12–14 grams.)

Any pregnant woman with an inadequate weight gain (less than two pounds per month), or a weight loss, or a woman who gains excessively (more than two pounds a week), or a woman who plans to breast-feed her baby—all face exceptional nutritional risk during pregnancy. They need to be certain that they have a nutritionally sound diet that includes the proper amounts of the nutrients known to be required during pregnancy.

Diet in pregnancy. Studies repeatedly have demonstrated that a healthy average weight gain during the course of pregnancy is 24 to 30 pounds. Furthermore, the pattern of weight gain should be relatively smooth—minimal in early pregnancy, then a steady increase of about one pound per week during the last two-thirds of the pregnancy. Because different women have different requirements, the exact number of calories needed will vary. However, every mother-to-be requires more calories than she did before pregnancy. She needs additional energy because her body is working constantly depositing both fetal and maternal tissues and sustaining their growth. Additional energy is also required for physical activity because the body weighs more.

Pregnant women synthesize complex new tissues at a rate greater than at any other time in their lives. To meet these needs it is recommended that they consume an additional 30 grams of protein a day, the amount of protein in a quart of milk. Surveys conducted with upper income pregnant women who tend to be healthy and have healthy babies show that their self-selected diets contain around 90 grams of protein per day. Women on therapeutic or rehabilitative diets may require even more protein. In some instances more than 100 grams per day have proven useful. The expectant mother also requires increased iron—iron tablets are recommended because it is extremely difficult to consume enough iron in the normal diet—and perhaps folic acid. Sodium is important for the healthy pregnant woman, so she should continue to use salt in ordinary amounts, not restrict it. Routine use of water pills to rid the body of salt is not recommended.

Teenage pregnancy. Pregnant teenagers, particularly those younger than 16, have, as a group, the most critical nutritional problems during pregnancy. The young mother-to-be must deal with the problems of transition from adolescence to adulthood, her forthcoming maternal role, and the physical and emotional changes that accompany adolescence and pregnancy.

The adolescent period, especially in girls, is a time of profound growth and developmental changes. Nutritional requirements approach the highest level of any age after infancy. When a growing girl becomes pregnant, added nutritional requirements are imposed. A further complication may be imposed by the girl's nutritionally poor but typically teenage eating pattern. Unfortunately, these vulnerable girls often make little or no change in their diets during pregnancy if left to their own resources. They particularly need the services offered by special programs for pregnant adolescents.

The girl and her family should participate in programs at school, churches, and community agencies designed to meet her social, educational, and vocational needs, as well as her health and nutrition requirements.

A sample meal pattern that meets the needs of a healthy pregnant woman is shown in the accompanying table. The quantities or serving sizes consumed should be adjusted to fit individual requirements.

SAMPLE MEAL PATTERN

Breakfast:	1 serving of fruits and vegetables rich in vitamin C
	1 serving of grain products
	1 serving of milk and milk products
Morning snack:	Optional
Lunch:	2 servings of grain products
	1 serving of protein foods
	1 serving of other fruits and vegetables
	1 serving of milk and milk products
Afternoon snack:	1 serving of protein foods
	½ serving of milk and milk products
Dinner:	2 servings of protein foods
	2 servings of leafy green vegetables
	1 serving of milk and milk products
Evening snack:	½ serving of milk and milk products

This is a sample meal pattern for the pregnant woman or the woman who is breast-feeding. For a guide to the serving sizes, refer to the basic food groups chart on page 442. Because pregnant women are synthesizing new tissue at a faster rate than any other time in their lives, each day they require about 30 grams more protein than the healthy nonpregnant woman. That is roughly the amount of protein in a quart of milk. A nonpregnant woman using this meal pattern could leave out one serving of protein food and one serving of milk or milk products.

Diet and oral contraceptives. There is laboratory evidence of biochemical changes associated with oral contraceptives. Their use appears to alter the blood levels of folic acid, vitamins B_2, B_6, B_{12}, and C, and certain trace elements. The meaning of these changes remains unclear. Women who take oral contraceptives should be assessed regularly for any signs of nutritional deficiency. Vitamin supplementation may be needed.

Infant Nutrition

As with diet and pregnancy, historically there have been many theories about infant feeding. But throughout history, the continuation of the human species always depended on the mother's ability to provide nourishment for the newborn infant until the child could feed itself.

In most developed societies, women have changed from a predominantly breast-feeding approach to a predominantly bottle-feeding society. In the last several years the trend has been slightly reversed. Most manufacturers of infant food have taken the view that mother's milk and commercially prepared formulas based on cow's milk are very much the same biochemically and nutritionally. But it should be noted that the two have differences, however slight. Further, commercial formulas contain a variety of added substances such as emulsifiers, thickeners, pH adjusters, and added oxidants, although these have never been shown to produce either ill or beneficial effects.

Advocates of breast feeding point out that human milk has been shown to be rich in host resistant factors, which help the baby ward off illness. Breast feeding, it is noted, and an avoidance of premature introduction to semisolid foods, may help to avoid food allergy in infancy. Another reason given for breast feeding relates to mother-infant bonding—the formation of a lifetime attachment between the mother and her infant. Bonding begins in the very sensitive first 24 hours of life, and is said to occur especially with breast feeding.

Still, for some infants, breast feeding is unsuitable. Those with certain genetic disorders may be unable to tolerate human milk and may need special diets. Mothers may be required to take certain drugs harmful to the infant if concentrated in the milk. Severely malnourished women are well advised to formula-feed the infant while replenishing their own nutrition. In any case, when breast feeding is unsuccessful for whatever reason, infant formulas provide a suitable alternative during the first year.

Introducing solid foods. The custom of introducing foods other than milk or formula before four to six months has evoked much criticism. It is now recognized that when a baby is given solids, it is usually determined by social practice, not nutritional needs. Properly, the introduction should occur when either formula or mother's milk no longer meets the infant's needs for growth and development. That is usually about midway through the first year.

Commercially prepared baby food. Commercial manufacturers now offer more than 400 varieties of prepared baby food. As a group, the producers have been criticized for including large amounts of modified starch and sucrose. Although these amounts have been reduced in many cases, it is feared that a diet of sweetened foods in infancy will imprint a taste for sugar that continues into adulthood. Some parents prepare baby foods at home in the belief that they are more nutritious and more economical.

Growth of the infant. A baby nearly triples the birth weight during the first year of life. Babies usually adjust their food intake by refusing food when they feel satisfied. The best guide to whether an infant is eating properly can be seen in the growth charts. If the child is gaining at a steady rate along the expected path, there is no cause for concern.

The growth of infants requires relatively high intakes of calories, protein, vitamins, and minerals. All of these needs are met by breast milk except vitamin D, which can be given simply and routinely. Vitamin D supplements may or may not be necessary in bottle-fed infants, depending on whether the milk or formula has been fortified with the vitamin.

Later, iron-rich foods such as infant cereals, meats, egg yolks, and greens can be introduced. Diets deficient in these elements, such as a milk-only diet can lead to scurvy, rickets, or iron-deficiency anemia. Iron-deficiency anemias are fairly common and result from the failure to add appropriate foods to an infant's diet of milk. Iron supplementation in various forms rapidly solves this problem.

Water. The water needs of an infant are relatively high, and in warm weather the requirement is increased. Infants are particularly vulnerable to losses of water and salts through diarrhea and vomiting.

Nutrition in Childhood

The major nutritional problems of childhood include the development and maintenance of sound food habits for later life. It has been shown that failure to eat breakfast can lead to poor classroom performance. Many schools now have breakfast programs in addition to the traditional school lunch. For older children and youths, nutrition education programs emphasize the importance of nutrition in life. The need for nutrition education for children and their families has been recognized as one of the important factors in establishing good life-long eating habits. A key lesson is that dietary needs do not have to be met each day because the body stores many important nutrients. This allows flexibility in planning menus.

Diet in the Middle Years

The 1969 White House Conference on Food, Nutrition, and Health pointed out that American society, particularly the affluent groups, is characterized by a series of excesses, especially for those in the middle years. Not much has changed since that report. Many middle-aged persons take in too many calories, with food choices that are not always the wisest. We eat too much fat and refined sugar, and our alcohol intake is too high. The conference report commented on our lack of exercise and our failure to develop habits to combat the ills of sedentary life. To these two problems could be added the growing recognition of the role of stress. All of these together are implicated in the common health problems of the middle years—obesity, diabetes, vascular disease, high blood pressure, and heart disease.

The goal of nutrition in the middle years should be to develop dietary and living patterns that are conducive to a more active life associated with a sustained healthy work capacity, physical fitness, and the maintenance of a desirable weight for both men and women. Experience has demonstrated repeatedly that a major factor in maintaining health in the middle years is motivation.

The best way to avoid becoming overweight is to consume only as much energy as is expended. Paradoxically, many persons with weight problems should increase their calorie intake. This increase in energy intake *must* be accompanied by a greatly increased energy expenditure, thus creating weight loss. Overweight people who try to lose by severely limiting their food consumption often suffer from lethargy and weakness. Any sound weight loss program must provide enough energy to support vigorous activity. Simply put, if a person doesn't have enough energy to exercise, he won't.

Many industrial organizations now make it possible for employees to engage in physical activities during the working day. This effort to combat the increasingly sedentary nature of our society will likely accelerate as time goes by.

Diet Among the Elderly

It has long been known that in some places in the world people reportedly live unusually long lives and remain vigorous even at advanced ages. The three best known places are portions of the Andes Mountains in Ecuador, the Himalayas in the Kashmir, and a relatively large area in the Caucasus Mountains of the Soviet Union. These locales have a num-ber of characteristics in common. They are all mountainous, and their residents have lived in mostly rural places. Throughout their long lives the people are characterized as being generally active, having a great capacity for self-aid, and continuing their interest in life. They are accustomed to strenuous physical activity. Indeed, their survival depends upon it.

Interestingly, dietary studies show great differences among the three regions. In the Andes and Himalayas, the people are mainly vegetarians, following a monotonous, rigid diet that is low in calories. Protein intake comes from beans, bread, and milk products. Sugar is seldom used. In the Caucasus the caloric intake is higher. About one-third of the calories come from meat and dairy products.

Apparently, the common characteristic of healthy elderly people is an energetic life and a controlled caloric intake to match. Perhaps

HEIGHT AND WEIGHT CHART

Height[a] (ft; in)	Men Acceptable Weight (lbs)[a] Range			Women Acceptable Weight (lbs)[a] Range		
	Average	Small Frame	Large Frame	Average	Small Frame	Large Frame
4 10				102	92	119
4 11				104	94	122
5 0				107	96	125
5 1				110	99	128
5 2	123	112	141	113	102	131
5 3	127	115	144	116	105	134
5 4	130	118	148	120	108	138
5 5	133	121	152	123	111	142
5 6	136	124	156	128	114	146
5 7	140	128	161	132	118	150
5 8	145	132	166	136	122	154
5 9	149	136	170	140	126	158
5 10	153	140	174	144	130	163
5 11	158	144	179	148	134	168
6 0	162	148	184	152	138	173
6 1	166	152	189			
6 2	171	156	194			
6 3	176	160	199			
6 4	181	164	204			

[a]Height without shoes, weight without clothes.

Approximate desirable weights for men and women are shown for small, medium, and large frames.

Comparison to desirable weights, however, is only one yardstick for measuring obesity.

the most helpful and beneficial feature in maintaining health in older age is the maintenance of physical activity.

The result of increased activity is that older people have an increased energy intake without becoming obese, and hence they can have a more varied, safer diet. Elderly people living alone should be encouraged to take advantage of group dining programs if they are available. One of the major causes of poor dietary intake among the elderly is boredom or loneliness.

FOOD, EXERCISE,
AND HEALTH

Years ago, nutritionists cautioned against such deficiency diseases as rickets, pellagra, and beriberi. They sought to tell the public how to abolish those diseases by selecting a diet containing the proper vitamins and minerals. Today, most nutritionists are faced with a problem far more pervasive: obesity.

Obesity is one of those matters that not everyone in medicine agrees on. Whether a person is obese remains a matter of who is doing the defining. One definition is that an obese person is 20 percent above the normal weight for his or her height (see the chart on page 446). But a professional football player may exceed that measure by a wide margin, yet not carry an ounce of fat; so overweight is not synonymous with obesity. Another definition says that a person is obese when 20 percent or more of the body weight is fat. But that doesn't recognize that women have a naturally higher proportion of fat than men.

In the absence of a single accepted standard, many physicians use four yardsticks: (1) the height-weight charts; (2) the pinch-fold test to see how much excess flesh can be grasped between thumb and forefinger at the waistline or back; (3) the "eyeball test"—people who look fat to others are fat; (4) and the "mirror test"—people who look fat to themselves are fat.

By all these standards, Americans make up perhaps the fattest population in the history of the world, excluding certain South Sea Islands where obesity is considered a mark of beauty. And this epidemic of obesity may account for our high incidence of diseases that obesity appears to be associated with—heart disease, still the nation's number one killer, and diabetes among older persons.

Dr. Jean Mayer, a respected authority on obesity, dates America's "fat period" from 1951. That year, he notes, featured the spread of a new product in the home—the television set. Schoolchildren decreased their after-school athletic activity and increased their sedentary rites in front of the television set, Dr. Mayer's studies show. This ritual often included extra calories in the form of snacks and soft drinks.

With the increasing sophistication of our technology, the average American worker can do his or her job with less physical effort, which means burning fewer calories, which in turn can mean a greater accumulation of fat. Decreasing caloric intake is one way to compensate for sedentary life. Exercise is the other.

Finnish lumberjacks, for instance, consume 4,700 calories daily compared to the recommended 2,700 for mature American males. Yet, these trim, hard-working lumberjacks have lower cholesterol levels than most American males even though their diets are about 50 percent fat. Their incidence of heart attack is lower, life-span longer, and appearance healthier. But things may be looking up for many Americans.

As the decade of the 1970s came to a close, this headline appeared in one of the nation's leading newspapers: "Decrease in Heart Attacks Baffles Medical Authorities." The report said that the rate of heart attack among Americans had shown a decrease for the first time in years. It also said that prominent physicians could not cite any single factor to account for this reversal. Perhaps the answer is too simple. Mere observation discloses that an increasing number of Americans are taking to the road, but without engines to drive them. Bicycling has become an increasingly popular alternative to the car. Jogging attracts millions. America, it would seem, is literally back on its feet. And the result? Fitter people, perhaps contributing to a lower incidence of heart attacks.

The miracle diet. Medical authorities, nutritionists, and well-meaning but ill-informed nutrition "experts" have written countless books on the subject of weight loss. There are diets for the "drinking man," diets that promise to burn off fat without effort, even diets that recommend eating synthetic protein (a definite health risk). Many diet books neglect the simplest, most miraculous step of all. This increasingly popular weight loss program includes an ample amount of a calorie-consuming ingredient. If this ingredient becomes a regular part of the daily routine, it will help burn away calories before they are converted to fat. This miracle ingredient is called exercise.

CALORIES BURNED PER HOUR IN EVERYDAY ACTIVITIES

Activity	Calories burned per hour
Light	**50–200**
Lying down or sleeping	80
Sitting	100
Driving an automobile	120
Standing	140
Domestic work	180
Moderate	**200–350**
Walking, 2½ mph	210
Bicycling, 5½ mph	210
Gardening	220
Golf	250
Lawn mowing, power mower	250
Bowling	270
Rowing a boat	300
Walking, 3¾ mph	300
Swimming, ¼ mph	300
Square dancing	350
Volleyball	350
Roller skating	350
Badminton	350
Vigorous	**over 350**
Table Tennis	360
Wood chopping or sawing	400
Ice skating (10 mph)	400
Tennis	420
Water skiing	480
Skiing, 10 mph	600
Squash and handball	600
Bicycling, 13 mph	660
Running, 10 mph	900

Five minutes of jogging will burn the calories in one large apple. To burn off a piece of cake, however, will take 18 minutes of jogging.

Exercise considerations. Every American should exercise. How much is right for you depends upon your physical condition, age, general health, and long-term goals. It would be wise for anyone about to embark on a new physical fitness program to consult a physician before doing so.

The goal of any sound exercise program is to improve the cardiovascular and respiratory systems. A strong heart and strong lungs are the basis for a lifetime of good health. However, not all exercise programs accomplish this goal. According to the American Heart Association's Committee on Exercise and Fitness, the heart and lungs are improved only by exercise that is sustained for 15 minutes or more. Thus, although tennis can call forth sporadic bursts of great energy, it also allows periods of rest. Distance running, on the other hand, provides continuous exercise for the cardiovascular and respiratory systems.

Of greatest importance, however, is that you choose an activity you enjoy. No one continues an exercise program that does not interest him or her. Benefits can be derived only when exercise becomes a regular part of your life-style. So find something you enjoy and stick with it. If you do, the results will stick with you.

Water and exercise. Body temperature is regulated by water. As we exercise, we increase our body temperature, producing sweat. The evaporation of sweat cools the body, thus maintaining our normal temperature. This "cooling system" is hampered by temperatures in excess of 90 degrees or humidity in excess of 40 percent. Under these conditions, sweat is not evaporating, and therefore is not cooling the system efficiently.

Two serious problems can occur under these conditions—sun stroke and heat exhaustion (see chapter 35, "First Aid"). In order to prevent them, drink plenty of water before, during, and after exercise. (Drinking water before exercise will enhance performance.) Never exercise in a "rubber suit" that does not allow the evaporation and cooling effect of sweat. Select clothing that allows air exchange between the skin and the air.

The other benefit of exercise. Many people who lead sedentary lives watch what they eat and still gain weight or remain overweight. When there is no program to burn off the excess, those unused calories turn to fat. Mealtime becomes one selection process after another in which the individual denies himself or herself a favorite food item because of its calorie content. We all have seen slender people who seem to have no trouble maintaining their weight even though they "eat like a horse." Only in unusual circumstances is this caused by natural or inherited tendencies. There are, of course, great variations among individual body structures, but it is safe to say that thinner people tend to lead more active lives. If you see a slender person who "eats like a horse," it is quite likely that he works (or plays) like one too.

Food as Medicine In the Ancient World

One of the great ages of discovery in medicine is almost completely unknown to us. Thousands—perhaps hundreds of thousands—of years ago man came to know that some berries are good for us, and that others are poisonous. He discovered that some foods contain medicinal properties that help treat specific diseases. Learning must have been a long process full of trial and error. How long did it take the North American Indian to discover that chewing the bark of the willow tree would relieve a headache, but not the bark of the oak, elm, or pine? For only the willow contains acetylsalicylic acid—the scientific name for aspirin.

From about 800 A.D. to 1000 A.D., medicine flourished in India. Two famous physicians of that period, Caraka and Susruta, learned that many medicines could be derived from plants. Caraka listed 500 medicinal plants and Susruta 760. But animal remedies also were practiced. They used milk from various animals, as well as bones for calcium. They also employed minerals such as sulfur, arsenic, lead, copper, sulfate, and gold in their formulations.

In those days, physicians gathered their own plants and prepared medicines from them. Some of these plants, such as cardamom and cinnamon, are still used today. (Cardamom can be used as a mild means of relieving gas pains in the alimentary canal. Cinnamon has been used for nausea and diarrhea.)

Even in those days the role of the diet in human health was being studied. Physicians recommended two meals a day, specified how much water was to be drunk before and after each meal, and even detailed the types of condiments to be used.

Similar discoveries were being made in ancient China. From the Chinese, Western medicine has adapted rhubarb, iron, castor oil, kaolin, aconite, and camphor. The Chinese have used the herb majuang for about 4,000 years. From this herb alkaloid ephedrine has been extracted and is used in the treatment of asthma and similar conditions. Reserpine, which is widely used in the treatment of high blood pressure, is the active principle of the Chinese plant Rauwolfia.

The most famous of all ancient physicians is Hippocrates. Born in Greece in the fifth century B.C., Hippocrates observed the body's tendency to cure itself. He said, "Our natures are the physicians of our diseases." He therefore recommended few drugs, laying greater stress on diet. His view of medical practice is strikingly contemporary, for he believed that the environment which surrounds the patient must be studied as well as the patient himself. This "ecological" emphasis is one of the cornerstones in the study and practice of contemporary medicine.

Hippocrates' influence on the course of nutrition and medicine was felt well into the Renaissance. A famous medical school was founded at Salerno, Italy, in the 12th century. Echoes of Hippocrates can be heard in the famous couplet written by Arnald of Villanova in Salerno:

"Use three physicians still, first Doctor Quiet, Next Doctor Merryman, and Doctor Diet."

The histories of food and medicine go hand in hand. Learning what to eat and what not to eat seems simple to us today, but only because we are the recipients of a great and long legacy of ancient "researchers" who laid the foundation for our modern scientific investigations of food, nutrition, and health.

This is not to recommend that you should go on a crash diet so that you can overindulge later. The yo-yo approach of fat to thin and back to fat again does more harm than good. After all, a "crash" diet doesn't even sound safe.

So along with promoting health, exercise can expand your food horizons. But don't think about the immediate results—"How will I look in three weeks?" Ask yourself, "How will I look in 10 or 20 years?" Set long-term goals for a healthy life, and make haste slowly.

If you're too thin. A more unusual nutritional problem is excessive leanness. Excessive leanness is often a sign of illness for which a physician should be consulted. A planned program for weight gain should be approved by the doctor. Gaining weight is sometimes as difficult as losing it, and success requires as much discipline as weight reduction.

What has been said about reducing diets is an excellent guide to what not to do in order to gain weight. A dietary program to increase weight aims to increase the daily intake of calories appreciably above caloric expenditure. This is done by eating more of all food groups, but particularly of foods high in calories.

The fundamental plan for a balanced weight-gain diet should adhere to the basic food groups outlined on page 442. From the milk group take four or more cups per day of whole milk, augmented by servings of cheese and ice cream. From the meat group one should eat two or more servings of meat, poultry, or fish, including the fatter cuts. One or more eggs per day and servings of the meat alternatives can add variety.

NUTRITION AND
GOVERNMENT

Federal food programs. Even in a country as food-rich as the United States, many people cannot afford a wholesome diet. The federal government has therefore created various food programs that focus on high-risk populations. These programs include the school lunch program, the food stamp program, the WIC program (Supplemental Food for Women, Infants, and Children), and Meals on Wheels, which delivers a hot, nutritious meal to shut-ins, the elderly, or the disabled.

State and local governments also sponsor nutrition programs. To learn whether these programs might help you in securing an adequate diet, contact your local health agency or local chapters of voluntary health organizations such as the American Heart Association or the National Foundation/March of Dimes.

Food monitoring. Since the Pure Food and Drug Act became law in 1906, the federal government has monitored the nation's food supply to see that foods and beverages are free of contamination.

Today, federal laws are intended not only to protect us from impurities in foods, but also from advertising which may be misleading and potentially unsafe.

In recent years, the government has enacted legislation which requires various kinds of food labeling.

Listing of ingredients. Government regulations called standards of identity define the composition of many foods, state which optional ingredients may be used, and specify which ingredients must be declared on the label. Examples of standardized foods are most canned fruits and vegetables, milk, cheeses, ice cream, breads, margarine, certain seafoods, sweeteners, and food dressings. Required or mandatory ingredients used in such standardized foods are exempt by law from label listings, although the Food and Drug Administration (FDA) has recommended that they be listed.

Earlier standards required that only a limited number of optional ingredients be listed because the special ingredients which could be used were named in the standard. Future standards can be expected to permit greater flexibility in the use of ingredients and, at the same time, require the listing of all optional ingredients. With the exception of certain spices, flavors, and colors, law requires the label to declare all ingredients in foods which are not standardized. Labels for all meat and poultry products, whether standardized or not, must list ingredients. Government regulations require that whenever ingredients must be declared on the label, they must be listed in descending order of predominance by weight.

Nutrition labeling is partly a voluntary program. It becomes mandatory only when a processor makes a claim on the label or in advertising about the food's nutritional value, or when the food is enriched with any essential nutrients. The program applies to foods regulated by the Food and Drug Administration. That includes most foods except meat and poultry which are regulated by the U.S. Department of Agriculture. The USDA also has

SIDE VIEW OF CEREAL BOX

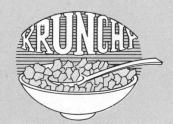

CORN FLAKES

**NUTRITION INFORMATION
PER SERVING**

Serving Size One Ounce (About 1 Cup) Corn Flakes
Alone and in Combination With ½ Cup Vitamin D
Fortified Whole Milk

SERVINGS PER CONTAINER 16

	Corn Flakes	
	1 Oz	With ½ Cup Whole Milk
Calories	110	180
Protein	2 g	6 g
Carbohydrates	25 g	31 g
Fat	0 g	4 g

**PERCENTAGE OF U.S.
RECOMMENDED DAILY
ALLOWANCE (U.S. RDA)**

	Corn Flakes	
	1 Oz	With ½ Cup Whole Milk
Protein	4	15
Vitamin A	25	25
Vitamin C	25	25
Thiamin	25	25
Riboflavin	25	35
Niacin	25	25
Calcium	*	15
Iron	10	10
Vitamin D	10	25
Vitamin B	25	25
Folic Acid	25	25
Phosphorus	*	10
Magnesium	*	4
Copper	2	2

*Contains Less Than 2 Percent of the U.S. RDA
 of These Nutrients.

Ingredients Milled Corn, Sugar, Salt, Malt Flavoring, Sodium
Ascorbate (C), Vitamin A Palmitate, Niacinamide, Ascorbic
Acid (C), Iron Pyridoxine Hydrocholoride (B_6), Thiamin
Hydrochloride (B_1), Riboflavin (B_2), Folic Acid and Vitamin
D_7, BHA and BHT Added to Preserve Product Freshness

**MADE BY KRUNCHY COMPANY
PIONEER, IOWA 99999 USA**

approved the use of the same type of labeling on many processed meat and poultry products. When a food label contains nutrition information, that information must be provided in a standard format that includes serving size and servings per container. For each serving the label lists the calories and protein, carbohydrates, and fat in grams, followed by protein and a minimum of seven specified vitamins and minerals in terms of the percentage of the U.S. Recommended Daily Allowances (RDAs). The quantities of other vitamins and minerals, sodium and potassium, cholesterol, and polyunsaturated and saturated fatty acids also may be included. The standardized way of presenting all this information is thought to be important to avoid confusing the consumer with multiple ways of expressing the same information.

Nutrition labeling can be of great importance to the consumer. It can help the cost-conscious shopper find the most nutritious product for the dollar and can help provide a well-rounded diet.

Food additives. Significant advances in the technology of food processing have made possible a variety of prepared or partially prepared foods, ranging from "mixes" to ready-to-eat frozen or packaged food. Common foods such as fats and bread now "keep" better. Many of these improvements stem from new and better packaging materials and the use of additives that prevent fat from becoming rancid (anti-oxidants), retard the development of molds in breads (mold inhibitors), and otherwise improve quality. Vitamin C, for instance, is added to peaches and other fruits during the freezing process to preserve the color of the fresh product.

The present-day use of chemicals in food (foods themselves are chemical substances) is regulated at federal and state levels. However, there are individuals and organizations who believe that adding chemicals to food is an unsafe practice. Indeed, debate over the safety of additives such as saccharin, an artificial sweetener, continues to flourish. The points of view cover a broad spectrum. Some people feel that any potentially hazardous food additives should be prohibited if the smallest risk can be determined. Others maintain that our food supply is almost hazard-free. However, it is likely that we will continue to monitor and test food additives, eliminating those that pose risks for society, and continuing to develop and use those that promote food safety.

CHAPTER 20   WILLIAM D. CAREY, M.D.,
RICHARD G. FARMER, M.D.

THE DIGESTIVE SYSTEM

Anything we eat, from the fastest fast-food snack to the most leisurely and elegant five-course dinner, starts a chemical process more intricate than that of the most sophisticated laboratory. Starting at the mouth, a bite of hot dog or spoonful of soup is transformed within the length of 26 feet into ever-simpler substances that can be used by the body for building, energy, and maintenance. Some parts of the meal have no nutritional value and are discarded. Others might harm the body and are neutralized. The useful substances pass into the bloodstream to be carried to the tissues. The remarkable set of organs that achieves this complex series of feats is called the digestive system.

Gastroenterologists, the medical specialists who study the digestive system and treat its disorders, usually classify the digestive system into two parts. They call the first the tubular gut. The tubular gut can be thought of as a long, flexible tube that begins at the mouth and ends at the rectum. Its length is doubled and coiled back on itself, much the way you can coil or kink a garden hose, so that a great length is compressed into a limited space. Along the route, the tube assumes different shapes that we give different names. The small intestine is cylindrical and less than an inch in diameter in places. The stomach above it is shaped like a wine flask and can expand into a two-quart sack to do its job as a food reservoir.

Although the general shape of the gut roughly resembles a garden hose, the similarity is more apparent than real. The garden hose's role is a passive one: It merely transports water from the faucet to the flower bed without changing it in any way. The intestinal tract, in contrast, plays an active part in the digestive process, transforming the food as it passes through to prepare it for absorption into the body tissues or for excretion. The hose's water provides its own pressure to move itself through the hose. The walls of the gut use a ceaseless process called peristalsis to move the inert contents from one point to another. These pressure waves can speed up or slow down, according to which is needed for food breakdown.

The second part of the digestive system consists of the solid organs, the pancreas and the liver. Grouped with the liver are a set of small tubes (bile ducts) and a sack (the gallbladder). All play a prominent role in digestion and are linked into the system high in the tubular gut, where the digestive process begins. Their chemicals help break down food as it passes from the stomach through the intestinal tract. They have other duties as well.

The pancreas manufactures a number of important digestive fluids. One of these is bicarbonate, which neutralizes the potent hydrochloric acid produced in the stomach. The pancreas also produces a number of digestive enzymes, chemicals essential to food breakdown in the intestinal tract. Specialized cells in the pancreas manufacture hormones that regulate certain body processes. The best known of these hormones is insulin, which helps keep the blood levels of the simple sugar glucose within narrow limits (see chapter 17, "Diabetes Mellitus").

The liver, a giant chemical factory, also contributes to digestion, but it has important non-digestive functions, too. It is the main location for production or synthesis of proteins, carbohydrates, and fats. It helps maintain the body's ecological balance, detoxifying potentially poisonous products of the body's normal metabolism. It cancels out harmful effects of the drugs we ingest. The liver also manufactures certain substances needed for blood clotting (and to oppose clotting) and is a storage place for vitamins.

A third "division" of the digestive system is only now coming to be recognized. It has recently been established that the intestinal tract is the largest endocrine organ in the body. The pancreas produces insulin and glucagon, also used in glucose regulation. At least 20 other hormones or hormone-like substances have been identified in the pancreas and in portions of the tubular gut.

The importance of many of these hormones is still unknown. Some are discussed later.

THE TUBULAR GUT

The tubular gut in primitive animals and in the human embryo is, in fact, a continuous tube, varying little in diameter or appearance throughout its length. As the fetus grows and develops, the lengthening tube differentiates into separate organs, each with a specific role to play in the process of digestion. We will refer to five major divisions of the gastrointestinal tract, several of which have their own subdivisions with their own tasks and functions. All have their own sets of muscles to help propel food along the tract. They also have purse-string muscles called sphincters, which can close them off from the next organ in the process. The organs are under control of the nervous system and are influenced by hormones secreted elsewhere in the body.

From top to bottom, the five structures are the mouth, esophagus, stomach, small intestine, and colon.

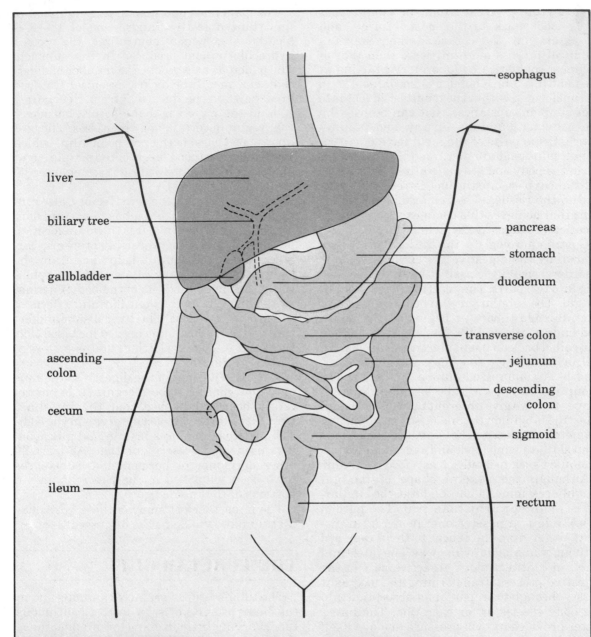

esophagus

liver

biliary tree

gallbladder

pancreas

stomach

duodenum

transverse colon

ascending colon

jejunum

cecum

descending colon

sigmoid

ileum

rectum

THE DIGESTIVE SYSTEM

The organs of digestion are shown in an exploded view. The shaded portions represent the stomach and small and large intestines, which make up the tubular gut and deal with digestion and absorption. The unshaded areas are the solid organs—the liver (with its associated gallbladder) and pancreas—where digestive enzymes and hormones are produced that help in the digestive process. Food is chewed into manageable pieces in the mouth, then passes down the esophagus into the stomach, where it is exposed to acid, pepsin, and some minor gastric enzymes. The food is churned into a

pasty substance by the motor activity of the stomach wall. The semi-liquid moves into the duodenum, where bile from the liver and gallbladder and pancreatic juices from the pancreas assist in the chemical breakdown. Usable nutrients are absorbed through the walls of the small intestine. The remaining substances pass into the cecum. Water is squeezed out as they are transported through the ascending colon, transverse colon, descending colon, and sigmoid colon into the rectum. The remaining materials, about a quarter pound a day, can then be excreted.

The Mouth

The mouth is obviously the beginning of the gastrointestinal tract, although we tend to think of it in terms of smiles and tastes. Its disorders are usually treated by specialists other than gastroenterologists. The mouth's assignment in digestion is called mastication, or chewing. Solid foods are broken up so they can pass into the narrow structures below. Liquid from the salivary glands is added to make swallowing easier. There are three types of salivary glands. The parotid, located in front of and below each ear, is the gland that swells painfully during a mumps infection. The sublingual and submandibular glands are in the floor of the mouth. All secrete saliva, usually in the presence of food, but they also may produce saliva when we merely think about food, or when we smell bacon frying. The salivary glands secrete enzymes, too, which help digest certain portions of food. However, salivary glands are more important in transporting food than digesting it.

Swallowing is so commonplace that it seems simple, but it is actually a complicated event. We start it consciously by thrusting the tongue against the hard palate, elevating the larynx, then moving the tongue backwards to force the food into the open throat. Once that has happened, however, the array of neurologic and motor activities that take place are largely involuntary, and the food proceeds in an orderly way through the system.

The Esophagus

The esophagus connects the mouth and the stomach. A muscular canal about nine to ten inches long, it begins at the throat, crosses the chest from top to bottom, and ends at the diaphragm, the large muscle that separates the chest cavity above from the abdominal cavity below. The esophagus passes through a small hole in the diaphragm called the hiatus in order to join with the stomach. A normal bit of food can traverse it in three to four seconds. But the esophagus is not merely a passive tube that delivers its cargo by force of gravity. Muscle fibers throughout its length propel food and liquid in an orderly fashion, the first example of the motor waves called peristalsis.

Like the organ below it, the esophagus can be closed off by specialized muscle fibers called sphincters, which circle it at top and bottom.

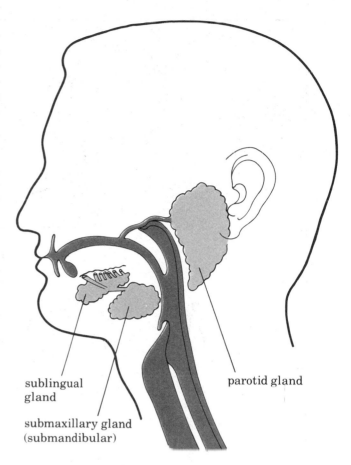

sublingual gland

parotid gland

submaxillary gland
(submandibular)

THE SALIVARY GLANDS

Three sets of glands produce saliva, which helps to liquefy food and ease its passage down the throat. They are the sublingual glands just beneath the tongue, the submaxillary (or submandibular) glands behind the sublinguals, and the parotid glands located in front of and below the ear. Saliva contains an enzyme that helps break down some starches, but the mouth does not play a prominent role in digestion.

These muscles are contracted at all times except during swallowing and vomiting. The upper esophageal sphincter prevents air from entering the esophagus during breathing. The lower esophageal sphincter, located at the level of the diaphragm, blocks irritating acid contents and ingested food from returning from the stomach back into the esophagus. Infants have a poorly developed lower esophageal sphincter, so they may regurgitate food quite readily when lying down. The opossum, on the other hand, has a highly developed lower esophageal sphincter and can hang by its tail without having stomach contents spill back into the esophagus.

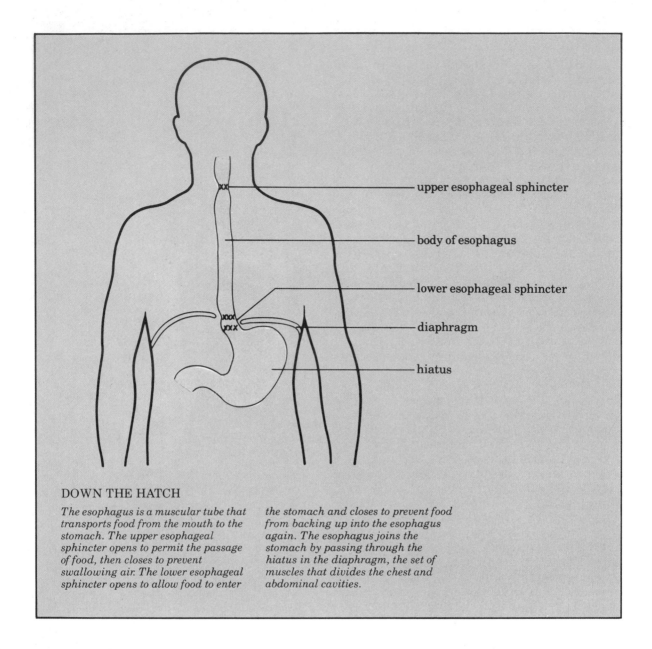

upper esophageal sphincter

body of esophagus

lower esophageal sphincter

diaphragm

hiatus

DOWN THE HATCH

The esophagus is a muscular tube that transports food from the mouth to the stomach. The upper esophageal sphincter opens to permit the passage of food, then closes to prevent swallowing air. The lower esophageal sphincter opens to allow food to enter the stomach and closes to prevent food from backing up into the esophagus again. The esophagus joins the stomach by passing through the hiatus in the diaphragm, the set of muscles that divides the chest and abdominal cavities.

The Stomach

The stomach, an expandable organ, is just a small wrinkled bag when empty. After a meal, its walls stretch, then slowly shrink again to a much smaller space between meals. These contractions are sometimes felt as what we call hunger pangs. The stomach is popularly thought to be located midway in the body, at about the waistline, but it lies higher than that, above the waist just below the diaphragm, to the right of the spleen and partially under the liver. It occupies the uppermost portion of the abdominal cavity.

In shape, the stomach resembles a wineskin turned upside down. The area where it joins the esophagus is called the cardia. The rounded portion at the top, located higher than the cardia, is the fundus. The main portion of the stomach is called the body. The tapered area where it narrows toward a union with the small intestine is called the antrum. The pylorus is the narrow passageway that leads into the small intestine.

The stomach has two openings, top and bottom. Both are controlled by strong sets of sphincter muscles. The cardiac sphincter at the top is the same sphincter as the lower esophageal sphincter. Its function is to prevent return of the stomach's contents back into the

SHAPE OF THE STOMACH

The stomach resembles an inverted wineskin, rounded at its upper end and tapering toward a neck (the pylorus). Joined with the esophagus through the hiatus opening in the diaphragm, the stomach lies in the upper portion of the abdominal opening. Food from the esophagus enters at the cardia and is stored in the fundus and upper body. Strong muscles in the walls of the body and antrum squeeze and knead the food as it moves toward the pylorus. The contents are then discharged at intervals into the duodenum.

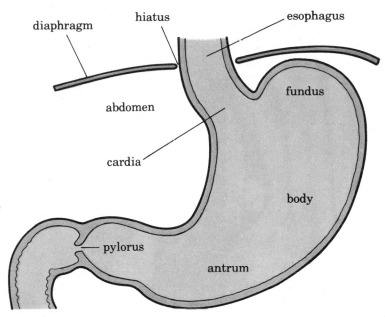

esophagus. The pyloric sphincter at the bottom regulates the amount of solids and liquids emptying into the small intestine, so the food does not overwhelm the digestive process.

There are three layers of smooth muscle fibers in the stomach, arranged longitudinally, laterally, and diagonally. The strong muscles are needed to move the stomach's contents along the path of digestion. The fundus and upper body of the stomach serve mainly to contain and break down food. Peristalsis, the pressure waves of the gut, begin in the lower portion of the body and continue in the antrum. The antrum's muscular activity performs an important mixing action, squeezing and churning the gastric contents somewhat the way a baker kneads bread dough. This prepares the material for easier passage into the intestine.

The stomach empties in a complicated way, controlled by gastrointestinal hormones and a large nerve called the vagus nerve. Liquids empty faster than solids (we get rid of soup in a hurry) and a built-in sensing mechanism regulates the rate according to the amounts of fats and proteins in the solids.

The stomach, like the rest of the intestinal tract, is lined by cells arranged in complicated and distinctive patterns. There are 35 million cells, with differing shapes and functions. Cells in some parts of the stomach have a tubular shape, others a columnar one. The shape and location of the cells are related to the substances secreted. For instance, the cells of the cardia produce mucus, which protects the stomach from damage caused by ingested substances or by the stomach's own potent secretions. Other substances found in the gastric (stomach) juices are pepsin, a potent digestive enzyme; rennin, the substance that causes milk to curdle; and acid. Acid in this case is the potent hydrochloric acid, in a concentrated form that will damage most tissues. Normally, mucus prevents it from harming the stomach.

What is the purpose of pepsin and acid in the stomach? For biological activity the pepsin requires the presence of an acid medium. The administration of a potent alkali such as sodium bicarbonate (baking soda) can easily inactivate it. Therefore, it seems likely that acid is found in the stomach to allow proper activity of pepsin. But the role of pepsin itself

pylorus   cardia   fundus

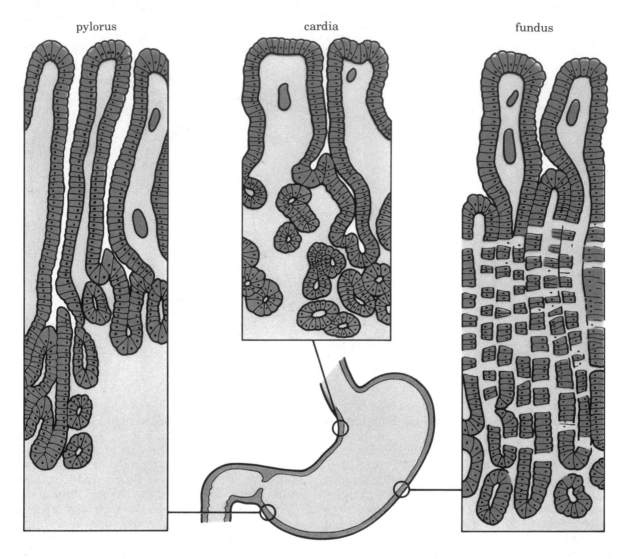

CELLS OF THE STOMACH

The 35 million stomach cells vary by location and function, as these magnified structures show. Special secretory cells of the cardia produce *mucus. Cells of the fundus produce pepsin and hydrochloric acid. Pylorus cells secrete mucus.*

is not clear. A person can digest food satisfactorily after a partial or even total removal of the stomach, when levels of both acid and pepsin are severely reduced. Although the role of pepsin and acid in normal digestion is poorly understood, both substances play an important part in ulcer disease.

Another important protein produced by the lining cells of the stomach is a hormone called gastrin. It originates in so-called G cells in the gastric antrum. Amino acids or proteins, alcohol, calcium, and possibly distention of the antrum by food all cause the release of gastrin.

One of the major effects of this hormone is to stimulate acid and pepsin secretion, making it important in the normal control of these substances. Certain very rare tumors can produce excessive amounts of gastrin.

Vitamin B_{12} is absorbed in the specialized area of the small intestine called the ileum. However, the vitamin is not absorbed unless acted upon by a protein called intrinsic factor, produced by mucosal cells in the fundus of the stomach.

Foodstuffs and liquids are not absorbed through the normal stomach wall. Therefore, unlike other portions of the intestinal tract, the lining cells of the stomach present a solid

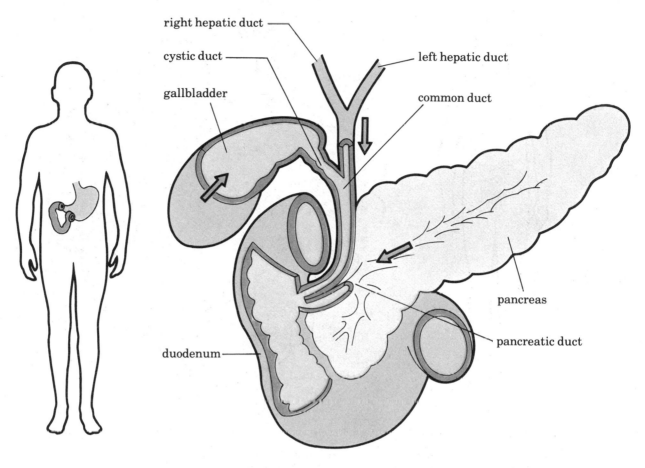

right hepatic duct

cystic duct

gallbladder

left hepatic duct

common duct

pancreas

pancreatic duct

duodenum

THE DUODENUM

The first 10 to 12 inches of the small intestine are an area of great chemical activity. The contents of the acid stomach move into the alkaline environment of the duodenum. Bile from the gallbladder and liver arrive via the cystic and hepatic ducts, which join in the common bile duct entering the duodenum. Digestive enzymes from the pancreas gland are secreted via the pancreatic duct. About 9 to 11 quarts of liquid are processed through the duodenum each day.

barrier to absorption. Essentially, no nutrition can be derived from food until it passes through the pylorus into the small intestine.

The Small Intestine

The entire portion of the tubular gut called the small intestine, or small bowel, is devoted to the breakdown and absorption of food, the absorption of fluids, and absorption of salts (electrolytes) contained in those fluids. The amount of fluid entering the small intestine from the stomach each day is between 9 and 11 quarts. This comes not only from the 1 to 1½ quarts we drink but from saliva, stomach secretions, pancreatic secretion, bile, and some secretion from the small intestine itself. Of this large volume all but a quart is absorbed through the intestinal walls by the time the contents have traveled the full length of the small intestine. This quart enters the colon.

The small intestine is divided into three portions: the duodenum (12 inches long), the jejunum, and the ileum. Although inspection reveals few differences among the various portions, certain features visible under the microscope distinguish them, and many functions are unique to each portion.

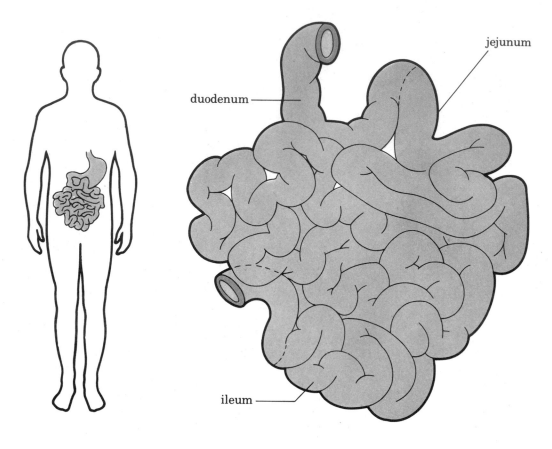

duodenum

jejunum

ileum

THE SMALL INTESTINE

Twenty-two feet or more of small intestine are compactly wound into the abdomen, where the process of absorption of nutrients takes place. Although the tube is continuous it consists of three portions—duodenum, jejunum, and ileum—which look similar at a glance but different under the microscope and perform different functions.

The surface area of the small intestine is many times greater than would be calculated simply by measuring its length (22 feet) and diameter. To allow for better absorption, the intestine's internal walls are pleated, like the folds of an accordion. When you extend an accordion to its full length, the pleats disappear, but when you compress it, the same amount of surface is folded into a much shorter distance. So it is with the small intestine. The accordion-like folds, called valvulae conniventes, are easily seen on a small-bowel X ray.

The area available for absorption is increased even further by the microvilli. These are tiny, hair-like projections on the intestinal wall that help move the contents through the gut. There are an estimated five million villi throughout the intestine, and they vastly increase its surface area.

Digestion and Absorption

Different parts of our diet are digested and absorbed in different ways. Food is comprised of carbohydrates, proteins, and fats (lipids). Additional nutrients include vitamins and minerals. Carbohydrates are sugars, and the major sugars are fructose, glucose, and galactose. Usually these simple sugars exist in combination. For example, table sugar is sucrose, made up of one molecule each of glucose and fructose. A special enzyme within the cells lining the tips of the microvilli breaks down sucrose into fructose and glucose. These simple sugars are then easily absorbed by the lining cells and transmitted into the bloodstream. The enzyme in this instance is called sucrase.

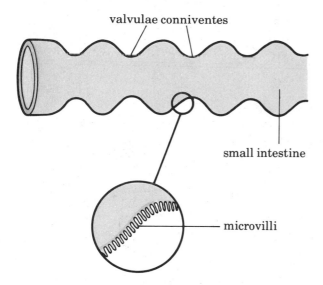

THE COMPACT INTESTINE

The surface available for absorption in the small intestine is increased many times by the accordion-like folds of the intestinal walls, called valvulae conniventes, and the five million hair-like microvilli, shown in the enlarged drawing.

The major sugar in milk is lactose, comprised of one molecule each of galactose and glucose, broken down by the enzyme lactase. Lactase activity is fully developed in infancy and throughout childhood. Humans are one of the few species that can tolerate much milk in the diet during adulthood. In fact, a high proportion of certain racial groups (particularly blacks and Asians) do not have as much lactase activity as others do, and cannot tolerate milk because of the gas, bloating, and sometimes diarrhea it produces. These people are lactase deficient.

Sixty percent of the carbohydrate in Western diets is comprised of starch. If we consider the simple sugars as links in a chain, then sucrose and lactose are chains with one link each. These are called disaccharides ("two sugars"). Starch, on the other hand, is more like a chain-link fence that contains hundreds or thousands of individual links of glucose. Starch is a polysaccharide (many sugars). The enormous polysaccharide molecules cannot be absorbed by the lining cells of the small intestine. To get around this problem potent enzymes (the principal one is amylase) are secreted by the pancreas to break down starch into much smaller pieces. These pieces then can be further broken down into simple sugars by the enzymes in the small intestinal villi before final absorption.

Protein absorption occurs in a similar fashion. Proteins are composed of amino acids. Two amino acids joined together are called dipeptides, three amino acids joined together are tripeptides. A few amino acids (number unspecified) linked together form an oligopeptide, and many linked together form a polypeptide. Proteins are merely large polypeptides. The pancreas secretes into the duodenum a fluid rich in enzymes (themselves proteins) which are able to break down complex polypeptides into simpler groupings. It was once thought that protein in the diet was completely broken down into amino acids before being absorbed. However, it has been shown that the small intestine is better able to absorb dipeptides and tripeptides than amino acids.

Fat absorption is more complex than absorption of carbohydrates or proteins. The basic difference is that proteins and carbohydrates can easily be dissolved in a water medium (the body is made up mainly of water), but fat does not dissolve readily. A greasy (fat containing) pan put under dishwater demonstrates that water and fat do not mix. For the energy in fat to become useful for the body it must be rendered soluble in water.

Fat is consumed almost entirely as triglycerides. Triglycerides can be thought of as being comprised of two different kinds of molecules. The backbone is glycerol. To the glycerol molecule can be attached one, two, or three fatty acid side chains. These fatty acid side chains can be short or long. Ninety percent of the triglyceride in food is comprised of glycerol molecules to which are attached three long-chain fatty acids.

The first step in fat absorption occurs in the stomach. Here the kneading process thoroughly mixes the food and assures that as much fat as possible will come in contact with the enzymes in the small intestine. One such enzyme, lipase, is capable of breaking off two of the three fatty acid molecules attached to the glycerol. This results in the formation of free fatty acids and a glyceride with one fatty acid attached, called a monoglyceride. But these substances still are not soluble in a water medium, so bile is needed. Bile is produced by the liver, stored by the gallbladder, and secreted into the duodenum in response to meals. Bile salts act exactly like the detergents used to clean a greasy pan. Bile salts surround the fatty acids and monoglycerides and make

1

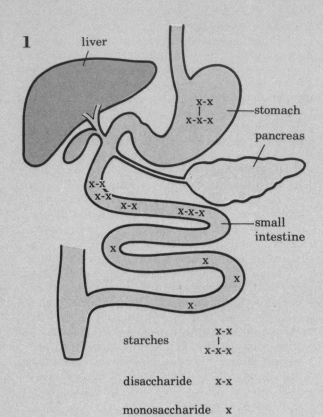

liver

x-x
|
x-x-x

stomach

pancreas

x-x
x-x

x-x

x-x-x

small
intestine

x

x

x

x

starches   x-x
                  |
                  x-x-x

disaccharide   x-x

monosaccharide   x

2

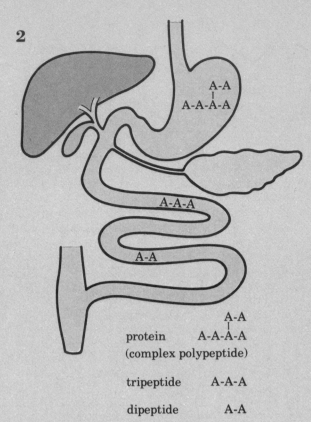

A-A
|
A-A-A-A

A-A-A

A-A

protein   A-A
(complex |
polypeptide)   A-A-A-A

tripeptide   A-A-A

dipeptide   A-A

ABSORPTION OF FOOD

The process of food digestion and absorption through the intestinal walls differs for carbohydrates, proteins, and fats. Carbohydrate absorption (drawing 1) depends on enzymes secreted by the pancreas to break down starches into smaller fragments called oligosaccharides (few sugars). These are further broken into simple sugars (monosaccharides) by enzymes in the lining cells of the small intestine. Simple sugars can be absorbed. Protein absorption (drawing 2) requires pancreatic enzymes to break down proteins (complex polypeptides) into dipeptides (two amino-acid chains) or tripeptides (three amino-acid chains). The dipeptides and tripeptides can be absorbed through the intestinal wall. Fat (triglyceride) absorption (drawing 3) depends on lipase from the pancreas to break off two fatty-acid side chains from the triglyceride molecule. The resulting fatty acids and monoglycerides are enveloped by bile salts from the liver so that they form units called micelles, which allow the fats to be absorbed through the intestinal walls. The bile salts are then recycled, being reabsorbed in the ileum.

3

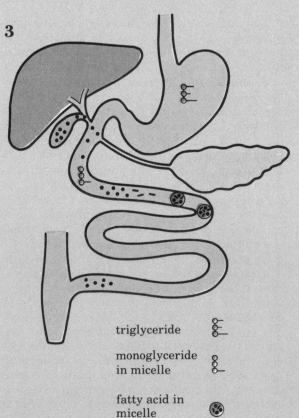

triglyceride

monoglyceride
in micelle

fatty acid in
micelle

them soluble in water. The combination of bile salt and fats (called micelles) is then delivered to the mucosal cells of the microvilli in the small intestine, where it can be absorbed into the cell itself. A new triglyceride molecule is formed within the cell, surrounded by a protein coat, and then transported not to the bloodstream but to the lymph spaces within the villi (the spaces are called lacteals). From there it passes into the lymphatic system and finally into the bloodstream.

Most absorption of carbohydrates, proteins, and fats occurs in the jejunum and the first portion of the ileum. Substantial amounts of small intestine can be removed without greatly hampering absorption. The small intestine obviously has a large reserve capability. However, certain elements are absorbed only in a single area, and diseases in these areas can result in specific absorption problems. For example, vitamin B_{12} is absorbed only in the lowermost portion of ileum. Extensive disease or surgical removal of the distal ileum can result in B_{12} deficiency anemia. Iron is absorbed primarily in the duodenum and folic acid in the upper jejunum. Disease in these sites may cause failure of absorption of these substances.

The Colon

The colon, or large intestine, can be viewed as a waste processor. Its principal function is to take the quart of fluid in which is suspended and dissolved the unabsorbed portion of the food, and reduce its volume as much as possible. Fortunately, the colon allows its owner freedom to eliminate this waste material intermittently and at his command, rather than continuously.

The large bowel begins in the lower abdomen on the right where the ileum enters into the first portion of the colon called the cecum. A small worm-like appendage four to ten inches long comes off the cecum and ends in a blind pouch. This is called the appendix. There is no known role for the appendix (and it often seems that its major purpose is to cause mischief). The next portion is the ascending colon, which comes up the right side of the abdomen and takes a 90-degree turn across the abdomen. The elbow of this turn is at the lower border of the liver (hepar), and is called the hepatic flexure. From the hepatic flexure the next segment of colon crosses the abdomen laterally—the transverse colon—and then makes another sharp turn downward near the spleen (splenic flexure). Now it becomes the descending colon. In the left lower abdomen,

the colon takes a series of S-shaped curves, so it is called the sigmoid colon. Next is the rectum, and the colon ends at the anus.

The total length of the colon is approximately three to four feet, but these measurements are more difficult to determine than one might think. The colon takes several turns and can be stretched a great deal when removed from the body. In a way, it resembles the coiled spring of a Slinky® toy. You could argue that the toy measures either a few inches (when completely compressed), or several feet. Fortunately, the precise length of the colon is rarely an urgent issue.

The muscular layers of the colon exert pressure waves. The major pressure waves are called segmenting waves. Unlike many other waves in the intestinal tract, segmenting waves do not propel the contents downstream. Instead, the segmenting wave tends to slow the speed with which the contents travel through the colon, allowing more time for the colon to process the contents.

The lining cells of the colon have the ability to absorb large amounts of fluid. In fact, the liquid contents which enter the colon are rendered solid in most individuals. The weight of the contents entering the colon per day is over three pounds, whereas the weight of the daily stool for most Americans is about a quarter of a pound.

The rectum is a specialized portion of the colon which serves as the stop-cock for the colon. The rectum's two sets of sphincter muscles keep it closed under normal conditions. The external sphincter is under voluntary control but the internal sphincter is not. The anus and rectum contain a number of blood vessels. The veins here can rather easily become defective from excessive pressures. In response to this, they may dilate like varicose veins in the leg. These are called hemorrhoids.

THE SOLID ORGANS

The Liver and Gallbladder

The body's largest internal organ, the maroon-colored, shiny-surfaced liver, weighs between five and six pounds. It lies on the right side of the upper abdomen, just beneath the diaphragm. The liver plays a key role in digestion and is important in many other bodily functions. It manufactures blood coagulants, stores vitamins and minerals, produces enzymes, cholesterol, and proteins, and neutralizes substances that would harm the body.

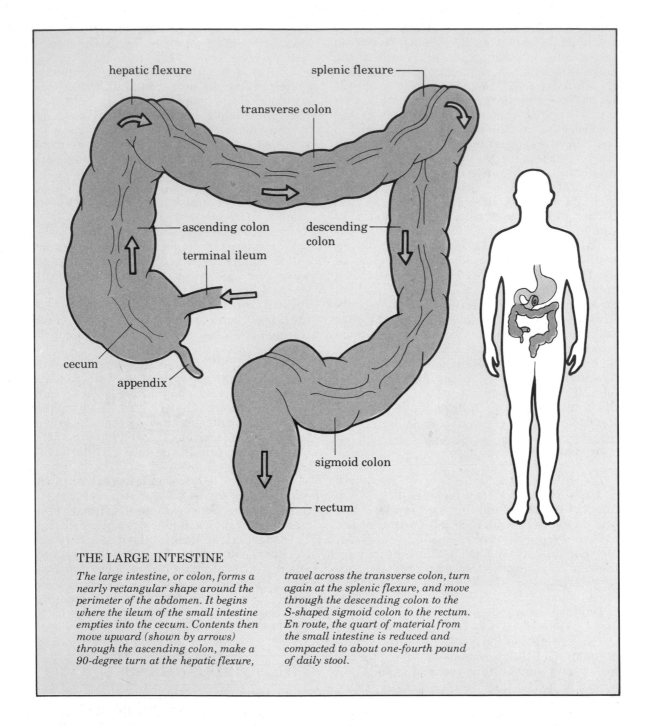

hepatic flexure

splenic flexure

transverse colon

ascending colon

descending colon

terminal ileum

cecum

appendix

sigmoid colon

rectum

THE LARGE INTESTINE

The large intestine, or colon, forms a nearly rectangular shape around the perimeter of the abdomen. It begins where the ileum of the small intestine empties into the cecum. Contents then move upward (shown by arrows) through the ascending colon, make a 90-degree turn at the hepatic flexure,

travel across the transverse colon, turn again at the splenic flexure, and move through the descending colon to the S-shaped sigmoid colon to the rectum. En route, the quart of material from the small intestine is reduced and compacted to about one-fourth pound of daily stool.

The working parts of the liver are the four lobes, the largest of which are the right and left lobes. Each lobe contains innumerable tiny lobules that can be seen under low magnification of a microscope. The lobules consist of row upon row of liver cells, radiating outward like spokes of a wheel. The hub of the wheel is a tiny vein called the central vein. At the periphery are the portal tracts, each of which consists of a minute artery, a tiny bile duct, and a branch of the portal vein.

Unlike other organs, the liver receives blood from two sources. The heart, eye, and kidneys, for instance, are fed by a single system of arteries that bring oxygen-rich blood to nourish the tissues. Another network of veins carries the blood away after the oxygen has been removed. In the case of the liver, the hepatic artery brings oxygen-rich blood and feeds it through tiny branches of the artery into each portal area. The blood courses along channels (sinusoids) dividing the cords of liver cells and provides the cells with oxygen. When the oxy-

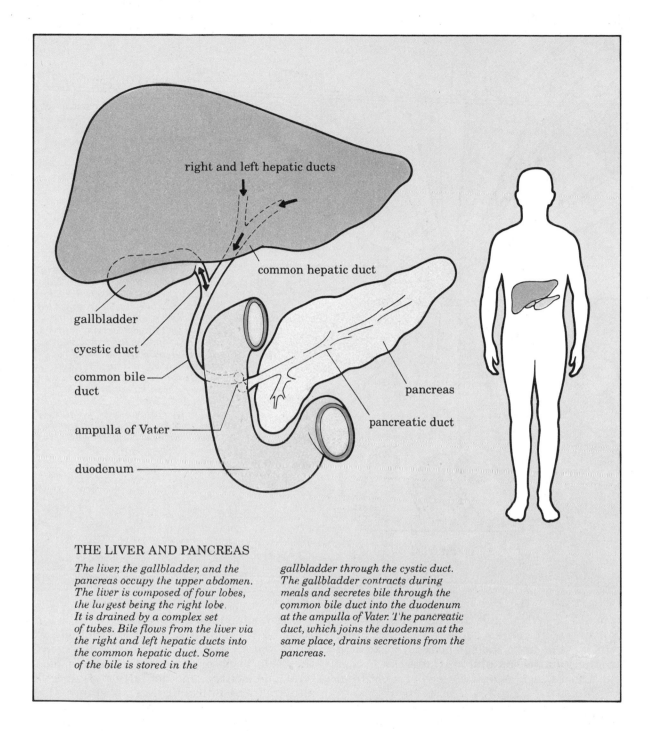

THE LIVER AND PANCREAS

The liver, the gallbladder, and the pancreas occupy the upper abdomen. The liver is composed of four lobes, the largest being the right lobe. It is drained by a complex set of tubes. Bile flows from the liver via the right and left hepatic ducts into the common hepatic duct. Some of the bile is stored in the

gallbladder through the cystic duct. The gallbladder contracts during meals and secretes bile through the common bile duct into the duodenum at the ampulla of Vater. The pancreatic duct, which joins the duodenum at the same place, drains secretions from the pancreas.

Labels in figure: right and left hepatic ducts; common hepatic duct; gallbladder; cycstic duct; common bile duct; ampulla of Vater; duodenum; pancreas; pancreatic duct

gen has been depleted, the blood passes into the central vein, then into a common hepatic vein and eventually back to the heart.

Meanwhile, another blood supply arrives via the portal vein and is fed into the liver cells via tiny branches. This blood carries less oxygen, but because the portal vein is formed from veins draining the intestinal tract, the blood is rich in nutrients. These are delivered to the liver cells for chemical manufacturing and processing, after which this blood, too, pours into the central vein of each lobule and is carried away through the hepatic vein for eventual transport back to the heart.

The main purpose of the second, or portal, blood supply is to allow the liver access to absorbed nutrients. But another important reason is that the nitrogen in the diet (mainly from proteins) is extremely toxic to the brain and other organs. If the blood leading from the intestinal tract were to bypass the liver, the result would be sleepiness, and eventually

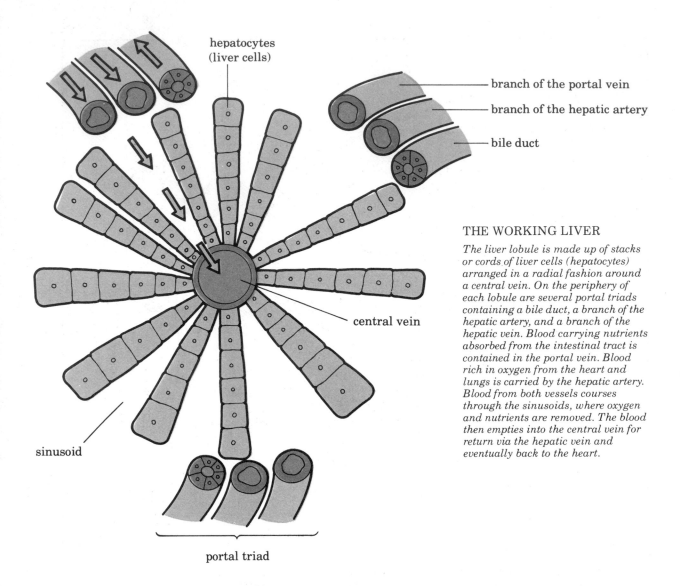

hepatocytes
(liver cells)

branch of the portal vein

branch of the hepatic artery

bile duct

central vein

sinusoid

portal triad

THE WORKING LIVER

*The liver lobule is made up of stacks
or cords of liver cells (hepatocytes)
arranged in a radial fashion around
a central vein. On the periphery of
each lobule are several portal triads
containing a bile duct, a branch of the
hepatic artery, and a branch of the
hepatic vein. Blood carrying nutrients
absorbed from the intestinal tract is
contained in the portal vein. Blood
rich in oxygen from the heart and
lungs is carried by the hepatic artery.
Blood from both vessels courses
through the sinusoids, where oxygen
and nutrients are removed. The blood
then empties into the central vein for
return via the hepatic vein and
eventually back to the heart.*

coma. The liver filters the nitrogen, rapidly converting it into a substance called urea, which is less toxic and can be readily excreted by the kidneys. Similarly, it detoxifies other substances such as medications brought from the intestinal tract by the portal vein.

In addition to building most of the body's needed protein, the liver also constructs the storage form of many energy sources (glycogen and fats, for example). The liver can also convert sugars into protein, protein into sugar, and fat into protein or sugar.

Perhaps the liver's best known product is bile. As noted earlier, bile plays a key role in fat breakdown and other digestive processes. The characteristics of bile are unmistakable: It is thick, orange-yellow, and bitter to taste.

Bile is manufactured in the liver cells and secreted via their tiny ducts. Its contents include water, salts, bile acids (the detergents that help to absorb fats in the diet), cholesterol, and lecithin, another fatty substance. It also contains bilirubin, the substance that gives it its characteristic yellow color. Bilirubin is produced principally from the hemoglobin of worn-out red blood cells, is changed chemically in the liver cells, then excreted via the bile. Many drugs and other toxic substances also are carried away via the bile. It is clear that bile has at least two purposes—digestion and excretion.

Bile finds its way into the digestive process through a complex system of tubes. After it is manufactured in the liver cells, it is secreted via the ducts in the portal system, which combine into gradually larger branches until they come together to form two major ducts, one from the right lobe and one from the left. These two merge into the common hepatic duct. A branch of this duct, the cystic duct, leads to the gallbladder, where bile is stored until needed. The main branch is called the common bile duct and enters the duodenum at the same point as the duct from the pancreas.

Since bile is produced continuously but meals are eaten only a few times a day, much of the bile production is diverted into the gallbladder. This flexible sac, about three inches long, is suspended from the underside of the liver. It modifies the bile chemically, concentrates it, and stores it. Much of the bile secreted during the night is shunted into the gallbladder. When you eat breakfast, especially if you eat eggs and butter, hormones cause the gallbladder walls to contract and expel bile to help digest your morning meal.

As can be testified by the millions of persons who have had their gallbladders removed, the organ is neither essential for life nor for normal digestive processes.

The Pancreas

The pancreas lies deep within the abdomen. It is so far toward the back that pain from this organ is usually reported as a combination of abdominal pain and backache. Just as the liver is a producer of many proteins, so too is the pancreas, primarily of the digestive proteins called enzymes. These include amylase (for breaking down starches), lipase (for breaking down fats), and a variety of enzymes that help to digest proteins. Curiously, it is proteins from the pancreas that are responsible for digestion of dietary proteins. The pancreas also secretes water and bicarbonate, which neutralizes the acid contents of the stomach. The main duct (pancreatic duct) joins the pancreas with the tubular intestinal tract and enters the duodenum at the same point as does the bile duct. This explains why diseases of the pancreas often affect the bile duct and diseases of the gallbladder or bile ducts cause inflammation of the pancreas (pancreatitis).

DIAGNOSING GASTRO-INTESTINAL DISORDERS

The years since 1960 have seen the development and widespread use of a great number of gastroenterological tests previously available in only a few research laboratories or not at all. Most of these tests cause a minimum of discomfort and can be well tolerated by the patient.

Endoscopy is a way of looking inside the body with the help of an optical device. The specialist in gastrointestinal disorders frequently uses an endoscope to examine the upper intestinal tract (the esophagus, stomach, and duodenum) or the colon. Upper intestinal endoscopy is sometimes referred to as esophagogastroduodenoscopy, a tongue-twisting term which merely designates the organs examined. Examination of the colon by means of endoscopy is called (more simply) colonoscopy.

The sighting device itself is a flexible tube composed of glass fibers that transmit high intensity light into the cavity to be examined and retransmit an image back to the eyepiece. Control knobs allow the scope's tip to be deflected for closer inspection. Attachments enable the operator to retrieve bits of tissue for microscopic examination. A cauterizing wire permits removal of polyps and other growths.

Because the modern endoscope is flexible and quite thin, passing it down the throat is not as uncomfortable as it might seem. The patient is usually given medication for relaxation and the back of the throat is anesthetized. He or she tips the head back, and the endoscope is carefully guided down the throat.

The bile ducts and pancreas can be examined by another form of upper endoscopy. This modification is called endoscopic retrograde cholangiopancreatography or ERCP. During the ERCP examination, a tiny tube, or catheter, is passed through the endoscope into ampulla of Vater, the area of the duodenum where the pancreatic duct and bile duct empty. A contrasting dye is injected through the catheter and X rays are taken. This is useful in diagnosing chronic inflammation of the pancreas, strictures and stones within the common bile duct, and certain tumors.

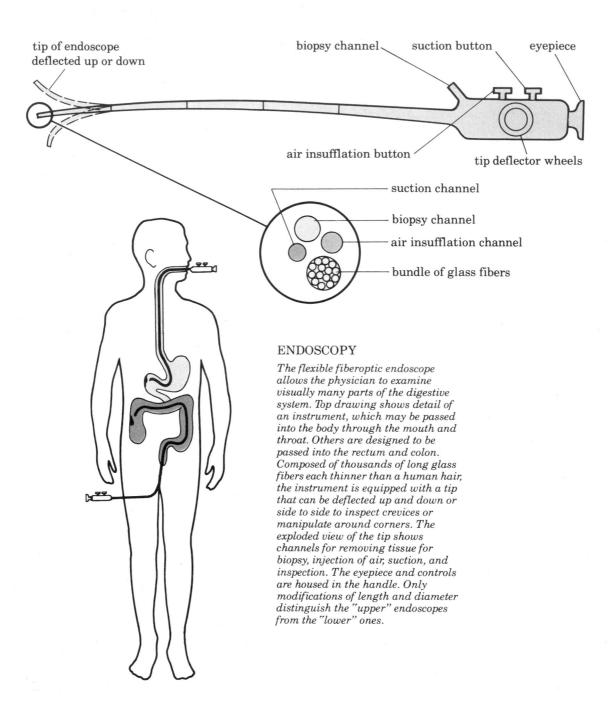

tip of endoscope deflected up or down

biopsy channel

suction button

eyepiece

air insufflation button

tip deflector wheels

suction channel

biopsy channel

air insufflation channel

bundle of glass fibers

ENDOSCOPY

The flexible fiberoptic endoscope allows the physician to examine visually many parts of the digestive system. Top drawing shows detail of an instrument, which may be passed into the body through the mouth and throat. Others are designed to be passed into the rectum and colon. Composed of thousands of long glass fibers each thinner than a human hair, the instrument is equipped with a tip that can be deflected up and down or side to side to inspect crevices or manipulate around corners. The exploded view of the tip shows channels for removing tissue for biopsy, injection of air, suction, and inspection. The eyepiece and controls are housed in the handle. Only modifications of length and diameter distinguish the "upper" endoscopes from the "lower" ones.

Peritoneoscopy (laparoscopy). Under certain circumstances, some of the intra-abdominal organs and the thin membrane covering them can be examined directly by means of laparoscopy, a procedure that stops short of a major abdominal operation. This is done by introducing a gas into the abdomen (usually carbon dioxide or nitrous oxide) to separate the abdominal wall from the internal organs. A small magnifying device can then be inserted into the abdominal cavity through a small incision to observe the liver, spleen, the outside of the stomach, portions of the small and large bowel, and the pelvic organs.

Laparoscopy is also used to diagnose and treat certain gynecological disorders. While examination by this means is not as complete as that obtained by exploratory surgery, it is much simpler and less expensive, and the patient can ordinarily resume normal activity a day afterwards. It is usually done under local anesthesia and the incision is about one inch long.

Esophageal motility study. By passing a suitable narrow tube into the esophagus, pressure waves can be recorded. This allows for the diagnosis of certain disorders of the esophagus which the examining physician is unable to evaluate by any other means.

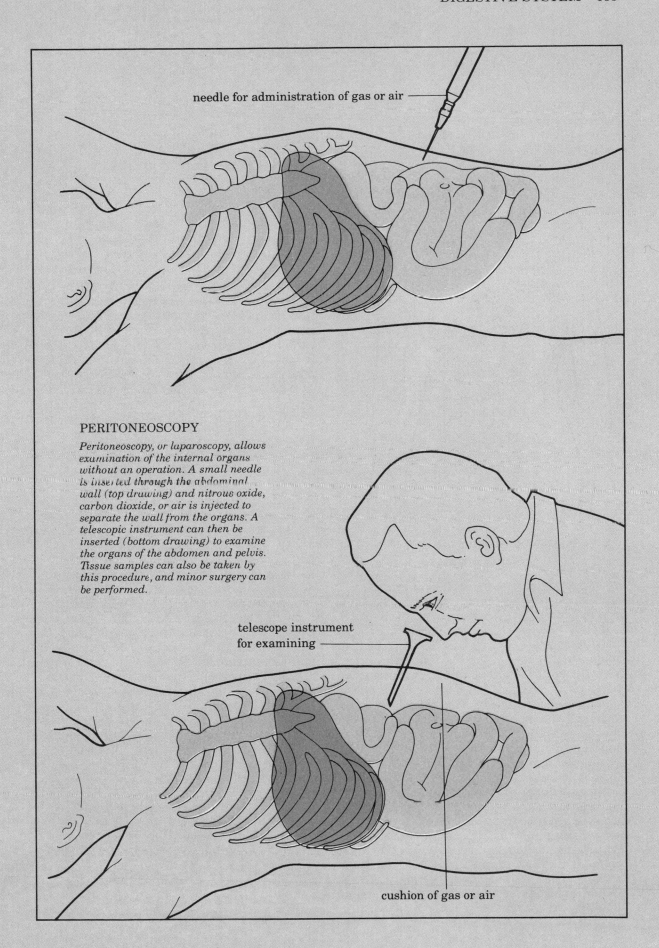

needle for administration of gas or air

PERITONEOSCOPY

Peritoneoscopy, or laparoscopy, allows examination of the internal organs without an operation. A small needle is inserted through the abdominal wall (top drawing) and nitrous oxide, carbon dioxide, or air is injected to separate the wall from the organs. A telescopic instrument can then be inserted (bottom drawing) to examine the organs of the abdomen and pelvis. Tissue samples can also be taken by this procedure, and minor surgery can be performed.

telescope instrument for examining

cushion of gas or air

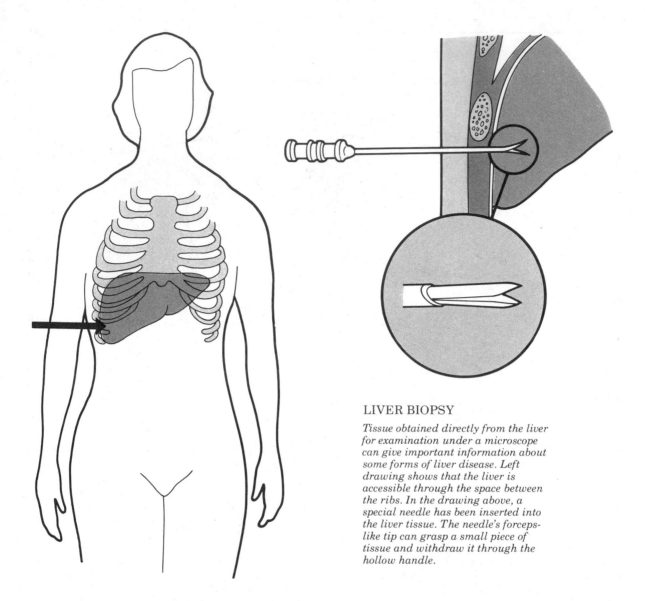

LIVER BIOPSY

Tissue obtained directly from the liver for examination under a microscope can give important information about some forms of liver disease. Left drawing shows that the liver is accessible through the space between the ribs. In the drawing above, a special needle has been inserted into the liver tissue. The needle's forceps-like tip can grasp a small piece of tissue and withdraw it through the hollow handle.

Liver biopsy. Obtaining a small fragment of tissue for biopsy is frequently important in diagnosing disorders of the liver. The tissue usually can be easily obtained by passing an extremely fine needle through the skin on the right side of the body. With the skin anesthetized, this is neither a difficult nor an unduly painful procedure. The most significant but uncommon complication is bleeding. As with laparoscopy, the chief value of the procedure is its relative simplicity.

Sigmoidoscopy (proctoscopy). This examination is another endoscopic procedure, but uses a rigid tube introduced into the rectum to allow inspection of the lining cells of the rectosigmoid area, the lower 10 inches of the colon. This is a common site for polyps and tumors. In some hospitals, the rigid tube is being replaced or complemented by a flexible device that resembles a short colonoscope.

Either way, discomfort is minimal, and the examination can be performed quickly. Its main value is to allow inspection of an area of relatively frequent disease easily and efficiently. Tissue for biopsies may be obtained by sigmoidoscopy and polyps are often removed.

Small bowel biopsy. In this test, a small catheter or flexible tube is swallowed by the patient and advanced through the esophagus, stomach, and duodenum until the tip reaches a suitable site for biopsy. The tube's position can be watched by use of a fluoroscope. Small bowel mucosal tissue is easily obtained without pain to the patient, and the tube is then withdrawn. Duodenal fluid may also be collected for examination for certain parasites.

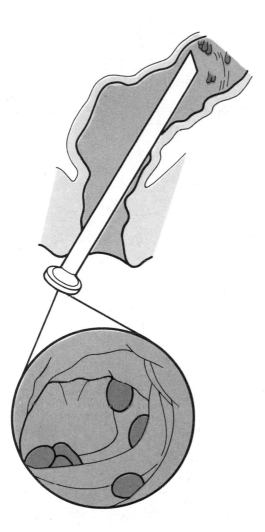

Proctoscopy, or sigmoidoscopy, allows direct examination of the inner lining of the lower portion of the large intestine. Drawing below locates the rectum and sigmoid colon, which can be seen with the instrument. The drawing at left shows the proctoscope in place and the exploded view reveals intestinal polyps as seen by the examiner. Because a large percentage of cancers develop in the last few inches of the colon, protoscopic examination can be valuable in detecting them before symptoms arise.

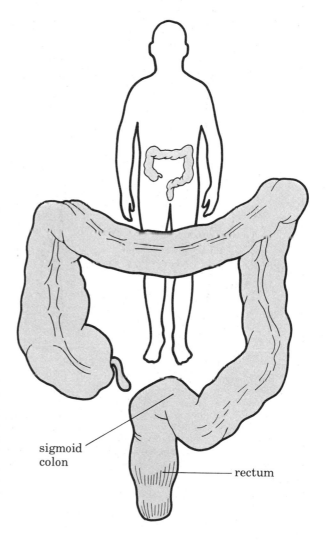

sigmoid colon

rectum

Gastric analysis. In certain situations, it is important to know the amount of acid output by the stomach. Passing a catheter into the stomach and collecting fluid allows for this measurement. The patient fasts from midnight the night before, and the test is usually performed between 8 a.m. and 10 a.m. Certain medications may be given intramuscularly or intravenously to stimulate acid production.

DISEASES OF THE

DIGESTIVE SYSTEM

In a system as lengthy and as complex as the digestive tract, things obviously can go wrong in many places and many ways. Gastrointestinal disorders range from the minor bellyache to much more serious complaints. The usual way to categorize them is from top to bottom: from mouth to colon, plus the solid organs. However, disorders within the mouth, even though they affect the digestive system, are usually treated by other specialists (see chapter 18, "The Teeth and Oral Health," and chapter 13, "The Ear, Nose, and Throat").

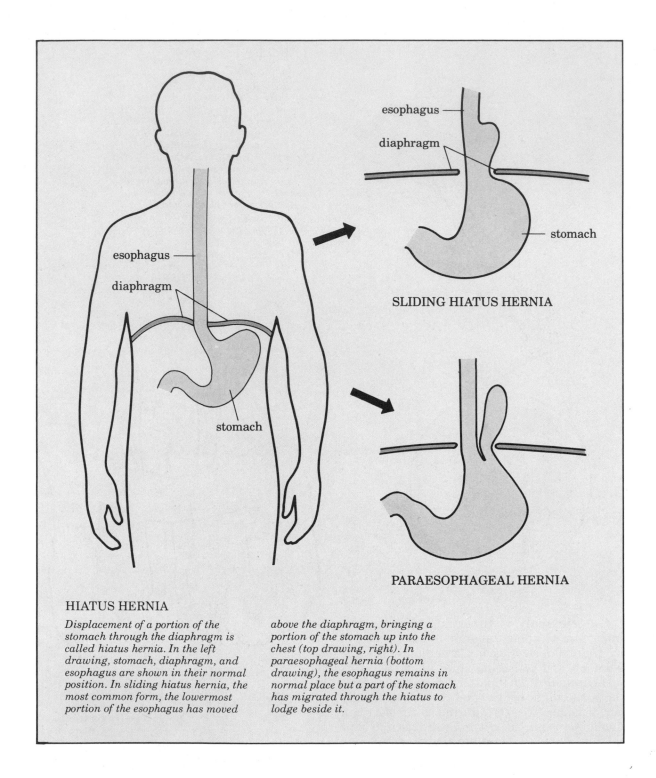

SLIDING HIATUS HERNIA

PARAESOPHAGEAL HERNIA

HIATUS HERNIA

Displacement of a portion of the stomach through the diaphragm is called hiatus hernia. In the left drawing, stomach, diaphragm, and esophagus are shown in their normal position. In sliding hiatus hernia, the most common form, the lowermost portion of the esophagus has moved above the diaphragm, bringing a portion of the stomach up into the chest (top drawing, right). In paraesophageal hernia (bottom drawing), the esophagus remains in normal place but a part of the stomach has migrated through the hiatus to lodge beside it.

The Esophagus

Hiatus hernia is common. Ordinarily the lowest portion of the esophagus (the area of the lower esophageal sphincter) is located at the point where the esophagus passes through the diaphragm. The opening that permits this passage is called the diaphragmatic hiatus. However, in many people the lower esophagus is not fixed at the diaphragmatic level but may rise considerably above the hiatus. Of course, when this happens, the uppermost portion of the stomach is not located below the diaphragm, but is pulled above it. This is called a hiatus hernia. (Hernia is the term applied when any organ or part of an organ protrudes

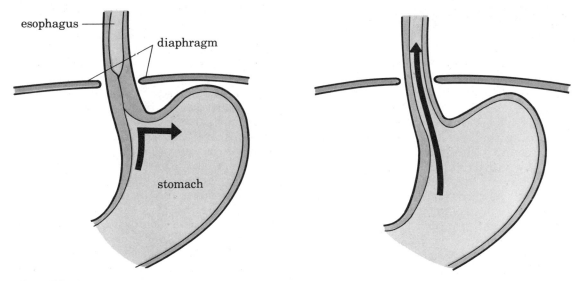

esophagus

diaphragm

stomach

HEARTBURN

Reflux esophagitis, which is commonly known as heartburn, occurs because a weakened esophageal sphincter muscle cannot close sufficiently to prevent the stomach's contents from flowing back into the esophagus. At *left, the normal closed channel prevents backflow from the stomach. At right, acid from the stomach easily gains entry into the esophagus, where it causes inflammation and burning.*

through the wall of the cavity that normally contains it.)

In some people the displacement is quite small. It may come and go depending on body position, pressure on the abdominal wall, food within the stomach, and other factors. A hiatus hernia that moves is called a sliding hiatus hernia.

A few people have a different type of hiatus hernia. For them, the lower esophageal sphincter is at the level of the diaphragmatic hiatus. However, a portion of the stomach slips up beside the esophagus, through the diaphragmatic hiatus, and into the chest. This type of hernia is called a paraesophageal hiatus hernia. An extreme and rare form of paraesophageal hiatus hernia occurs when most or even all of the stomach slides up alongside the esophagus. This is referred to as an intrathoracic stomach and can be a dangerous condition.

What symptoms are caused by a typical sliding hiatus hernia? Surprisingly, most experts agree that few if any symptoms are produced by the hernia's mere existence. In past years the simple diagnosis of a sliding hiatus hernia was considered sufficient to warrant surgery. This is no longer felt necessary. It is true that many people with a sliding hiatus hernia com-

plain of heartburn (pyrosis). However, it is now clear that heartburn is caused not by hernia but by reflux into the esophagus of the stomach's contents, including potent hydrochloric acid. The reflux rather than the hernia is the cause of the symptoms. Moreover, not all patients with a hiatus hernia experience reflux, and not all patients who experience reflux (heartburn) have a hiatus hernia. Attributing heartburn to a sliding hiatus hernia is a little like blaming bad weather on the weatherman.

Reflux esophagitis is the technical name of the heartburn-causing condition described above. Heartburn occurs because the enzyme pepsin and hydrochloric acid secreted by the stomach irritate the lining cells of the esophagus. When reflux bathes the esophagus in acid, most people feel a hot, burning sensation behind the breastbone. But acid is not the only cause of heartburn. A patient whose stomach has been surgically removed also may experience it, presumably due to reflux of bile and other contents of the small intestine. Nevertheless, acid and pepsin are the usual offenders, so the condition is sometimes referred to as peptic esophagitis.

The burning sensation is sometimes accompanied by a hot, sour liquid in the back of the throat (water brash) and by chest pain. As might be expected, reflux into the esophagus is more likely to occur while lying down or bending over, when gravity, which ordinarily promotes drainage from the esophagus into the stomach, no longer exerts that influence. Increased abdominal pressure, either because of overweight or the use of a tight belt or girdle, also helps to promote reflux.

Why don't we all have reflux into the esophagus when we lie down? Fortunately, the lower esophageal sphincter ordinarily protects us, keeping the lower end of the esophagus closed despite high intra-abdominal pressure. Patients who do suffer from reflux esophagitis usually have a weakened lower esophageal sphincter. Lowered pressure within the sphincter can be shown clearly by an esophageal motility study. Certain chemicals contained in medicines or foodstuffs also may reduce pressure in the sphincter. Chocolate, coffee, cola drinks, tobacco, and certain drugs all may make reflux esophagitis symptoms worse.

The diagnosis of reflux esophagitis can often be made simply on the basis of characteristic symptoms. The physical examination provides no clue to the diagnosis. Barium X rays may demonstrate reflux when pressure is exerted on the abdominal wall. Most commonly, however, when additional tests are necessary the doctor will perform esophagoscopy to look for inflammatory changes in the lower esophagus and to take biopsies for confirmation. It is also possible to insert into the esophagus a special tube with a probe at the tip which can detect the presence of acid in the esophagus. This is probably the most sensitive way of making the diagnosis.

Treatment of reflux esophagitis is geared to the severity of symptoms. Practically everyone suffers from heartburn occasionally. The most effective treatment in most cases is simply to recognize and eliminate the sources that trigger attacks. The overweight patient is encouraged to lose weight, the smoker is advised to give up tobacco; chocolate is discontinued, along with cola drinks, coffee, and tea. Because symptoms often become worse soon after going to bed, the person is urged to elevate the head of the bed with blocks, not to eat large meals, and to eliminate bedtime snacks. Men are encouraged to wear suspenders instead of tight belts and women advised to avoid girdles.

Antacids usually provide temporary relief. Additional drugs are occasionally necessary. But some patients fail to benefit from any of these treatments and are candidates for surgical correction of the reflux problem. Operations to correct reflux esophagitis are commonly referred to as hiatus hernia repair operations (see chapter 31, "Understanding Your Operation"), which only adds to the confusion about the two conditions. In fact, the principle of the operations performed today is to strengthen the lower sphincter. This usually involves bringing the lower esophageal sphincter down into the diaphragmatic hiatus, but this is not always necessary.

Stricture is a localized area of narrowing. Within the esophagus, strictures can occur anywhere. Most often, however, narrowing occurs in the lower esophageal area and stems from longstanding inflammation caused by reflux esophagitis. As one might expect, the principal symptom of a stricture is a feeling that food is sticking in the throat. Indeed, many people can point to the exact location of the stricture. Precise diagnosis is usually made by a combination of X ray and esophagoscopy. Aside from their troublesome symptoms, strictures are a major concern because the physician must always be on guard to distinguish a benign peptic stricture from a narrowing caused by a cancer within the esophagus. That is why most physicians think it is important to perform a biopsy before treating most strictures.

The treatment of benign esophageal strictures is most often to enlarge or dilate the narrowed area. A variety of dilators are available. The most common are mercury-filled rubber tubes that are introduced in sequence, beginning with a small diameter tube and gradually progressing to larger and larger tubes. Occasionally dilation must be done with the patient in the operating room and under general anesthesia, but most often it can be accomplished with the patient awake. After dilation, the stricture normally remains open. However, repeated dilations may be necessary if the stricture recurs.

Uncommonly, surgical treatment of a stricture may be necessary. It is important to treat the underlying cause for a stricture, such as reflux esophagitis.

Esophageal varices, or dilated veins in the esophagus, resemble varicose veins in the legs. When they appear in the lower esophagus they are a major threat because they may bleed massively and repeatedly.

Esophageal varices usually occur because of high pressure in the portal vein leading to the liver, most commonly caused by advanced liver disease (cirrhosis).

Esophageal varices produce no symptoms until they bleed, but are sometimes found before bleeding at the time of an upper gastrointestinal X ray or during endoscopy. The treatment of bleeding varices includes immediate hospitalization, blood transfusions, attempts to stop the bleeding by medication and by directly plugging up the lower esophagus with a balloon (esophageal tamponade). Sometimes a doctor using an endoscope can inject certain medicines directly into the area of bleeding to cause the blood to clot. After the bleeding has stopped and the patient has been stabilized, an operation is often recommended to prevent further bleeding. These operations usually succeed in preventing further bleeding episodes, but postoperative complications can be serious, particularly mental confusion (hepatic encephalopathy). Also, many patients have such severe underlying liver disease that surgery is impossible.

Tumors. Most tumors of the esophagus are malignant. The most common benign tumor of the esophagus is called a leiomyoma, a tumor of smooth muscle that usually causes no symptoms and is discovered by accident.

Malignant tumors of the esophagus constitute about four percent of all fatal cancers in humans. Thus, although not exactly rare, esophageal cancers fortunately are uncommon. Their incidence follows an odd pattern. Esophageal cancer is more common in industrial cities than in rural areas. Whether this represents differences in genetic or environmental factors, such as diet, is unknown. Use of cigarettes and alcohol is known to be associated with an increased likelihood of esophageal cancer as well. About three times as many men as women suffer from esophageal cancer. They are generally between the ages of 55 and 65.

The most frequent symptoms of cancer of the esophagus are weight loss and swallowing difficulty (dysphagia). Such symptoms, of course, are not limited to cancer. The patient with a benign stricture may have them, too. However, in the case of a stricture, the individual usually has a long history of heartburn accompanied by gradually worsening swallowing difficulty. The patient with esophageal cancer, on the other hand, most often has less than a six-month history of food sticking, and often there has been no background of severe heartburn at all.

X ray of the esophagus may be the key to diagnosis but it is confirmed by a biopsy during esophagoscopy. Cancers can occur anywhere in the esophagus, and treatment depends on their location. Cancers in the upper one-third of the esophagus are so close to other vital structures that surgery is rarely feasible. When the cancer involves the lower two-thirds of the esophagus and there is no evidence that it is widespread, surgery is most often undertaken, although radiation therapy may be used. Unfortunately, the odds are poor for long-term survival after any form of therapy.

Motor Disturbances of the Esophagus

Motor disturbances of the esophagus occur either when the muscle becomes unable to perform its function (or performs it in irregular fashion) or when the nerves supplying the muscles are abnormal in some way.

Achalasia is an unusual disorder characterized by failure of the lower esophageal sphincter muscles to relax. Normally, relaxation occurs during swallowing. In achalasia, however, not only is the pressure within the lower esophageal sphincter region high, but relaxation does not occur. The sphincter muscles may also thicken.

Achalasia usually is slowly progressive. Earliest symptoms are vague, often nothing more dramatic than just slowness in eating. Gradually, the esophagus above the lower esophageal sphincter often dilates, sometimes to enormous proportions. Late in the course of the disease the patient may have difficulty swallowing both liquids and solids, or may complain of regurgitation, especially when lying down or bending over. Occasionally, the esophageal contents spill backwards into the respiratory tract and the patient may have a variety of lung complaints such as wheezing, asthma, or recurrent pneumonia. X ray of the esophagus is often highly characteristic. Usually, endoscopy is performed to establish that no cancer is present.

Two forms of treatment are available for achalasia. The first is called pneumatic dilatation. A deflated balloon is placed in the narrowed esophagus, and then it is suddenly inflated under pressure, separating the thickened muscles. The other treatment is to separate the muscles surgically. There may be a higher risk of cancer in persons with long-standing, untreated achalasia.

Scleroderma is a disease of the collagen tissues, which most commonly causes the skin to take on a stiff, thick, leathery appearance (see chapter 15, "Arthritis and Related Diseases"). The intestinal tract is often involved, although not necessarily sufficiently to produce symptoms. In the esophagus, the disease may attack the muscles of the lower esophageal sphincter, so that they cannot tighten properly. Accordingly, pressures are low and the barrier to reflux of gastric contents is weakened, causing heartburn. The principal symptoms are those of severe reflux esophagitis. Treatment of the symptoms is the same as for reflux esophagitis. Scleroderma itself may be slowly progressive, and does not respond well to treatment.

Esophageal spasm is a motor abnormality that results in multiple high-pressure waves being generated at the same time in many different portions of the esophagus. Instead of the waves progressing in an orderly way from top to bottom, the entire esophagus is in spasm. The symptoms are often provoked by drinking very hot or very cold liquids. There is severe chest pain which closely mimics that of a heart attack. Further confusion may exist between esophageal spasm and heart disease because the pain due to esophageal spasm is often improved by nitroglycerin, the same drug that reduces heart pain. At times a gastroenterologist sees a patient referred by a cardiologist who has discovered normal coronary arteries in a patient complaining of severe chest pain. The treatment is to avoid substances that bring on spasm. Nitroglycerin or Isordil® may be prescribed as well. Surgery is rarely necessary.

Esophageal diverticulum is an outpouching of the esophagus. One type may result from repeated forceful contractions of the esophagus, so-called pulsion diverticulum. When these contractions occur the doctor often will look for an associated motor abnormality.

Inflammation of organs near the esophagus may push the esophagus out of normal position and cause a so-called traction diverticulum. Esophageal diverticula usually require no treatment, but if they produce symptoms, they may require surgical removal. Correction of the underlying motor abnormality, if one exists, is often undertaken at the same time.

Webs are congenital, membranous bands that partially block the esophagus. Symptoms may not occur until adulthood when food begins to stick in the throat. Webs usually are diagnosed by X rays and are easily treated by dilating the esophagus.

Esophageal atresia is a congenital failure of a portion of the esophagus to develop normally. It is always diagnosed in childhood, usually within the first hours or days of life. Atretic infants have a thread of fibrous tissue connecting normal portions of the esophagus, often with additional connections between esophagus and windpipe. Surgery usually brings good results.

The Stomach and Duodenum

Gastritis simply means inflammation of the stomach. There may or may not be pain associated with it. It is important to distinguish between acute gastritis and chronic gastritis. Acute gastritis is commonly caused by ingestion of substances that break down the protective barriers of the stomach. Aspirin and alcohol are perhaps the most common offenders. A number of other medications, particularly those taken for arthritis and related conditions, can act as gastric irritants. Tobacco and possibly coffee may also contribute.

Acute gastritis may cause no symptoms, but when it does it actually causes a burning, gnawing sensation in the upper abdomen. Since this pain is promptly relieved by antacids, milk, or food, it is often confused with ulcer disease. Occasionally, the degree of inflammation is so intense that lining cells of the stomach are damaged and there may be erosions or even hemorrhage. The person may then vomit blood (hematemesis) or pass it in the stool (melena). The diagnosis is often made solely on the basis of history, sometimes accompanied by gastroscopic inspection of the stomach. Interestingly, X-ray examination of the stomach often will not disclose gastritis.

Treatment of acute gastritis rests primarily on recognizing and avoiding precipitating causes. Antacids or drugs to inhibit acid production also may be prescribed. The outlook is good, although some people bleed profusely and even require surgery.

Chronic gastritis usually produces no symptoms. The most common type of chronic gastritis is chronic atrophic gastritis. In this condition, the normal furrows and ridges of the stomach are absent, with thinning of the membranes lining the stomach. The stomach may be unable to produce intrinsic factor, a substance essential for the normal absorption of vitamin B_{12} (see page 458). Over a long period the body's stores of B_{12} may be depleted and a potentially serious form of anemia called pernicious anemia may occur. However, if recognized, pernicious anemia can be treated satisfactorily (see chapter 6, "The Blood"). Patients with chronic atrophic gastritis are not able to secrete acid normally, and thus are less likely to suffer from ulcer disease.

A much less common form of chronic gastritis is chronic hypertrophic gastritis. In this condition, the folds in the stomach are much more prominent than usual. There may be secretion of a protein-rich fluid into the stomach. Occasionally, excess acid is produced and ulcer disease may result.

Patients with chronic gastritis often require no treatment. Pernicious anemia may be treated with injections of vitamin B_{12}. If the hypertrophic gastritis is associated with protein loss or with ulceration, surgery is sometimes necessary.

Peptic ulcers. Ulcers are miniature excavations in the mucus membrane. They resemble the divot a Sunday golfer carves in the fairway. Why ulcers develop is not known, despite a great deal of research. People whose stomachs cannot produce hydrochloric acid—those with chronic atrophic gastritis, for instance—never have typical ulcers, so attention has been focused on a possible link between acid and ulcers. However, when acid is present in the stomach, the powerful enzyme pepsin is present, too, so pepsin may be just as important in ulcer production. Possibly, ulcers result when there is a breakdown of the natural defense mechanisms that balance the destructive potential of acid and pepsin. (Remember, almost everyone produces acid and pepsin, yet only a few people get ulcers.) Mucus and other substances may play a major role in preventing ulcers, too.

Peptic ulcers most often occur in the stomach (gastric ulcers) or duodenum (duodenal ulcers). About 80 percent of all ulcers are duodenal. On the average, patients with gastric ulcers produce less acid than normal people, and those with duodenal ulcers produce more acid. Agents incriminated in the formation of gastric ulcers include aspirin and

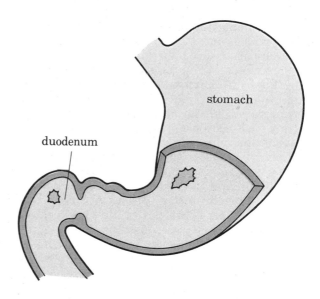

ULCERS

Peptic ulcers may occur in the stomach, duodenum, or esophagus. Above, a gastric ulcer is shown in the stomach wall and a duodenal ulcer in a common location in the wall of the duodenum. Ulcers may erode the stomach or duodenal wall to various depths. Perforation enables contents to seep into the abdominal cavity.

tobacco. A multitude of agents such as cortisone, alcohol, indomethacin, phenylbutazone, and others have been blamed for the formation of gastric ulcers although some doubt remains as to their role. Folklore portrays the tense, hard-driving executive as ulcer-prone, but the link between personality and ulcers has been largely discredited.

Symptoms produced by peptic ulcers, whether in the stomach or duodenum, are burning, gnawing, upper abdominal pain. The pain usually gets worse during fasting and improves after snacks or meals. It is also promptly relieved by antacids. The symptoms are usually periodic, with weeks or months of no symptoms interspersed with symptomatic periods. Some patients are awakened by pain in the night. Symptoms vary from patient to patient. Those with gastric ulcers are more likely to have unusual symptoms than those with duodenal ulcers.

Occasionally, patients first are made aware of an ulcer by the complications. The major complications are bleeding, intestinal obstruction (which will produce profuse vomiting), perforation (causing sudden, severe abdominal pain with nausea and vomiting), or penetration of the ulcer into a nearby structure such as the pancreas (producing severe abdominal pain, often back pain as well).

The diagnosis of ulcers often can be made on the basis of a history and a known tendency for the individual to harbor ulcers. Ulcer disease tends to be chronic. This does not mean that the same ulcer is present in the same location over a long period of time, but that the individual is prone to develop an ulcer which heals, only to have a new ulcer form nearby. When the history is not characteristic, an upper gastrointestinal X ray is performed. This usually will reveal about 90 percent of peptic ulcers. If the X ray is negative despite a convincing history or if the X ray is difficult to interpret, another means of diagnosing an ulcer is esophagogastroduodenoscopy (see page 467). In some hospitals this procedure has replaced upper gastrointestinal X rays for diagnosis of ulcer disease.

The treatment of peptic ulcer disease involves the elimination of agents thought to be important in the formation of ulcers. Avoidance of coffee, smoking, alcohol, and aspirin is usually recommended. The use of bland diets, although still widespread, does not have proven value. It is prudent to avoid foods that regularly produce gastric disturbances, but lists of prohibited foods should be individualized. Additional measures for control of ulcer disease include the use of regular antacids. Antacids act by neutralizing (buffering) acid produced in the stomach. In addition to lowering the acid content this also inactivates the enzyme pepsin.

In the late 1970s a new class of drug for the treatment of ulcer disease was introduced. Cimetidine (Tagamet®) was the first compound available in this class. These drugs are different from antacids because they do not buffer acids. Instead they turn off the acid-producing capability within the cells in the stomach. Cimetidine is potent and has been found to be remarkably free of serious side effects. It is of interest, however, that this class of drugs has not been shown to be superior to the regular use of a strong liquid antacid. The main advantage of cimetidine lies in its convenience. It is easier to remember to take a single pill four times a day rather than take antacids according to a complex schedule.

Follow-up of ulcer treatment is important. Ulcers in the duodenum are virtually always benign. Once in a while, however, ulcers in the stomach are not due to peptic ulcer disease but are ulcerations within a cancer. For this reason, it is important to see that all gastric ulcers heal completely to be sure that they are not cancerous. This healing can be assessed by X rays or gastroscopy. Many specialists prefer to use gastroscopy in all cases of gastric ulcers so that biopsy material may be obtained. Whichever method is used, the important thing is that all gastric ulcers must heal within a certain time. If not, surgery probably will be necessary.

Surgery in ulcer disease. There appears to have been a decline in the incidence and severity of ulcer disease over the past 50 years. Nevertheless, ulcer surgery is often necessary. A number of operations have been devised. The fact that there are several procedures suggests that none is perfect.

Perhaps the most common operation for duodenal ulcer is cutting the vagus nerve (vagotomy). This nerve regulates acid flow in the stomach, so the operation reduces the acid-producing potential. However, the operation also reduces normal motor activity, so it is often necessary to combine the vagotomy with pyloroplasty, a procedure to promote drainage from the stomach. The combination is frequently referred to as "V and P." More recently it has been discovered that if only certain branches of the vagus nerve are cut, the gastric emptying function can be retained and pyloroplasty is not necessary. This is called a superselective vagotomy. Other operations include the removal of a portion of the stomach, sometimes combined with vagotomy. Other options may be employed under special circumstances.

Post-gastrectomy syndromes. Despite medical treatment, many persons require surgery for gastric or duodenal ulcers. Of these, about 10 percent develop post-surgical problems. Consequently, surgeons are searching for improved ulcer operations that will prevent recurrent ulcers while minimizing side effects.

A common complaint of patients who have had a portion of the stomach removed is an overly full sensation after meals. The stuffed feeling generally diminishes with time.

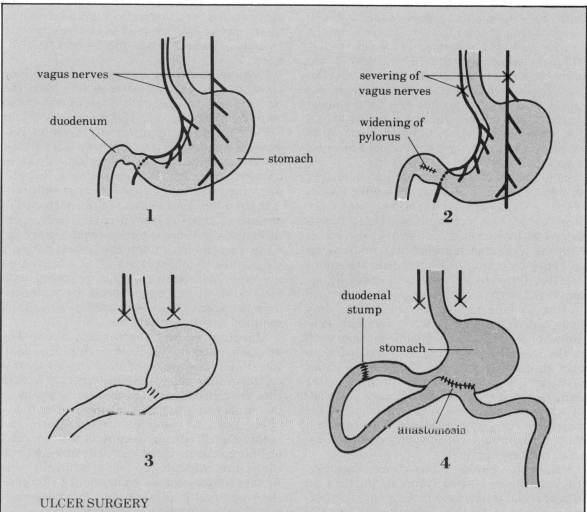

vagus nerves

duodenum

stomach

1

severing of
vagus nerves

widening of
pylorus

2

3

duodenal
stump

stomach

anastomosis

4

ULCER SURGERY

Various operations are performed for treatment of peptic ulcers. First drawing shows the normal relationship of the stomach and duodenum, and the anterior and posterior vagus nerves, whose branches to the stomach stimulate secretion of acid and pepsin. An operation called vagotomy and pyloroplasty, referred to as V and P (second drawing), is sometimes performed to sever the vagus nerves and reduce secretion of acid and pepsin. Because the operation sometimes slows emptying of the stomach, the pylorus opening may be widened at the same time to speed drainage. No portion of the stomach is removed. In partial gastrectomy (third drawing) the antrum of the stomach is removed and the stomach remnant sewed directly to the duodenum. The vagus nerves may be severed at the same time. In another type of partial gastrectomy (fourth drawing), the antrum is removed and the stomach remnant is sewed to a new opening created in the small intestine, usually in the jejunum. The duodenum stump is sewed closed. The vagus nerves usually are severed in this variation.

However, after surgery to sever the nerves controlling the motor activity of the stomach, the emptying of solid foods from the stomach may be slowed. Collections of food particles, called bezoars, may form. These may cause nausea or vomiting, or completely obstruct the stomach, so that additional surgery is required. Bezoars sometimes can be managed successfully, however, by drugs aimed at enhancing their digestion. Other drugs help to restore normal activity of the stomach muscles in such patients.

Some patients may complain following surgery of abdominal symptoms after meals, including abdominal bloating, sweating, nausea, diarrhea, and rapid heartbeat. Physicians refer to this constellation of symptoms as dumping syndrome. It probably stems from the too rapid emptying of liquids into the small intestine from the stomach and resulting attempts of the small intestine to dilute the food substances delivered. Hormonal changes may result as well. Persons with dumping syndrome must reduce fluid consumption with meals. Restriction of carbohydrates (particularly simple sugars) may help. Eating small meals or lying down 15 to 20 minutes after eating also may be of benefit. Occasionally, additional surgery needs to be considered if the symptoms become intolerable. For most patients the symptoms of dumping syndrome resolve spontaneously.

Stomach cancer has been declining gradually in the United States during the past 50 years, and it now accounts for only five percent of cancer deaths. The reasons are not clear, but speculation is that it may be related to changes in the American diet. The incidence remains high in a number of other countries, notably Japan, Austria, and nations of Eastern Europe. Immigrants from these countries and their first-generation descendants have more stomach cancer than other Americans, indicating that other factors, including genetics, play a part.

Malignancies of the stomach are of several types. The most common symptoms are upper abdominal pain, loss of appetite, frequent fatigue, and weight loss. A physical examination may reveal a tumorous mass in the upper abdomen or in adjacent organs such as the liver. An upper gastrointestinal X ray often discloses the tumor. Gastroscopy can confirm its presence and obtain biopsy tissue for microscopic examination. Surgery can control bleeding, obstruction, and relieve pain, but the cure rate is low. Even when the surgeon has removed all visible tumor, the likelihood of distant spread or recurrence remains. X-ray treatment is ineffective. Chemotherapy with special anticancer drugs may be beneficial for a few.

Pyloric stenosis, narrowing of the pyloric opening, may be congenital or acquired. The congenital form is usually seen in male newborns (see chapter 27, "Taking Care of Your Child"). Affected infants may vomit in projectile spurts, and often a hard mass can be felt in the upper abdomen. The pylorus must be opened surgically. The operation is usually performed within the first few weeks of life.

In the adult, the pylorus is often narrowed as a result of scarring from prolonged, recurrent ulcer disease. Vomiting and weight loss are the most prominent symptoms. Most patients have a history of repeated ulcer attacks over the years. Although vigorous treatment with ulcer medications may reopen the narrowed area in some persons, surgery is usually required within a short time.

Marginal ulcer (anastomotic ulcer). The area where the stomach is sewn to the small intestine in the course of an ulcer operation is called an anastomosis. New ulcers may form in this area. Because of the deformity produced by surgery, the upper gastrointestinal X ray often fails to disclose these ulcers and esophagogastroduodenoscopy is the best way of finding them. Until recently, marginal ulcers were difficult to treat medically and further surgery was often necessary. However, the drug cimetidine (see page 478) may permit more successful medical treatment.

THE LIVER

Although the liver is the largest organ inside the body, its importance does not lie in its size. Indeed many persons have survived after more than half of the liver has been removed. However, total breakdown of the liver is fatal. Experimental animals lapse into coma within a few hours after its removal. Moreover, the liver's functions are so myriad that disorders of the liver may manifest themselves in all parts of the body.

Jaundice

Jaundice is caused by abnormal accumulation of the pigment bilirubin (see page 466) in the blood and body tissues. This yellow-brown substance, which is produced from breakdown of old blood cells, is metabolized by the liver and excreted into the bile to be passed out of the body via the intestinal tract. Bacterial action on bilirubin in the gut is what gives the stool its normal brown color. When bilirubin cannot be passed off by the normal means, it accumulates in the liver and tissues throughout the body. The stool may become very pale, almost colorless, and a yellowish cast develops in the skin and in the whites of the eyes. This is why jaundice used to be referred to as "yellow jaundice."

Jaundice commonly occurs when a blockage of the bile duct causes a backup of bile and thus of bilirubin. But there are other causes as well. A severely inflamed or damaged liver may not be able to process the bilirubin delivered to it. Or production of bilirubin by the rapid destruction of red blood cells may become excessive, and the capacity of the liver may be overwhelmed. In examining a jaundiced patient the doctor must decide whether the patient has excess bilirubin production (hemolysis of red blood cells), defective metabolism of the bilirubin within the liver (seen in hepatitis), or defective flow of bile because of a bile-duct blockage. It is sometimes easy to distinguish between these possibilities, but in about 15 to 20 percent of the cases it is quite difficult.

Doctors often classify jaundice into two types: surgical jaundice (caused by blockage of the bile ducts) or medical jaundice (hemolysis, hepatitis, etc.). Persons with surgical jaundice usually are relieved of their symptoms promptly by surgery, but those with medical jaundice will not benefit from (and may be harmed by) an operation. Recently it has become considerably easier to look at bile ducts to establish whether they are blocked without resorting to surgery. Endoscopy has provided us with a test called endoscopic retrograde cholangiopancreatography (ERCP) (see page 467). An endoscope is passed into the duodenum to the area where the bile ducts and pancreatic duct enter the duodenum. A small catheter or flexible tube is inserted into this opening (called the ampulla of Vater) and dye is injected into the ducts. When successful, this procedure clearly discloses the bile ducts and can show the nature of any obstruction. Ultrasound waves also can be used to examine obstructed ducts, as can a CAT scanner (see chapter 32, "X Rays and Radiology"). Finally, the bile ducts may be examined by inserting a very thin needle through the skin into the liver until a bile duct is punctured, after which dye is injected. These tests ordinarily are not all ordered simultaneously for a single patient, but are options.

Hepatitis

Hepatitis means inflammation of the liver tissue, which may be caused by toxins, drugs, radiation, or most commonly, viral infection (see chapter 28, "Infectious Diseases"). The illness may occur in epidemic form, and the culprit is usually the so-called hepatitis A virus. Victims are often extremely ill, but the disease rarely causes severe destruction of the liver, liver failure, or the degenerative changes of cirrhosis. It is rarely, if ever, fatal.

Spread by oral ingestion of the virus, hepatitis A is highly contagious. Because of its epidemic nature, it is often easy to diagnose. If a number of people develop hepatitis simultaneously, hepatitis A is usually suspected. The patients may complain of weakness, fatigue, dark urine, light stools, itching skin, and jaundice. Blood tests reveal a characteristic pattern of liver abnormalities. It is sometimes possible to test the blood for the presence of antibodies to hepatitis A. Treatment consists of "taking it easy," but bed rest is not necessary. A nutritious diet is recommended, but some patients are so nauseated that they can eat very little. Hospitalization is rarely necessary. Strict hygiene is warranted. The patient should use separate plates and utensils and a separate bathroom, if possible. However, the patient with hepatitis A is at his most infectious just *before* his illness becomes apparent. When the telltale signs of jaundice appear, the virus particles are no longer present in the patient's stool and he can no longer infect persons around him.

Hepatitis B is often indistinguishable from hepatitis A at first glance. The same symptoms and the same pattern of liver test abnormalities occur. There are, however, several specialized tests that can detect hepatitis B virus in the blood. The most common test is for the hepatitis B antigen (Australia antigen).

Antibodies developed by the patient after contact with the hepatitis B virus can also be determined.

The route of infection by hepatitis B is almost always different from that of hepatitis A. Hepatitis B is usually caused by transfusion (or other inoculation) with contaminated blood. There is also increasing evidence that the disease may be spread by sexual contacts. A mother with hepatitis B at the time of labor and delivery stands a chance of transmitting the virus to the baby. Other people at risk are illicit drug users who share needles used by infected people.

Treatment for hepatitis B is the same as for hepatitis A. The outcome is generally just as favorable, but an occasional patient will develop severe liver disease with liver failure. Further, patients who have hepatitis B may go on to develop a chronic form of hepatitis.

Not all cases of hepatitis transmitted by blood transfusions are caused by the hepatitis B virus. One or more additional viruses obviously exist. The disease caused by these other viruses is referred to as non-A, non-B hepatitis (or hepatitis C). The best designation, however, seems to be simply post-transfusion hepatitis. The disease produced by these organisms is quite similar to that produced by hepatitis B. Several other viruses are occasional causes of hepatitis. Active research is being carried on in this field.

Chronic active hepatitis, unlike acute hepatitis, implies a long-term illness characterized by continued inflammation and gradual destruction of the liver. Some cases are caused by drugs, some by hepatitis B, some by post-transfusion hepatitis, but most have an unknown cause. Chronic active hepatitis may begin with a typical attack indistinguishable from acute viral hepatitis. In other cases, however, the illness begins gradually with a sense of fatigue, muscle or joint aches, nasal bleeding, easy bruising, or simply as the gradual discoloration of jaundice. The diagnosis is often delayed because of the mild, nondescript nature of the symptoms. A multiple-channel blood test that shows abnormal liver enzymes will be a tip-off. The diagnosis must be confirmed by a liver biopsy. The more severe cases are treated with cortisone-like drugs. The outcome is frequently favorable.

Chronic persistent hepatitis does not produce significant disease. Its major importance lies in possible confusion with chronic active hepatitis. The persistent form causes only a minor inflammation in the liver that does not progress. The liver biopsy is the only sure way of establishing whether a patient is suffering from chronic active hepatitis, which requires treatment, or from chronic persistent hepatitis, which requires no treatment.

Alcohol and the Liver

Alcohol is one of the most common causes of severe liver injury in the United States. This does not mean that every social drinker suffers liver damage, for the liver can adjust well to moderate amounts of alcohol, and not all persons are equally susceptible. However, alcohol-related damage to the liver has become one of the nation's leading causes of death.

Changes in the liver brought about by alcohol occur in sequence. The earliest change is the fatty liver. The liver becomes large and pale, with a yellowish hue, and on autopsy the cells are found crammed with fat. This change produces no symptoms and few, if any, laboratory abnormalities. Continued heavy drinking can bring on inflammation of the liver tissue and death of some of the cells. This stage is called alcoholic hepatitis and does cause symptoms, primarily fever, jaundice, and abdominal pain. If the person stops drinking, the injury may be reversible. However, there is also a possibility that scarring of the liver (cirrhosis) may occur, regardless of whether drinking is stopped. Sometimes cirrhosis appears after a single episode of alcoholic hepatitis; sometimes it occurs after repeated episodes. The symptoms in this stage are fatigue, loss of energy, and swelling of the legs and abdomen.

Cirrhosis of the Liver

Although heavy use of alcohol is the leading cause of cirrhosis in the United States, the term cirrhosis is not the same as alcoholic liver disease. There are many forms and many causes of cirrhosis. The disease is characterized by extensive scarring within the liver substance. In addition, there are areas of liver tissue where cells have regenerated to replace those damaged by the disease. The anatomical arrangement of these cells is abnormal. The new arrangements, called regenerative nodules, function normally but block the normal pattern of blood flow through the liver.

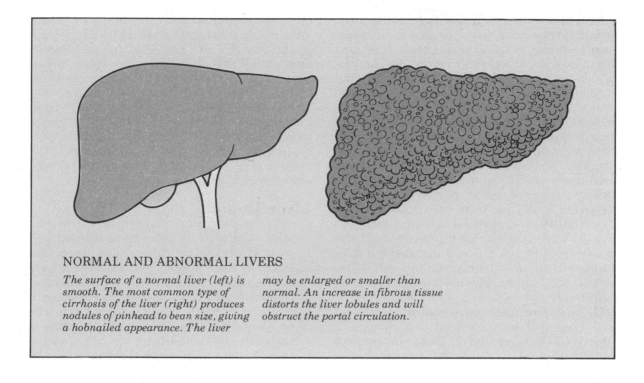

NORMAL AND ABNORMAL LIVERS

The surface of a normal liver (left) is smooth. The most common type of cirrhosis of the liver (right) produces nodules of pinhead to bean size, giving a hobnailed appearance. The liver may be enlarged or smaller than normal. An increase in fibrous tissue distorts the liver lobules and will obstruct the portal circulation.

Cirrhosis can produce a variety of symptoms, depending on the cause of liver damage and on the severity of the cirrhosis itself. The most prominent symptoms are salt retention, portal hypertension, and encephalopathy.

Salt retention occurs because of poorly understood mechanisms whereby the kidneys of a cirrhotic patient do not excrete salt properly. The usual result is swelling of the ankles and legs. Sometimes the abdomen also swells, a condition called ascites. The treatment is to restrict the amount of dietary salt. Sometimes diuretic medications are given to enhance the kidney's ability to rid the body of sodium.

Portal hypertension usually becomes apparent when dilated veins at the lower end of the esophagus begin bleeding (see page 474). Treatment is not generally undertaken until after bleeding occurs. In some patients, an operation can be performed to shunt blood from the portal system into the general circulation to reduce the varices. Others are treated by directly injecting medications that clot the vessels and stop bleeding.

Encephalopathy may be the principal problem in cirrhosis. The term means deranged function of the brain. In the patient with cirrhosis this may take the form of loss of memory, disorientation and confusion, or even coma. In all but the milder forms of this complication some treatment is required, usually a low-protein diet and medications to decrease the absorption of ammonia from the gut.

Certain forms of cirrhosis present their own pattern of symptoms and require special treatment.

Alcoholic cirrhosis, also known as micronodular cirrhosis or Laennec's cirrhosis, produces an irregular surface of the liver known as hobnail liver. Its cause, as the name implies, is a high consumption of alcohol over many years. The first step in treatment is to stop drinking, after which the doctor concentrates on managing the disease's complications.

Posthepatitic cirrhosis, or macronodular cirrhosis, is a form of progressive liver injury that occurs in a few people after a viral hepatitis attack. The condition is usually marked by gradual fluid accumulation. Victims may also have jaundice, abdominal pain, and other symptoms if inflammation and destruction continue. Treatment is similar to that for other forms of cirrhosis. If the hepatitis is still quite active (as judged by liver tests and liver biopsy) a cortisone-like drug may be used.

Primary biliary cirrhosis (cholangiolitic hepatitis) is a relatively rare form of liver disease, the cause of which is unknown. It is most commonly found in women over 30. The disease is characterized by destruction of the tiny branches of the bile ducts within the liver substance. There is also an abnormality of copper metabolism. Tissue copper levels within the liver are often strikingly elevated. The first signs are usually skin itching and progressive jaundice. In recent years many cases have been discovered at an early stage, thanks to multiple-channel analyzers which provide the physician with liver tests even when no liver abnormality is suspected. Cortisone is ineffective in this disease. Using drugs to remove the copper from the liver has been tried but is of unproven value. Cholestyramine can often control the itching. The disease is often fatal within five years.

Hemochromatosis (pigment cirrhosis) is a disease of iron overload (see chapter 6, "The Blood"). Excessive amounts of iron are found not only in the liver but in many other tissues. Patients with hemochromatosis sometimes show the signs of liver disease, but just as often they show evidence of tissue destruction in other organs, particularly the pancreas (diabetes), the heart (electrical abnormalities), or the gonads (impotence). Although this condition is uncommon, it often runs in families. Males are far more likely to be affected than females, partly because women lose sufficient iron during their reproductive years through pregnancy and menstruation so that abnormal amounts cannot accumulate. Hemochromatosis is suspected by finding high iron levels in the blood, and confirmed by demonstrating increased iron content in the liver. The treatment consists of removal of blood (phlebotomy). This is done usually at weekly intervals until enough iron has been removed to halt the destructive process.

Wilson's disease (hepatolenticular degeneration) is an inherited disease that usually strikes members of affected families between the ages of 10 and 25. It results from defective copper metabolism, associated with an inborn abnormality of the protein that normally binds copper. The metal accumulates not only in the liver but in the brain, eye, and other tissues. The victim may either have neurological symptoms—bizarre behavior, slurred speech, staggering gait, and muscle contortion— or evidence of liver disease, including jaundice, fatigue, and hepatitis-like symptoms. Wilson's disease is progressive and is fatal if untreated. It can be treated with D-penicillamine to remove the accumulated copper from the brain and liver. The treatment brings good results, although damage cannot always be reversed. The disease is inherited in an autosomal recessive pattern, which means that offspring of two carrier parents have about a 25 percent chance of developing the disease. Early testing of susceptible family members is important.

Liver Tumors

Tumors of the liver can be cystic (fluid-filled) or solid. Cystic tumors are seldom important except that they may be confused on a liver scan with more serious growths. An occasional cyst may be caused by a parasite ingested with food or through the skin that lodges in the liver. These are rare in the United States. Cysts of any type usually grow slowly over the years and eventually surgical removal may be necessary.

Solid tumors of the liver may be primary (arising within the liver) or secondary (spread to the liver from some other source). Benign primary tumors of the liver can arise spontaneously. However, it has become apparent that prolonged use of female hormones, including birth control pills, may lead to the formation of these benign tumors.

Hepatomas are malignant tumors originating in the liver. These usually arise in a previously scarred cirrhotic liver, but also may develop after other liver injury. Evidence suggests that the hepatitis B virus is important in the formation of these tumors. Patients with hemochromatosis or alcoholic cirrhosis also face higher risk of developing a hepatoma. Any age may be affected. When a hepatoma arises in a young person without underlying cirrhosis, surgical removal is sometimes attempted. In the older patient this is seldom feasible. Other more uncommon primary malignant tumors also exist.

Cancer in the liver is frequently spread from a source elsewhere. Cancers of the colon, lung, breast, stomach, and pancreas are just a few of the tumors that may involve the liver. When a secondary tumor is diagnosed in the liver, drug treatment is generally used instead of surgery.

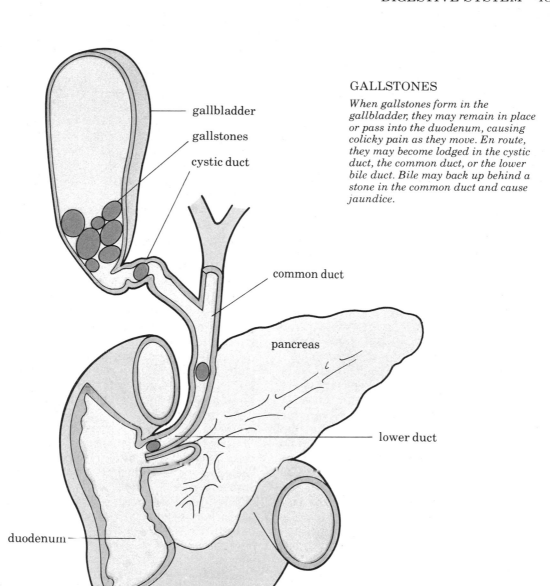

gallbladder

gallstones

cystic duct

common duct

pancreas

lower duct

duodenum

THE BILIARY TREE

The biliary tree is another name for the bile ducts and the gallbladder. The bile ducts are conduits that carry bile from the liver to the intestinal tract. The gallbladder is the storage organ where bile is retained until needed.

Stone disease is the most common problem of the biliary tree. The formation of crystals or pellets can block the normal bile flow and cause acute pain. Stones found in the gallbladder are called gallstones; those that occur elsewhere in the tree are called duct stones. Together they afflict an estimated 10 to 15 million Americans. More than 400,000 gallbladder removals are performed each year.

The stones themselves may be made up of a number of substances. The bulk are composed mainly or exclusively of cholesterol. A smaller number, containing almost no cholesterol, are made of calcium and bilirubin.

Many persons have gallstones without being aware of it. When a gallstone blocks the cystic duct, however, an attack of acute cholecystitis occurs and the pain can be memorable. Typically, it strikes suddenly with an acute, severe stab in the upper abdomen, usually under the lowest rib. Sometimes it may be felt in the back under the shoulder blade. The pain characteristically lasts two to ten hours and soreness may persist for several days afterwards. Attacks often occur at random, with no set relationship to meals or time of day.

Some people have chronic cholecystitis, which means major and minor attacks of "biliary colic" occurring over months or years. Some of them say that their symptoms often follow meals at a predictable interval. However, the notion that fatty foods are likely to provoke attacks is probably not true. Nor is fatty food intolerance a reliable symptom of gallbladder disease.

Some gallstones remain in the gallbladder. Others are able to pass from the gallbladder but lodge in the common bile duct. The blockage may cause jaundice as well as the typical symptoms. Infection may arise in the backed-up bile, causing pain, fever, and chills.

Although the symptoms of gallbladder disease are characteristic, diagnosis is usually made by X ray. Sometimes it is necessary to do an ultrasound examination, too. When typical symptoms are present and gallstones are verified, surgery is almost always the preferred treatment. The operation involves removal of the gallbladder (cholecystectomy) and exploration of the common bile duct if there is evidence of duct stones. A hotly debated question is what to do for a patient who has stones but no symptoms. Surgery is often recommended for the younger patient in good general health because there is a 50 percent risk he or she will eventually develop an inflamed gallbladder (acute cholecystitis). When stones are discovered in patients over the age of 50 or with underlying disease, such as heart disease or diabetes, surgery is less often recommended. Medication to dissolve the gallstones may then be considered.

Post-cholecystectomy syndrome refers to abdominal pain that persists even after removal of the gallbladder. Occasionally, this pain represents a genuine bile duct disease. Most often, however, the pain probably comes from a different source. Not all abdominal pain occurring in patients with gallstones originates in gallbladder disease. Irritable bowel syndrome, for example (see page 496), may be responsible. Unfortunately, it is often impossible to prove that pain is *not* coming from the gallbladder until the organ has been removed. This is particularly true if the initial symptoms were not typical of biliary colic. Thus, many patients labeled as having "post-cholecystectomy syndrome" are really patients whose pain has always derived from sources other than the gallbladder. Although they may achieve temporary benefit from gallbladder surgery, the pain usually returns within six to twelve months. Further surgery on the biliary tree is then seldom helpful. On the other hand, the biliary tree can develop a recurrent stone or a stricture. Care must be taken to rule out these developments in the patient who fails to improve after surgery for stone disease.

Cholangitis is a bacterial infection of the biliary tree. It most commonly occurs behind an obstruction in the duct. It is treated with antibiotics, plus surgery to clear the obstruction.

Sclerosing cholangitis is a chronic change in the bile ducts, resulting in a thickened ductal wall with areas of irregular narrowing. The change may occur after recurrent episodes of bacterial cholangitis. It also may be associated with certain bowel diseases such as chronic ulcerative colitis (see page 494). Or it may occur without any known underlying abnormality. The symptoms are the fever, chills, and pain characteristic of recurrent infections in the biliary tree. Diagnosis is made by X ray of the bile ducts. Surgery can occasionally relieve a local area of obstruction and decrease the incidence of infection, but there is no cure.

Stricture (narrowing) of the common duct most often results from prior surgery on the biliary tree. It also may occur as a result of stone disease. If not treated it may cause chronic changes in the liver and ultimately cirrhosis. Surgery is the treatment.

Cancers of the biliary tree usually give symptoms of jaundice. The patient also may complain of severe skin itching. X rays of the bile ducts may disclose a characteristic defect, but sometimes it is difficult to distinguish between cancer of the bile ducts and a benign stricture. The cancerous area must be removed surgically. Cancers of the bile ducts grow slowly so significant improvement can occur even when surgical cure is not possible.

Cancer of the gallbladder is rare. Unfortunately, it is also rare for these cancers to be diagnosed before spread of the tumor has made surgical cure impossible.

THE PANCREAS

Disorders of the pancreas can arise from either of its two sets of functions. As an endocrine gland, it produces hormones, particularly insulin used in regulating blood sugar. Disorders in the hormone-producing cells can result in endocrine disease (see chapter 16, "The Hormones and Endocrine Glands" and chapter 17, "Diabetes Mellitus"). The other parts of the pancreas, which produce digestive enzymes, are affected by different disorders.

Pancreatitis

Pancreatitis (inflammation of the pancreas) may be classified as either acute or chronic, but these classifications have slightly different meanings than they have in other diseases. Acute pancreatitis means one or more attacks of inflammation of the pancreas, after which the organ returns to its normal function. Even the occurrence of many attacks of pancreatitis over many years is considered acute if there is no progressive destruction of the pancreas. Thus a single attack of pancreatitis is termed acute pancreatitis; many attacks with normal function between are termed relapsing acute pancreatitis. Chronic pancreatitis, on the other hand, implies gradual deterioration of pancreatic function. Attacks of pain over the course of many years are associated with gradual destruction of the pancreas so that it can no longer perform its endocrine or enzyme-producing function. Diabetes and inability to absorb food nutrients are the end result of chronic pancreatitis, but not of relapsing acute pancreatitis.

Acute pancreatitis. Most attacks of acute pancreatitis are caused either by gallbladder disease or by alcohol intake. High levels of blood fats, pregnancy, and certain drugs also have been implicated. The characteristic symptom is a severe stabbing pain in the upper abdomen, which may then move to the back. There may be sweating, fever, nausea, and vomiting, too. Most cases of acute pancreatitis produce only swelling within the pancreas. These attacks are less likely to develop complications. Occasionally patients develop severe acute pancreatitis with bleeding and destruction of the pancreatic gland. This form is far more serious and can even be fatal.

The diagnosis of acute pancreatitis can often be made on the basis of the history. Differentiation from ulcer disease and gallbladder disease is important. Laboratory confirmation of the diagnosis often involves finding elevated levels of certain enzymes.

The first step in treating acute pancreatitis is to stop the use of alcohol, drugs, or other possibly harmful substances. Medications to reduce pain, intravenous fluids, and rest are usually prescribed, and sometimes a thin tube is placed through the nose and throat into the stomach to drain its contents. Surgery is not recommended unless required by specific complications, and it may do more harm than good.

Abscesses or cysts often form in the pancreas after an acute pancreatitis attack. Draining abscesses used to be quite difficult but today their contents can often be sucked out with the guidance of ultrasound or CAT scan. Pseudocysts (accumulations of pancreatic fluid) used to mean automatic surgery, but with the relative ease of diagnosing them by ultrasound or CAT scan, the usual policy is one of watchful waiting. Most pseudocysts diagnosed early clear themselves without incident, but may have to be drained surgically if the person makes a slow recovery.

Chronic pancreatitis often begins with repeated attacks of abdominal pain diagnosed as acute pancreatitis. With gradual loss of pancreatic tissue, diabetes may occur. When about 90 percent of the organ's enzyme output has been lost, serious disturbances of digestion follow, and the patient may show evidence of weight loss with increased amounts of fat and other nutrients in the stool. X ray of the abdomen may reveal multiple calcifications within the pancreas, most commonly in alcoholic pancreatitis. The diagnosis can be confirmed by demonstrating diabetes and maldigestion of fat along with the decreased pancreatic enzymes. ERCP examination (see page 467) is helpful in many cases because the pancreatic duct changes are highly characteristic.

The treatment of chronic pancreatitis involves the avoidance of alcohol. Pain medications are often necessary. Surgery may help, particularly if the ERCP examination shows a narrowed area or a stone in the pancreatic duct. If diabetes is present, it must be treated, usually with insulin. For digestive problems, pancreatic extract tablets are given regularly with meals. Patients with chronic pancreatitis often continue to have symptoms and the long-term prognosis is poor.

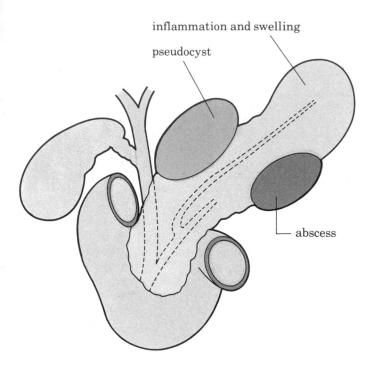

inflammation and swelling

pseudocyst

abscess

PANCREATITIS

Pancreatitis causes characteristic changes in the organ, as well as complications. Uncomplicated acute pancreatitis is caused by escape of normal digestive enzymes, which then attack the pancreatic tissue and cause inflammation and swelling. Accumulations of uninfected fluid rich in pancreatic enzymes are called pseudocysts and often distort or obstruct nearby structures. Abscesses are accumulations of pus that may cause pain and fever. In chronic pancreatitis, diabetes mellitus and malabsorption also may occur.

Pancreatic Tumors

Benign tumors of the pancreas are rare. Occasionally a benign tumor of the pancreas will develop and secrete one or more hormones. The symptoms are those of hormone excess.

Insulinomas are benign tumors that contain insulin-secreting cells. Since insulin causes the blood sugar to fall, it is not surprising that patients with insulinomas have symptoms similar to diabetics who have been given too much insulin (causing an "insulin reaction"). Symptoms of nervousness, irritability, sweating, and rapid heartbeat may occur. Because the low blood sugar level stimulates the appetite, patients often gain weight. In severe cases the blood sugar may fall low enough to cause seizures or coma. The treatment is surgical removal of the tumor.

Gastrinomas are tumors that secrete gastrin, a potent stimulator of acid output by the stomach. This produces severe ulcer disease that resists treatment. Patients not only have common ulcer symptoms, but complications of ulcer disease such as hemorrhage, perforation, and obstruction. They also may have diarrhea and lose weight. Measurement of the serum gastrin level helps to confirm the diagnosis.

Treatment revolves around a curious fact about tumors that produce gastrin or other hormones. Although many such tumors are benign and single, the majority are multiple and behave as malignant tumors of low virulence. Therefore, if a single tumor is suspected, surgery may be performed. But only about 15 to 20 percent of these tumors can be removed successfully by surgery, so many doctors do not even attempt such an operation. Instead they remove the stomach, the target organ for gastrin, so that ulcer formation is prevented. Since most gastrin-producing tumors, even malignant ones, spread very slowly, the patient may live many years in relatively good health.

With new drugs capable of suppressing acid production, even when there are elevated levels of gastrin, total removal of the stomach is less common today in the treatment of gastrin-producing tumors. Many patients are successfully managed with large doses of cimetidine, often in combination with other medications.

Cancer of the pancreas has been gradually increasing in frequency in recent years. The reasons are not known. More men than women are affected but the increase has involved both sexes.

Malignancies in the pancreas produce different symptoms depending on their location. Cancers developing in the head of the pancreas are at a critical point where they may obstruct both the pancreatic duct and bile duct, causing jaundice and thus leading to their early discovery.

Pancreatic cancer occasionally arises in the ampulla of Vater, the point where the pancreatic duct and the bile duct enter the duodenum. The outlook for patients with tumors here is somewhat better than for patients with cancers elsewhere in the pancreas.

When the cancer originates in the body or tail of the pancreas, there are ordinarily no symptoms until the tumor has progressed too far to be operable. The first symptom is usually upper abdominal pain which often radiates into the back. The patient may lose weight and develop diabetes. A profound change in mood, usually depression, is common. The increase in pancreatic cancer has not been matched by more successful treatment. The diagnosis is usually confirmed when surgery is performed. Widespread use of ultrasound and CAT scans has improved diagnosis but has not improved survival. Only about one percent of persons survive five years after diagnosis.

THE SMALL INTESTINE

Afflictions of the small intestine are common. They range from structural problems present at birth to progressive disease, and from mild symptoms to distressing ones.

Congenital atresia and stenosis. Occasionally, a section of the small bowel fails to develop into a tubular structure. A segment of fibrous cord occurs instead. This is referred to as atresia and becomes evident soon after birth. If the involved portion forms a tube that does not reach sufficient diameter to allow passage of foodstuffs, the narrowing is termed stenosis. In either event, the symptoms will be those of intestinal obstruction, notably vomiting and a distended abdomen. The stenosis must be repaired surgically.

Meckel's diverticulum, an outpouching of the small intestine producing a finger-like pouch, is the most frequent congenital abnormality of the intestinal tract. It usually occurs near the junction of the small bowel and colon. Such abnormalities may produce no symptoms throughout life. When they do cause symptoms, it is usually before the age of two. Complications of Meckel's diverticulum include hemorrhage, intestinal obstruction, and inflammation.

Ileus is a temporary inability of the small intestine to propel foodstuffs along its length so that absorption can take place. There are two types of ileus. Paralytic ileus occurs when any damage to the abdominal cavity or the nerves leading to the gut is severe enough to halt intestinal action. This may happen, for instance, immediately after surgery, when the bowel is silent. There are no propulsive waves and little if any absorption can occur. If a patient is fed too soon, he may have a bloated abdomen, become nauseated and vomit. Paralytic ileus may also be caused by a perforation of the bowel or infection in the abdominal cavity. The treatment is to put the intestine at rest, stopping all food by mouth and draining the stomach with a tube passed through the nose. The underlying condition that caused the ileus must be treated as well.

Mechanical ileus occurs when blockage prevents the normal flow of intestinal contents. This is also referred to as intestinal obstruction. A common cause of mechanical ileus is an adhesive band that develops across the bowel. In an attempt to get beyond the obstructed segment the intestine increases its propulsion activity with more forceful contraction of the intestinal walls. This causes severe cramping abdominal pain. After a time the abdomen enlarges and vomiting begins.

Other causes of mechanical small bowel obstruction include intussusception, volvulus, and stricturing from inflammatory disease. Intussusception is a condition in which a portion of the small intestine telescopes within the adjacent portion of intestine. Volvulus, on the other hand, exists when a segment of bowel twists upon itself like a knot. Strictures are areas of narrowed bowel. The treatment of almost all forms of small bowel obstruction is surgical. One exception is intussusception of the colon occurring in children (see chapter 27, "Taking Care of Your Child"), where a gentle barium enema is not only diagnostic but usually serves to reduce the intussusception.

Hernia is a general term applied when any organ or part of an organ protrudes out of the cavity that normally contains it. Hiatus hernia (see page 472) occurs when a part of the stomach slides upward through the esophageal passageway in the diaphragm. Similarly, parts of the small intestine may protrude through the abdominal wall. These hernias are given different names according to their location. They include inguinal hernia (common in men), femoral hernia (common in women) and ventral hernia (through the abdomen's forward wall).

Hernias also are referred to as reducible, incarcerated, or strangulated. A reducible hernia is one in which the displaced portion of the intestine can be pushed back into normal position, usually with simple pressure of the fingers. An incarcerated hernia cannot be restored to its proper place. A strangulated hernia is an incarcerated hernia in which the blood supply to the intestine is pinched off by the narrowness of the opening. This dangerous condition is a medical emergency.

Inguinal hernia accounts for more than 80 percent of all hernias. The condition occurs when a loop of the bowel passes through the inguinal opening, the passageway through which the male spermatic cord passes to the scrotum. The cause is usually weakening of

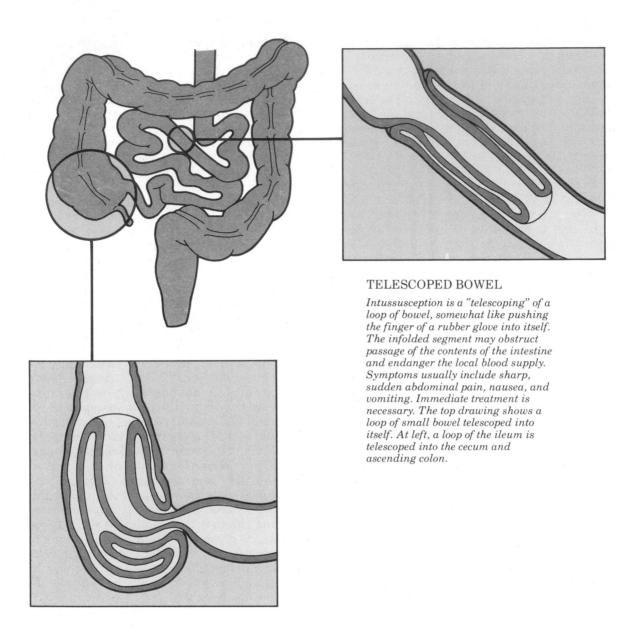

TELESCOPED BOWEL

Intussusception is a "telescoping" of a loop of bowel, somewhat like pushing the finger of a rubber glove into itself. The infolded segment may obstruct passage of the contents of the intestine and endanger the local blood supply. Symptoms usually include sharp, sudden abdominal pain, nausea, and vomiting. Immediate treatment is necessary. The top drawing shows a loop of small bowel telescoped into itself. At left, a loop of the ileum is telescoped into the cecum and ascending colon.

the abdominal muscles with age, but sometimes the opening has been widened by the strain of improper lifting or even a violent coughing attack. One or both sides may be affected. The hernia may develop gradually or suddenly.

Typically, an inguinal hernia shows itself with a bulge in the groin, accompanied by mild pain. An incarcerated hernia may cause bowel obstruction and greater pain. Even though an inguinal hernia may be reducible, elective surgery is usually recommended because of the danger of eventual incarceration and strangulation (see chapter 31, "Understanding Your Operation"). However, an elderly patient may be satisfactorily treated with a truss, a garment designed to support the abdominal wall and keep the hernia reduced, rather than undergo the risk of surgery. Surgery is also recommended for femoral and many ventral hernias.

Regional enteritis (Crohn's disease) is a disease of unknown cause characterized by inflammation in the intestinal tract. It most commonly involves the distal ileum, the lowermost portion of the small intestine. The disease may occur primarily in the small bowel, primarily in the colon, or in both. Uncommonly, it may involve the esophagus, stomach, or duodenum.

Symptoms vary because they depend on the location of the inflammation and its complications. Indeed, it is not uncommon for a patient to have early symptoms of regional enteritis for many months or even years and be thought to have simple indigestion or irritable bowel syndrome (see page 496). When the inflammation is in the distal ileum, the symptoms are usually crampy lower abdominal pain, diarrhea, and weight loss. Afflicted children may grow more slowly than normal and are often underweight. They may have fever, nausea, and vomiting. Severe inflammation may leave scars that narrow a segment of small bowel and cause intestinal obstruction.

Regional enteritis involves many systems of the body, so that symptoms and signs outside the intestinal tract may occur as well. They may include eye disease, canker sores, arthritis and muscle aches, red, raised, tender nodules on the skin of the legs, or even skin ulcers. Fissures, abscesses, or fistulae of the rectum are common. When the inflammation primarily affects the colon, diarrhea is common and there is frequently rectal bleeding.

Crohn's disease is treated with drugs of the cortisone family, such as prednisone, and with sulfasalazine if the colon is involved. The disease usually can be managed with medication successfully for a period of time, although a majority of patients eventually require one or more operations to remove affected portions of the bowel. Why not operate as soon as the disease is diagnosed? The problem with early surgery is that even when all apparent disease has been removed, a recurrence in the remaining intestine is common. If a long segment of bowel has been removed and disease occurs in the remaining bowel, severe nutritional problems may occur. Therefore, medical treatment is continued as long as it is successful and complications have not occurred.

In Crohn's disease, X-ray examination of the small intestine usually will show characteristic abnormalities in the distal ileum. Instead of its normal ringed pattern, the intestine has irregularities resembling a cobblestoned surface. Long areas of the narrowing also may be seen. When only a trickle of barium can get through this narrowed area, it may look like a string. Doctors call this the "string sign."

Occasionally, a child is operated upon because of a sudden onset of signs and symptoms characteristic of acute appendicitis, and the surgeon finds instead an inflamed distal ileum. This is referred to as "acute ileitis." Often, the surgeon will remove the appendix in any case because he knows the patient may have subsequent similar episodes of pain, and

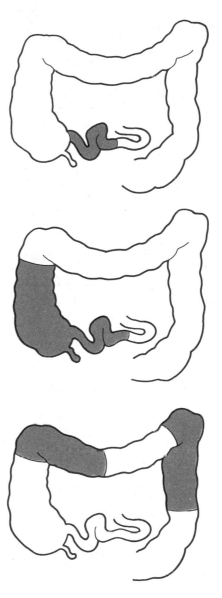

CROHN'S DISEASE

Regional enteritis, or Crohn's disease, may affect any part of the large or small intestine, and less commonly, the esophagus and stomach. Three common patterns of disease are shown here. Disease confined to the small intestine (enteritis) (top drawing) almost always involves the last portion of the ileum. Additional areas of the small intestine may be involved, sometimes with disease-free areas between. In the enterocolic variety (center drawing) both the small intestine and colon are diseased. Colonic Crohn's disease may involve the entire colon, a segment, or multiple segments (bottom), but the small bowel is spared.

with the appendix gone there will be no future confusion. On the other hand, if the cecum and the appendix are very inflamed, the appendix is not removed because of healing difficulty afterwards.

Malabsorption syndrome results from a number of diseases that prevent the small bowel from absorbing nutrients properly. Although any class of nutrients may be involved, the most striking symptoms usually result from an inability of the intestine to absorb fats. The cardinal symptom of fat malabsorption is the daily production of a large, bulky, foul-smelling stool. The stool is usually pale and very sticky. The toilet may have to be flushed two or three times. Oil globules may be seen in the toilet water. Patients who have had malabsorption for many months or years have weight loss (or failure to grow, in the case of children), easy bruising, weakness, and fatigue. Sometimes they also have cramps and diminished night vision.

Several diseases of the small intestine may produce malabsorption syndrome. Celiac disease, also called nontropical sprue, is usually a disease of children, but also may occur in adults. It is caused by a sensitivity of the intestinal tract to gluten, a protein present in many grains, including wheat flour used in bread. The child fails to grow properly and may have diarrhea, malnutrition, and a bleeding tendency. X ray and small bowel biopsy will confirm the diagnosis. The child improves on a gluten-free diet, usually within weeks or months, but must follow the diet for an indefinite period, possibly for life. Extensive disease in the small bowel, such as regional enteritis, may also result in malabsorption. Other causes include chronic intestinal infection such as giardia and the tropical infection known as tropical sprue. Surgical removal of part of the small bowel also may cause absorption problems. Because pancreatic enzymes are necessary for the breakdown of fats, severe pancreatic disease also may result in malabsorption.

Tumors of the small bowel occur in various types but they are uncommon. Symptoms are obstruction and sometimes bleeding. A mass may be felt in the abdomen, which may be confirmed by small bowel X ray. The tumor is usually removed surgically, particularly if the intestine is obstructed. Lymphatic cancer of the intestine is sometimes treated successfully with irradiation or chemotherapy.

Carcinoid tumors are peculiar growths of the intestinal tract that frequently begin in the small bowel but also may occur in the appendix, cecum, or other areas. These tumors occasionally secrete hormones, most commonly serotonin. A benign carcinoid tumor is limited to the intestinal tract and the serotonin is rapidly neutralized in the liver, so it produces no symptoms. Malignant carcinoid tumors may spread to the liver, and from there large amounts of serotonin may be released into the general circulation. This may produce a group of symptoms including flushing, sweating, rapid heartbeat, and diarrhea. Anti-tumor drugs and other medications reduce the symptoms. Sometimes all or most of the tumor can be removed surgically.

THE COLON

Like the small intestine, the colon is subject to disease throughout its length, malformations, and structural abnormalities. The more common malformations of the colon include imperforate anus and congenital megacolon.

• **Imperforate anus** may be a partial or complete blockage of the waste material's final passageway to the outside. A partial imperforate anus is really a narrowing of the rectum. It is discovered soon after birth. The infant may be unable to pass stool normally, and may have an enlarged abdomen and the crampy pain associated with colic. Sometimes there is also an abnormal connection between the colon and the genitourinary system. If the problem is only narrowing, daily dilatation may enlarge the rectum to the proper dimension. If the normal passage has not formed or is blocked, an operation will be necessary.

• **Congenital megacolon** (Hirschsprung's disease) occurs because of faulty development of the nerves that control the rectum (see chapter 27, "Taking Care of Your Child"). The nerves may be markedly reduced or even absent. Consequently, the colon does not move its contents forward and an obstruction develops. Megacolon usually becomes apparent shortly after birth when the obstructed colon grows to giant proportions, swelling the abdomen, and the infant passes no stool. The condition can be corrected surgically.

Inflammatory Diseases of the Colon

Appendicitis is a term familiar to almost everyone. It refers to an inflammation of the appendix, that unexplained blind loop of tissue suspended from the cecum. The inflammation may be caused by obstruction of the appendix, although there are other causes.

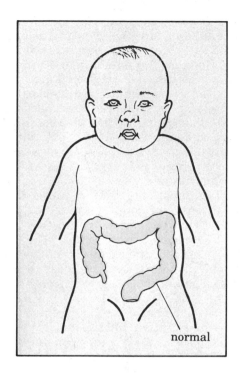 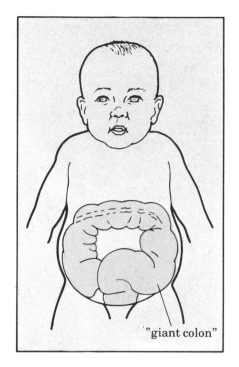

MEGACOLON

Megacolon ("giant colon") occurs because of faulty development of the nerves that control the rectum. It is present from birth. The colon cannot move its contents forward, normal stimulus to have a bowel movement is absent, and the backed-up fecal matter may greatly dilate and enlarge the abdomen, as in the child in the right drawing above. The condition usually is discovered in the first few days of life when the infant's abdomen enlarges and he passes no stool. It can be corrected by an operation.

Appendicitis is rare before the age of five and seldom occurs after 50. The typical symptoms are pain, nausea or vomiting, tenderness in the lower right portion of the abdomen, and fever. Often the pain is felt first in the center of the abdomen, then shifts to the lower right portion after several hours.

If appendicitis is suspected, prompt surgical intervention is necessary. Apart from the location of pain, an important clue is sudden onset of symptoms in a child or young person who previously has been healthy. It is important not to give the person food or laxatives, or to apply heat. Surgical removal of the inflamed appendix is a relatively simple procedure (see chapter 31, "Understanding Your Operation").

When the symptoms are characteristic, appendicitis is unmistakable. However, many bizarre forms of the inflammation can occur. It can be particularly confusing if the appendix or cecum is not in the normal location. Several other diseases, including acute inflammation of the lymph nodes in the area of the appendix, kidney disease, and inflammation of the pelvic female organs, often mimic the symptoms of appendicitis.

Inflammatory bowel disease of the colon is a general term for inflammation of the lining cells of the colon. Causes include infection, types of dysentery, tuberculosis, and gonorrhea. Certain parasites cause inflammation of the bowel. It has recently been recognized that an inflammatory disease of the colon called pseudomembranous colitis may result from treatment with certain antibiotics. This disease, which may be quite serious, is probably caused by a toxin produced by an uncommon strain of *clostridia* (a relative of the bacteria that cause gas gangrene). Radiation for treatment of pelvic tumors also may cause inflammatory changes and bloody diarrhea in some patients.

large intestine

cecum

appendix

APPENDICITIS

The vermiform appendix is a small, narrow, blind tube projecting from the cecum. A distended and inflamed appendix may rupture, release toxic contents, and cause peritonitis. The inflammation also may impair blood supply in the single artery serving the appendix. Gangrene may result. Although an inflamed appendix classically produces pain in the lower right abdomen, symptoms vary, especially in young persons. Do not give laxatives and pain-killers to persons with abdominal pain.

However, the most common forms of inflammatory bowel disease in the United States are those whose cause is unknown. There are two distinct types, Crohn's colitis (granulomatous colitis or regional enterocolitis) and ulcerative colitis. Crohn's colitis is the same basic disease as regional enteritis (see page 490) except that it occurs in the colon. When both colon and small bowel are affected, the diagnosis usually is made easily. However, when the colon alone is involved it is sometimes difficult to distinguish Crohn's colitis from ulcerative colitis. Barium enema X ray and colonoscopy help to distinguish them.

Chronic ulcerative colitis is characterized by recurrent bouts of rectal bleeding usually associated with diarrhea. If disease is limited to a few centimeters of the rectum, it is termed ulcerative proctitis. More extensive disease may include the entire colon. The diagnosis is usually made by proctoscopic examination, the process of inserting a lighted scope into the rectum. In ulcerative colitis the rectum is almost always involved. A colonoscope may be used to determine extent of the disease and to assess the risk of cancer.

The treatment of ulcerative colitis depends on the intensity of symptoms and the extent of disease. Some persons with proctitis can be treated with medicated enemas. When medication is needed, it is usually sulfasalazine. Cortisone-like drugs may be added, either as enemas if only a short segment is involved, or as pills.

Surgery ordinarily is considered in the patient with ulcerative colitis under any of three circumstances: toxic megacolon, severe symptoms that fail to respond to medical treatment, and longstanding disease with pre-cancerous changes. When surgery for ulcerative colitis is necessary, the entire colon usually must be removed and the ileum attached to the skin (ileostomy) for emptying intestinal contents into a bag.

Toxic megacolon is an uncommon complication of ulcerative colitis. Patients with this disorder are very sick with fever, abdominal distension, and even mental changes. The abdomen is distended and X ray of the abdomen shows a tremendously enlarged colon. There is danger that the colon may perforate. If medication does not bring prompt improvement, surgery is undertaken.

A patient with severe and unresponsive symptoms but without megacolon is treated first with medications. If there is no improvement after several months, surgery is usually recommended.

Finally, surgery may be undertaken in some patients who have had their disease more than 10 years because the risk of colon cancer is increased, especially among those whose disease began in childhood and whose entire colon is involved. How to treat such patients remains controversial. At the present time, treatment is individualized and may be based on biopsy findings. It is important to perform colonoscopic examinations periodically to take biopsies and look for abnormal cells.

Tumors of the Colon

Benign polyps make up the majority of tumors of the colon. These are localized over growths of tissue in the colon mucosa. Most are in or near the sigmoid colon. Some polyps have a fibrous stalk connecting the tumor with the colon. These are referred to as pedunculated polyps. A polyp without a stalk is called sessile. Polyps usually cause no symptoms. The treatment of most polyps, whether they cause symptoms or not, is removal. This is because of evidence that polyps may occasionally degenerate into cancer if left unattended for a long time.

Most colonic polyps can be removed without an operation. The polyp is located by sigmoidoscope or colonoscope. A wire snare advanced through the scope is looped around the base (around the stalk if the polyp is pedunculated). Electrical current applied through the wire can cut through the tissue and simultaneously seal off any bleeding vessels. The severed polyp is then retrieved and examined for malignancy. There are a number of rare familial polyposis syndromes where the polyps are widespread and the risk of cancer approaches 100 percent. The usual treatment for these patients is removal of the colon.

Malignant tumors of the colon are frequent. In fact, cancer of the colon is the second most frequent malignancy in both men and women, with about 100,000 new cases detected in the United States each year. Approximately 50,000 Americans die of colon cancer annually.

The cause of colon cancer, as with many cancers, is unknown. Some evidence suggests that the American diet plays an important role, either because it is low in dietary fiber, or because Americans eat too much animal (particularly beef) fat. There is no reason to think that colon cancer has only one cause. There are marked geographic and cultural differences in the incidence of colon cancer that may be explained by differences in diet, but other factors may be involved.

The location of colon cancer often determines its symptoms. Cecal cancers often produce only vague symptoms, such as weakness, weight loss, and vague abdominal pain. They do not obstruct the flow of colonic contents because the contents are liquid and can pass through even a narrowed space with relative ease. Cecal cancers often bleed intermittently. Colon cancers occurring in the sigmoid colon closer to the rectum are more likely to obstruct the passage of stool. They also are more likely to bleed, and therefore give earlier warning of their presence. Most cancers occur in the sigmoid or descending colon.

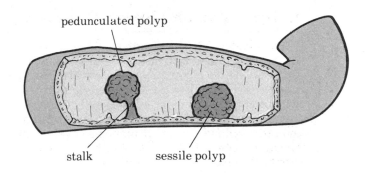

peduculated polyp

stalk   sessile polyp

COLONIC POLYPS

Two types of polyps that may develop in the colon are called pedunculated if they have a stalk and sessile if they have no stalk. Differences in tissue, seen under the microscope further divide them into adenomatous and villous. Some colonic polyps apparently lead to the development of cancer. Large polyps are more dangerous than small ones, and villous polyps more dangerous than adenomatous.

Colon cancers often can be diagnosed either by finger examination of the rectum or by sigmoidoscopy (at which time a biopsy can be taken). Cancers higher up in the bowel can be detected by colon X ray. Many times visual inspection with a colonoscope is required to make the diagnosis.

The treatment of most colon cancers is surgical. Unlike tumors in most other portions of the gastrointestinal tract, colon cancers often provoke symptoms early enough so that the diagnosis is established and treatment undertaken at a time when good results are possible.

When the tumor is limited to the lining of the colon, the survival rate after surgery is 70 to 80 percent (without tumor recurrence) five years later. More extensive tumor invasion produces a much lower five-year survival rate. When the tumor occurs close to the rectum the surgeon must remove the rectum as well as the tumor. This requires the patient to have a colostomy in which a loop of bowel is brought through the skin of the abdomen. Stool passes through the loop and is collected in a bag for disposal. Most cancers occurring higher up in the colon can be removed (with a margin of normal colon on either side) and the ends of the colon reattached. These patients will not require a colostomy and have normal bowel function afterwards.

Other Colon and Rectal Disorders

Hemorrhoids are dilated veins occurring in the rectum. Actually, almost any symptom involving the rectum may be falsely attributed to hemorrhoids because everyone is familiar with this term. Hemorrhoids usually cause no symptoms and require no treatment. Occasionally a blood clot or thrombosis develops in the hemorrhoid, but this is usually treated by a sitz bath (sitting in warm water with the legs out) or suppositories. Surgical removal of the thrombosed hemorrhoid is occasionally necessary. Surgery also may be performed if the ring of hemorrhoids becomes large and bulky. The other problem caused by hemorrhoids is bleeding. Hemorrhoidal bleeding turns the toilet water red and stains the toilet tissue. Repeated bleeding may be an indication for surgical treatment.

Irritable bowel syndrome is the most common diagnosis made in a gastroenterology clinic. The condition causes substantial suffering and loss of work, yet is surprisingly poorly understood. It is also difficult to categorize. Symptoms vary. Most often, the person complains of pain in the lower abdomen but pain may occur anywhere in the abdomen. There is frequently a pattern of disordered bowel movements: Some patients complain of constipation, others of diarrhea, while most have alternating constipation and diarrhea. There are few of the symptoms of other intestinal disorders. This disorder does not produce fever, chills, weight loss, or rectal bleeding. People with irritable bowel syndrome are seldom awakened at night by symptoms.

The disorder often begins in late adolescence or early adulthood. Many factors may contribute to it. Tension, anxiety, and worry are some. It is not, however, a "psychological disorder," because objective changes in colon activity can be found. All standard gastrointestinal tests are normal. The diagnosis is established by finding the characteristic symptom pattern and excluding other possible explanations.

The treatment of irritable bowel syndrome consists of a careful explanation of symptoms. A surprising number of people with irritable bowel symptoms improve substantially when they learn that their pain does not represent cancer or some other feared disease. Often a doctor will suggest that the patient follow a diet high in fiber, and may suggest that he or she supplement it by adding bran or other fiber sources at the table. Drugs to quiet the bowel's spasms are sometimes prescribed. Psychotherapy is seldom necessary, unless there are emotional problems apart from the disease.

Irritable bowel syndrome may be a chronic disorder. Fortunately, however, it does not lead to other serious problems within the gastrointestinal tract.

Diverticulosis and diverticulitis. There is considerable confusion concerning the differences between diverticulosis and diverticulitis. The former is common, the latter is less so. Diverticulosis simply means the presence of one or more diverticula in the colon. A diverticulum is an outpouching through a weakened area in the wall of the bowel. Such outpouchings are extremely common in people over 50. In general, diverticula cause no symptoms. The patient who has irritable bowel syndrome and diverticula is sometimes referred to as having "painful diverticulosis," but this designation is unnecessarily confusing. Occasionally, a patient with diverticulosis will develop a complication, usually bleeding, infection, or inflammation.

The patient with a bleeding diverticulum develops sudden, copious, red rectal bleeding. The onset is so dramatic that the patient wastes no time in seeking medical attention. Treatment is to replace lost blood. If the bleeding does not stop spontaneously, surgery is necessary.

The infected diverticulum is referred to as diverticulitis. Diverticulitis begins as a rather abrupt onset of lower abdominal pain, a change in bowel habits (usually constipation), fever and sometimes chills, and sometimes rectal bleeding. If diverticulitis is suspected, diagnostic studies are not ordinarily undertaken early in the course of the illness for fear that installation of barium under pressure may cause the outpouch to perforate. Acute diverticulitis is treated with antibiotics. Fluids are given intravenously and diet is restricted. After an acute episode is over a high-fiber diet is often recommended to prevent further bouts of diverticulitis. Most attacks of acute diverticulitis clear up successfully. Only an occasional patient requires surgery, usually because of one or more attacks.

Fistula. A fistula is an abnormal connection between adjacent structures. A rectal fistula usually forms between the skin around the rectum and the rectum itself. A symptom of a fistula is an abnormal drainage, often from a lump located at a variable distance from the anus. The drainage is often pus but may also resemble stool. The treatment is surgical to remove the connection. It should be kept in

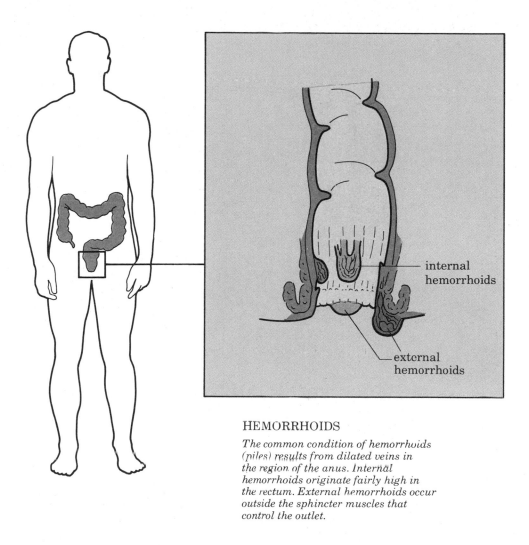

HEMORRHOIDS

The common condition of hemorrhoids (piles) results from dilated veins in the region of the anus. Internal hemorrhoids originate fairly high in the rectum. External hemorrhoids occur outside the sphincter muscles that control the outlet.

mind that a fistula may be the first manifestation of Crohn's disease involving either the small or large bowel.

Perirectal abscess usually begins with throbbing, constant pain around the rectal area. A tender mass may be found, either near or within the rectum. If the abscess is large, the patient may also have fever. The abscess must be removed surgically. As with fistulas, repeated perirectal abscesses are often associated with Crohn's disease.

Anal fissure is a tiny tear in the mucous membranes and skin at the anus. It is an extremely painful disorder that may afflict infants, children, and adults. There is often a conscious effort to avoid having a bowel movement, because bowel action makes the pain worse. If the fissure has been present only a short time, the treatment generally includes pain medicine, warm sitz baths, and medicines to soften the stool. If the fissure has been present for some time, it may be necessary to repair it surgically.

Pruritus ani is not a disease but a symptom, and a common one. It is an intense itching sensation at the rectum. It is not caused by hemorrhoids. A number of diseases are said to be responsible, but most cases are of unknown cause. Since bile salts will produce itching when injected under the skin, it is sometimes thought that excess bile salts in contact with inflamed rectal skin may be the cause. This remains unproven. In any event, relief of symptoms is usually obtained by good (but not overly aggressive) anal hygiene. Pruritus ani is not a serious malady, but it is certainly a humbling one.

CHAPTER 21   PETER F. KOHLER, M.D.

ALLERGY AND THE IMMUNE SYSTEM

A housewife sneezes repeatedly each time she goes into her dusty attic. A young boy playing in a garden is stung by a wasp and collapses, gasping for air.

Despite their differences, both of these are examples of allergic reactions, or allergies. Allergies occur in more than 20 percent of Americans at some time during their lives. The symptoms vary from the housewife's slightly irritating one to the life-threatening reaction of the young boy.

Exactly what are allergies? The accepted definition is that they are harmful immunologic occurrences or diseases in which a person reacts abnormally to an everyday stimulus that would cause no problems in most other persons. Hay fever is an allergy; so is eczema; so is asthma. The abnormal immunologic reaction can affect many different systems of the body or all of them. Some allergies cause intestinal upsets, some cause skin rashes, some cause breathing difficulties. Anaphylaxis, the technical name for what happened to the child stung by a wasp, can be fatal.

Immune responses normally protect us from infections caused by bacteria, fungi, parasites, and viruses, and from developing cancer. The immune system consists of protein molecules called immunoglobins (antibodies) that combine specifically with substances called antigens, the allergens that are foreign to the body. These antigens are present on the numerous infectious agents that enter the body through the skin and through the mucous membranes that line the respiratory and gastrointestinal tracts. By combining with the antigens, the immunoglobins destroy them. The immune system also plays an important role in recognizing antigens on potentially malignant cells and eliminating these early cancers.

Certain white blood cells called lymphocytes are also part of the immune system. There are two types of lymphocytes. B lymphocytes produce immunoglobins, the antibody proteins that combine with antigens. T lymphocytes regulate production of antibodies and participate in immune reactions.

The most important elements of the immune system are illustrated at right. Lymphocytes originate in the bone marrow, circulate in the blood and lymph vessels, and reside in the thymus gland, spleen, and lymph nodes. They travel continuously between the blood and lymph vessels, ready to react to any invading antigen by producing antibodies or regulating their production. Immunoglobins (Igs) are found in plasma, the clear part of the blood, and also bathe the tissues.

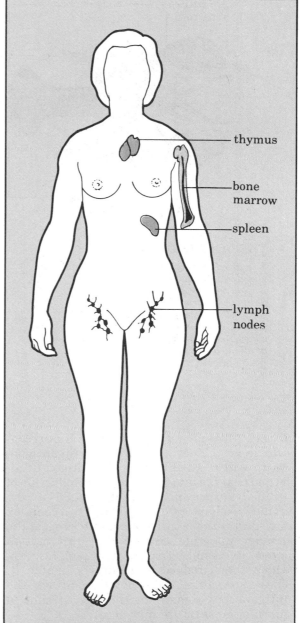

THE IMMUNE SYSTEM

Important elements of the immune system, which protects us against disease, are distributed throughout the body. Antibodies, which combine with invading substances and destroy them, are formed by highly differentiated lymphocytes called plasma cells, which originate in the bone marrow. T lymphocytes develop in the thymus gland under the breastbone. B lymphocytes are converted into plasma cells in the spleen. Both types of lymphocytes are stored in the lymph nodes, ready to react to any invader by traveling through the blood and lymph vessels.

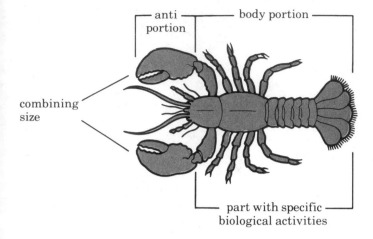

anti portion — body portion

combining size

part with specific biological activities

THE "ANTI-BODY"

The structure of an antibody can be visualized as a lobster. The "body" portion determines the function of the antibody molecule and is different for each of the five major types. The "anti" portion, comparable to a lobster's claws, combines only with an antigen or allergen that provides a precise fit. Each antibody is specific for only one allergen and no others.

Each antibody has specific sites that recognize and combine only with a certain antigen. An Ig will react only with the antigen or allergen that fits into the sites. The production of antibody in the presence of antigen, as described in chapter 6, "The Blood," is a complex one. Certain cells called phagocytes ingest the invader molecule and transfer information about its composition to the lymphocytes, which then produce antibodies to match it. These specialized cells not only attack the antigens but remain in the bloodstream to guard against future invasions.

One way to think of an antibody is to view it as a lobster, with the "anti" or combining sites represented by the claws. The antibody will react only with the specific antigen that fits into the claws.

The structure of the "body" portion determines how each antibody functions. Five types or classes of antibodies exist, each with a different body structure. They are designated IgG, IgA, IgM, IgD, and IgE. The functions of each class differ considerably.

IgG is the only type of antibody that can cross the human placenta from mother to fetus, and at birth the majority of a newborn infant's antibody proteins are provided by the mother's IgG.

IgA antibodies are transported to the external surfaces of the respiratory, gastrointestinal, and urinary tracts, and also into breast milk. IgA serves as the first line of defense against viruses such as polio and against bacteria on mucosal surfaces. Breast milk protects infants from infection because of its high concentration of IgA.

IgM is the first antibody produced in response to infections or immunizations.

IgD's function is uncertain but it may be involved with T lymphocytes in the control of antibody production.

IgE is the chief offender in the conditions we think of as allergies. It is responsible for hay fever, asthma, and anaphylaxis (see page 505).

Normally antibodies are produced that react only with foreign or "non-self" antigens. However, antibodies to "self" (autoantibodies) can be produced which react with and injure the individual's own tissues. This is called an autoimmune disease.

IgE-TRIGGERED ALLERGIES

Just a small amount of IgE is present in blood plasma, one part per million (the concentration of IgG is 100,000 times higher). But that amount is extremely potent. IgE is responsible for most of the common allergic reactions, including hay fever, asthma, hives, eczema, and acute anaphylaxis.

The steps by which IgE triggers allergic symptoms are illustrated on page 501. The immunoglobin binds to the surface of special cells called mast cells, which are particularly abundant around small blood vessels in the nose, lung, intestine, and skin. The tail of an IgE molecule attaches firmly to receptors on the surface of the mast cell. A single mast cell can bind more than 100,000 IgE molecules. Each mast cell is packed with granules that contain potent chemicals called mediators, so named because they represent an intermediate step between trigger and symptom. Histamine is the best-known of these mediators.

When an allergen combines with its corresponding IgE antibody on the surface of a mast cell, the contents of the granules are released. The histamine and other mediators cause nearby blood vessels to dilate and leak fluid through their walls. The result is swelling of tissues, increased mucus production, spasm of

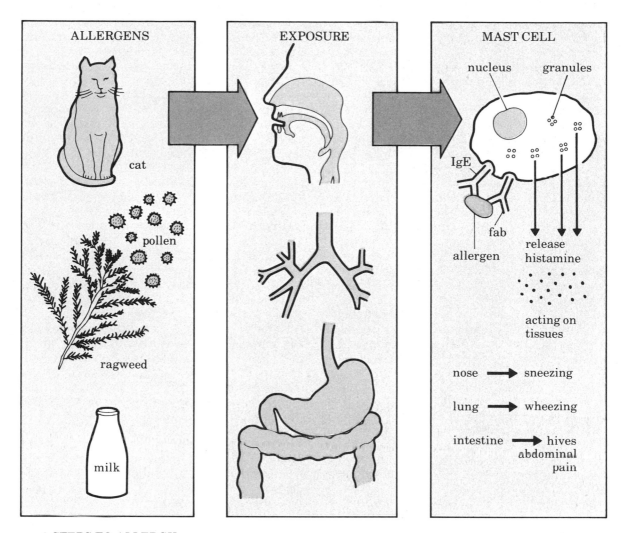

ALLERGENS

cat

pollen

ragweed

milk

EXPOSURE

MAST CELL

nucleus   granules

IgE

fab

allergen

release
histamine

acting on
tissues

nose ➔ sneezing

lung ➔ wheezing

intestine ➔ hives
abdominal
pain

3 STEPS TO ALLERGY

The essentials of an allergic reaction occur in three steps. Allergens are substances that originate outside the body. Animal dander, plant pollens, and foods are examples. They usually enter the body through the nose and mouth, although some enter through the skin. They affect the mucous membranes of the nose, throat, and respiratory and digestive systems. When they combine with immunoglobin E (IgE), attached to the small mast cells in these areas, the cells release histamine and other substances that act on the tissues to produce symptoms such as sneezing, wheezing, and hives.

smooth muscles, itching, and an accumulation of inflammatory cells called eosinophils and neutrophils. The symptoms may be mild or severe, and vary depending on the location and extent of the allergen-IgE-mast cell reaction.

The mast cell is like a bomb filled with explosives. IgE is the trigger for the bomb, and the allergen is the finger that squeezes the trigger. The "explosion" of the released mediators results in the allergic symptoms.

The sequence of events that produces allergic symptoms has only recently become fully known. But for hundreds of years, people have realized that they sneezed, wheezed, coughed, or developed itchy, watery eyes at certain times of the year or when they approached certain animals. Folklore attributed these symptoms to substances borne by the wind that were inhaled and directly irritated the tissues of the nose and lung. Not until about 1920 was it recognized that some substance in the blood also is necessary to provoke allergic symptoms. The discovery came when a New York City resident who had never shown symptoms of asthma received a blood transfusion for treatment of severe anemia in a New York hospital. Afterwards, he rode in a horse-drawn hansom cab through Central Park and developed the characteristic asthmatic wheezing for the first time. Even closer contact with horses in the past had caused no breathing difficulty. The wheezing stopped after he left the cab, but returned each time he approached a horse again. His physician traced down the blood donor and found the man had a long history of asthma triggered by exposure to horses. This suggested that an element in the donor's blood had been transferred to the recipient.

Several years later, two German medical investigators, one of whom developed hives when he ate cooked fish, performed a related experiment. Serum from the physician who was allergic to fish was injected into the skin of his colleague, who normally could eat fish without incident. A day later, the nonallergic physician ate a meal of cooked fish and developed a large, itchy hive where the serum had been injected. This conclusively demonstrated that allergy was caused by an element in the blood. In each case, the allergic donor's IgE had attached to the recipient's mast cells. On exposure to horse dander in the anemic patient and fish in the German physician, the mast cells released their allergic mediators and symptoms occurred.

Nearly 50 years passed, however, before these suspicions could be confirmed. Because of its low concentration in the blood, it was not until 1966 that the offending element (IgE) was isolated, and the exact mechanism of action was not determined until the 1970s.

Asthma

Allergic asthma occurs when certain inhaled antigens or allergens combine with IgE antibodies on mast cells in the lungs. The combination brings on attacks of airway obstruction, which is completely reversible but occurs repeatedly. About 9 million American adults and children have asthma, and it is a major cause of school absenteeism and of time lost from work. Almost 500 million sick days are recorded each year because of asthma.

How does asthma occur? In normal breathing, air passes through the nose or mouth and into the throat, then through the voice box (larynx) into the trachea, the large tube leading into the lung. Then the air progressively travels into smaller branching air tubes called bronchi. These air tubes are surrounded by smooth muscle cells and glands that produce mucus. The larger bronchi divide progressively into smaller branches (thus the term "the bronchial tree") and terminate in clusters of tiny air-filled sacs called alveoli. The exchange of inhaled oxygen for carbon dioxide, the waste gas produced by the body, occurs in the alveoli (see chapter 8, "The Lungs.")

During an asthmatic attack, the mediator released from mast cells causes spasm of the bronchial smooth muscle, narrowing the airways and limiting air flow. Excess mucus secretion further clogs the passages. Thus the asthmatic wheezes because the passageways are not clear, coughs as he tries to clear them, and is short of breath because he cannot completely fill the alveoli.

In the majority of child asthmatics, IgE-mediated reactions are the major causes of the disease. By age 16, however, about half of children with allergic asthma become symptom-free spontaneously. Why this occurs is not understood. It may be related to a decreased exposure to the allergens that trigger asthma, or to fewer respiratory virus infections, which often combine with IgE and allergens to produce asthma.

Allergic asthma is often referred to as "extrinsic," meaning that its stimuli come from outside the body. In many adults, however, there is no evidence that attacks are triggered by external allergens. The asthma more often appears to be related to chronic respiratory infections or exposure to nonspecific irritants such as fumes, strong odors, cold air, and ingestion of aspirin-containing drugs. These patients are said to have "intrinsic" (nonallergic) asthma. The basis for airway spasm in these persons is less well understood. They have one characteristic in common, however: All patients with asthma, whether allergic or not, have extremely reactive airways that go into spasm easily.

Vigorous exercise often precipitates asthmatic attacks in nonallergic cases, apparently because heat and moisture are lost during rapid and deep breathing. Thus, running on a cold day with low humidity is much more likely to induce asthma than running on a warm humid day. If a runner keeps the mouth closed, asthma is less likely to occur. Conversely, swimming often is good exercise for asthmatic patients because of the air's warm temperature and high moisture content. Several asthmatics have competed successfully as U.S. Olympic swimmers.

Recognizing and preventing attacks. The telltale indication of asthma is its characteristic wheeze upon exhaling, but this sound is not always noticeable to the asthmatic or those around him. It is therefore important to emphasize that cough, a tight or uncomfortable sensation in the chest, and shortness of breath also may indicate asthma, particularly if they occur in combination and if they occur after exercise. Recognition of asthma is particularly important because steps to deal with it should be taken immediately.

Relief from asthma falls into two categories. First is avoidance of allergens such as animal dander, dust, or pollens. Respiratory irritants such as tobacco smoke, strong perfume, or cooking odors also should be avoided, because the asthmatic's extremely sensitive airways respond not only to inhaled allergens but to less specific irritants as well. The second step is the use of medication to relieve and prevent attack. Extremely effective medications are available, which, if taken by mouth on a regular basis, minimize both bronchial muscle contraction and excess bronchial secretions.

The chart at right summarizes the steps that should be taken to help asthmatics. It is important that measures to reduce allergens and prevent bronchial spasm both be included in the care program.

Hyperreactivity of the bronchi underlies both allergic and nonallergic asthma, and the longer asthma persists the more difficult it is to reverse. So the immediate goals are to reduce the increased irritability by avoiding irritants such as tobacco smoke and by using medicines that dilate the bronchial tree. On the other hand, avoidance of allergen exposure will effectively prevent the allergen's interaction with IgE. As long as IgE cannot combine with allergen, there can be no release of the mediators, which would result in narrowing of the airways, increased secretions, and the asthmatic symptoms.

Commonsense Care of Asthma

General health measures:
- A nourishing, nonallergenic diet.
- A large intake of fluids to keep respiratory secretions thin.
- Adequate rest and sleep to avoid excess emotional and physical fatigue.
- Regular physical activity.

Avoid:
- Physical and mental fatigue and stress.
- Irritating fumes from tobacco smoke, volatile solvents, and strong perfumes.
- Extremes of temperature.
- Occupational irritants and smog.

Control allergen exposure by avoiding:
- Airborne pollens and molds.
- Animal hair and danders (pets).
- House dust, including stuffed toys, uncovered mattresses, feather pillows.

Psychological and emotional aspects:
- An understanding family in a pleasant home environment.
- Regular visits with an understanding physician.
- Avoidance of resentment or guilt by parents and an overprotective attitude.

Allergic Rhinitis (Hay Fever)

The most common IgE-mediated allergy is allergic rhinitis, popularly known as hay fever. More than 20 million Americans, 10 percent of the population, are familiar with its symptoms, which include congestion, swollen nasal membranes and obstructed breathing, itching and inflamed nostrils, and sneezing. Some persons have itching, watery eyes as well. The bouts occur either periodically (seasonal) or continuously (perennial) if there is a constant exposure to allergens. Seasonal rhinitis is twice as common as the perennial form of rhinitis.

As in other IgE-mediated allergies, the symptoms occur as chemicals are released from mast cells by the combination of allergen with IgE antibody. In this case, the offending mast cells are in the nose.

Often the symptoms of allergic rhinitis are mistakenly attributed to a "summer cold." But the difference is usually apparent. Typically, colds do not last more than a week and are accompanied by a painful, burning sensation in the nose and a thick yellow nasal discharge. The discharge of allergic rhinitis, in contrast, is clear and watery. Of course, allergy and infection are not the only causes of nasal stuffiness. Congestion also occurs in the last months of pregnancy. It usually disappears after delivery. Overuse of nose drops and sprays also causes chemical irritation in the nose that often is mistakenly attributed to allergies. Symptoms do not improve until the nasal medication is stopped. Reserpine and propranolol, used for the treatment of hypertension, can cause nasal obstruction. Persons with aspirin intolerance often develop overgrowths of nasal tissue (nasal polyps), which cause chronic obstruction (see chapter 13, "Ear, Nose, and Throat"). After accidental ingestion of aspirin, profuse nasal discharge and obstruction develop. Aspirin acts directly on the mast cells of intolerant people without involving IgE.

Hives and Giant Hives (Urticaria and Angioedema)

Almost everyone has "broken out" in hives (urticaria) or giant hives (angioedema) at some time. In many cases IgE is responsible.

The distinction between the two forms is more than size. Hives occur primarily on the skin in the form of raised red welts that itch. Although annoying, they are seldom life-threatening. Giant hives most often occur beneath the skin. They can affect the respiratory and gastrointestinal tract. The swelling that results can interfere with body functions and in severe cases closes off the larynx, causing death.

The two forms of hives sometimes occur together, but frequently giant hives occur independently of urticaria, and can be particularly dangerous because outward signs are lacking.

There are several IgE-related causes of hives and giant hives, including penicillin, rubbing against a pollinating plant, being licked by animals, or stung by insects. Food allergies also cause hives, although allergic persons are usually able to recognize the asso-

ciation without the help of a physician. Hives also occur in association with certain infections, probably as part of the normal immunologic response to the infectious agent. For example, up to 30 percent of persons develop hives during the early or incubation phase of viral hepatitis.

Physical factors also induce hives. In these cases, IgE allergy is not involved. Pressure urticaria, for example, occurs when tight belts or brassiere straps cause histamine to be released from mast cells by simple pressure alone. The result is a line of raised welts precisely where the garment pressed. Indeed, in some persons histamine is released from mast cells so easily that it is possible to write on their skin with a fingernail. The letters appear in raised, pink tracery. This is called dermatographism.

Exposure to cold can cause an outbreak of giant hives. This can be a particularly serious problem if it occurs while swimming. The cold water can cause a massive release of histamine, causing an abrupt decrease in blood pressure similar to acute anaphylaxis (see page 505).

Chronic urticaria (hives lasting over six weeks) occurs in only a very small number of persons but often is a significant problem because of the appearance and bothersome itching. It is often difficult to identify the cause, but foods and drugs, especially aspirin, are always prime suspects. Food additives such as dyes and preservatives are also possible causes.

Hives can be aggravated by emotional stress, but there is no evidence that they are caused by it.

The most effective treatment for hives is to avoid the recognized factors that cause the symptoms. In physical urticarias, this is usually done by avoiding tight clothing and shoes. People with cold urticaria must avoid cold places, especially cold water. Fortunately, both pressure and cold urticaria may last for years, then disappear spontaneously.

Eczema

The skin rash known as eczema (atopic dermatitis) affects one to three percent of the U.S. population. It is more common in infants and young children than adults. Usually a person with eczema also has a history of allergic rhinitis or allergic asthma. Often another member of the family has eczema.

The infantile form usually begins before one year of age with a reddened rash on the cheeks and ears which then spreads to the backs of the arms and fronts of the legs. Eczema is often the first sign of a tendency to develop IgE-mediated respiratory allergies. The skin problem frequently disappears about one year of age but may recur in a childhood form between the ages of three and five. At this age the rash is characterized by intense itching in the elbow and knee creases and the sides of the neck. The intense itching induces scratching, which makes the rash worse and establishes a vicious scratch-itch cycle that is difficult to break.

The skin of eczema patients is easily irritated, just as the membranes of the nose and lungs are in patients with hay fever and asthma. For this reason, it is essential to minimize the use of strong soaps. The skin is characteristically dry, too, which further contributes to the vicious scratch-itch cycle. Thickening of the skin also develops after vigorous and prolonged scratching.

Scratching plays a central role in eczema. If it can be stopped or reduced, eczema will improve, which in turn reduces the itching. This is dramatically shown when the involved skin cannot be scratched. If a child with eczema breaks an arm and a cast is applied for several weeks, the rash under the cast will disappear. In children, it is important to keep fingernails trimmed to minimize the damage of scratching.

Treatment of eczema depends on severity. Patients with extensive skin involvement should be cared for by a physician, usually in consultation with an allergist or dermatologist. Although high IgE levels are often found in persons with eczema, and hay fever or asthma is frequently present, it is usually not possible to implicate specific allergens. Hyposensitization, attempting to sensitize the person with small amounts of the suspected allergen (see page 513), has not been shown to be effective and occasionally even causes a flare in the itch-scratch-rash cycle.

Anaphylaxis and Insect Stings

Anaphylaxis is the least common but most serious IgE-mediated allergy. It is a life-threatening emergency that requires prompt treatment. Symptoms begin within seconds to minutes after the sting of an insect or the ingestion of medications or foods that combine with IgE antibody on mast cells. There is a widespread (systemic), massive release of histamine and other mediators in contrast to the localized release that occurs in allergic rhinitis or asthma. This results in leaky blood vessels

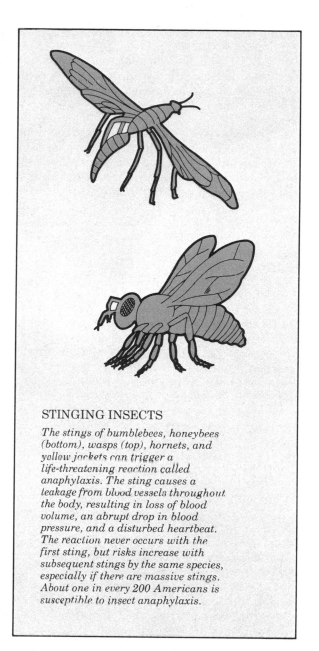

STINGING INSECTS

The stings of bumblebees, honeybees (bottom), wasps (top), hornets, and yellow jackets can trigger a life-threatening reaction called anaphylaxis. The sting causes a leakage from blood vessels throughout the body, resulting in loss of blood volume, an abrupt drop in blood pressure, and a disturbed heartbeat. The reaction never occurs with the first sting, but risks increase with subsequent stings by the same species, especially if there are massive stings. About one in every 200 Americans is susceptible to insect anaphylaxis.

throughout the body, with loss of blood volume, a fall in blood pressure, and frequently a disturbed heartbeat. Accompanying acute anaphylaxis may be generalized skin itching, hives and giant hives, nasal discharge, sneezing, itchy eyes and tearing, and asthmatic symptoms.

About 40 percent of the persons who have had anaphylactic reactions also have a history of allergic rhinitis, asthma, or eczema, compared to 20 percent of the general population. This means that people with IgE antibody to inhaled and ingested allergens are more likely to develop anaphylaxis. However, it is important to note that 60 percent of the reactions occur in persons who do not have the common IgE-mediated allergies. Males and persons under 20 years of age are at greater risk, probably because of increased exposure to allergens.

Anaphylaxis was first described in hieroglyphics on the wall of an Egyptian pharaoh's tomb. He had died after an insect sting in 2621 B.C. About one in 200 persons in the United States has IgE antibody to stinging insects and runs the same risk as the pharaoh. At least 40 deaths a year are caused by insect stings in the United States.

There are two main groups of stinging insects: honeybees and bumblebees, which only sting when provoked, and vespids (wasps, hornets, and yellow jackets), which often sting without provocation. Wasps build honeycomb-type nests under the eaves and in rafters of buildings, while hornets build nests in trees and shrubs. The yellow jacket is the most common source of dangerous stings and builds its nest in the ground under logs.

On the first sting, there are no symptoms except local discomfort and swelling at the site of the sting. After IgE antibody has been produced to the injected venom, subsequent stings by the same species of insect will result in the chain of events leading to the generalized allergic symptoms.

The only sure way a susceptible person can prevent reactions is to avoid the insect stings. Outdoor activities should be done with caution. Areas where insects have been seen should be avoided. Shoes, long pants, and shirts should be worn when walking in woods and fields. Gloves and a protective net to screen the neck and face should be used while gardening. Cosmetics, perfumes, and hair sprays should be avoided because these odors attract bees and vespids. Bright clothes, particularly whites and pastels, attract insects and should not be worn.

If an allergic person is stung, prompt treatment is essential, but the victim is usually many minutes away from a physician's office or a hospital emergency room. Therefore the insect-allergic persons should carry emergency medication kits containing adrenalin and antihistamine as well as an identification bracelet or necklace describing their allergy.

The kits allow administration of adrenalin simply by pressing the dispenser against the side of the leg, without the necessity of injection. This allows the victim to treat himself, or the medication can be given by another person without medical training.

The insect-allergic person never has a systemic anaphylactic reaction on the first sting, but a greater-than-normal reaction should not be ignored. Precautions should be taken to avoid further stings.

Food Allergy

The onset of vomiting, diarrhea, abdominal pain, and particularly hives and angioedema after eating a specific food suggests an IgE-mediated allergy. Symptoms primarily arise in the digestive tract where the food allergen-IgE-antibody-mast cell reaction is occurring. These usually develop within two hours after eating. A skin test usually shows IgE antibody to the specific food. As discussed earlier, investigation of the German physician's symptoms after eating fish was the first step in the discovery of IgE.

Food allergy is more frequent in the young and in older people who lack IgA antibody. This is because IgA blocks the action of food allergens by combining with the allergens, such as milk and egg proteins, in the digestive tract. IgA is normally absent at birth and gradually increases during childhood to normal levels by age 10. In 0.2 percent of the population (1 in 500 persons) a deficiency of IgA persists throughout life along with an increased risk of developing IgE-mediated allergies.

For many years allergists had suspected that food allergens were absorbed more easily by infants and that allergic symptoms could be reduced by modifying the diet early in life. Recently a study in England compared two groups of babies who were considered likely to develop allergies because both parents had IgE-mediated symptoms. One group of 23 babies was fed only breast milk until six months of age. Only two (13 percent) developed eczema by one year of age. In contrast, eczema developed in nine of the 19 babies (47 percent) who were not breast-fed and whose diets included cow's milk plus eggs and cereals before six months of age. Whether breast feeding influences the development of allergic rhinitis, asthma, or urticaria is not known. Further studies are needed of this "breast is best" theory of reducing eczema in babies to confirm the results.

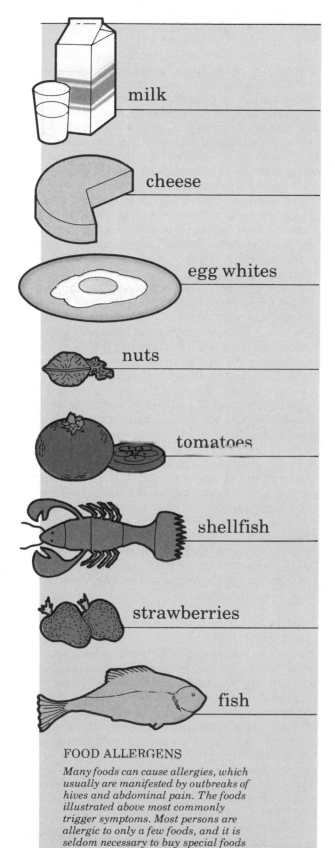

milk

cheese

egg whites

nuts

tomatoes

shellfish

strawberries

fish

FOOD ALLERGENS

Many foods can cause allergies, which usually are manifested by outbreaks of hives and abdominal pain. The foods illustrated above most commonly trigger symptoms. Most persons are allergic to only a few foods, and it is seldom necessary to buy special foods or follow a severely restrictive diet.

ALLERGENS

What are allergens, those mysterious substances that can cause the body to react in so many different ways? A variety of ordinary substances fall into this category, and they enter the body by a number of different routes. Allergens are swallowed, inhaled, injected, or applied directly to the skin. They are in the air we breathe, the ground we walk on, the animals and plants around us, the medicines we take, the food we eat. There is continuing controversy about which substances cause harmful immunologic reactions and which do not, particularly in the area of food and food additives.

Food

Which foods cause allergies? Virtually any food has the potential to cause an allergic reaction. Those most frequently responsible include cow milk and other dairy products, such as ice cream and cheese; egg white; pipped fruits such as tomatoes and strawberries; beef; nuts of various kinds; fish and shellfish, especially shrimp and lobster. Wheat is often blamed for allergic reactions, but is only rarely responsible.

Identifying the food responsible for the allergic symptoms is often easy. Since the symptoms occur within such a short time, the most recent foods eaten are obviously suspect. The presence of IgE antibody to that particular food can usually be confirmed by skin or RAST test (see page 511). Most persons are found to be allergic to only one or two foods, not to the entire spectrum shown at left.

Avoiding the food, however, may be more of a problem than identifying it. Many foods are used in small amounts in recipes where one might not expect to find them. Shrimp, for instance, is used in small amounts to provide flavor in Chinese dishes and in certain soups. It is easy to avoid whole milk, butter, and ice cream, but milk also turns up in such foods as margarine and packaged luncheon meats. Eggs (and milk, too) are found in baked goods and in the batter used for fried chicken.

Cooking odors provoke allergic reactions in some persons. The aroma of frying fish carries enough protein to set off an IgE reaction in the mast cells of the nose.

The allergy is sometimes not to the entire food, but to some natural chemical within it, or to some chemical produced in the breakdown of foods in the gastrointestinal system. In these cases it may be more difficult to identify the offender. When the offending allergen is not obvious, some physicians suggest keeping a food diary in which the person records all foods eaten over a given period in an attempt to establish a pattern that will identify the cause. An elimination diet also can be used. In this diet suspected foods gradually are added to the person's menu one at a time until symptoms occur. Elimination diets are particularly useful in identifying the source of allergies in small children, whose diets can be more easily controlled.

In the case of food additives, about 20 percent of those who cannot tolerate aspirin show an adverse reaction to tartrazine, a food dye (FDA Yellow Dye No. 5). Although the dye is not always apparent, sensitivity usually can be demonstrated by test. The relationship of other additives to allergy has not been proven, and many tests purporting to show a relationship are not scientifically proven.

Food allergy causes discomfort for a great many people, but its significance should not be overstressed. A multimillion dollar industry promotes the consumption of "natural" and "nonallergenic" foods as a way to prevent allergy, but it is seldom necessary for a person, even with a demonstrated sensitivity, to follow such a totally restrictive diet. There is no evidence that such foods will prevent development of allergic reactions in persons who do not have them. In fact, the diet may do more harm than good.

In addition, not all gastrointestinal symptoms that occur after eating a specific food can be attributed to allergy. If the abdominal pain is not accompanied by hives, the chances are that another cause is responsible. For instance, a child who has abdominal pains and bloating after drinking milk may have a deficiency of enzyme that breaks down milk sugar (lactose). This condition is relatively common among black and Asian children. The undigested lactose, not IgE, causes the symptoms.

Pollens

Outside the home, the most important allergens are pollens from trees, grasses, and weeds. Pollens are small microscopic grains that are the male germ cells of plants and are essential for plant fertilization. Not all pollens cause IgE allergies. Colorful scented flowers, such as roses and lilacs, have pollens that are large and sticky. Rather than being distributed by the wind, they are carried from plant to plant by insects. Trees, grass, and weeds, on the other hand, are pollinated by the wind. Their pollen, produced in large quantity, is small, light, and easily transported in the air. For example, ragweed pollen has been detected hundreds of miles out in the Atlantic Ocean. A single ragweed plant can produce a million grains of pollen a day, making ragweed pollen virtually impossible to eradicate. In addition to being produced in large amounts, pollens must be capable of causing IgE antibody formation in susceptible patients. Although the pine tree produces a large amount of airborne pollen, it is rarely the cause of allergic symptoms.

There is a relatively constant pollinating season for each species of tree, grass, and weed, depending on climate. The individual's symptoms develop only when the particular pollen that reacts with his or her IgE is in the air. At any given time, the amounts of sunlight, rain, and wind determine the amount of airborne pollen. Trees pollinate in the spring from February to April in the north. In May and June grass pollens are present. In August and September until the first frost, weed pollens are prevalent. Weed pollens produce the most significant symptoms. Many patients are allergic only to ragweed and have symptoms on the East Coast and in the Midwest from mid-August until late September. In northern climates where a definite frost develops, the typical allergic patient's seasonal symptoms may last from March through the first frost when pollination ends, while in southern locations pollens and symptoms can be present almost the entire year.

Molds

Another important airborne allergen is mold spore. In the northern United States, particularly in the Midwest, molds grow in large quantities on plants, foods, and other living matter. Molds are microscopic in size and produce large amounts of spores even smaller than pollens that are easily disseminated in the air. In northern states, spores begin to appear in the air in May and increase through June and July. In the South, molds are present throughout the year and are major causes of respiratory allergen for more than nine months of the year.

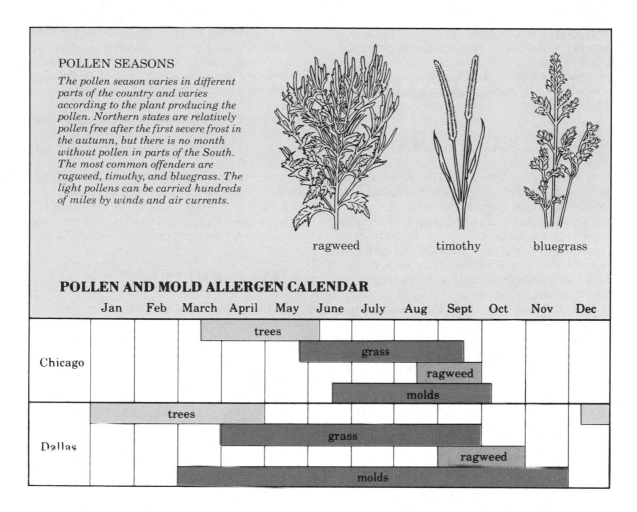

POLLEN SEASONS

The pollen season varies in different parts of the country and varies according to the plant producing the pollen. Northern states are relatively pollen free after the first severe frost in the autumn, but there is no month without pollen in parts of the South. The most common offenders are ragweed, timothy, and bluegrass. The light pollens can be carried hundreds of miles by winds and air currents.

ragweed   timothy   bluegrass

POLLEN AND MOLD ALLERGEN CALENDAR

	Jan	Feb	March	April	May	June	July	Aug	Sept	Oct	Nov	Dec
Chicago				trees		grass		ragweed		molds		
Dallas	trees			grass				ragweed		molds		

Molds are more likely to cause allergic asthma than pollens, which more often produce allergic eye and nasal symptoms. This is because the smaller size of the mold spores allows easier entrance into the lungs. Mold allergies are common in southern and midwestern farm areas, where mold concentration is much higher than in the Atlantic and Pacific coastal states. Molds inside the home may cause year-round allergic symptoms if moist conditions promote growth. Individuals who develop respiratory symptoms while mowing grass more often have allergy to mold spores, which grow on grass, than to grass pollen. Most persons who are sensitive to molds also will be allergic to pollens.

Household Allergens

Other allergens in the home and workplace produce significant year-round allergy symptoms. The primary offender is house dust, which is a mixture of a large number of potentially allergenic materials. Mold spores, food particles, insects, hair and dander from household pets, and decaying organic matter from pillows, mattresses, toys, furniture, and fibers are often found in house dust.

When pets are kept indoors, a considerable amount of dander and hair is distributed throughout the household. Cats and dogs are major causes of allergic symptoms. There is no particular breed of cat or dog that can be considered "nonallergenic." All breeds shed dander, the trigger for IgE production. Veterinarians and laboratory research workers who handle mice, rats, rabbits, and guinea pigs frequently develop IgE antibody and respiratory symptoms after exposure to the specific animal. Anaphylaxis after bites of experimental animals is also common in allergic laboratory personnel.

Drugs and Medications

With the increasing use of medications, drug allergy is assuming more importance. The ancient proverb, "One man's medicine is another man's poison," is illustrated strikingly by the fact that 10 to 20 percent of patients experience some type of adverse drug reaction while hospitalized. The majority of these reactions are not related to an immunologic response (allergy), although IgE-mediated reactions to penicillin are frequent, occurring in about one percent of all patients. Penicillin allergy is the most frequent cause of acute anaphylaxis in the United States.

WHO GETS ALLERGIES?

Why does 20 percent of the population develop IgE antibodies to certain inhaled or ingested allergens while the other 80 percent does not, even though everyone is inhaling and ingesting the same substances? The reason is the tendency to produce IgE to allergens that touch the mucosal surfaces of the respiratory and gastrointestinal tracts. That tendency is the common characteristic shared by persons with eczema, allergic rhinitis, and asthma.

Three related factors appear to determine who carries this sensitivity and who does not. First, an inherited predisposition is usually present. Between 60 and 70 percent of infants whose parents both have a history of IgE allergies will develop some allergic symptom before two years of age. Fortunately, these symptoms do not always persist. When one parent is allergic the figure falls to less than 10 percent.

The second obvious factor is exposure to the specific allergen that stimulates IgE antibody formation. This exposure begins immediately after birth in the form of foods and airborne allergens such as house dust and animal hair and dander. Breast-feeding reduces IgE to foods and reduces the risk of developing eczema.

The third factor is viral respiratory infection, which is being recognized more and more as an important initiating event in the development of allergic asthma. Very often the first episode of wheezing in an infant begins during a viral infection, usually diagnosed as asthmatic bronchitis. The virus infection allows, in a poorly understood manner, the production of IgE antibodies to environmental allergens either by increasing allergen penetration into the lining of the respiratory and gastrointestinal tract or by interfering with the T lymphocyte suppressive mechanisms that normally control IgE production.

This interplay of heredity, stimulation of the immunologic system by allergen, and virus infection is under intensive investigation at several asthma and allergic disease research centers across the United States. These studies may yield practical benefit. For instance, if respiratory virus infection could be prevented by vaccinations, perhaps production of IgE antibody to environmental allergies also could be blocked.

It is important to emphasize that IgE production does not persist without continued exposure to allergens. If steps are taken to remove the allergens, the chain of events leading to allergic symptoms can be interrupted.

WHAT GOOD IS IgE?

Anyone who has or knows someone with IgE-triggered allergies must wonder what advantage, if any, IgE provides. This question is difficult to answer. There is increasing evidence that IgE is necessary for protective immune reactions to parasitic infections of the stomach and intestines, which are common in underdeveloped countries. What advantages IgE confers in other situations is only speculation. For instance, IgE-triggered sneezing or wheezing could discourage persons from prolonged contact with allergens that produce even more serious illnesses.

TESTING FOR IgE

The presence of intermittent or seasonal nasal or chest symptoms strongly suggests the possibility of allergic rhinitis or asthma. When symptoms are present throughout the year without any seasonal fluctuation and do not disappear when a person moves to another city or a different type of environment, the probability that an IgE-triggered allergy causes the symptoms is much lower.

Confirmation is required before a definite diagnosis of allergic rhinitis or asthma can be made. This is usually done by allergy skin testing, in which a minute amount of the suspected allergen is introduced into the superficial skin by a puncture or an injection. If IgE antibody is present, a raised, itchy, red wheal or hive resembling a mosquito bite will appear within minutes. The larger the size of this reaction, the greater the amount of IgE antibody is present. The reaction is the allergic response in miniature and mimics what occurs in the nose

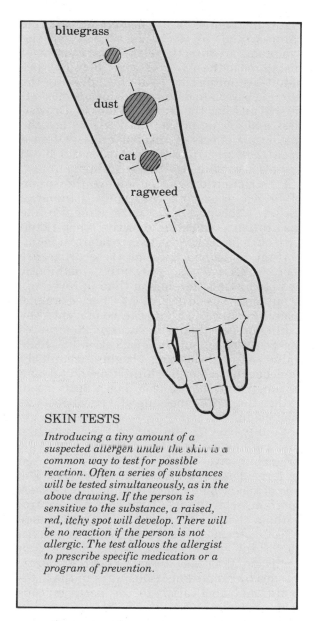

SKIN TESTS

Introducing a tiny amount of a suspected allergen under the skin is a common way to test for possible reaction. Often a series of substances will be tested simultaneously, as in the above drawing. If the person is sensitive to the substance, a raised, red, itchy spot will develop. There will be no reaction if the person is not allergic. The test allows the allergist to prescribe specific medication or a program of prevention.

or bronchial tree when mediators are released by the interaction of the inhaled allergen and the IgE on the mast cells. The skin test is the most rapid and sensitive method of detecting specific IgE antibody. It is useful in pollen, mold, animal dander, and house dust allergies, and also in diagnosing penicillin allergy. Often, the person is tested for all these allergens simultaneously in a series of injections in one or both arms. The allergist then gets an immediate picture of the spectrum of a person's allergies.

Skin testing for IgE allergy to penicillin is recommended when the patient has a history of a suspected allergic reaction. In circumstances when another antibiotic would be less effective, skin testing with penicillin will establish whether IgE antibody exists. If the test is positive, the patient faces a high risk of experiencing anaphylaxis even from a normal amount of penicillin. If negative, the risk of an immediate allergic response is ruled out and penicillin can be administered safely. Unfortunately, penicillin is the only drug in which skin testing is of value in predicting allergic responses.

Recently, tests have been developed that use serum for the detection of IgE antibodies without the necessity for skin testing. These depend on the use of a highly sensitive radioimmunoassay procedure called RAST (radioallergosorbent test), which measures the amount of IgE to specific allergens in test tubes. This procedure is sometimes indicated in small children in whom skin testing is difficult or in persons with extensive skin rash. It is also used to monitor changes in IgE antibody levels during treatment.

High levels of IgE to specific allergens usually mean the person will produce symptoms on exposure to the allergen. The results of skin or RAST testing for IgE antibodies must be related to the individual's symptoms to determine the relevance of the test results. If high concentrations of allergens are used in skin testing, many people will show positive skin reactions, even though they do not have the same reaction when they inhale the allergen. It is extremely important that the history, physical examination, and results of IgE testing be considered together before a reliable diagnosis of allergy can be made and an appropriate treatment program can be started.

PREVENTION & TREATMENT OF IgE ALLERGIES

Avoidance. The first and most important step in treatment is to minimize exposure to the offending allergens. This is often the easiest, usually the least expensive, sometimes the most effective, and always the safest treatment. Avoiding allergens in the home is the best way to improve symptoms in patients with IgE allergies to house dust, animal danders, and feathers. The table on page 503 outlines steps that will substantially reduce the intensity of allergen exposure in the home. Frequently, decreasing the allergen exposure will significantly reduce or even eliminate the distressing symptoms.

It is impossible to avoid exposure to pollens and molds in the atmosphere. Exposure can be reduced, however, by removing weeds around the home and by keeping doors and windows closed as much as possible. Home air conditioners are beneficial because doors and windows can be kept closed, preventing the entrance of airborne pollens and molds. Allergens themselves are not removed by air conditioning. The effectiveness of expensive air purifiers for removing home allergens remains controversial. Forced-air heating systems that recirculate the air increase the amount of dust, molds, and animal hair and dander in the air, so it is important to vacuum the air ducts thoroughly before use in the fall, and to install and change frequently the filters in the furnace. If possible, the air ducts in the room of the person with allergic symptoms should be taped shut and the room heated by simply keeping the door open. If this is not possible, a filter at the entrance of the air duct into the room may help.

Animals should never be allowed in the allergic person's bedroom, and animals should not be permitted in the house. This is often extremely difficult once an emotional attachment to a pet has been established, but is the most effective way to reduce allergic symptoms caused by dander. It must be stressed that the animal hair and dander will persist in the home for weeks to months after the pet is removed so that immediate benefits may not be obvious. The pet should never be allowed back in the house just because improvement has not occurred, particularly when the allergic person has positive skin tests to animal hair and dander.

Medications. The overuse of aerosol spray medications for allergic rhinitis or asthma can aggravate nasal and lung symptoms by irritating the tissues. Overzealous advertisements encourage the use of these nonprescription drugs, which in some cases perpetuate rather than relieve the problem.

Antihistamines are effective in allergic rhinitis and hives because most of the symptoms are directly related to the action of histamine in the nose and skin. Different types of antihistamines are available, allowing the allergic person to determine which is most effective and has the least side effects. Drowsiness and drying of the nasal tissues are the major side effects of antihistamines. Often a drug that constricts the dilated nasal blood vessels is combined with the antihistamine.

Prescription drugs that relieve the spasm of bronchial smooth muscle in asthmatics include theophylline and adrenalin-like medications, which are effective when taken by mouth for as long as twelve hours. It is important to emphasize that these drugs are more effective in preventing asthmatic symptoms from developing than in reversing symptoms already present. For example, exercise-induced asthma can be prevented by taking bronchodilator medication 20 minutes before exercise, but the medication has little value after wheezing begins. Similarly, someone with allergic rhinitis should take an antihistamine before cleaning a dusty room rather than after sneezing and nasal obstruction begin.

Finally, corticosteroid or cortisone-like medications are very effective anti-allergic drugs but have significant side effects if used in large doses and for prolonged periods. The use of cortisone by mouth on an every-other-morning schedule has been shown to control asthma effectively without producing the side effects associated with prolonged daily use. An important improvement is the delivery of cortisone-like drugs directly onto the allergic tissues by inhaled aerosol sprays in the asthmatic and application to the nasal mucous membranes in patients with rhinitis.

Emotional factors. While emotional stress can frequently aggravate allergic symptoms, emotions are never the sole cause of allergic rhinitis or asthma. Frequently, asthma and eczema will be intensified during periods of stress, such as when a child is disciplined or the parents have an argument. But a combination of factors is necessary to provoke an attack, and emotional stress can only cause symptoms during a specific pollen season. There is no firm evidence that a particular personality type predisposes to either eczema or asthma, nor is there evidence that asthmatic patients have more emotional problems than nonasthmatics before the onset of their lung symptoms. Once symptoms begin, however, it is clear that emotional factors can be important in triggering episodes of bronchospasm, and this must be recognized if the asthmatic patient is to receive maximum benefit from treatment.

At present, knowledge about the inherited aspects of allergies is not solid enough to make recommendations about genetic counseling. If both parents have allergic symptoms, the child is at high risk of developing some form of allergy at some time. In the future it probably will be possible to identify persons who face increased risk of developing serious allergic symptoms such as asthma. It is enough to say that a predisposition for allergies is often contributed by both parents equally and heredity is only one factor in the development of allergy.

Immunotherapy. If significant allergic symptoms caused by IgE persist despite medication and preventive steps, the physician may suggest a program of hyposensitization or immunotherapy, better known as "allergy shots." This consists of injecting increasing amounts of the allergen to which the patient has high IgE antibody levels as shown by skin tests and symptoms. Initially, a minute amount of allergen is injected, then a gradually increased dose is repeatedly given at intervals of several days to a week. Injections should be administered only in a physician's office because a serious reaction (anaphylaxis) can occur.

Immunotherapy should be used only in conjunction with avoidance and preventive medications. Benefits are not apparent until after six to twelve months of treatment. It has been shown conclusively that the majority of persons receiving immunotherapy for ragweed hay fever have significantly fewer symptoms and require less medication. In 20 percent of patients, allergic symptoms will disappear entirely. On the average, a 50 percent reduction in symptoms occurs.

A number of important changes in the immune system apparently explain the relief produced by immunotherapy. Usually, levels of IgE antibody increase after the pollen season, but in patients under treatment a decrease in IgE occurs. Also, increases in IgG anti-pollen antibody are produced by the therapy, which blocks the combination of the allergen with IgE and thereby prevents release of mediators and symptoms. Immunotherapy with purified venoms is particularly effective in preventing the severe life-threatening reactions in persons allergic to bee, hornet, and wasp stings.

Can you move away from allergies? Patients frequently ask whether moving to another climate would improve their allergies. The theory sounds reasonable, but in fact moving is seldom worthwhile, because most persons with allergies develop IgE to allergens no matter where they live. No part of the world is entirely free of potential airborne allergens except for the North and South Poles. Therefore, like the student from Asia who arrives in the Midwest and develops allergic rhinitis to ragweed after two seasons of exposure, the ragweed-allergic patient who moves from Baltimore to Arizona is equally likely to display allergic symptoms to Bermuda grass pollen after several years in his new location, although ragweed is no longer present. Because of the frequently harmful economic, social, and psychological effects of such a move for both the patient and relatives, it is rarely recommended. Before a final decision is made, a trial period of one to three months in the new location is advised.

OTHER ALLERGIC DISEASES

Although most allergic reactions can be attributed to IgE antibody, the other immunoglobins are sometimes responsible. They cause a variety of respiratory symptoms, skin disorders, even damage to such organs as the kidneys and blood vessels.

Allergic (Hypersensitivity) Pneumonia

Allergic pneumonia is caused by immunologic reactions in the tiny air sacs of the lung. Many people are exposed to high concentrations of dusts from organic material at work or in the home. The particles are less than five millionths of a meter in size, six times smaller than most plant pollens, so they can be drawn deeply into the lung and reach the tiny air sacs where the exchange of oxygen and carbon dioxide occurs. When exposure continues for long periods, IgG antibody and specific T lymphocytes are produced. They interact with the dust allergen within the air sacs and cause inflammation.

Symptoms of allergic pneumonia are different from those of asthma. In contrast to the immediate response in allergic asthma, symptoms are delayed until six or more hours after exposure. The person who has previously felt and breathed well develops chills, cough, shortness of breath, and fever. The symptoms closely resemble those of infectious or bacterial pneumonia and a chest X ray may show shadows in the lung. The patient may even be hospitalized with a diagnosis of bacterial pneumonia and treated with antibiotics. Within a day or two, symptoms begin to disappear and the chest X ray improves, seeming to confirm that an infection was present. However, on return to the dusty environment, symptoms recur. With repeated episodes of allergic pneumonia a progressive, irreversible loss of lung function occurs.

Sometimes the presence of allergic pneumonia is less obvious and does not show acute symptoms. A slow progressive loss of lung function occurs over many years, and if the exposure to dust continues, the lungs become unable to transport enough oxygen to the blood.

Allergic pneumonia has been recognized for 50 years in farmers who handle spoiled or moldy hay during the winter while feeding cattle in closed barns, where millions of mold spores are inhaled per minute. Poor farmers who could not afford to discard the moldy hay were particularly afflicted. Recently, similar symptoms have been observed in executives in office buildings where the central air conditioning system is contaminated with molds. These men and women are perfectly well on weekends, but on returning to the air conditioned office on Monday they experience cough, fever, and chills, which continue through the work week. Repeated exposure causes them to develop IgG antibody to the molds that were inhaled after being dispersed by the contaminated air conditioning system. This type of allergic pneumonia has been called "Monday morning fever."

Homemakers can also develop allergic pneumonia. This usually occurs when home humidifiers attached to the furnace or hot air heating system are turned on without being thoroughly cleaned. In one series of cases treated at the University of Colorado, the humidifiers had been installed several years previously and had functioned satisfactorily. One fall, however, the women became ill with fever, chills, cough, shortness of breath, and an abnormal chest X ray. Antibiotics were given for presumed infectious pneumonia. Symptoms disappeared in the hospital only to return within hours after return home. Examination of fluid in the humidifiers disclosed heavy contamination with bacteria and molds, and IgG antibody to both mold and bacterial allergens was found in the women's blood. To confirm the diagnosis of allergic pneumonia, the women inhaled small amounts of aerosolized humidifier fluid, which reproduced the symptoms in a milder form. This "inhalation challenge" was done so that the source of the allergen could be identified and eliminated to prevent further lung damage. By simply removing the humidifier system, these women were no longer exposed and no longer had attacks of pneumonia.

The estimated number of Americans with this allergic problem is less than 10,000, compared to the 35 million with IgE-mediated allergies. However, allergic pneumonia frequently is not recognized, which is unfortunate because it can be prevented.

The clues that help differentiate the allergic illnesses from other common respiratory illnesses are shown on page 515.

Skin Rashes (Allergic Contact Dermatitis) and Cosmetics

Allergic contact dermatitis, or skin rash, is more common than any other allergic reaction (see chapter 7, "The Skin"). The outbreak of redness, small raised papules, and blisters occurs because small chemical allergens called haptens, which do not induce an allergic reaction by themselves, combine with skin proteins and become allergenic. This moist reaction distinguishes contact dermatitis from the usually dry, thickened skin of eczema. This reaction is delayed, occurring up to a day after exposure to the chemical, compared to the immediate reactions caused by IgE. Many chemicals or haptens are capable of inducing this reaction. Cosmetics are often a source. Reactions to poison ivy, poison oak, and poison sumac also fall into this group. These affect at least half the U.S. population.

DISTINGUISHING ALLERGIES FROM RESPIRATORY ILLNESS

	Allergic Rhinitis	Common Cold	Sinusitis	Bronchitis	Asthma*
Length of illness	Weeks or months, usually seasonal	At least 5–7 days; self-limiting	Days; months if not treated	1–2 weeks	Seasonal (allergic) to constant (non-allergic)
Cough	None, unless caused by post-nasal drip	Dry, hacking; mucus, if any, is clear	None	Severe; productive of purulent sputum	Plus wheezing and shortness of breath
Fever	None	Low-grade (if any)	Over 100°F; variable	Over 100°F; variable	None
Nasal discharge	Clear	Clear, copious	Purulent, thick, tenacious, yellow-green nasal discharge	No nasal discharge, discolored (purulent) sputum	No nasal discharge unless rhinitis is present; variable cough & sputum production
Pain	None	None, or headache and muscle ache at onset	Pain over involved sinuses	In chest, on coughing or drawing deep breath	Discomfort or tightness rather than pain in chest
Sore throat	None	Should be gone within 3 days	None	None	None
Other	Constant symptoms indicate allergen in the home or at work	1 to 3 episodes yearly common even in healthy persons	Sore throat may occur due to sinus drainage	Very common in cigarette smokers	Exercise and aspirin precipitate the episodes

*Consultation with your family physician is recommended.

After the first exposure to the offending chemical, allergic sensitization develops over seven to ten days. On reexposure a blistering rash develops at the sites of contact. The reaction is a cell-mediated response dependent on T lymphocytes reacting with the hapten-protein combination that makes up the allergen. Immunoglobulins such as IgE are not involved. The sensitizing potential of the chemical depends on its ability to combine with skin proteins, the concentration of chemical touching the skin, and the area of skin contacted. The length of contact is also important. Contact on injured skin is much more likely to cause sensitization than on normal skin. Therefore, the use of ointments and medications applied directly to diseased or damaged skin may be followed by the development of contact sensitivity persisting as long as the medication is used.

In addition to cosmetics and plants, medications and perfumes often cause contact sensitivity. Many occupational exposures also are to blame. Contact dermatitis is one of the leading causes of work-related illness. The location of the skin rash is often a clue to the cause. A rash on the ear lobes suggests sensitivity to the metal in earrings, particularly if the ears are pierced, or to hair dye and perfumes. Cosmetics frequently cause rashes about the eyelids and lips. A rash on the toes may indicate a reaction to the dyes in shoe leather. Rashes about the belt line may be caused by elastic bands in clothing.

It is important to discover which chemical substance is causing allergic contact dermatitis because the rash will persist unless the allergen is scrupulously avoided. This can be done by careful history, which will suggest the possible offenders, and by patch testing. Patch testing is done by applying a small, non-irritating amount of the suspected chemical to a gauze bandage and attaching it to normal skin on the back or arm. In 24 to 48 hours the patch is removed. If the person is sensitive to the chemical, a localized reddened spot of varying intensity will be present. The offending substance should be avoided.

Once contact dermatitis develops to one chemical, the person is more likely to develop sensitivity to others. The capacity to develop this type of allergy is much more common than IgE-mediated symptoms. It is estimated that with sufficient exposure, more than nine out of ten persons could develop contact sensitivity. Persons with IgE-mediated allergies do not have a greater predisposition to develop allergic contact dermatitis, but because persons with eczema frequently apply medications to the skin, they more often develop contact sensitivity on the basis of increased exposure.

As with other allergies, the best treatment is to minimize or completely avoid the allergenic chemical. Women sensitive to rubber gloves can substitute plastic gloves when washing dishes. Nickel, present in jewelry, is a common cause of sensitivity. Once this sensitivity is recognized, it is relatively easy to avoid earrings, bracelets, rings, and necklaces containing nickel. The problem is particularly difficult in occupational exposures. Rubber sensitivity is caused by chemicals added to natural rubber gum. Because rubber use is widespread, rubber is much more difficult to avoid than materials such as cosmetics,

deodorants, perfumes, and synthetic glues. It may be necessary for a worker to change jobs.

Extensive contact dermatitis may require the use of cortisone-like drugs by mouth. Locally applied cortisone ointments are among the few medications that can be safely used for rashes of any sort without running the risk of causing contact sensitivity.

The rash of contact dermatitis is self-limited and only involves areas of the skin touched by the chemical. The rash does not leave scars unless a secondary infection occurs. Infections can follow intense scratching that introduces bacteria into the open sores of the skin. It then becomes important to see a physician immediately. The use of nonprescription lotions for allergic contact dermatitis is ineffective and frequently will produce additional sensitization to chemicals contained in the lotion.

Poison Ivy, Poison Oak, and Poison Sumac

When the English colonists reached Virginia, the Indians told Captain John Smith about a skin rash acquired by touching plants. Smith's description was the first recorded evidence of allergies in America, and poison ivy, poison oak, and poison sumac have been plaguing Americans ever since. In this case, the offending agent is a plant oil called urushiol, which causes severe rash, intense itching, and blistering where it touches the skin.

The three species of urushiol-containing plants have distinct appearances. Poison ivy has glossy green leaves which grow in groups of three, and small light green flowers and berries. It usually grows as a vine and occasionally as an erect shrub. It is common in the central and eastern portions of the United States. Poison oak closely resembles poison ivy, but grows as a shrub with leaves resembling oak leaves. It is common on the West Coast of the United States. Poison sumac is found in swampy locations where it grows as a small tree with green berries. It can be distinguished from harmless sumac plants, which have clusters of red berries.

It is often difficult to avoid these plants because poison ivy and poison oak grow almost everywhere, including suburban backyards and pastures. The oil is often spread by pets who do not react to it but may carry it on their fur. When recognized in the yard, the plants should be eliminated by digging out the roots extremely carefully. The plant should then be buried and not burned, because smoke from the plants can carry the offending oils great distances.

Although some persons claim to be "immune" to the plants' effects, this is seldom the case. Touching the plant usually does not produce a rash on first exposure, but repeated exposures increase the likelihood of outbreak. Persons with a history of sensitivity should always keep well covered when exposure is possible, wearing trousers and long-sleeved shirts, for instance, when walking in the woods.

For those who work outdoors, avoiding the plant may be impossible. Immunotherapy can be attempted before the plant season begins. This treatment, too, derives from the American Indians. They recognized that sensitization to the plant could be prevented by swallowing the leaves. However, the injection method is only useful to prevent sensitization before it has developed. It can be dangerous once sensitivity is present. Currently, only research groups are using this method.

ALLERGIC VASCULITIS AND GLOMERULONEPHRITIS

Immunologic injury of blood vessels (vasculitis) and the kidney (glomerulonephritis) occurs when complexes of allergen and antibody are deposited in the tissues and cause an inflammatory reaction. Henoch-Schonlein purpura is an example, manifested by bleeding into the skin and digestive tract and by kidney abnormalities. IgA and IgM antibodies can be identified in biopsies of injured skin and kidney, and sometimes the allergen can be identified. In addition to the hemorrhagic skin rash, abdominal pain often is present because of vasculitis in the digestive tract. Henoch-Schonlein purpura frequently follows respiratory tract infections and viruses may be the allergens. In a study of more than 100 patients with this type of allergic vasculitis, food could be shown to be the allergen causing the vasculitis in only one patient while infectious allergens were identified in 20 percent.

AUTOIMMUNE DISEASES

Most allergic diseases are caused by immunologic responses to allergens from outside the body that are inhaled, eaten, injected, or touched. Autoimmune diseases are produced by harmful immunologic reactions to the body's own tissues. While IgE-mediated allergies and allergic contact dermatitis are more common in males, the autoimmune diseases are much more common in females. Far fewer people develop autoimmune diseases than allergies to external (foreign) allergens. However, these "allergic to self" diseases are frequently life-threatening or associated with chronic severe symptoms and are being recognized with increasing frequency.

It is important to recognize that the autoimmune or autoallergic reaction is against normal tissues. There is considerable evidence that the normal, protective immune response can recognize early changes in cells that may develop into malignant tumors. This type of response to altered tissue, called "immune surveillance," is an important defense mechanism against cancer. It also appears that very early in life and in the elderly, the peak ages of cancers and leukemias, there is a relative deficiency of immunity.

Rh Disease of the Newborn

One of the triumphs of modern immunology is the prevention of what was, until the early 1970s, an often fatal disease of newborns. It occurred in babies with Rh-positive blood who were born to mothers with Rh-negative blood. The Rh factor is an antigen on the surface of red blood cells and is present in 85 percent of the population. Those people are classified as Rh-positive. The remaining 15 percent lack the antigen and are Rh-negative. They will produce anti-Rh antibody if transfused with Rh-positive blood. If an Rh-negative woman conceives by an Rh-positive husband, there is a good chance that the child will be Rh-positive. In one in 20 Rh-negative women carrying an Rh-positive baby, sensitization by the baby's red cells will trigger the development of IgG antibody against the Rh blood group. This usually occurs after delivery of the first Rh-positive baby and causes no health problems or difficulty for the woman.

In subsequent pregnancies in which the fetus is Rh-positive, however, dire consequences can occur. Since IgG antibody can cross the placenta from mother to baby, it combines with baby's Rh-positive red blood cells and rapidly destroys them. The resulting anemia may be so severe that the fetus develops heart failure and may die before delivery unless early induction of labor or a cesarean section is performed. The problem does not end with delivery, either, because red cell destruction continues and the accumulated breakdown products cause jaundice and can damage the baby's brain. An exchange transfusion is then necessary to remove all the baby's Rh-positive blood, plus the harmful antibody, and replace it with Rh-negative cells.

Fortunately, there has been a happy ending to the story of Rh disease. It is now possible to prevent sensitization of the Rh-negative mother by the Rh-positive baby by treating the mother within 72 hours after birth of her first Rh-positive baby with IgG anti-Rh antibody from another person. This keeps her from producing IgG anti-Rh antibody. With this simple, inexpensive, and safe treatment, the problem of Rh hemolytic disease of the newborn is being eliminated.

Autoimmune Hemolytic Anemia

Autoimmune hemolytic anemia occurs when a person produces antibodies against his or her own red blood cells, resulting in their destruction. The anemia is similar to that of the newborn with Rh disease. The cause of the illness is unknown. Often it is associated with a viral infection that can alter the membrane of the red blood cell. Autoimmune hemolytic anemia can be transient and mild in nature and go unnoticed. However, in the majority of patients, treatment with cortisone-like drugs is necessary to decrease the immunologic destruction of red blood cells. If cortisone is not effective, the spleen may be removed. Splenectomy has several effects. One is to remove the site where antibody-coated red cells are destroyed. Another effect is elimination of a tissue that produces the harmful antibody. A new treatment for autoimmune hemolytic anemia is similar to that used in Rh disease. It is called plasmapheresis and involves removing plasma, the portion of blood containing the IgG antibody, then returning the red cells to the patient (see chapter 6, "The Blood").

Hyperthyroidism

It is now recognized that hyperthyroidism is an autoimmune disease caused by an IgG antibody which directly stimulates the thyroid gland to release excessive amounts of its hormone (see chapter 16, "The Hormones and Endocrine Glands"). Hyperthyroidism usually develops in women and is characterized by enlargement of the thyroid gland in the neck. Excess thyroid hormone release causes the entire cellular machinery of the body to function at an accelerated rate. The person becomes nervous and upset, loses weight in spite of a good appetite and food intake, and feels warm even in cool surroundings. Additional symptoms include bulging of the eyes, sweating, and tremor. Hyperthyroidism is often associated with other autoimmune diseases. Treatment includes medications to block the production of the thyroid hormones, administration of radioactive iodine that accumulates in the thyroid gland and destroys thyroid tissue, and the surgical removal of portions of the enlarged, overactive gland. Even though IgG antibody is recognized as the cause of hyperthyroidism, there is no safe and effective way to stop its production.

Myasthenia Gravis

Myasthenia gravis (grave weakness) is an autoimmune disease manifested by muscle weakness. In contrast to hyperthyroidism, myasthenia gravis occurs when IgG autoantibody blocks the communication between the nerves and muscle cells. The consequence is weakness in specific sets of muscles. It is predominantly a disease of women aged 20 to 40, but in another affected group, those over 60, males are more commonly affected.

Myasthenia occurs when an IgG autoantibody combines with the receptor of the nerve signal responsible for muscle action. This signal is provided by the neurotransmitter acetylcholine, a chemical released from the nerve ending that normally links with its receptor on the muscle. This linkage is a signal for the muscle to contract. IgG autoantibody interferes with the linkage, and muscles respond only weakly. The weakness intensifies with continued muscle activity. Symptoms vary from double vision (weakness of the eye muscles) to generalized muscle paralysis with inability to swallow or breathe. In 70 percent of myasthenia gravis patients, the thymus gland is enlarged. Tumors of the thymus gland occur in an additional 15 percent. The overgrowth is related to the development of the IgG antibody to the muscle receptor for acetylcholine.

Myasthenia gravis may be treated with oral medications to prolong the action of acetylcholine. Surgical removal of the enlarged thymus also results in improvement, particularly in young women. More recently, a transfusion technique similar to that used for Rh babies has been developed. This method removes the IgG antibody by completely exchanging the blood.

Systemic Lupus Erythematosus

Systemic lupus erythematosus (SLE) occurs eight times more often in women in the childbearing ages than in men. SLE patients develop a wide range of symptoms often without obvious physical changes. Thus it may not be diagnosed until several years after initial symptoms occur. The first clues usually are fatigue and muscle and joint pains. The joint pain often occurs without obvious swelling or destruction of the joints. Patients with SLE produce autoantibodies that react with their blood cell membranes and other cell parts. The antibodies to the cell membrane cause direct damage as in autoimmune hemolytic anemia. Other antibodies injure tissue by combining with self antigens. The resulting complexes are deposited in the kidney and blood vessels, causing inflammation.

Until the 1970s, SLE was described in medical textbooks as a fatal disease of young women. At the present time, however, more than 95 percent of patients with SLE are alive and often feel well ten years after diagnosis. It is likely that the outcome of SLE is even better than this, but newer treatments have not been used long enough to establish their long-term benefits. SLE remains a potentially life-threatening illness, but significant progress has been made in the diagnosis and treatment of the disease.

The cause of SLE is not known. An inherited predisposition appears important, although not as important as in IgE-mediated allergies. Development of autoimmune disease appears to be related to a loss of the normal regulatory control of the immune response so that the response in the form of antibody is directed against the body's own tissue. Another factor appears to be an environmental trigger. This can be a viral infection or exposure to drugs or toxins that upset the normal controls of the immune system.

PROGRESS AGAINST ALLERGY

Enormous progress has been made since 1970 in understanding the events that lead to the development of harmful allergies, to diseases caused by immunologic responses to external substances in the environment, and to the less well-defined autoimmune diseases.

Because these recent advances are not widely known, considerable misunderstanding and outright ignorance exists about allergies and their treatment. It is tragic to see many illnesses labeled as "allergies" when, in fact, they are not. Also, highly questionable "allergy" treatments, ranging from such severely restricted diets that dangerous weight loss occurs, to living like a hermit, are harmful. Rarely does an allergic person have IgE antibody to more than a few foods. An even more bizarre so-called allergy treatment is injections of a person's own urine. There is no valid scientific evidence whatsoever for urine injections as a treatment for allergies. It is a dangerous practice because antigens from the kidney are present in normal urine. When this urine is injected back into the patient, a definite risk arises of producing autoantibody which could damage the kidney. This has occurred in experimental animals.

For the most part, allergic diseases can be controlled when a sensible and commonsense approach is taken by the patient and family. Medications are used under the guidance of the family physician or a specialist in allergic and autoimmune diseases. The National Institute of Allergy and Infectious Diseases, Bethesda, Maryland, the Allergy and Asthma Foundation of America, New York City, New York, and the Arthritis Foundation, Atlanta, Georgia, can provide updated information about allergic and autoimmune diseases.

CHAPTER 22   **CALVIN M. KUNIN, M.D.**

THE KIDNEYS AND URINARY SYSTEM

We think of the human body as solid, but in fact a large proportion of it is liquid. The fluid we call blood, pumped by the ceaseless work of the heart, reaches every extremity of the body. Fluids surround and bathe the cells. The conversion of food to energy or to the substances that form the body's building blocks produces other chemical fluids and wastes. It is the task of the kidneys to monitor and control these fluids, to keep them within rigorously narrow limits. Without the kidneys, we would drown in fluid or die of the accumulation of poisonous waste.

The kidneys can be thought of as the circulatory system's quality control department. The heart works blindly and untiringly, pushing the blood through its chambers into the arteries of the body without regard to its makeup. The kidney, as sophisticated as any computer, ensures that volume and composition are precisely right. It filters out substances that are in excess and removes those that might be harmful. The job is prodigious and endless. Every time we eat or drink, the composition of the fluids is changed. Metabolism steadily produces acids and waste products and feeds them into the body fluids and bloodstream. Several hundred chemicals are present in the body, and delicate balances must be maintained for each of them.

We all know the kidney's method for ridding the body of waste. Urine, a supersaturated solution of salts, is formed in the kidneys, drop by drop. It is funneled down a tiny conduit called the ureter, then into a storage organ called the bladder, and finally, when a half pint or more has been collected, it is carried outside the body via another conduit, the urethra. The organs that transport urine out of the body are known as the urinary system.

Of course, urine is only one way the body disposes of salts and water. The ordinary process of breathing gets rid of water vapor and carbon dioxide. Salt and water pass through

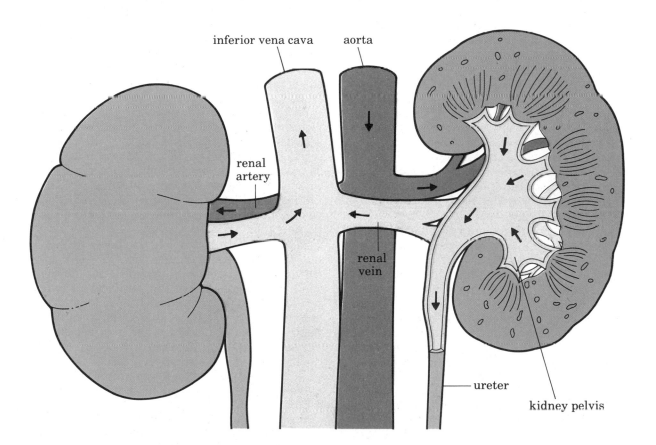

THE KIDNEY IN ACTION

About 400 gallons of blood flow through the kidney each day, arriving via the renal artery and leaving via the renal vein. Black arrows show the blood pathways. As shown in the cutaway drawing (right), the delicate workings of the kidney filter materials from the blood and concentrate about 1½ quarts of urine daily. Urine is collected in the kidney pelvis and passes down the ureter to the bladder.

the skin by evaporation and perspiration, with the losses greatly increased during hot weather, exercise or fever. Prolonged vomiting and diarrhea rob the body of large amounts of fluid and salt. The ever-vigilant kidney must adjust for these losses by retaining salt and water when intake is inadequate to keep up with losses or when excretion is excessive. At times of injury or blood loss, the kidney must protect the volume of the blood in circulation. It does so by holding water and salts and returning them to the bloodstream. This is the body's first line of defense against shock.

A LOOK AT THE KIDNEYS

The kidneys are a pair of maroon-colored, bean-shaped organs, each weighing about half a pound. They are so distinctive in shape that if we describe a swimming pool or sofa as kidney-shaped, listeners know immediately what we mean. Located behind the abdominal cavity, they lie at the base of the rib cage. The right kidney is a little higher than the left. It rests just beneath the liver, and the left kidney rests beneath the spleen.

Renal arteries connect the kidney directly to the aorta, the main artery of the body, and bring its blood supply. After blood has passed through the kidneys, it returns to circulation through renal veins linked to the vena cava, the body's main vein. As urine is formed in a kidney, it flows into the renal pelvis, a funnel-shaped structure that covers the small ducts leading from the kidney. Each pelvis is connected to a ureter, which feeds into the bladder.

The kidneys receive about one-fourth of the blood pumped into the aorta with each thump of the heart. Some simple arithmetic shows what enormous work these organs silently perform. The heart of a healthy adult at rest beats about 60 to 70 times a minute. Each beat expels about two ounces of blood into the aorta. This adds up to about a gallon of blood a minute, 60 or more gallons an hour, more than 1,440 gallons a day. The kidney receives about 25 percent of that total—360 to 450 gallons a day. Each drop is filtered carefully, then returned to circulation. For all of that, only one to two quarts of urine is manufactured a day.

The kidneys are protected by a pad of fat that holds them in place and cushions them against injury. They are hardy organs, with a remarkable backup reserve. Removal of one kidney leaves function virtually intact. The remaining kidney slowly enlarges to compensate for the loss of its partner. Even when up to 90 percent of function in both kidneys has been destroyed by disease, the kidneys still can maintain normal blood volume and adjust the composition of body fluids to sustain life. In fact, some persons are born with a solitary kidney and the fact is never realized until the absence is disclosed by X ray or autopsy.

When all kidney function is destroyed, however, death follows inevitably. Toxic substances and acids produced by the cells accumulate in the body. The tissues become overburdened with salt and water. The clogged organs are no longer able to work properly. The gradual process of disturbed organ function caused by kidney collapse is called uremia. Left untreated, it progresses to convulsions, coma, heartbeat irregularities, and finally death.

The Functioning Kidney

If you were to slice open a kidney from top to bottom and examine it microscopically, you would see a million or more tiny microscopic tubes called nephrons. These nephrons are the working parts of the organ. Each is a miniature kidney in the sense that it draws blood from the arteries, filters fluid out of the blood, returns some of the fluid back to the bloodstream, and collects urine at its terminal end. The nephrons are aligned alongside each other in a semicircular pattern, which gives the kidney its distinctive shape. Each nephron performs the same specialized task as its neighbor.

The kidney itself is no bigger than your fist, but the nephrons are quite long. It has been estimated that some of their capillaries, if they could be stretched out and laid end to end, would extend for 50 miles. Like a strand of spaghetti dropped on a plate, however, the nephron bends back on itself in a series of curves and hairpin turns so it covers a great deal of distance in a compact space.

At the beginning of each nephron is a specialized, indented, spherical structure called a Bowman's capsule. Its shape is roughly what you would get if you punched your fist deeply into a soft rubber ball—cup-shaped with two thicknesses of wall. The cup contains a lacy filigree of small capillaries called the glomerulus. A tiny artery brings blood into the glomerulus, and another tiny vessel carries the excess back into circulation.

The relationship between the glomerulus and the mitten-like Bowman's capsule forms a microscopic filtration plant. Blood pressure is its driving force. Pressure pushes the components of the blood, except blood cells and most protein, through the walls of the capillaries into the space between the glomerulus and Bowman's capsule and then through the thin wall of the capsule. The resulting fluid, or filtrate, then flows into the tubule, the hollow tube of the nephron.

About 180 quarts a day of the filtrate pass through this filtration plant. Most of it is water, but it also contains many dissolved materials. Some are indispensable for the body's welfare, and some are harmful. Obviously if all this fluid were lost, we would be in a state of perpetual thirst and so starved for essential

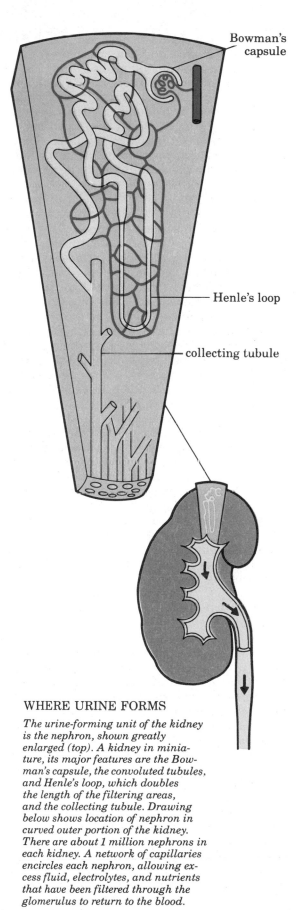

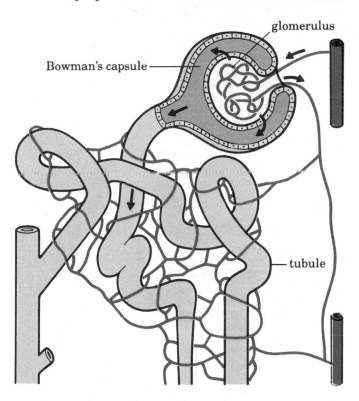

THE FILTRATION PLANT

The kidney's filtration system has three basic elements: the cup-shaped Bowman's capsule, the glomerulus, which is a tufted network of capillaries within the capsule, and the convoluted tubule. Blood arrives via the capillaries and is filtered through their walls and into the space between the double walls of the capsule. The filtrate then passes down the tubule, where most of the water and some other substances are reabsorbed and the remainder is concentrated as urine. Arrows show direction of flow. After filtration, blood returns to circulation.

WHERE URINE FORMS

The urine-forming unit of the kidney is the nephron, shown greatly enlarged (top). A kidney in miniature, its major features are the Bowman's capsule, the convoluted tubules, and Henle's loop, which doubles the length of the filtering areas, and the collecting tubule. Drawing below shows location of nephron in curved outer portion of the kidney. There are about 1 million nephrons in each kidney. A network of capillaries encircles each nephron, allowing excess fluid, electrolytes, and nutrients that have been filtered through the glomerulus to return to the blood.

chemicals that death would soon result. The task of the tubule is to reduce the huge filtered load to a quart a day by reabsorbing most of the water and essential chemicals back into the circulatory system. Down its convoluted course the fluid is gradually concentrated and the excess water squeezed out, until only a small amount of fluid carrying unneeded or unwanted chemicals remains. This product, emerging from the distant end of the nephron, is urine.

Meanwhile, the kidney also can draw certain chemicals from its surrounding network of capillaries. This process, called active transport or secretion, helps the kidney keep acid-base, fluid, and electrolyte balances in the body within proper limits. Thus the kidney can exchange acid, which is the hydrogen ion, for sodium or potassium and manufacture ammonia to neutralize excess acid.

The electrolytes, which are a major concern of the kidneys, are dissolved salts or ions that are needed in the body's chemical processes. The most familiar one is sodium, an element of common salt. About 2½ pounds of salt pass through the tubules daily, but not even a third of an ounce is excreted in urine. If the body contains too much salt, or if the kidneys cannot excrete it, the tissues become waterlogged and fluid-filled, a condition called edema. On the other hand, if the salt balance falls too low, from profuse perspiration during physical exertion in hot weather, salt depletion may cause dehydration and "heat cramps." Similarly, the kidney keeps many other electrolytes in balance. Its sophistication has never been matched by even the most complex man-made substitutes.

The Composition of Urine

The liquid that trickles from the base of the nephron is quite different from the blood that entered at the top. Urine ordinarily is entirely free of red and white blood cells and platelets, and contains only small amounts of blood protein. It resembles serum, the watery portion of the blood in which salt and certain other compounds are dissolved. The major substances carried by the urine are sodium, potassium, chloride, and hydrogen-ion (acid); minor ones are calcium, magnesium, phosphates, and sulfates.

Urine is acid or alkaline, depending on diet and the products of cell breakdown. A diet high in animal protein tends to produce an acid urine. A deficiency of animal protein produces an alkaline one. Urea, the waste product left when proteins and their amino acid building blocks are broken down, and creatinine, a

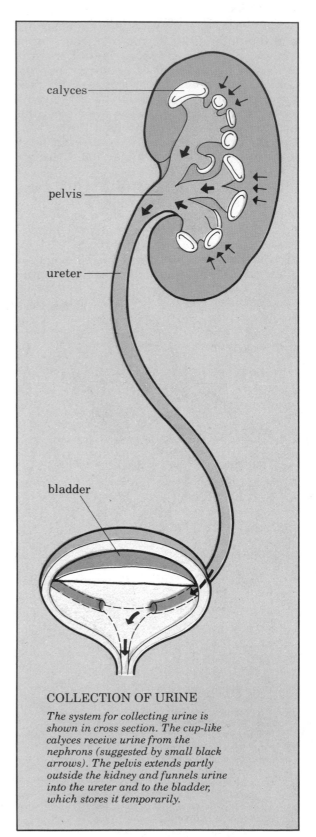

COLLECTION OF URINE

The system for collecting urine is shown in cross section. The cup-like calyces receive urine from the nephrons (suggested by small black arrows). The pelvis extends partly outside the kidney and funnels urine into the ureter and to the bladder, which stores it temporarily.

product of the normal breakdown and repair of muscle, also are excreted into the urine. Urine composition further depends on water intake, and loss via sweating or breath vapor. Exercise, fever, disease, and drugs may alter how much blood is delivered to the kidney, and the quantity of water or chemicals returned to the blood or excreted into the urine.

Although the composition of urine is highly variable, it provides certain clues to kidney disease. Among the warning signs are white or red blood cells or cells shed into the urine from the kidney itself. Large amounts of protein in the urine may indicate kidney damage. Crystals in the urine warn of the possibility of other diseases. Glucose or acetone may appear in the urine of diabetics, and bile in that of persons with liver diseases.

Urine is sterile when formed in the body and stored in the bladder. The presence of bacteria, viruses, or yeasts is distinctly abnormal.

The Collecting System

The urine collecting system operates on the principle of gravity and is simplicity itself. After the clear fluid has been manufactured by the tubules, it flows into a series of microscopic collecting ducts that merge into several funnel-shaped structures, the papillae, then into cup-like calyces, which feed into larger calyces until finally all pour their products into a large single cavity, the kidney pelvis. The pelvis is partly inside and partly outside the kidney and is drained by two tube-like ureters, one for each kidney. The pressure of the urine and the force of gravity carry the urine down the ureters into the bladder.

The bladder is a storage organ. It is elastic, built of a strong network of muscle fibers that allow the wall to stretch as urine collects. The outlet at the base is surrounded by sphincter muscles that tighten like purse strings and keep the liquid from escaping until it can be disposed of. That occurs when nerves within the walls send signals to the spinal cord and brain that the bladder is ready to be emptied, usually when about a half-pint of urine has been collected, although as much as a quart can be retained. Messages relayed back to the bladder stimulate the organ to contract and simultaneously relax the purse-string muscles, so that urine can pass freely into the urethra. This final passage out of the body is relatively short in women—one to two inches long—but measures eight to nine inches in men. The midportion of the male urethra is surrounded by the prostate gland (see chapter 23, "The Male Reproductive System").

The Kidney Hormones

In addition to their other duties, the kidneys produce three hormones that are released into the bloodstream and regulate other body functions.

Renin is a large protein that acts as a catalyst to activate another protein, angiotensin, which is made in the liver. In one of the body's exquisite feedback systems, angiotensin then acts on the cells of the adrenal cortex, the exterior of the adrenal gland atop the kidney, to produce another hormone, aldosterone, which "tells" the kidneys to retain salt and water. Thus the kidney senses when the body is threatened by excess loss of fluid or blood, and releases renin to warn the body. Aldosterone returns the message to hold back salt and water to protect the blood volume.

Erythropoietin is sent by the kidney through the blood to the bone marrow. There it stimulates the production of red blood cells. One reason persons with severely damaged kidneys are also anemic is that production of erythropoietin is reduced.

Vitamin D, the "sunshine vitamin," normally is manufactured in the skin or provided in the diet. But kidney action transforms it into an enormously more potent form, 1,25 dihydroxy metabolite, which assumes the role of a hormone. Secreted into the bloodstream, this "enhanced" vitamin helps control absorption of calcium from the digestive system and the laying down of calcium in the bones.

During episodes of uremia or severe kidney failure, the bones may soften (a condition called renal osteomalacia or "sick bones") because of a drop in production of this enhanced vitamin D and a resulting loss of calcium.

In severe kidney disease, calcium is often lost in the urine and phosphate retained. Blood levels are low in calcium and high in phosphate. The body responds by releasing a hormone from the parathyroid gland in the neck, which mobilizes calcium from the bones. Unfortunately, this calcium may not restore blood levels but instead may crystallize in muscles or skin. This so-called metastatic calcification is another complication of kidney failure and sometimes causes further softening of the bones. The potent form of vitamin D has been synthesized and is now available commercially to treat this condition.

Congenital Abnormalities

Like teeth and fingerprints, kidneys are highly individual. Probably no two persons in the world have kidneys exactly alike. Most differences are unimportant and do not affect kidney function. The tracery of creases on the kidney surface, called fetal lobulations, are an example. Malformations normally do not affect kidney performance, but may produce a problem if the kidney becomes overburdened because of injury or disease. For this reason it is important to know whether abnormalities exist and whether the kidneys are functioning properly.

Horseshoe kidney is one of the more common abnormalities. The two kidneys are linked across the top or bottom into a single mass of tissue in the shape of a capital U. Sometimes the bridge between the two does not contain functioning tissue. Sometimes the two kidneys act as one.

Double ureters also are relatively common. Instead of the customary single ureter draining each kidney, some persons have duplicates on one or both sides. This is usually harmless.

Ectopic kidney ("out of normal place") occurs because the fat pad that normally surrounds and protects the kidneys is missing, allowing one or both to move out of position. Sometimes both are found on the same side of the body. The malformation may cause a kink in the ureter, damming the urine behind it and leading to swelling of the pelvis, a condition called hydronephrosis.

Fibrous bands in the kidney pelvis also may obstruct the urine flow. These, too, may cause hydronephrosis. The bands must be removed surgically.

Solitary kidney, which is a single kidney from birth or two kidneys fused so that they function as one, may go unnoticed for years because of the tremendous reserve capacity a kidney has. As long as the kidney is healthy, there is no problem. But a solitary kidney leaves the person without a spare. It is important to know before a kidney operation, because one cannot count on an extra kidney to take over.

Polycystic kidneys develop before birth and reflect improper linkage of the newly formed nephrons to the collecting system. The kidneys contain hundreds of tiny blister-like cysts that collect fluid and have no outlet. In children they may fill to enormous size and may be felt in the abdomen. Sometimes the cysts rupture and bleed or may become infected. The condition, which has a tendency to "run in families," is slowly progressive and can lead to gradual kidney failure.

Vesico-ureteral reflux is the name given to backflow of urine into the ureters instead of into the urethra during urination. It is common in young children, tending to disappear with age. Normally, ureters enter the bladder by tunneling into its wall. As the bladder fills with urine, pressure tends to clamp off the ureters so that flow is automatically downward into the urethra. When the tunnel is abnormally short, however, the ureter is not completely closed and urine backs up into it. If not outgrown or corrected, the condition can cause pressure damage to the kidney called reflux nephropathy. Fortunately, severe cases can be repaired.

Urethral valves, which are bits of membrane-like tissue growing from the lining of the urethra, may obstruct the flow of urine in young boys. They can be removed surgically.

Hypospadias and epispadias are male abnormalities in which the urethra does not end at the tip of the penis, but elsewhere along the shaft. In hypospadias it emerges on the bottom side of the penis; in epispadias it emerges on the top. Both abnormalities can be corrected by a urologic surgeon.

Tests and Instruments

Techniques for studying the functions of the kidney and visualizing the urinary tract have been extensively developed in recent years. Important information can be obtained with highly refined instruments, chemical analyses, X rays, and special function tests.

Urinalysis. Urine is readily obtained and easily studied in the laboratory. From a clean specimen of about two to three ounces, most standard tests for kidney disease can be performed. These include examination for protein, glucose, concentration, acidity (pH), blood and pus, crystals, and bacteria.

Small amounts of protein are always present in urine. Their presence is referred to as proteinuria or sometimes as albuminuria because the principal blood protein that appears in urine is albumin. The finding of small amounts of albumin in the urine is not alarming. Most of the commonly used laboratory tests for protein are so sensitive that they detect even normal amounts in the urine. Most nephrologists do not consider protein in the urine to be abnormal unless one or more grams are excreted into the urine in a day.

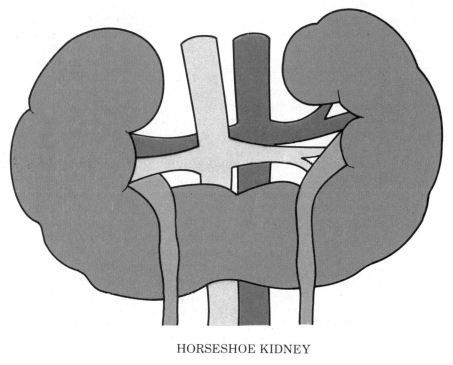

HORSESHOE KIDNEY

POLYCYSTIC KIDNEYS

cysts

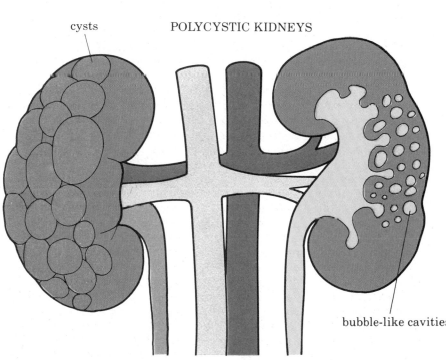

bubble-like cavities

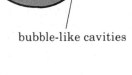

KIDNEY MALFORMATIONS

Kidney malformations are not uncommon. At top is a horseshoe kidney, so-called because the kidneys are joined in the shape of the letter U. Below, polycystic kidneys are covered with blister-like cysts and have bubble-like cavities inside. Outline drawing shows location of a solitary kidney. Because of the great reserve capacity kidneys have, many persons live all their lives with a malformation and never become aware of it.

Small amounts of glucose also are found in urine of healthy persons. Fortunately the routine tests detect only abnormal amounts. An excess of glucose, a condition called glycosuria, may be a sign of diabetes but may also result from severely damaged kidneys. The kidneys usually retain glucose so well that even when 99 percent of kidney function has been lost, glycosuria is a distinctly unusual finding. Hospitalized patients who are receiving intravenous solutions containing glucose often have spillover into the urine, but this is simply caused by overload.

Victims of severe kidney disease often cannot produce a concentrated urine. This can be detected by measurement of a specific gravity, just as one can test the amount of antifreeze in a car radiator. The amount of salt is slight relative to the amount of water. Of course, a person who drinks large amounts of fluids also excretes a highly dilute urine to rid the body of excess water. Therefore, measurement of specific gravity is meaningful only when the amount of fluids consumed beforehand is known. Urine is usually highly concentrated while fasting during sleep. A dilute urine in the first voided specimen of the day suggests possible kidney damage.

The acidity (pH) of the urine depends largely on diet. Urine is usually acid in carnivores (meat eaters) and alkaline in herbivores (vegetable eaters). It is acid during starvation, because muscle is being broken down to supply energy to the body. Persons with infections of the urinary tract caused by bacteria that split urea to ammonia often have an alkaline urine. And for all of us the urine sometimes becomes alkaline for a short time after a heavy meal when the kidney must compensate for loss of stomach acid.

Blood or pus in the urine is abnormal and calls for investigation. During menstruation, there may be some mixing of the menses with urine. Women should always inform their physician if they are menstruating so the doctor will not be confused by an abnormal urine test.

When urine is cooled below body temperature, crystals form and the fluid becomes cloudy. This is normal and no cause for alarm. Crystals tend to obscure blood and pus cells so that fresh urine must be examined to see them clearly under the microscope.

Because bacteria are picked up by the stream as it passes over the external tissues, their presence in urine does not necessarily signify infection. Only when large numbers of bacteria are found in freshly obtained urine in several consecutive tests does one have "significant bacteriuria."

The nitrite test allows persons to test for urinary tract infection at home. The test is based on the principle that small amounts of nitrate from the diet are excreted in the urine. When nitrate is exposed to large numbers of bacteria for about six to eight hours, nitrite is formed and will produce a pink color when mixed with the chemicals impregnated onto filter paper in the test strip. When the strip is moistened with or dipped into the urine, the color changes within a few seconds if nitrite is present. A first morning voided urine sample must be used because it represents urine that has incubated in the bladder overnight.

Properly used, the nitrite test has about a 70 percent chance of detecting infection. If performed on three consecutive days, the odds rise to 90 percent. The test is inexpensive and can be used by mothers to screen their children for infection, or for follow-up to determine whether treatment was effective.

Inexpensive home tests to culture and identify bacteria are also available commercially. For example, with "dip-slide" tests, the slide covered with nutrient for the bacteria is dipped into the urine, then put into a sterile plastic container and brought to the physician's office for interpretation. Or a well-instructed layman can incubate and interpret the test at home with as much accuracy as more expensive cultures done in hospital laboratories.

Blood tests and timed urine collections are used together as measures of kidney function to determine the efficiency of the remaining nephrons. The test usually measures amounts of urea or creatinine, the products of protein and muscle breakdown. Sometimes inulin, a sugar polymer, is measured for even more accurate determination.

Essentially, blood tests assess how well the kidney extracts substances from the blood and excretes them into the urine, calculating the volume of the substance cleared per minute. Other indicators in the blood of kidney insufficiency are concentrations of calcium and phosphate, and concentrations of the electrolytes sodium, potassium, and chloride. Low levels of sodium are associated with muscle cramps and convulsions. High levels of potassium are associated with rhythm disturbances of the heart. If excess albumin is lost, hypoalbuminemia (low blood albumin) and collection of fluid in the tissues may result.

X rays. The kidneys often can be outlined on X rays of the abdomen. They can be seen best by intravenous pyelogram. In this test, a radiopaque dye (one that X rays cannot penetrate) is injected into the veins, then is rapidly excreted by the kidneys. X rays every few minutes show the kidney shape, the collection of dye in the pelvis, ureters and bladder. Doctors can even determine whether the bladder empties properly by waiting until it is filled with dye, then X-raying after voiding to see whether dye is left behind.

If kidneys are too severely damaged to excrete dye from the blood, dye can be introduced into the bladder and the ureters via a catheter. This is called a retrograde pyelogram because the dye is introduced upward. The dye and X-ray combination outlines the bladder more

distinctly and can show whether the dye refluxes into the ureter during urination.

A renal arteriogram is used to examine the blood vessels of the kidney. Radiopaque dye is injected into the aorta near the renal arteries by threading a fine catheter through the arterial circuit. An arteriogram is particularly useful for determining blood flow in the kidney and visualizing tumors or cysts.

Computerized axial tomography (CAT scan) gives a finely detailed X-ray "slice" of the body (see chapter 32, X Rays and Radiology). It is useful to detect tumors, collections of pus, and blood in the kidney region.

A catheter is a rubber or plastic tube used to drain urine from the bladder, relieve obstruction, or inject dye and measure resistance to passage. It also can be used to test for resid-

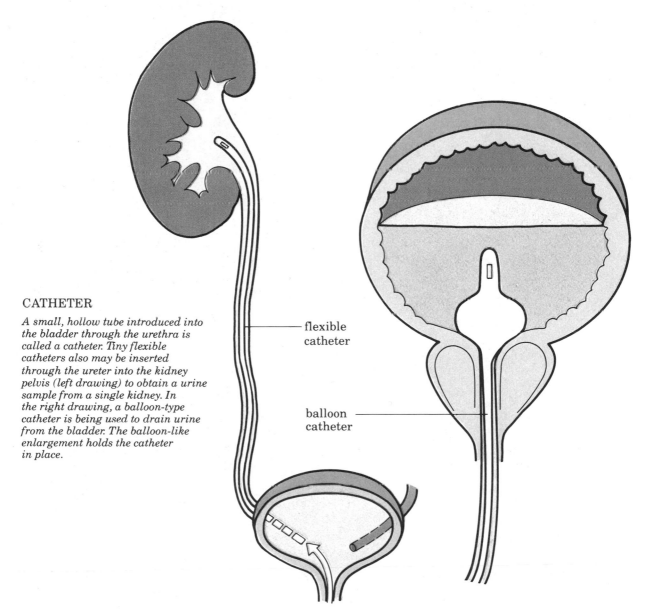

CATHETER

A small, hollow tube introduced into the bladder through the urethra is called a catheter. Tiny flexible catheters also may be inserted through the ureter into the kidney pelvis (left drawing) to obtain a urine sample from a single kidney. In the right drawing, a balloon-type catheter is being used to drain urine from the bladder. The balloon-like enlargement holds the catheter in place.

flexible catheter

balloon catheter

ual urine. In this test, the subject voluntarily passes all the urine he or she can void. A well lubricated catheter is then inserted to drain off the remaining urine. This provides an excellent measurement of the ability of the bladder to empty.

Catheters sometimes carry bacteria with them into the bladder, but they may be life-saving if they relieve obstruction or permit emptying of bladders that are poorly controlled because of disease of the spinal cord. When a catheter is left in place for long periods, it is anchored by a soft rubber balloon at the tip, and attached to a closed sterile plastic drainage bag to prevent infection.

A cystoscope is a lighted, flexible, tube-like instrument with a magnifying lens that can be inserted through the urethra into the bladder to allow the urologist to inspect the bladder visually. He or she can thus detect points of bleeding, tumors, or bladder stones. About the diameter of a fine pencil, the cystoscope often is equipped with tiny attachments that can lift out small stones, burn off tumors, or snip bits of prostate to relieve obstruction.

Drugs

Many drugs can alter blood supply to the kidney or enhance the flow of urine. Those that promote urine production are called diuretics, and in their simplest form are known as osmotic diuretics. This means they draw water with them when excreted by the kidney. The most common examples are urea and mannitol, a compound similar to the sugar glucose that the body does not metabolize.

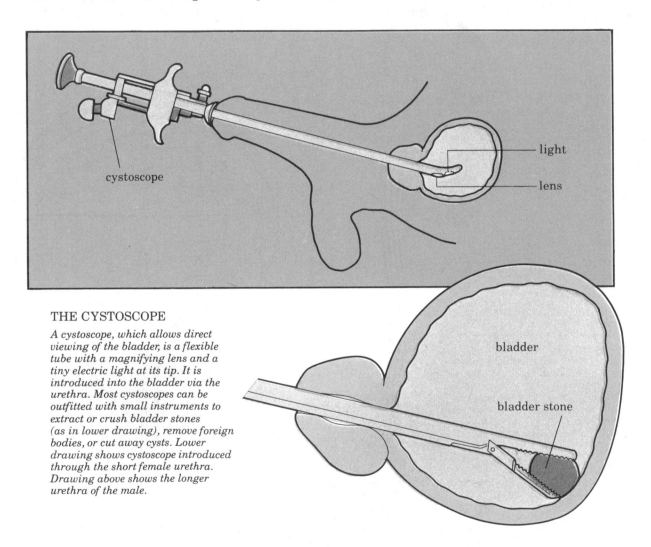

cystoscope

light

lens

bladder

bladder stone

THE CYSTOSCOPE

A cystoscope, which allows direct viewing of the bladder, is a flexible tube with a magnifying lens and a tiny electric light at its tip. It is introduced into the bladder via the urethra. Most cystoscopes can be outfitted with small instruments to extract or crush bladder stones (as in lower drawing), remove foreign bodies, or cut away cysts. Lower drawing shows cystoscope introduced through the short female urethra. Drawing above shows the longer urethra of the male.

Other drugs directly alter the function of the tubules. Spironolactone, for instance, limits the action of the hormone aldosterone, causing excretion of sodium and water and retention of potassium. Mercurial diuretics, very rarely used today, interfere with reabsorption of sodium and chloride by the kidney. Acetazoleamide interferes with exchange of bicarbonate and chloride in the kidney and produces an alkaline urine. Thiazide, ethacrynic acid, and furosemide, all commonly used, are known as high-ceiling diuretics because they produce the greatest increase in loss of water and sodium of any known diuretics. Excessive use can lead to dehydration and low body stores of sodium and potassium.

DISEASES OF THE KIDNEY

Kidney diseases are often classified according to the portion of the kidney that suffers the most damage, either the glomerulus or the tubules. Actually, many diseases involve both portions and are grouped as glomerulonephritis. Another name is "Bright's disease," named for Dr. Richard Bright, an English physician who first described the disease in 1827 before the microscopic anatomy of the kidney was well understood.

The nephrotic syndrome of childhood, also known as minimal glomerular disease or lipoid nephrosis, is the most common disease affecting the glomerular tissue only. Many of the victims of the disease are under four years old. The cause is unknown. Unlike many other forms of kidney disease, there is no inflammation of the kidney and no abnormal findings can be seen under the microscope. The disease is characterized by leakage of blood protein into the urine, apparently because tiny pores enlarge in the glomerular membrane and allow protein molecules to pass through. The concentration of the blood protein albumin falls, and there is massive edema as fluids are lost from the blood into space around the cells.

Sometimes the first symptoms are puffiness around the eyes, or difficulty putting on the child's shoes. Later the small body, particularly the abdomen, may be swollen with fluid. In addition, the disease liberates fats into the blood, so that the serum becomes milky instead of crystal clear. Droplets of fat in the shape of a Maltese cross appear in the urine.

Fortunately, childhood nephrosis often disappears spontaneously or can be treated effectively with corticosteroids or other drugs. Nephrosis can leave the young kidney damaged, however, and it can recur. A similar nephrotic condition occurs in adults and can cause extensive damage to the glomeruli.

Fanconi syndrome, a rare disease, affects only the tubules. They become unable to adjust the levels of amino acids and salts properly, losing them into the urine in excessive quantities. The disease requires careful control of the diet.

Most of the diseases that progressively damage the kidney and ultimately lead to kidney failure are forms of glomerulonephritis. The cause is not understood. In some cases the inflammation seems to result from an immune reaction in which the body mistakenly attacks its own tissue (see chapter 21). A fraction of the cases occur after infection with certain strains of Group A hemolytic streptococcus, the family of bacteria implicated in some sore throats, scarlet fever, and skin rashes. Antibodies produced by the immune system form a complex with antigens that damages the glomerular membrane and allows protein to leak through.

Acute glomerulonephritis, fortunately, is self-limiting in 95 percent of all cases. More common in children than adults, it usually begins with blood in the urine, puffiness in the cheeks and face as fluids are retained, and a sharp rise in blood pressure. Most glomerulonephritis cases that occur after a streptococcus infection fall into this category. Acute glomerulonephritis usually disappears even without treatment, although hospitalization may be required to provide a special diet and to monitor blood pressure. Most patients, especially children, recover completely without kidney damage and rarely have a second attack.

Chronic glomerulonephritis refers to long-standing, persistent inflammatory kidney disease. Most cases are of unknown cause, although the immune reaction likely is implicated here, too. The disease can occur at any age, but is more common in adults than children. Because it is relatively rare and develops slowly in most cases, the disease usually is not detected until the person begins to complain of feeling weak, has aches in the region of the kidney, or is found to have high blood pressure. Blood studies reveal anemia and increased concentrations of urea and creatinine, the protein and muscle wastes. The urine may contain large amounts of protein and red blood cells and casts (protein and cells that solidified in the renal tubules).

The rate of progression of chronic glomerulonephritis varies. Some people may have the disease for five to ten years without needing treatment by artificial kidney (see page 541). Others deteriorate in a few weeks or months. Although some cases can be treated, most persons who eventually require artificial kidneys or kidney transplant have had their kidneys destroyed by these diseases.

Alport's syndrome is an inherited form of glomerulonephritis. It is often accompanied by deafness.

Interstitial nephritis refers to any condition that produces inflammation and damage to the kidney tubules and spaces between them. Among the causes are overuse of analgesic medicines (see page 543) and allergy to such drugs as penicillin and sulfonamides.

Infections of the Kidney and Urinary Tract

Because urine ordinarily is sterile until it is passed through the urethra, bacterial growth in the urine is abnormal. But it is by no means uncommon. At any time, about one percent of the girls in the preschool and school years have asymptomatic bacteriuria, which is silent growth of bacteria in the urine. Thereafter the frequency increases by about 1 percent for each 10 years of life. About one-third of all women will acquire asymptomatic bacteria during their lifetimes. In contrast, the condition is rare in males except during infancy and when the prostate begins to interrupt the flow of urine in later years.

The presence of bacteria in the urine indicates that any of the structures bathed in urine—kidney, bladder, or tract—may become infected, and perhaps damaged before the infection is discovered. Fortunately, cases without symptoms are usually benign, seldom causing serious disease of the kidneys except in persons who have obstruction of the tract caused by stones or malformations, and in those who cannot urinate normally because of bladder paralysis caused by neurological or other diseases. Diabetics also may develop complications. And when asymptomatic bacteriuria is detected early in pregnancy, it must be treated vigorously to prevent symptoms from developing later.

Although not generally alarming, bacterial infections of the urinary system can be distinctively painful and unpleasant, depending on the severity and area affected.

Cystitis (inflammation of the bladder) may be produced by drugs, radiation, or foreign objects, as well as by bacterial infections. Regardless of the cause, the symptoms are often the same: burning on urination, frequent urination, pain in the lower abdomen over the bladder and cloudy, sometimes bloody, urine. In bacterial infections, pus cells and bacteria may be seen when urinary sediment is examined under the microscope. Many antibiotics are available to treat bacterial bladder infections.

Urethritis refers to inflammation of the urethra, also from a variety of causes including (but by no means limited to) gonorrhea or other venereal organisms. As with cystitis, urination is painful and sometimes pus is passed. Bacterial cases can be treated with antibiotics.

Pyelonephritis is the term for bacterial infections of the kidney. In acute pyelonephri-

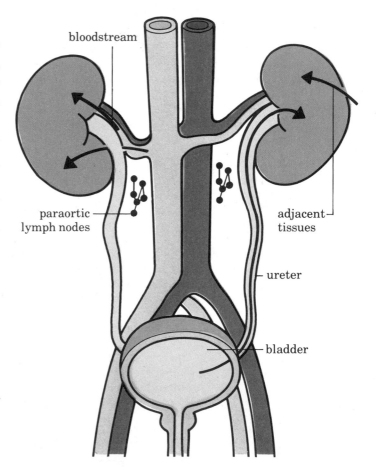

KIDNEY INFECTIONS

Infections arrive in the kidney via various routes; ascending infection from the bladder and ureter, from adjacent tissues, from the bloodstream, and from the lymphatic system.

bloodstream

paraortic lymph nodes

adjacent tissues

ureter

bladder

tis the patient often develops fever and flank or loin pain (over the kidneys below the ribs), and may become acutely ill. Urine contains pus cells and bacteria. The infection may be caused by bacteria migrating up the urinary tract. Some people have both cystitis and acute pyelonephritis at the same time. Most cases of acute pyelonephritis improve gradually, but antibiotics hasten the healing process.

Chronic pyelonephritis indicates either a continued, smoldering infection of the kidney (active) or simply old scars of healed infection (inactive). In severe cases, large portions of the kidneys may be destroyed and the infection may even spread to the tissues surrounding the kidney. Many severe chronic or recurrent pyelonephritis cases occur in persons with diabetes, kidney stones, or obstruction of urinary flow. Their cases may lead to end-stage kidney failure.

Most women with urinary tract infections do not have major anatomic defects of the urinary tract, as X rays show. Those with recurrent infections can often be given a bedtime dose of antibiotics or other drugs.

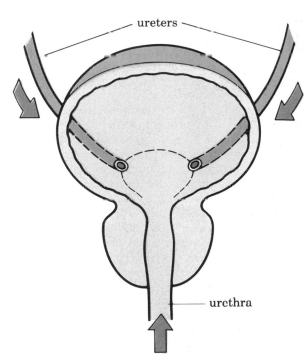

ureters

urethra

CYSTITIS

Inflammation of the bladder (cystitis) usually is caused by bacteria migrating up the urethra, and occasionally by downward migration from the upper urinary tract. Drugs, radiation, or foreign objects also may be responsible.

Sources and symptoms. The source of bacteria in presumably sterile urine is something of a mystery. Bacteria probably are introduced in small numbers into the female bladder periodically (no one knows how often) and rapidly shed by the urine stream during voiding. The event is not detectable since urine passed through the urethra always picks up a few bacteria, and tests cannot determine where the bacteria originated. Sexual intercourse and methods of wiping the genitalia after voiding are thought by some to be important means of introducing bacteria into the bladder, but this has been difficult to document scientifically. Furthermore, urinary infections are common in sexually inactive schoolgirls and are more common in elderly women than sexually active females.

There is no clear evidence that a change in sexual habits will reduce the frequency of urinary tract infections. Oral contraceptives do not increase the frequency of urinary tract infection in young women. Most urinary infections are caused by bacteria commonly found in the bowel. Occasionally, however, organisms present on the skin (staphylococci) can cause urinary infections.

Men who develop urinary tract infections often have been catheterized. Many women can also trace their first infection to catheterization to drain the bladder before delivery of a baby, which is no longer standard practice. The catheter may introduce bacteria into the tract.

Urinary tract infections produce many of the same symptoms of painful and frequent urination as vaginal and venereal infections and are often confused with them. But the infections are quite distinct, caused by different organisms. Bacteria and yeasts responsible for vaginitis do not thrive in the bladder. And there is no evidence that the bacteria that cause urinary tract infections can be transmitted to a partner during intercourse.

Kidney and Bladder Stones

Urinary stones generally are categorized by their primary location either as renal (kidney) stones, technically called nephrolithiasis or renal calculus, or bladder stones. These hard bits of crystalline material precipitated into the urine may obstruct the flow of urine from the kidney and cause kidney damage. More often, stones lodge temporarily in one or both of the ureters and produce severe pain and blood in the urine. Or they serve as a location for persistent infection of the urinary tract. Sometimes they arise as a result of blockage caused by the infection.

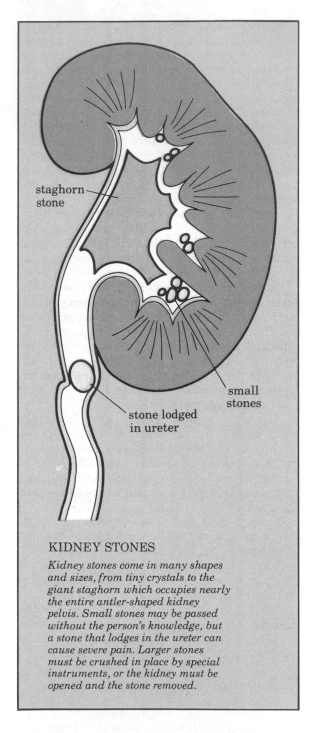

KIDNEY STONES

Kidney stones come in many shapes and sizes, from tiny crystals to the giant staghorn which occupies nearly the entire antler-shaped kidney pelvis. Small stones may be passed without the person's knowledge, but a stone that lodges in the ureter can cause severe pain. Larger stones must be crushed in place by special instruments, or the kidney must be opened and the stone removed.

staghorn stone

stone lodged in ureter

small stones

Stone disease has been recorded since the earliest times. Hippocrates, the father of medicine, for example, cautioned physicians not to "cut persons laboring under the stone, but leave this to be done by men who are practitioners of this work." Nonetheless, the incidence of stone disease still has some puzzling features. In the 18th and 19th centuries, bladder stones were common, but they are rarely seen in Europe and America today. In one English hospital between 1772 and 1816, one in every 38 patients admitted had a bladder stone. These stones were mostly composed of urate crystals and probably were related to diet. Similar epidemics of bladder stones were reported in male children in Thailand and India. The British navy has found a higher frequency of stones among seamen stationed in tropical or semitropical regions, among those who are overweight, among cooks, and among those with sedentary jobs.

In the United States, urinary stone disease (mainly kidney stones) accounts for about one in 1,000 hospital admissions, or more than 200,000 cases per year. This does not include patients who consult physicians about the spasmodic pain of renal colic or "passing gravel," in which small sand-like particles can be seen in the urine. Incidence rates are about the same in both sexes.

Kidney and bladder stones may be divided into several distinct types according to chemical composition. Treatment varies according to their makeup.

Calcium-containing stones account for about two-thirds of stone cases in the United States. They are generally composed of calcium oxalate or calcium oxalate mixed with calcium phosphate. Why calcium oxalate stones develop is not known in most cases. Some occur in persons who show elevated calcium levels in blood or urine, but the reasons for the elevation are not known, either. Stones appear in Americans of both sexes, and are far more common in adults than children. "Stone making" seems to run in families. There is no clear link to diet in the United States, but persons who regularly drink three or more quarts of milk a day, take megadoses of more than 300 units of vitamin D daily, or use large quantities of bicarbonate of soda for indigestion relief run a higher risk of developing stones.

A small number of calcium-containing stones occur as a consequence of other diseases such as sarcoidosis or hyperparathyroidism. Prolonged immobilization because of illness or injury also accounts for some cases, as the body robs the bones of calcium and causes increased excretion of calcium into the urine.

Struvite or infection-induced stones make up about 15 percent of all cases of kidney stones. They are composed of magnesium ammonium phosphate and occur mainly in patients with chronic urinary tract infections containing urea-splitting bacteria. These bacteria convert the urea to ammonia, making the urine alkaline and favoring formation of

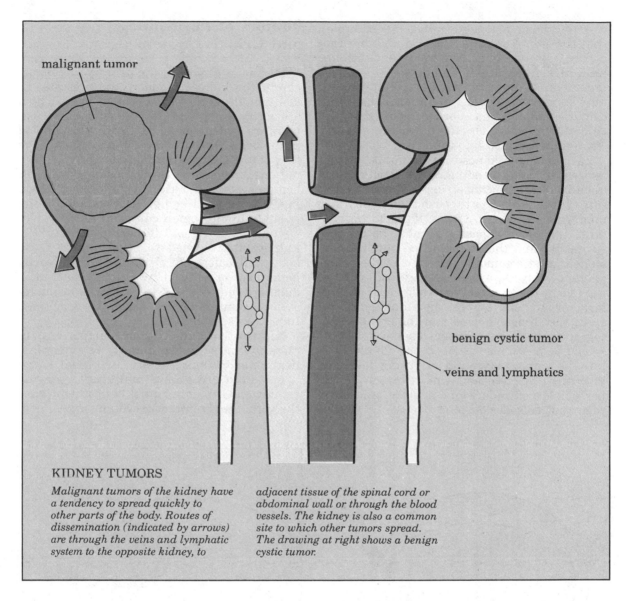

KIDNEY TUMORS

Malignant tumors of the kidney have a tendency to spread quickly to other parts of the body. Routes of dissemination (indicated by arrows) are through the veins and lymphatic system to the opposite kidney, to adjacent tissue of the spinal cord or abdominal wall or through the blood vessels. The kidney is also a common site to which other tumors spread. The drawing at right shows a benign cystic tumor.

large crystals and stones. Bacteria and cellular debris become incorporated in the stone, which may grow so large that it fills the entire renal pelvis, extending around the papillae and forming an antler-like shape that gives it the name "staghorn" calculus. The growth eventually may fill the pelvis and obstruct the kidney completely.

Many victims of infection-induced stones are paraplegics or other invalids who require long-term use of a catheter to drain the bladder. Other cases are associated with structural abnormalities of the urinary tract that are difficult to correct and promote chronic nesting places for infection.

Uric acid and cystine stones make up about 10 percent of all cases. Uric acid stones result from gout; cystine stones from a hereditary disease that interferes with the handling of an amino acid in proteins.

Many persons pass tiny stones and are never aware of it. Others are emphatically notified by blood in the urine or by painful urination as gritty bits of sand pass along the urethra. The pain of kidney colic can be excruciating and unforgettable. It occurs when a stone enters one of the ureters and works its way down, gouging as it goes. The pain is felt sometimes in the back, sometimes in the pelvic area. And the pain may be accompanied by nausea, vomiting, chills, and fever.

Treatment of stones. Because the treatment differs by type of stone, a person who suspects he or she has urinary stones should attempt to collect a sample by urinating through a fine strainer. The stones can then be given to a physician for analysis.

A physician may determine, for example, that the stone contains uric acid and that the person has gout, requiring treatment with alkali, high fluid intake, and drugs such as allopurinol. In contrast, calcium oxalate stones may be prevented by use of antacids that bind calcium and phosphate, or by the drug hydrochlorothiazide, which cuts down the amount of calcium excreted into the urine.

Large bladder stones that cannot be passed and cause pain, bleeding, or obstruction are usually treated by inserting a special cystoscope into the bladder to crush them. The fragments are then flushed away. If this technique fails, the urinary passages must be opened surgically and the stones lifted out. Kidney stones, most commonly situated in the renal pelvis or calyces, are exceedingly difficult to remove by the tube method. In the case of very large or staghorn stones, the kidney must be split, the stone removed and the organ sewn together. Smaller stones sometimes can be dissolved by passing a catheter through the skin into the kidney pelvis and irrigating the stone with an acid solution. Unfortunately, some persons are chronic "stone makers" and have recurrent episodes of stone disease.

Tumors of the Kidney and Urinary System

The major tumors of the urinary system occur in the kidney, bladder, and prostate. In addition, the kidney is a common site to which other tumors spread. Early symptoms of tumors are destruction of tissue leading to blood in the urine (hematuria) or obstruction of the flow of urine. But often there are other explanations for these symptoms. Kidney stones or benign cysts of the kidney can produce blood in the urine, and benign enlargement of the prostate in older men can obstruct flow. Unfortunately malignant tumors (cancers) of the kidney often spread to other parts of the body well before they reveal themselves by hematuria or other local signs. The initial diagnosis may be made in such cases by microscopic examination of tissues to which the tumor has spread.

Kidney cancer. The most important tumors that arise in the kidney are embryonal nephroma (Wilms' tumor) and renal carcinoma. Both are highly malignant, growing rapidly and spreading quickly to other organs through the lymphatic system and blood-

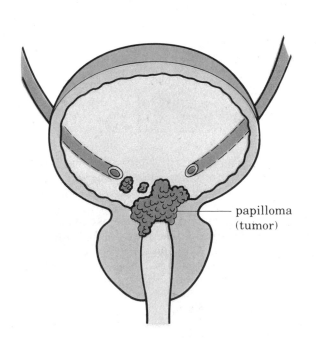

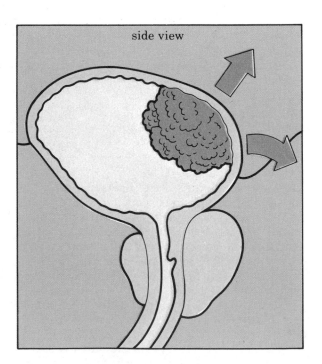

side view

papilloma (tumor)

BLADDER TUMORS

Bladder tumors frequently reveal themselves by bloody or cloudy urine. At left, a papilloma tumor completely blocks the entrance to the urethra. At right, a malignant tumor on the rear wall of the bladder does not interfere with urinary outflow. Unless detected and removed early, malignancies may spread via the lymphatic system to nearby tissues.

stream. Common secondary sites are the lungs, bones, or the central nervous system, so that kidney tumors may be first detected by X rays of the chest or a painful bone site. Large tumors may be felt in the upper abdomen and flanks.

Wilms' tumor is one of the most common forms of cancer in children under five years and accounts for about one-fourth of all childhood cancers. It appears to arise from abnormal development of kidney cells before birth. This is intriguing to cancer researchers because most other cancers apparently result from changes in well differentiated, mature cells. Because of its origin early in development, most Wilms' tumors occur in children under 2 and rarely after age 5.

The tendency to develop Wilms' tumor appears to be inherited, associated with an absence of a specific chromosome. Recent research indicates that it may be detected shortly after birth by absence of the iris of the eye, which is caused by lack of the same chromosome. Fortunately, Wilms' tumor is a form of cancer that responds well to treatment. Radiation therapy and chemotherapy have achieved an 80 percent two-year disease-free survival rate, even when the cancer is widespread on discovery.

Carcinoma of the kidney accounts for about two percent of adult cancers. It is more common in men than women and strikes most frequently between ages 45 and 60. The incidence has increased slightly in recent years, possibly because the U.S. population is growing older.

Kidney cancer may first show itself with confusing symptoms such as unexplained fever, a high white blood count, weight loss and fatigue. Some tumors produce large amounts of hormones such as erythropoietin, causing sudden polycythemia (increased mass of red blood cells). Blood in the urine and flank pain are late symptoms.

Kidney cancer usually develops in a single kidney. If the cancer is detected before it has spread to nearby organs, the diseased kidney can be removed surgically. The other kidney takes over function and chances of recovery are relatively high. In a distressingly high percentage of cases, however, the cancer is widely spread before discovery, and chances of successful treatment are slim.

Bladder cancer accounts for about six percent of male cancers in the United States and two percent of female cancers. In certain geographical areas and in certain occupations, however, these percentages are much higher. Workers exposed to aniline and other dyes used in the textile, paint, and rubber indus-

tries, and residents of certain industrial areas show an increased rate of bladder cancer. The disease also appears linked to cigarette smoking. Outside the United States, the cancer is common in tropical regions, as a result of the infectious disease schistosomiasis caused by worm eggs deposited in the bladder wall.

Bladder tumors arise mostly in the cells lining the urine collecting system. Similar tumors occur in the renal pelvis, ureters, and urethra, but are less common. Apparently the bladder is a particular target because urine is stored there, increasing the bladder's exposure to potential cancer-inducing substances in urine.

The Kidney Specialists

A physician who specializes in kidney diseases is called a nephrologist. One who deals primarily with surgical problems of the bladder and urinary tract is called a urologist. A urologist also may treat problems of the male genitals, which are closely associated with the urinary system. Most general physicians however, can readily manage the common problems associated with diseases of the urinary tract and will call on specialists for complicated problems.

Fortunately bladder tumors tend to bleed and thus may give early warning of their presence before the disease has invaded the bladder wall or spread to regional lymph nodes. Localized tumors often can be cut or burned out by a cystoscope inserted through the urethra. Even if the cancer has progressed into the organ wall, it often may be treated successfully by removing a segment of the wall. In more severe cases, the entire organ may be removed surgically.

Prostate cancer is the second most common tumor in males, after lung cancer. It accounts for 16 percent of all male cancers, mostly in men over 65, and is often found during autopsy in older men who have died of other causes. Because benign prostatic hypertrophy also occurs in this age group, cancer may be found incidentally during operations on the prostate. The physician often suspects it if he feels a "rock hard" mass in the prostate region during rectal examination.

As with other cancers of the urinary tract, prostatic cancer may spread rapidly to regional lymph nodes and through the bloodstream to bone and lung. The first sign may be pain in the hip or back caused by its spread to bone. The enzyme acid phosphatase, manufactured in the prostate, often is elevated in the blood of prostate cancer patients and is a useful indicator of the disease. Surgical removal of the prostate is the customary treatment.

Injury

The kidneys are well protected by thick layers of muscle in the back, a tough surrounding membrane called the renal capsule, and a cushion of fat called the perinephric fat pad. They are much less likely than the liver or spleen to be damaged during injury to the abdomen. In a violent impact, however, the kidney may be torn and bleed profusely. Blood pours into the capsule, pooling in surrounding tissues and back muscles, a condition called a retroperitoneal hematoma.

The condition is not limited to injury or wound victims, however. Patients taking anticoagulant drugs or who have a tendency to bleed because of low blood platelets or hemophilia also develop hematomas, not always easily recognized because the kidneys are located so deep in the body. Massive bleeding into the urine can produce blood clots that obstruct the flow of urine. More often, however, kidney injuries result in only slow bleeding into the urine.

Athletes, including runners and joggers, sometimes find blood in their urine after long periods of exercise. This "jogger's hematuria" appears to arise from the bladder, not the kidneys. It is not serious and usually disappears until another episode of running.

One of the major complications of abdominal surgery is accidental severing or tying of the ureters. This occurs because the tiny conduits are difficult to differentiate from blood vessels. When the ureter is cut urine leaks into the abdomen, producing swelling. Fortunately, the severed ureter can be repaired surgically.

The bladder and urethra also may be torn during injury to the pelvic bones in severe crush injuries. This requires prompt measures to redirect the flow of urine by placing tubes into the ureters or the kidney pelvis.

Obstructions to Flow

Besides stones, clots, and abnormalities, urinary flow in males may be blocked by enlargement of the prostate gland, which surrounds the midportion of the urethra (see chapter 23, "The Male Reproductive System"). The prostate gland always enlarges with age, but seldom enough to interfere with urinary flow until after age 60. The enlargement is called adenomatous hyperplasia and strictly speaking is a benign tumor because the growth remains localized.

Early symptoms of prostatic enlargement are difficulty in beginning to urinate, less forceful urination, a narrower stream and dribbling of urine at the end of voiding. If the obstruction increases, a man will have to urinate frequently, often being awakened during the night. Although distressing, prostatic enlargement is not dangerous unless urine accumulates in the bladder and cannot be voided. Ordinarily a male can nearly empty the bladder until less than a teaspoonful of urine remains. When obstruction is severe, as much as several quarts of urine may accumulate, producing reverse pressure which sends urine back up the ureter, increases the pressure in the kidney pelvis, and causes swelling, or hydronephrosis. If left untreated, hydronephrosis can result in uremia and severe kidney damage.

Diseases That Alter Flow

The major nerves that control emptying of the bladder can be blocked by many drugs. In general, drugs that mimic the action of the parasympathetic nerves tend to enhance emptying. Drugs that block transmission of impulses from the parasympathetic system tend to delay it. Thus older men with hypertrophy of the prostate may have even greater difficulty in urinating when taking certain drugs. These include atropine, phenothiazines, antihistamines, and drugs used to treat Parkinson's disease.

Any disease or injury that damages the spinal cord also can severely affect the bladder. These include severing of the cord by injury (paraplegia), multiple sclerosis, and other neurologic diseases and tumors.

Children born with spina bifida and meningomyelocele also may have severe malfunction of the spinal cord and poor bladder emptying. Because of damaged nerve connections the bladder may become large and flaccid and retain huge volumes of urine. Reverse pres-

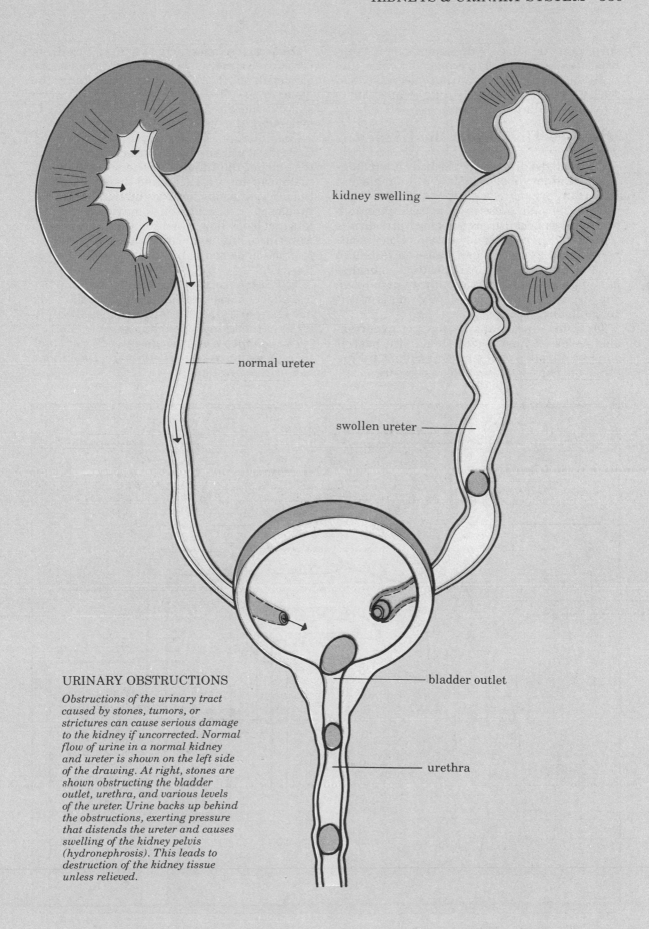

kidney swelling

normal ureter

swollen ureter

bladder outlet

urethra

URINARY OBSTRUCTIONS

Obstructions of the urinary tract caused by stones, tumors, or strictures can cause serious damage to the kidney if uncorrected. Normal flow of urine in a normal kidney and ureter is shown on the left side of the drawing. At right, stones are shown obstructing the bladder outlet, urethra, and various levels of the ureter. Urine backs up behind the obstructions, exerting pressure that distends the ureter and causes swelling of the kidney pelvis (hydronephrosis). This leads to destruction of the kidney tissue unless relieved.

sure may produce hydronephrosis. In contrast, the bladder may become shrunken and tightened, with a substantially decreased capacity. In either case resistance to infection is markedly reduced.

Diseases That Affect the Kidney

Generalized diseases in the body often damage the kidneys or choose these vulnerable and important organs as a particular target.

Hypertension presents a special threat to the kidneys because proper blood pressure is crucial to their filtering action. Consistent, heightened pressure can cause severe and lasting damage to the delicate membranes of the glomerulus. Fortunately, hypertension can usually be detected readily and is a correctable disease.

Toxemia of pregnancy, a form of hypertension, is less common today than in the past. It can be controlled by restricting salt and taking other measures to lower blood pressure.

Diabetes, particularly when it has been present for many years, may damage the glomeruli of the kidney by thickening the membranes. This condition, called Kimmelstiel-Wilson disease, allows blood protein to leak out of the blood vessels into the urine.

Gout disrupts the kidney in several ways. Crystals of gout-induced uric acid may form in the cells of the tubules or the space between them, causing irritation and disturbing function. Crystals may form in the channels of the tubules, or uric acid stones may dam the ureters and block flow. Flushing the kidneys with water or using medications that reduce acid production or neutralize it with alkali lowers the risk.

Arteriosclerosis, or hardening of the arteries, affects blood vessels throughout the body, but is a particular threat to the small capillaries of the kidney (see chapter 5).

The collagen diseases, described in chapter 15, also can have serious effects on the kidney and urinary system.

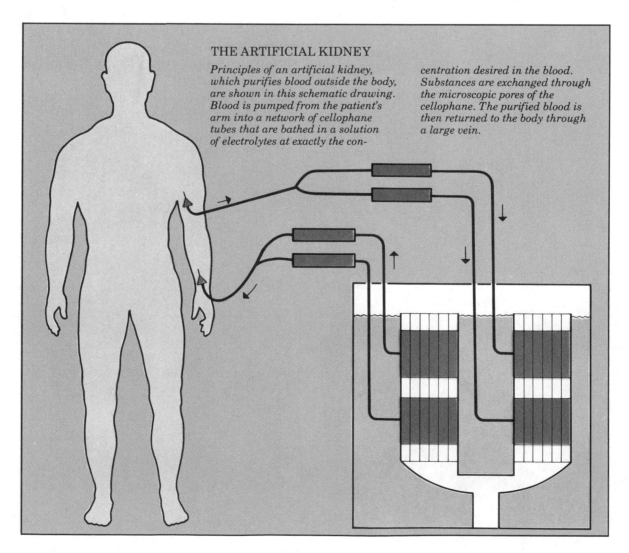

THE ARTIFICIAL KIDNEY

Principles of an artificial kidney, which purifies blood outside the body, are shown in this schematic drawing. Blood is pumped from the patient's arm into a network of cellophane tubes that are bathed in a solution of electrolytes at exactly the con- *centration desired in the blood. Substances are exchanged through the microscopic pores of the cellophane. The purified blood is then returned to the body through a large vein.*

Artificial Kidney

Although the term has become part of the language, there is no such thing as an "artificial kidney." Man's best efforts have not been good enough to duplicate the complex organ discussed in this chapter. But medical techniques and machines can take over temporarily for a damaged kidney too weak to fulfill its function. This artificial means of removing wastes and restoring proper fluid and electrolyte balance to the blood is called dialysis.

Dialysis is required when the kidneys reach the stage of renal insufficiency. This means that the kidneys no longer are able to filter all the wastes from the blood. The wastes accumulate in the body and can lead to damage and ultimately to death if not corrected. If the condition is temporary, resulting from acute illness or injury, dialysis is needed only until the kidney recovers, which usually occurs swiftly. More often it is a result of gradual, long-term destruction of the kidney by disease. Dialysis is now widely used and has kept many victims of end-stage kidney failure alive for years.

Hemodialysis is what most people mean when they say "artificial kidney." It refers to a machine that purifies the blood outside the body. Blood is pumped from an artery into a vast length or series of cellophane tubes that are bathed in a solution of electrolytes at exactly the concentration desired in the blood. Salts and water pass through the microscopic pores of the cellophane from blood to bath and back. Waste molecules are washed away as they are diluted in the bath, while desired electrolytes pass from bath to blood. Excess water is removed by raising the resistance to blood flow in the circuit. After purification the blood is returned to the body via a large vein.

Long-term hemodialysis patients usually are fitted with a shunt (see illustration) in the forearm, tying into an artery and a vein. This simplifies connecting them to the system at each visit. During dialysis they are given an anticoagulant such as heparin to prevent the blood from clotting. The anticoagulant is neutralized afterwards by protamine to return clotting to normal.

The first artificial kidney was invented in the 1950s by Willem Kolff, a Dutch physician. It has undergone steady revision and improvement since. The original model was about the size of a small bathtub. The filtering tubes, about an inch in diameter, were wrapped around a large drum which rotated in the bath. A built-in pump assisted blood flow. More recent dialyzers are smaller and simpler, and can be used in the patient's home. Commonly, they use a bath of about two to three quarts with hundreds of thread-sized cellophane tubules arranged in parallel, the fluid passing between them. Sometimes the blood is filtered through pellets of activated charcoal.

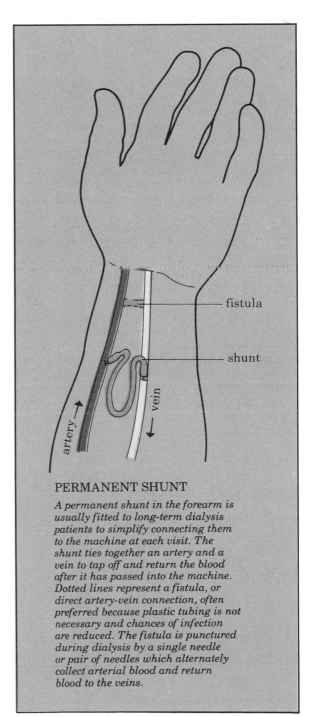

fistula

shunt

artery

vein

PERMANENT SHUNT

A permanent shunt in the forearm is usually fitted to long-term dialysis patients to simplify connecting them to the machine at each visit. The shunt ties together an artery and a vein to tap off and return the blood after it has passed into the machine. Dotted lines represent a fistula, or direct artery-vein connection, often preferred because plastic tubing is not necessary and chances of infection are reduced. The fistula is punctured during dialysis by a single needle or pair of needles which alternately collect arterial blood and return blood to the veins.

Peritoneal dialysis uses the thin membranes of the abdominal cavity to substitute for the filtering membranes of the kidney. A solution similar to that used in hemodialysis is fed into the abdomen via force of gravity, draining through a long plastic tube from a large bottle suspended over the patient. The fluid bathes the surface membranes of the abdomen, exchanges waste molecules for the electrolytes in the solution, then drains off into an outflow bottle placed on the floor. The process is repeated until blood composition has reached proper levels. Excess water is removed by increasing glucose in the fluid, so that it draws water out of the body into the outflow bottle.

Like hemodialysis, peritoneal dialysis has become simpler and more automated since it was first devised. Regular dialysis patients now wear a special adapter or plastic plug in the abdominal wall so that a needle need not be threaded through the abdomen on each dialysis visit. Bottles can be hooked up so that a fresh bottle of fluid is tapped automatically each time another has been used and the waste drained away.

Both dialysis processes require about six to eight hours and must be performed two to four times a week, depending on the condition of the patient's kidneys. Some persons require close supervision at a hospital center, but thousands of others now perform either peritoneal dialysis or hemodialysis at home. Many hold jobs, tend to household tasks, and lead a relatively normal life. Some women have even become pregnant and borne children while undergoing long-term dialysis. A network of dialysis centers around the country trains patients and families to perform dialysis, including how to monitor blood levels and administer drugs if necessary.

Life on the artificial kidney calls for strong motivation. After all, many people are lax about even simple acts of self-care such as brushing the teeth properly or adhering to a diet. The demands on the dialysis patient are infinitely more difficult and time-consuming, and the consequences of neglect are immediate and far more serious. Not surprisingly, some patients feel imprisoned by the machine. And dialysis is not always without complications.

Bleeding, infection, and chronic anemia are among them. Some persons continue to accumulate wastes that cannot be disposed of completely. Depression and discouragement are common. Some dialysis centers provide professional counseling and guidance for patients. Family support is critical, too.

Kidney Transplant

For young people with end-stage kidney disease, and for older ones who face long-term treatment on the artificial kidney and who do not have other major diseases, a replacement kidney donated by another person is the ultimate hope. Kidney transplant has been performed successfully only since about 1960, but has become the most common of all organ transplant operations. In the first 20 years of the procedure, more than 16,000 persons were returned to full, active life-styles after receiving a new kidney to replace one riddled by disease.

The most successful transplants are from one identical twin to another. Obviously, only a few persons are in this select group. Close relatives are the next best choice, and many relatives have willingly donated a kidney to a loved one. Most donated kidneys, however, come from healthy persons who have died suddenly, often in accidents, and who have willed the organs or whose survivors have agreed to the donation.

Transplanting an organ as sensitive as a kidney is a delicate procedure, calling for skill and speed (for surgical details, see chapter 31, "Understanding Your Operation"). Donor and recipient must be carefully matched by tissue and blood type. The donated kidney must be removed rapidly, within minutes of death, and kept alive in special solutions until it can be installed in place. Special teams transport the donated kidney from hospital to hospital or by airliner to other parts of the country.

As in all transplant operations, the most difficult problem in kidney transplant is to prevent rejection of the new organ by the immune systems of the body. Despite careful blood and tissue typing, a perfect match is seldom possible, and the recipient of the kidney must be treated with drugs to suppress the normal immune response against an invader. This immunosuppressive treatment may continue several months to allow the new kidney to "take." This can lower the body's defenses against other infections, so close follow-up by specialized physicians is required.

Keeping the Kidneys Healthy

Although there are many over-the-counter nostrums purporting to promote good health by flushing out the kidneys and urinary system, these vital organs usually require no special medicines or attention. The system of urine production and disposal works automatically if there is an adequate daily intake of water, nutrients, and salt. For most persons, that means about two to three quarts of fluid a day and about two grams of salt. The amount varies, of course, with temperature, exertion, illness, thirst, and desire for salt.

Normal blood pressure is important to the health of the kidneys. Hypertension can severely damage the delicate capillaries, so it is important to keep close watch on blood pressure and to treat it promptly and effectively when detected.

Overuse of aspirin and other pain relievers also can harm the kidneys. This condition is called analgesic nephropathy. These drugs should be used sparingly and only when needed. Large amounts of bicarbonate of soda or antacid may lead to calcium deposits in the kidneys. Their use, too, should be minimized.

Severe blood loss from injury elsewhere in the body or shock leading to a drop in blood pressure can harm the kidneys by causing them to shut down their blood flow and depriving the cells of the kidney of their blood supply. Structural damage to the kidney and acute kidney failure can result. First-aid measures in the event of injury or accident should deal with shock first in order to prevent the complication of kidney failure.

Diarrhea and vomiting rob the body of salts and water. If they are not replaced, kidney shutdown may follow. No matter how bad you feel, it is important to take plenty of fluids in the event of illness. Because the functional reserve of the kidney tends to diminish with age, the need is particularly acute in older people.

Bed-wetting

Our culture places great importance on the privacy of urination and defecation. Parents are pleased by children who are toilet trained early and distressed by those who can't control their urinary or bowel movements. Thus the young child (or grandparent) who wets the bed is considered difficult and troublesome.

Enuresis, or urinary incontinence, is a common condition of childhood. It appears to run in families, and is surprisingly widespread. One study indicated that 20 percent of six-year-olds and 10 percent of seven-year-olds had never experienced a full month without an episode of bed-wetting. Even one in 20 twelve-year-olds had not had a dry month. The bed wetters were about equally divided between boys and girls.

A majority of children are reliably dry at night by the age of four. The remainder gain nighttime control as they grow older. A few are successfully nighttime trained, then relapse and wet their beds again. A psychological upset (such as the birth of a brother or sister) or a urinary infection may be the explanation for these secondary cases. Physical abnormalities rarely play a part if the child can control the bladder during the day.

The specific cause of bed-wetting is not known. The child usually has a normal-sized bladder. Because it appears to run in families, one possible explanation is a congenital delayed maturation of nerves controlling the bladder. Some but not all bed wetters visit the bathroom more often during the day.

Remedies are not wholly satisfactory because the cause is not known. Most stress decreasing the anxiety of parents and children through counseling. Limiting fluids at bedtime may help. You can help the child with bladder-training exercises and by rewarding success.

Alarm systems work for some children. A pad-and-buzzer method consists of two layers of foil or wire mesh separated by a layer of cloth and connected by wires to a battery and bell or buzzer. Wetting on the cloth completes the circuit, sounds the alarm and wakes the child. The repeated association of bed-wetting and being rudely awakened is said to condition children to greater bladder control within two to ten weeks in most cases.

CHAPTER 23   GERALD P. MURPHY, M.D., D.Sc.

THE MALE REPRODUCTIVE SYSTEM

The male reproductive system is closely involved with the urinary system. In large measure, the male and female apparatus for ridding the body of wastes are alike. The kidneys, ureters, and bladder are the same in both sexes. The resemblance ends with the urethra, the pipeline that carries urine outside the body. In women the urethra is about 1½ inches long and its main purpose is discharge of urine. The male urethra is about nine inches long, running the full length of the penis. It carries off urine, but is also the passageway through which the male reproductive materials travel en route to their possible union with those of the female.

Disorders or abnormalities of both the male reproductive and urinary systems are dealt with by urologists or urologic surgeons. The entire system is sometimes spoken of as the genitourinary system. The most prominent parts of that system include the prostate gland, through which the urethra passes and where the seminal fluids are produced; the testes (male sex glands), where spermatozoa and male hormones are produced; the vas deferens, which conveys spermatozoa to the urethra for ejaculation; the penis; and the scrotum, the sac containing the testes.

THE MALE URETHRA

The meatus in the penis is the external opening of the urethra. It is the end of the urinary system which begins with the kidneys. For purposes of description, the continuous male urethra is divided into two anatomic areas. The portion that begins at the bladder outlet and runs through the prostate gland is referred to as the posterior or prostatic urethra. The remainder is called the anterior urethra and is located primarily in the shaft of the penis. The posterior urethra contains openings through which the ducts of the surrounding prostate gland empty secretions. These secretions are carried away during urination. Also located within the male urethra are the openings of the ejaculatory ducts, which carry spermatozoa from the testes, where they are formed, to the urethra to be carried to the outside. Spermatozoa are the male cells which unite with the female egg to form a new life. The anterior urethra also includes certain small glands, the so-called "glands of Littre," which help keep the urethra lubricated, particularly during sexual intercourse. The two

Cowper's glands also secrete a lubricating fluid and empty into the anterior urethra. Thus the anterior urethra directs two different forms of urologic traffic: (1) carrying the urine and (2) providing materials for reproduction.

Defects and Narrowings of the Urethra

A stricture, which is an abnormal narrowing of the passageway of the posterior urethra, can be present at birth (congenital) or can occur later in life. The congenital type is usually a defect of the bladder. Birth defects of the urethra are essentially gaps in the construction of the tube itself and are primarily related to the anterior urethra.

Hypospadias is a failure of the urethra to close on what is considered the underside of the penis. It is like an open trough or a tube with large openings. Ordinarily, the defect does not extend into the posterior urethra, so that the sphincter muscles that control urination function normally and the patient is able to contain his urine. However, the trough-like external opening interferes with the normal delivery of the urinary system and with the transport of semen to the outside. The defect can be corrected surgically, and the operation usually is attempted early in childhood.

Epispadias is a comparable but less common defect in which a portion of the upper side of the urethra remains open. It can be a slit or a roofless channel running a short distance from the end of the penis on its upper surface. In some cases it traverses the shaft of the penis more extensively. Sometimes the opening begins and ends at the base of the penis. In that case, normal sexual intercourse and delivery of semen is not possible. Occasionally, the posterior urethra is involved, too. Malformation of the bladder's sphincter muscles prevents the person from controlling urination, although the bladder surface is normally formed. The problem for the urologic surgeon is to restore urinary control and then to form a new tube from the sphincter area to the outside. Usually the prostate gland, testes, and scrotum are not involved in the operation.

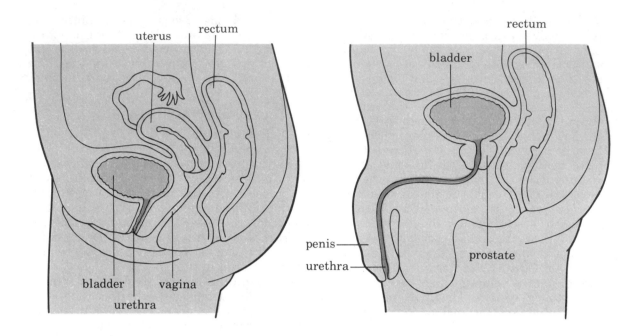

FEMALE AND MALE URETHRA

In both men and women, the urethra is the passageway through which urine is carried outside the body. The female urethra (shaded area, left drawing) is only about 1½ inches long, whereas the male urethra (shaded area, right drawing) is about nine inches long. In addition to urine, the male urethra carries reproductive materials outside the body.

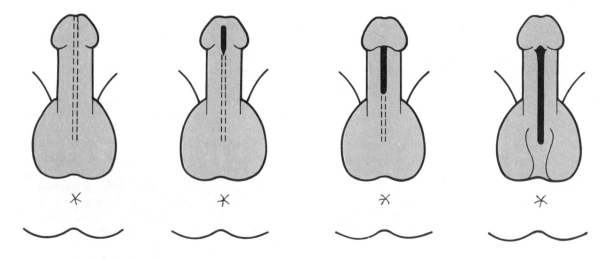

HYPOSPADIAS

An imperfect closure of the urethra on the underside of the penis is called hypospadias. The normal urethra is a closed tube hidden from direct sight, as shown at left. In the second drawing the terminal portion of the urethra has failed to close. In the third drawing there is imperfect closure of half of the urethra. In the far right drawing the urethra is open its entire length. Hypospadias usually can be corrected surgically.

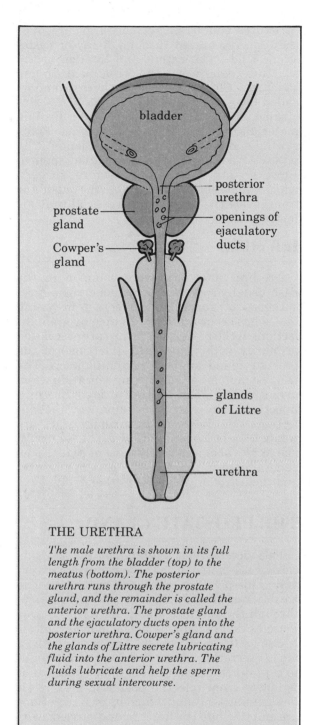

THE URETHRA

The male urethra is shown in its full length from the bladder (top) to the meatus (bottom). The posterior urethra runs through the prostate gland, and the remainder is called the anterior urethra. The prostate gland and the ejaculatory ducts open into the posterior urethra. Cowper's gland and the glands of Littre secrete lubricating fluid into the anterior urethra. The fluids lubricate and help the sperm during sexual intercourse.

Injuries

Injuries to the male urethra are serious for two reasons. First, the urethra is rich in blood vessels, which are subject to recurrent engorgement and changes in size during sexual excitement. Injury to an organ so well supplied with blood can cause severe hemorrhage, pooling of blood under the surface, and extensive blood loss. Because the urethra is a conduit for urine, any injury that breaks the pipeline will permit urine to seep into the surrounding tissues where it can cause inflammation and other damage.

If the injury is in the posterior urethral region, urine can seep into the area between the anus and scrotum or into the tissues around the bladder. The presence of the urine may not be obvious on initial physical examination. It is more difficult to recognize, and therefore more dangerous than urinary seepage in the so-called anterior urethra. Posterior seepage can create a serious situation rapidly unless drainage and repair are carried out.

Anterior seepage is usually recognized quickly because there are no sphincter muscles to hold back the blood or other fluids, and bleeding is almost constant from the external opening of the urethra. Furthermore, when the patient voids, an alarming swelling of the penis and scrotum usually is noticed and immediately brought to the physician's attention. Early repair of such tears or cuts or traumatic damage is achieved by sidetracking the urine to bypass the injury until the conduit is reconstructed. This is usually necessary to avoid severe disability and even more serious consequences. Unfortunately, such damage often occurs in company with other injuries and may be missed. Thus, the damage to the urinary tract frequently has to be dealt with later because of other lifesaving emergencies.

Tumors

Malignant tumors of the posterior urethra are rare unless they arise in the prostate gland. Malignant tumors of the anterior urethra are extremely rare. Blood in the urine and constriction of the urethra with difficulty of urination are general, nonspecific symptoms. Although they could be caused by a tumor, more frequently the cause is stricture, obstruction, or other nonmalignant conditions. If a tumor is suspected and then diagnosed, surgical removal of the tumor usually is recommended. Radiation is occasionally used.

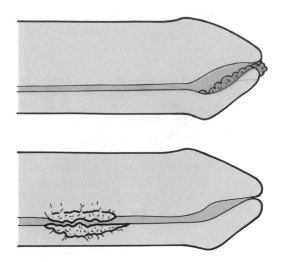

STRICTURES

An abnormal narrowing of the urethra is called a stricture. Congenital strictures cause children to have difficulty in urination. In top drawing, an abnormal growth in the urethra has caused constriction near the terminal opening. At bottom, infection has narrowed the urethral channel. Strictures can be dilated with instruments or opened surgically.

Strictures

Following injury or infection, a stricture of the urethra may develop. A stricture is any abnormal narrowing of the channel which impedes the free flow of urine or in extreme cases blocks it completely. Symptoms of stricture are general slowing of urinary flow, a desire to urinate frequently, and, occasionally, dribbling at the end of urination. The same symptoms, however, are produced by prostate enlargement or obstruction at the bladder neck.

Among the underlying causes of urethral strictures are physical and chemical injuries, birth defects, and inflammations. There are three common areas of stricture. One is at the bladder neck, usually as a result of an operation near the junction of the posterior urethra and the bladder. This can result from a transurethral resection of the prostate gland (see page 552). The second common area is the bulbous urethra where the anterior urethra begins. The third common area is the meatus or external opening. Strictures of the meatus and contractions of the bladder neck may be present at birth and make it difficult for children to urinate. In fact, bladder neck contracture is more common than was once thought.

Strictures can be corrected surgically once they are recognized through X ray or cystoscopic study. The extent and location of the stricture determine the treatment. Some strictures can be dilated with instruments called bougies, or urethral sounds. These instruments include both rigid and flexible materials designed to pass by the area of narrowing and permit careful expansion of it by progressive dilation with lubrication applied. However, other strictures require surgery, which can be accomplished from the outside or from inside the urethra with special urologic instruments.

Infections

Urethral infections were common in the past, usually stemming from gonorrhea. A resurgence of gonorrheal infection in young males has occurred today. In men over 45, infections of the posterior urethra are associated primarily with nonspecific infections of the prostate gland and are not uncommon. The usual symptoms are a burning sensation when urinating and frequent urge to do so. Urethral infections are treated the same way that infections elsewhere in the urinary tract are treated: by establishment of adequate drainage, removal of any dead tissue or scar tissue, general care to improve the patient's health, and the use of antibiotics or other drugs.

THE PROSTATE GLAND

This accessory sex gland of the male is closely associated with the lower urinary tract and is the primary concern of urologists. The posterior or prostatic urethra forms a channel through the prostate gland. Its wall contains muscles that hold urine in the bladder until it is ready to be expelled. The prostate is a mucus-secreting gland and has been thought to contain three continuous major lobes that completely encircle the posterior urethra. It has openings through which its own secretions are emptied into the urethra and carried away during urination or during the sexual act.

The prostate is a sex gland that develops under the influence of male hormones. It is normally rudimentary in infants, although hormonal influence during pregnancy is possible. The ejaculatory ducts that carry male germ cells (spermatozoa) from the testicles enter the prostate and open into the urethra.

The scrotal sac contains two testes (testicles). Spermatozoa mature in enormous numbers in certain tissues of the testes. Other testicle cells produce male sex hormone which enters the bloodstream. Spermatozoa travel through the seminal ducts from the testes to the region of the ejaculatory ducts, where there is a reservoir-like structure called the seminal vesicle. The seminal vesicle empties on ejaculation into the posterior urethra through the two openings of the ejaculatory ducts. Simultaneously, the prostate gland contracts and empties its materials into the urethra. The combined substance, called semen or ejaculate, is then expelled by a wave-like motion in which the frontal part of the urethral sphincter opens and the posterior portion closes to prevent secretions from backing up into the bladder.

The prostatic secretion supplies substances necessary to maintain spermatozoa in their long course through the female genital tract. The secretions contain acid-base substances, sugar, and other nutrients.

Diseases of the prostate gland are very common and are very important. Congenital abnormalities of the prostate are extremely rare unless they are associated with other abnormalities. The prostate is prone to two major ailments, infections and tumors. The tumors can be benign or malignant.

Examining the Prostate

Examination of the prostate by a urologist or physician is important and has a special diagnostic function. The patient is generally asked to bend over with hands on knees or to support himself on a chair or table. The doctor inserts a lubricated, rubber-gloved index finger into the rectum. By feeling the prostate through the rectum, the doctor can tell a good deal about its condition. The doctor's sense of touch will detect whether the prostate is firm, or soft and boggy, or stony hard, or hard in a few areas, all significant findings.

A complete prostate examination usually includes a prostatic massage to obtain prostatic secretions for study later. A few strokes during the rectal examination expel secretions from the prostate through the urethra. The secretions are then collected on a glass slide, a cover slide applied, and studied under the light microscope. If pus is found, it may indicate an infection. Other elements also help in the diagnosis. Prostatic massage also is useful to empty the prostate and relieve congestion.

Urine specimens (usually three) are obtained. If the first specimen contains pus or bacteria but the next two are clear, infection is probably limited to the urethra. If all three specimens in the so-called "three-glass test" show infection, the condition is more widespread, probably involving the prostate, urethra, bladder, and perhaps other portions of the urinary tract.

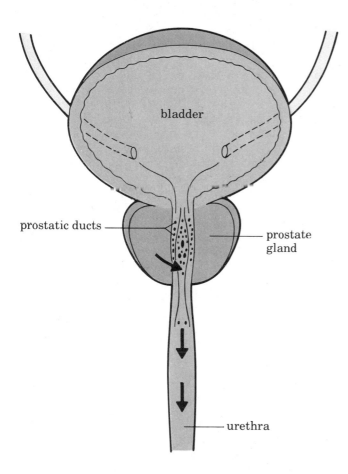

PROSTATE GLAND

The prostate is an accessory male sex gland that surrounds the urethra at the bladder outlet. Its secretions are discharged into the urethra through tiny openings called the prostatic ducts. Spermatozoa from the seminal vesicles are also discharged into this portion of the urethra.

Prostatitis

Infections of the prostate gland, called prostatitis, are not uncommon. In younger men the infection is usually caused by particular organisms such as those of gonorrhea (see chapter 28, "Infectious Diseases"). In these cases, an infection that travels up the urethra to the prostate may also spread beyond it. In older men, prostatitis is usually nonspecific and nongonorrheal, associated with a urethritis that has spread upward to the prostate. Prostatic infections also can be blood-borne from a focus of infection elsewhere in the body, such as the nasal sinuses, tonsils, or teeth.

Acute prostatitis is encountered less frequently since the modern era of antibiotics. Symptoms are acute indeed: high fever plus an urgent and frequent need to urinate, an urge that goes unrelieved. There may be blood in the urine at the beginning and end of urination. Sitting may be uncomfortable because of pain in the genital area.

Chronic prostatitis is seldom accompanied by fever. Urination is frequent, both day and night, and urine may be cloudy and contain blood at the beginning or end of urination. Usually there is no history of acute prostatitis. Respiratory infections or abscessed teeth may be contributing factors, but usually are not identified. In many cases there are few significant symptoms or none at all. Some older patients have a variety of complaints in the presence of chronic inflammation, such as diminished sexual drive, incomplete erection, or premature ejaculation.

Management of prostatitis is essentially the same as management of infection elsewhere in the body: establish good drainage, remove the source of infection, and destroy the infecting organisms. Because chronic prostatitis is almost always associated with cystitis or bladder inflammation, the primary cause may be in the bladder, possibly a stone or tumor. Prostatitis can be the first evidence of such a lesion in the bladder. Nevertheless, acute prostatitis has a variety of identifiable but difficult-to-culture bacterial causes in addition to others that can be transmitted by sexual contact. Treatment depends on accurate diagnosis, selection of antibiotic therapy, and careful follow-up by a urologist.

Benign Prostatic Enlargement

In medical language a benign tumor is one that is not cancerous and does not invade other parts of the body. Symptoms of a benign tumor, however, can be anything but benign in the patient's estimation. This is usually true of tumors of the prostate, called adenomatous hyperplasia of the prostate. This condition is a result of an overgrowth (hypertrophy) of the prostate gland associated with aging. It is rarely found before age 40. The incidence increases with age. It is estimated that two-thirds of the men between 60 and 70 have some degree of prostatic enlargement. The overgrowth may become so large that it causes a narrowing of the urethra or obstruction that interferes in the emptying of the bladder.

The outstanding symptom of prostatic enlargement is urinary obstruction. Most lesions that obstruct the neck of the male bladder are located in the prostate. But no matter where the obstruction is or how severe it is, the

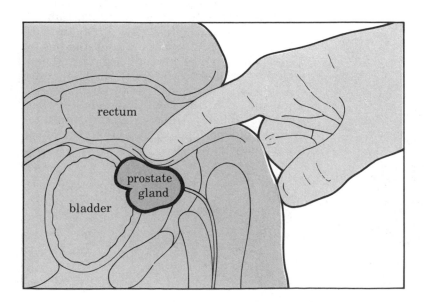

rectum

prostate gland

bladder

PROSTATE EXAMINATION

A side view of the pelvis shows the technique for examining the prostate by a finger in the rectum. Firmness, bogginess, or hardness of certain areas of the gland can be detected by this method. Regular prostate examinations are recommended for men over 50.

symptoms are the same. There is an increased frequency of urination, especially at night, and the act of urination may require more effort or may take several efforts. The urinary stream may be slow to start, less forceful, decreased in caliber, and end in dribbling.

Operation. Factors such as the extent of enlargement, how well the kidney is functioning, and hazards to the upper urinary tract are taken into consideration by urologists in deciding whether surgery is advisable. An operation is usually designed to fit the particular problem. A slight enlargement of the prostate gland can be detected early in the man who has regular examinations. Bladder neck obstruction requires an operation. Unrelieved obstruction usually results in dilation and weakening of the bladder wall. The retained urine can inflate the upper urinary tract and inflict serious damage, even causing kidney failure with uremia. A patient with severe obstruction is susceptible to infections that can result in serious complications.

There have been many advances in surgical care of bladder neck obstruction. These include improvements in diagnosis and better recognition of the changes in the urinary tract and kidneys. Measurement of the amount of urine retained in the bladder, the so-called "emptying test," is of value. Such a test uses a catheter

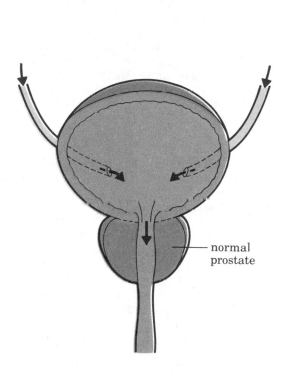

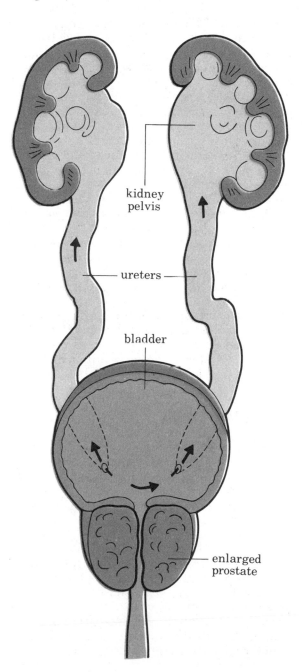

kidney pelvis

ureters

bladder

enlarged prostate

normal prostate

PROSTATE ENLARGEMENT

An enlarged prostate can cause serious damage to the upper urinary tract by obstructing the flow of urine. Drawing above shows the normal ureters, bladder, and urethra. At right, an enlarged prostate compresses the bladder outlet. If the obstruction is not relieved, the bladder dilates and weakens. Backed-up urine enlarges and weakens the ureters and can dilate the kidney pelvis. Continued pressure can severely damage the kidney tissue.

inserted into the bladder to determine how much urine remains in the bladder after urination should have emptied it completely. Obstruction can be relieved by a urethral catheter to achieve slow and gradual decompression of a chronically distended bladder. The damage caused by the obstruction (essentially infection and damage to the kidneys, ureters, and bladder) usually must be corrected later. The surgery for the condition is never an emergency, so there is time to prepare the patient for the best possible result.

There are four standard techniques of prostatectomy for relief of this benign condition. Three are considered "open" procedures in which the area is approached through an outside incision. The fourth, which employs a route through the urethra, is called transurethral resection. The open techniques are termed suprapubic prostatectomy, retropubic prostatectomy, and perineal prostatectomy, although the procedures are not in truth prostatectomies, but rather removal of the overgrown portion of the prostate gland. The prostate capsule and its remaining components are generally left behind. Meticulous care of bleeding, drainage, and postoperative problems are keys to the success of this surgery (see chapter 31, "Understanding Your Operation"). The operations are not without hazard and should not be considered lightly.

In selected cases the transurethral resection of the prostate gland is a safe and acceptable alternative to the so-called open operations. Since it is accomplished without an incision, some doctors believe the transurethral resection is superior because the length of stay in the hospital and degree of discomfort to the patient may be less. The size of the prostate and other considerations best evaluated by the operating physician influence which procedure is selected.

Prostatic Cancer

After cancer of the lung, prostate cancer is the second most common cancer to afflict the American male. It is not uncommon in men 40 to 50 years of age. The incidence increases steadily with age, and is high in men over 70. An estimated 20 percent of all men over 60 have prostatic cancer in some form. The estimates stem from careful postmortem studies of men of this age group who have died from other causes. In contrast to benign prostatic hypertrophy, which at an early phase can produce evidence of urinary obstruction, prostatic cancer is not likely to provide early signs or symptoms. Prostatic cancer that grows in the outside region of the prostate gland does not always immediately involve the bladder outlet or the urethra. That means there may be no early warnings such as impediment of urinary flow or consequences of obstruction such as infection and kidney problems. The cancer is often present for some time without being suspected.

Prostatic cancer in early stages can be suspected as the result of a routine rectal examination. The presence of a stony-hard area in the prostate will arouse suspicion. Conditions such as prostatic stones and certain chronic infections are difficult to distinguish from cancer by rectal examination alone, so it is necessary to remove a small piece of prostatic tissue from the suspicious area for study under the microscope to confirm or rule out cancer. This procedure can be completed with a short hospital stay and in some cases does not require hospitalization at all.

The American Cancer Society now recommends that every man over age 50 have a rectal examination annually. If a suspicious area is detected in the prostate, an early biopsy can be obtained. When prostate cancer is recognized early and treated by surgery or radiation, the cure rate is high.

New methods of radiotherapy for prostate cancer involve insertion of radioactive isotopes such as iodine or gold. Proponents believe these methods are as effective as surgery or external radiation, although long-term results are not yet available. At any rate, there are a variety of surgical and radiotherapy techniques for treating prostate cancer that render potentially excellent results. However, when it is discovered late, the cure rate is low.

Hormones. For more than 30 years doctors have known that prostate cancer is susceptible to hormones that influence its natural course. As in female breast cancer, this is one of the malignancies that on occasion are "hormone dependent." Male sex hormones are believed to have an accelerating effect on the growth of prostatic cancer. For a variety of reasons, female hormones (diethylstilbestrol [DES] or its derivatives) have an opposite effect that inhibits its growth. Prostate cancer patients sometimes benefit from the administration of so-called female sex hormones or from removal of the male hormone effect by castration (removal of both testes). Alteration of the secreting powers of the anterior pituitary, which controls the male sex glands (see chapter 16,

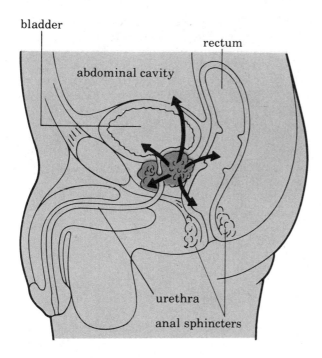

PROSTATE CANCER

The arrows show how prostate cancer spreads. Organs and structures that may be invaded are the abdominal cavity, rectum, bladder, anal sphincters, and urethra. Early prostate cancer causes few symptoms, so a physician's examination is the best method of detection.

"The Hormones and Endocrine Glands") is also believed to have a beneficial effect. No patient is ever cured by such hormone treatment, but the growth of the tumor can be controlled or limited for months, perhaps even two to three years, in cases of prostate cancer that has spread to organs such as bone marrow.

Hormones, of course, produce side effects, including effects on potency and sexuality. The operation for prostate removal may disrupt ejaculation. The ejaculate no longer travels through the anterior urethra because the posterior portion of the urethra is left open. As a result, the material is delivered into the bladder and voided later during urination.

Precautions against prostate cancer. Although prostatic cancer management has advanced strikingly with hormone therapy, because of its silent onset and sometimes insidious growth, late discovery is still a problem. Men in the susceptible years must be made aware of the need for annual physical examinations with routine rectal inspection and biopsy if necessary. Questions you should ask the examining urologist, regardless of the presence or absence of benign or malignant prostate conditions, include the following:

• Doctor, what are the results of my prostate examination?
• Did you also check for rectal cancer? What are the results?
• What drugs are you prescribing and why? Are there any side effects?
• If you recommend surgery or a procedure, will it affect my ability to have erections and to ejaculate? What would be the long-term or lifelong effects?
• Why do you prefer this particular procedure? Are there alternatives? Are there any side effects?
• Is the test you recommend necessary and what are the benefits and risks to me?
• Is there alternative treatment for solving my problems? What are the benefits? What are the risks?
• What are the changes in my body that I should expect in the next five years?
• Are there any other symptoms or abnormalities I should be aware of and watch for?
• What are the proportions of the four prostate operations that you perform? How many of these are open and how many use the closed transurethral technique?

OTHER DISORDERS

The seminal vesicles containing seminal fluid lie next to the prostate. The associated organs are the vas deferens, which is the excretory duct of the testis, and the epididymis, a portion of the seminal duct. Except for rare congenital abnormalities, infections are the principal disorders of these organs. Infection usually results from infection of the prostate. Treatment usually involves drainage via catheter and medication. Sitz baths or hot compresses provide comfort.

THE TESTES

Hormone-producing interstitial cells of the testes, also known as the cells of Leydig, are independent of the organ's spermatozoa-producing department. Tumors of these cells are extremely rare. Changes in the part of the testes that forms the spermatozoa also are relatively rare and usually are associated with various forms of intersex.

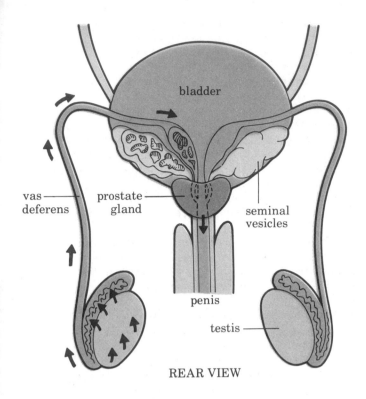

vas deferens

prostate gland

seminal vesicles

penis

testis

REAR VIEW

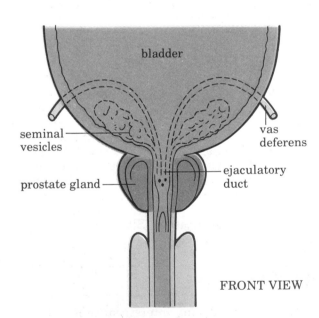

bladder

seminal vesicles

vas deferens

prostate gland

ejaculatory duct

FRONT VIEW

MALE REPRODUCTIVE ORGANS

The system for delivery of spermatozoa into the urethra is outlined in the rear view (top). Spermatozoa are manufactured and stored in the testis, pass through the vas deferens, and are mixed with secretions from the seminal vesicles and prostate gland before being ejaculated into the urethra. The lower drawing, a front view, shows the relationship of bladder, seminal vesicles, and prostate.

Intersex. In rare cases a person can have both male and female gonads which secrete both male and female hormones. The opposing organs may "cancel out" and prevent the production of spermatozoa. In some genetic deviations the patient appears to be male anatomically and yet is genetically female. Determining the sex of an infant appears to be simple, and indeed usually is. At times, however, the external organs vary in some way from the normal, yet appear to be unmistakably of one sex or the other. Major distortions will be recognized but lesser ones may not be. If a genetic male is brought up as a female, or vice versa, adult life may be anything but wonderful for the patient. Some intersex conditions are correctable to a satisfactory if not total extent by timely surgery in selected cases. There are many gradations and puzzling anatomical variations that frequently require exploratory surgery.

In recent years there have been tremendous advances in understanding of genetic mechanisms involved in sex differentiation. Certain of the heredity-transmitting chromosomes are duplicated, missing, or combined in abnormal ways to produce various degrees of male-female elements and even infertile "super females" who have an excess of X chromosomes. It is possible to determine sex by studying the nuclei of body cells.

Undescended testis or cryptorchidism is a condition in which one or both testes fail to descend from the abdomen, where the organs grow during fetal development, into the scrotum. The defect may be genetic and congenital, it may be mechanical, or endocrine factors may interfere with migration of the testicle relatively late in individual development. If only one testis is involved, the defect is probably mechanical in origin, but if both are involved the underlying problem may be hormonal, such as a poorly functioning pituitary gland. Sometimes, improving function by administering pituitary extracts, or marking time until puberty, will ease the testicle into its proper position. However, surgical correction may be necessary. If surgery is needed, doctors generally agree that the operation should be done before age five, and certainly before the onset of puberty. A fully functioning testicle capable of producing spermatozoa requires an environmental temperature lower than that of the internal body. The scrotum, with its relax-

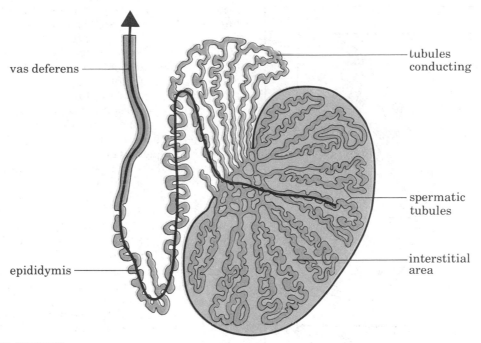

THE TESTES

This is a cross section of a testis, the gland that produces spermatozoa and male hormones. Sperm are produced in the spermatic tubules, and hormones are produced in the interstitial area. The conducting

tubules are part of the epididymis, a portion of the seminal duct lying upon and behind the testis. The vas deferens leads to the urethra. The path of the spermatozoa is indicated by arrows.

ing and contracting "thermostatic" muscle response, adjusts to this environment. It is not clear why sperm-producing tissues cannot function normally in the heat of the body.

Tumors of the testicle are not unusual. They are highly malignant and can occur at any age, but are most common in the early teens and 20s. Any mass in the testicle, especially if it is not associated with fever, should be suspected of malignancy. Treatment is extensive surgical excision and, depending on the type of tumor, irradiation or other therapy.

Removal of the tumor is achieved through an incision in the groin. The clamped spermatic cord and the testis are then carefully removed. Depending on the grade and appearance of the tumor, additional treatment may be given. In some cases the lymph nodes that drain from the testis and pass through the back part of the body cavity are also removed. The area sometimes is treated with external radiation therapy. After surgery or irradiation, additional treatment with multiple drugs may be prescribed.

Hydrocele is an accumulation of fluid in the scrotum and cystic dilation of the coverings of the testis. The swelling is obvious, varies in size, and can be painful. Hydrocele frequently is associated with hernia. Spermatocele is a similar cyst involving the sperm-conducting apparatus. The treatment is removal.

IMPOTENCE

Increasing levels of sexual awareness and the development of satisfactory penile prostheses for impotence are factors that have increased the number of patients who come to doctors for diagnosis and treatment of sexual problems. Impotence, something seldom talked about in an earlier era, now can often be treated.

Normal erections can be expected if there is an anatomically normal penis, adequate arterial blood flow, and intact nerve supplies. All of these can be determined by a physician. If no physical cause for impotence is apparent, a careful interview with the patient and preferably his sexual partner in a professional setting might reveal a psychological explanation. The patient usually is urged to present the problem in his own words and to describe the treatment he has had. Some physicians use a

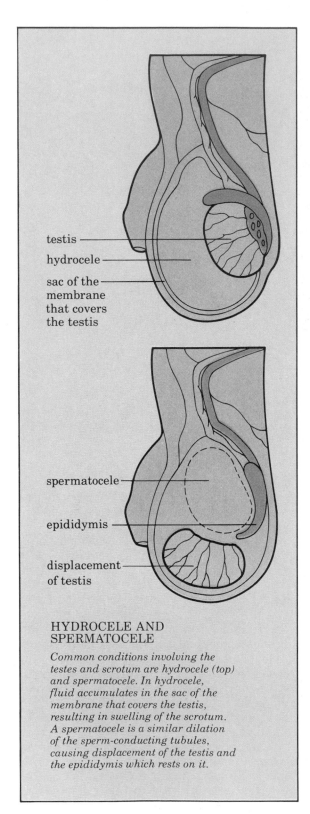

testis

hydrocele

sac of the
membrane
that covers
the testis

spermatocele

epididymis

displacement
of testis

HYDROCELE AND SPERMATOCELE

Common conditions involving the testes and scrotum are hydrocele (top) and spermatocele. In hydrocele, fluid accumulates in the sac of the membrane that covers the testis, resulting in swelling of the scrotum. A spermatocele is a similar dilation of the sperm-conducting tubules, causing displacement of the testis and the epididymis which rests on it.

sexual function questionnaire. One important question the doctor usually asks is whether the failure to achieve erection is situational, occurring under some circumstances but not others. Impotence can have a psychological explanation. It is not always caused by situational or anatomical problems.

The quality of erections and the presence or absence of orgasm and ejaculation must be determined. Erection is not necessary for either orgasm or ejaculation. In fact, orgasm can occur without erection in diabetics and in men who have had radical pelvic or retroperitoneal surgery. Medications or diseases can cause impotence, medicine for high blood pressure can interfere with the ability to achieve erections because of decreased sex drive (libido). Diabetes mellitus is often associated with what are termed nerve deficits. Tranquilizers can decrease sex drive or cause a nerve blockage. Antidepressants can be the culprit. Hypothyroidism or hypogonadism are associated with decreased sex drive. The classical history of testosterone deficiency (male sex hormone deficiency) is one of lack of sexual interest followed by decreased ejaculatory volume followed by loss of erection. Cancer chemotherapy can cause generalized weakness. Estrogens for prostate cancer can decrease the sex drive. Narcotics can decrease libido. Prior surgery is a possible factor. Psychological or organic nervous conditions and alcoholism are other causes.

Since implantation of a penile prosthesis is the most common surgical cure for impotence, it is important to determine the sexual partner's attitude about prosthetic surgery. Many women are less than enthusiastic about artificial erections. The implantation is usually preceded by a series of tests for physical abnormalities of the penis or painful inflammatory lesions. Tests also will be made for interference with the penile blood supply, hernia, prostatitis, and other conditions that might interfere with intercourse or with satisfactory implantation of a prosthesis.

Some implants are of a rigid or semiflexible nature. Others include an inflatable device and connecting tube that can be implanted under the skin, then inflated or deflated by pressure on the inflate/deflate mechanism. This mechanism is connected to the inflatable device by a surgical procedure and the control button and operative section can be placed under the skin in the pubic area.

Understandably, the selection of a candidate for this procedure involves a careful evaluation of psychological and sexual needs for the man and his partner. Emphasis on care of selection has increased over the years as experience with the devices has been gained. The implantation procedure has been extended in recent years to include patients with spinal cord injuries.

INFERTILITY

Semen analysis in the study of infertility or in routine endocrine surveys sometimes reveals a very low sperm count. The sperm under microscopic inspection may be of unusually poor quality or show lack of movement, or may be completely absent. In cases of poor sperm counts without evidence of endocrine problems, the administration of small doses of the hormones testosterone or chorionic gonadotropin can be helpful. This usually helps for patients who have had high fever, mumps, or viral disease. Other forms of male infertility have been attributed to a so-called slackening of gonadal function. In men there is no true, identifiable counterpart of the menopause, although it has been documented on occasion in some men. This is characterized as a symptom of loss of self-confidence and associated behavior, poor memory, insomnia, loss of libido, apprehension, and nervousness. Occasional cases respond to testosterone therapy. Among men who have low sperm counts and difficulty in conception, it is not uncommon to find a varicocele, which is a varicose vein of the spermatic cord. Removal of such varicose lesions, which are usually localized, can lead to recovery of sperm count levels and successful conception.

VASECTOMY

Surgical interruption of the vas deferens, which normally carries sperm from the testes to the urethra, has become an increasingly popular method of contraception. It is frequently performed under local anesthetic in a physician's office or clinic. The operation consists of a small incision on either side of the groin. The vas is then lifted forward and severed and the two ends are cauterized to seal them off, or sometimes tied with ligatures. The healing process is said not to be painful, and sexual performance ordinarily does not suffer.

For a period of weeks afterwards, however, it is necessary to use another form of contraception until all sperm are cleared from the vas.

Although regarded as minor surgery, the procedure is not without problems. These include bleeding at the site of surgery, inflammation at the site of surgery (this is usually at a later period), and autoimmune or other reaction to leftover sperm at the site of surgery. In some cases the operation fails to obstruct the passage of sperm, or the passageway later reopens, resulting in pregnancy.

More recently, some men who had vasectomies have sought to have fertility restored by having the severed vas reunited surgically, or reanastomosed. Many of these procedures have failed because of the inability to open the passageway. A few surgeons have reported success on a limited number of patients. The success rate may be improved by the introduction of microsurgery techniques that allow the tiny canals to be rejoined under enormous magnification.

CIRCUMCISION

Shortly after birth, many male children throughout the world undergo what is termed prophylactic circumcision to remove some of the foreskin on the penis. For some the procedure has both a medical and religious significance, and is sometimes performed according to strict ritual. Medically, hygiene is usually given as a reason for circumcision. It is also said that the incidence of cervical cancer is lower in women whose sex partners have been circumcised. These contentions are disputed, however, and the medical value of circumcision is a matter of debate. The position of the American Academy of Pediatrics is that infant circumcision is not required medically.

Circumcision in the adult is sometimes performed for medical reasons, including the avoidance of infection, the presence of conditions that make infection likely (such as diabetes), or a history of irritation. Another reason is to avoid cancer of the glans of the penis, because most cases of penile cancer worldwide are found in uncircumcised men. In adult circumcision, extra care must be taken to avoid postoperative pain and blood loss. The operation is performed under local, spinal, or general anesthesia. There is no evidence that adult circumcision affects potency.

THE FEMALE REPRODUCTIVE SYSTEM

Gynecology, which comes from the Greek words for "women" and "study," is the specialty of medicine that deals with female reproductive organs. Obstetricians and gynecologists, who specialize in this area of medicine, care for pregnancy and delivery of the child and treat infertility, endocrine disorders, and medical and surgical problems of the female reproductive tract.

THE FEMALE ORGANS

The reproductive organs in both sexes are among the earliest to form in the prenatal period. Although they are fully developed anatomically at birth, they do not mature until puberty. Throughout life (and indeed, before birth) the organs are under the influence of hormones from the pituitary gland (see chapter 16, "The Hormones and Endocrine Glands"), which orchestrates their maturation and what they do, readying the body for possible pregnancy and childbirth.

The basic female organs are the ovaries, uterus and fallopian tubes, vagina, and external genitalia. The ovaries, walnut-sized sex glands on each side of the pelvis, contain the female eggs (ova). A girl is born with several million eggs in her ovaries, but the number dwindles to about a half million by the onset of puberty. After puberty, one egg (rarely more) matures each month, and ovulation, the release of the ovum from the ovary, takes place. Pregnancy ensues if the egg is fertilized by a sperm.

The ovaries also produce the female hormones estrogen and progesterone. Estrogen is responsible for breast development, maturation of the genitals, body hair distribution, and redistribution of body fat. Estrogen also prepares the other organs of the reproductive system for the possible events of pregnancy.

The fallopian tube (oviduct) is the passageway through which the ovum moves en route to possible fertilization. Conception, if it takes place, occurs in the upper third of this tube. Fluid movement in the tube and microscopic, hair-like projections called villi help to move the ovum along the canal's length. If fertilization of the ovum does not occur, the ovum is shed with the lining of the uterus, the process known as menstruation.

The uterus lies in the center of the pelvis. It consists primarily of muscle bundles and can expand to many times its size with a growing pregnancy. The tapered end of the uterus, known as the cervix, has a canal leading into the vagina below.

The interior of the uterus is covered with a tissue known as the endometrium. Under the influence of the female hormones this layer thickens and enriches each month to provide a bed for the possible pregnancy. If the egg released by the ovary is fertilized by a sperm, the fertilized egg implants in the enriched endometrium and grows there throughout the pregnancy. If no fertilization occurs, the layer breaks down and is washed away in the menstrual flow.

The vagina is also known as the birth canal. It is the entry through which sperm reach the female organs to fertilize the ovum and is the outlet through which the baby passes at birth. The vagina is sometimes described as a "potential space" because its walls actually touch, but the tissues can expand to accommodate the birth of a child.

Gynecological Examination

Most adult women see a gynecologist routinely about once a year. The most important reason, but by no means the only one, is for a Pap smear. This procedure, named for its originator, the late Dr. George Papanicolaou, checks for changes in the cervix that could lead to cancer. The test is simple. A wooden spatula is used to scrape the external surface of the cervix. In some instances a cotton swab is used to obtain cells from just inside the cervix. Smeared on a microscope slide, the cells are then examined for evidence of change. The change itself does not mean cancer, but early detection by this means has sharply reduced the formerly high death rate from cervical cancer (see page 569).

In addition to the Pap smear, the yearly examination usually includes a patient history, examination of the breasts, examination of the abdomen, and a pelvic examination. A pelvic exam consists of an inspection of the external genitalia, after which a speculum, a long-handled instrument, is inserted in the vagina for visual examination of the cervix. The speculum is then removed and the vaginal walls inspected. A bimanual examination is also performed. Two fingers are inserted into the vagina while the other hand palpates the uterus, fallopian tubes, and ovaries. A rectal examination determines the position of the uterus, ovaries, and fallopian tubes. None of these procedures involves more than minor discomfort for the woman.

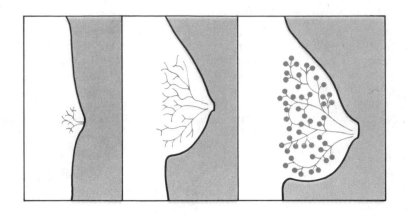

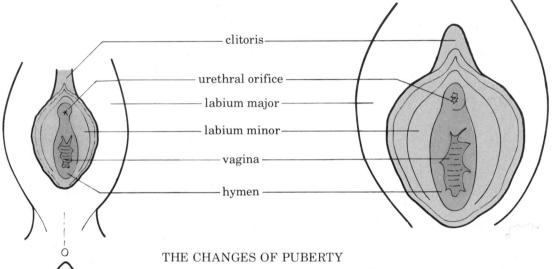

clitoris

urethral orifice

labium major

labium minor

vagina

hymen

THE CHANGES OF PUBERTY

Influenced by the hormones, the breasts and external genitals undergo change at puberty. The top drawings show normal breast development. At left, only rudimentary milk ducts are present during infancy and childhood.

In the center drawing, the ducts elongate and tissue develops in early stages of puberty. At right, the adult breast includes milk-secreting lobules. Lower drawings show the external genitalia of a child (left) and of an adult.

Many women consult a physician less frequently when they have finished childbearing but they should not. The yearly pelvic examination and Pap smear remain important. Women should ask questions of their physicians, particularly if they have concerns about procedures. If she has doubts, a woman should seek a second opinion.

NORMAL PUBERTY

Usually by the age of 12, a female begins the physical and behavioral transition from childhood to adolescence. She notices changes in her body that will continue for about four years. Puberty is characterized by a series of changes such as a sudden spurt in the rate of growth,

maturation of the breasts (thelarche), the appearance of secondary sexual hair in the armpits and pubic area (pubarche), and the first menstruation (menarche).

Breast development begins with darkening of the area around the nipple at an average age of 11 years, although it could begin as early as age 8 and be considered normal. Pubic hair growth begins at an average age of 11½ and usually reaches adult quantity by age 14. Growth of axillary hair, such as under the arms, ordinarily begins two years after the appearance of pubic hair. The first menstrual period occurs any time from age 9 through 17. If a girl does not begin breast development or growth of secondary sexual hair by the age of 15 and has not had a menstrual period by the age of 16, she should seek medical attention.

MENSTRUATION

Menstruation is a cyclical discharge of blood, secreted fluids, and degenerated tissue from the uterus. A menstrual cycle, calculated from the first day of one menstrual episode to the first day of the next, is usually 28 days, but varies from 24 to 32 days, both among individuals and from period to period. Blood flow usually lasts three to seven days, with an average total blood loss of about one ounce per period (30 cubic centimeters). Menstrual periods usually occur each month (except during pregnancy) through the age of 48 or 50, although they can occur irregularly. Menstrual bleeding that occurs less frequently than normal is called oligomenorrhea and menstrual bleeding that occurs more frequently than normal is called polymenorrhea.

The degenerated tissue in the menstrual substance is shed from the lining of the uterus as a result of a timed series of events directed by the endocrine system. Normally, once a month the follicle-stimulating hormone (FSH) is secreted from the pituitary gland in the brain and stimulates an ovary to develop one or two eggs (ova). In turn, the tissues and cells around the ova produce the hormone estrogen, which stimulates the growth of the lining of the uterus. At the same time, the estrogen inhibits the secretion of FSH and causes the release of luteinizing hormone (LH), which triggers ovulation, the discharge of the egg from the ovary into a position where it can be fertilized. Following ovulation, the tissues around the ovum's former site produce not only estrogen but the second female hormone, progesterone, which causes the lining of the uterus to issue secretions. Some women complain about a large amount of clear mucus discharge at the time of ovulation, when the glands of the cervix secrete mucus in abundance to facilitate sperm penetration and fertilization of the ovum. If fertilization does not occur, however, the tissue around the ovulation site undergoes degeneration, the estrogen and progesterone levels in the circulation fall, and the lining of the uterus is shed.

Menstruation requires normal body functions, a normal pituitary gland, a responsive ovary, and a normal uterus. Defects in any of these can prevent the start of menstruation or cause menstrual periods to stop even if they have been regular. The term used to describe the lack of onset of menstruation is primary amenorrhea. The term describing when menstrual periods stop for some reason is secondary amenorrhea.

Absence of Menstruation

Vaginal causes. The most common reasons why menstruation fails to begin in otherwise normally developed women are abnormalities of the vagina and uterus. These abnormalities range from an imperforate hymen—the hymen is the piece of tissue that narrows the opening of the vagina—to incomplete development of the uterus. The hymen varies greatly in form, but it is rarely imperforate, which means that there is no opening through the tissue at all. The absence of an opening is diagnosed by a pelvic examination and treated by incision. The incision allows trapped menstrual blood to escape from the vagina and thereby corrects the lack of menstruation. In a few women a dividing wall called a septum is positioned across the vagina higher than the hymen. This partition does not allow the menstrual blood to flow through the vagina and must be opened surgically.

Uterus. The absence of the uterus or of a portion of the vagina is rare, but when it does occur the vagina ends as a blind pouch. The woman does not have menstrual periods, but the vagina usually is of adequate length and caliber to allow for normal sexual relations. However, sometimes a dilator must be used to enlarge the vagina. If this fails, the woman must undergo surgery. These women are unable to have children but can marry and lead normal sexual lives.

Ovaries. Lack of onset of menstruation also can be caused by failure of the ovaries to develop. Because these organs produce estrogen and progesterone, which are responsible for making the uterus secretory during ovulation, the shedding of the lining of the uterus (menstruation) does not take place. Women with this condition also lack breast development and other secondary sexual development at puberty.

Gonadotropins are substances that stimulate the gonads, or reproductive glands, such as the ovaries. The pituitary gonadotropins FSH and LH are integral to the menstrual process. A low production level of these hormones can result in a lack of menstruation. Low gonadotropin levels stem from a number of causes, some of which are associated with

HORMONE LEVELS DURING MENSTRUAL CYCLE

A cyclical series of endocrine events controls ovulation, menstruation, and conception. At the beginning of the cycle, follicle-stimulating hormone (FSH) is secreted by the pituitary gland. Under its stimulation, an ovum (egg) matures and estrogen is secreted. Estrogen inhibits the flow of FSH but triggers a second pituitary hormone, luteinizing hormone (LH), which causes ovulation, the release of the egg for possible fertilization. Cells around the ovulation site then secrete the hormone progesterone, which enhances the preparation of the uterine lining for implantation of the fertilized ovum. If conception does not occur, estrogen and progesterone levels fall and menstruation takes place.

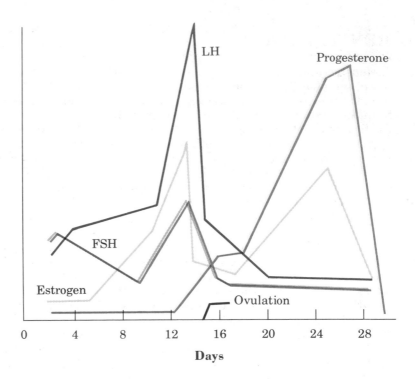

tumors or disease of the pituitary gland or injury to the hypothalamus above it. On occasion, the condition is associated with chronic diseases, including diabetes mellitus, kidney failure, and extreme weight loss.

Irregular Uterine Bleeding

Bleeding without ovulation. It is not unusual for young women to have irregular bleeding when they first start menstrual cycles. They frequently skip one, two, or three monthly cycles, then bleed intermittently. Irregular bleeding occurs during the early cycles because they are not ovulatory cycles. It is not considered abnormal at this time of life. Cycles in which the woman is not ovulating are seldom profuse or frequent enough to cause anemia, but if anemia is suspected, the woman should see a physician. Irregular bleeding often disappears spontaneously as ovulatory cycles ensue, but in cases of anemia the cycles may have to be regulated with hormones for a short time. Once ovulation occurs on a regular basis, menstrual cycles are relatively consistent throughout reproductive life until the menopause, when many women bleed but do not ovulate.

Ovulatory bleeding. There may be spotting or slight bleeding at the time of ovulation, which occurs about 14 to 16 days before a menstrual period. This is prompted by a slight decrease of estrogen, which is secreted during ovulation. The spotting lasts one or two days.

Spotting before menstruation. A menstrual period may be preceded by several days of spotting because of decreased hormonal levels and consequent irregular shedding of the lining of the uterus. These cycles may persist for several months before subsiding or reverting to normal cycles spontaneously. The bleeding pattern usually occurs intermittently, but if it persists and becomes annoying, it can be treated.

Bleeding without ovulation, mid-cycle bleeding, and irregular shedding are termed dysfunctional uterine bleeding, meaning abnormal bleeding that occurs in the absence of pregnancy or any pathologic condition. Profuse cyclic or irregular menstrual bleeding can also be a sign of a pathologic condition and should be investigated if it persists. In older women, abnormal bleeding before or after menopause, the period when menstruation naturally ceases, should be investigated by taking a sample of the lining of the uterus for examination under a microscope.

Menopause

Signs and symptoms. The menopause begins when ovulation stops. The average age for this event is 51. After ovulation stops, irregular menstrual periods and times of lack of menstrual periods are not unusual. Next comes a decrease in the production and secretion of estrogen, accompanied by signs and symptoms of the deficit in the organs dependent upon estrogen, such as uterus, cervix, vagina, and breasts. The only signs and symptoms that are truly characteristic of the postmenopausal period are hot flashes and shrinking (atrophy) of the genital organs. Symptoms such as inability to sleep, irritability, or depression, commonly considered by many women to be part of the menopause, are much more difficult to attribute to reduction of estrogen. In fact, estrogen levels in many postmenopausal women often are not even low. As many as half the women who have experienced menopause have adequate estrogen levels.

The vasomotor symptoms, those that affect the blood vessels and produce hot flashes and sweats, are quite distinct and are troublesome in as many as 60 percent of menopausal women. Some women, if not most, experience severe symptoms for a few months to two years. Others suffer for an even longer time. Estrogen deficiency also causes a gradual reduction and eventual loss of the thickness of the vaginal wall. Similar changes, although not as pronounced, occur in the bladder. The result is increasing dryness in the vagina. When the deficiency is severe there is vaginal irritation, itching, and sometimes pain during intercourse. Administration of estrogen restores the normal thickness of the vagina and corrects the symptoms.

Osteoporosis is the term for reduction of bony material in the skeleton and increased fragility of all bones except the skull. It is primarily age-related and occurs because of a loss of calcium in the bone and gradual decrease in bone formation. Osteoporosis may be related to the menopause. Studies have shown a correlation between accelerated osteoporosis and decreased estrogen secretions. This is significant for the female population because about 25 percent of women over 60 have spinal fractures resulting from osteoporosis. Women also have a 2½ times greater risk of hip fractures than men do.

Treatment. Estrogen replacement therapy for the postmenopausal women is beneficial for relieving involuntary hot flashes, sweats, and symptoms attributed to atrophy of the vagina. However, the benefits of estrogen replacement should be weighed against the possibility of adverse effects. For instance, the possibility of an increased incidence of cancer of the endometrium in postmenopausal women using estrogens is a concern. Although a definite cause-and-effect relationship is not proven,

one is suggested. While investigations continue, judicious use of estrogen therapy may be considered if the benefits outweigh the risks.

Before starting estrogen therapy the woman should have a thorough evaluation, including a complete history and physical examination to discover any factor that may place her in a position of higher risk. If estrogen therapy is chosen, it is advisable to prescribe the smallest dose that will relieve the symptoms. The program should be cyclical, such as taking the medication for three consecutive weeks, then going without it for the fourth week. The individual should be examined at regular intervals so that blood pressure, breast, and pelvic examinations can be performed. If irregular bleeding occurs at any time, a sampling of the endometrium and microscopic examination of the tissue is mandatory.

INFECTIONS

Infections of the female reproductive tract involve both the external and internal genitalia. Infections of the vulva and vagina are not life threatening and are among the most common gynecologic complaints of women. Infections of the internal genitals, however, can be more severe and can lead to infertility and surgical removal of the organs.

External Infections

Vulvitis. Most of the time, inflammation of the vulva results from profuse vaginal discharge caused by vaginal infection. However, a primary infection of the vulva called vulvitis can occur secondary to a herpes virus infection, a form of inflammatory skin disease. Symptoms are evident two to seven days after exposure to herpes virus, type II (see chapter 28, "Infectious Diseases"). Blisterlike sacs of fluid called vesicles form on the vulva and evolve into small ulcers covered by a white colored fluid of cell debris. The ulcers become infected, red, and swollen, but tend to heal in seven to ten days. In some women, the ulcers are recurrent even with treatment. The condition is extremely painful and therapy usually is aimed at alleviating the symptom associated with the pain. The pain can become severe enough to warrant hospitalization.

Vaginitis. The most common forms of vaginitis, which means infection of the vagina, are yeast or monilial vaginitis, trichomonas vaginalis vaginitis, and hemophilus vaginalis vaginitis. All produce similar symptoms—irritation of the external genitalia, itching, frequent urination, and occasional pain when urinating or during intercourse. Despite the similarity, it is important to identify the responsible organism because treatment differs for each.

Yeast vaginitis. Yeast or monilial vaginitis is caused by a fungus known as *Candida albicans.* The infection also is known as candidiasis or moniliasis. It occurs during pregnancy, and it also occurs among women who take oral contraceptives. Yeast vaginitis can also follow treatment with broad-spectrum antibiotics because the antibiotics change the types of bacteria normally found in the vagina, thereby permitting infection with other bacteria. The treatment requires insertion of suppositories or cream in the vagina.

Trichomonas vaginalis vaginitis. The organism responsible for this type of vaginitis is *Trichomonas vaginalis,* an oval one-celled organism with a tail-like appendage that gives it great motility. Infection is usually associated with vaginal discharge, irritation of the vulva, itching, and pain during intercourse. The diagnosis is made by taking a smear of the thin, foamy discharge and examining it under a microscope. The most effective treatment is metronidazole (Flagyl®), a compound taken orally that requires a physician's prescription. Good results follow a single course of treatment. Since trichomonads can be harbored in the male urinary tract and be transmitted during intercourse, a person can be reinfected by a sexual partner, so it is recommended that sexual partners seek medical attention and therapy simultaneously.

Hemophilus vaginalis vaginitis produces less severe itching and burning than the other infections of the vagina. The diagnosis is made by microscopic examination of the vaginal discharge or by laboratory culture of the organism, which is a process of allowing the sample of the discharge to grow so the organisms are more visible. Treatment of this type of vaginitis involves the use of vaginal antibiotic creams.

Internal Infections

Cervicitis is an inflammation of the cervix, the lower end of the uterus. It is detected microscopically and usually is of no clinical consequence, although it is accompanied by a discharge. It requires treatment in some women, especially when it produces erosion, a zone of infected tissue around the cervical opening that has become red and irregular. Since some cancers of the cervix can have a similar appearance, an examination is important to rule out a malignancy. All cases of cervicitis should be investigated with Pap smears. A biopsy of the cervical tissue sometimes is necessary. Usual treatment of chronic cervicitis is application of antibiotic vaginal cream. Some conditions require treatment with electrocautery, a method of destroying tissue with heat, or with cryosurgery, the destruction of tissue by freezing.

Gonorrhea is one of the most common sexually transmitted (venereal) diseases (see chapter 28, "Infectious Diseases"). It infects the internal genital tract organs—the uterus, fallopian tubes, and ovaries—and is associated with a general feeling of ill health and fever. As many as 80 percent of the women who contract the disease have no symptoms except a heavy, white discharge from the vagina. For others, the symptoms often begin near the end of or after a menstrual period. The woman urinates frequently or experiences pain while urinating. As the infection extends up to the uterus and fallopian tubes, she may have abdominal pain with fever. Sometimes the lower abdominal pain is more severe on one side than the other and is mistaken for appendicitis. Prompt antibiotic treatment brings a return to normal temperature and clears the abdominal signs. In spite of the patient's recovery from the acute attack, there is always the possibility of adhesions in the fallopian tubes that could result in infertility.

DISORDERS OF REPRODUCTIVE ORGANS

Pelvic Relaxation

Pelvic relaxation results from a weakening of the supporting tissues of the bladder, the upper walls of the vagina, the uterus, and the rectum. The organ or part of the organ then can move out of normal position or alignment in the same way as a hernia or protrusion of an organ or tissue. Although pelvic relaxation is thought to be a result of childbirth, it occurs in women who have not had children. Symptoms vary depending on the structure involved. It may create a sense of pressure in the vagina or feel as if a structure is protruding from the vagina. Other symptoms include pelvic pain and inability to control urination while pushing, laughing, coughing, or at times of stress.

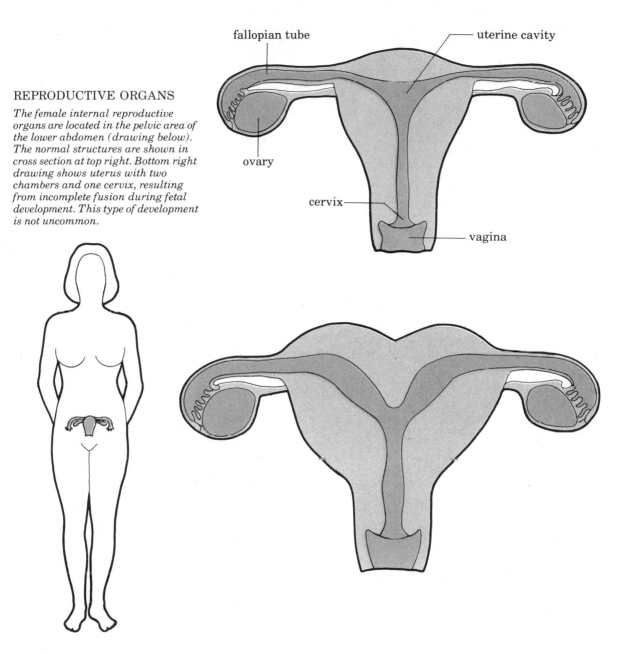

REPRODUCTIVE ORGANS

The female internal reproductive organs are located in the pelvic area of the lower abdomen (drawing below). The normal structures are shown in cross section at top right. Bottom right drawing shows uterus with two chambers and one cervix, resulting from incomplete fusion during fetal development. This type of development is not uncommon.

Uterine prolapse. Prolapse is a term for falling down or sinking. Uterine prolapse occurs when the supporting ligaments of the uterus are stretched or injured and permit the uterus to descend into the vagina. The prolapse can be so severe that the entire uterus protrudes beyond the vaginal opening. Discomfort stems from having the uterus in the vagina, and irritation results from the uterus being exposed to the outside. The bladder is attached to the uterus and frequently prolapses along with the uterus. Uterine prolapse can be treated with a pessary, which is a supporting device inserted in the vagina to hold the uterus in place. A pessary is used for women who are not candidates for hysterectomy, or surgical removal of the uterus. Suspension of the uterus can be attained by shortening the supporting ligaments, but this is rarely done and only if the woman desires children.

Vaginal wall relaxation. Relaxation of the front wall of the vagina results in cystocele and urethrocele, a bulging of the bladder and the urethra, which leads from the bladder to outside the vagina. This loss of support stems from a weakening of the vaginal bands of tissue called fascia. The symptoms consist of a bearing down sensation and protrusion of the organs outside the vagina. Frequently there

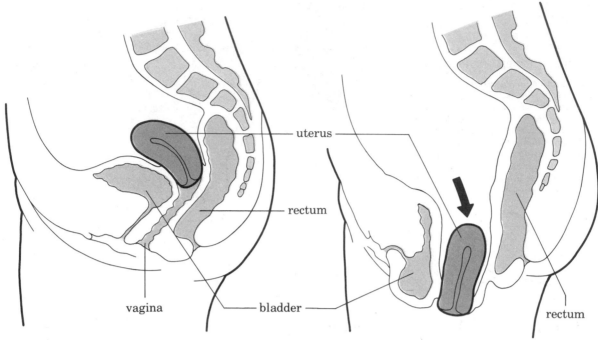

uterus

rectum

vagina

bladder

rectum

PROLAPSE

Prolapse occurs when the supporting ligaments of the uterus are stretched or injured. The left drawing shows a uterus in normal position. In the drawing at right the uterus has prolapsed into the vagina. The condition can be so severe that the *entire uterus protrudes beyond the vagina, causing discomfort and inflammation. The condition is usually repaired surgically, but sometimes a supporting device is inserted in the vagina.*

is a loss of urine when coughing, sneezing, laughing, and at other times of increased abdominal pressure. Some women must wear protective clothing because of the possibility of unplanned expulsion of urine that could cause embarrassment. Cystoceles and urethroceles are not life threatening. Surgery can relieve the symptoms in most cases, depending upon the severity.

Relaxation of the back wall of the vagina creates a protrusion of the rectum into the vagina called a rectocele. A minimal amount of rectocele usually does not produce symptoms, but a considerable protrusion pushes the bowel into the herniated sac. A common complaint with this disorder is that the woman must apply pressure around or inside the vagina to stimulate a bowel movement.

Simultaneous surgical repair of the front and back walls of the vagina usually corrects a cystocele, urethrocele, or rectocele.

Benign Lesions of the Uterus

Fibroid tumors, also known as myomas, are encapsulated benign tumors of the uterus composed of muscle and fibrous tissue. They are the most common pelvic tumors. It is estimated that one of every five women over 35 years of age has uterine fibroid tumors. Myomas frequently produce no symptoms and are found during pelvic examination. The fibroid tumors may be located outside the uterus on the exterior surface and may protrude inside the uterus to the mucosal surface. There may be multiple growths of varying sizes.

Although most myomas do not produce symptoms, they can cause abnormal bleeding, particularly if they protrude into the cavity of the uterus. The most common form of abnormal bleeding associated with myomas is excessive or prolonged menstruation. Depending on the size and location, myomas also press on other organs. For instance, pressure on the bladder by myomas produces urinary frequency. Pain is not common but occurs if the tumors degenerate.

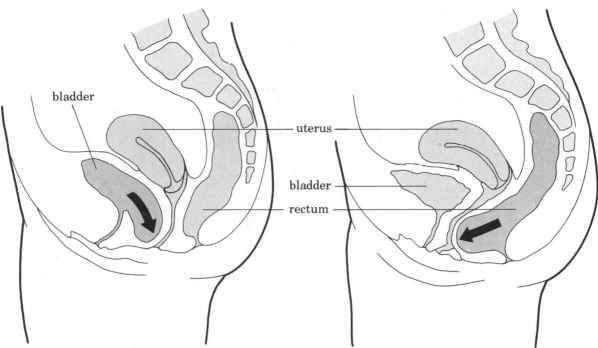

RELAXED VAGINAL WALL

Weakening of the vaginal wall allows adjacent organs to change position. Relaxation of the front (anterior) wall causes bulging of the bladder (cystocele) and urethra, as shown by the arrows in the left drawing. This can cause loss of *urinary control. Relaxation of the posterior wall allows the rectum to protrude into the vaginal space (rectocele), as shown in drawing at right. Both cystocele and rectocele can be repaired surgically, depending upon the severity of the case.*

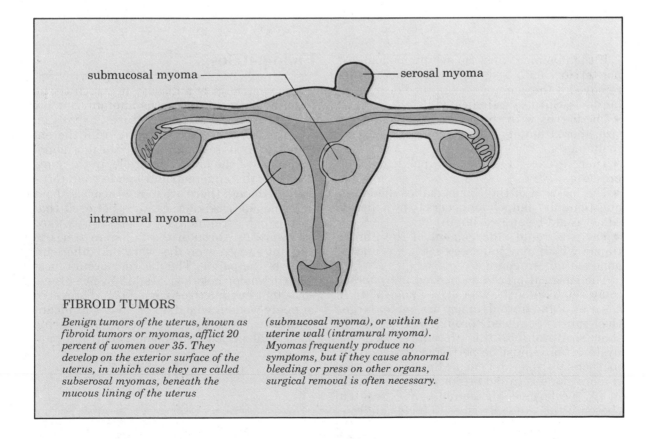

FIBROID TUMORS

Benign tumors of the uterus, known as fibroid tumors or myomas, afflict 20 percent of women over 35. They develop on the exterior surface of the uterus, in which case they are called subserosal myomas, beneath the mucous lining of the uterus *(submucosal myoma), or within the uterine wall (intramural myoma). Myomas frequently produce no symptoms, but if they cause abnormal bleeding or press on other organs, surgical removal is often necessary.*

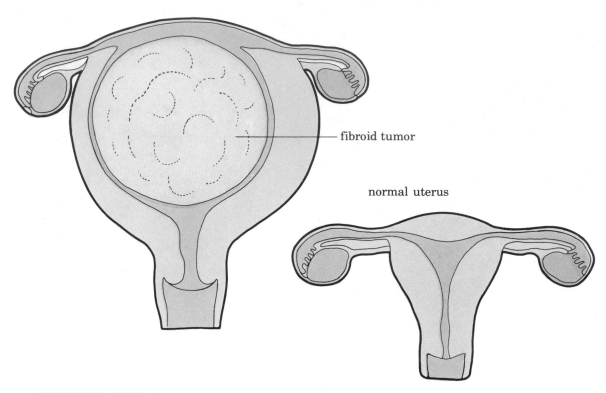

fibroid tumor

normal uterus

ENLARGED MYOMA

Although many tumors (also known as myomas) are small, there can be multiple growths or one can become so large that it distends the uterine cavity (left drawing). The entire uterus may have to be removed surgically. If the woman wishes to have children, then only the tumor will be removed, and it will be done abdominally, a procedure called myomectomy.

If the myomas cause no symptoms and are not terribly enlarged, they do not need to be removed if the woman is examined on a regular basis. Surgery is indicated if:
• The uterus with the myoma is of sufficient size, approximately 8 to 10 inches (20 to 25 cm) in diameter.
• There is excessive bleeding, pelvic pain, or pressure.
• The location of the tumor makes diagnosis questionable, and what appears to be a fibroid tumor could be an ovarian tumor.
• There is rapid enlargement of the fibroid tumor, which may indicate that it has undergone malignant changes.

The surgical procedure needed is hysterectomy, removal of the uterus (see page 579). If the uterus and fibroid tumors are not too large, they can be removed through the vagina. If their size prohibits this procedure, then the hysterectomy must be performed through an incision in the abdomen. Removal of the tumors alone is called myomectomy. It is commonly performed abdominally and is often chosen if the women wishes to have children.

Endometriosis

Endometriosis is a disease in which tissue from the lining of the uterus implants outside the uterus on the pelvic structures, usually on the ovaries. Since the tissue is from the endometrium, it responds to all the hormonal variations of the menstrual cycle, in the same way that the endometrium inside the uterus does. Although there are many theories about how endometriosis arises, it is believed that endometrial fragments of the uterus flow backward up through the fallopian tubes to implant and grow on the ovary and other surfaces in the pelvis. The disorder occurs most often in women between 20 and 35 years of age. Although endometriosis has been discovered in many women who did not have significant symptoms, it can cause severe pain during menstrual periods (dysmenorrhea) and pain during intercourse (dyspareunia). Infertility sometimes leads a patient to see a physician and in the course of the evaluation endometriosis is found.

The treatment of endometriosis is determined by age and by whether the woman is seeking medical care because of infertility. Therapy is often aimed at relieving the symptoms yet conserving the organs necessary for childbearing if the woman plans to have children. Hormonal therapy using combinations of estrogens and progestogen has been used for many years to suppress ovulation, creating a pseudopregnancy that allows the endometrial glands to atrophy. If there is significant disease and adhesions have formed secondary to the endometriosis, conservative surgery is performed to remove the endometrial implants and free the adhesions. Radical surgery to remove the ovaries is done only in women who are beyond the childbearing age or when the disease is severe and has not responded to hormonal therapy and conservative surgery.

Ovarian Cysts

An ovarian cyst is a closed cavity or sac. Some are fluid-filled, some are in a semi-fluid state, and others are solid. Cysts are usually small. They occur in women of all ages and produce symptoms only when they create pressure on other organ systems. A cyst can become large enough to increase the size of the abdomen before it is noticed. An ovarian cyst is not painful unless it twists, in which case it can cause acute pelvic pain. If it ruptures and hemorrhages into the abdominal cavity, it also will cause pain. Any twisting or bleeding of an ovarian cyst must be treated immediately by surgery.

Ovarian cysts are usually removed surgically. If the cyst is small, appears to be functional, and occurs in a menstruating woman, it may be observed through at least one menstrual cycle, because it will probably subside. If it persists, however, it is an abnormal growth of tissue that should be removed. The likelihood of a malignancy of all ovarian tumors and ovarian cysts is between 15 and 25 percent, depending upon the woman's age. The extent of surgery required cannot be determined in advance because it is largely based on findings during the operation. Treatment may be as uncomplicated as excision of the cyst while conserving the remainder of the ovary, or it may be necessary to remove one or both ovaries as well as the uterus if the tumor is malignant.

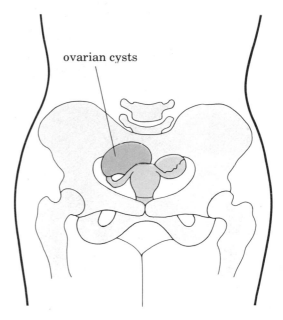

ovarian cysts

OVARIAN ENLARGEMENT

An enlargement of an ovary can be cystic, filled with fluid, or solid. It may cause no symptoms until it is large enough to press on adjacent organs, as in the drawing above, or until it is twisting or bleeding, in which case it must be removed surgically.

Cancer of the Reproductive Tract

Cancer of the cervix is the most common cancer of the reproductive tract, occurring in 45,000 women a year in the United States. The earliest recognizable indication is dysplasia, a change in the superficial cells of the covering (epithelium) of the cervix. Theoretically, if dysplasia remains untreated it will progress into preinvasive cancer of the cervix. When the cancer progresses past the preinvasive stage by spreading from the site of origin to invade the tissue beneath the epithelium, it is called invasive cancer. The average age for cancer confined to the cervix is 38. Women with dysplasia or preinvasive cancer of the cervix do not have symptoms as a rule and frequently the diagnosis is suspected by a positive Pap test obtained during a routine examination. The Pap test is highly successful in detecting the cancer and allows treatment at a stage when cure is certain.

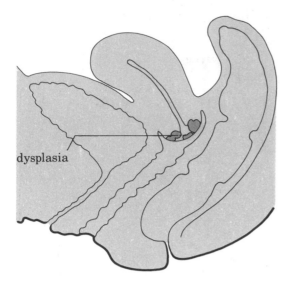

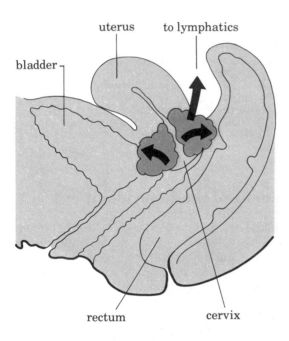

CANCER OF THE CERVIX

The most common cancer of the female reproductive tract is cancer of the cervix. It can be cured if detected early. The first indication is likely to be a distinct change of cell structure, called dysplasia, at the cervical opening (upper drawing). The cells are obtained and tested by Pap smear. Although not all dysplasias become cancerous, if not identified and treated, they can progress to become invasive cancer, which spreads to nearby structures (lower drawing) and may be too far advanced for cure.

If a Pap smear yields abnormal results, colposcopy is the next step. Colposcopy is a technique of viewing the cervix magnified through an instrument similar to a microscope. If the epithelium is abnormal, the abnormality can be seen with the colposcope. The colposcope also helps determine where a specimen of tissue of the cervix should be obtained by biopsy for laboratory diagnosis. Colposcopy can help differentiate invasive cancer from noninvasive or inflammatory lesions of the cervix.

Removal of preinvasive cancer is done by an operation or by cryosurgery. Selection of treatment is influenced by whether the woman wants to have children. If she does, a cone biopsy of the cervix or cryosurgery is recommended. For the patient who is beyond childbearing years or who considers her family complete, the selected treatment may be hysterectomy. The cure rate of preinvasive cancer of the cervix is virtually 100 percent.

Symptoms of invasive carcinoma of the cervix include irregular bleeding, bleeding after intercourse, pain, and weight loss. A woman who experiences irregular spotting should seek medical attention immediately because the possibility of curing invasive carcinoma decreases markedly in advanced stages. The treatment selected for invasive cancer of the cervix depends upon the extent of the disease, which can be classified from stage I to stage IV, with stage IV being the most advanced. If the invasion is in stage I, treatment will be either radiation or radical surgery, an extensive hysterectomy which includes some tissue around the cervix. If the carcinoma has invaded the cervix, the tissues around the cervix, or the vaginal wall, the treatment chosen is often radiation. The cure rate for advanced cases is less hopeful, however, than for preinvasive cancer or cancer confined to the place of origin (in situ).

Cancer of the uterus. About three-fourths of all cases of endometrial cancer (cancer of the lining of the uterus) are found in women beyond the menopause. The average age of occurrence is between 50 and 60. Because the primary symptom is bleeding, any bleeding in a woman who is past the menopause should be investigated thoroughly to rule out the possibility of endometrial cancer. The diagnosis is made by obtaining tissue from the inside of the uterus, either by dilation of the cervix and curettage of the endometrium, the procedure known as D&C (see page 578), or by taking a biopsy of the endometrium. The treatment for cancer of the uterus is removal of the uterus, fallopian tubes, and ovaries. In some patients radium is inserted in the uterus before surgery. In others, depending upon the extent of the disease, X-ray therapy is administered after surgery. As with most cancers, the cure rate correlates with the extent of the disease, but the outlook for cancer of the endometrium is favorable, particularly because it remains localized for a long time.

Cancer of the ovary is the fourth leading cause of death from cancer among American women, after breast cancer, lung cancer, and colon-rectal cancer. About 60 percent of all malignant ovarian tumors occur in women 40 to 60 years old, 20 percent occur in women under 40, and the remainder occur in women over 60. Because of the silent growth of the tumor and the fact that the ovary is not readily available for tissue diagnosis, many women have advanced disease when they seek medical help for the first time. Periodic pelvic examinations can help in early diagnosis, but the final diagnosis must await surgical exploration. Treatment involves drug therapy, X-ray therapy, or surgery. The basic operation for cancer of the ovary is a total abdominal hysterectomy with removal of the fallopian tubes and ovaries. If the disease is extensive, the surgery is often followed by X-ray therapy and various drug therapies.

Cancer of the vulva comprises only a small percentage of the malignancies of the reproductive tract. In most cases, it occurs in women 60 to 70 years of age. The most common symptom is itching. The diagnosis is made by taking tissue for microscopic examination. The treatment is usually surgical.

Exposure to DES

In 1970, there was a report of seven cases of rare vaginal adenocarcinoma (cancer) in young women. After these cases were investigated completely, six of these seven women were found to have been exposed to the synthetic hormone diethylstilbestrol (DES) before they were born. A study of additional cases also showed that this rare disorder occurred in other young women whose mothers took the hormone while pregnant to prevent miscarriage. Results showed benign abnormalities of the vagina and cervix, with the most common

lesion being vaginal adenosis, defined as the unusual presence of gland-like epithelium in the vagina. There are also some abnormalities occurring in the cervix.

All young women who suspect that they have been exposed prenatally to DES should have gynecologic examinations by age 14 or shortly after the first menstrual period. This is especially important for the individual whose mother took the hormone before the eighth week of pregnancy, which places the daughter at an increased risk. Ordinarily, the examination includes inspection of the vagina and cervix, a Pap test, and colposcopy. Another way to detect the benign changes attributed to DES exposure is a staining technique performed at the time of the vaginal examination.

INFERTILITY

A couple is considered infertile when they have been unable to conceive children although they want to. Primary infertility exists when there have been no conceptions. Secondary infertility exists when a couple has an infertility problem after one or more previous pregnancies. Simultaneous investigation of both sexual partners is preferred in infertility cases. Infertility presents a problem for 10 percent of married couples. About 40 percent of infertility problems stem from a defect in the male partner.

Conception depends upon normal female ovarian function, meaning that ovulation must occur. The hormones from the ovary must prepare the uterus so that if fertilization occurs, the fertilized egg can implant in the uterine lining and grow. The male must deposit a sufficient number of motile spermatozoa in the vagina because the sperm have to migrate through the cervix and the uterus to the fallopian tubes before fertilization can take place. In the course of a fertility evaluation, all of these aspects have to be examined.

A general history and physical examination of the woman should be accomplished. A semen analysis is done on the male partner to see if he has enough motile spermatozoa. Whether ovulation occurs on a regular basis can be determined by keeping a chart of the woman's basal body temperature (which will rise slightly at ovulation), by sampling the lining of the uterus, or by hormone assays. A hysterosalpingogram can be performed to be sure there are no abnormalities of the uterus. Hysterosalpingogram is an X-ray technique that involves instilling a radiopaque dye in the uterus. The dye outlines the cavity of the uterus and the fallopian tubes to show whether the tubes are open or blocked. The possibility of tubal disease or abnormalities inside the pelvic cavity is evaluated through laparoscopy (see page 577). If tubal disease has blocked the tubes, surgery may be necessary. If ovulation is not occurring, drugs are available to induce it. If the natural hormones are not of sufficient levels to prepare the lining of the uterus, hormonal therapy is prescribed.

CONTRACEPTION

Methods of avoiding pregnancy have been used for centuries. Although breast-feeding reduces the risk of pregnancy and is a method that has been used historically, it is not highly effective. Oral contraceptives and intrauterine devices are newer methods of family planning. The use of a contraceptive reduces the statistical probability of pregnancy, but it is important to remember that no method of contraception is 100 percent effective because all are subject to biological or human failure. Generally, the effectiveness of contraceptives has been measured by means of the Pearl formula, which defines effectiveness in terms of pregnancy rates per 100 woman-years of exposure. Some methods are more effective than others. The range of effectiveness is wide and varies from less than one pregnancy in 100 women per year with oral contraceptives to between 10 and 40 pregnancies in 100 women per year using the rhythm method. It is expected that if 100 women were to have regular intercourse for one year with no form of contraception, 80 to 90 of them would become pregnant, most in the first three to four months.

The Rhythm Method

During the menstrual cycle, there are days of absolute infertility, days in which the woman is potentially fertile, and days when pregnancy is unlikely but possible. A number of procedures have been devised to help identify the time of maximum fertility so intercourse can be avoided to decrease the likelihood of pregnancy.

The best way for a woman to determine her infertile period is to record the durations of 12 cycles. A cycle is determined from the first day of one menstrual period to the first day of the next. Ovulation occurs 14 to 16 days before the next menstrual cycle. Allowing for about 72 hours of survival time for both the ovum and the sperm, the unsafe time for intercourse is

Approximate number of pregnancies per 100 woman-years*	
Method	Pregnancies
Rhythm	13
Condom	3–5
Diaphragm (with spermicide)	2–3
Intrauterine device	1–2
Oral contraceptive	0.5
Vasectomy	0.15
Tubal ligation	0.04
*Assuming method of contraception is used correctly and consistently.	

The effectiveness of contraceptive methods is usually compared in terms of woman-years, which means the number of women who would become pregnant in a year while using the method correctly and consistently. The most effective method of preventing pregnancy is tubal ligation, a form of female sterilization. The least effective is the rhythm method.

between 11 and 18 days before the next period begins. To allow for variation in cycle length, the first unsafe day is determined by subtracting 18 from the number of days of the shortest of the last 12 cycles. The last unsafe day is determined by subtracting 11 from the number of days in the longest cycle. If the shortest of the last 12 cycles is 23 days, and the longest is 33 days, then the calculation is 23 minus 18, which equals 5; and 33 minus 11, which equals 22. Thus, conception is considered possible from day 5 up to and including day 22.

The rhythm method sometimes is coupled with methods to identify the time of ovulation more precisely. One way is to chart basal body temperature, which rises when ovulation occurs. Another way to identify time of ovulation is to monitor changes in the body, including a marked increase in the volume of mucus secreted by the cervix. Both improve the effectiveness of the rhythm method.

The rhythm method becomes most effective when it is part of the life-style of the couple, when the couple is well-motivated and the woman's menstrual cycles are regular. This method of contraception is not suitable for women who have irregular menstrual cycles.

Condoms

The condom, or rubber prophylactic, is one of the common contraceptive methods. It can be effective if used properly. Failures are recorded at five pregnancies per 100 woman-years when used correctly. The condom has the advantage of being widely available, and it decreases the likelihood of transmitting venereal disease. The condom is put on the penis when full erection occurs and before the penis enters the vagina. Failures can occur if the condom is not put on soon enough. Following intercourse it may be necessary to hold the condom in place when the penis is removed from the vagina so the condom does not slip off. Using a chemical spermicide in the vagina as well as the condom further lessens the chance of pregnancy.

Barrier Methods: Diaphragms

Diaphragms are satisfactory methods of birth control for many women. The diaphragm is a rubber cup attached to a metal circular spring, which must be fitted for a patient by a physician. It is positioned in the vagina so that it covers the cervix, being large enough to fill the vagina yet not cause discomfort. A spermicidal jelly or cream is placed within the diaphragm so that there is both a mechanical and chemical barrier. When used diligently, the diaphragm has an effectiveness in the range of 2 to 15 pregnancies per 100 woman-years. Popular in earlier eras, it is now being used again because of women's increased awareness of complications that can result from hormonal contraceptives and intrauterine devices. Although reliable and without serious side effects, the diaphragm does require a high degree of patient motivation. It must be inserted in the vagina before intercourse and remain there at least six to eight hours for the spermicide to be effective.

Preparations that kill sperm are available as foams, creams, jellies, and vaginal suppositories. They work in two ways: First, the inert chemical base that holds the spermicide acts as a barrier to the entry of the sperm into the cervix. Second, the agent contains a spermicidal chemical that immobilizes and kills the sperm. The failure rate of using spermicidal preparations alone, without a diaphragm, can be as low as five pregnancies per 100 woman-years for women who are motivated to use them. However, the failure rate increases to 30 pregnancies per 100 woman-years when a large number of users are analyzed. Failures sometimes result because a woman does not use enough foam or cream, or does not have it available when it is needed. Its effectiveness is increased by also using a barrier method such as a condom.

Intrauterine Devices (IUDs)

Intrauterine devices (IUDs) are usually made of steel and plastic. The sizes, shapes, and types of IUDs vary. Some have copper wire wound around them and some contain a hormonal material. They are inserted into the uterus by a physician and normally remain there until removed or expelled.

How IUDs work is not completely known. When tested in laboratory animals it appears to vary by species. Originally, studies performed with rhesus monkeys indicated that the device caused a more rapid transfer of the ovum from the ovary to the uterus, but later studies did not substantiate this explanation. It is now believed that in humans the intrauterine device creates an environment in the uterus that is not conducive to early growth of the embryo or interferes with the sperm as they pass through the uterus to fertilize the ovum in the fallopian tube. The theoretical effectiveness of most IUDs is one to two pregnancies per 100 woman-years. Once the device is inserted, the patient need not worry about contraception. If an IUD is tolerated well for several months, subsequent expulsion or removal because of pain or bleeding is markedly decreased. However, as many as 20 to 30 percent of users discontinue within the first year.

The IUD is inserted during menstruation to reduce discomfort, but most women experience cramping for a short time. The device should not be used if the woman is pregnant, has abnormal bleeding, or has pelvic infection in the uterus or fallopian tubes. Infection in the vagina usually does not rule out IUD use. Some physicians will not prescribe an IUD for a woman who has never given birth, primarily because of the increased pain and increased frequency of expulsion. Side effects that occur with intrauterine devices include bleeding, usually at the time of insertion. IUDs usually do not cause a change in the menstrual cycle. However, there may be occasional bleeding between periods, and menstrual periods may be increased in amount of flow and duration. Uterine cramps may recur and increase during menstrual periods. The potential for expulsion varies with the type of device. Most expulsions occur in the first three months after insertion.

Complications that result from use of the intrauterine device include perforation of the uterus and pelvic inflammatory disease. Perforation of the uterus commonly occurs at the time of insertion. The likelihood of perforation depends on the skill of the inserter and the type of device. Pelvic inflammatory disease (bacterial infection of the reproductive organs) occurs in about two percent of the users. Although most cases are mild, it can be severe enough to cause infertility.

When pregnancy occurs with an intrauterine device in place, the risk of spontaneous abortion (miscarriage) is increased. Because the IUD is in the uterus, this type of abortion is associated with infection. If the woman wishes to continue the pregnancy, the IUD should be removed gently.

Oral Contraceptives

Hormonal contraception ("the pill") became widely used in the 1960s. It has since had vast ramifications in all parts of the world because of its simplicity and its high rate of reliability. Most hormonal contraceptive preparations consist of estrogens and progestogens, which are synthetic derivatives of estrogen and progesterone. The combinations vary. The optimum dose for each woman is the lowest amount of each hormone that will produce the desired effect.

Pills are normally prescribed for 20, 21, or 22 days in a row. The woman takes one each day, then abstains for seven days. They are often packaged in reminder packets, with one for each prescribed day and vitamin or iron tablets for the "off days." During the seven days a woman is not taking the contraceptive pill, she normally has withdrawal bleeding.

Contraceptive pills act by altering the neuroendocrine system that controls the hypothalamic-pituitary-ovarian relationships, thus inhibiting ovulation. They also induce change in the reproductive tract by making the cervical mucus thick and tenacious so that it prevents sperm migration, and they affect the endometrium and tubal function in a way that is detrimental to conception. If ovulation occurs—and it can in the presence of a low dose pill—pregnancy rarely results because the reproductive tract is unfavorable for sperm migration and ovum transport.

The theoretical effectiveness of using the combined pill is 100 percent, with a failure rate of only 0.1 pregnancies per 100 woman-years. When patient errors are included, the effectiveness becomes approximately five pregnancies per 100 woman-years. The failure rates are attributed to women forgetting to take the pills regularly or discontinuing them before instituting another method of contraception.

Side Effects of Oral Contraceptives

Endocrine effects. Estrogen and progestogen mixtures in oral contraceptives alter the secretion of natural sex hormones as they tend to replace the normal ovarian function. Also, sometimes the function of the thyroid gland is affected in a way that mimics the state of pregnancy.

Fertility effects. Women who stop taking oral contraceptives usually become pregnant afterwards as readily as other women in their age group who have never taken oral contraceptives. A small percentage of women who cease taking oral contraceptives do not resume regular ovulatory cycles and should be evaluated by a physician for an endocrine problem. A woman who has not borne a child before using oral contraceptives should realize that her ability to become pregnant is uncertain. For this reason some physicians are cautious about prescribing oral contraceptives for young women who have not had children. Physicians used to recommend that a woman discontinue oral contraceptives for two or three cycles after following the regimen for two or four years, but this is no longer recommended because research has not indicated it will alleviate the problem.

Thromboembolism. Use of oral contraceptives during the 1960s yielded reports of users who experienced medical complications secondary to blood clotting, or thromboembolism. Cases were reported of women having blood clots in the lungs, the brain, and the arteries of the heart. Continued investigation showed that users over 35 years of age face a greater risk of blood clot problems than younger women, and that the risk is not related to the duration of use of oral contraceptives, but to the content and dose of estrogen in the oral contraceptives. Preparations containing more than 75 micrograms of estrogen were suspected of creating a greater risk than those with lower amounts. Consequently, the risks of blood clots decreased markedly when preparations containing 30 to 50 micrograms of estrogen were introduced. A tablet containing 30 micrograms of estrogen has since become available. It does not appear to be associated with any increase in pregnancy rate and possibly reduces the blood clot risk even more.

Cancer. There is no evidence to support the hypothesis that oral contraceptives contribute to an increased risk of developing cancer of the uterus, the breasts, or the cervix.

Metabolic changes. Glucose tolerance is reduced with the use of oral contraceptives. A woman who has had an abnormal glucose tolerance test should be considered at risk of developing diabetes and should be watched carefully by her physician if she is prescribed oral contraceptives. Most women with diabetes are advised to choose another method of contraception.

Hypertension. Hypertension can be a reason to avoid the use of oral contraceptives. If a woman has a normal blood pressure before taking oral contraceptives and her blood pressure rises after taking the tablets, it is recommended that she discontinue the pill and use another method (see chapter 4, "Hypertension"). It is especially important for women who are over 35 years of age to be watched closely for signs of elevated blood pressure and to stop taking oral contraceptives if a significant rise in blood pressure occurs.

Changes in lactation. High doses of estrogen prescribed for women immediately following childbirth can inhibit the production of breast milk (lactation). Most doctors believe that once lactation is under way, it is unlikely that continued lactation will be affected. Traces of the hormones are secreted in the mother's milk, yet there have been no harmful effects noted in breast-fed babies.

Other side effects that can occur from taking oral contraceptives include nausea, slight weight gain (probably caused by fluid retention), headaches, decreased flow, and occasional missed periods. Many of these effects diminish or disappear as the individual continues to take the pill. In some women, side effects are decreased if the prescription is changed to a smaller dose or a different combination of ingredients.

Other hormonal contraceptive agents include progestogen-only oral preparations, composed of small doses of progestins and no estrogens. These so-called minipills are often recommended for women who cannot tolerate the estrogen side effects such as headache, weight gain, or pigmentation of the skin. The theoretical effectiveness of the nonestrogen tablets is less than that of combined oral contraceptives, but is in the same range as intrauterine devices. The average pregnancy rate is about 2.5 per 100 woman-years.

"Morning-After" Pills

The administration of estrogens after intercourse interferes with pregnancy. The estrogens must be taken shortly after intercourse before the fertilized egg implants in the uterine wall. Large doses of estrogen, usually in the form of diethylstilbestrol (DES), are given daily for five days, beginning within 24 to 36 hours after intercourse. Some women experience nausea, vomiting, and possible disturbances of the menstrual cycle. The "morning-after" administration of estrogens is considered an emergency measure, not a routine method of contraception.

STERILIZATION

Sterilization as a means of fertility control is the most popular form of contraception for couples over 35 years of age who have achieved their desired number of children. In either sex, the objective is to prevent egg or sperm from uniting by interrupting their route permanently by surgical means. Because the reversible methods of contraception are not sufficiently predictable to assure that a woman will never conceive, it may be desirable for one member of the couple to be sterilized as a more certain method. It is essential, however, that a couple understand the consequences of a sterilization procedure, and realize that it should not be undertaken unless they are absolutely certain they desire no more children. No one should undergo sterilization intending to reverse the procedure later.

The type of sterilization procedure selected for a woman depends on the skill of the surgeon, the type of anesthesia that will be used, and the type of equipment available. Before the procedure, the patient's medical history is recorded and she is given a general physical and a pelvic examination. If the examination reveals an accompanying gynecologic problem, a hysterectomy (removal of the uterus) may be recommended. For example, hysterectomy is likely to be preferred for a woman who has multiple myomas and excessive vaginal bleeding and who wants to be sterilized. Other types of sterilization close the fallopian tubes but leave the uterus intact.

LAPAROSCOPY

Laparoscopic tubal sterilization is a method of severing or closing off the fallopian tube so that sperm and ovum cannot unite. Two small incisions are made in the abdomen (below) to allow insertion of the laparoscope (right), which is a sighting device, and an instrument to cut or cauterize the tube. A section of tube is usually removed and the ends sealed. Afterwards, sperm migration is blocked by the closed tube. Although ovulation continues, fertilization does not occur.

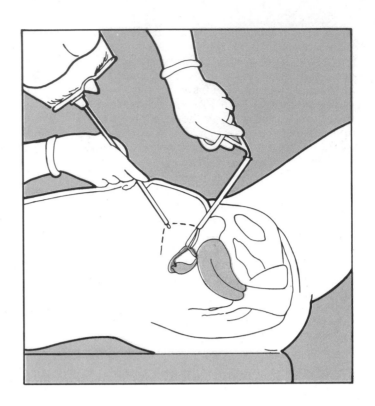

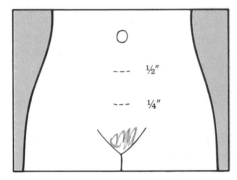

½"

¼"

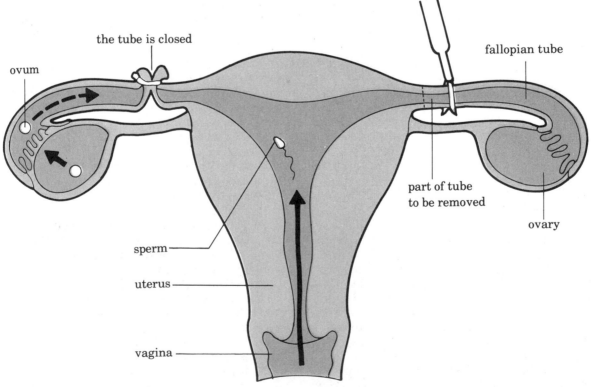

the tube is closed

ovum

fallopian tube

part of tube
to be removed

ovary

sperm

uterus

vagina

Vaginal total sterilization is begun by making an incision in the vagina to the rear of the cervix and into the pelvic cavity. The fallopian tubes are visualized through the incision, then grasped and tied with suture, and a portion is removed. In most instances this procedure is done under general anesthesia and requires a 48-hour hospital stay. Using the vaginal approach for tubal sterilization is dependent upon the mobility of the uterus and the skill of the surgeon. Not all gynecologic surgeons are practiced in vaginal surgery.

Postpartum sterilization. Immediately after a woman has had a child, the uterus is enlarged and a postpartum tubal sterilization can be carried out quickly and easily. The procedure is usually performed through a small abdominal incision just below the navel. The incision is usually two to four centimeters (about 1½ inches) in length. The technique most commonly preferred is the Pomeroy, in which the fallopian tubes are identified and ligated with absorbable suture, and a portion of the tube is removed. The procedure ordinarily does not prolong the new mother's hospital stay, although some are detained one extra day. This procedure is sometimes done at the time of a cesarean birth.

Minilaparotomy is the term used to describe sterilization performed through a small abdominal incision in a nonpregnant woman. It is done under general or local anesthesia. A small incision of three to four centimeters is made just above the pubic area. When the procedure is not done shortly after birth of a child, the uterus is usually deep in the pelvis, and an instrument must be placed in the uterus to elevate it and visualize the fallopian tube. The tubes are then closed off in the same manner as in postpartum sterilization. If the procedure is performed under local anesthesia, the woman can be discharged the same day. If it is done under general anesthesia, she is hospitalized one to two days.

Laparoscopic tubal sterilization can be accomplished under general anesthesia or local anesthesia. In many instances it can be done in an outpatient facility so that the patient can be admitted in the morning and go home in the late afternoon. A laparoscope is a long cylindrical instrument with a lens and a light system that is used to visualize the abdominal structure. It is less than one-half inch in diameter, about the size of a pencil, and is inserted into the abdominal cavity through a small incision below the navel.

The surgeon inserts a needle into the abdominal cavity. Through this needle, carbon dioxide or nitrous oxide gas is introduced. The gas raises the abdominal wall from the abdominal contents, and allows the insertion of a sharp instrument, known as a trocar, and a cannula into the abdominal cavity through a small incision. The trocar is then removed and the laparoscope is inserted through the hollow cannula, allowing the surgeon to observe the abdominal organs. Frequently, a third incision is made above the pubic hairline so that another instrument can be inserted to grasp each fallopian tube separately and close it off, or occlude it. Occlusion can be accomplished by placing a tight band around each tube, or by cauterizing (burning) a midsection of each tube. After the pelvic organs are inspected again with the laparoscope, the gas is allowed to escape from the abdominal cavity, the laparoscope is removed, and the incisions are sutured.

The procedure is considered safe, although complications include injury to the intestines, injury to other abdominal organs, bleeding from the incisions, or problems resulting from the anesthesia. In general, there are no significant long-term effects.

INDUCED ABORTION

Induced abortion, the deliberate interruption of a pregnancy, can be brought about in several ways. The technique used is usually dictated by the nature of the case, but all patients fall into either a low-risk or a high-risk group.

A low-risk pregnancy is when the woman is healthy and has been pregnant fewer than 12 weeks from the first day of her last menstrual period. The pregnancy usually is terminated surgically, requires a short outpatient visit, and is associated with a low rate of complications or death. When abortion is performed early in the pregnancy, it can be a relatively simple operation.

Abortion during this first trimester (the first 12 weeks of gestation) is performed under local, spinal, or general anesthesia. Local anesthesia, or paracervical block, is preferred and consists of injecting an anesthetic in each side of the cervix. Additional pain medication or a tranquilizer is sometimes administered.

The technique is similar to dilatation and curettage (see page 578), which involves visualization of the cervix, followed by gradual dilatation through the use of dilators increasing in size. Once the cervix is dilated, a hollow cannula or tube is inserted in the uterus and its contents are removed through vacuum aspiration. The entire procedure takes about 15 minutes.

In some instances, the removal of the tissue is performed with special forceps and a curette, a process similar to the tissue-removal procedure of D&C.

A high-risk pregnancy is one in which a woman is in her second trimester, meaning she is between 12 and 24 weeks pregnant. This advanced stage of gestation, or perhaps some other complication associated with the woman's health, necessitates that she be hospitalized one or two days. The second trimester abortion can be accomplished by several techniques, but any surgery on the high-risk patient carries a hazard.

The techniques used in most instances after the twelfth week involve amniocentesis. This is the act of inserting a needle through the outer wall of the abdomen into the amniotic sac, or the bag of waters (see chapter 26, "Pregnancy and Childbirth"). A drug is then instilled which produces uterine contractions and results in a spontaneous abortion (delivery of the fetus and placenta) in 12 to 36 hours. In addition to increased risk, the disadvantage of this technique is that the woman consciously experiences the labor and expelling of the fetus. In about one in four cases, this method results in an incomplete delivery of the placenta and curettage must be performed to remove it. There are also some risks involved for the woman in the instillation of the drug into her circulation.

Another pregnancy termination technique is the use of a suppository or drug that is placed in the vagina and is absorbed through the vaginal mucosa. It, too, induces labor contractions that result in the delivery of the fetus and the placenta. The suppository method has the same disadvantages as amniocentesis, those of undergoing labor and risking incomplete abortion, which could necessitate curettage to remove the retained placenta. However, it has the advantage of being easier to administer.

The chance of complications for the high-risk group rises rapidly as the stage of the pregnancy advances. The immediate risks are perforation of the uterus, laceration of the cervix, or hemorrhage. Complications that occur within one week of the procedure include infection and hemorrhage. The risk of these complications is as high as 20 to 25 percent when the pregnancy is between 12 and 20 weeks. The risk is less than five percent for the first trimester abortions. It is therefore important to remember that the length of a pregnancy is the most significant factor in an abortion. An abortion of a pregnancy less than 12 weeks from the last menstrual period is surgically much easier, emotionally much easier, and is much safer for the patient.

OPERATIONS

Operations through the Vagina

Dilatation and curettage. Cervical dilatation and uterine curettage (D&C) is done to diagnose abnormal uterine bleeding and, in some instances, to control hemorrhage. It also is used following inevitable or incomplete abortion (see page 616) or to obtain a tissue sample for biopsy. D&C is one of the most commonly performed gynecologic operations.

This procedure can be done under local anesthesia with the woman awake. She is given a minimal amount of medication to relieve discomfort. The local anesthesia is injected in the vagina on either side of the cervix. Less commonly, it is done under general anesthetic.

D&C begins by locating the cervical canal into the uterus with a small probe. The position of the uterus is identified by inserting a probe (an instrument used to dilate) through the cervix to the uterus. Dilators are inserted into the cervical canal and gradually increased in diameter until a long-handled metal scraping instrument called a curette can be inserted into the cavity of the uterus. The curette is a rather firm instrument and has a spoon-shaped loop at one end for removing tissue.

Cervical biopsy involves taking a small amount of tissue from the cervix to confirm or rule out the possibility of cancer. The procedure usually is conducted when a woman has a positive Pap smear or when a growth or lesion can be identified. The tissue is sent to a pathologist for microscopic analysis. The tissue is obtained by taking many small "bites" with a punch biopsy, or by conization biopsy, which means taking a whole wedge or section. Conization biopsy requires hospitalization, incision, and suturing of the cervix.

Cauterization and cryosurgery. Cauterization of the cervix is performed to relieve chronic infection of the cervix or the cervical glands. Although cauterization is usually done with a hot probe or a caustic substance, it is not necessary to anesthetize the patient. After cauterization, the infected tissue degenerates and is replaced by healthy tissue. An alternative is cryosurgery, which involves freezing the tissue. Anesthesia is not necessary for the procedure, in which a super-cold probe is applied to the cervix for several minutes.

Vaginal hysterectomy. Removal of the uterus through the vagina (vaginal hysterectomy) is recommended when the uterus is associated with uterovaginal prolapse, or vaginal wall relaxation (see page 564). The vagina is the preferred route for removal of the uterus if the uterus is not too large. Vaginal hysterectomies are generally reserved for benign circumstances, although some operations for cancer of the cervix (see page 569) can be performed safely through the vaginal canal. Vaginal hysterectomy should not be done when other organ systems are jeopardized, such as when the uterus is excessively enlarged, when there are multiple adhesions to the uterus, or when there is a possibility that the uterus or the ovaries are malignant. Vaginal surgery is also useful in obese patients because it avoids problems associated with abdominal operations.

The technique of removing the uterus begins with incision of the vaginal mucosa. The attachments of the uterus are then divided and sutured. Next, the bladder and the anterior wall are displaced and an opening is made into the peritoneal cavity at a point between the uterus and the rectum. The uterus is removed, the peritoneal cavity is closed, and the vaginal mucosa is closed. The procedure is done under general or regional anesthesia.

Operations through the Abdomen

Abdominal operations can be performed through either a vertical or a transverse (side to side) incision in the skin. Vertical incisions usually are located in the midline and extend from the navel to slightly above the pubic hairline. All of the abdominal wall components are incised vertically and the vertical incision is carried through the abdominal wall into the abdominal cavity. A vertical incision is preferred over a transverse incision when malignancy is suspected and surgical exploration of the upper abdomen is recommended. A vertical incision is also done when the uterus or an ovarian mass is so large that removal is impossible through a transverse incision.

Transverse incisions usually begin in the line of skin cleavage just above the pubic hair. The transverse incision is carried through the skin, the fatty layers, and through some of the coverings of the muscle. The area between the muscles of the abdominal wall is split and the incision follows a vertical path underneath the muscle into the pelvic cavity. A transverse incision produces a negligible scar, which is preferred by most women, but the incision can be a disadvantage to the surgeon because it limits exposure of the organs.

Abdominal hysterectomy. An abdominal hysterectomy is performed using a vertical or transverse incision, depending on the need for the hysterectomy and the size of the uterus. An abdominal hysterectomy is chosen over a vaginal hysterectomy if there is a questionable malignancy, if abdominal exploration is suggested, if the uterus is excessively large, if the woman has a history of inflammatory disease, if severe adhesions are suspected, or if an ovarian cyst could be malignant.

Reasons for hysterectomy include uterine myoma (fibroids), cancer of the body of the uterus, cancer of the ovary, and chronic inflammation or infection of the fallopian tubes. Ovaries are not routinely removed from young women who still have ovarian function.

Myomectomy. For women who are young and wish to bear children, myomectomy—removal of the uterine fibroids—is preferred over removal of the entire uterus. This is usually done through the abdominal route and requires incising fibroids located in the uterine wall, shelling them from the area, and repairing the uterine wall.

Salpingectomy, the removal of a fallopian tube, is performed when there is an ectopic (tubal) pregnancy (see Chapter 26, "Pregnancy and Childbirth"), when there is an infection in the fallopian tube, when the tube has become a fluid-filled sac, or in combination with oophorectomy or hysterectomy.

The most common reason for removal of a fallopian tube is tubal pregnancy. If the tube is unruptured, an attempt is made to remove the pregnancy without disturbing or removing the tube. If the tube is ruptured, it is removed.

Ovarian cystectomy. In cases where there is a benign cyst of the ovary, the cyst can be shelled out of the ovary, leaving the ovarian tissue in place. This is referred to as an ovarian cystectomy and is a highly successful procedure if malignancy is not suspected. Frequently, the ovary regains normal function.

Oophorectomy. A persistent tumor in the pelvis that is suspected of being ovarian in origin is a reason for oophorectomy, the abdominal removal of an ovary. It is recommended if the tumor is benign. With few exceptions, if malignancy is present, the operation is extended to include bilateral salpingo-oophorectomy and complete hysterectomy regardless of the patient's age.

CHAPTER 25   WILLIAM J. SPANOS, JR., M.D.

CANCER OF THE BREAST

Cancer of the breast is the most common cancer affecting women. The incidence of breast cancer has been increasing gradually over the years that doctors have been keeping accurate statistics. Approximately one out of 14 American women will develop breast cancer at some point during her lifetime. Because of the large number of women affected and the physical and psychological factors often associated with it, breast cancer is one of the most exhaustively studied human cancers. Yet there remain a number of misconceptions and unknowns about it.

THE NORMAL BREAST

To understand breast cancer it is valuable to have an understanding of the normal anatomy and function of the breast.

The breast is a complex structure of glands that respond to stimulation by various hormones, particularly in relationship to reproduction and nourishment of an infant. In our society the breast also plays an important appearance and self-image role for many women.

Development

The breast goes through a number of significant developmental phases during a woman's life. It originates before birth from a special band-like thickening of tissue, extending from under the arm to the groin region. This is known as the milkline. Sometimes regions of the milkline apart from the normal breasts develop into breast tissue, and a woman may have what are known as accessory breast glands. From birth until the approach of puberty, the breast changes very little. Near the onset of puberty, the breast enlarges due to an increase in glands, ducts, and fat.

After a girl begins to menstruate, a change in the breast takes place with each period. During the premenstrual phase, there is an increase in blood supply, as well as an increase in the size of the glands. In the postmenstrual phase, the glands become smaller and the breast remains inactive until the next premenstrual phase.

The breast is in its most active form at the time of pregnancy. It visibly enlarges after the second month. The duct system develops during the first six months, and the glands develop during the last three months. This increased activity of the breast continues throughout the nursing period.

Structure

The gland cells are the primary component of the active breast. They are arranged to form microscopic sacs called alveoli. These cells, when called upon, secrete milk for breast-feeding. The alveoli are arranged in clusters called lobules, which empty their contents into a duct or small canal. A number of these small ducts join to form larger ducts. These multiple ducts eventually lead to the main ducts, of which there are approximately 15 to 20 converging at the nipple.

Interspersed around the glands and ducts and between the lobules is a fibrous tissue that supports the breast. Within this fibrous supportive tissue are nerves, blood vessels, and lymphatic vessels.

Lymphatics. Lymphatic vessels are an integral part of the body's complex system required for normal cell function. Lymph vessels are channels that carry exchange fluid and by-products from cellular activity, cast-off cells, bacteria, and other matter for the body to reprocess. The lymphatic fluid containing this material flows into lymph nodes. The lymph nodes act as screening mechanisms to determine if anything potentially harmful or foreign to the body is present that requires the attention of the body's immune system. The lymphatic vessels and lymph nodes become an important consideration in the pattern of spread for breast cancer.

The lymph nodes draining the breast are found in the axilla (underarm area), the supraclavicular fossa (hollow above the collarbone), the internal mammary region (along blood vessels beneath the breast bone), and scapular regions (at the back of the chest wall).

Nonmalignant Breast Abnormalities

The breast is very responsive to hormonal changes. The hormones affect not only the glandular tissue but the fibrous tissue as well. Because of the continual changes in the breast, it is not uncommon for either glandular tissue or fibrous tissue to become more prominent, producing a lump in the breast. Fibrous tissue can develop, producing fibrous lumps.

BREAST STRUCTURES

The basic structures of the breast are shown in horizontal and vertical cross section. The lobules are clusters of microscopic sacs, or alveoli. Their milk gland cells secrete milk for breast-feeding. The alveoli empty into small ducts that form larger ducts and then connect to the 15 to 20 main ducts converging at the nipple. The vertical view shows how fibrous tissue is interspersed throughout the breast to provide support.

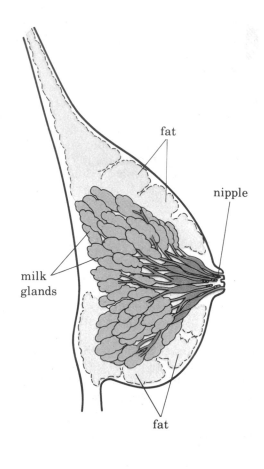

fat

nipple

milk glands

fat

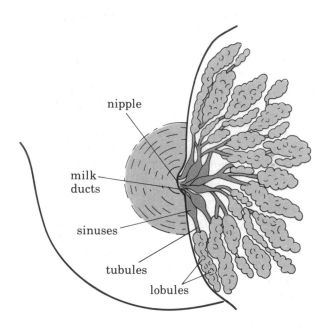

nipple

milk ducts

sinuses

tubules

lobules

Glandular tissue can proliferate or become cystic, also producing abnormal lumps. Often the two occur together. These lumps are not malignant, and usually do not represent any threat to a woman's health. However, they are often difficult to distinguish from malignant tumors. Frequently, the only way to know with certainty whether one of these lumps is benign or malignant is to perform a biopsy procedure, which involves taking a small sample of tissue from the lump and examining it microscopically for signs of malignancy.

BREAST CANCER

The term "cancer" applies to an abnormal growth of cells that can invade surrounding tissues. These cells also have the property of being able to travel via the lymphatic fluid or blood to distant parts of the body and can start new colonies there. Cancers are generally divided into two main categories: carcinomas and sarcomas.

Carcinomas arise from the cells covering the body, or from cells that line the body tracts leading outside the body (for example, the gastrointestinal tract or the respiratory tract), or from cells that line glandular structures (breast, salivary glands, thyroid).

Sarcomas arise from the connective and supportive tissues of the body.

More than 95 percent of breast cancers are carcinomas. They start predominantly in the cells lining the ducts and less commonly in cells lining the alveoli. Breast cancer spreads predominantly in three ways: local extension, lymphatics, and blood vessels.

Initially, cancer grows by local extension. As the cancer cells break through the membrane surrounding the duct or lobules, they gain access to other structures and the connective and supportive tissue that may allow further spread. Structures commonly involved include the lymphatics. As cancer cells are deposited in the lymphatics, they are free to travel to the lymph nodes where they may lodge and grow.

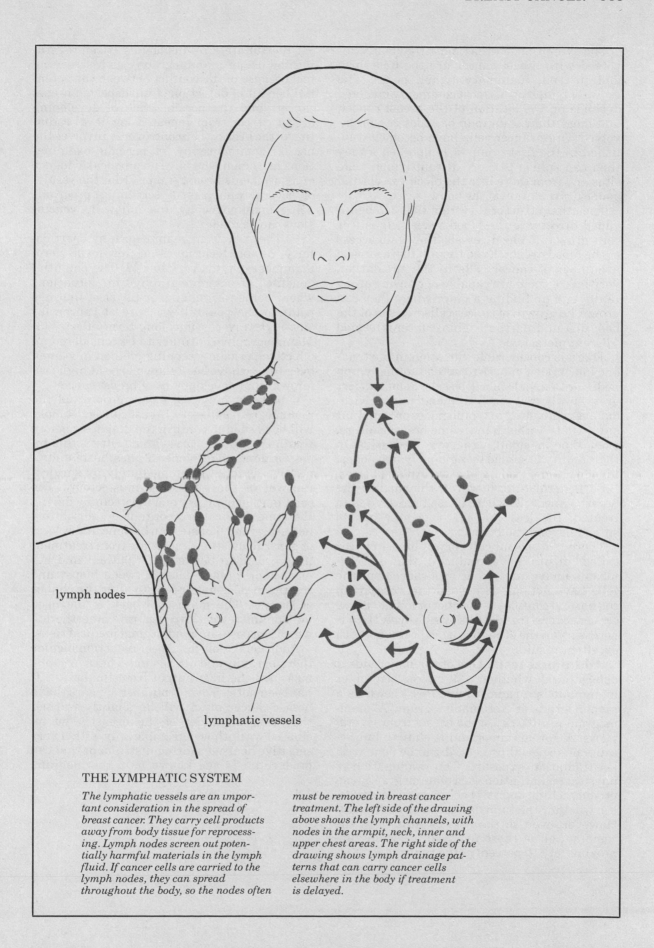

lymph nodes

lymphatic vessels

THE LYMPHATIC SYSTEM

The lymphatic vessels are an important consideration in the spread of breast cancer. They carry cell products away from body tissue for reprocessing. Lymph nodes screen out potentially harmful materials in the lymph fluid. If cancer cells are carried to the lymph nodes, they can spread throughout the body, so the nodes often must be removed in breast cancer treatment. The left side of the drawing above shows the lymph channels, with nodes in the armpit, neck, inner and upper chest areas. The right side of the drawing shows lymph drainage patterns that can carry cancer cells elsewhere in the body if treatment is delayed.

The lymph node areas most frequently involved with breast cancer are the underarm and internal mammary lymph nodes. The group of lymph nodes most commonly involved depends on the location of the breast cancer, and more than one group of nodes can be involved. Once cancer cells have become established in the first group of lymph nodes they then can spread to more distant lymph node sites and from there into the blood vessels and general circulation of the body.

The other structural system that can be invaded directly is the blood vessels. If cancer cells grow into blood vessels, they gain access to the bloodstream. Even though there may be a number of cancer cells in the circulation, very few of them are capable of growing or actually end up finding a place where they can grow. The growth of cancer cells in a site of the body distant from the original cancer is termed "distant metastasis."

There is considerable variation in the tendency for breast cancer to spread to the lymph nodes or to invade blood vessels. Some cancers grow slowly and reach tremendous size without ever spreading to lymph nodes or to distant sites. On the other hand, some breast cancers, even though small, are very aggressive in their ability to spread to regional lymph nodes, invade blood vessels, and grow in distant sites. As a general rule, however, the smaller the breast cancer is when it is discovered and treated, the less chance the cancer has to spread beyond the breast.

There is a special category of breast cancer called "in situ" or "intraductal" that is recognizable under microscope as a cancer, but the cells have not spread beyond their origins in the normal confines of the duct or lobule. These cancers can be treated less aggressively than is necessary in the other breast cancers, yet with excellent results.

Additional tests. One of the major aids in determining whether a lump is benign or malignant is a radiographic tool known as a mammogram or xeromammogram. A mammogram is an X ray of the breast from several views. A xeromammogram is similar, but because of a special process, it can be done with less radiation exposure. The combination of physical examination with mammography can produce a high degree of accuracy in determining whether the lump is benign or malignant. However, even in the best of situations, the combination of these tools can be wrong approximately 10 percent of the time.

Unfortunately, confusion has arisen regarding the use of mammography as a screening tool because of the conflict between the potential benefit of detection of unsuspected breast cancers and the possible risk of developing breast cancer from repeated low-level radiation to the breast. The controversy involves the use of mammography for periodic examinations in women who have no physical evidence of a suspicious breast lump. From the results of several analyses of screening programs using mammography, the following conclusions can be made:

(1) The risk from mammography (particularly newer techniques of low-level xeromammography) is very low. (2) The potential benefits of mammography in situations where benign symptoms or physical findings point to the possibility of breast cancer far outweigh any possible long-term effects. (3) Mammography continues to be considered an effective periodic screening method in women over 40 who have been shown to be at high risk for eventual development of breast cancer.

If both the physical examination and the mammogram suggest a breast cancer, a biopsy will be needed to confirm the diagnosis before treatment can be carried out. Often, this biopsy is done under general anesthesia and, if positive, is followed immediately by surgical removal of the breast, or mastectomy. The combination of biopsy and mastectomy during the same surgical procedure is not absolutely necessary, and biopsies can be done under local or general anesthesia separate from treatment if agreed upon between the patient and her physician. A short delay between biopsy and treatment does not appear to alter the chance of success. The main drawback is the need for administering two separate anesthetics, which can pose slight additional medical risks.

Additional tools for cancer detection include thermography and ultrasound. Thermography measures the heat output from the breast. It has been noticed over a number of years that a breast cancer often will be slightly warmer than the remainder of the breast. The increased warmth is detectable only with a very sensitive heat-measuring instrument that can produce an image known as a thermogram.

However, many noncancerous breast changes may cause increased heat resulting in an abnormal thermogram, and small cancers may not produce enough heat to be detected. For these reasons, thermograms, if used, are usually combined with other diagnostic methods.

Ultrasound uses reflected high-frequency sound waves to map the inside of the breast. It is being investigated as a method of detecting small breast cancers without radiation.

If a malignancy is confirmed, additional tests are recommended to evaluate the possibility of distant spread. Among the more useful and frequently employed examinations are: chest X ray, serum enzyme levels (blood test), blood count, bone scan (use of mildly radioactive materials to take pictures of bone activity), and bone survey (X rays of most of the bones). Even with all of the tests available and the use of the most accurate of techniques, the majority of distant growths can be detected only when they are fairly large (more than one-half inch in diameter).

Who Is at Risk?

All women past the onset of menstruation face the potential risk of breast cancer. However, the incidence of breast cancer in women below the age of 25 is so low as to have no practical importance. Significant risk begins at 30 and steadily increases through the remainder of a woman's life. Regardless of the fact that the risk increases with age, keep in mind that the total risk throughout the lifetime of a woman is only approximately 7 percent.

By studying large groups of women where accurate and complete records have been kept, factors can be analyzed to see whether they are associated with the increased occurrence of breast cancer. Of course, any analysis done in this manner only shows a relationship between numbers—and does not imply that the factor is a direct cause of an individual breast cancer. These are only sign posts to point out which groups of women face a higher risk than others of the development of breast cancer.

The most important factor associated with a higher risk of breast cancer is a family history of the disease. In general, the closer the affected relative with breast cancer, the higher the risk. Breast cancer in a mother or sister is associated with a much higher risk than breast cancer in a cousin or aunt. The highest risk occurs where two or more close relatives have had breast cancer. This is true even if the relatives are on the father's side. A strong family history of breast cancer also points to possible development of breast cancer at an earlier age. If relatives have been affected early, before menopause, the risk is also increased.

Women with previously treated breast cancer are at a higher risk for development of a second breast cancer in the opposite breast, especially if there is a family history of cancer in both breasts.

Weaker risk factors include obesity, lack of pregnancies or pregnancies late in life, an unusually long menstrual life, failure to breast feed, and following a high-fat diet. Suspected factors, such as use of estrogens, use of birth control pills, and presence of fibrocystic disease, have not been reliably shown to be associated with an increased risk of the development of breast cancer.

If you find yourself in a high-risk category—especially if you have close relatives with breast cancer—more frequent periodic professional examinations are recommended in addition to your regular self-examination, particularly after 40. In these situations, mammography may be suggested as a screening tool.

Treatment

Treatment for breast cancer has always been controversial. While there have been important advances in the methods, no treatment program is 100 percent effective. There are a number of reasons why the best treatment for breast cancer is difficult to define clearly.

Part of the problem has to do with medicine's inability to determine accurately how extensively breast cancer has spread. Effectively treating the local breast cancer without recognizing and treating involved regional nodes will allow the regional nodes to grow, producing a recurrence, or will allow them to spread, producing distant cancerous growths. In the same light, effective treatment of the local cancer and the regional nodes without recognizing already existing distant spread will not affect the eventual development of these distant growths. Ideally, if information could be accurately obtained regarding whether each potential group of lymph nodes was involved and whether distant spread had already occurred, the treatment program could be tailored for that case.

Even if the cancer could be accurately located when there is spread beyond the breast, the unknown amount of tumor at each location can limit the effectiveness of a treatment program. And there are other less well understood factors that limit the ability to plan an ideal treatment.

Breast cancer in most situations is a fairly slow growing tumor. Often, at least five years, and preferably ten years, are required before a new treatment program can be adequately analyzed by physicians so that they can become confident of the results. Not all of the factors that influence the outcome of breast cancer are known.

Yet there are three main treatments, used alone or in combinations, in current programs. They are surgery, radiation, and chemotherapy.

Surgery. Surgery was the first successful way to treat breast cancer, and historically the standard surgical approach has been radical mastectomy. To describe the radical mastectomy procedure, it is necessary to review some additional anatomy.

Between the breast and the chest-wall ribs are two muscles overlying each other. The larger muscle, closest to the breast, is known as the pectoralis major. The smaller muscle, which lies beneath the pectoralis major, is known as the pectoralis minor. The pectoralis minor muscle is hidden by the pectoralis major. The pectoralis major muscle can be identified by placing your hand on your hip and pushing inward. With your other hand you can feel a tenseness in the area of the chest wall just behind and above the breast and in the fold of tissue that forms the anterior fold covering the underarm. In a radical mastectomy, the breast is removed along with both the pectoralis major and pectoralis minor muscles. As the breast and muscles are removed, the axillary chain of lymph nodes in the underarm are removed up to the level of the clavicle or collar bone. A wide section of skin overlying the breast tumor also is taken with the breast, and in some situations when there is not enough skin remaining to close the gap, a skin graft is used.

An alternate surgical procedure frequently used is called modified radical mastectomy. The primary difference between the two procedures is that even though one of the chest-wall muscles (the pectoralis minor muscle) is taken, the major muscle, which gives most of the contour and form to the chest wall and fold of the axilla, is left in place. For most situations, there does not appear to be any difference in the results between radical and modified radical mastectomies.

More modified surgical procedures may be used when they are combined with radiation. These include total mastectomy with (or without) removal of the axillary nodes. In both situations, both the pectoralis major and minor muscles are left in place. A procedure known as a subcutaneous mastectomy (removal of breast tissue while leaving the skin intact) is sometimes used in benign breast diseases, but it has no place in the treatment of breast cancer. However, it is sometimes performed on the unaffected breast of women who have had one breast removed. The operation is an elective one requested by the patient.

Recently, plastic surgery has been used to reconstruct a breast-like form in the chest wall following mastectomy. There have been significant advances in the capability and success of this procedure in selected cases. If you have had a mastectomy and are interested in this possibility, you should discuss it with your physician. Many surgeons recommend waiting at least six months and preferably two years before reconstruction. These recommendations will vary depending on the surgeon.

Yet the overwhelming majority of women who have had a mastectomy wear a prosthesis, an artificial breast worn inside a bra. Thanks to a wide variety of prosthetic materials, most women can achieve a natural appearance after surgery by this method.

A form of surgery known as segmental mastectomy or wedge resection has become more common because of its use in conjunction with radiation treatment of breast cancer without a mastectomy. This type of surgery involves removing a wedge or segment of breast tissue surrounding the breast cancer. This procedure can be done with no more change in the form of the breast than would be expected from an excisional biopsy.

Radiation. Radiation is one way to treat breast cancer after the cancer has been removed by wedge resection (without removing the entire breast). In the early era of cancer treatment with radiation, the only breast cancers radiated were those in which the woman refused a mastectomy. Following the promising results from those early cases, the methods of treatment have become more refined and more systematic. Evidence has indicated that when carefully done, wedge resection and radiation are just as effective for cure of early breast cancer as radical mastectomy.

The amount of radiation necessary to eradicate the cancer depends on the size of the tumor. It also is known that when a tumor mass is surgically removed, a dose of radiation treatment to the microscopic residual tumor is very effective, leaving the breast soft and normal in appearance. A number of programs have used this procedure on a growing number of patients, and the results indicate that following local removal of the breast cancer, radiation to the breast and regional lymphatics can provide local control and freedom from distant spread equivalent to the results obtained with radical mastectomy. In addition, the cosmetic appearance of the breast is preserved and, with careful radiotherapy, the consistency of the breast remains soft with essentially no visible changes. This approach is suitable for breast cancers that can be removed without creating a large distortion of the breast and when only a few lymph nodes are involved. Often, it is helpful to know whether axillary nodes are involved. A limited surgical sampling of the axilla can be done at the same time the breast cancer is removed.

This type of treatment usually requires five to six weeks of radiation following surgery. The radiation has only minimal side effects and is given on an outpatient basis.

Two of the lymph node groups other than the axilla are frequently involved with breast cancer. They are the internal mammary chain and the supraclavicular chain of lymph nodes. Neither of these regions is removed in any of the surgical procedures. In breast cancer cases with high risk of spread to these nodes, radiation to these regions is frequently used in conjunction with mastectomy. There can be various combinations of surgery and radiation, depending on a number of factors including tumor size, location in the breast, surgical procedure, and the number of axillary nodes.

Chemotherapy. Despite adequate treatment of both the local tumor and the regional lymph node distribution, undetectable distant spread of a cancer may have already taken place. It is impossible to tell who does or does not have very small distant cancerous growths at the time a breast cancer is diagnosed and treated. Some factors, such as degree of lymph node involvement, correlate with a high risk of eventual development of distant spread. Because of this high risk in some patients, there has been a great deal of interest in additional forms of treatment that would affect these distant cancer cells before they had a chance to grow large enough to become detectable. This additional treatment, known as adjuvant chemotherapy, has undergone a considerable amount of study and clinical use since the early 1970s.

As mentioned earlier, the natural development of breast cancer in individuals is long, and a relatively long observation time is needed to accurately assess any new treatment programs. The final results of adjuvant chemotherapy trials are not complete, but preliminary results appear to indicate decreases in the occurrence of distant spread of cancer cells in some high-risk groups of women.

Adjuvant chemotherapy has taken several forms over its years of development. It initially started with single drugs, but for the most part multiple drugs are now being used. The most effective drugs and the most effective combinations of drugs are still being investigated.

Hormonal therapy also is being used in cancer treatment. Some breast cancers have been shown to be responsive to the level of male and female hormones in the body. These hormones also have been used alone as adjuvants, or in conjunction with adjuvant chemotherapy following surgery and radiation. These studies have been encouraging.

YOU AND BREAST CANCER

The most important fact to remember from this brief overview is that you are your own best insurance policy against breast cancer. Although there are exceptions, monthly self-examinations can detect breast cancer at the early stages of growth when there is low risk of regional or distant spread. This type of cancer is easily treated and the treatment has a high chance of success. The treatment of breast cancer also has evolved to a point where it can be tailored to individual needs to some degree without compromising the final result. If appearance is an important factor, mastectomy may not be necessary, depending on the size and extent of the cancer. Even when there is spread to regional lymph nodes, combinations of treatment have improved chances of success, and there is continuing evidence of potential advances.

When a breast cancer is found, a woman should always discuss the particulars of the disease (and its spread, if any) with her physician. In addition, she should learn about and discuss the doctor's recommendations and the alternatives in treatment.

BREAST SELF-EXAMINATION

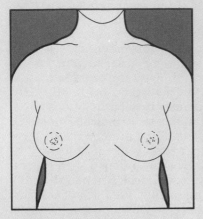

Look into a mirror with both arms relaxed at your side. Compare the breasts for size, color, and position. Note any ulceration, scaling, discharge, nipple changes, skin puckering, or shrinkage.

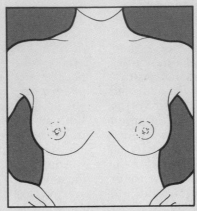

Place your hands on your waist and press inward. Turn from side to side and note any of the changes mentioned at left.

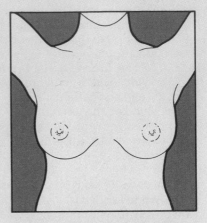

Place your hands behind your head, pressing firmly. Turn from side to side and again look for any changes. Relax your hands at your sides. You are now ready to feel the breasts.

You are the most important person in discovering a breast cancer while it is still small and the risk of its spreading is low. Approximately 90 percent of all breast cancers are found by women themselves. Often the discoveries are accidental, occurring when you brush your hand across the breast and touch a lump, or feel a lump while showering, or notice a dimpling of the skin of the breast while dressing. More early breast cancers are found when women regularly examine their breasts. A number of these early cancers are in-situ or intraductal tumors, which have not spread beyond the point of origin and which are easier to treat than advanced tumors.

It is not difficult to understand why self-examination is so important. You can examine yourself much more frequently than a professional examiner, and repeated examination has the benefit of allowing you to become so familiar with your breast anatomy that early changes quickly come to your attention.

Breast self-examination should be done with a relaxed attitude. Keep in mind that your breast may normally be somewhat lumpy. Do not become alarmed if you feel a distinct lump. Most breast lumps are benign.

If you should discover a lump, a thickening, a dimple, a discharge, or any other change in feel or appearance, bring it to the attention of your physician for further evaluation. Even though most lumps are benign, abnormalities should be promptly evaluated. Unnecessary delay only defeats the advantage of careful self-examination.

When a physician examines your breast, he or she either will tell you that the lump is not suspicious and that you should continue with your own self-examinations and periodic clinical checks, or the doctor will consider the lump suspicious enough to perform additional tests.

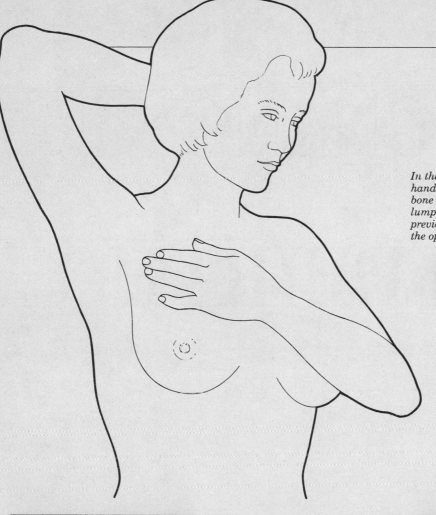

In the shower or bath, run a wet soapy hand down one breast from the collar bone to the nipple, feeling for any lumps or thickening or changes from previous exams. Repeat the process on the opposite breast.

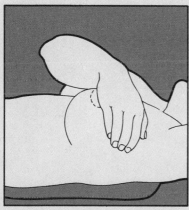

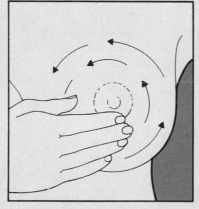

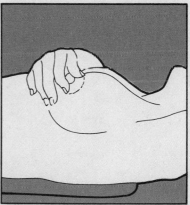

After bathing, lie down. Place a pillow beneath your left shoulder and place your left hand behind your head. Use the palm of your right hand to examine the left breast. Gently move it in a circular motion around the entire breast. A small amount of lotion or oil will make your fingers more sensitive to the feel of the breast.

Then, move your fingers in toward the nipple and repeat the circular motion. Do this until the entire breast is covered. Notice the firm ridge of tissue in the lower portion of the breast.

Gently squeeze the nipple between the thumb and middle finger. Look for any discharge. Gently depress the nipple to check for a lump beneath the nipple area. Repeat this process on the other breast.

CHAPTER 26   HARLAN R. GILES, M.D.

PREGNANCY AND CHILDBIRTH

A healthy pregnancy culminating in a healthy child is so commonplace that most of us take it for granted. Yet in our grandparents' day, death in childbirth was not unusual, and up to one-fourth of all pregnancies ended in miscarriage, premature delivery, or death of the infant. Today, more than 90 percent of expectant mothers can look forward to a routine and uneventful nine months, followed by delivery of a robust son or daughter. The majority of adverse outcomes can be traced to a minority of women designated as "high risk." Even in these cases, advances in obstetrical and newborn care have had a favorable impact. Most pregnancy complications can be readily identified and dealt with.

The events of conception and pregnancy are familiar to most of us. Beginning at puberty and for the next 35 to 40 years, women undergo a process called ovulation at approximately monthly intervals. Under the influence of hormones secreted by the pituitary gland in the brain, the ovaries prepare one of literally hundreds of thousands of egg cells, each no bigger than a pinpoint, for the process of starting a new life. Tissues around the chosen egg nourish and ripen it, and form a protective covering around it. On cue from the pituitary, the egg erupts from this protective follicle. In a normal menstruating woman, this occurs about 14 days before the beginning of her next menstrual cycle. In a woman with a 32-day cycle, ovulation can be pinpointed on day 18.

Although this event has occurred countless times throughout history, the details thereafter are still poorly understood. The female sex hormones, estrogen and progesterone, prepare the lining of the uterus, called the endometrium, for the possibility of conception. The hormones also affect the mucous lining of the cervix, which is the lower portion of the uterus, so that it becomes receptive to sperm. The egg, meanwhile, moves into the fallopian tube. During intercourse, millions of spermatozoa are ejaculated into the vagina, each capable of fertilizing the waiting egg. The spermatozoa traverse the cervix and the uterus and pass into the fallopian tube. Sperm and egg each have a fertile life-span of at most 72 hours. If they meet and unite during this period, conception takes place. If not, the egg degenerates and is washed away along with the nourished uterine lining, the familiar process known as menstruation (see chapter 24, "The Female Reproductive System").

If sperm and egg do meet under the proper circumstances, they unite in the upper third of the tube. A single sperm penetrates the outer covering of the egg, gradually working its way toward the nucleus. Each of the cells carries a blueprint for the new life in the form of 22 dark-colored, rod-shaped bodies called chromosomes, which contain submicroscopic units called genes. As explained in chapter 2, "Medical Genetics," these 22 chromosomes incorporate characteristics passed down from previous generations, determining such matters as the child's skin color, hair color, body build, and whether he or she will develop certain diseases. A twenty-third chromosome decides whether the child will be male or female. In the ovum the sex chromosome is always X, or female. In the sperm it can be X (female) or Y (male). An XX combination produces a girl, an XY a boy.

When the sperm reaches the nucleus of the egg, the two are contained in the same envelope. The single cell then begins a process of division, first into two cells, then four, then eight. Over the next seven days, the division continues as the new body gradually moves down the tube and through the uterus. At last it implants in the lush, thick wall of the endometrium, where it can be nourished from the mother. The cells differentiate into those that form the embryo, later called the fetus, and those that form the placenta, or "afterbirth," which helps nourish the growing life through the pregnancy. The fetus is surrounded by a membrane within a membrane, and the space between those two is filled with fluid, the so-called bag of waters in which the fetus will float and move for the next nine months. The fetus is joined to the nourishing placenta by the umbilical cord, a long, coiled structure that passes through the membrane, carrying oxygen and food from placenta to fetus and waste products in the reverse direction to be passed off through the woman's urinary system.

From conception to normal birth requires about 40 weeks or 280 days from the first day of the last menstrual cycle, popularly rounded off to nine months. Doctors usually divide gestation into three-month periods, known as the first, second, and third trimester, although in fact it is a continuous period. A delivery that covers the full 280-day period is said to be a birth at term, and the child is referred to as a full-term baby.

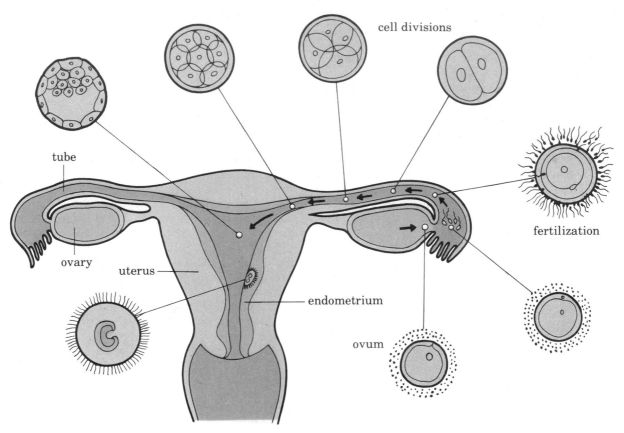

FERTILIZATION AND IMPLANTATION

The sequence of ovulation, fertilization, and implantation of the fertilized egg is a multi-step process. The process begins when the ovary releases a ripened ovum (egg) from its follicle. If the ovum encounters spermatozoa in the fimbrian end of the tube, fertilization occurs. The male and female cells unite into a single cell, which then undergoes a series of divisions during a slow three- or four-day descent down the tube. The cell cluster, now called a morula, then floats free in the uterine cavity for several days before it embeds itself in the endometrium, the lining of the uterus, which nourishes it.

SYMPTOMS OF PREGNANCY

How does a woman know when she is pregnant? In a healthy woman who previously has menstruated regularly, a delayed period is the best indicator. Because of the usual variation in menstrual cycle length, however, this sign is not always reliable until the anticipated menstrual period is 10 to 14 days overdue. When a second period is missed, the probability of pregnancy becomes much stronger. However, pregnancy occasionally occurs in the absence of previous menstruation, such as in the nursing mother or in the young teenager who has just began to ovulate.

There are explanations other than pregnancy for failure to menstruate or delayed menstruation. Women who are particularly underweight or overweight are more prone to miss a cycle, and those with chronic disease such as diabetes or thyroid dysfunction are susceptible to irregularity. Benign cysts of the ovaries sometimes interfere with normal menstruation. So do factors such as climate, travel, or work-related stress. Perhaps one of the more common causes of menstrual delay is emotional distress or anxiety, including the fear of pregnancy itself.

Besides menstrual changes, there are other early signs of pregnancy:

Nausea and vomiting. Disturbances of the digestive system are experienced by most pregnant women. The most common problem is "morning sickness," which often begins in the early part of the day and subsides by afternoon, although nausea and vomiting occur without relation to meals, activity, or time of day. The reason for this symptom is not known. Some doctors believe that nausea results from a direct hormonal change brought about by the pregnancy, while others believe that the gastrointestinal tract is affected by changes in sugar metabolism. The problem usually subsides spontaneously after 12 to 14 weeks.

Fatigue. Many women find that they tire easily and lack pep during early pregnancy. The decreased energy levels may be related to increased circulating levels of progesterone, a hormone produced by the placenta. Some women require extensive rest and sleep, but the majority are able to overcome the fatigue and carry on normal levels of activity at work or at home.

Urinary disturbances. Direct pressure from an enlarging uterus and congestion of the blood vessels within the pelvis create an almost constant sensation of bladder fullness and lead to frequent urination, even in the middle of the night. Interestingly, the amount of urine produced is usually not increased. This symptom, too, usually subsides after four or five months, but may recur near term as the fetus begins to descend into the pelvis in preparation for birth.

Some patients note occasional leakage of urine when they cough, sneeze, or attempt to lift heavy objects. This, too, results from increased pressure within the pelvis and usually resolves itself a few weeks after delivery.

Breast changes. During early pregnancy, the breasts increase in size and weight. The increase is more pronounced than the increase before a regular menstrual period. The breasts may become exquisitely tender and the glands under the nipple area may enlarge. A little later in pregnancy, the pink-brown area around the nipple (the areola) darkens in color. These changes are also brought about by the elevated levels of hormone in the circulation produced as a result of the pregnancy.

Appetite. There are many jokes about the pregnant woman's sudden and insatiable craving for unusual foods or food combinations, such as pickles and ice cream, but this symptom is very real for a number of women and requires some to modify their diet. An aversion to alcohol or to cigarette smoking also occurs in early pregnancy in some women.

Quickening. One of the last symptoms noted by most pregnant patients is quickening, the awareness that the fetus is moving, even though fetal motion is present as early as six to seven weeks. In a woman who is pregnant for the first time, quickening is felt on the average of 19 weeks after the onset of the last menstrual period, plus or minus two weeks. In subsequent pregnancies, quickening usually is noted one to two weeks earlier, but there is considerable variation among individuals.

Physical findings. A physician usually can diagnose pregnancy two to three weeks after the first missed menstrual period. Further laboratory testing is normally unnecessary unless the continuation of the pregnancy is in doubt or there is some pressing medical complication.

Although many women perceive abdominal enlargement in the first few weeks of pregnancy, it is usually related to bloating rather than expansion of the uterus. By 12 weeks after the date of the last menstrual period, the uterus has attained the size of a large grapefruit and can be felt by external examination of the abdomen. Before this time, the physician must rely on other clues.

During the pelvic examination, the physician may notice a bluish tinge about the vagina and cervix. This is called Chadwick's sign, named for the physician who first observed it. Chadwick's sign is related to congestion within the pelvis that develops in the first few weeks of pregnancy. The area around the junction of the cervix (the mouth of the uterus) and the body of the uterus itself usually feels soft to the touch, a characteristic known as Hegar's sign. In some patients, there is softening of the uterus over the area of implantation.

The nonpregnant uterus is roughly the size and shape of a small pear. Enlargement of the uterus is detectable as early as six weeks in a woman pregnant for the first time, and usually no later than seven to eight weeks in patients who have had previous pregnancies. By carefully outlining the size and shape of the uterus, an experienced doctor can estimate the duration of the pregnancy within 1½ weeks. If the examination is carried out in early pregnancy, a cyst of the ovary may be found which ranges from the size of a golf ball to the size of a tangerine. This represents the corpus luteum, which maintains the pregnancy during the first 10 to 11 weeks of gestation.

Between 12 weeks and delivery, the uterus can be felt through the abdomen. By measuring the height of uterus, it is often possible to estimate the stage of the pregnancy. Beyond 28 weeks, the wide variation in infant birth

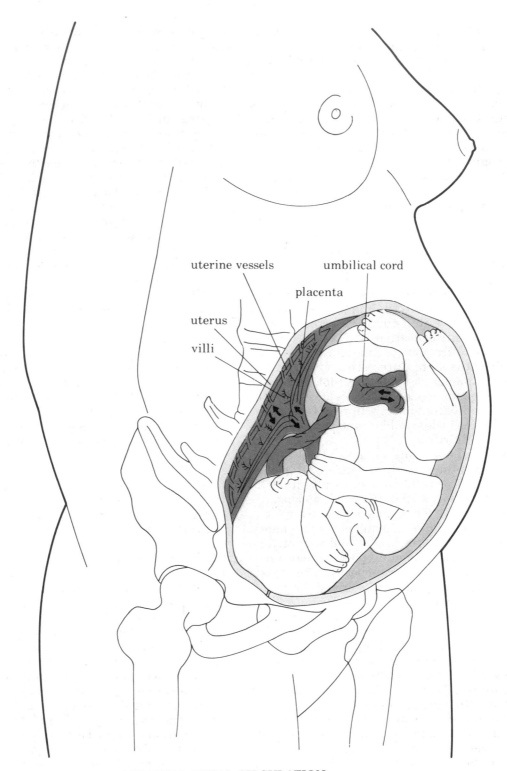

uterine vessels

umbilical cord

placenta

uterus

villi

MATERNAL-FETAL CIRCULATION

The circulation of the mother and fetus are closely interlocked, as this cutaway drawing shows. Arrows show how the blood vessels of the mother's uterus carry nourishment and oxygen from her body into the placenta, then through the umbilical cord to reach the developing baby. The

reverse set of arrows traces the path of the baby's wastes, which are disposed of through the mother's body. Fingerlike villi (center) help transport substances through the placenta. The so-called placental barrier helps remove substances that might harm the developing child.

weights makes this impossible. Instead, during the last three months the obstetrician can only attempt to estimate the fetal weight rather than the stage of the pregnancy.

In the past the detection of fetal heart tones was a relatively late physical finding. Using the conventional fetoscope, which is a bell-shaped stethoscope worn on the head, the obstetrician could not detect the heart tones until about 19 or 20 weeks. This is too late to be helpful in determining whether a woman is pregnant, although it helps in estimating the delivery date. Today, small ultrasonic stethoscopes called Doppler units detect the heart tones much earlier. Using the principle similar to that of sonar in a submarine, these battery-powered devices beam high-frequency sound waves into the uterus and trace their echoes. They pose no hazard to the fetus, and pick up heart tones as early as nine or ten weeks in most patients and by the twelfth week in all but the most obese women.

Diagnostic Tests

Not so many years ago, laboratory confirmation of pregnancy required injection of a urine sample from the woman into a laboratory animal such as a frog, mouse, or rabbit. If the woman was pregnant, in two or three days the animal's ovaries changed in a characteristic way. Because these tests were expensive, time consuming, and frequently inaccurate, they were not often requested unless there was considerable doubt about the pregnancy.

Today, the accuracy of pregnancy testing is greatly improved. The procedures are simplified and relatively inexpensive, and results are obtained in a few hours at most.

Hormonal tests. Most of the new urinary pregnancy tests are designed to detect human chorionic gonadotropin (HCG), a hormone secreted by placental tissue that rapidly enters the mother's circulation after conception. The individual test methods vary in their sensitivity to human chorionic gonadotropin. Almost all of these tests will detect a pregnancy 10 to 14 days after the missed menstrual period, and a few are capable of doing so even before a

period has been missed. A home pregnancy test based on this principle is available, but considerable care should be exercised in taking the test and interpreting the results.

Regardless of the type of test, the first morning sample of urine is preferable because it is usually more concentrated. The concentration can be enhanced by reducing intake of fluids the night before the test.

Blood tests. In certain situations, a woman wants to know as quickly as possible whether she is pregnant, even before the next period is expected. A test using a blood sample rather than a urine sample measures even the most minute concentrations of HCG circulating in the blood. This analysis, called a beta subunit HCG determination, is so sensitive and specific that pregnancy can be detected just a few days after conception. It is especially useful in suspected cases of ectopic pregnancy (pregnancy outside of the uterus), medical complications, or unwanted pregnancy.

Ultrasound. Diagnostic ultrasound involves transmitting low-energy, high-frequency sound waves into the patient's abdomen and displaying the returned echoes as a two dimensional image on a television screen. The procedure causes no discomfort to the patient. It involves no radiation, and studies have found no harmful effects.

The echoes from the amniotic sac form a distinctive circle or ring that can be seen as early as four to five weeks after the last menstrual period or two to three weeks after conception. Echoes representing the fetus can be seen at six weeks. Motion of the fetal body and beating of the fetal heart can be visualized in most instances between seven and eight weeks.

Although ultrasound is used occasionally to confirm that a woman is pregnant, its greatest asset lies in assuring the viability of a pregnancy, particularly when there is a great discrepancy between the size of the uterus and the presumed duration of the pregnancy, or when bleeding is complicating the early pregnancy. Some fetal abnormalities can be recognized by ultrasound, but not until 16 weeks or more have passed. Multiple pregnancy is easily diagnosed at an early stage.

X ray. In the past, conventional X rays of the abdomen were used to confirm pregnancy when the diagnosis was in doubt, usually after 14 to 16 weeks. The technique has been abandoned in favor of diagnostic ultrasound.

PHYSICAL CHANGES
IN PREGNANCY

Changes in the uterus. The most dramatic physical changes in pregnancy involve the uterus. The weight of uterine muscle increases 10-fold, while the capacity of the uterine cavity increases more than 500-fold. It is amazing that an organ smaller than an average pear must enlarge to the size of a watermelon to accommodate the full-term fetus, placenta, and amniotic fluid. The enlargement is possible because muscle fibers become longer and thinner, and numerous new muscle fibers are formed. Supporting ligaments are stretched significantly as the organ expands, which can cause discomfort. Throughout pregnancy, the muscle fibers of the uterus contract, sporadically at first, then more frequently and regularly as labor approaches. In late pregnancy, this phenomenon is referred to as Braxton-Hicks contractions.

The blood flow to the uterus increases, too. To accommodate the growing demands, the blood flow must increase from one-half ounce per minute in early pregnancy to more than one pint per minute when birth is near.

Cervical changes. Changes in the cervix accompany those of the uterus. As the pregnancy advances, the muscle fibers of the cervix are stretched upward into the lower portion of the body of the uterus. This makes the cervix shorter and thinner in preparation for labor. The cervix also rolls out and softens, becomes pliable, and sometimes bleeds on contact. Mucous glands are stimulated by the hormonal influence of the pregnancy and often give rise to an excessive vaginal discharge.

As a rule, the corpus luteum matures as a single cystlike structure on one of the ovaries. The blood vessels of the tubes and ovaries dilate markedly, and this congestion often contributes to a sense of fullness in the pelvis.

Skin. Skin changes are prominent during pregnancy. Increased hormone levels cause darkening of the nipples and genitalia, and "stretch marks" (stria) are often noted in the skin of the abdomen. On the other hand, skin conditions such as acne often improve during pregnancy. Superficial veins, particularly in the legs, may become more noticeable and may become painful or tender. These conditions should be reported to the physician at once.

Metabolic changes and weight gain. The average woman gains 24 pounds during the nine-month period. Of this amount, 19 pounds are accounted for by the pregnancy itself: the fetus about 7½ pounds, the placenta

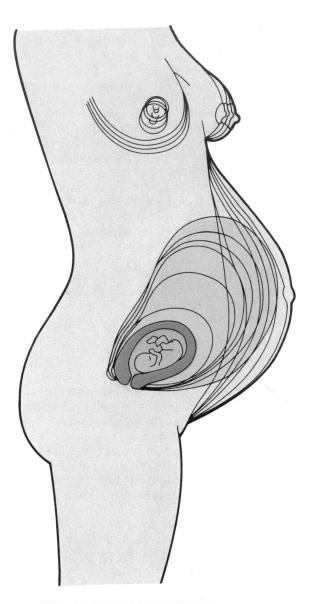

THE GROWING PREGNANCY

The contours of the breasts, uterus, and abdomen change steadily during the nine months of pregnancy. The uterus reaches progressively higher levels in the abdomen until about the middle of the last month. At that time, the baby's head tends to settle deeper into the pelvis, an event known as lightening because it decreases the sensation of abdominal distention.

The Delivery Date

The average length of pregnancy has been established at 281 days calculated from the first day of the last normal menstrual period. The simplest method of estimating the expected date of delivery is to count back three months from the first day of the last menstrual period, and then count forward seven days.

A woman whose last menstrual period began on January 19 would count back three months to October 19, then forward seven days to October 26. The majority of pregnant patients will deliver two weeks before or after this date, or 38 to 42 weeks after the first day of the last normal menstrual period.

1 pound, the amniotic fluid 2 pounds, added weight of uterus 2½ pounds, increased weight of breasts 2 pounds, and increased blood volume 4 pounds. The rest of the weight is accumulated fats and fluids retained by the body but which will be lost after birth. It is important that the woman gain at least this amount, because restricting weight gain can result in a baby of low birth weight, which poses a greater risk of complications. Gains up to 35 pounds are considered normal.

Hormonal changes of pregnancy produce dramatic changes in water metabolism. This means that the woman's tissues retain more water, a phenomenon related to an increased retention of sodium, a decrease in the protein content of the blood plasma, and an increased tendency of fluid to leak from the small blood capillaries. The functional capacity of the kidneys appears to increase during pregnancy, primarily because of an increase in the rate of blood flow directed through the kidneys.

Protein metabolism is changed to allow an accumulation of amino acids, the building blocks for fetal growth and development. (Increased protein requirements in pregnancy and lactation are discussed on page 604.)

Carbohydrate and insulin metabolism. Pregnancy can be thought of as a diabetic stress to the pregnant woman. Carbohydrate metabolism is altered, and greater demands are imposed on the mother's pancreas. Some women develop diabetes during the course of pregnancy, then revert to a normal state of sugar tolerance after the delivery. For patients already known to be diabetic, the additional stress of pregnancy requires stringent dietary control as well as an increase in the daily dosage of insulin. The increased insulin requirements are primarily attributed to placental hormones, which not only antagonize the action of insulin, but which can cleave the insulin molecule and render it ineffective.

Cardiovascular system. Although the volume of the heart enlarges only 10 percent during pregnancy, the heart's function changes significantly. It pumps as much as 40 percent more blood than in a nonpregnant woman. This occurs for two reasons: Each stroke of the heart pushes out more blood, and the heart rate itself increases. These changes are necessary to supply the increasing demands of the growing pregnancy.

Blood pressure, essentially unchanged during the first trimester, drops somewhat because of decreased blood vessel resistance in the second trimester, then returns to near normal levels in the third trimester. In some women, changes in the kidney and blood vessels lead to higher blood pressure and a condition known as toxemia or preeclampsia (see page 619).

Respiration. Increased oxygen demands during pregnancy increase the mother's breathing rate as well as the tidal volume (the amount of air moved during each cycle of inhalation and exhalation). The total capacity of the lungs is not significantly changed, but the rising diaphragm, pushed upward by the expanding uterus, can diminish the overall lung capacity. Consequently, the mother feels short of breath, especially during the eighth month. The condition ordinarily subsides once the fetal head has descended into the mother's pelvis.

Gastrointestinal tract. Besides the nausea and vomiting of early pregnancy, the stomach and intestines are significantly compressed by the enlarging uterus as pregnancy progresses. Constipation is frequent, caused by both mechanical and hormonal factors that decrease the movement of food through the gastrointestinal tract. Relaxation of the muscle around the entrance to the stomach leads to reflux of stomach acid into the esophagus and the woman often experiences heartburn.

Musculoskeletal changes. Increased weight of the pregnancy tends to shift the center of gravity forward. In most women, the curve of the spine compensates in late pregnancy to shift the weight back, giving rise to a characteristic swayback stance. Increased joint mobility, also under hormonal influence, contributes. These changes produce discomforts ranging from dull aches to sharp pains in the back, pelvis, and legs.

Some women experience impaired muscular coordination during the last trimester and the first few weeks after delivery. The cause is uncertain, but pregnant women should be aware of this possibility in planning their physical and recreational activities.

Emotional changes. As a major event in the life of any woman, pregnancy obviously has a significant emotional impact. Mild emotional upsets are common in pregnancy and should be understood as a part of adaptation to motherhood. Anxiety in pregnancy is even more common, generally related to concern for the normality and well being of the infant. It must be remembered that the father is by no means immune to the emotional impact.

PRENATAL CARE

Pregnancy should not be considered a disease. On the contrary, it represents the ultimate state of hormonal balance and maturation of the female reproductive system. Unfortunately, the demands and metabolic stresses engendered by the pregnancy may bring about disturbances in body function, and on occasion they make previous medical problems worse. A doctor must consider not only the impact of pregnancy on a disease process, but also the effect of a disease on the pregnancy.

The overall objective of prenatal care is simple: a healthy mother and a healthy baby. For the mother, that means maintaining or improving her physical and emotional health, reducing complications through prompt identification and treatment, and improving standards of care for the labor and delivery process.

For children the goals of care are reduction of mortality during birth and the early days of life, and the reduction of birth defects such as cerebral palsy. Unfortunately, many pregnant women today receive no medical attention before delivery, and the importance of prenatal care to the health of the child is not generally appreciated. Even women who do receive care often come to the doctor late in the pregnancy. A comprehensive prenatal program of medical and educational care is needed to provide the greatest service for mother and child.

The initial visit. The woman who suspects she is pregnant should schedule a visit to an obstetrician after she has missed a second menstrual period. Most doctors like to begin care when the woman is about eight weeks pregnant. By then the symptoms of pregnancy are usually recognizable, but it is still early enough to outline a full program of care. Visits to the obstetrician after the first are commonly scheduled at one-month intervals until the woman is 32 weeks pregnant, then at two-week intervals for a month, and then each week until delivery. However, the schedule varies according to the woman's needs and the doctor's practice.

The visit usually begins with a comprehensive health history, which is taken by the doctor or another member of the medical staff. The woman's entire obstetrical history is reviewed. This covers problems in past pregnancies such as miscarriage, premature delivery, or hypertension, any of which require special attention. A history of large infants or stillbirths suggests the possibility of diabetes, and a history of prolonged labor or obstetrical hemorrhage calls for special precautions.

The doctor will ask about the pregnancy, with particular attention to nausea and vomiting, headache, visual disturbances, swelling of the feet or face, urinary and bowel problems, vaginal bleeding, uterine cramps, or other symptoms. The woman will be questioned about her past medical and surgical history, especially any chronic illness. Previous surgery, particularly in the abdomen, requires careful follow-up. Other questions cover illness in the immediate family, plus information about her occupation (and its possible impact on her pregnancy) and about the emotional and financial support available to her.

More than half of the patients with "high-risk" pregnancies—those presenting a danger to either mother or child—can be identified by historical criteria alone. From the outset, these women can be given special care.

If the history uncovers any previous medical or obstetrical problems, the doctor probably will request detailed copies of medical records. Details the patient may be unaware of can have substantial importance in a pregnancy.

Physical examination. A meticulous physical examination is an integral part of the first visit to the doctor. Weight, blood pressure, pulse, and respiration are recorded. The eyes, ears, nose, and throat are inspected, and the thyroid gland examined for evidence of enlargement. The heart and lungs are checked

Fetal Development

If you could peer inside the uterus a month after conception, you would hardly believe that the tiny bit of tissue before your eyes could grow into a breathing, squalling baby. The diminutive figure measures only a quarter of an inch long—less than the length of a newborn's fingernail—and weighs perhaps one one-hundredth of an ounce. You would see no human face, no arms, no legs—just a small rudimentary tail.

Yet the most complex and vital organs already are forming. The month-old fetus has a microscopic brain, a threadlike spinal cord, and a crude nervous system. A U-shaped tube two millimeters long forms the heart and is pumping blood through primitive arteries. Another tube leading from the mouth is a rudimentary digestive tract, and a bulge midway in its length marks the spot where the stomach will develop.

A month later, there is no mistaking the human characteristics. Eyes, a nose, mouth, and ears give it a decidedly human countenance. Arms and legs have developed, complete with fingers, toes, elbows, and knees. Sex organs have become apparent, although it is still difficult to distinguish male from female. And the fetus has grown. It now measures a full inch from head to heel and weighs one-thirtieth of an ounce.

At the end of the third month, the baby is three inches long and weighs a full ounce. Fingernails and toenails show, and the buds of baby teeth appear in the jawbone. An observer can detect the presence or absence of a uterus. A rudimentary kidney excretes waste into the amniotic fluid. The fetus moves, but too slightly for the mother to feel.

At four months, nearly all vital organs are formed, yet the fetus is not ready to live alone. It is now about six and a half inches long and weighs about four ounces. Fine hair covers the body, and a few hairs appear on the head. More active now, the baby waggles tiny arms and legs. Using an amplified stethoscope, the doctor can hear the fetal heartbeat—a rapid 140 beats per minute, faster than that of the mother.

By five months, the fetus has developed hair, eyebrows and lashes, and even facial expressions. The father can hear the fetal heartbeat by placing an ear against the mother's abdomen. And the fetus now moves vigorously and frequently; the mother can "feel life." The baby is now nearly a foot long and weighs almost a pound and a half.

At six months, the fetus is 15 inches long, weighs two and a half pounds, and is growing rapidly. For the first time the fetus looks like a miniature human being. The skin is covered with fuzz and a creamy substance called vernix caseosa ("cheesy varnish"), a one-eighth-inch-thick layer that protects the skin from the fluid environment.

At seven months, the fetus is 16½ inches long and weighs four pounds. Development now is mainly a process of fine-tuning, getting ready for independent existence. The intricate biochemistry governing many bodily functions begins to evolve; production starts on the body's 20,000 enzymes. The nerve cells mature, and the fetus fattens.

During the last two months, the fetus gains a half pound per week, accumulating layers of fat to increase its ability to survive in the outside world. At eight months, the fetus weighs six pounds; at full term it weighs seven and one half.

The last organs to be fine-tuned are the lungs. Even though the child appears fully mature, the respiratory system is not ready. The lungs cannot function until acted upon by chemicals that are among the last to be produced. Some doctors believe normal birth can begin only when the fetal respiratory system has completed this maturation.

Prior to the end of the seventh month, an infant has only an outside chance to survive if born prematurely. The chances increase with each additional day or week in the womb. Despite an old belief that a seven-month baby has a better chance to live than an eight-month baby, no evidence confirms that notion. However, at eight months, the chances of survival are nearly as good as if the baby had completed the full term of pregnancy.

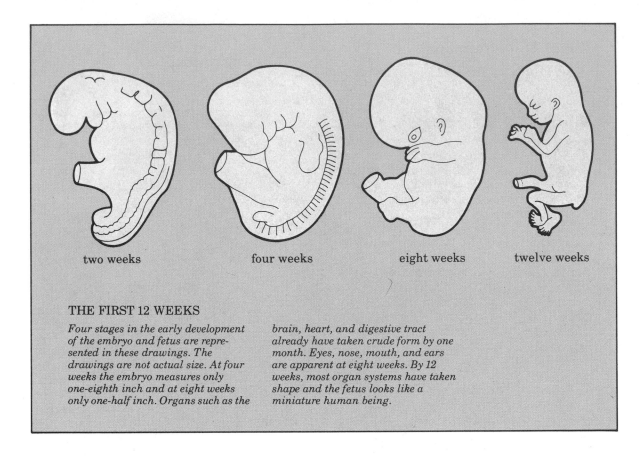

two weeks   four weeks   eight weeks   twelve weeks

THE FIRST 12 WEEKS

Four stages in the early development of the embryo and fetus are represented in these drawings. The drawings are not actual size. At four weeks the embryo measures only one-eighth inch and at eight weeks only one-half inch. Organs such as the

brain, heart, and digestive tract already have taken crude form by one month. Eyes, nose, mouth, and ears are apparent at eight weeks. By 12 weeks, most organ systems have taken shape and the fetus looks like a miniature human being.

for function, rate, and rhythm, and for evidence of airway obstruction. The breasts are examined for glandular distribution, the suitability of the nipples for nursing, and for possible cysts or tumors. The general examination helps the doctor to recognize changes if they occur later.

Abdominal examination. Abdominal examination is carried out to assess enlargement or abnormality of the liver, spleen, or kidneys. If the pregnancy has progressed beyond 12 weeks, the height of the uterus is measured, and fetal heart tones are recorded (see page 595). The arms and legs are evaluated for evidence of swelling, and for the presence of varicose veins.

A thorough pelvic examination is carried out, including examination of the external genitals, vagina, and cervix. A Pap smear of the cervix is obtained to test for malignancy. In most instances a culture of the cervix is taken to test for gonorrhea. The ovaries are also examined for ovarian masses.

The doctor will measure the three bony planes of the pelvis—the inlet, midpelvis, and the outlet. These are indirectly measured manually or by using calipers to determine their dimensions, which will help later in managing the conduct of labor. Only on rare occasions, such as following pelvic injury, is the structure so compromised in shape or dimension that it mandates a cesarean delivery, through the abdominal wall. In most instances, even with slightly reduced pelvic dimensions, the doctor will try first to have the baby delivered vaginally.

Laboratory tests. In addition to the Pap smear and the cervical culture, a number of other laboratory tests usually are obtained during the first three visits.

One is a blood sample. The red blood cell counts such as the hemoglobin or hematocrit indicate whether the woman has anemia, which would require treatment. The white blood cell count reflects any chronic underlying illness, either viral or bacterial. The blood group (A, B, AB, or O) is determined routinely, as is the Rh factor (see chapter 6, "The Blood").

Approximately 80 percent of the U.S. population carries the Rh factor. Those people are classed as Rh-positive. About 14 percent do not carry it (Rh-negative). An Rh-negative woman pregnant by an Rh-positive father may carry antibodies in her bloodstream to Rh-positive blood. If her child is Rh-positive, the antibodies can cross the placental barrier and adversely affect the unborn child. Although this is seldom a problem in a first pregnancy, all Rh-negative patients should undergo testing in later pregnancy to protect the child against this danger.

Many states require a blood test for syphilis. At this same time, the doctor will usually request a rubella titer to determine exposure and resistance to German measles, even if the woman has been vaccinated. Mothers with a low titer will usually receive rubella vaccine following delivery of the baby. Antibody levels achieved by vaccine are rarely as high as after the natural disease, and vaccine may need to be readministered after several years.

Many physicians obtain a blood glucose or sugar level. An abnormal value on this test indicates previously unrecognized diabetes, or at least the need for further testing. Because of the shift in carbohydrate metabolism, some women develop diabetes during pregnancy but return to normal afterwards. The condition requires careful follow-up.

Finally, a sample of the woman's urine is examined for protein and sugar content, and a small portion is examined under the microscope for pus cells and bacteria, which might reflect an infection of the urinary tract.

COMMON PROBLEMS
IN PREGNANCY

Because pregnancy is not an illness, the overwhelming majority of women are not incapacitated and carry on with their normal lives virtually throughout the nine-month period. Most of them, however, have minor discomforts and complaints that seldom require a doctor's attention.

"Morning sickness." Nausea and vomiting are often the first clues that a woman is pregnant, and often persist in mild form throughout the early part of pregnancy. The symptoms begin as early as four to five weeks and usually subside spontaneously by the twelfth to fourteenth week. This is related to hormonal changes associated with the pregnancy, so there is little cause for concern.

The nausea and vomiting usually can be controlled by minor changes in diet. Dried fruit or crackers, particularly in the morning, help to coat the stomach and minimize gastric distress. It also helps to eat six or seven small meals rather than three larger ones. (Snacks should be nutritionally balanced, not consisting of sweets and carbonated soft drinks.) A hurried schedule or emotional pressure can increase nausea, and "taking things easy" sometimes calms the queasiness. If nausea and vomiting are severe, the physician should be informed. He or she can prescribe medications to provide relief. Occasionally, vomiting becomes so frequent that no food is retained. If this persists for more than a day or two, dehydration and nutritional deficiency occur. This condition, known as hyperemesis gravidarum, threatens the fetus as well as the mother and requires immediate medical attention, often in the hospital.

Constipation is common in early pregnancy. Most of the time it is easily corrected by drinking plenty of water and other fluids, such as fruit juices. Bran cereals will increase the bulk of intestinal contents and are helpful in establishing normal bowel habits. Mild laxatives such as milk of magnesia, senna products, or mineral oil will not harm the fetus in any way.

Heartburn, a hot aching sensation just below the breastbone, is common during later pregnancy. One reason is pressure on the stomach caused by an enlarging uterus (see page 596). Another reason is relaxation of the muscular valve between the esophagus and the stomach. The combination allows stomach acids to back up and irritate the sensitive lining of the lower esophagus. Highly seasoned foods accentuate the problem, as do late-night dinners, because acid refluxes more easily when lying down. Milk or over-the-counter antacids are usually helpful. Because heartburn is often most noticeable at bedtime, using pillows to elevate the head also helps.

Gas. Gas production in the bowels increases during pregnancy, often resulting in excessive belching or passage of gas. Gas-producing foods such as baked beans, chili, cabbage, or cauliflower are best avoided during later pregnancy or should be eaten in small quantities.

Diarrhea also results from bowel changes associated with pregnancy. The problem usually subsides spontaneously. During episodes of diarrhea, liquids or bland foods are advisable. If the problem persists, over-the-counter preparations of kaolin-pectin may be used safely. Doctors also prescribe paregoric or codeine derivatives, with no adverse effects for the baby.

Hemorrhoids are large swollen veins that emerge around the anus and cause considerable discomfort, particularly during the bowel movement. They stem from the increased back pressure on the veins created by the large pregnant uterus and can be aggravated by constipation. The discomfort usually can be relieved by topical commercial preparations or by washing the area with cotton balls soaked with witch hazel. The doctor may prescribe suppositories. To prevent hemorrhoids, a woman should try to avoid constipation by following the diet described earlier. Although hemorrhoids occasionally cause bleeding during bowel movements, the blood loss is rarely great enough to cause anemia.

Pica. Some pregnant women develop a craving for strange foods or even for substances generally considered inedible, such as laundry starch, baking flour, clay, or refrigerator frost. The reasons for these unusual appetites are not known. The substances do not harm the fetus directly, but may result in considerable nutritional deficiencies for the mother.

Salivation. Pregnant women are sometimes bothered by an annoying increase in production of saliva, which may accentuate the nausea and vomiting in early pregnancy. A reduction of starchy foods sometimes provides partial relief.

Fatigue. Especially in early pregnancy, a woman is likely to tire easily and feel sleepy. She is not able to tolerate as much exercise as before pregnancy. Most women need more rest during pregnancy, a fact that should be taken into account when planning recreation or work.

Backache. Discomfort in the lower back is common during pregnancy. In the early months, this is likely to be related to stretching of the ligaments supporting the uterus. In later months it often results from the stress on the spine by the enlarging abdomen.

Most pregnant women find that sitting on firm, straight chairs is preferable to soft couches or "free form" furniture. A firm mattress provides support for some women, while others prefer a water bed. Some patients note significant back discomfort when driving an automobile. If discomfort is severe, driving should be curtailed and rest stops should be frequent.

Simple exercises of abdominal and back muscles help decrease back pain. Hot baths and aspirin also are helpful. If severe pain persists, it should be reported to the physician, because some chronic conditions of the spine become initially apparent or worsen during pregnancy.

Light-headedness. Episodes of light-headedness or even fainting are not unusual during pregnancy. The increased hormones cause a relaxation of the blood vessels so that they are often less responsive to changes in posture. In a few instances, low blood sugar levels are responsible.

Rapid changes of posture should be avoided. The pregnant woman should rise from bed gradually and use caution in getting up abruptly from a chair. Pregnant women are particularly prone to faint after emerging from a whirlpool, sauna, or very hot tub bath. Exposures to such high heat conditions should be restricted to a brief time or curtailed entirely.

Insomnia. Anxiety or concern for the welfare of herself or her child may make if difficult for a pregnant woman to fall asleep. Physical discomforts can make it difficult to find a comfortable sleeping position. Avoiding late-night meals, a daily exercise program, and continual reassurance from the physician or nurse are sometimes all that is needed to correct the problem. A glass of milk before retiring is sometimes helpful. If the loss of sleep is severe, mild sedatives may be prescribed.

Varicose veins. The pregnant uterus may significantly impair the return blood flow from the legs toward the heart, causing the superficial veins in the legs or groin to swell. Some women also develop pain and tenderness in these vessels, a condition called varicose veins (see chapter 5, "Blood Vessel Disorders").

Varicose veins are seldom a problem in a first pregnancy, but the risk increases as subsequent pregnancies further weaken the vein walls. The tendency appears to be inherited. Sufficient bed rest and sitting with the legs elevated are the most important steps in avoiding or reducing the severity of varicose veins. A woman who must be on her feet a great deal should wear properly fitted support stockings. Such stockings should fit snugly and extend to the waist. The best way to put them on is to elevate the leg above the rest of the body and roll the stocking on from the foot.

Prepared Childbirth

A variety of childbirth preparation classes are available in almost every community. Although several formats are offered—Lamaze, Bradley, Childbirth Education Association (CEA), and Leboyer—the factual content of most parent education programs is similar. The differences are philosophical.

Most obstetricians strongly advise that both parents take these classes to prepare for labor and delivery. They are offered as part of the hospital's prenatal service, or by a local Y, by adult education centers, or community colleges. There are usually six classes, beginning about the seventh month of pregnancy. The classes are taught in groups of 20 by a trained childbirth education instructor.

Classes usually include information on pregnancy, labor and delivery, the postpartum period, and introduction to parenting. Most classes stress an understanding of the physical and hormonal changes of pregnancy, body conditioning exercises, relaxation and breathing techniques, birth mechanisms, and the role of support personnel in the delivery process. Information is provided on the stage of labor, medications, and potential complications of childbirth.

Initially, the goal of childbirth education was to minimize the pain associated with labor and delivery. Today, however, childbirth education also seeks to improve the quality of the childbearing experience. Objectives include:
● To help expectant parents establish realistic goals and plans for their childbearing experience. Parents who have set attainable goals are more likely to have a satisfying childbirth.
● To help expectant parents cope with childbirth and daily life as a parent.

● To promote the concept of family-centered maternity care, whereby the woman, her coach, the doctor, and other medical staff members work together as a team.

Four types of breathing exercises are taught in childbirth education classes:
● Deep-chest breathing is used in the early stages of labor. It consists of a deep-cleansing breath taken in through the nose until the lungs swell and the abdomen rises, then exhaled through the mouth. Deep-chest breathing should be timed to coincide with contractions, which can be up to 60 seconds long. The breathing rate should be about six per minute.
● Shallow, accelerated breathing is used as the contractions become more intense. It begins with deep breathing, followed by short, shallow breaths from the chest only. They should be fast, light, effortless, in through the nose and out through the mouth. As the contraction subsides, the pace of breathing should be slowed, followed by a deep breath.
● Panting is used when the delivery is imminent. It enables the woman to hold or resist the urge to push until the appropriate time, which is usually when the doctor asks. Breaths are taken in and out through the mouth in a regular panting rhythm. Exhaling should be forceful but not too forceful, like blowing out a candle. After the urge to push has abated, return to deep breathing.
● Expulsion or delivery breathing is used during pushing. It consists of two slow, deep breaths, followed by a push. During the push, breath is held as long as possible, then another deep breath is taken. Pushing and delivery breathing are done only during contractions.

If a vein becomes tender, swollen, or inflamed, or if severe pain develops, the physician should be contacted immediately. Because of the increase in clotting factors in pregnancy, inflammation of the vein (phlebitis) is much more common and must be recognized and treated promptly.

Varicose veins usually subside six to eight weeks after delivery. Surgery is rarely necessary during pregnancy.

Muscle cramps are a common nuisance in pregnancy but are of no particular significance. Moderate exercise helps to relieve them, but overexertion must be meticulously avoided. A few women benefit from supplemental calcium, but most receive an adequate intake of calcium from a balanced diet. Hot tub baths can provide relief.

Vaginitis. Inflammation of the vagina and external genitalia is somewhat more common during pregnancy because of altered hormonal balance. Although monilia or yeast infection is the most common type of vaginitis, the physician should be consulted so that a proper diagnosis can be made and treatment begun. Most cases of vaginitis are easily correctable without adverse effects on the baby.

Headache. It is not unusual for a pregnant woman to develop a headache occasionally because of fatigue, tension, or anxiety. Because of concern over drugs and their effect on the fetus, patients are often reluctant to take any medication. However, two aspirin or acetaminophen can and should be taken if needed with complete safety for the baby. Persistent headache, particularly in late pregnancy, requires medical evaluation.

PERSONAL CARE

AND HYGIENE

Nutrition. For each fetus there is a genetically determined ideal weight that can be achieved only if the mother consumes adequate protein and calories in her diet during pregnancy. This is especially important for the woman who enters pregnancy at less than her ideal body weight, for the woman who has poor nutritional status, or the woman who inadequately gains weight during pregnancy. In addition to adequate protein and caloric intake, certain vitamins and minerals must be increased during pregnancy. The most notable are iron and folic acid, which are rarely adequate in the pregnant woman's diet and are routinely supplemented by prenatal vitamins.

In the woman whose prepregnancy diet is adequate, the additional requirements of pregnancy can be completely met by the addition of one quart of milk per day to the diet. Three meals a day are important. A balanced diet that includes citrus fruit or orange juice, eggs, meat, fish, bread, vegetables, and potatoes in addition to eight ounces of milk at each meal should ensure adequate nutrients for both mother and the developing child.

A recommended diet for pregnant women is shown in chapter 19, "Nutrition."

A woman's pattern of weight gain is a good indicator of her nutritional status. She should gain about 10 pounds during the first 20 weeks, then three-quarters of a pound to a pound each week thereafter until delivery. The gain should be steady, as shown in the illustration on page 605. Women who gain at a substantially lower rate face an increased risk of a problem with fetal development.

Strictly vegetarian diets that exclude dairy products, or fad diets that markedly restrict essential nutrients (such as protein, iron, or certain vitamins or minerals) are hazardous during pregnancy. The physician or clinic providing a woman's prenatal care can usually answer specific questions about diet.

Women who are planning to breast-feed require a weight gain of four to seven pounds more than the recommended average gain of 24 pounds. This extra weight is for fat stores that help the initiation and maintenance of lactation. This weight can be lost again after breast-feeding is ended.

Clothing. The general rule about maternity garments is that they should be loose and nonconstricting. Girdles and tight garters probably should not be worn after the first trimester. Because the breasts increase in size during pregnancy, a comfortable brassiere that provides good support is important.

Bathing. Bathing habits need not be changed during pregnancy. Contrary to an old wives' tale, bath water does not readily enter the vagina, nor does it pose a threat of infection to the fetus. Individual preference for tub bath or shower should prevail. However, a pregnant woman should exercise caution in entering or leaving the tub, especially in later pregnancy, because her off-balance posture increases the danger of a fall.

Exercise. Regular exercise is important in pregnancy, and there are few restrictions on the form it takes. Many women choose daily routine calisthenics. Walking, swimming, golf,

MOTHER'S WEIGHT GAIN

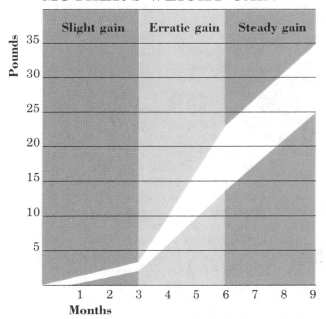

WEIGHT GAIN

The pregnant woman should gain at least 25 pounds during pregnancy, but the rate of gain is more important than the amount. As the bottom line of the chart shows, she should gain about 10 pounds during the first 20 weeks, then about three-quarters of a pound a week until delivery. Women who gain at a lower or higher rate run a higher risk of birth complications. A sudden spurt in weight is a danger signal, indicating that the body is retaining fluid.

and tennis provide equally good exercise, as long as all are carried out in moderation. A period of time set aside each day for exercise is highly desirable. About an hour of exercise is a reasonable goal.

Pregnancy exerts an adverse influence on neuromuscular coordination, so sports requiring a high degree of reflex coordination should be avoided or restricted. The list includes water skiing, snow skiing, diving, and ice-skating. Although scuba diving is somewhat controversial, most authorities believe there is no deleterious effect from it.

Women with pregnancy complications such as vaginal bleeding or uterine cramps may need to avoid exercise altogether.

Travel. In the past, pregnant women were often restricted to short trips, and then only in the first two trimesters. Recent data has confirmed that travel, no matter what the mode and distance, has almost no detrimental effect on the pregnancy. Thanks to the pressurized cabin, air travel is considered safe, too. (During the ninth month, however, most airlines require a statement from the physician saying that it is safe for the woman to travel, and giving the estimated date of delivery.) The only major drawback to travel in any form is the tendency for blood to pool in the lower extremities during prolonged sitting. A woman who travels during pregnancy should stop at least every one to two hours to stretch her legs. This is important to minimize the possibility of cramps or phlebitis.

In the last few weeks of pregnancy, long trips should be avoided if possible, because an early labor might find the woman in unfamiliar surroundings or without ready access to obstetrical care. A woman who must travel during the last few weeks should make it a point to carry photocopies of her prenatal records, including all laboratory tests and records of physician visits. This information would be of vital importance to the medical team assuming responsibility for care at the distant location.

Many women continue to drive an automobile on short trips virtually throughout pregnancy, and there is no reason not to do so if it can be done comfortably. Whether driving or a passenger, a pregnant woman should wear a seat belt with a shoulder harness. The belt should be placed snugly about the hips and should not be allowed to ride high on the abdominal wall.

Of course, in individual cases, complications might arise that would restrict or rule out travel. Women should discuss their plans in detail with the physician.

Smoking during pregnancy has harmful effects. Infants born to smoking mothers are significantly smaller than those born to nonsmokers, and the reduction in average birth weight appears to be directly proportional to the number of cigarettes smoked per day. There may be an association between smoking and premature labor, and a few other complications of pregnancy are more frequent in mothers who smoke. The long-term effect on the ultimate physical and mental development of the child is still under study.

There has never been a beneficial effect noted from cigarette smoking in pregnancy, so pregnancy is an ideal time to quit. A pregnant woman at least should make an effort to reduce the number of cigarettes smoked per day, because nicotine, carbon monoxide, and other potentially toxic products associated with smoking readily cross the placenta and enter the fetal circulation.

Alcohol. Until the late 1970s, little significance was attributed to drinking during pregnancy, even though alcohol consumed by the mother appears rapidly in the fetal circulation, and the fetal blood level of alcohol approximates the mother's level.

In recent years, however, the fetal alcohol syndrome has been recognized and widely publicized. Infants born to mothers who drink regularly or heavily (at least two or more drinks per day) have an increased chance for mental and motor retardation. These babies often have flattened features in the midface, resembling a child whose face is pressed tightly against a store window. Information is still being gathered, but the severity of the fetal alcohol syndrome appears to be directly proportional to the amount of alcohol consumed (see chapter 33, "Drugs and Medicines").

Although absolute guidelines have not been developed, it appears that there is little harm in an occasional drink or glass of wine. In no case should a mother consume more than two drinks on a daily basis. Apart from potential fetal damage, drinking can make the pregnant woman unsteady on her feet and increase the risk of a fall.

Medications. In the early 1970s, studies revealed that the average pregnant woman was exposed to 13 different medications during pregnancy. Then, because of presumed harm to the fetus, patients were generally advised to take no medication during pregnancy unless absolutely mandatory. Today, most obstetricians feel that a variety of medications necessary for the mother's health or comfort have been demonstrated to have no adverse fetal effects. There is no reason why a mother should deny herself two aspirin when she has a severe headache, nor refrain from the use of antihistamine for a severe cold. Obviously, it is advisable that the patient discuss any and all of these medications with her physician and abide by recommendations.

LABOR AND DELIVERY

In the normal, uncomplicated pregnancy, spontaneous labor begins about 40 weeks, plus or minus two weeks, from the first day of the last normal menstrual period. (In other words, the average length of a normal pregnancy is between 38 and 42 weeks.)

Research has shown that the fetus itself, not the mother, is responsible for starting normal labor. This is brought about by a series of hormonal changes in the fetal endocrine glands, which triggers the formation and release of hormones called prostaglandins from the membranes lining the mother's uterus. The prostaglandins cause the uterus to contract at rhythmic intervals.

As labor approaches, most women appreciate a general sense of well being. In a process called lightening, the fetal head descends into the maternal pelvis, and most patients suddenly find that their shortness of breath is substantially alleviated. Because the volume of amniotic fluid normally decreases as delivery approaches, the fetus usually moves less frequently and with less vigor.

There are three possible indications that labor is approaching. Not all women experience all three indications, although some experience them without being aware of it. They can appear in any sequence.

Contractions of the uterus can be detected as early as seven to eight weeks of pregnancy, but usually are not felt until the second or third trimester. These irregular, infrequent tightenings of the uterine muscle, which gradually prepare the lower portion of the uterus and the cervix for labor, are known as Braxton-Hicks contractions. They generally increase in frequency and duration as term approaches and often are mistaken for early labor. Braxton-Hicks contractions are relatively painless and sometimes are experienced as backache or merely increased pressure in the lower abdomen and pelvis.

As labor begins, they are felt more intensely and may occur at regular intervals. The first sensation is sometimes a mild backache, followed by a slight abdominal cramp. The initial contractions usually last for only 10 to 20 seconds and come 20 to 30 minutes apart. The interval gradually narrows, and the duration and intensity increase.

The beginning of contractions may dislodge the plug of mucus that has closed off the uterus during pregnancy. There is a scant amount of bleeding, often so slight that it goes unnoticed. This phenomenon is called "show." Labor may begin shortly afterwards, or may be delayed up to 72 hours.

About 10 percent of women experience premature rupture of the amniotic membranes. This means that the bag of waters surrounding the baby has broken before the start of active labor. Depending on the size and location of the break, there may be a gush or a trickle of fluid from the vagina. In most women near term, labor can be expected to begin within 24 hours. If it does not, most physicians try to stimulate contractions to minimize the risk of infection to the child.

Although all three signs are considered normal, any heavy bleeding or leakage of any large quantity of fluid through the vagina should be reported immediately to the physician. Most patients are asked to come to the hospital when there has been any significant bleeding, leakage of fluid, or regular contractions at intervals of five minutes or less.

Labor Progress

Labor is the start of regular contractions of the uterus that produce a change in the cervix. For the woman having her first child, active labor can range from six to 14 hours or more. For subsequent pregnancies, however, labor is generally shorter, ranging from three to 10 hours. However, it is not unusual for some to experience longer labor with subsequent children, depending on the shape of the pelvis and the size and the relative position of the fetus during labor. Prolonged labor can be detrimental to both mother and child. On the other hand, labors lasting only one to two hours are equally undesirable and are associated with a higher incidence of fetal distress.

Labor Assessment

When a woman arrives at the hospital or clinic in suspected labor, a general physical examination is performed. The medical team's first step is an abdominal and pelvic examination to assess the progress of the labor. This is what the medical team looks for:

Presentation. The doctor or nurse must determine whether the baby is arriving head first or bottom first. Rarely, the fetus tries to deliver shoulder first, face first or brow first. Labor may then be obstructed.

Dilation refers to the diameter of the opening of the cervix. The size is recorded in centimeters ranging from 0 to 10 (0 to 4 inches). Because the average fetal head measures 9.5 centimeters in diameter at term, the opening must dilate to 10 centimeters to allow for easy passage. Before labor, the cervix may appear closed, or may be as much as 4 to 6 centimeters dilated. This varies greatly from one patient to another. In early labor, the first few centimeters of dilation usually require more time than the last several centimeters.

Effacement. Before labor, the cervix measures about three centimeters (more than an inch) in length and is said to be uneffaced. Before labor or during the early phase of active labor, the cervix continues to thin out and shorten, a process called effacement. Progressive degrees of effacement are estimated in percentages, with 100 percent representing full or complete effacement. The cervix that is completely effaced may range from several millimeters in thickness to the thickness of tissue paper. The position of the cervix in the pelvis and its general consistency is also important. Obviously, a softened cervix will efface and dilate more rapidly than a firm one.

Station is the term used to designate how far the fetal head has descended within the pelvis. A pair of bony landmarks called the ischial spines represent the plane of the midpelvis. When the leading part of the baby's head has reached the midpelvis, the patient is said to be at station zero. In the majority of cases this means that the widest portion of the baby's head has successfully negotiated the inlet to the pelvis. If the head has not reached the level of the spines, the station is measured in minus centimeters from that point. If the head has descended below the spines, the station is referred to as plus centimeters. For most patients, station plus 3 or plus 4 means that the head is visible in the vagina and the baby is ready for imminent delivery.

Position. Even if the baby appears head first, the doctor or nurse usually determines whether the baby is looking at the ceiling or the floor, because this is directly related to successful progress in labor.

In some instances, it is not possible in the preliminary examination to determine whether active labor is under way. If the labor is false, the woman may be discharged, often with a mild sedative to help her rest.

In cases of active labor, the woman is generally transferred to a private labor room with a trained obstetrical nurse or resident physician in attendance. An external or internal electronic fetal monitor (page 610) is often attached to follow the progress of labor.

Past practice was to shave the pubic hair completely. While originally thought to decrease the chance of infection, this was not borne out by scientific study. Most patients today receive only a clip or shave of the hair between the vagina and the rectum for a vaginal delivery. For a cesarean delivery, pubic hair is shaved only to the level of the pubic bone or perhaps the upper portion of the labia.

If a patient is in early labor, a gentle enema may be given. This serves to stimulate the uterus to contract and also evacuates the rectum to provide greater room in the pelvis.

NORMAL BIRTH

At the end of "transition" labor, the baby's head emerges from the birth canal, gently assisted by the obstetrician's hands. Most babies are born facing toward the floor. The obstetrician will rotate the head slightly to ease the passage of the shoulders through the opening.

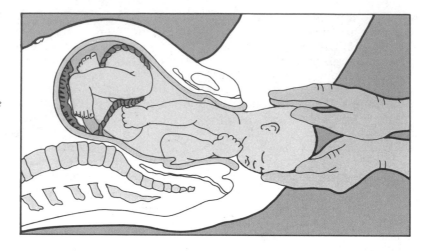

Stages of Labor

Labor is commonly classified into three and sometimes four stages, although in fact they are a continuous series of events.

The first stage begins with dilation of the cervix and ends when it has become fully dilated. This is the longest stage of labor. For women having their first baby, labor often proceeds no more rapidly than a single centimeter of dilation per hour. In subsequent pregnancies the cervix usually dilates 1⅓ to 1½ centimeters per hour.

During the first stage, the intensity of contractions gradually increases. Under this pressure, the membranes containing the amniotic fluid may rupture. If they do not, the doctor may suggest rupturing them artificially in hopes of accelerating the delivery.

When the cervix is almost fully dilated, the patient enters a stage called transition. At this time, there is a great sensation of pressure in the pelvis and pressure or discomfort in the region of the bladder or rectum. The woman may feel the urge to have a bowel movement. More often she feels a tremendous urge to push. The physician or nurse will help her to restrain this urge, because pushing too early can cause a tear in the cervix.

The second stage begins with full or complete dilation of the cervix and ends with delivery of the infant. For first pregnancies this stage requires from 30 minutes to two hours. For subsequent pregnancies the second stage varies from as brief as a few minutes to an hour at most. During this time the baby's head must travel another three to five centimeters to pass through the birth canal. If difficulty occurs during descent of the fetus, the doctor may have to intervene, either through use of forceps or by cesarean section.

The third stage of labor begins with the birth of the infant and ends with the delivery of the placenta or afterbirth. The placenta is usually passed spontaneously within several minutes of delivery, but sometimes 15 to 30 minutes elapse. If the placenta is retained a half hour or more, the obstetrician may need to remove it manually under a brief general anesthetic.

Fourth stage. The first hour after delivery is regarded by some to be a "fourth stage of labor." Regardless of terminology, this is a time of great importance for the mother. Vital signs, especially the blood pressure, must be recorded frequently and the amount of bleeding must be carefully recorded. One of the most common problems encountered during this time is atony, or relaxation of the uterus, which may bring on increased bleeding. The doctor or nurse can massage the uterus through the abdomen or give hormonal medications to correct the problem.

Delivery

A woman who has borne children is taken to the delivery room at or before full dilation of the cervix according to how fast her labor is progressing. Most first-time mothers remain in the labor room until the baby's head is visible at the entrance of the vagina. When the visible portion reaches the size of a quarter, the patient is ready to be moved to a delivery area.

The modern delivery room is a fully equipped operative theater with provisions for

EPISIOTOMY

The episiotomy is a small incision in the margin of the vagina to widen the opening and allow the baby's head to pass through more easily. The procedure helps to minimize torn vaginal tissue. It is usually performed under local anesthetic at the time of delivery if the obstetrician believes it is needed. The incision is closed afterwards with absorbable sutures that need not be removed.

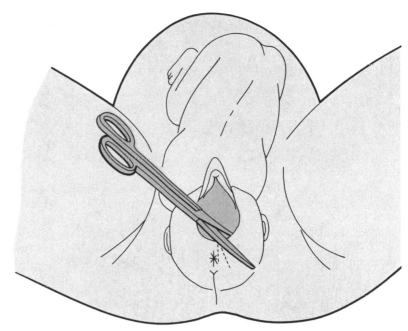

any type of delivery. Equipment is available for immediate evaluation, resuscitation, and treatment of the newborn.

Most mothers are placed on the back on the delivery table, with the legs in metal stirrups for support. This position allows the greatest flexibility for the obstetrician to assist delivery. The genital area is cleansed with a local antiseptic, and the legs, abdomen, and buttocks are covered with sterile drapes.

When delivery is imminent, most patients will benefit from an episiotomy. This is an incision in the outer part of the vagina extending toward the anus. It allows more room for an easy delivery. In addition to reducing pressure on the fetal head, episiotomy helps prevent stretching and tearing of the muscles. It also decreases the incidence of bowel and bladder problems caused by lack of vaginal support in later life. The decision for or against episiotomy should be discussed with the doctor during the last trimester, but it is usually a decision that must be made at the last moment before birth.

At birth, most babies arrive with the face looking toward the floor. As the head emerges, the mother is often asked to refrain from pushing or to pant like a puppy to allow greater control of the delivery process. The head usually rotates left or right as the shoulders make their way through the maternal pelvis. A gush of amniotic fluid or blood then occurs. Infants who are born looking toward the ceiling may require assisted rotation with use of forceps.

After the baby enters the world, the nose and mouth are gently suctioned and the baby is dried briskly with gauze sponges or cloth towels. The majority of infants breathe and cry promptly on their own, and the custom of spanking the buttocks or feet is rarely used today. If there is no difficulty, the infant can be placed on the mother's abdomen while the cord is clamped and cut. The infant is then swaddled in warm blankets and cradled in the mother's arms or placed nude in an infant warmer beside the delivery table.

Most infants delivered today receive an Apgar score or rating of their well-being, first at one minute and then five minutes of life. Up to two points each are awarded for heart rate, respiratory rate, pink color, muscle tone, and response to stimulation. Although a perfect score of 10 is seldom achieved, most healthy newborns have a score of at least 7 by five minutes of age. Infants with low Apgar scores (0 to 5) may require substantial evaluation, support, and resuscitation.

The newborn infant must have a thorough physical examination, either in the delivery room or in the nursery. The eyes, ears, nose, palate, heart, lungs, and abdomen are carefully examined. Birth defects are sought and ruled out. A tube is passed into the stomach and the rectum is checked to assure that the gastrointestinal tract is open.

The infant is weighed and the length and head circumference measured. Silver nitrate or another antibiotic ointment is applied to the baby's eyes to prevent infection by gonorrhea. This is compulsory in most states and does not imply infection of either parent.

FAMILY-CENTERED CHILDBEARING

Not so many years ago, pregnancy and childbirth were considered strictly a woman's concern, not a family matter. Little consideration was given to the father or other children in the family. Hospital and clinic protocol often banned them from participation in the experience, and even from visitation afterward.

Today, most obstetrical and health-care professionals not only recognize that it is important for the mother to hold her child in her arms shortly after delivery to promote the process called bonding, but they stress the emotional and psychological preparation of the family for the arrival of the baby. Many nurses and obstetricians today encourage family attendance at prenatal visits. Being allowed to hear the fetal heart tones or feel the mother's abdomen helps a child become part of the pregnancy process and helps diminish sibling rivalry after birth. It also has educational value, especially if the child is encouraged to ask questions.

The hospital birthing room has become a welcome option for many families although regarded skeptically by some medical personnel. Here the father or other significant support persons can be present throughout labor and delivery. At the discretion of parents, children may attend.

The modern birthing room is pleasingly decorated and comfortably furnished. The patient is allowed to labor and deliver in the same bed without transition to a formal delivery room. The newest technology, such as fetal monitoring, is available, and in the event of an emergency, fully equipped delivery rooms are only a few steps away.

Family oriented care is the choice of many persons, but it should not necessarily be considered superior to conventional labor and delivery management. In fact, unless basic elements of care and monitoring are followed, the risk to mother and infant can be somewhat increased in such a setting.

ELECTRONIC FETAL MONITORING

The normal process of labor presents a significant stress even to a healthy, full-term fetus. If the infant is premature or if there are medical complications, the risk of injury or death from lack of oxygen is increased. Although the overwhelming majority of infants today are delivered safely and without handicap, the first and second stages of labor represent the most hazardous period in a person's entire life. Close surveillance during labor and delivery is essential to the delivery of a healthy baby. That surveillance is now carried out electronically in most hospitals.

Before the advent of electronic fetal monitoring, the fetal heartbeat was obtained by a stethoscope, and the rate of the fetal heart in beats per minute was recorded, with a normal range of 120 to 160. However, the fetal heart rate rarely remains constant, changing many times over the course of one minute. For more than two decades doctors have realized that the variability of fetal heart rate and its response to stimulation such as uterine contractions are far more important as indicators of the baby's health than the average fetal heart rate. This information is only available through the use of a monitor that is capable of continuous and instantaneous display of the fetal heart and measuring each interval from one fetal heartbeat to the next. The electronic fetal monitor also provides a graphic display of uterine contractions. During normal labor, the fetal monitor graph generally shows significant variation of the fetal heart rate during each minute, with no particular correlation with uterine activity. Fetal distress generally results from a diminished flow of oxygen to the fetus, which is most marked during a uterine contraction. It can be detected on the monitor graph by a loss of heart rate variability and by a periodic slowing of the fetal heart rate just after the peak of each uterine contraction. In most cases, fetal distress can be alleviated by changing the mother's position or by giving her oxygen to breathe by mouth. If it cannot be relieved, the doctor may advise speeding the delivery by means of low forceps or by cesarean section.

There are two simple methods of electronic fetal monitoring. During early labor and before rupture of the membranes, two belts are placed over the mother's abdomen to record fetal heart rate and uterine contractions. When labor is well established after rupture of membranes, a tiny lead can be applied directly

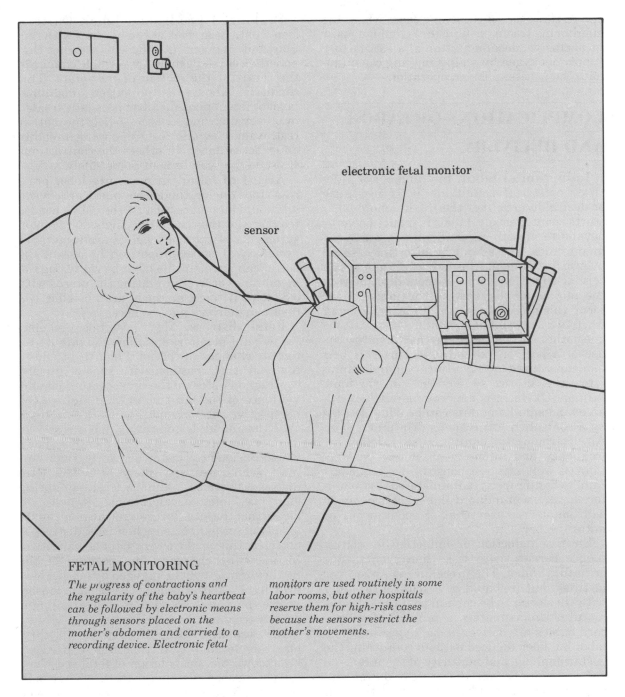

FETAL MONITORING

The progress of contractions and the regularity of the baby's heartbeat can be followed by electronic means through sensors placed on the mother's abdomen and carried to a recording device. Electronic fetal monitors are used routinely in some labor rooms, but other hospitals reserve them for high-risk cases because the sensors restrict the mother's movements.

electronic fetal monitor

sensor

to the fetal scalp, and a small plastic tube is inserted past the cervix to measure the duration and intensity of uterine contractions. Although the belt method is cumbersome and imposes certain restrictions on the mother's movement, neither method carries any significant risk or discomfort for the mother or baby.

Electronic fetal monitoring is available in the majority of hospitals today. In some delivery units, electronic fetal monitoring is made available to all patients. In others, monitoring is reserved for patients known to be at increased risk. When used routinely, electronic monitoring often offers the expectant couple greater reassurance and helps the health care team to follow routine labor progress.

Fetal scalp sampling. Another method of diagnosis for fetal distress is the direct sampling of blood from the fetal scalp. In this way, the concentration of oxygen and carbon dioxide can be measured directly. Oxygen lack also causes a buildup of acid in the fetal bloodstream, and this can be measured directly from a fetal scalp blood sample.

In most cases of fetal distress, the diagnosis can be made by electronic fetal monitoring alone. However, in those few cases where the monitoring tracing is unusually ambiguous or inconclusive, documentation of a satisfactory supply of oxygen by scalp sampling can eliminate the necessity for an operation.

COMPLICATIONS OF LABOR AND DELIVERY

Induction of labor. In a number of high-risk obstetrical conditions it is necessary or desirable to deliver the infant before labor starts spontaneously. Labor is induced near or beyond term with an artificial rupture of the membranes, carried out by inserting a small plastic instrument through the vagina and cervix. This can be done without discomfort to the mother or jeopardy to the infant. Near term, this procedure alone can bring on labor in 70 to 80 percent of patients.

Another method of induction involves the use of a hormone called oxytocin. This hormone, produced by the pituitary gland, stimulates the uterus to contract in rhythmic fashion. Oxytocin is now commercially available, and small amounts can be administered by a controlled intravenous drip into a vein. An electronic fetal monitor is used to follow the frequency and intensity of uterine contractions as well as the response of the fetal heart rate. When properly administered and monitored, oxytocin-induced labor carries little additional risk over that of spontaneous or natural labor.

Elective induction or induction for convenience carries more risk than spontaneous or natural labor. The procedure is sometimes justified, but it should be discussed carefully with the doctor to be certain that the infant is mature. Unfortunately, a number of premature babies are delivered each year in which labor has been induced without confirming the gestational age and maturity of the infant.

By a vaginal exam, the nurse or doctor usually can determine whether an induction will proceed smoothly. Sometimes X-ray measurements are needed. When the cervix is soft, effaced, and partially dilated, induction is more likely to succeed. If the cervix is not ready, two or three days may elapse from induction to delivery.

Prolonged prodromal labor. On occasion a patient arrives at the hospital with regular and frequent uterine contractions that nonetheless result in no appreciable change in the cervix or the station of the infant. This condition, known as prolonged prodromal labor or latent phase of labor, is usually treated by observation and sedation to help the mother rest. After adequate rest some women readily enter active labor. In others the contractions stop and they can be sent home safely.

Arrest of labor. Infrequently, labor progress stops during the active phase of cervical dilation. This occurs because the baby's head is too large for the size of the pelvis. X-ray measurements of the bony pelvis are sometimes necessary. If no disproportion is shown, the doctor can augment the labor by rupturing the membranes or by stimulating the uterus with oxytocin. If these methods are not effective, cesarean delivery may be necessary.

Fetal distress. Most hospitals use electronic fetal monitors to follow the minute-to-minute changes in the fetal heartbeat and to correlate their pattern with that of uterine contractions. Most of the time, continuous surveillance of the fetal heart rate assures the prospective parents and the health care team that the infant is tolerating the stresses of labor well. Occasionally, the monitor shows rates consistently faster or slower than normal. Such rates are likely to reflect fetal distress. The most ominous fetal monitoring sign is late decelerations, which indicate that the fetus is receiving an inadequate supply of oxygen. Even when fetal distress is detected, this can be corrected in a majority of instances by changing the position of the mother or by giving her oxygen by mask. However, if these patterns do not respond to conservative measures, cesarean delivery might prove necessary.

Rh sensitization. Rh disease (erythroblastosis fetalis) is a condition caused by breakdown and destruction of fetal red blood cells by antibodies from the mother. The condition is only seen in Rh-negative women who bear Rh-positive infants (see chapter 6, "The Blood").

At delivery, Rh-positive fetal cells can accidentally leak into the mother's circulation. The mother's immune system recognizes the Rh-positive fetal cells as foreign and generates an antibody directed against those cells. Most of the time, leakage of fetal cells into the maternal circulation occurs only during the delivery, and consequently only the next pregnancy is affected. If antibodies to Rh-positive cells are present, they will leak across the placenta and attack the baby's circulation.

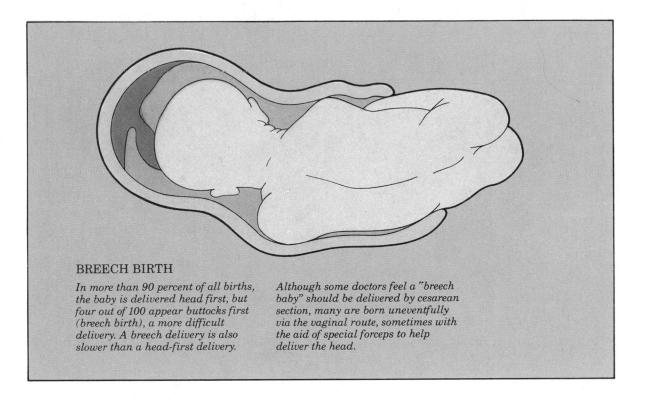

BREECH BIRTH

In more than 90 percent of all births, the baby is delivered head first, but four out of 100 appear buttocks first (breech birth), a more difficult delivery. A breech delivery is also slower than a head-first delivery.

Although some doctors feel a "breech baby" should be delivered by cesarean section, many are born uneventfully via the vaginal route, sometimes with the aid of special forceps to help deliver the head.

Infants affected with Rh-positive disease are badly swollen with an excessive accumulation of fluid in all of the soft tissues in the abdomen. Fetal heart failure is not uncommon when the process is severe. Management of the problem consists of early delivery, often by cesarean section, or intrauterine fetal transfusion whereby Rh-negative blood cells compatible with the mother's blood are placed directly into the fetal abdomen to sustain life until the baby can be delivered.

In 1968, Rh immune globulin was introduced to be given to all Rh-negative women after delivery of an Rh-positive infant. This medication effectively prevents antibody formation in the mother, in effect making every pregnancy a first pregnancy. Patients who miscarry or whose pregnancies are terminated should also receive Rh immune globulin when the fetal blood type is unknown.

Breech delivery. In about four percent of all deliveries, the infant appears buttocks first, a so-called breech delivery. The incidence is higher in premature deliveries, ranging up to 12 to 15 percent at 26 weeks.

For some time it has been realized that the breech vaginal delivery carries increased risk factors for mother and infant. In the frank breech configuration, the baby's legs are extended and the feet are tucked up beside the ears. This position is most favorable for vaginal delivery. In a complete breech position, the knees are flexed and the infant is literally sitting with feet over the cervix. The incomplete breech position refers to the appearance of one or both feet at the entrance to the vagina, with the buttocks high above the pelvis. In this position, the infant is literally standing up. This is the highest risk presentation for vaginal delivery because of the increased opportunity for kinking the umbilical cord and the decreased effectiveness of a foot or leg, as opposed to head or buttocks, in dilating the cervical opening.

During the late 1970s many obstetricians began to perform cesarean sections routinely on all breech births out of fear of adverse outcomes. That approach is not totally justifiable medically, but continues for legal reasons. There is little doubt that these infants are at increased risk. Yet a number of breech infants, both full term and premature, could and probably should deliver normally, because cesarean delivery also carries a distinct increase in risk to the mother. This is an issue that a woman should discuss with her obstetrician, carefully comparing maternal discomfort and risks with risks to the baby.

In the vaginal delivery of a breech, X rays are usually performed to determine whether the pelvis is adequate for delivery, and to determine the relationship between the presenting part and the pelvis.

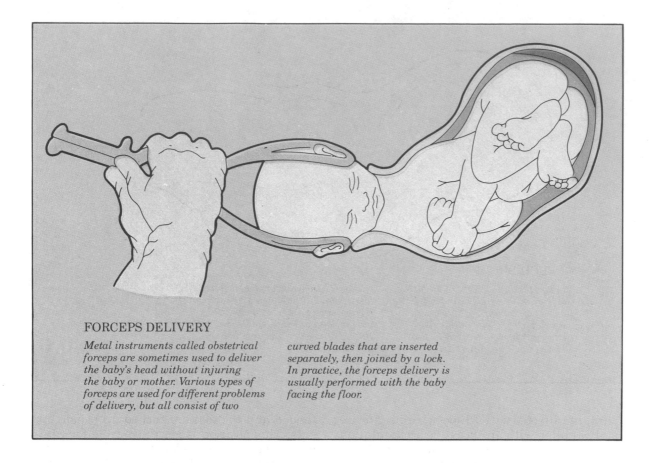

FORCEPS DELIVERY

Metal instruments called obstetrical forceps are sometimes used to deliver the baby's head without injuring the baby or mother. Various types of forceps are used for different problems of delivery, but all consist of two curved blades that are inserted separately, then joined by a lock. In practice, the forceps delivery is usually performed with the baby facing the floor.

The time of labor in breech presentations is ordinarily longer than in a head-first delivery. General obstetrical practice is to leave the membranes intact as long as possible to dilate the cervix more effectively. Once the cervix is fully dilated, the second stage is prolonged in the effort to bring the buttocks down.

As the buttocks emerge from the vagina, an episiotomy is performed. Then the obstetrician gently guides the delivery of the shoulders. Delivery of the head is accomplished manually or by using special forceps designed for the purpose.

Forceps delivery. Occasionally the position of the baby or ineffective labor make spontaneous delivery difficult, if not impossible. In other instances the delivery time is unnecessarily prolonged. In these circumstances, the doctor uses curved stainless steel instruments called forceps to assist in the delivery of the fetal head. Most forceps have a cup-shaped blade to precisely fit the head's contours and are shaped to traverse the mother's pelvis safely.

Forceps have been used to assist deliveries for several hundred years. Although some patients might be frightened by the thought of such an instrument, a skilled obstetrician can often bring about delivery with greater ease and safety than a spontaneous birth. Indeed, a number of obstetricians use forceps routinely to minimize fetal trauma and the risk of tearing the mother's tissue.

A number of different types of forceps are available. Special forceps assist the baby from the outlet when the mother is too tired to push. Others are designed for application in mid-pelvis and are especially helpful in rotating a fetus who is in poor position for delivery. Forceps are particularly useful if there is fetal heart rate distress, massive bleeding, or meconium (green stool) staining of the infant. This hastens the delivery of the infant and permits prompt resuscitation of the child.

When the second stage of labor is progressing poorly, most obstetricians consider a trial of forceps. If the instruments cannot be easily applied or if there is difficulty in extracting the fetal head, the procedure is abandoned and cesarean delivery is selected as the safer alternative.

Forceps deliveries are generally classified into low- and mid-forceps procedures. Low forceps are used when the leading part of the baby's head is visible at the vaginal opening. The most common reason for using low forceps is to help a mother who has become overly fatigued from pushing in the second stage of labor. In other instances, low forceps are useful in achieving better control over a delivery, thus minimizing the risk of torn vaginal tissue. Today, low forceps are routinely used in the delivery of the premature infant, whose skull bones are soft and unable to withstand the compression associated with spontaneous vaginal delivery. Low forceps are also useful in expediting delivery when there is evidence of fetal distress.

Mid forceps are most commonly used to rotate the fetal head to a normal postion for delivery. Infants usually are born looking straight down toward the floor. If the baby's head is turned, it may fail to descend properly through the mother's pelvis, and delivery is obstructed. With the mid forceps instrument, the head is first rotated to the normal position, then extracted by gentle pressure. This procedure ordinarily is accomplished under a low spinal or a general anesthetic to achieve maximum relaxation of the muscles of the pelvic floor.

High forceps, which for years were associated with increased trauma to the infant and the mother, are rarely used in modern obstetrics. If the infant is too large or the pelvis too small, the infant is today more easily and safely delivered by cesarean section.

Cesarean birth. A cesarean section was for many years considered tantamount to obstetrical defeat and was performed only in desperate situations. More recent information about fetal distress during labor and the ultimate risk to the infant from a traumatic delivery has caused obstetricians to liberalize their thinking on cesarean birth. Improved surgical technique and the availability of blood and antibiotics to combat infection has dramatically reduced maternal risk. Still, the maternal risk with cesarean delivery is never as low as that associated with vaginal birth. For that reason, cesarean delivery should never be considered the easy way out.

Since the mid-1970s, cesarean sections have been performed at a rapidly increasing rate. In some hospitals, the incidence of cesarean birth ranges as high as 20 to 25 percent of all deliveries. Although repeat cesarean deliveries account for many of such procedures, occasionally the convenience factor for the physician or precaution against possible lawsuits has taken precedence over sound obstetrical judgment.

However, in the overwhelming majority of cases, cesarean delivery is chosen because it is the safest option for mother and child.

The most common reason for cesarean delivery is cephalopelvic disproportion, which means that the infant is too large or the pelvis too small for a safe vaginal delivery. Although measurements of the maternal pelvis are usually carried out in early pregnancy, it is often impossible to confirm cephalopelvic disproportion until a trial of labor ends in a failure of labor to progress. The second most common reason for cesarean birth is fetal distress, which is most often detected by a persistent pattern of the fetal heart rate on the electronic monitor or by a loss of the normal beat-to-beat variation in the fetal heart rate. Fetal distress can often be corrected by changing the mother's position or by giving her oxygen. However, the fetus is in jeopardy if it fails to respond, and delivery must be accomplished quickly.

There are many other reasons for cesarean section, including abnormal position of the fetus, low implantation of the placenta, premature separation of the placenta before delivery, and certain cases of Rh sensitization. Although most patients who previously have delivered by cesarean section are admitted for repeat cesarean delivery, a number of patients today are given a trial of labor under rigorous supervision despite a previous cesarean birth.

In most instances, the reasons for cesarean delivery are relative rather than absolute. Hospital policy in many institutions requires an obstetrical consultation (a second opinion) before a first cesarean delivery is performed.

The operation is performed by incising the skin and fatty tissue, then the fascia or tough connective tissue. The lining of the abdominal cavity (peritoneum) is entered and the uterus exposed. The skin incision is made vertically from a point below the navel to a point just above the pubic bone, or else a slightly curved "smile" incision is performed from side to side just above the pubic hairline. Advantages and disadvantages of each type of incision should be discussed with the obstetrician.

The lining of the uterus is incised crosswise in the lower part of the uterus just above the bladder. The bladder is pushed downward to avoid injury. An incision is made in the muscular wall of the uterus just above the bladder and extended from side to side. After the bag of waters has been ruptured, the infant is carefully delivered by hand or by forceps through the incision. The placenta is removed manually and the uterus is closed by a locking suture in either two or three layers. For patients desiring voluntary sterilization, the fallopian tubes can easily be tied and divided at this time, extending the operating time by only a few minutes (see chapter 24, "The Female Reproductive System").

Most patients experience significant abdominal discomfort after the procedure, but pain usually can be controlled with medications for the first few days. Patients are generally encouraged to sit up in a chair and walk a short distance the day after surgery. If not overdone, exercise often hastens the recovery. The usual stay in the hospital after a cesarean delivery is four to five days. How soon a woman can return to full activity is highly individual and ranges from two to six weeks.

Although the risk of cesarean delivery increases slightly with each procedure, there is no limit to the number of cesarean deliveries a woman can undergo. One patient is recorded as having had 10. Occasionally, it is necessary to make an incision high on the uterine wall. This poses an additional risk of separation of the uterine scar during subsequent pregnancy and requires meticulous obstetrical supervision.

When cesarean delivery is repeated electively, there is always the danger of delivering the infant before it is mature. Consequently, the physician may ask to perform amniocentesis, a sampling of the amniotic fluid with a small needle before scheduling the delivery. Tests can be performed on the small sample of fluid to find out whether the baby is indeed at full term and whether the lungs are mature enough to survive in the outside world. If there is uncertainty regarding the due date, the physician is likely to choose to wait for spontaneous labor to begin and then perform elective cesarean section. Although sometimes inconvenient for the patient, this nonetheless provides additional assurance of the infant's maturity. If sizes and dates are consistent during the pregnancy, and the fetal head growth as measured by ultrasound is also consistent with dates, additional testing is not necessary.

PREGNANCY COMPLICATIONS

Miscarriage. Between 10 and 15 percent of all pregnancies end in miscarriage. The majority of these occur early, before the twelfth week, sometimes before the woman is even aware she is pregnant. However, loss of pregnancy can occur at any time in the second trimester. Research has shown that the majority of spontaneous abortions result from genetic defects in the fetus or abnormal implantation of the placenta. If spontaneous miscarriage never occurred, a far greater number of children would be born with severe mental or physical handicaps.

Most mothers experience a mild degree of cramping during the first trimester. Severe cramping, especially when associated with vaginal spotting or bleeding, must be considered a threat to miscarry and should be reported to the doctor at once. Several different terms are applied to different types of early miscarriage. Incomplete abortion means that the products of the pregnancy have been partially expelled through the cervix. In an inevitable abortion, no tissue is passed, but bleeding and cramping are so great that they rule out continuation of the pregnancy. The term missed abortion refers to a halt of uterine growth in the absence of bleeding, cramping, or passage of tissue. Whether miscarriage is inevitable, incomplete, or missed, a dilatation and curettage (D&C), a minor operation (see chapter 24, "The Female Reproductive System"), is almost always necessary to remove the products of pregnancy and reduce the risk of bleeding or infection. A complete abortion implies spontaneous expulsion of all fetal and placental tissue, and then a D&C might not be necessary.

Molar pregnancy, a rare condition, is not actually a true gestation. Instead, placental tissue proliferates and fills the uterus in the absence of a fetus. It is initially suspected as a pregnancy, but the uterus often enlarges more rapidly than normal, and fetal heart tones cannot be heard. Vaginal bleeding or passage of grape-like tissue clusters may occur. With molar pregnancy there is an increased incidence of toxemia (see page 619) and some patients become seriously ill.

The diagnosis is easily confirmed by ultrasound, and a dilatation and curettage is necessary. In less than three to four percent of patients, the condition persists after D&C, and in rare instances it becomes malignant. Although this cancer can spread to involve multiple organ systems, the overwhelming majority of patients are cured by chemotherapy.

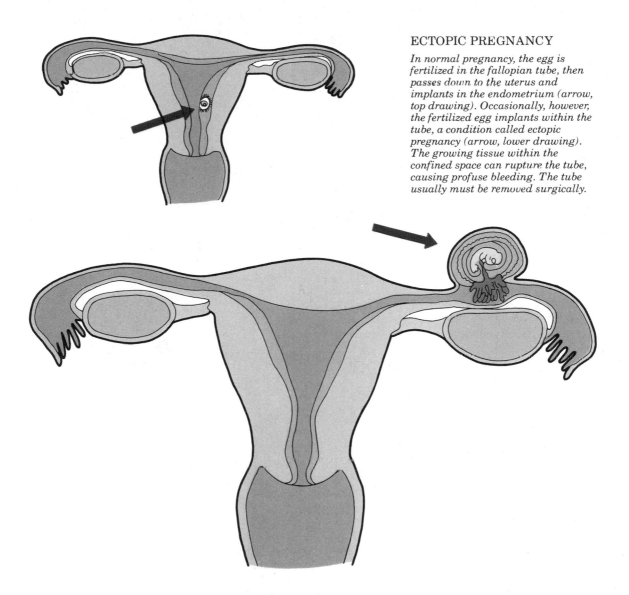

ECTOPIC PREGNANCY

In normal pregnancy, the egg is fertilized in the fallopian tube, then passes down to the uterus and implants in the endometrium (arrow, top drawing). Occasionally, however, the fertilized egg implants within the tube, a condition called ectopic pregnancy (arrow, lower drawing). The growing tissue within the confined space can rupture the tube, causing profuse bleeding. The tube usually must be removed surgically.

Ectopic pregnancy. In rare cases the fertilized ovum is obstructed in its travel from the fallopian tube to the uterus, and implantation takes place in the wall of the tube itself. Although capable of some expansion, the tube itself is quite narrow. As the pregnancy enlarges, the tube ruptures causing profuse bleeding into the abdomen. Symptoms of ectopic pregnancy vary but usually include pain (often limited to one side) and irregular vaginal bleeding. Common symptoms of pregnancy are not always present, and a urine test is negative in almost half of all cases.

Pelvic examination may reveal a lump or mass beside the uterus. Diagnostic ultrasound can visualize the mass and at the same time rule out pregnancy within the uterus.

Despite these methods, the diagnosis of ectopic pregnancy often remains inconclusive, and a surgical procedure known as laparoscopy must be carried out. With the woman under general anesthesia, a lighted optical device is inserted through a small incision below the navel. If the ectopic pregnancy is confirmed, the abdomen is opened and the affected tube excised. In rare instances, it is possible to attempt to salvage the damaged tube, but the complication rate for bleeding, infection, and recurrent ectopic pregnancy is high.

Women who have had pelvic inflammatory disease, major pelvic or bowel surgery, or previous ectopic pregnancy face an increased risk of ectopic gestation.

Placental problems. Any bleeding during the second or third trimester must be considered abnormal whether it is mere spotting or bright red flow. Although the bleeding could be caused by minor injury to the cervix or vagina, the physician must be notified at once. It could be an early warning of a major placental complication.

Placenta previa results when the pregnancy is implanted low in the uterine wall. As the pregnancy develops, the outlet of the uterus can become completely covered by the placenta, thus blocking the safe passage of the fetus. This condition is known as central placenta previa. Marginal placenta previa results in incomplete or partial blockage of the uterine outlet. In either case, profuse bleeding may result as early as 24 to 26 weeks. In some patients, heavy bleeding does not occur until the onset of labor.

Although the bleeding is usually painless, immediate hospitalization and bed rest is mandatory. If bleeding is profuse, premature delivery by cesarean section is necessary. If the bleeding is relatively slight and the mother's blood level can be maintained by transfusions, delivery often can be postponed until the fetus reaches maturity. Meticulous obstetrical management usually results in a healthy mother and baby.

Women who have malformations of the uterus, fibroid tumors, a history of multiple births, or who have had previous cesarean delivery are statistically predisposed to low implantation and placenta previa. The diagnosis of placenta previa is easily made by ultrasound. Pelvic examination is always deferred in the patient with possible placenta previa because of the risk of causing profuse hemorrhage.

Abruptio placenta. Premature detachment of the normal implanted placenta from the uterine wall occurs in about one in 200 pregnancies. The term abruptio is reserved for severe degrees of separation involving half the surface area of the placenta. This is associated with severe pain and a rigid, enlarging uterus. Immediate cesarean section is the only hope for saving the baby. With smaller areas of separation, there is increased risk of fetal distress, although labor may proceed to vaginal delivery with intensive fetal monitoring.

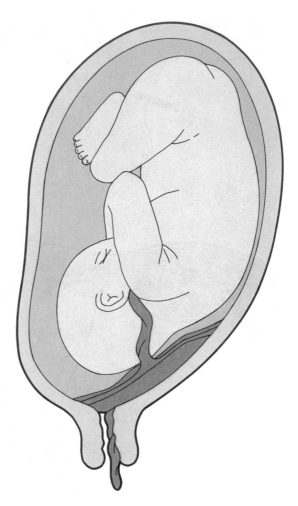

PLACENTA PREVIA

The embryo usually implants high in the uterine wall, but sometimes implantation takes place in a lower location. As the placenta grows, it can partially or completely cover the outlet of the uterus, blocking safe delivery of the fetus. Premature delivery is sometimes necessary. In other cases placenta previa can be overcome by hospitalization and bed rest, allowing the delivery to be postponed until the fetus is more mature.

Major areas of placental separation can be seen by an ultrasound scan, yet in a majority of instances, the ultrasound reveals nothing more than a normal site of implantation.

Premature labor. In the United States today, premature labor is the leading cause of death, ranking higher than heart disease, cancer, or stroke. Almost one in ten infants born today is significantly premature—less than 37 weeks gestational age or weighing less than 2,500 gms (5½ lbs.).

Even though all organ systems are present in the premature newborn, the majority are not mature enough for full function. This is especially true of the lungs, where the tiny air sacs lack stability and tend to collapse. The result is known as respiratory distress syndrome and usually requires mechanical support of breathing with a respirator.

With improved techniques and equipment an intensive neonatal care nursery can help infants to survive even as early as 25 or 26 weeks. Such infants are best delivered at a medical facility capable of providing immediate intensive obstetrical and newborn care and many patients who appear likely to deliver prematurely need to be transferred to such a hospital if the local facility is inadequate. Where premature labor is exceedingly rapid, delivery occurs unexpectedly and necessitates infant transport in an incubator.

A long list of factors predispose to prematurity. Twin pregnancy, placental accident, uterine fibroids, maternal illness, and excessive amniotic fluid all increase the likelihood of a premature birth. Yet in 50 percent of premature labors there is no known cause.

In recent years, medications have become available that can dramatically suppress uterine contractions. In fact, the majority of labors can be stopped through a specific action on the muscle cells of the uterus, averting premature delivery. In addition, a cortisone-like drug may be administered to the mother prenatally to stimulate and mature the premature fetal lung. Although not effective in all patients, the medication has been shown to benefit the majority of infants from 26 to 35 weeks and has no major maternal or fetal side effects.

If premature labor cannot be halted, or if there are maternal reasons why labor cannot be stopped, careful electronic fetal surveillance is required. The premature fetus is much more susceptible to the stresses of labor than a full-term baby. Vaginal delivery is usually accomplished with forceps to protect the delicate head from the sudden compression and decompression associated with its emergence from the vagina.

Preeclampsia and eclampsia. Years ago, preeclampsia and eclampsia were called toxemia and were thought to arise from a toxic substance circulating in the maternal blood. Today, the two conditions are still incompletely understood, despite modern technology and research. However, no toxic substance has ever been isolated.

Preeclampsia is a condition of the latter half of pregnancy characterized by hypertension, swelling of the feet, hands, legs or face, and the appearance of protein in the urine. Without prompt medical intervention, the condition progresses to eclampsia, characterized by convulsions and a state of coma. Preeclampsia and eclampsia are a significant threat to the life of mother and infant, and a major thrust of prenatal care is early detection and prompt management of these conditions.

The only cure is delivery of the infant. The first step in management is absolute bed rest, which is usually best accomplished in the hospital. If the hypertension is mild, delivery can be delayed from a few days to several weeks to allow the fetus to mature. During this time, the mother's blood pressure is continually monitored, and urine and blood are collected to observe kidney function. Although the patient can be given a mild sedative for comfort, no medication has been shown to be effective in curing the disease, and diuretic medications sometimes impede the circulation of blood through the placenta.

If the mother's condition worsens, immediate delivery is required, either by induced labor with intravenous oxytocin or by cesarean birth. Magnesium sulfate usually is used intravenously during labor and delivery to control the blood pressure and to prevent seizures.

Although preeclampsia and eclampsia are most common in young women having a first baby, the condition can appear in any pregnancy regardless of the woman's age or number of children. A patient who has had the problem with prior pregnancies is more likely to repeat it in subsequent pregnancies. Preeclampsia and eclampsia are also more frequent

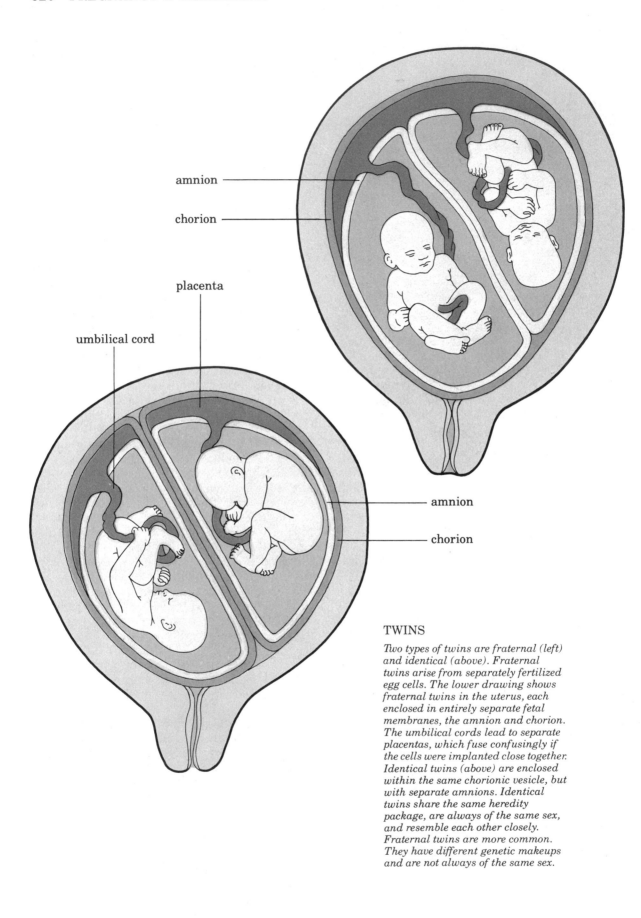

amnion

chorion

placenta

umbilical cord

amnion

chorion

TWINS

Two types of twins are fraternal (left) and identical (above). Fraternal twins arise from separately fertilized egg cells. The lower drawing shows fraternal twins in the uterus, each enclosed in entirely separate fetal membranes, the amnion and chorion. The umbilical cords lead to separate placentas, which fuse confusingly if the cells were implanted close together. Identical twins (above) are enclosed within the same chorionic vesicle, but with separate amnions. Identical twins share the same heredity package, are always of the same sex, and resemble each other closely. Fraternal twins are more common. They have different genetic makeups and are not always of the same sex.

in women with underlying hypertension, chronic kidney disease, diabetes mellitus, or multiple pregnancy.

Multiple births. Twins occur in the United States about once in every 93 pregnancies, and triplets once in 8,500. The diagram on page 620 illustrates a twin pregnancy with entirely separate fetal membranes and a shared placenta.

Multiple gestation immediately shifts any pregnancy to a high-risk category. There is a markedly increased risk of premature birth, and in fact the average duration of pregnancy is three weeks less than for single pregnancies. There is also an increased incidence of labor difficulties, and the necessity for cesarean delivery is increased. Nonetheless, a healthy outcome can be expected in most cases with increased bed rest and meticulous care in the last trimester.

Identical twins originate from an early division of a single fertilized ovum. The process almost always occurs on one of the first several cell divisions following conception. Such twins are not only identical in sex and physical appearance, but the genetic information carried in their chromosomes is also precisely the same.

Fraternal twins originate from two separate ova fertilized by two separate spermatozoa. These implant separately in the uterus and growth and development occur independently, even though the twins may share a common fused placenta. Fraternal twins are not necessarily of the same sex, because the sex of each is determined independently by chance.

Statistically, about two-thirds of all twin pairs are fraternal and one-third are identical. At birth, the obstetrician is not always able to determine with certainty whether the infants are identical or fraternal, but a microscopic examination of the membranes after the delivery usually resolves the question. If two layers are identified under the microscope, the twins are usually identical. If there are four layers, they are fraternal. If any doubt remains, blood studies can be carried out at about six months of age to determine genetic identity.

Twins are most often diagnosed by rapid uterine enlargement. The diagnosis is easily confirmed by diagnostic ultrasound, even as early as nine to ten weeks of pregnancy. Early detection is important to reduce the risk of prematurity.

MEDICAL RISK FACTORS IN PREGNANCY

Maternal age. It is interesting that the greatest pregnancy risk is seen in mothers at either end of the reproductive age spectrum. Teenage mothers face increased risk of miscarriage, prematurity, toxemia, and ineffective labor patterns resulting in an increased incidence of cesarean birth. Mothers in their 30s and 40s are at risk for these same problems and are more prone to deliver infants with genetic defects. The level of chromosomal defects rises from one-half percent when a mother is in her 20s to 1½ to two percent at age 35, three to four percent at age 40 and five to eight percent at age 45. All mothers close to age 35 are offered prenatal diagnosis by amniocentesis. By inserting a small needle into the uterus and withdrawing a sample of fluid and cells, chromosomal defects can be detected.

Maternal weight. Patients with a pre-pregnancy weight of less than 100 pounds or greater than 200 pounds also face greater risk of prematurity, retardation of fetal growth within the uterus, and irregular, ineffective labor patterns. Nutritional or dietary consultation is particularly important for women in this category to aid fetal growth.

Diabetes. Pregnancy itself exerts a considerable stress on maternal glucose metabolism. A number of women develop diabetes during pregnancy, then revert to normal afterward.

A woman with diabetes should consult her internist, obstetrician, and nutritional counselor before conception if possible, and certainly as soon as pregnancy is suspected. Caloric requirements are increased in pregnancy, so the insulin requirements are usually increased, too. Meticulous control of blood sugar is essential for the baby's well being and must be maintained throughout the pregnancy. Hospitalization at intervals is sometimes necessary to reestablish control.

In some cases, early delivery is necessary, particularly when the mother's glucose level has been poorly controlled. Although there are more cesarean births among diabetics, the majority of patients deliver vaginally.

Insulin requirements for diabetic mothers usually decline rapidly for a few days after delivery, and insulin must be managed carefully during this period.

Hypertension. Chronic elevated blood pressure also increases prenatal risk. Retarded fetal growth, immaturity, partial separation of the placenta, and fetal distress during labor increase in patients with hypertension. A thorough diagnostic evaluation and regulation of the blood pressure should be achieved before conception if possible. During the pregnancy, the diastolic blood pressure should be held between 85 and 100. Several medications effectively lower the mother's blood pressure while consistently sparing the circulation to the uterus and placenta.

In the third trimester and in labor, there is an increased incidence of toxemia of pregnancy. The diagnosis is made more difficult by the underlying hypertension, but nonetheless necessitates management for toxemia in cases of doubt. In addition to improving fetal outcome, careful control of the blood pressure during pregnancy will prevent damage to the mother's kidneys.

Thyroid disease. Patients who have markedly excessive or insufficient thyroid hormone function rarely become pregnant. However, many women with less pronounced degrees of thyroid imbalance do conceive and require rigid medical surveillance.

Patients with hyperthyroidism (Graves' disease) have such excessive thyroid hormone production that they are predisposed to thyroid "storm." This is a life-threatening condition characterized by severe hypertension, nervousness, irregular rapid heartbeat, and occasionally heart failure. It is usually controlled by medication designed to reduce the output of thyroid hormones. Less frequently, partial or total surgical resection of the thyroid gland becomes necessary.

Women with a low thyroid function who are maintained on thyroid preparations generally find it necessary to increase dosage somewhat to compensate for the increased demands of pregnancy. Medications are usually adjusted on clinical grounds, because pregnancy itself interferes with the routine laboratory evaluations of thyroid function.

The fetal thyroid gland is usually capable of producing all necessary thyroid hormones by the tenth or eleventh week of gestation. Thus fetal thyroid function is independent of the mother.

Cardiac disease. Women with a history of rheumatic fever or congenital heart defects face increased risk during pregnancy. During the late second and third trimester, the blood volume is dramatically increased, and the strain on the heart and lungs can be enough to cause congestive heart failure.

Even with normal heart function, patients with damage to the heart valves may benefit from antibiotics given as a preventive measure during labor and delivery.

A woman with heart problems should discuss risk factors and medical management in advance with both a cardiologist and obstetrician. The risk that the infant will inherit a heart defect is not dramatically increased compared to the general population.

Infectious disease. A number of infections, both viral and bacterial, can exert a profound influence on maternal and fetal health. Rubella, perhaps the best known example, is associated with an increased incidence of ear, eye, and heart defects in the infant when the mother is exposed during the first trimester. Cytomegalovirus, toxoplasmosis, and encephalitis are associated with an increased risk of fetal death or genetic handicaps. Coccidiomycosis carries an increased risk of widespread dissemination during pregnancy and requires aggressive treatment (see chapter 28, "Infectious Diseases").

For most short-term viral illnesses and for the overwhelming variety of bacterial infections, risk to the baby is not dramatically increased if aggressive treatment is carried out. Urinary tract infections, especially infections of the kidney itself, carry an increased risk of premature labor.

AFTER THE DELIVERY

The six week period after delivery is known as puerperium. During this time, the hormonal changes associated with pregnancy subside, and the organ systems of the body slowly return to the prepregnant level. The majority of these changes are complete after six weeks, when most obstetricians schedule a checkup visit for the mother.

Bleeding. Most patients continue to bleed lightly for three to six weeks or more after delivery. Generally the vaginal flow (lochia) changes from dark red to dark brown and finally to an almost clear mucuslike substance. Heavy flow with bright red bleeding or large clots should be reported to the physician immediately. Cramping should also subside gradually.

Episiotomy care. Most physicians prefer to repair an episiotomy with absorbable, nonreactive sutures that do not require removal. Although these usually dissolve within the body tissues over several months, occasionally small fragments are expelled from the vagina. This should be no cause for alarm unless it occurs in the first three or four days after delivery. Many patients find hot tub baths or the use of an anesthetic spray helpful in minimizing episiotomy discomfort. Intercourse should be avoided for at least three to four weeks to allow proper time for healing of the vaginal tissues. When intercourse is resumed, some discomfort is not unusual and the problem generally resolves itself in a short time.

Bowel habits. Constipation is common after delivery, and a woman would be wise to increase her daily fluid intake as well as the roughage in her diet, with vegetables and bran cereals. She should not hesitate to use a mild laxative whenever necessary.

Exercises. An exercise program can be started on a gradual basis the first few days after vaginal delivery. Women who have delivered by cesarean section should delay for about two weeks or as instructed by their physician. The obstetrician may suggest special exercises for tightening the muscles of the pelvic floor and for preventing subsequent problems with bowel or bladder function. The exercise program should be aimed at restoring the strength of the rectus muscles across the lower abdomen. Almost any exercise program followed conscientiously will help the woman to regain her normal prepregnant posture. Usually, weight will return to prepregnant levels by the sixth week.

Rest. A decrease in energy levels is the rule rather than the exception for the woman who has just delivered a baby. Fatigue is even more pronounced in the patient recovering from cesarean birth. The new mother should allow at least an hour or two during the day for a short nap or a period of uninterrupted rest with her feet elevated.

Breast-feeding. Although the choice between breast and bottle must be an individual one, an ever increasing number of mothers today are electing to breast-feed. Recent emphasis on bonding with the infant and the social acceptability of breast-feeding in public have contributed to this trend.

There are a number of distinct advantages to breast milk. The nutritional component of breast milk is ideal for the human infant. Antibodies against diseases pass freely from the mother to the infant and confer a degree of immunity during the first few months of life. Statistically, infants who breast-feed are less likely to develop gastrointestinal problems such as colic or diarrhea (see chapter 21, "Allergy and the Immune System").

Of primary importance is the mother's attitude toward breast-feeding and her motivation to succeed. Opinions of relatives and friends, although sincerely offered, generally should be discounted. If during early pregnancy the patient decides she will breast-feed, the nipples can be prepared through massage and creams long before delivery. If the decision is made after delivery, breast-feeding still can be accomplished easily with appropriate nipple care.

In most obstetrical settings today, the healthy term infant is allowed to suckle in the first few minutes of life, even while the mother remains on the delivery room table. No milk is obtained at this time, but the liquid that comes from the breast, called colostrum, contains antibodies beneficial to the infant, and the stimulation to the nipple activates a reflex that helps the uterus contract. The infant should be put to the breast on a regular basis thereafter, generally five to ten minutes on each side. On the second or third day after delivery, the breasts become engorged or swollen and there is a let-down of milk.

Before each nursing session, the nipples and breasts should be washed carefully with soap and water or mild antiseptic to prevent infection. If milk production is low or inadequate to satisfy the infant, the mother should force fluids and continue breast-feeding. Relatively few women are unable to produce enough milk to meet the nutritional needs of the infant.

Many breast-feeding mothers notice a delay in the return of normal menstruation after delivery. Some patients notice no menstrual flow whatsoever during the time they are breast-feeding, while others have irregular or infrequent bleeding episodes. Ovulation is difficult if not impossible to predict in the breast-feeding mother, and contraceptive requirements should be discussed with the doctor.

While breast-feeding, a woman should remember that almost all medications will cross from the maternal circulation into the breast milk and reach the circulation of the infant. Use of over-the-counter preparations should be minimized, and prescription drugs should be cleared with the obstetrician or pediatrician (see chapter 33, "Drugs and Medicines").

Occasionally, the breasts become engorged with milk. This problem is usually relieved by manual expression of milk or temporary use of a breast pump. In severe cases, ice packs or binders applied tightly to the breasts are necessary. Mastitis or infection of the breasts occurs rarely. This most often produces pain and redness across the breasts, and a low-grade fever. Usually, mastitis can be treated without the need to discontinue breast-feeding entirely, but the patient should alert her physician to these symptoms and follow recommendations.

Infections. Patients who recently have delivered an infant should be alert for the onset of fever, severe pain, or abnormally heavy bleeding. These warning signs often indicate the presence of infection. Discomfort and frequency of urination may indicate an infection of the bladder, while cramping pain and fever are the earliest indications of an endometritis, infection of the cavity of the uterus. The breasts become swollen and tender from mere engorgement, but redness of the breasts and fever herald the onset of mastitis or breast infection.

Six-weeks checkup. Most physicians like to have their patients return for examination about six weeks after delivery. At this time the breasts are examined for masses, a Pap smear and pelvic exam are performed, and contraceptive requirements are considered. This is also an opportunity for the patient to review with her physician any problems encountered during the pregnancy, labor, delivery, or postpartum period.

Although the mother's weight has often returned to prepregnant levels by this time, an increase of five or ten pounds might be of concern to the patient. A carefully planned diet may help her return to her desired weight range.

Not infrequently, a woman will fail to menstruate after six weeks. This is particularly true of breast-feeding mothers, but a variable delay is normal after delivery and represents no cause for alarm. However, if periods fail to resume several months after delivery or after breast-feeding stops, additional hormone treatment may be necessary.

The postpartum visit is a time to discuss the timing of the next pregnancy, medical or genetic risk factors, and a discussion of the desired intervals between pregnancies. A variety of contraceptive methods are available that allow couples to space their children (see chapter 24, "The Female Reproductive System").

PAIN MEDICATION
IN CHILDBIRTH

Not so many years ago, mothers were often put to sleep by general anesthetic for an uncomplicated vaginal delivery. The procedure not only delayed infant bonding, but the general anesthetic was often unnecessary and in fact increased maternal risk. Today a variety of techniques are available for pain relief during the labor and delivery process. These methods are generally discussed quite thoroughly in childbirth education classes, and individual preferences should be discussed with the doctor before delivery. Although a knowledge of medications and techniques is helpful, the patient should not attempt to decide what she will or will not require before the onset of labor. Not only is each labor a unique process, but each patient has a different threshold for pain. It is not unusual for women to require substantially more or less pain relief than they anticipated.

Several of the most common techniques for pain relief are:

Education. Women who are thoroughly informed about what discomfort to expect in all stages of labor and delivery are prepared to deal with it and usually require less relief than patients who are unprepared. Fear or anticipation of the unknown often heightens the impression of the level of pain experienced.

Narcotics. Narcotics such as Demerol® or morphine can be injected through an intravenous line or directly into the muscle of the patient. The level of pain relief is easily controlled by adjusting the dosage. Although these medications do not put the woman to sleep, they do take the edge off the discomfort associated with contractions, and allow her to rest or doze between contractions. In controlled doses, such medications rarely cause any problem for the baby if it is near term. Premature infants, however, are more susceptible, and these medicines should be decreased or eliminated during premature labor. An antihistamine-like drug is commonly used in combination with the narcotic to enhance its effect and to reduce the total narcotic dosage to the fetus.

Paracervical block. After the cervix has begun to dilate, the physician may inject a small amount of local anesthetic on either side of the cervix. This is designed to block the pain associated with dilation, and it is reasonably effective for most patients. Infrequently, slowing of the fetal heart rate results. Because of this, patients receiving a paracervical block are usually checked by external or internal electronic fetal monitoring.

Pudendal block. Shortly before delivery, the obstetrician may inject a small amount of local anesthetic through the side wall of the vagina to block the pudendal nerve. This nerve carries pain sensation from the lower portion of the vagina, and the area of the intended episiotomy between the vagina and the rectum. This block is designed to reduce discomfort resulting from birth of the head, and to anesthetize the tissues for repair of the episiotomy. It is the most commonly used method of anesthesia for vaginal delivery.

"Twilight sleep." In past years, Scopolamine was used with narcotic agents to produce a "twilight sleep" state. Although this did not appear to pose great risk to the infant, the mother was unable to cooperate or participate in the delivery. Mothers often failed to remember the labor or delivery itself. Today, twilight sleep is rarely used except in patients suffering intense emotional distress or in patients whose infants have died in the uterus, making amnesia a desired effect.

Epidural anesthesia. The greatest degree of pain relief in labor can be achieved by a continuous epidural anesthetic. The anesthesiologist places a small plastic catheter in the hollow of the lower back just outside the spinal sac. A local anesthetic is then injected continuously throughout labor and delivery for pain relief. Under epidural anesthesia, patients experience an almost complete numbness of the lower abdomen, legs, and external genitalia. Although the incidence of operative delivery is somewhat increased, the technique carries little additional risk for mother or baby. The degree of analgesia is even satisfactory for cesarean delivery if necessary.

Spinal block or "saddle block." In preparation for an operative delivery, the obstetrician may advise the use of a low spinal or "saddle block" anesthetic. Like an epidural, but at a lower level, this results in a loss of sensation in the pelvis, external genitals, and legs. The saddle block or low spinal is satisfactory for vaginal deliveries, and the spinal placed at a higher level provides excellent anesthesia for cesarean delivery. Both epidural and spinal anesthetics wear off gradually over a period of hours after delivery, depending on the type of anesthetic used and the dose administered.

General anesthesia. Except in midforceps deliveries, general anesthesia is rarely used for vaginal birth. A few patients wish to be asleep for delivery and should advise the attending physician as early as possible. Patients who are to undergo general anesthesia are often asked to consult with the anesthesiologist before their delivery to assess their history and to anticipate potential problems.

For cesarean delivery, in most cases the patient is free to choose between general, spinal, or epidural anesthesia. Occasionally, medical risk factors such as hypertension make one technique safer or more desirable than another. In these cases, the obstetrician or anesthesiologist will explain the need. Otherwise, the choice is a simple matter of whether the patient wishes to be asleep or awake during the birth process.

CHAPTER 27   ROBERT J. HAGGERTY, M.D.

TAKING CARE
OF YOUR CHILD

Pediatrics is the branch of medicine dealing with prevention and cure of disease in children. Dramatic changes have occurred in the past century in child health. At the turn of the century, one in three children died by age five, largely because of infectious diseases such as measles, diarrhea, diphtheria, and pneumonia. Today, as a result of public health advances such as pure water, food, and milk, and immunizations against infectious diseases, most children born alive will survive childhood. Antibiotic treatment of bacterial infections and other medical advances have helped, but most medical "miracles" affect only a few children, while public health measures have had an impact on millions.

Two-thirds of the deaths of children today occur in the first month of life and are related to being born too small, too early, or malformed. This most hazardous period of life has been termed "The Valley of the Shadow of Birth." Today parents can be assured that if a child is born at term with no malformations, the chances that he or she will survive to adulthood are 99 percent. By far the most common cause of death after the newborn period is accidents. The emphasis in child health has shifted from illnesses that are potentially fatal to those that are nonfatal and to prevention.

The major non-fatal health problems of children today are acute infections (colds, ear infections, sore throat, skin infections), accidents, and chronic illnesses (asthma, vision and hearing problems, epilepsy, and mental retardation). In addition, problems of behavior and learning have surfaced as among the most disturbing to children and parents. It is not likely that behavior and school learning disturbances are much more common today than in years past, although they may be different now when children must cope with a complex, mechanized society that has great expectations for its young. But serious physical diseases have declined so much that behavior problems stand out as disturbing and perplexing. Most acute illnesses such as colds, and most chronic problems such as behavior disturbances, will pass with time without any serious or lasting consequences.

Most children are well most of the time. Most problems that do arise can be thought of as normal processes. In only a few instances do serious complications occur. The challenge to parents and physicians is to recognize the difference between normal processes and complications, to learn not to worry needlessly about those that will clear with no specific therapy, and to avoid harmful interventions and anxiety. At the same time parents must learn to act effectively when those few important problems, both physical and behavioral, do occur. A good motto for parents is the old prayer: "God give me the serenity to accept those things that cannot be changed, the courage (and knowledge) to change those things that can be changed, and the wisdom to know the difference."

NORMAL PROCESSES

"Normal processes" are frequent, and they rarely lead to harmful long-term consequences unless they start a vicious cycle of anxiety and guilt or dangerous treatments. It helps parents if they know the range of normal variation and how to deal with minor deviations. As an example, breast-feeding, which is normally the best way to feed babies, can be difficult for some women. Failure can lead to a permanent sense of insecurity and lack of self-confidence. With help most problems can be overcome before that. It is important for parents and children to overcome and pass through such stages of "normal processes" with success. Each victory leads to increased ability to handle the next.

Parents have great wisdom and skill to handle these normal processes. However, they sometimes carry over fears of former times, when so many children did die, and they have had confidence in their own wisdom shaken by the development of experts and specialists. Parents sometimes feel that someone (the expert) must know how to handle a given problem of growing up better than they do. This chapter is dedicated to parents and their children, with faith that parents know more than they think they do about bringing up children, and that with a little knowledge and reassurance, plus the availability of a physician for occasional help, they will be the best parents for their child. For those few families faced with serious child illness, this chapter will discuss the more common and well-known examples, but the emphasis is on the normal, recognizing that self-reliance and time are great problem solvers. Unneeded interventions, both physical and behavioral, can have harmful consequences. Sometimes it is wise to "just stand there, don't do anything!"

Babies are individuals. We now recognize what parents have long known—that babies have different temperaments. Some are slow to warm up, others irritable, many are easygoing. There is a good deal of evidence that temperament tends to be present at birth and to persist. It helps to recognize the type of baby you have and adjust to him or her. Problems sometimes arise when parents wanted a placid baby but ended up with an irritable one. But each personality type has its strengths and weaknesses. One of the most difficult but important tasks for parents is to recognize the strengths of children and encourage these strengths, yet at the same time exert responsible influence to guide the children into habits the parents value.

Growth and development characterize children. Therefore their illnesses differ from adult illnesses mainly because they occur in developing or changing individuals. The same illness—pneumonia, for example—can be quite different for infants, in whom it may produce very little cough or sputum, compared to adults, in whom cough and sputum are characteristic. This chapter emphasizes growth and development because knowledge of this topic is essential to understand children's health problems and to distinguish the normal processes from the abnormal. Not every illness or deviation from normal growth and development can be covered. Many will be found in other chapters.

NORMAL PROCESSES THAT OFTEN CAUSE CONCERN

Feeding

In proportion to their life-span, humans have the longest period of childhood of any species. This is presumably to allow for growth and maturation of the brain, the distinctively large part of human anatomy. Growth of brain and body requires two major factors: food and sensory stimulation. The infant must grow from about seven pounds at birth to 21 to 28 pounds at one year (a three- to four-fold increase) and only to 120 to 180 pounds by maturity over the next 20 years. The absolute growth of 14 to 21 pounds in the first year of life is rarely exceeded in any other year.

"Breast is best" refers to the fact that breast milk by itself meets this incredible growth requirement for the first three or four months of an infant's life, and nearly completely meets it for the first six to eight months. But while breast-feeding is best for nutritional and psychological reasons, parents—yes, both parents—must be allowed to make the decision to breast-feed or not to breast-feed without coercion. The decision is best made before birth because there is so little time and so much happening after birth. But parents should not feel obligated to continue breast-feeding if it is not successful. Whatever the decision, babies can be fed safely and well with breast or formula. Neither choice should provoke feelings of guilt.

Breast-feeding has the advantage of providing all known nutritional requirements and probably some we do not know about. The one exception is vitamin D, which is often given as a supplement to breast milk. In nature enough vitamin D was produced in the skin through interaction between hormones and sunlight. But with clothing, northern climate, and indoor living, production sometimes is not sufficient. Even without supplemental vitamin D, however, few children show signs of deficiency. Breast-feeding is clean, provides protection against many infections, and can be provided easily as needed. This may result in somewhat irregular intervals compared to the four-hour schedule often prescribed for bottle-fed babies. But human infants were not made to feed regularly at four-hour intervals, and the breast is always ready for the irregular hunger or sucking needs, while even pre-bottled formula requires some preparation and cannot be adapted quite so easily to the individual baby.

Breast milk is also less likely to cause allergy and may result in less obesity later in life. Just as important, the physical contact between a breast-feeding mother and a nursing baby promotes bonding, a necessary first step in normal human development. Bonding of babies to mothers and fathers is a process of attachment. Although difficult to define, indicators of bonding in newborns include fondling, kissing, cuddling, and prolonged gazing. Artists have often captured this feeling better than writers. These behaviors, known to be essential to human survival and development, flow back and forth between parent and baby with each influencing the other. Bonding, of course, is as old as the human race and has been a major reason for its survival. There is debate over when it occurs. Some argue that the first few hours are crucial, but humans probably have much greater flexibility than that. If reasons do not permit contact in the first few hours, mothers can make up for it later. It can occur equally well no matter what type of feeding is used, but the physical contact of baby and breast helps.

Yet none of the advantages of breast-feeding are absolute. All can be compensated for if you decide to feed a formula. Most formulas are made from cow's milk. They are diluted with water to bring the higher protein concentration of cow milk closer to that of human milk, then sugar is added to increase the calories back to the level of breast milk.

One major advantage of bottle feeding is that the father can help feed the baby. In addition, the mother can have more freedom and the parents have the assurance of knowing how much milk has been taken.

Techniques of feeding. If you are planning to breast-feed, learn everything you can about the subject beforehand. Reading books on breast-feeding will help. So will personal advice from your physician or nurse practitioner, from other mothers, and from the La Leche League, a group that advocates and supports breast-feeding.

The baby should be put on the breast as soon as possible after delivery. The first feedings will yield a substance called colostrum rather than true milk, but this is an important source of antibodies to protect the baby against infections. True milk will not "come in" until three to five days after birth. With the 24- to 48-hour hospital stays that are now common after birth, this event usually occurs after the mother has returned home. Nonetheless, the baby should be fed during the hospital stay. Many hospitals now provide for "rooming in," in which the baby remains in the room with the mother. This not only allows the mother to become accustomed to caring for her new child, but also to feed him or her when crying occurs. Sucking stimulates milk production and can then be provided as needed. The baby will lose weight until milk comes in. The weight loss is normal and no cause for worry.

Nursing can be done sitting up or lying on your side, whichever is more comfortable. Place the nipple near the corner of the baby's mouth and he or she will turn to it (the rooting reflex) and start to suck. It is wise to alternate the breast offered first at each feeding. In the beginning, feedings are short but frequent.

Later the baby will settle into a more regular pattern of feeding every two to four hours for about 20 to 30 minutes, half on each breast. Some babies are fast feeders, others slow. Some feed more often than others. Remember that different babies have different temperaments, but rarely will one feed with clockwork regularity every four hours. Some feed as often as every two hours, although more frequent feedings than that should be avoided after the first few weeks, mainly because they tie the mother down. The schedule of feeding by bottle is similar.

Babies vary the amount they take at a feeding. Breast-fed babies stop feeding naturally when satisfied, but parents of bottle-fed babies sometimes become concerned when the child takes less than expected. Merely because the doctor has prescribed five ounces at a feeding does not mean that the baby will take this amount each time. Let the baby be the guide.

Sterilization of formula was formerly a big process. Now parents can buy prepared and sterilized formula in cans or bottles. It needs no refrigerated storage nor even warming before feeding (room temperature is fine). Be sure to store a bottle that has been partly used, however, because the bacteria from the baby's mouth will enter the bottle and grow at room temperature. You can keep a partly used bottle in a refrigerator for three to four hours, but it is best to discard it after that.

"Solid foods" for babies are really soft purees. They are usually started at about three or four months. There is no need to give a baby any foods except milk until that time. The one exception is orange juice, which can be started at three to four weeks. (Some babies develop a slight rash about the face after taking orange juice. This is rarely an allergy, but is more likely caused by contact with the slightly acidic juice. It is not a sign that orange juice should be discontinued.)

Some parents give thin cereal by bottle as early as six weeks, in the belief that it encourages the baby to sleep through the night. If longer intervals of sleep occur, it is probably because parents are reassured that the baby has had enough food and they then tolerate short periods of wakefulness without getting up to feed the baby.

When solids are begun, single-grain cereals such as rice or barley are the usual first choice. If the baby is being fed cow milk formula, cereals with added iron are preferable because less iron is absorbed from cow milk than human milk. The first serving is usually about one or two teaspoons, mixed with either formula or breast milk. The quantity can be gradually increased. A new food may then be added to the baby's diet every two to three weeks. A common sequence is fruits, then vegetables, then meats. Egg yolk is usually withheld until six to eight months, particularly if there is a family history of allergy. After nine to twelve months, babies can eat small mashed-up portions of whatever you eat. From six to nine months the baby can learn to drink from a cup and then can be switched to whole cow milk and weaned from breast to bottle, although some mothers prefer to continue to offer the breast, especially for solace, which both they and the baby receive, even after the first birthday.

Feeding and growth after the first year. In the second year, the incredible weight gain of the first 12 months slows and the baby's food intake diminishes. The decrease is perfectly normal and is no reason for alarm. Let the baby set his or her own intake, and do not enter into a struggle over feeding.

Most children appear chubby at one year, then gradually slim down until at four to six years they appear skinny. During this process, they eat much less avidly. In early adolescence girls in particular may appear fat again. A common complaint of parents when a child is five years old is "Why is he or she so skinny?" At 14, for the same child, the question becomes "Why is he or she so fat?" In fact, both stages are normal. If the child is gaining, growing, and feels well, differences in size are not important.

Parents are often more concerned about eating patterns of adolescents than of babies. Social pressure, seeking of independence from the family, altered daily life schedules, and availability of quick snacks outside the home lead to parental worry about irregular eating hours, junk foods, and adolescent fads. Little is known about the long-term effects of these commonly used foods, but in the short term if the child is not gaining more than expected or is not losing weight, there is little evidence that irregular eating schedules or junk foods are harmful.

Growth in Infancy

Physical growth has two dimensions: height and weight. Individual babies have different rates of growth but these rates are usually steady. That's another way of saying some babies grow faster than others. Doctors find it useful to plot height (really length in infants since it is measured lying down) and weight on charts that express various normal rates. These charts are constructed by measuring a group of well children at different ages. The bottom line is called the third percentile. A child growing steadily along this line is perfectly normal, even though he or she may be considerably smaller than one growing along the 97th percentile line. To say that a child is on the third percentile line means that of every 100 normal babies, three are smaller. If the child is on the 97th percentile, 97 percent of normal children are smaller. When a child is on the 50th percentile line, half of normal children are smaller and half larger. But all are *normal* growth patterns.

Body proportions change remarkably from birth to maturity. Legs are short in proportion to trunk at birth, and the head is large compared to the rest of the body. At birth, the head is about one-fourth of body length; at puberty, it is only one-seventh. Despite the head's size at birth, it still has a lot of growing to do, mostly in the first year of life. Your doctor will measure and plot the circumference of the head on the same growth charts as height and weight. A head that grows too fast or too slowly demands a thorough medical checkup.

These differences in growth simply emphasize the wide but normal variation among humans. A child growing along the 25th percentile line compared to one on the third will be three pounds heavier at one year, although both may have started at the same birth weight. Growth can only be meaningful when it is compared over time, and when height and weight are studied together. There is nothing intrinsically more healthy about a 97th percentile child than a third percentile child, any more than there is about a child with blond hair compared to a brunette. In most children, both height and length are near the same percentile, and heredity is the main determinant. Unfortunately, because Americans tend to feel that bigger is better, parents of a smaller child tend to become worried. Steady growth along any one percentile is one of the best signs of good health, no matter what the percentile.

Underweight and Overweight

Parents are often worried about the five- or six-year-old child who appears skinny and eats little. Plotting height and weight over the years is the most useful test of whether this is reason for concern. If growth has followed a steady pattern, there is usually no abnormality. A five-year-old can be expected to gain only four to five pounds a year compared to 14 to 18 in the first year of life. Naturally one needs to eat less to gain less. Unless there are other signs of illness, children at five who eat little yet are slow but steady gainers are normal. Children who lose weight while eating well, or who fall from one percentile to another in height and weight, should be evaluated by a physician.

A much more important problem in the Western world is overweight, which usually becomes apparent in adolescence and persists into adult life. There are no simple answers, however, to prevention or treatment of obesity. Since obesity is ultimately caused by too many calories or not enough exercise, it is wise to help adolescents develop skills and pride in activities that demand some amount of exercise, and to maintain examples at home of balanced, regular, and moderate-calorie meals. So-called glandular troubles (too little thyroid hormone) do not cause obesity. The obese child is usually taller than average in early adolescence, while the hypothyroid child is usually shorter. Successful weight loss or obesity prevention is almost always the result of individual, family, and peer interaction, not the physician's magic or pill. Peer group weight-reduction programs for adolescents and adults have been successful, but rapid weight loss should be avoided because it almost always is followed by regaining of excess weight. Managing obesity is a lifelong process.

Adolescent Growth

Adolescence is a time when every boy and girl feels different and is very sensitive to the differences. It is quite natural that slightly earlier or later onset of growth spurt or puberty will cause great anxiety. The exact reason why the growth spurt of adolescence starts is not known, but heredity and nutrition play important roles. Girls start their growth about two years before boys, and there has been a trend to increasingly early onset of puberty in both sexes over the past 100 years, probably as a result of better nutrition.

As early as age eight, girls may begin to have breast enlargement, although ten to twelve years is more common. The first menstrual period usually occurs two years later. On average, girls in the United States begin to menstruate at 12.4 years today, but many start as young as 10.

In boys, no similar dramatic event announces the arrival of puberty. However, from 10 to 14 years, growth of the penis, pubic hair, underarm, chest and facial hair, and muscle mass occur. Most of the questions raised by boys and girls concern late or inadequate growth and development of breasts and penis, although in rare cases a girl's increase in height to six feet or more worries parents and the girl a great deal. Such growth can be stopped with female sex hormones, but such therapy is rarely needed and must be supervised carefully by a physician (see chapter 16, "The Hormones and Endocrine Glands").

Late onset of puberty is a major social problem for both boys and girls. While sex hormones can expedite the customary sex changes, they are rarely needed and can have harmful side effects. The best advice for adolescents who fail to start puberty as soon as their peers, or who feel too tall, too short, too big, or too little, is to see a doctor to be sure that no treatable disease is responsible, then to accept that size differences are normal and one of the things that make humans so interesting.

Development: A Wholistic Approach

Growth is increase in size, while development is an increase in complexity of function. Mostly, that means neurological and psychologic function, and most of our measures of development in children are expressed in neurologic or psychologic ways—walking, talking, or thinking. Rapid changes in function as well as size are characteristic of childhood. But it is important to recognize the relationship between development and health in children, and to recognize that we cannot separate humans into separate spheres of physical and psychological development or illness. All illnesses in children have developmental implications, and development in turn affects when, how, and sometimes whether a child becomes ill.

CHILD DEVELOPMENT LANDMARKS

MONTH	NORMAL VARIATION	ACCOMPLISHMENT	
1	2 weeks	Smiles	
2	2 weeks	Coos	
3	2 weeks	Holds head up	
4	3 weeks	Grasps object	
5	3 weeks	Rolls from back to front	
6	3 weeks	Sits alone	
7	3 weeks	Crawls	
8	3 weeks	Uses pincer grasp	

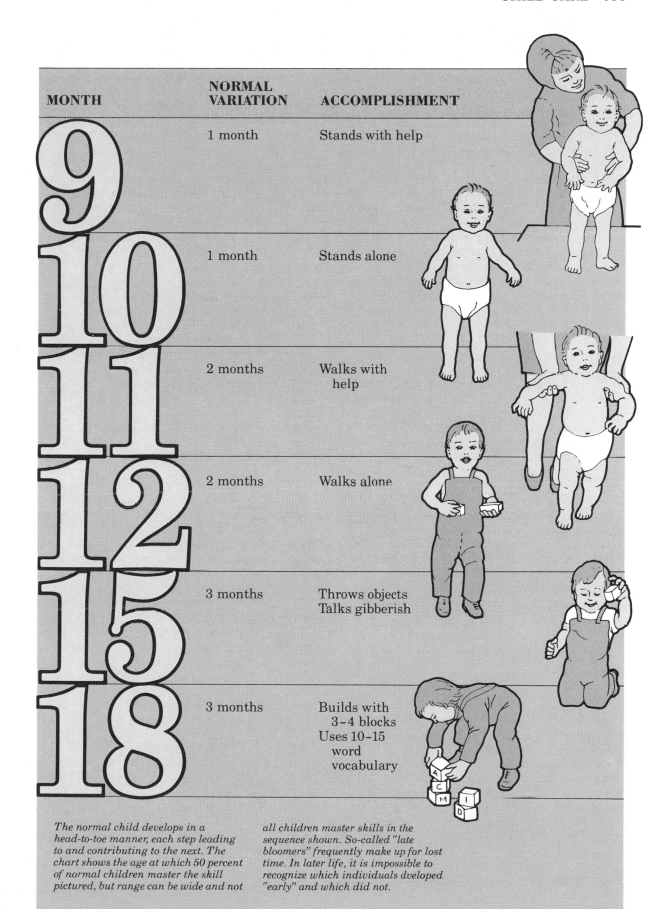

MONTH	NORMAL VARIATION	ACCOMPLISHMENT
9	1 month	Stands with help
10	1 month	Stands alone
11	2 months	Walks with help
12	2 months	Walks alone
15	3 months	Throws objects Talks gibberish
18	3 months	Builds with 3–4 blocks Uses 10–15 word vocabulary

The normal child develops in a head-to-toe manner, each step leading to and contributing to the next. The chart shows the age at which 50 percent of normal children master the skill pictured, but range can be wide and not

all children master skills in the sequence shown. So-called "late bloomers" frequently make up for lost time. In later life, it is impossible to recognize which individuals dveloped "early" and which did not.

The process of development. Development proceeds in a head-to-toe sequence. The first parts of the nervous system to increase complexity of functioning after birth are the brain and the cranial nerves.

The first evidence of a new skill in a baby is the ability to smile, a function that helps ensure survival of the human race. The smile that comes in response to a mother or father at two to four weeks of age or earlier "hooks" the parent. The bonding process that starts at birth is then cemented. Each new stage is exciting to watch, but is just as much an interaction with the baby's environment as the first smile. The chart on page 632 lists easily observed developmental tasks of the first 18 months and the average age when they are accomplished. As with physical growth, there are wide variations. But note that during the first year the characteristic new skill added each month takes place lower and lower on the body, an example of head-to-toe development.

There are many other important developmental tasks as more complex motor skills develop together with language, social interactions, personality, and moral-ethical development. We now recognize that development goes on throughout life. The pace slackens in adulthood and becomes more difficult to change. However, change is a biological characteristic.

A delay in development that occurs early in life is likely to be more profound and have greater consequences than delays that occur later. Thus a physician will test the baby's development at each visit to assess progress. Any unusual delay needs to be evaluated. Some are caused by lack of stimulation in the environment. Others are caused by diseases, either congenital or acquired.

Common Developmental Concerns

A number of symptoms that often concern parents should be considered separately from disease because they are variations of normal development and rarely, if ever, lead to any persistent problem.

Constipation is a condition of excessively hard stool with difficulty of passage, sometimes leading to painful rectum. It is not defined by the frequency of stools. A soft stool passed without difficulty, even at intervals of every second or third day, is perfectly normal. The importance of a daily bowel movement has been overemphasized in the past. Consistency of the stool, not frequency, is the criterion.

Children are frequently constipated after an acute illness because they drink and eat less and thus have fewer fluids. Others are chronically constipated as a result of a diet containing little fiber. An all-milk diet may lead to hard stools in babies. Usually all that is necessary to relieve constipation is to add fruits and vegetables to the diet. Children should avoid laxatives, suppositories, or enemas. In early infancy, great difficulty in passing stool that is unrelieved by adding fruit to the diet should be brought to the attention of the physician.

A common problem is constipation related to toilet training (see below). Some children rebel against the compulsory or threatening environment, hold in their stool, and finally produce a large and hard stool. The stool is hard because the water it normally contains has been reabsorbed by the bowel. Passage may cause a small, painful fissure in the rectum, which sets up a cycle of further stool withholding, pain, and more fissures. If this problem occurs, see your physician.

Toilet training is an important stage of development that is not always accomplished serenely and can be exhausting for both parent and child. Fortunately the conflicts rarely have lasting effects.

Bowel training usually comes before bladder training. It is usually begun about the middle of the second year, but individual children vary in when they are ready. Most children have a reflex some 20 minutes after eating that stimulates their bowels to move. They usually give some indication—grunting, straining—that the reflex is occurring. When the parents recognize the sign, the child can then be placed on the potty chair.

It seems best to use a small, free-standing potty chair rather than a seat attached to a full-size toilet, because the height and flushing action frighten some children. The child should be left on the chair for five to ten minutes at most, then removed if there is no result. Don't scold, push, wheedle or coax, or show that the child can irritate you by withholding the bowel movement.

Bowel training occurs at a time when children are normally going through what is called "the terrible twos." Problems arise if parents allow the normal two-year-old struggle for independence to carry over to bowel training. Withholding a bowel movement is a way a child can show a parent who is boss. Playing with feces is another expression of independence.

MAJOR EVENTS OF ADOLESCENCE

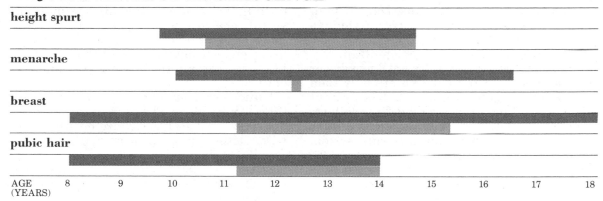

height spurt

menarche

breast

pubic hair

AGE (YEARS)   8   9   10   11   12   13   14   15   16   17   18

The four major events of female adolescence are height spurt, breast development, growth of pubic hair, and onset of menstruation. The orange bars show the ages at which the events occur for the average girl. The brown bars represent the range of ages at which the events may occur in other normal girls.

Breast development in the average girl covers four years, hair growth about three years. The figures on the bars represent stages of each. The average age of first menstruation is 12.4 years. First menstruation is normally a late event in puberty, occurring after the growth rate has slowed.

KEY

Brown— Range of ages at which events occur

Orange—Average age span of occurrence

Bladder training usually occurs after bowel control has been achieved, although in some children both developmental achievements occur simultaneously. The process of bladder training is the same as with bowel training. When a child indicates that he or she is about to urinate by moving about or holding the genitals, or at regular intervals after meals, help him or her to the potty. However, if urination does not occur, don't get upset, even if the child urinates immediately after you have buttoned his or her clothing. Most children achieve daytime urine control by three or four years, although there is wide variation among individual children. The keys are patience, praise for success, and attention to the child's signs of readiness.

Nighttime bladder control takes longer. One reason may be development of bladder capacity. The bladder needs to be large enough to store the urine produced overnight. About 10 percent of children do not achieve nighttime dryness by age six.

Some now advise a "one day" stimulus-response or behavior modification approach to training. It has been successful for parents who are able to follow the plan. It should be emphasized that most children train successfully without this effort and there is no evidence that different methods of training or early or late training makes much difference in the long run. Use the training method that seems natural and discuss it with your physician if you have questions.

Bed-wetting or enuresis is a troublesome issue that occurs at some time in most children (see chapter 22, "The Kidneys and Urinary System"). A child who has previously been dry often may regress to bed-wetting after an illness, after moving to a new home, or after the arrival of a baby in the family. Some extra time and attention for the child are all that is needed for this temporary setback.

There has been considerable debate about causes of persistent bed-wetting. Allergy, diabetes, abnormalities or infections of the urinary tract, or serious psychiatric problems are sometimes held responsible. These are doubtful explanations in the absence of other symptoms, and extensive laboratory studies for bed-wetting are seldom justified. A simple urinalysis is sufficient. Bed-wetting is a developmental problem, like late walking or talking. The nerves that control the bladder muscles may be slower to mature than in other children. The fact that bed-wetting runs in families supports this explanation. In any case, the majority of otherwise normal children who are bed wetters pass through this developmental problem without signs of other difficulties. But the tolerance of a mother who has to change a wet bed morning after morning is limited, and the sense of insecurity provoked in a child explains why parents seek any solution and doctors are willing to try anything to help. The secondary reactions usually are far more damaging than the symptom itself.

Treatment is not necessary until age five or six, because so many children are only then developing nighttime control. The parent should avoid blame or scolding, but place responsibility with the child. Restricting fluids before bedtime, and using a reward system (stars on a chart, praise, or other rewards) for dry nights may help. Some parents awaken the child after two to three hours, or set an alarm for the child. Mild medications and alarm systems can be prescribed by your doctor.

Breath-holding. Some small children suddenly hold their breath when punished, hurt, frightened, or when denied some request. They stop breathing for what seems an eternity to the frightened parent. Some even turn slightly blue around the mouth. Then with a few deep gasps, they resume breathing normally. There are no ill effects, except that the worried parent quite naturally may give in to the child's wishes. The attacks cease when the child is about four years old.

Temper tantrums are similar to breath-holding spells. Under stress of being refused, punished, or frustrated, the child will appear to lose control with stamping, shouting behavior. Tantrums appear to be part of the process of achieving autonomy for two-year-olds, and cease by four or five (although we all know adults who use similar tactics to achieve their ends). Firmness, consistency of punishment, and at times isolating the child in his or her room until the attack subsides are useful.

Head-banging and rocking. Many children go through a period of rhythmical movements of the head against a solid object such as a crib, mattress, or headboard. Or they may rock the entire body, usually in bed before going to sleep. It usually occurs in the one- to three-year-old and appears to be a pleasurable experience. Most of these children are entirely normal and outgrow the practice with no treatment and no consequences. Sometimes it is useful to pad the crib or to secure the bed to prevent it from moving. If the practice persists after three, or if it is accompanied by lack of social interaction, failure to play with other children, or self-stimulating behavior such as compulsive masturbation, it is useful to talk to a physician.

Thumb-sucking, nail-biting, and hair-pulling. For some children, these almost universal behaviors become persistent and seem to be a way of relieving tension. It is wise to avoid punishment for these common behaviors, but to reward the absence or elimination of them.

Colic is common in babies during the first three months of life. The causes are not known, but colicky babies usually are healthy otherwise, despite prolonged periods of crying, usually at night. There is no way to tell whether the baby is in pain, although many may draw up their legs, turn red in the face, and sometimes strain as if about to have a bowel movement. Hunger may be a cause, although sucking seems to be more of a need than actual hunger. Try a pacifier, swaddling, feeding, burping, rocking, and carrying. Sometimes when the parents' sleep loss is great, doctors prescribe medication, although there is little evidence that it does much good other than to reassure the parents. It seems as if this is part of temperament. Many babies with colic are irritable, vigorous, and hard to soothe; yet, these same traits when they grow up become important for success. Indeed, colicky babies do seem to grow up to be more driving. The main problem is the parents' sense of guilt and failure. The condition seldom persists beyond the first six months.

Cradle cap is a common skin condition of babies. The cause is unknown. The condition appears as a thick scaling or crusted patch on the scalp, and is not related to frequency of bathing. It probably stems from oil glands of the scalp that are not developed fully (see chapter 7, "The Skin"). Cradle cap is treated by removing the scab or crusts by softening with baby oil or petroleum jelly (yes, oil on oil!), gently combing out the scales with a fine-tooth baby comb, then shampooing. Most babies need a shampoo only twice a week, but a baby with cradle cap may benefit from daily shampoos. The condition clears completely with time, although such a child may have oily skin in adulthood, too.

Diaper rash is caused by the irritant effect of urine-soaked diapers on the baby's sensitive skin. Changing diapers often, leaving the baby "open to the air," and using talc, corn starch, or baby powders all help (but be sure the baby doesn't inhale the talc). Occasionally, the raw wounds of the rash become infected with bacteria, in which case antibiotic ointments and soaks may be needed.

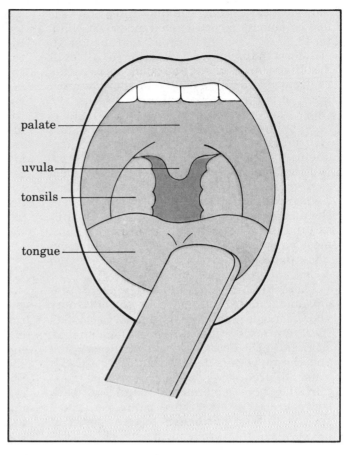

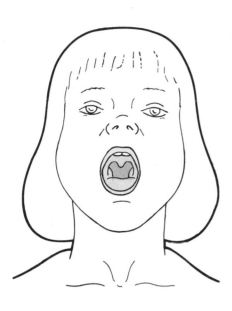

ENLARGED TONSILS

Swollen and inflamed tonsils in the throat can readily be seen, especially when the child's tongue is depressed (right drawing). The enlargement usually occurs during and after periods of infection, because tonsils are part of the body's system for fighting disease. Sometimes the tonsils themselves become infected. Bouts of "tonsillitis" usually decline as the child grows older, and removal of the tonsils and adenoids, which are related tissue at the back of the nasal passages, is less common than in the past.

Teething usually begins about six months of age and proceeds until the 20 primary teeth are in place, generally by age two years (see chapter 18, "The Teeth and Oral Health"). Some children are cranky during teething, but this normal process does not cause fever, convulsions, or other problems previously attributed to it. Rather the teething child is simultaneously being exposed to common infections, which are the cause of the fever and irritability. Since teething goes on almost continuously from 6 to 24 months, infections and teething are sometimes bound to coincide. Rubbing the gums with a finger or providing teething biscuits, a chilled rubber ring, or plastic teething devices that can be filled with water and chilled in the refrigerator are all that is needed.

Thrush is a mild fungus infection of the mouth that produces a cheesy gray-white material that sticks to tongue and cheeks. The fungus (monilia) is often acquired from the mother's birth canal during delivery and therefore manifests itself during the first few weeks of a baby's life. It can be easily treated with a mild fungicide prescribed by a doctor. The baby's mouth should be cleaned with water after feedings.

Tonsils and adenoids. Most parents do not think of tonsil and adenoid conditions as normal processes. Yet most alleged disorders of these organs are really normal, and removing them by operation, previously the most common surgical procedure in the United States, is less commonly recommended today (see chapter 13, "Ear, Nose, and Throat" and chapter 31, "Understanding Your Operation"). All children have large tonsils and adenoids as part of their normal development. These organs play a key role in defense against infections. Because the preschool and school-age child is repeatedly exposed to strange bacteria and viruses, the tonsils and adenoids are frequently enlarged and may become infected. But removal merely for frequent throat infections is not needed and will not reduce the frequency of infections. As children grow older, the number of infections drops as their immunity builds. Therefore, after a tonsillectomy, most children will have fewer throat infections, but so will children of the same age who do not have the operation.

There is still considerable difference of opinion among doctors as to when tonsillectomy and adenoidectomy are justified. Some feel there are no legitimate reasons for removal, citing also the potential risks of surgery and anesthesia. Others believe that there are still some children who benefit. There is no question that there is increasing scepticism about the operations. Fewer are being performed each year. With antibiotics to treat bacterial infections of the throat (primarily streptococcal sore throat), few children have complications of tonsillar infection, which leaves one less reason to consider removal of tonsils. Only when tonsils and adenoids are so large that they obstruct breathing is removal indicated. Even then, waiting several months will usually bring enough improvement that no operation is necessary.

If your doctor recommends tonsillectomy or adenoidectomy, you may want to ask for a second opinion. Physicians have honest differences about this issue.

Sleep disturbances in children are common. Infants vary in when they begin to sleep through the night. Usually it occurs around six to eight weeks (to the great relief of their parents). During the second year of life, many children resist going to bed or awaken during the night, frequently coming into the parents' bed. It can be safely stated that no child ever suffered from sleep deprivation at this age, although parents surely have. It is advisable to establish a quiet routine for bedtime and a firm deadline for going, with no wavering response to requests for "one more drink of water." Similarly, when a child awakens in the night, go to the bedside once to assure yourself that everything is in order, then firmly ignore the crying after that. This may cause a very unhappy household for a day or two but the child soon learns to go back to sleep after 10 to 15 minutes. Nothing can make otherwise normal parents become disturbed more quickly than loss of sleep night after night, but avoid giving sleeping medicine of any kind for this distressing situation.

It is also important to recognize that children vary in the amount of sleep they need, just as they vary in other ways. There is nothing magic about any given amount of sleep.

COMMON PROBLEMS

It is useful for parents to realize that temporary disruptions such as diarrhea, vomiting, and respiratory infections are common, affecting virtually every child at some time in life. These common problems are only slight deviations from normal processes, and rarely have any long-term consequences. Parents need to understand how to manage these temporary upsets, yet be aware of the rare instances when they should seek advice from a physician.

Diarrhea

Development occurs in the biochemical reactions of the body as well as in the nervous system. Certain enzymes are poorly developed at birth, but increase with age. Kidney function at birth is quite different than it is later, because the newborn's kidneys do not concentrate their urine (do not conserve water) as much as those of adults. This enables the baby to lose some of the water present at birth. Infants have a larger proportion of their body composed of water (nearly 80 percent) than at any other time in life, so aging can be thought of as a gradual process of drying out. But if a baby develops diarrhea in the first weeks of life, he or she has greater trouble conserving water as a result.

A baby also has a much smaller margin of safety in water needs and water reserves than does an adult. A 10-pound baby has more than three quarts of water in the body, but takes in nearly one quart a day, whereas an adult weighing 150 pounds has nearly 50 quarts of body water, but takes in only two to three quarts of fluid daily. If water intake is diminished or if the water loss is increased by vomiting or diarrhea for only a day, the infant can quickly become dehydrated. The smaller the baby, the greater the danger.

All babies get diarrhea occasionally. Most instances in the United States are caused by common viruses, for which there is no specific treatment. The main requirement is to supply fluids to the baby until the infection has run its course. Commonly used treatments such as paregoric or kaopectate are of no value in babies' diarrhea, and may do harm by lulling the parent into a sense of complacency that the disease is being treated while neglecting the needed fluids.

Most children with diarrhea, even if it is combined with vomiting, can take small amounts of fluid repeatedly to maintain the vital balance. Cola, ginger ale (with the fizz out), apple juice, or weak tea are all good ways to provide fluids. A baby up to two years of age needs 2½ to 3 ounces of fluid per pound of body weight each 24 hours. Watching the behavior or vigor of the baby, the urine output, and weight are all important in treatment and evaluation of the baby with diarrhea. If the baby loses weight, decreases urine output, becomes listless, or if there is bloody diarrhea, a physician should be called.

Breast-fed babies frequently have very soft, yellow stools. This is not diarrhea. Green stool is of importance only because it signifies more rapid passage of stool before the green bile has had a chance to be changed to brown or yellow. It is the water loss, not the color of the stool, that is important.

Vomiting

Vomiting in infants and children is another common symptom associated with a variety of conditions, because it is one of the few ways that infants can respond to disease. The most common causes are bacterial infections, sometimes with diarrhea, or ear or general viral infections. If vomiting begins suddenly in a previously healthy child who remains alert and who has not had a head injury, the treatment is to withhold everything by mouth until vomiting stops and for one to three hours thereafter. Then give small amounts of clear fluid every 20 minutes, starting with one-half tablespoon and gradually increasing to one-half ounce. The frequency then can be decreased and amounts increased. For older children, cracked ice or popsicles are good

Preparation of Children for Hospitalization

When hospitalization is planned, children should be fully prepared so they avoid psychological trauma that may lead to night fears afterward and even delay recovery. Children of ages one to five fear separation from home and familiar surroundings most, while five- to ten-year-olds fear the trauma of surgery and tests. Most hospitals now permit a parent to stay with a young child to minimize this trauma. Many hospitals also offer day surgery. The child is admitted to the hospital in the morning, the operation is performed, and the child is sent home later in the day when the anesthesia has worn off. Recovery occurs at home and separation trauma is avoided.

Telling the child a few days before hospitalization what to expect, reading from one of the many excellent books available to prepare children for hospitalization (ask your doctor for suggestions), staying with your child in the hospital, and providing recreation programs (often called child-life programs) in the hospital have been shown to prevent the potentially harmful effects.

sources of fluids. Almost all children with simple infectious causes of vomiting will respond in 24 to 36 hours. In babies under one month, or when vomiting is accompanied by such symptoms as drowsiness or abdominal pain, you should call a physician.

Vomiting, like diarrhea, is a common symptom, usually easily managed with no serious consequences. However, the task of parents and the child's physician is to distinguish the rare instance that indicates a more serious problem from the great bulk of cases in which children recover promptly. Medicines are sometimes prescribed but are of less importance. Simple treatment to prevent dehydration is the most effective approach.

Fever

Fever in childhood differs from fever in adults. Children can be thought of as being born immunologic virgins. Babies inherit antibodies from the mother against most infections, but the immunity ends by four to six months of age. For the next 10 years, children develop their immunity by acquiring infections. Each child must have about 100 immunizing infections before growing up. That means about 10 to 12 common infections per year on the average for the first 10 years of life. Not all of these produce symptoms. Some occur without the parent (or child) being aware of them. But most make their presence known. Runny nose, cough, or diarrhea are common, but the cardinal symptom is fever, a marked increase in body temperature above the "normal" reading of 98.6 Fahrenheit.

Parents should learn to take a child's temperature by rectum (up to age six years), but not become a slave to the thermometer. If the child is active and alert, high fever by itself usually does not warrant treatment. Most parents and many doctors like to give aspirin or acetaminophen, an aspirin substitute, the amount dependent on age. One reason is to ward off a complication of high fever unique to children—a febrile convulsion or fit. Five percent of children will have a febrile convulsion sometime in life, most commonly between two and four years. We now know that treating fever once it appears is unlikely to prevent these convulsions. Most occur early in the course of the fever, but convulsions, even brief ones, are worrying to all. This worry leads most of us to use a medicine to bring down fevers, something more useful for comfort than to prevent convulsions.

If the child is active, is taking fluids well, and (for older children) does not complain of headache or muscle ache, aspirin is not recommended merely for fever. It is much more important to determine whether there are uncommon symptoms or complications requiring a physician's attention.

The best guide for a parent, one experienced pediatricians learn to use, is how well or sick the child looks. A parent is in the best position to judge how a child acts with a fever compared to the normal state. Even with a temperature of 103 to 104 degrees, a child who is alert and eating well is rarely seriously ill.

Treatment of fever. If fever makes a child uncomfortable, aspirin (60 milligrams per year of age every four hours) can be given safely. Baby aspirins come in 75 milligram size and are safe for children 10 to 12 months of age. Liquid preparations of acetaminophen are also good as a fever-reducing agent. The dose is the same as for aspirin. With either preparation, it is extremely important to prevent overdose. Children's dose strength should be used for anyone under five years of age. Follow the di-

rections carefully. If the child is under one year of age you should consult your physician for dosage.

Always return the fever medicine to a safe storage place after each use. If it is left on a bedside table, the sick child or another child may accidentally ingest them. It takes only 12 adult-size aspirin to produce serious poisoning in a two-year-old child. Safety caps help, but sometimes parents leave the cap off between doses and accidents occur.

The best treatment of most fever is time. Suppositories of aspirin, alcohol or water sponging, enemas, and other time-honored ways of lowering fever are not very effective and a few are dangerous. Sponging a child with alcohol can be painful if there are cuts, and the alcohol can be absorbed through the skin. Of the old methods, the best is to place the child who is old enough to sit without support into a tub of tepid (not cold) water and gently sponge the entire body. This treatment will reduce fever and promote comfort.

Upper Respiratory Infections

The common cold is the most common illness of children. Familiar to all, the symptoms can include the well-known running nose, slight fever, headache, muscle ache, and slight cough. There is still no known treatment, except aspirin to reduce fever and ease muscle ache, and time. The nasal congestion may produce noisy, somewhat difficult breathing in small babies. It is best treated with an infant nasal aspirator, a small rubber bulb to remove the secretions by suction. Nose drops (¼ percent neosynephrine) and oral decongestants are widely used but are unwise in babies under six months of age because they can cause stimulation. There is no evidence that they benefit older children, but if used as directed they do no harm and appear to make some children feel better temporarily.

Upper respiratory infections may lead to ear infections or pneumonia if air passages become obstructed and elimination of bacteria is decreased. In some children with allergies, ear infection may be associated with wheezing and sometimes is the first clue to what later becomes asthma. However, the vast majority recover completely without consequences.

Bronchiolitis is a common infection in babies, usually those under two years of age. It is caused by several different viruses. The signs are wheezing (like asthma), cough and slight fever. Most babies have one or more bouts of bronchiolitis when growing up, the vast majority with no serious consequences.

THE NEW THERMOMETER

The traditional thermometer measures body temperature via a column of mercury in a glass tube. It is illustrated, along with directions for its use, in chapter 35. Several new types of thermometers have been introduced, one of which is shown here. When the instrument is placed in the mouth, yellow dots of chemicals change to a molten form and turn red. The Celsius type shown here gives a reading within 60 seconds and is easier to read than three-minute glass types. However, it cannot be used rectally. Other types use chemically impregnated strips that are placed on the forehead. Although traditional glass models are said to be more accurate, precise readings are seldom critical in home care.

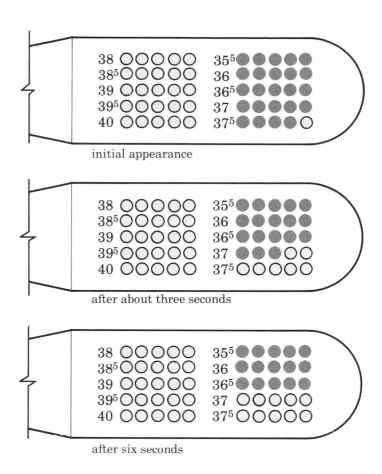

initial appearance

after about three seconds

after six seconds

There is no effective treatment but time. Rarely, children will become fatigued as a result of the labored breathing and require hospitalization for oxygen and even breathing assistance. A good home remedy, as it is for croup, is to take the child into a bathroom, turn on the shower to produce mist, and sit in a chair with the child in your lap in the mist-filled room.

Common Contagious Diseases

There are a few common contagious diseases against which we have no immunizing agent.

Chickenpox (technically called varicella) is contracted by all children at some point, although in a few instances the encounter may be delayed until young adulthood. A vaccine is being developed but is not yet available. The illness is caused by a type of herpes virus, which also causes shingles in adults. In fact, the virus lives in the body after childhood ex-posure to chickenpox, then is reactivated years later to produce shingles. The incubation period of chickenpox is 12 to 19 days after exposure. Symptoms are fever (usually mild) and headache, followed in a day or two by the characteristic rash which starts as a small red spot, rapidly progressing to a pinhead size blister which turns to a scab in three or four days. The amount of rash varies in different children. Some have only one or two blisters, while others have a mass that covers the entire body, sometimes including the scalp and inside of the mouth. The blisters are itchy and secondary infections occur as a result of scratching. Any commercial preparation of calamine lotion or an antihistamine may reduce the itch. The disease usually ends in a week.

Roseola is a contagious disease for which the cause has not been identified. It occurs largely in children six months to two years, starting with a high fever and irritability. After three to five days the fever drops to normal and in a few hours there is a characteristic rash—pink flat spots, especially on the trunk. This rash rarely lasts longer than 24 hours.

Roseola is a mild disease, but a puzzling one because of the high fever without other telltale signs. Once the rash appears the fever has disappeared, the child feels better, and parents and doctors are relieved to have a diagnosis. Treatment consists only of the methods to reduce fever. Rarely does the disease recur.

Several other contagious diseases also produce rashes. They are usually milder than roseola and may have characteristic symptoms or signs.

Erythema infectiosum produces a rash, largely on the cheeks—a "slapped cheeks" look. This occurs largely during school years.

Other rash diseases are nonspecific and must be labeled as "another virus." Most are benign. It sometimes helps to call your doctor, who will know what is "going around" in your community and be able to advise you on its cause or severity.

Conjunctivitis ("pink eye") is inflammation of the whites of the eye and the eyelids. It may accompany one of the viral diseases described above, it may be the only symptom of a virus infection, or it may result from an allergy, foreign body, or bacteria (see chapter 12, "The Eyes"). Itching is common in allergy-caused conjunctivitis but not in the other cases. Bacterial conjunctivitis usually causes more pus. Treatment of common viral conjunctivitis is not usually necessary. Mild eye washes may bring comfort, but if pain or pus is present, consult your physician.

Immunizations. With the exception of sanitation and pure food, immunizations have produced more improvement in the health of children in the past 100 years than any other scientific advance. Among once-prevalent diseases for which we now routinely immunize are diphtheria, pertussis (whooping cough), tetanus, measles, mumps, rubella, and poliomyelitis. (The immunizations commonly given, with the standard age of administration, are listed on page 644.)

All immunizations use the same principle: A small dose of killed germs, a modified toxin, or a weakened live virus is administered to build the body's natural defenses against the disease. There is a slight risk involved, but there are risks with all treatments. Risks for the standard immunizations are small and benefits far outweigh them. In the case of smallpox, immunization has wiped out the disease, and now the small risk of reaction to the vaccine is greater than the risk of the disease, so the vaccine is no longer given.

In addition to the standard immunizations, vaccines are sometimes given for specific diseases under special circumstances, such as influenza vaccine during epidemics or pneumococcal vaccine for children with poor defense against the germ. Children (and adults) are immunized before travel to certain parts of the world.

The most important thing for parents is to see that their baby receives the usual full immunizations at the proper time and that they keep their own record.

While it is important for doctors to know the signs and symptoms of these diseases against which we now immunize children, there is no need to list them here. The parent whose child is immunized will never need to know symptoms of these once common diseases.

Certain immunizations, such as the one used against poliomyelitis, cause very rare reactions. Polio vaccine uses a live but weakened virus, and it does cause illness in one or two persons per 10,000,000, mainly adults. The combined diphtheria-pertussis-tetanus inoculation, known as DPT, causes frequent but mild swelling at the site of injection, along with fever and irritability. If the child is uncomfortable after an immunization, aspirin or acetaminophen can be given and you should inform your physician before the next dose.

SERIOUS ACUTE ILLNESSES

Most acute childhood illnesses are self-limited, cause no long-term consequences, and require no treatment. A few acute illnesses, however, mostly infections, do not follow this rule. They require prompt diagnosis and treatment, which may be life-saving. Croup and meningitis are two examples. Others are milder, but effective treatment is available and they should not be ignored. Ear infections and pneumonia are in this group. Another category is the acute problems of the newborn.

Croup is marked by noisy breathing when inhaling (in contrast to asthma or bronchiolitis, which involve wheezing during exhaling). Most cases are caused by an acute infection which causes swelling in and around the larynx. Since the child's larynx is smaller than an adult's, even a very slight swelling can cause noisy breathing. As the larynx grows, croup becomes less common and cases are rare after age five. Some children have repeated attacks without much fever or other signs of a cold or infection. When there is little fever and only mild in-drawing of the chest with each breath, treatment with steam is usually sufficient. Take the child into the bathroom, turn

Common Misconceptions About Infections

Colds, sore throat, and diarrhea do *not* result from getting wet or chilled, although other stressful events do reduce resistance in some children. All are caused by germs, mainly common viruses. In addition to cases in which symptoms make the illness evident, many more children carry the germs but show no signs or symptoms. Most immunity, in fact, comes from these asymptomatic infections. Thus when your child has a mild upper respiratory infection but otherwise feels well, you can send him or her to school, for he or she poses no greater risk to others than the many asymptomatic children carrying the same germ. The same situation holds in reverse. There is no point in keeping your child home to prevent exposure to children with one of these common infections. Your child is as likely to catch a cold from an asymptomatic playmate as from one who has symptoms.

on the hot shower, sit, and hold the child. The comfort of being held reduces anxiety and helps lower the need for air. If a child has recurrent attacks, a cold-mist vaporizer is a worthwhile investment. It has been traditional to use syrup of ipecac to produce vomiting and relieve the symptoms, but vaporizers have become so much more efficient that ipecac is rarely used today.

Some patients with croup have more serious acute obstruction of breathing and require a physician's attention promptly. If the croup does not subside in half an hour with steam or mist, if it increases in intensity, if it is associated with fever of more than 103 degrees or with drooling, call your doctor or go immediately to a hospital emergency room. Children with severe croup sometimes require life-saving measures to provide an airway. Severe croup is one of the most serious problems of childhood.

Pneumonia is still a common disease of children but it is most often caused by bacteria and can be successfully treated with antibiotics at home. Even viral pneumonias, which do not respond to these drugs, rarely cause serious disease. Symptoms include fever, cough, and rapid breathing. In small babies, the cough may be absent and only a grunting breathing is present. Older children with pneumonia, like adult victims, produce sputum, which is sometimes rusty or blood-tinged. If these symptoms are present, call your physician. Occasionally a foreign body, such as a peanut, is aspirated and causes chronic pneumonia in an area of the lung.

Meningitis is an inflammation of the membranes surrounding the brain and spinal cord (see chapter 9, "The Brain and Nervous System"). Several types of bacteria can cause it, including those responsible for ear and general bloodstream infections. Early symptoms are difficult to distinguish from those of a self-limiting infection. Most cases occur between ages six months and four to five years. In addition to fever and vomiting, any child with lethargy or unresponsiveness, poor color, stiff neck, a rash (which occurs only with one type), or convulsion should be suspected of meningitis. These symptoms are an emergency, warranting a prompt call to your doctor. Although these symptoms occur in many children without serious problems, they call for evaluation.

Usually, the doctor will be able to reassure you by an examination, but on occasion may need to perform a spinal tap. This is a frightening-appearing test in which a needle three to four inches long is inserted in the middle of the lower back to obtain a few drops of spinal fluid. It is much more frightening to see (or imagine) than it is painful for the patient, for whom it constitutes little more than a pinprick. The most difficult part is for the child to remain still long enough. In small infants, this requires holding the child firmly, which increases his or her anxiety.

Meningitis can be successfully treated today if the diagnosis is made promptly. If allowed to continue untreated, it has such severe consequences, including retardation, deafness, cerebral palsy, and hydrocephalus, that mere suspicion merits emergency measures. Meningitis is still rare, however, affecting only 1 in 2,500 children. Even if the question is raised about your child, chances are it will be resolved in the negative with reassurance for all. Occasionally, meningitis occurs in epidemics in schools, and antibiotics may be prescribed as a preventive measure.

Streptococcal sore throat, often called "strep throat," is common among school-age children. It rarely occurs before age three years. At any time, as many as 20 percent of school-age children harbor a streptococcus bacterium in their throat without symptoms.

ROUTINE IMMUNIZATIONS

Age	
2 Months	DPT (Diphtheria, Pertussis, Tetanus) and Oral Polio
4 Months	DPT and Oral Polio
6 Months	DPT and Oral Polio
15 Months	Measles, Mumps, Rubella (one injection)
18 Months	DPT (Booster) and Oral Polio
4–6 Years	DT (Booster) and Oral Polio
10–12 Years	Rubella (for females with a blood test that shows little or no immunity)
Every 10 Years	TD—(adult tetanus and a weak diphtheria toxic)

Immunization against infectious disease should be given at appropriate intervals in infancy and early childhood. This is the schedule recommended by the American Academy of Pediatrics. Thanks to widespread immunization, many of the "childhood diseases" of the past have virtually disappeared.

Hence, virtually all children are exposed to this common germ and most will have several bouts while growing up. There are dozens of different strains of "strep." Infection with any one of them produces immunity only to that particular strain. Regardless of strain, symptoms are similar: fever, severe sore throat, difficulty swallowing, and swollen lymph glands in the neck. There also may be vomiting and abdominal pain. Certain strains produce a rash. This variety is called scarlet fever.

The importance of strep throat is that untreated cases occasionally may lead, about two weeks afterward, to rheumatic fever, which can result in heart damage. Treatment with penicillin almost always prevents this.

If your child has symptoms, your doctor may want to take a throat culture to prove the presence of streptococcus, because other causes of sore throat are difficult to distinguish by examination alone. Penicillin must be given for 10 days to adequately eliminate the germ—a tedious procedure if given by mouth, because the child usually feels well after two or three days. To ensure adequate length of therapy, some doctors administer the penicillin by injection, using a long-acting form of the drug. The disadvantage is the pain of injection.

As with many areas of life, one must weigh the risks and benefit of these two ways of administering penicillin. Penicillin by mouth is as effective as injection if continued for ten days, but injection ensures the proper length of therapy.

Ear infections (otitis) are familiar to every parent. They occur when germs commonly present in the throat pass up the small eustachian tube to the middle ear. Congestion may trap the germs there and allow them to proliferate, causing inflammation (see chapter 13, "Ear, Nose, and Throat"). Symptoms include fever, irritability, pain in the ear (which can be severe), and vomiting. Small children who cannot describe the pain may hold the affected ear, pull at it, or rock the head. The physician usually diagnoses the infection by examining the tympanic membrane (ear drum) with an otoscope, an instrument with a light and small tube that allows him to look in the ear. Sometimes the tympanic membrane ruptures and fluid runs out of the ear canal. You should consult your physician for either type of symptom because treatment with antibiotics is necessary and effective. Aspirin can reduce the fever and pain. Many doctors also prescribe other medicines to decrease congestion in the eustachian tube, although there is debate over the benefit of these drugs.

Chronic fluid behind the ear (serous otitis media) or scarring of the ear drum are common results of otitis and can cause diminished hear-

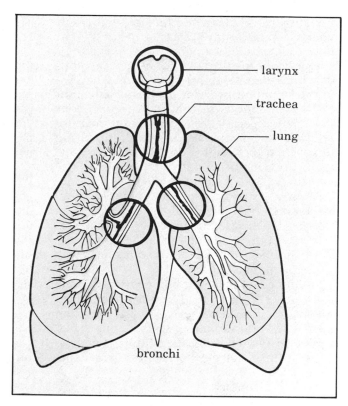

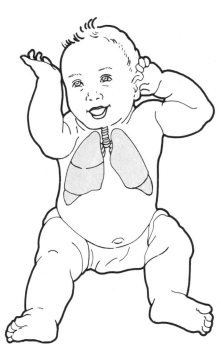

CROUP

Noisy breathing and a ringing cough are characteristic of croup, which results from a swelling in and around the larynx. It is usually caused by an acute infection. Secretions of thick mucus also can clog the larynx, bronchi, and trachea and further obstruct air passage to and from the lungs. Croup may be accompanied by high fever. Mild cases may be relieved by steam inhalation or a cold-mist vaporizer, but severe croup is a medical emergency and victims should be taken to a hospital emergency department immediately.

ing. Your doctor will want to see your child after an ear infection for follow-up to determine if this complication has occurred, because further treatment is necessary to prevent hearing loss. The doctor may prescribe drugs to reduce the fluid, or surgically insert a tiny polyethylene tube through the drum to allow the fluid to drain and air to enter. This "PE" tube operation, done under general anesthesia, has become one of the most commonly performed operations. While the tubes are in place, a child should not swim.

As a child grows older, ear infections, like most infections, become less frequent.

Sudden infant death syndrome (SIDS). Nothing strikes fear in the heart of a parent more than the threat of a previously healthy child being found dead in the crib. In recent years, this feared problem has been recognized as a distinct syndrome accounting for as many as 8,000 deaths per year in the United States.

Typically a baby of four to ten months who has been well is found dead in his or her crib. In the past, when small babies often shared their mother's bed, the cause of death was thought to be smothering. That is clearly not the cause, but the precise cause, or more likely multiple causes, are not clear. Sudden infant death syndrome does occur more often in premature babies and is thought, in part, to be related to immaturity of the central nervous system and the breathing center in the brain.

Some surviving babies are now recognized to have been "near-misses"—that is, they have been observed to stop breathing and then have been resuscitated by stimulation. This has given rise to the widespread use by apprehensive parents of apnea monitors, electronic devices that sound an alarm if the sleeping baby stops breathing. The use of any such device should be undertaken only after a thorough discussion with your physician. Such monitors have their bad side effects, such as labeling the child sick or vulnerable and raising parental anxiety. Lack of sleep and tension that result when the family stays alert for the bell night after night are other potentially harmful effects. But the monitor may prevent a susceptible child from stopping breathing. The best advice for parents worried about sudden infant death syndrome is to talk it over with your physician, especially if you have a premature baby who has had pauses in breathing lasting longer than six to eight seconds, or if you have had a previous SIDS baby or near-miss. The chance of a second such baby in the same family is only 2 percent. However, this is 50 times the average rate for all babies.

If you have suffered such a loss, other parents now stand ready to help and counsel you. You should ask your doctor for advice on how to contact a parents' group.

The danger of sudden infant death syndrome is obviously frightening, but it is important to put the problem in perspective. The condition is still very rare, occurring in about one in 500 to 1000 births. The average pediatrician, who cares for 100 to 200 newborns a year, will experience such an event only once in every five to ten years of practice.

It is also important for parents of victims, who often accuse themselves of neglect or culpability, to recognize that they are not to blame for the death. Research is advancing understanding of the syndrome rapidly. In the future we hope to have the knowledge to prevent one of the last great causes of death in children.

Acute problems of the newborn. The newborn child must adapt to several new conditions upon entry to the "outside" world. In the womb, temperature is controlled by the mother's body heat. Oxygen and food are provided from the placenta, and the baby is protected from most infections. At birth, this sheltered existence abruptly changes. The baby must maintain his or her own temperature, start breathing with lungs that have never been used, and within a few days take nourishment by mouth. The remarkable thing is that for most babies this series of momentous transitions occurs smoothly.

The major problems of the newborn period result from premature birth, when the abilities to adapt may not be fully developed. Control of temperature is difficult and handling of infections inefficient. Therefore, small babies are placed in incubators to stabilize body temperature, and to protect them from infections. They often must be fed by tube or intravenously. But the most life-threatening problem for small newborns is the immaturity of their lungs, which results in a condition called respiratory distress syndrome (RDS).

The baby cannot absorb oxygen and rid the body of carbon dioxide adequately. Breathing is rapid and the baby may die from exhaustion and lack of oxygen. Treatment of this condition has improved so much since 1970 that nearly half of all babies weighing less than two pounds at birth can be saved, although twenty years before only 1 percent survived. Today, most babies weighing more than 2½ to 3 pounds survive.

Usually, the baby's breathing is assisted by placing a tiny tube in the trachea. Blood, oxygen, carbon dioxide, and sugar are carefully monitored, and any metabolic abnormalities are treated.

The babies usually are cared for in neonatal intensive care units with sophisticated equipment and specially trained doctors and nurses. Because these units cannot be maintained at every hospital, regional perinatal centers have been developed in most large cities. Specially equipped ambulances transport the babies from the hospital of birth to the regional centers. Often obstetricians can identify a high-risk mother who is likely to have a small or premature baby and will arrange for delivery in such a regional center (see chapter 26, "Pregnancy and Childbirth").

Babies with respiratory distress syndrome usually recover in three to five days. Most are then normal, although a few have persistent lung disease. Major efforts are being made to prevent the birth of babies prematurely and to increase the maturity of their lungs before birth. Since respiratory distress syndrome is the largest single cause of death in all of childhood, prevention and effective treatment are leading to a continued decrease in infant mortality.

Premature babies are observed closely for signs of infection. If caused by bacteria, the infection usually can be treated successfully. However, a variety of infections (mostly viral) acquired by the baby from the mother while still in the uterus cannot be treated and may have serious effects. Cytomegalovirus infection is the most common now that German measles has been reduced by immunization. It can produce mental retardation.

Improved methods of feeding premature babies, and the advances in treatment and prevention of respiratory and infectious diseases of the newborn, have focused attention on their later intellectual and emotional development. Intellectual development of even very small babies, if they are cared for optimally, is surprisingly good. The long period of incubator care in the past often led to difficulty in establishing a normal mother-child bond after the baby's discharge from the hospital. Most nurseries now encourage mothers to visit the intensive care unit to touch and look at the baby. With sophisticated technical care, early attachment of mother and baby, and stimulation of the baby after discharge, the outlook for even very tiny "preemies" is now very good.

CHRONIC DISEASE

Chronic disease is defined as any illness that lasts three months or more. Pediatrics, until recently, was consumed with the burden of acute illness. Now that many of the more serious acute illnesses can be controlled or prevented, chronic disease has become a major focus of pediatric care. There are, of course, hundreds of different chronic diseases. This section will concentrate on what is common to such problems in children and briefly discuss the most common ones. Many of the specific diseases are dealt with elsewhere in this book.

Psychological Aspects

Sometimes the broader points of caring for a child with chronic disease are forgotten in the pressure of getting laboratory tests or giving drug therapy, yet they can provide a great deal of help to improve the functioning of both child and family. Chronic illnesses in children are often more alike than different. Here are some problems that these families face.

Guilt. Parents and the child, too, if old enough, often feel responsible for causing an illness. "Did I do anything that caused it? Is there anything I didn't do that could have prevented it?" are almost universal questions. While occasionally some act was responsible (such as having taken a toxic drug during pregnancy), it does no good to avoid the question. Ask your doctor. Recognize that everyone feels guilt, and guilt can produce depression, marital bickering, and difficulty in dealing honestly with your child. Hereditary diseases create special problems of guilt but often are erroneously attributed to one side of the family. In fact, many are inherited from both sides. Learning about inheritance can be very helpful (see chapter 2, "Medical Genetics").

Competence, or one's sense of worth, is always susceptible to damage in the child with a chronic illness, as well as in the parent. The mere fact that a child is labeled as having a disease, or has to take medicines, makes the child feel differently from others. Parents of children with chronic disease should know this and help their child develop strengths. Nothing overcomes feelings of unworthiness so much as succeeding at something. Success breeds success. Most chronic diseases produce more dysfunction through the secondary effects on the child's feeling of competence than through the disease itself.

Family relationships. Chronic illness in children is a family affair. Parents and siblings are all affected. Some families retreat into social isolation once a child is diagnosed as having a chronic illness. Some parents ignore their children who are well. Care of some chronic illnesses is time-consuming and physically wearing. Parents may have less time for each other. Recognizing these pressures and normal responses leads to making time for siblings, getting baby sitters, and going out periodically for parents or obtaining help with the housework. It is better to give the children, both sick and well, your own time and obtain help in the household than try to do everything and neglect spouse and children.

Children with chronic disease also have the normal problems of childhood. Discipline, recognition of individual differences, dealing with developmental stages such as toilet training, feeding, or school all occur in children with chronic illness just as they do in other children. It is frequently difficult for parents who have dealt with these normal processes competently with their other children to deal with them in a child with chronic illness. It is difficult to treat a child who has diabetes or asthma the same way you treat other children when the ill child has a temper tantrum or fails in school. It is easy for the child unconsciously to use the illness as an excuse and for parents to feel guilt about setting limits.

It is easy to say "try to treat a child with a chronic illness the same way you treat your other children," but difficult to do. Yet, that is the goal. Setting limits and allowing independence to develop are just as important in children with chronic illness as in healthy ones, perhaps more so. If you have dealt with and resolved your guilt about the illness, it is easier to confront these normal developmental issues in your child with a chronic illness.

Denial is a defense we all use to deal with unpleasant facts of life. At times, it is a useful defense. But to deny to the child that he has a handicap or illness, or to deny to yourself that the child has a chronic problem, often leads to greater problems. When leukemia was universally fatal, many parents denied the illness, never told the child the diagnosis, and as a result created, by a "conspiracy of silence," greater anxiety in the child. We now know that children can face the truth quite well, however harsh it may be. In diseases such as leukemia, where there is now hope for long-term survival, there is every reason for parents to be honest.

Common Chronic Diseases

The following are brief descriptions of several common chronic illnesses of childhood. They are not designed to tell you all you need to know about the illness. If the illness is covered elsewhere in this text, the chapters are listed. In addition, you should ask your physician for more information. He or she may suggest further reading.

Asthma is the most common chronic physical disease of childhood. It affects three to five percent of all children. Asthma is characterized by attacks of wheezing because of obstruction of the small air passages of the lung. The causes include allergy to pollens, dusts, or fumes, cold air, emotions, infections, and occasionally other agents. Severity varies from mild, occasional attacks to severe, frequent ones. Many treatments, including drugs, avoidance of allergens, and desensitization, can help most children with asthma lead fully active lives.

Allergy may also manifest itself by hay fever, eczema, hives, or occasionally other means (see chapter 21, "Allergy and the Immune System," and chapter 8, "The Lungs").

Birthmarks are common and result from enlargement of blood vessels in the skin or from extra pigment in the skin. The cause is unknown, but is not related to frightening events during pregnancy. Several types of birthmarks are seen, most having their origin before birth.

Hemangiomas, or strawberry marks, are not present at birth, but appear after the first two to four weeks of life. They are caused by a collection of small blood vessels in the skin. Hemangiomas all shrink with time, lose their color and disappear, although the process may take several years. Treatment by surgery, X ray, or dry ice produces more scars than if time is allowed to eradicate the lesion. If they occur on the face, the major problem of hemangiomas is the anxiety they cause parents, but only in extreme situations should anything but time and reassurance be used. Another of the most common types of hemangiomas is a light salmon pink flat patch, common on forehead or back of the neck. A common name is "stork bite." These, too, disappear without treatment.

Moles are permanent pigmented spots (see chapter 7, "The Skin"). Everyone has several moles and those in children require no special care. If they are large and occur in highly visible areas, moles can be removed by surgery or covered with cosmetics. Those present at birth should be seen by a doctor for removal.

Port wine stains are a special type of birthmark with purple stain and small blood vessels on the skin. Treatment is limited to cosmetic coverings. Some dermatologists can cover them with a neutral tattoo.

Cancer is far less common in childhood than in adults and yet, because of the low overall death rate in children, it is the second most common cause of death. Two general forms occur: solid tumors of many organs and leukemia, a cancer of white blood cells (see chapter 29, "Cancer").

The symptoms of cancer can be multiple because any organ may be involved. The important point is that even though it is a leading cause of death, cancer in childhood is still uncommon. Great advances in treatment have occurred since 1960, and most childhood cancers have a good-to-excellent outcome. Leukemia, which before 1970 was almost universally fatal, now can be "cured"—that is, victims will survive five years or more—in 50 percent of all cases. In others, life is extended. Dealing with the child with cancer is one of the most difficult tasks for any parent. Suggestions for how to handle honestly the guilt, denial, and other common reactions, are covered on page 647.

Convulsions are frightening. Nearly five percent of children have one convulsion (also called a seizure or fit) by the age of five. Most follow a high fever and are called febrile convulsions. The child suddenly loses consciousness, rolls up the eyes, then twitches all over rhythmically. The episode is followed by a general relaxation and apparently deep sleep. The convulsion may be over in a few seconds or may persist for several minutes.

Almost all convulsions cease by themselves before medical help arrives. There are a few ways to prevent complications. Fever can be brought down later by the methods outlined on page 640, but this will not help in the acute stage. Do not place the child in a cold bath or ice bath. Call your doctor. He or she will want to determine whether a treatable illness is present.

A few children tend to have recurrent seizures with high fever until they are four or five years old. Physicians disagree about whether seizures can be prevented by an anticonvulsant drug such as phenobarbital given daily for two to three years. Most now believe that the side effects (hyperactivity and reduced attentiveness) are more dangerous than the small risk of recurrence. The most important point is that a febrile seizure in an otherwise healthy child almost always produces no harm in the long run.

Chronic or repeated seizures are called epilepsy (see chapter 10, "Epilepsy"). Even the word brings terror to parents. We now know more about this group of disorders than in the past. We recognize different types of epilepsy, ranging from the typical major motor seizure, which is much like a febrile convulsion, to much less obvious "spells," lapses, or even periodic uncontrolled types of behavior. A brain wave test or electroencephalogram EEG, a measuring of the electrical current of the brain), plus biochemical, X ray, neurological, and psychological tests, help doctors to define the cause. Thanks to new drugs, almost all types of seizures can be controlled. The psychological consequences to both child and family are often the most difficult part of the disorder, but most children with epilepsy can now lead relatively normal lives.

Cystic fibrosis (CF) is one of the more common inherited conditions, affecting about 1 in 1,000 children (see chapter 2, "Medical Genetics"). Cystic fibrosis affects mucous glands in the body, producing thick secretions. The most common symptoms occur in the respiratory tract where small airways are blocked by the secretions, resulting in chronic infection, cough, wheezing, and shortness of breath. There are often intestinal symptoms caused by blockage of secretory glands in the pancreas, resulting in poor digestion of food, loose foul-smelling stools, and failure to gain weight.

Children with cystic fibrosis also lose salt through their sweat glands in excessive amounts. This has given rise to the most common test to establish the diagnosis—the sweat test, which measures the amount of salt in perspiration.

Treatment must be continued for life, but has successfully extended the life of these children into adult years.

Diabetes mellitus is a common disease of adults. The juvenile form is less common. Sugar metabolism is altered, because the islets of Langerhans in the pancreas don't produce enough insulin. The resultant high blood sugar leads to loss of sugar in the urine, frequent and copious urination, and weight loss despite increased appetite. The onset is usually sudden. Acute complications include accumulation of acids in the body (acidosis), while the long-term chronic complications include hardening of the arteries, diminished kidney function, and visual problems. Since insulin was introduced in 1922, the acute stage can be successfully treated by daily injection, coupled with sensible diet and exercise, and blood sugar levels can be controlled. There is still debate about whether the late complications can be overcome (see chapter 17, "Diabetes Mellitus") but most now believe that careful clinical control decreases the risk of late complications.

Failure to thrive is a special problem of infancy, characterized by poor growth. The most common pattern is for the weight to increase less rapidly than height, or there may be weight loss. The most common cause worldwide is lack of food. However, in America, the more likely cause is some disturbance in the mother-child relationship that prevents the mother from feeding the child adequately. Some babies are more difficult to feed. Depression in the mother, especially common in the period after birth, problems in the household, such as marital strife, unsteady employment, and poor techniques of feeding, which often result from poor care the mother herself received as a baby, all contribute to a vicious cycle. A baby who is a slow or difficult feeder or a mother with little experience who develops minimal bonding with her baby early in the baby's life also may contribute. There are less common causes, such as a congenital abnormality of the heart, nervous system, or kidney, a chronic infection, or an inborn abnormality of the baby's metabolism. Most of these cause the baby to have a slowing of length as well as weight. Any baby who is not growing well should be seen by a physician. If there is a congential problem, it is best treated early. If the problem is mother-child interaction, the sooner help is given the less likely there is to be a permanent sense of failure in the mother, and treatment for the baby is more likely to be effective.

Treatment of mother-child interaction problems includes practical help in the home and a visiting nurse or social worker to help the mother to learn feeding techniques and to counsel her about her psychological problems. Occasionally, short hospitalizations are helpful to establish the diagnosis and to break the cycle.

Heart defects and heart disease cause great anxiety among parents, but serious heart disease is quite uncommon, occurring in about 1 in 200 children. Children have two types of heart disease, congenital and acquired. The congenital types can be diagnosed with great precision and many can be completely corrected with surgery. There are few greater examples of the benefits of modern scientific medicine than the diagnosis and successful treatment of congenital heart problems. In older children, congenital heart disease is often recognized by discovery of a heart murmur. Younger children and babies usually show some symptoms, although babies have only limited ways to demonstrate heart disease. Some are blue (cyanotic) because venous blood from the right side of the heart mixes with arterial blood from the left, the result of an opening between the two sides. Other symptoms are easy fatigue shown by slow or interrupted feedings, and rapid breathing. Some congenital heart conditions appear only after two to three weeks of life. Treatment with digitalis to strengthen the heart muscle, diuretics to remove excess fluid, and surgery have saved the lives of many such children. Sometimes a palliative surgical procedure is necessary when the baby is very small, delaying the corrective procedure until the child is older (see chapter 3, "The Heart and Circulation" and chapter 31, "Understanding Your Operation").

The major acquired heart disease in children is rheumatic heart disease, a complication of rheumatic fever. The symptoms and signs of rheumatic fever are fever, joint pains or arthritis, involuntary jerky movements called chorea, and heart disease. Rheumatic fever usually follows a streptococcal infection. With prompt treatment of "strep throat" (see page 643) and prevention of second attacks of rheumatic fever by daily penicillin therapy, the heart damage and the heart failure that formerly were consequences of rheumatic fever have been almost totally prevented. Prevention of rheumatic heart disease is one of the major accomplishments of penicillin.

Heart murmur. As many as 40 percent of all children have a heart murmur sometime during childhood. Most are of little consequence. The difference between that 40 percent figure and the 0.5 percent (1 in 200) who have serious heart disease indicates how frequently "innocent" or functional murmurs occur. Murmurs stem from turbulence in the flow of blood, much like the noise made by rapids in a river. Abnormal heart valves can cause murmurs because they create turbulence in the blood flow inside the heart. Most functional (innocent) murmurs arise outside the heart because of slight turbulence in the flow of blood through veins. In children, with their thin chest walls, these murmurs can be easily heard. Growth temporarily changes the relation of chest wall to blood vessels underneath and contributes to murmurs. Murmurs are also heard during episodes of fever. Your physician usually can tell the difference between functional and organic heart murmurs by their location, timing, and character. On occasion, the doctor may need a chest X ray, electrocardiogram (ECG), or other tests. Most heart murmurs in children are not a cause for worry. Even when they are caused by organic heart disease, it is not the murmur itself that is the problem, but the heart function. Restriction of activity is not required in functional murmurs in children.

Hernias are small openings in the abdominal wall with ballooning of a bit of intestine through the opening.

Umbilical hernias occur at the navel and are common in babies. They may range in size from the diameter of a small pencil to as big as a finger. Umbilical hernias practically never cause harm. As the abdominal muscles become stronger, the hernias close by themselves. In the past, taping the bulge or even operations were used, but it is now recognized that umbilical hernias should be left alone.

Inguinal hernias occur in the groin or scrotum. They may occur at any time in life. If the intestine cannot be pushed back into place (reduced) the hernia may strangulate as the blood supply to the intestine in the sac is pinched off. While strangulation is uncommon, it is the main reason to operate on all children found with an inguinal hernia. Hernia operation, even in the very young, is simple and effective (see chapter 31, "Understanding Your Operation").

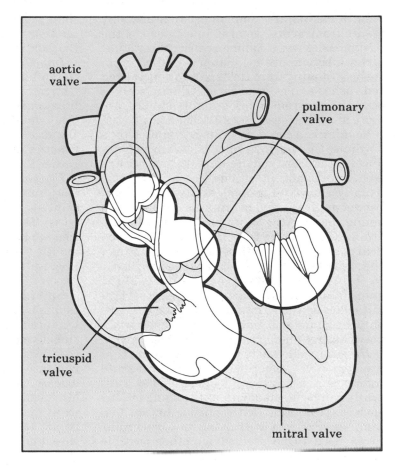

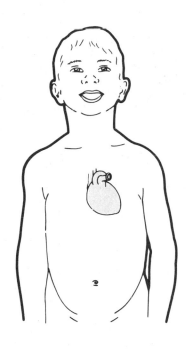

HEART MURMURS

Abnormal noises accompanying the heartbeat, known as "murmurs," occur in two out of five children and are seldom a cause for worry. A very few indicate damaged heart valves, either from birth (congenital) or as a result of disease (acquired). Rheumatic fever, an aftermath of strep infection, is the leading cause of acquired damage to the heart valves. Its particular targets are the mitral and aortic valves (right drawing). Valvular damage as a result of rheumatic fever does not always become apparent until adulthood. With antibiotics to treat strep infection, rheumatic fever is less common than it was in earlier years.

Hydrocele is a collection of fluid in the scrotum. It may look like a hernia and in some instances is associated with a hernia. You should see your physician to distinguish between the two. In infants with only a hydrocele, no treatment is necessary.

Intussusception is an emergency seen in children under two. It occurs when one part of the intestine telescopes into another. The blood supply of the internal portion may be cut off, leading to gangrene of the bowel.

Symptoms occur suddenly with crying, repeated attacks of abdominal cramps, vomiting, and blood in the stool (often appearing as "currant jelly"). This is an acute emergency. Many hospitals now are able to reduce the bowel with manipulation under fluoroscope with barium in the large bowel. At times, surgery is necessary.

Pyloric stenosis stems from enlargement of the circular muscle at the end of the stomach, which obstructs the passage of food out of the stomach. It occurs much more commonly in first-born boys than girls, appearing mainly during the first two months of life. The major symptom is vomiting after feeding, often so forcefully that the material spurts several inches out of the baby's mouth (called projectile vomiting). A doctor usually can feel the mass of muscle, although an X ray may be necessary. A simple operation to cut the enlarged muscle fibers cures the condition.

Skin rashes are common in children. Many result from acute general infections. In the past measles was a common cause. Many other virus infections are associated with short-term rashes, ranging from tiny spots to generalized red rashes and even to hives. Others, such as eczema, recurrent hives, scabies, and lice, are more chronic (see chapter 7, "The Skin").

Scabies is a contagious disease caused by a tiny mite that burrows under the skin and produces irritation and itching. It has become epidemic again in recent years. The rash usually shows up around wrists and ankles, between fingers, and in any skin crease, but in young babies the eruptions may be generalized. The severe itching may trigger a good deal of scratching, with secondary infection of the scratches. Diagnosis can be made by looking for the mite or its eggs in scrapings of the skin. Treatment is application of one of several mitacides to the skin, but should be done for only 12 hours at a time with at least a week between treatments to avoid possible toxicity.

Hives are pale red to white raised areas that are very itchy, sometimes caused by an acute infection, more often by allergy. They generally can be treated with anti-itching lotions such as calamine with phenol or antihistamines. Patients with recurrent or chronic hives need to be studied for other possible causes (see chapter 21, "Allergy and the Immune System").

Lice of different species infest the hair of the head, the body, or the pubic area. Head lice in children are most common. Itching is fierce and the scratching that follows produces infected lesions. Lice are diagnosed by finding tiny pearly nits or eggs on the hair. Insecticide shampoos or lotions such as Kwell® are applied for treatment and infected clothes should be thoroughly washed.

Impetigo is a bacterial infection of the skin that often follows insect bites, mite or lice infections, or eczema because scratching and breaking of the skin allow bacteria to enter. In other children it is seen as a primary disease. Because the bacteria are deep in the skin, antibiotics must be given by mouth or injection rather than applied to the skin surface.

Fungus diseases of the skin include athlete's foot, fungus of the hair and scalp (tinea capitis), and fungus of the body (tinea corporis). There are several effective medications, some to be applied locally and some taken by mouth. Good hygiene helps fight athlete's foot because fungus lives in dead moist skin between the toes.

Suicide in children is now the third most common cause of death among adolescents (after accidents and cancer). Girls attempt suicide more often, but boys more often succeed. Girls use overdoses of drugs more often; boys use guns. While suicide is not a chronic disease, the act itself is acutely disturbing to all. It usually occurs in children who are chronically disturbed and depressed. Two important points for parents: (1) Never take lightly a threat of suicide. It is a call for help, and consultation should be obtained. Let experts help you and your child sort out the problems. (2) Be alert to early warning signs. Adolescents without friends, those who are blue or depressed, and those who suddenly develop school failure or have a personal crisis are a greater risk. Most adolescents with suicidal attempts can be helped to complete recovery.

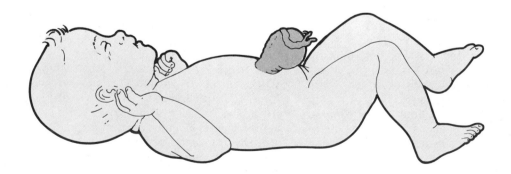

UMBILICAL HERNIA

Protrusion of a portion of the intestine through an opening in the abdominal wall is called a hernia. Umbilical hernia near the navel is relatively common at birth but usually closes without difficulty as the muscles of the abdomen strengthen. In rare cases a hernia may be of such size (as shown above) that it requires surgery.

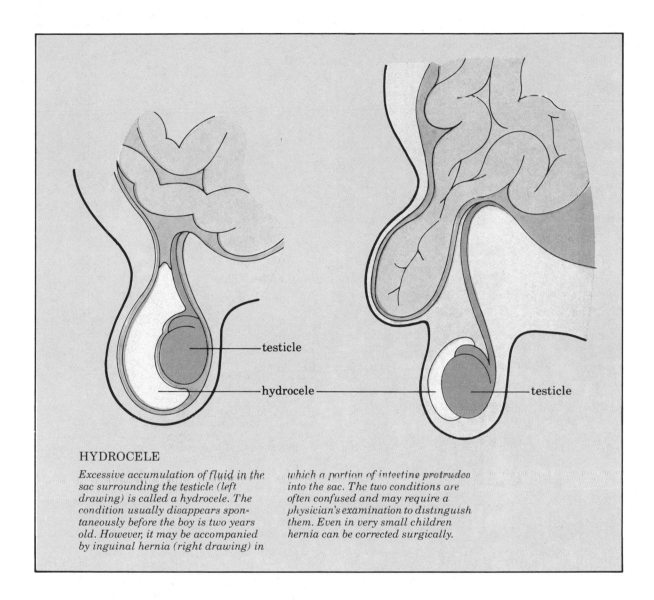

HYDROCELE

Excessive accumulation of fluid in the sac surrounding the testicle (left drawing) is called a hydrocele. The condition usually disappears spontaneously before the boy is two years old. However, it may be accompanied by inguinal hernia (right drawing) in which a portion of intestine protrudes into the sac. The two conditions are often confused and may require a physician's examination to distinguish them. Even in very small children hernia can be corrected surgically.

Intellectual Development Problems

Mental retardation is a problem now brought "out of the closet." In the past many parents felt as stigmatized by a retarded child as one with venereal disease. Retarded intellectual development has many causes and a wide range of seriousness. Few children are so severely retarded that they cannot become self-sufficient adults. The causes of severe retardation are many but all are quite rare, such as inborn errors of metabolism (phenylketonuria) or severe birth injury. Tests performed on newborns can diagnose such problems soon after birth. Most tests are done by analyzing a drop of blood taken by heel prick. Other problems, such as the chromosome abnormalities causing Down's syndrome, can be diagnosed by analyzing fluid from the uterus during pregnancy (amniocentesis) (see chapter 26, "Pregnancy and Childbirth," and chapter 2, "Medical Genetics").

Much more common are the milder forms of retardation, the vast majority of which are more of a handicap during school years when ability to memorize is important. Most children with mild retardation grow up able to function effectively in the workplace. One fairly common cause of mild retardation is lack of infant stimulation. The same sort of factors that are responsible for physical failure to thrive occur here. Mothers overwhelmed with other problems or who have themselves suffered from a difficult young life may not be able to give their child enough time, social contact, and verbal stimulation to bring out the latent potential in the youngster.

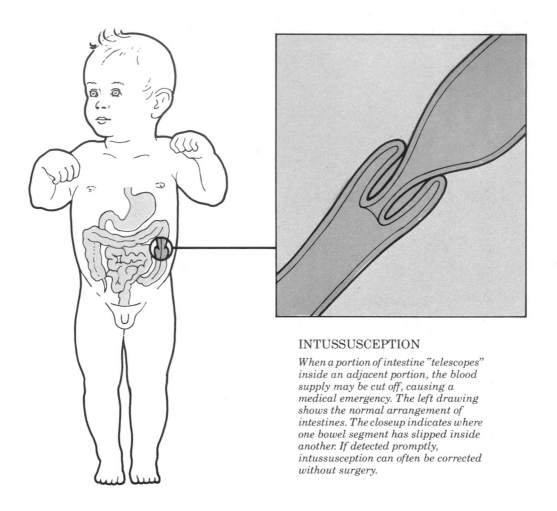

INTUSSUSCEPTION

*When a portion of intestine "telescopes"
inside an adjacent portion, the blood
supply may be cut off, causing a
medical emergency. The left drawing
shows the normal arrangement of
intestines. The closeup indicates where
one bowel segment has slipped inside
another. If detected promptly,
intussusception can often be corrected
without surgery.*

It is always difficult to talk about this subject in a book directed at parents because it appears to place blame on parents and has the potential to cause anxiety in parents whose children are normal but not developing as fast as parents might wish. On the other hand, one of the great advances in the past two decades has been our understanding of how children who fail to develop are often victims of a generational cycle that can be broken with proper intervention. It is important to bring this issue out in the open in order to diagnose these conditions early and treat them effectively.

If your child is not developing as you believe he or she should, or if your doctor finds such delays, it is important to have further tests performed to determine the amount of delay, the most likely cause, and to set up a program of help. In almost all types of developmental delay, some improvement can be obtained by treatment. This may involve helping the mother to develop her own life and skills, offering the child stimulation in the form of reading or playing special games, providing developmental day care center for part of the day, and counseling the parents. Sometimes simple changes in the household routine, such as a supportive friend to talk with the mother, can bring about improvement.

Something can always be done to help the slow child and his or her parents and siblings. Human intelligence is a spectrum. There is no sharp precise cut-off point between normal and abnormal. Many children with low IQs can grow up to be productive and happy adults.

Many factors of human development exist in addition to intellect. Social and interpersonal skills, creativity, compassion, manual dexterity, and other skills are not necessarily linked to IQ. Any child with developmental delay needs an assessment of these other facets of development, in part to determine what strengths he or she has that can be developed.

Failure in school or learning problems are sometimes the first evidence of developmental difficulties. Understanding of this field has developed rapidly. It is important to recognize that failure in school is not necessarily caused by low IQ. Several different causes are now recognized, although considerable confusion still exists. Dyslexia (inability to read), hyperactivity syndrome, attention deficit, and emotionally disturbed are some of the terms used for various causes. School is so important for a child's sense of worth and for his or her future that a child who fails in school should be studied by a team of educators, psychologists, and physicians to determine the cause. As with other forms of developmental disabilities, much can be done to help those in difficulty but a precise evaluation is necessary first.

Many of these problems with school, development, and behavior are outside what has traditionally been the responsibility of medicine. There are some who argue that medicine should not be involved, but the distress to child and parents is great.

Physicians offer one of the few open doors for people in trouble, especially for the preschool child. Some of the causes are physical or have physical consequences, and the child's physician is the one professional who follows the child from birth to maturity and can provide the "long view." Physicians cannot deal with many developmental delays alone, but they should be a part of the evaluation and plan of management.

A federal law now mandates that every child with a problem likely to lead to difficulty in schooling, either because of physical or mental handicap, must be evaluated and have a plan of management organized before school age. If you are concerned about your child's development, consult your doctor. If the child is in school, consult both doctor and teacher.

Hyperactivity, with its usual accompanying symptom of school learning difficulty, may affect as many as 5 to 15 percent of children in grade school. The majority are boys. There are many causes and many claims of successful treatments about which physicians disagree, so parents, teachers, and children faced with the problem are confused. Another name used for the condition is minimal brain dysfunction syndrome, an unfortunate name, because it makes many parents believe that the child is brain damaged. The characteristics include normal (or higher) intelligence but poor school performance, hyperactivity, disorders of attention (short span and distractible), impulsiveness, and several types of specific problems with reading, spelling, arithmetic, or coordination. Diagnosis and management should be done by a team that includes the child's physician, school representatives, and specific therapists for reading or emotional upsets as needed. Allergy to food dyes, chocolate, and other items has been widely touted as a cause and large numbers of such children are treated with elimination diets. Careful studies have not shown a great deal of benefit. Drugs that increase attention span have been useful in some children, although they should be used only as part of a total plan of management and only under a physician's guidance.

Hyperactivity and learning problems are a specific problem mainly in relation to schooling. Many of these children, once they pass this hurdle, do well during the rest of their lives when short attention span and learning difficulty may have less relevance. As with other chronic diseases, it is important to keep the child's sense of worth high. Praise for what he or she can do rather than blame for what cannot be done is a good approach.

PREVENTION: KEEPING CHILDREN HEALTHY

Pediatrics traditionally has been more concerned with prevention than most branches of medicine. Indeed, about one-half of a pediatrician's time is devoted to prevention. Some of pediatrics' greatest contributions to child health have been in prevention, especially the development of immunizations.

Prevention can occur at several stages in the cycle of disease. The first phase is health promotion, developing the environment and habits that prevent disease. It includes diet, exercise, hygiene, and the ability to cope with stress. The second phase is specific disease prevention, such as immunizing against a specific disease. The third phase is early diagnosis and treatment before a disease has caused damage. Screening in the newborn period for phenylketonuria is an example of this phase, as is the physical exam your doctor gives at each visit on vision and hearing screening.

At each visit your doctor will provide four types of preventive service: (1) health assessment (history, examination, and tests); (2) specific prevention (immunizations); (3) anticipatory guidance (helping you anticipate

KEEPING CHILDREN SAFE

Typical Accidents	Normal Behavior Characteristics	Precautions
First Year		
Falls, inhalation of foreign objects, poisonings, burns, drownings.	After several months of age can squirm and roll, and later creeps and pulls self erect. Places anything and everything in mouth. Helpless in water.	Do not leave alone on tables, etc. from which falls can occur. Keep crib sides up. Keep small objects and harmful substances out of reach. Do not leave alone in tub of water.
Second Year		
Falls, drowning, motor vehicles, ingestion of poisonous substances, burns	Able to roam about in erect posture, goes up and down stairs, has great curiosity, puts almost anything in mouth, helpless in water.	Keep screens in windows. Place gate at top of stairs. Cover unused electrical outlets. Keep cords out of easy reach. Keep in enclosed space when outdoors and not in company of an adult. Keep medicine, household poisons, and small sharp objects out of sight and reach. Keep handles of pots and pans on stove out of reach, and containers of hot foods away from edge of table. Protect from water in tub and pools.
2 to 4 Years		
Falls, drowning, motor vehicles, ingestion of poisonous substances, burns	Able to open doors, runs and climbs, can ride tricycle, investigates closets and drawers, plays with mechanical gadgets, can throw ball and other objects.	Keep doors locked when there is a danger of falls. Place screen or guards in windows. Teach about watching for automobiles in driveways and in streets. Keep firearms locked up. Keep knives, electrical equipment out of reach. Teach about risks of throwing sharp objects and about danger of following ball into the street.
School Age		
Falls, drowning, burns, pedestrian auto accidents	Adventuresome	Safe school playgrounds, supervised swimming pools, helmets and leg and arm pads for skateboarding, play off streets.
Adolescent		
Auto accidents, falls	Peer pressure, athletic drive	Seat belt use, safe driving, no driving with alcohol, supervised sports in age appropriate competition, use of helmets for motorcycles and bicycles.

normal development, such as the decrease in appetite in the second year of life); and (4) counseling (teaching about diet, exercise, life-style, etc.). Promotion of healthy habits for life is one of the most important aspects of child care and development.

Accident Prevention

Accidents are the leading cause of death among children who have successfully passed the first month of life. The causes vary by age. Burns, falls, and poisonings are major causes in the preschool period, while drowning and motor vehicle accidents (both as a pedestrian and rider) are major causes during school ages. In adolescence motor vehicle accidents (including motorcycles) are by far the major cause of death and serious injury.

There are generally two approaches to accident prevention. One is to make the environment safe, and the other is to teach children to practice safe habits of living. By far the first approach has been most successful to date. Examples are child-resistant caps on medicines and household poisons, grills on windows of buildings to prevent falls, flame retardant nightwear, and motorcycle helmets. The most successful accident prevention measure, the 55 mile per hour speed limit, has been accompanied by nearly 10,000 fewer deaths annually in the United States since it was begun. Some safety measures such as seat belts and infant car seats are effective but it has been difficult to convince people to use them.

When children are small parents must act for them. For older children it seems wise to instill safe habits by precept (putting on your own seat belt) rather than by preaching.

On page 656 is a list of common accidents and accepted preventive measures by age groups. Accident prevention is another good example of the need for a concept of developmental stages. Poisoning is largely a problem from one to three years of age, drowning largely from five to ten. Each age has its own risks and its own priority for prevention. It is obviously foolish to wait until the child is three years old to poison-proof your home. Timing the prevention to the developmental stage and providing a good example of safe living is the best preventive approach.

Life-Style to Promote Health

In recent years, it has been recognized that medical care for illness has limited effectiveness. Even the specific preventive services such as immunizations do not deal with the major illnesses of adult life—heart disease, stroke, cancer, arthritis. The ways we live, eat, exercise, handle stress, and use alcohol and tobacco have been found to be important in determining how healthy we are as adults (see chapter 1, "A Preventive Approach To Health"). Most of these habits have their origin in childhood and in the family. To be truthful, we do not know much about how to teach children healthy life-styles except by precept. Sermons do little good. Facts may help. For instance, children should learn that smoking increases the risk of heart disease and is the major factor responsible for cancer of the lung and chronic obstructive lung disease. They should know that excess weight and lack of exercise are causes of heart disease. Ability to deal with stress has been studied less, but many studies now show that people with more stressful life events—job change, marriage, divorce, accidents—have more illness of all types. Although many of these stresses cannot be avoided, everyone should learn to space those that can be. For instance, changing jobs or moving shortly after the death of a parent or spouse is not wise. In addition, all should learn how to handle symptoms of stress through relaxation and coping with the stress. Going to a quiet room once or twice a day for ten minutes and repeating a simple number or word, even "one, one, one," has been shown to lower blood pressure. Although these procedures are not practical for small children, adolescents can begin to learn stress-reducing techniques. Teaching children stress and coping skills is one of the frontiers of medicine.

Healthy children are one of the greatest legacies one generation can leave the next. We have made great strides in treating major illness in children, but in most instances elimination of a disease has only been achieved by prevention. Immunizations are one of the great success stories of medicine. It is likely that in the future more improvement in child health will be achieved by changes in health habits and improvements in the environment than by advances in physician care. This does not diminish the importance of highly competent, humane medical care for conditions we cannot prevent. The more parents and children know about health and illness, the more effective they will be in prevention and as partners in treatment of illness.

CHAPTER 28   JULIA A. WALSH, M.D.
EDWARD H. KASS, M.D., Ph.D.

INFECTIOUS DISEASES

The greatest revolution in the history of human health occurred during the past century. During the early 1900s, infectious diseases were the major causes of death. Typhoid fever, cholera, plague, smallpox, scarlet fever, measles, pneumonia, and similar acute infections produced dread in families and communities alike when they appeared. They accounted for millions of deaths annually. Since then, acute infectious diseases have declined dramatically as causes of death in industrialized countries. Tuberculosis has fallen to the point where it has become a relatively rare disease. Scarlet fever and streptococcal infections are now considered relatively mild and easily treatable except in unusual instances. Typhoid fever is rare, smallpox has been eradicated, and so on.

Nonetheless, infectious diseases are still more common in underprivileged groups than they are in more affluent segments of the population, and they remain major causes of death in most of the world. Africa, Asia, and South America still record large numbers of deaths from the same diseases that were major killers in the industrialized countries only a few decades ago. In many parts of Africa and Asia 25 percent or more of all children die before age 5, and infectious diseases account for most of those deaths.

What has caused the remarkable decrease in common infections in the industrialized world is not entirely clear. Improved sanitation, improved water supplies, improved housing, the spread of better information about hygiene, and the spread of better information about the preparation, marketing, and storage of foods have undoubtedly played a large role. To add to these important environmental changes, science has developed over the past several decades powerful antimicrobial drugs and equally important vaccines and antiserums (serum obtained from immunized persons) that have made it possible to prevent many illnesses and to treat many others that previously were untreatable. To those who can recall the havoc caused by many infections—the sudden appearance of fever followed by death in a day or two, the prolonged treatment and convalescence for chronic infections such as tuberculosis, the disfigurement and disability that followed many other infections—the present situation borders on the miraculous. Nevertheless, important infectious disease problems remain, and researchers are seeking to overcome them.

WHAT ARE INFECTIOUS DISEASES?

Infectious diseases are illnesses caused by germs. Germs are tiny living cells, so small they can be seen only with high-powered microscopes. Germs invade the tissues of our bodies, where they grow, multiply, and interfere with the normal functions of cells. Some of these germs manufacture and release poisons.

However, it should be kept in mind that the number of bacteria and other germs in the universe is large and most are not harmful.

In this chapter we shall concern ourselves almost entirely with that small minority of germs (otherwise known as microbes, from the Greek word for smallest living things) that cause disease. Such microbes are single-celled organisms and are divided into several different categories, including bacteria, protozoa, and viruses. Bacteria are exceedingly small, about 1/25,000th of an inch long, and can be seen only with the highest magnifications of the ordinary light microscope. It is a continuous wonder that such tiny organisms could produce so much disease in hosts the size of mammals.

Bacteria normally are found in certain areas throughout the body. As might be expected, those areas in contact with the environment, such as the skin, the mouth and nose, the intestinal tract, the openings to the ears and to the genital organs, all normally have bacteria present. Such bacteria ordinarily are not the type to produce disease, although occasionally they invade the tissues under circumstances described on page 660. Some bacteria are spread from individual to individual, such as the types of streptococci ("strep") commonly involved in some sore throats. Streptococci and other unwanted bacteria inhabit the noses and throats of many persons without necessarily producing disease, and are spread via droplets of moisture exhaled in breathing. Therefore, certain disease-producing bacteria are carried in people who are apparently healthy, yet the bacteria are able to produce disease in them or in others, particularly if resistance is lowered.

Bacteria differ in their capacity to produce disease, a capacity referred to as their pathogenicity. Similarly, individuals differ in their relative resistance to infection, both in resistance present at birth and in terms of varying levels that occur at different times throughout life. There are times when resistance is lowered and times when resistance is at its peak. We know all too little about how to influence the body's resistance except that cleanliness, good nutrition, and hygiene play a large role in keeping resistance up and minimizing the spread of pathogenic bacteria.

Bacteria come in different sizes and shapes. Some are cigar shaped or shaped like small cylinders. These are referred to as bacilli or rod-shaped bacteria. Some occur singly and others in long chains. Still other bacteria are small spheres or cocci. Some cocci divide in only one direction so that they form pairs or chains of cocci, while other bacteria may form clusters because they divide in different directions. The long-chained cocci are known as streptococci (Greek for chains of spheres) and the clusters are known as staphylococci (grape-like clusters). Some bacteria, quite curiously, divide in one direction once and at exactly right angles in the next division, and tend to appear in packets of four. Still another group of cocci divide at right angles in three dimensions so that they always appear in tiny packets of eight. The diversity in size and shape is seen in still other bacteria that tend to form comma-shaped structures. Still others form spirals. Some spirals are loosely formed, much as a snake would look while lying in the grass, while others are tightly coiled, almost like a spring.

Precisely why and how these different shapes have evolved is not known, but the shape of bacteria is a genetic characteristic that tends to give each bacterium its own appearance and its own way of multiplying. In addition, different bacteria use different types of materials in the environment that can change some of the chemicals around them. All these characteristics have been used by microbiologists to identify bacteria.

Just as with other living things, bacteria can be put into broad classifications. The classifications can be used by microbiologists to isolate microorganisms, identify them, and thereby give some indication of what has been learned about them, about their properties,

the manner of spread, and the antibiotics that are most likely to kill them. Identification is the purpose of the bacteriological culture that is often taken during an illness. Certain bacteria will produce certain diseases that are quite characteristic. The more we learn about how the body reacts to bacterial products, the more it is clear that the body can react to them in only a limited number of ways. That is why it is often necessary to isolate the particular bacterium causing a disease to determine which drugs affect it and what other approaches might be used to control the infection.

Certain bacteria are known as the higher bacteria because they tend to form branching cells and to appear as multicellular groups instead of single cells. Some of these become much like the smallest and simplest plants in their appearance. Some of these more complex bacteria also cause disease. Still larger and more complex are certain primitive plants that are known as fungi, the name given to common mushrooms and molds. Certain fungi also cause disease under certain circumstances. On the other hand, many of the higher bacteria and the fungi have been powerful sources of antibiotics. It is a curious phenomenon of nature that many bacteria and fungi manufacture substances that kill off other bacteria. In recent years these substances have been discovered, isolated, and purified. Many of them turn out to be useful as medicines to kill disease-producing bacteria. When these antibiotics (substances produced by one living thing that are antagonistic to other living things) have been chemically isolated and purified, it has been possible at times to change the chemical molecule and produce still more powerful and more beneficial antimicrobial substances.

Other types of microbes that are larger than bacteria are the protozoa, the smallest animal cells. In nature there are large numbers of protozoa. They are found in soil, in ponds, on plants, in the body, and elsewhere. The amoeba and paramecium are known to every schoolchild and are examples of common protozoa. Some protozoa can produce disease. Still larger organisms that can produce disease are certain worms that become parasites. Parasites draw all of their nutrition from the host and live in or on the host. The ideal parasite does not kill the host so it can continue to live there. This is true of many worms.

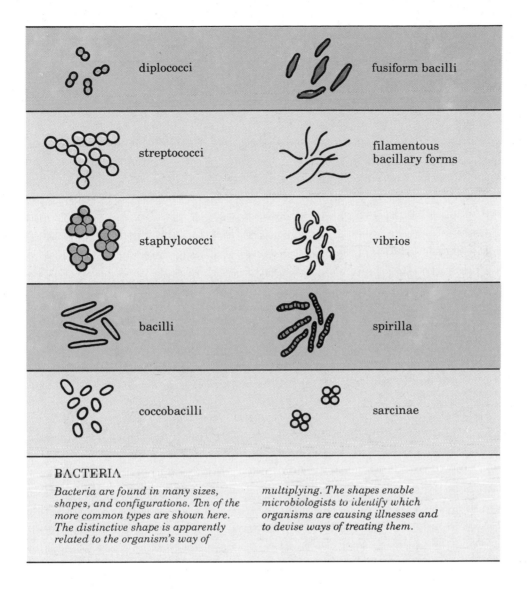

diplococci		fusiform bacilli	
streptococci		filamentous bacillary forms	
staphylococci		vibrios	
bacilli		spirilla	
coccobacilli		sarcinae	

BACTERIA

Bacteria are found in many sizes, shapes, and configurations. Ten of the more common types are shown here. The distinctive shape is apparently related to the organism's way of multiplying. The shapes enable microbiologists to identify which organisms are causing illnesses and to devise ways of treating them.

Biological scientists discovered early in their research that there are materials that produce disease even when passed through filters so fine that they hold back all bacteria. The term filterable viruses emerged, a term suggesting there was something in the filtered material that could produce disease, yet was too small to be seen by the ordinary microscope. In time this group of filterable viruses was detected using more advanced microscopes, such as the electron microscope, and it is now clear that the diversity among viruses is as great as among bacteria. Viruses, although much smaller than bacteria, also come in a wide variety of shapes—rods, spheres, and tiny, multi-sided crystal-like structures. It has become possible to study these viruses chemically, and we have discovered that some are quite complex, others less so. In contrast to most bacteria, viruses cannot multiply outside a living cell. Scientists who work with viruses either must pass them through a suitable host or must grow them in a tissue culture. The knowledge of how to grow viruses in tissue cultures played a major role in the study of viruses and the development of more and better vaccines.

Not only do some viruses attack animals and large plants, but other viruses attack bacteria. These tiny viruses are known as bacteriophages. Bacteriophages enter bacterial cells and multiply, causing the bacterial cells to burst. Many attempts have been made to use bacteriophages to kill bacteria in infected humans. Unfortunately, this approach has not been highly successful, partly because not all bacterial cells are killed by bacteriophages, and because the bacteriophages are often inhibited by body substances.

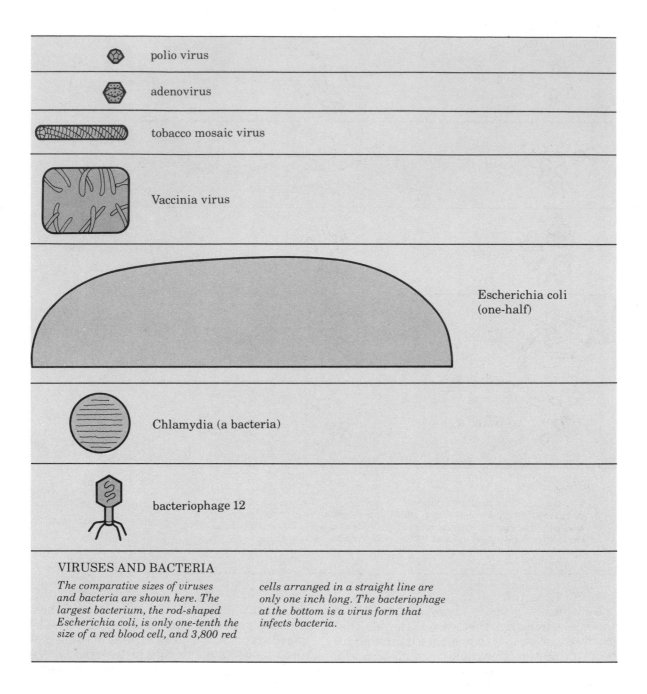

polio virus

adenovirus

tobacco mosaic virus

Vaccinia virus

Escherichia coli
(one-half)

Chlamydia (a bacteria)

bacteriophage 12

VIRUSES AND BACTERIA

The comparative sizes of viruses and bacteria are shown here. The largest bacterium, the rod-shaped Escherichia coli, is only one-tenth the size of a red blood cell, and 3,800 red cells arranged in a straight line are only one inch long. The bacteriophage at the bottom is a virus form that infects bacteria.

What then are infectious diseases? They are diseases caused by tiny microbes that invade the tissues of a host or release poisons. Some microbes such as viruses multiply within a cell and destroy that cell. The polio (poliomyelitis) virus destroys certain cells of the brain or spinal cord, producing the paralysis that is polio's frightening feature.

Certain bacteria, such as those that cause tetanus or diphtheria, produce and secrete powerful poisons (toxins) that spread throughout the body. An unusual example of the effect of bacterial poisons is botulism, a disease produced not by bacteria invading the body but by eating poisons that have been secreted into food by these bacteria. Improper sterilization of food permits these bacteria to survive. (The disease was first associated with improperly prepared sausages, hence its name, from the Latin word for sausage.)

Still another way that bacteria produce disease is by interfering with normal body functions. The bacteria that cause diarrhea disturb the functions of the intestinal tract so that large amounts of water and salts escape without being reabsorbed. Other bacteria can destroy tissue and cause vital organs, such as the brain or liver, to function improperly. Un-

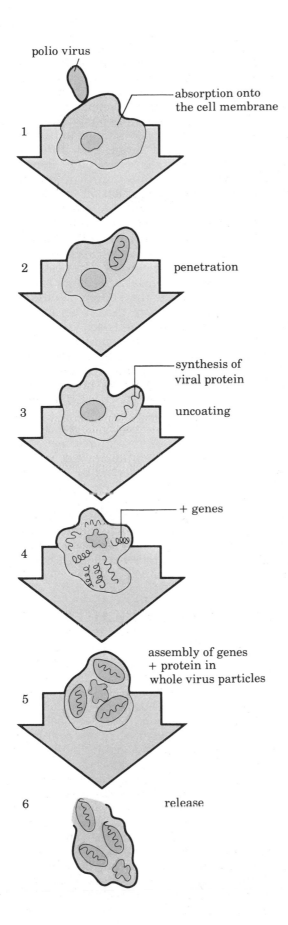

polio virus

1 — absorption onto the cell membrane

2 — penetration

3 — synthesis of viral protein / uncoating

4 — + genes

5 — assembly of genes + protein in whole virus particles

6 — release

INVADING A CELL

The six steps in the multiplication of a virus are charted here, with the polio virus used as an example. In step one the virus attaches itself to a living cell. Step two is penetration: the virus passes through the cell membrane into the cell body. The virus then sheds its outer covering, the capsid (step three). In step four it uses the protein of the living cell to form new viruses containing the genes for further multiplication (step five). In step six the new organisms pass back through the cell membrane to penetrate other cells. Unlike bacteria, viruses are not able to replicate themselves outside living cells. In the process, the cell may be altered or destroyed.

fortunately, the ways that all bacteria produce disease are not understood.

When bacteria or viruses are present in a susceptible host, certain steps must take place before disease occurs. In most cases, the organisms must attach themselves to host cells. Viruses must then penetrate into the cell and be able to multiply. Certain bacteria have attachment preferences for certain cells of the body. Some prefer to attach themselves to teeth, others to the cells of the nose and throat, still others to the cells of the bladder, and so on. This preferential attachment helps explain why some bacteria are found in certain parts of the body more often than in other parts.

Once bacteria have attached themselves, the body tries to defend itself in many ways. One way is through inflammation. During the course of inflammation, the blood vessels enlarge and more blood flows to the area where the bacteria are producing irritation. The blood brings antibodies, protective cells, and other substances to the area, including cells that can "eat" (ingest) the bacteria. These cells are known as phagocytes (cells that eat) (see chapter 6, "The Blood").

Phagocytes are more efficient at ingesting if the bacteria are first coated with antibodies, proteins made by the body in response to foreign substances. In some instances bacteria can be killed by antibody, assisted by other substances in the blood known as complement. Some bacteria are susceptible to the combined action of antibody and complement. Other bacteria resist this combined action but can be killed by phagocytes after being coated with antibody and complement. When bacteria have been attacked by antibiotics, the bacteria stop multiplying and are more easily killed by phagocytes or by antibody and complement.

HUMAN POLIOMYELITIS

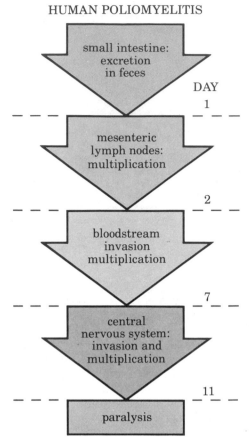

small intestine:
excretion
in feces

DAY
1

mesenteric
lymph nodes:
multiplication

2

bloodstream
invasion
multiplication

7

central
nervous system:
invasion and
multiplication

11

paralysis

4 percent of those with disease
develop paralysis

THE DAMAGING VIRUS

*The spread of a virus and its
consequent damage cover several
days. In this chart of the action of a
polio virus, the organism is swallowed
and it enters the small intestine, where
it invades the cells and multiplies.
The invasion spills over to the
mesentery, which supplies blood to
the intestine, and the cells spread
throughout the body via the lymphatic
system and bloodstream. About a
week after exposure they reach the
brain and spinal cord. Depending on
which cells are affected and the extent
of damage, paralysis of various
body functions can result after about
11 days. If the person has been
vaccinated or had a previous mild
infection, antibodies circulating in the
bloodstream neutralize the invading
viruses, which are then excreted
harmlessly. Only four percent of polio
infections in unvaccinated persons
result in paralysis.*

Even tiny amounts of antibiotics that do not kill bacteria can injure them enough to make them susceptible to the protective activities of the body. Often antibiotics can kill bacteria without the need for other defenses, but in most instances antibodies and phagocytes are critical in helping the body withstand infections. Antibiotics act differently on different bacteria, and the manner of use and their effectiveness vary from infection to infection. Understanding the interaction of antibiotics and body defense mechanisms is one of the skills physicians need to treat infections.

Everyone has experienced inflammation and has noticed that an inflamed area becomes reddened, swollen, and painful. The best way to reduce inflammation is to treat its cause. Occasionally, however, the degree of inflammation becomes so severe that it becomes a threat in itself, and steps then need to be taken to reduce the inflammation. Some bacteria kill so many cells of the host in a small area that the dead cells and tissue fluids accumulate and become pus, a combination of broken-down cells and components of the blood that have been carried to that area to defend the body. Often the pus also contains the bacteria that caused the inflammation. Sometimes the bacteria have been killed but the pus is still present and cannot be absorbed by the body. Judging when the bacteria have been killed, when the pus is safe to remove, and when removing it will spread the infection are aspects of medicine that require understanding and skill. Simply draining pus by squeezing the infected area or by putting a needle in it can be unwise and dangerous.

HOW THE BODY REACTS
TO INFECTION

The first feelings of illness are headache, body ache, weakness, fatigue, listlessness, and poor appetite. As the illness worsens, more severe symptoms develop. The face becomes flushed, the skin and mouth dry, and confusion and even delirium can develop. If the illness is prolonged, there can be weight loss.

The hallmark of infectious diseases is fever. Not all infectious diseases are associated with fever, but most are. There are many causes of fever other than infectious diseases, but when fever is present infection is the most likely source. Fever is caused by certain bacterial products and also by chemicals made by cells other than those of the host in response to the infection. The normal body temperature ranges between 97 and 99 degrees Fahrenheit

(36.5 to 37.5 degrees centigrade). Higher temperatures represent fever. However, "normal" body temperature varies depending on age, sex, and individual differences, so each person's temperature pattern must be taken into account before fever is considered to be present.

Fevers are not dangerous unless the temperatures rise above about 106° Fahrenheit (42° centigrade). They are even beneficial, because some microbes are sensitive to higher temperatures and body defenses may be more active at temperatures higher than 37° centigrade. Fever is even caused by physical activity on hot days, or by diseases in which the metabolism of the body is greatly increased, causing the body to make heat faster than it can lose the excess.

Sweating and heat loss through the skin are among the most useful ways the body can lose excess heat. Aspirin, as everyone knows, can induce sweating in persons with fevers, which causes the temperature to fall because of evaporation. Other substances also can produce sweating and lower body temperature.

It is not always necessary or desirable to reduce the temperature. Except in mild infections such as common colds, aspirin or related drugs should not be used without medical advice, because abrupt changes in temperature can sometimes be harmful. At other times the artificial removal of fever interferes with attempts to determine its cause. For feverish persons who are uncomfortable, or in whom the temperature has risen high enough to be a concern, sponge baths with cool water or alcohol can lower body temperature as well as aspirin or related drugs.

When aspirin is used in mild infections on medical advice, it is recommended that the drug be given regularly every few hours to avoid fluctuations of body temperature.

HOW INFECTION SPREADS

There are many ways that infections spread from one person to another. Respiratory spread occurs when people cough or sneeze, sending into the air infected particles that carry bacteria or viruses to other persons. But inhaled infectious particles do not necessarily come directly from other persons. They come from soil, as in coccidioidomycosis (see page 693), or from bacteria-contaminated fluids such as cooling tower and air conditioning water, as has occurred in instances of Legionnaires' disease. However, person-to-person transmission of infected particles is the most common method of spreading the microbes that cause disease.

Another method of spread has to do with close contact. Many of the viruses that cause common colds are spread this way. A person with a cold can transfer the virus to someone else by touching that person with hands that have acquired the virus from rubbing the nose or eyes. The virus that causes infectious mononucleosis does not spread readily from one individual to another except by quite close contact. That is why the disease has sometimes been nicknamed "the kissing disease."

Infectious agents also can be transmitted by the bites of insects. Mosquitoes transmit malaria, viral encephalitis, and yellow fever. Ticks transmit several diseases.

Water and food are methods of transmission, too. Water-borne infections occur primarily in areas of poor sanitation, when bacteria leave the body and enter the water supply. Spread by food occurs relatively infrequently in industrialized countries, except when contaminated food is improperly prepared or stored before being eaten. If bacteria that cause food poisoning are deposited in a food and if the food is insufficiently cooked and improperly refrigerated, the bacteria will multiply and produce disease in persons who eat it.

Many methods have been developed to prevent the spread of infectious agents from the environment and from other people to susceptible hosts. Common rules of hygiene are among the most important. Careful hand washing, thorough cooking, and proper refrigeration are important in preventing the spread of disease by food. Care is necessary to see that water supplies are not contaminated by sewage and body excretions, particularly in rural areas or in areas with poor sanitation. Isolation of sick persons is sometimes necessary with highly contagious or dangerous diseases, and it is a regular practice to isolate those with tuberculosis until it can be demonstrated that they are no longer shedding bacteria in a manner that can be a hazard to others.

Vaccinations are widely used to stimulate the body's defenses against a particular virus or bacterium. This is a method of giving a mild dose of an infection, which then produces immunity against the organism. Immunity produced by vaccination may last for several years or for life. The degree of immunity differs for different vaccinations, so your immunization record should be reexamined regularly by your physician. Many childhood diseases can be prevented by vaccination. Measles, mumps, German measles (rubella), diphtheria, whooping cough (pertussis), and tetanus are examples of diseases that could be virtually eliminated if the highly successful vaccines against them were widely and properly used. The extraordinary success of smallpox vaccination has been a stimulus to everyone preparing vaccines. (Once a major cause of death and serious illness, smallpox has been completely eradicated.)

Contaminated materials can be sterilized by boiling or by soaking in water with strong soaps or detergents. Soaps and detergents are good sterilizing agents but cannot penetrate and therefore cannot sterilize large amounts of adherent food particles or other dirt and contamination.

Sometimes a physician or health worker will advise that all materials that have been in contact with an ill patient be sterilized before they are handled by others. The sterilization procedure depends on the type of illness.

DIAGNOSING INFECTIOUS DISEASES

Several different microbes can produce similar illnesses. The organism must be identified so the right drug can be given. For example, the common sore throat usually is caused by viruses for which no antibiotic treatments exist. However, some sore throats are caused by types of streptococci, and antibiotics are available to treat them. A throat culture can be taken to detect the presence of the bacteria, which are usually those known as hemolytic streptococci (streptococci that break down red blood cells when added to certain bacterial culture media). Viral sore throats can be sufficiently severe that it is almost impossible to be certain whether a streptococcus or a virus is the cause without a bacterial culture.

Diarrhea also can be caused by several organisms, including viruses, bacteria, protozoa, and even worms. The stool must be examined to identify the cause so the best treatment can be prescribed. A drug used to eradicate worms will have no effect on amoebas, bacteria, or viruses. After treatment is completed, follow-up tests are sometimes necessary to be sure that the cause of the infection has been eliminated.

Identification of the infecting microbe is important in dealing with the spread of an epidemic. An outbreak of influenza might encourage public health authorities to introduce mass immunization campaigns or to close schools to inhibit further spread. Individuals might be advised to avoid extended contacts with large groups of people, such as in theaters, churches, or other gathering places.

A tissue culture is performed by taking a sample or specimen from the infected person. This is usually done by swabbing a small amount of secretions from the throat, although sometimes a specimen of urine or stool is used. The specimen is then placed in a culture medium, a chemical solution in which bacteria will grow.

Different types of culture media are used for different microorganisms, and most bacteria will grow out rapidly and can be identified within a few days. However, the bacteria that cause tuberculosis may take several weeks to grow out and be identified. Viruses are more difficult to culture because they require living cells. A laboratory sometimes needs several weeks to identify certain viruses. Because this is an expensive and demanding procedure, it is not usually performed for mild infections unless there are strong public health reasons.

Other methods of diagnosing infecting microbes have been developed. Skin tests are particularly useful in certain infections. For example, purified extracts of the organisms that cause tuberculosis, if injected into the skin, will indicate whether a person has been infected at some time with tuberculosis bacteria by producing a distinctive rash at the injection site. Related tests have been developed using various ways of introducing these extracts, known as tuberculin. A positive tuberculin test does not necessarily indicate active tuberculosis, only that exposure has occurred sometime in the past. Further tests, X rays, and careful clinical examination are needed to determine whether there is active disease. Often, antituberculosis therapy will be given if the test is positive, even without more evidence of active disease if the physician feels the person runs the risk of developing active disease later. Such therapy has been shown to be effective, particularly in high-risk individuals.

Blood tests are widely used to diagnose infectious diseases. The most common test is to look for antibodies against the microorganisms or their products that have been involved in producing the infection. The body begins to produce specific antibodies a few days after an infection begins, and by about two weeks antibodies are detectable in most infections. However, in some infections, such as toxoplasmosis or infectious hepatitis, an-

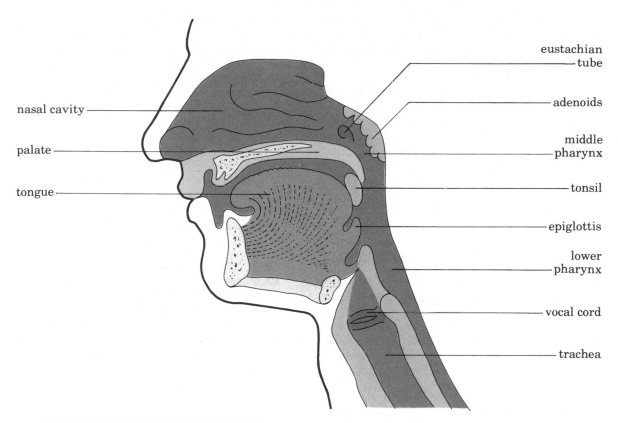

UPPER RESPIRATORY INFECTIONS

Respiratory infections are the most common human ailments. A variety of viruses and some bacteria are responsible. Once these organisms have been inhaled, they can reproduce and spread throughout the interconnecting structures shown here, causing inflammation and swelling. This illustrates why a person with a common cold can have inflamed nasal tissues, a sore throat, a hoarse voice, plugged ears, earache, difficulty swallowing, and perhaps tonsil and adenoidal symptoms. The infections are spread by personal contact and by droplets of moisture that contain the offending organism.

tibodies sometimes do not appear for several additional weeks. In those cases the doctor is likely to ask for more blood later.

Antibodies remain in the body after infection subsides. They often protect against a recurrence of the same infection, but not always. Sometimes, as in influenza, the virus changes from year to year so the previous antibody offers limited or no protection.

RESPIRATORY INFECTIONS

Respiratory infections are the most common infectious diseases. The symptoms and signs for the common upper respiratory infections are well known: running nose, stuffiness, headache, sneezing, general feeling of illness, occasional cough, and fever. These usually last five to seven days, but in more severe infections caused by certain viruses, symptoms are likely to persist for two or three weeks and then disappear slowly.

The Common Cold

The common cold is caused by a great variety of different viruses. That is why the same person may have so many different attacks, and why the symptoms may be a bit different from one attack to another. Some immunity develops after repeated exposure, so adults get fewer colds than children.

Colds are contagious. They spread by personal contact more than by droplets, but droplets are to some degree infectious, too. Most colds in families occur because schoolchildren come into close contact with one another, allowing an infection to spread rapidly and to be brought to the home. Viruses also can be transferred by touching contaminated objects that have been handled by infected persons, although once objects have been dried and cleaned the amount of virus disappears rapidly.

Exposure to cold or wet weather has nothing to do with "catching a cold." There probably are more colds in winter because colder temperatures keep people indoors and in closer contact with one another. The feeling of chill that many persons experience is usually the first sign that a cold is developing. The chill does not cause the cold.

At the first sign of a cold, try to avoid contact with others. Colds are most contagious during the early period when the cold is developing and during the first day or two after the symptoms have appeared. For milder forms of the common cold, aspirin and related compounds can relieve the fever and general feeling of ill health. Other drugs can help to dry the nasal congestion and give some comfort. These measures provide comfort but do not hasten recovery. The usual cold lasts five to seven days regardless of treatment.

The most important complications of common colds are secondary bacterial infections, which appear in the form of sinusitis, pneumonia or bronchitis, and tonsillitis. In general, if a cold is not getting better, or if it becomes abruptly worse after it appeared to be improving, medical attention should be sought.

Influenza

Many respiratory infections are labeled "flu," but true influenza is caused by a specific group of viruses that produce a characteristic pattern of disease. True influenza comes on suddenly, with fever, chills, muscle aches (particularly in the back), fatigue, and weakness that can be severe. In contrast to the common cold, there is a dry nose and dry cough, but the eyes can be quite red. The lack of energy may continue for several weeks, particularly in older people, and the disease is particularly severe in the elderly. Influenza spreads rapidly through a school or community. In fact, one of the ways of determining whether an outbreak of respiratory infection is influenza is to look for rapid spread of these symptoms.

Although each attack of influenza means most of the victims produce enough antibody to protect them from a new infection with the same virus, the organism has a tendency to change (mutate) every few years. The changes usually are minor, so that those who were ill the previous "flu season" tend to have some immunity to the new virus. Periodically, perhaps every decade or so, the virus undergoes a striking change, radical enough that even those who have experienced the previous attacks are not immune to the new variety. The appearance of new viruses accounts for the worldwide influenza epidemic of 1918 and 1919, the "Asian flu" of 1957, the "Hong Kong flu" of 1966, and the "Russian flu" of 1978, all of which are named for the areas in which the virus was first identified.

Because the "flu" virus has a propensity to change, public health authorities have established laboratories in various parts of the world to try to isolate the responsible virus whenever an outbreak occurs. The newly isolated virus is then compared with those that have caused previous epidemics. If they are different, attempts are made to produce and distribute vaccines as quickly as possible, particularly to those who face increased risk, such as pregnant women, infants, the elderly, and those with cardiac or respiratory disease. The vaccine generally is harmless, producing only redness and occasional pain at the site of injection. However, it is prepared from fertilized eggs, and persons allergic to egg proteins should receive the vaccine only under close medical supervision.

Influenza is usually spread by the inhalation of infectious virus particles that have been coughed and sneezed into the air. Once an outbreak has begun, individuals should avoid crowded places and contact with those who have the infection. Because influenza is a viral disease, antibiotics are not effective against it.

The best treatment is bed rest, fluids, and aspirin or related compounds to relieve the ache and fever. Persistent fever or worsening of symptoms may herald the onset of pneumonia, the most feared complication of influenza. Sometimes the complication is caused by the influenza virus itself, which penetrates the lung and causes severe pneumonia, damaging cells throughout the larger air passages. More often, the preceding viral infection decreases the lung's resistance to bacterial infection, and bacterial pneumonia occurs. Under the latter conditions, antibiotics should be instituted promptly. Influenza is a dangerous disease, particularly to those in the high-risk category.

Sinusitis

The sinuses are air-filled spaces within the facial bones. The most important sinuses are shown on page 296. They are connected through small passages to the nose or mouth, and the linings of the sinuses secrete a mucous substance that drains through these passages. Bacteria and viruses enter the sinuses upward through these connections, and if the connecting ducts become inflamed, the sinuses will fail to drain either mucus or the products of inflammation. They can then become severely inflamed, painful, and swell.

Usually, sinusitis begins with a common upper respiratory infection, after which painful swelling occurs over one or more of the sinuses. Thick mucus and pus sometimes drain through the passages into the nose or the back of the mouth. There may be fever, fatigue, and soreness, tearing, and sometimes reddening of the eyes. The pain may be severe over the afflicted sinus. In rare instances the infection spreads from the sinus to surrounding bone or even to the eye or brain. Acute sinusitis must be recognized and treated promptly with antibiotics.

Treatment is directed at restoring drainage of the sinuses by using drugs that kill the microbes and drugs that shrink the tissues of the connecting ducts. It is sometimes necessary to provide drainage surgically.

Sore Throat

Often, when a common cold or influenza is coming on, mild discomfort occurs in the throat and back of the mouth, along with feelings of tiredness and chilliness. The throat becomes reddened, swollen, and painful as the organisms spread in the tissues and multiply. In some cases the soreness is severe.

Most sore throats stem from the common respiratory viruses. A minority of sore throats are caused by the common bacterium hemolytic streptococcus (see page 666).

Bacterial sore throats can have symptoms and signs that are difficult to distinguish from viral sore throats, and sometimes they are more severe. Viral sore throats tend to get better within a few days without treatment. However, a "strep" throat should be treated with antibiotics to help prevent spread by destroying the organisms promptly, and to prevent the complication of rheumatic fever.

Before antibiotics, rheumatic fever was a common disease in childhood, particularly affecting underprivileged populations. Joint pain and swelling, sometimes accompanied by complications of the heart, appeared in about three percent of the children about two weeks after a streptococcal infection. An additional complication was Sydenham's chorea, also known as St. Vitus' dance, marked by uncoordinated, jerky movements. Many children with rheumatic fever suffered permanent scarring of the heart valves. The victims of rheumatic heart disease were more often women than men, for reasons not clear.

In recent years, the incidence of rheumatic fever has fallen strikingly, possibly because of antibiotic treatment for bacterial sore throats, possibly because the population is generally healthier and less crowded. However, "strep throat" still can be serious because the streptococci can spread from the throat into other tissues or into the bloodstream. Streptococcal infections should be treated for a minimum of 10 days. If they are treated for a shorter time, there is a greater likelihood of recurrence of the infection and of the development of rheumatic complication.

Certain kinds of hemolytic streptococci are associated with a kidney disease called acute glomerulonephritis. Antibiotics do not appear to prevent glomerulonephritis from occurring in infected persons, but they do appear to be helpful in limiting the spread of streptococci, so they reduce the likelihood that close contacts will develop the infection. Fortunately, glomerulonephritis usually heals itself and only rarely produces severe kidney trouble later. However, during the acute illness, the kidneys can be so affected that the person develops high blood pressure, swelling of the face and other tissues, and other serious complications. The telltale clue is blood in the urine. If this symptom follows streptococcal infection, it should receive prompt medical attention.

Tonsil infection. Occasionally, sore throats progress and the streptococci invade the tonsils and surrounding tissues, producing acute tonsillitis or quinsy sore throat, which is abscesses around the tonsils or in the throat. These complications are characterized by persistent high fever, severe sore throat, and difficulty in swallowing. Usually an enlarged or displaced tonsil can be seen in the area of inflammation. Antibiotics are effective if administered early. Occasionally, if pus is present, the infection must be drained surgically. Tonsillectomy is sometimes recommended if infections occur repeatedly.

Diphtheria in its mild form can look like other sore throats. In its severe form, the throat is covered with a gray inflammation that can be so severe that it interferes with breathing as it spreads down to the vocal cords and the bronchi. The bacteria that cause diphtheria are not themselves highly invasive, but they secrete a powerful poison (toxin) that can damage heart muscle and the nervous system. Diphtheria is uncommon in the United States now that most children are immunized, but it still occurs in populations that have not been immunized, and remains common in underdeveloped countries. Occasionally, it strikes adults who were immunized in childhood, but whose immunization no longer protects them, so booster "shots" at least every 10 years are recommended. However, in affluent populations where there is no contact with diphtheria, the risks are tiny.

Treatment for diphtheria involves antitoxin to neutralize the bacterial toxin and antibiotics to kill the bacteria so they cannot produce more toxin. Killing the bacteria alone has no effect on the toxin already released. If the swelling in the throat becomes so severe that the person cannot breathe, it is necessary to insert a tube in the throat (entubation) or make an opening into the trachea leading to the lungs (tracheostomy) for breathing assistance until the disease is brought under control.

Laryngitis

Inflammations of the larynx, the area of the throat containing the vocal cords (see illustration on page 667), are common and often associated with acute respiratory illnesses. Some hoarseness accompanying a common cold is well known to all. However, the hoarseness occasionally becomes more severe, particularly in children. The cough may become deep and barking, and worsen at night. Bacteria sometimes cause laryngeal infections, but more frequently the offenders are viruses, spread in the same manner as common cold viruses.

When laryngitis is caused by bacteria, antibiotics are helpful, but for viral infections there is no treatment except to rest the vocal cords, drink fluids, and take analgesics if necessary. If the person has difficulty breathing, prompt medical attention is essential.

A common form of laryngitis in young children is called croup. It often comes on suddenly when a child has an upper respiratory illness. A barking cough and hoarse voice indicate that the child's larynx has become inflamed.

The inflammation and swelling narrow the airway and can impair breathing, making croup a serious disease. Steam relieves the swelling and eases breathing. Because children are often frightened by the change in voice and the difficulty in breathing, a reassuring way to help is for an adult to hold the child while sitting in a closed bathroom with a shower of hot water running into a cold bathtub or into a bathtub in which there is a small amount of cold water.

Pertussis (Whooping Cough)

Infants and children have the most severe form of this bacterial infection. They experience long episodes of coughing so severe that they must take a huge inward breath which produces the characteristic whoop. The mucus in the bronchi is thick and sticky. That makes it difficult to cough up, so the coughs come in paroxysms, or may be so long and fierce that the infant turns blue and vomits. However, asphyxia does not seem to occur. The most life-threatening complication is pneumonia that sometimes follows whooping cough. The pneumonia usually can be treated with antibiotics, as can pertussis. Exposure to warm, moist air, good nutrition, and medical attention to remove the thick mucus are helpful.

Once common in the United States, pertussis has been nearly eliminated through widespread immunization. The vaccine is usually given in two doses, often combined with the vaccines for diphtheria and tetanus, so that the combination is known as the "DPT" shot (see chapter 27, "Taking Care of Your Child," for recommended schedule of immunizations). Immunity conferred by the vaccine generally decreases after seven to ten years, and there have been a few small outbreaks of whooping cough among adults. Fortunately, infection in adults is generally mild.

In populations not immunized, as many as five percent of the children who get whooping cough die of the disease. They are found mostly among the underprivileged in the United States and in the developing countries.

Pneumonia

Pneumonia is an infection of the lung. The infection may be limited to one area of the lung, or may involve several portions. Because the lungs are needed to transfer oxygen from the air into the blood, lung disease can reduce oxygen supply to the rest of the body. Another danger is that the bacteria causing the infection can spread from the lung to other parts of the body. For these reasons, pneumonia can be one of the most serious infections and must be treated carefully.

There are two lungs, one on each side of the chest. The left lung is divided into two sections called lobes. The right lung is divided into three lobes. If an entire lobe is involved, the pneumonia is referred to as lobar pneumonia. Sometimes more than one lobe is involved at the same time. If patches of the lung but not an entire lobe are involved, the condition is called bronchial pneumonia. Often pneumonia and bronchitis occur together.

Symptoms of pneumonia are cough, fever, rapid breathing, pain in the chest, and production of sputum. There is often a shaking chill. The sputum is whitish-yellow or brown-gray and sometimes is bloodstained, depending on the severity of the disease and the size of the lung area involved.

Many different kinds of bacteria and viruses can cause pneumonia. In highly susceptible individuals, almost any of the common bacteria or viruses can be responsible. New bacteria continue to be discovered as causes.

The pneumococcus or *Streptococcus pneumoniae* is the most common cause of bacterial pneumonia, both lobar and bronchial. The disease begins when a small number of these germs are inhaled into the lung tissue. Often a previous viral respiratory infection has lowered resistance to superimposed bacteria. Some persons carry pneumococci in the throat for long periods without contracting disease. It is not clear why bacteria sometimes trigger severe disease and at other times cause no ill effects.

Other bacteria besides pneumococcus cause pneumonia. It is important to try to determine exactly which type of bacterium is responsible, because different strains require different treatments. It is not always possible to make this determination precisely, so the physician will make the best judgment he or she can, based on the probabilities and the clinical appearance of the patient, the sputum, and other findings. If the initial judgment brings less than satisfactory results, the treatment often will be changed because different bacteria may be involved that require different antibiotics. Most forms of bacterial pneumonia respond to the proper antibiotic, usually in about two weeks. No antibiotic cures the viral form, but it is usually less severe.

A pneumococcal vaccine has been developed to prevent certain kinds of pneumonia. It consists of bacterial products isolated from the 14 types of pneumococci that are the most common causes of pneumonia. The value of the vaccine is still under investigation, but it is clear that individuals who have unusual susceptibility benefit substantially from it. Whether the vaccine should be used more widely is not clear.

Legionnaires' Disease

In the summer of 1976, 182 persons who attended a convention of the American Legion in Philadelphia or who were near the conference center became ill with severe pneumonia, and 29 died. However, the pneumonia did not spread to members of the family or to others in close contact with the patients.

After months of investigation researchers found that the pneumonia was caused by a bacterium never before identified. It has since been named *Legionella pneumophilia,* a term that combines the American Legion connection with the Greek words that mean "love of the lung."

Since this group of microorganisms was first isolated, other outbreaks of illness caused by them have been recognized. Two major forms of the illness are now known. In the most severe, there is a rapidly progressive pneumonia with dry cough, fever, muscle pains, and diarrhea, which begin a week to three weeks after exposure. This form, which is particularly severe for the elderly, has sometimes been traced to sprays from water towers and air conditioning units in which the organism has multiplied.

A less severe influenza-like illness lasting two or three days, marked by fever and a general feeling of illness but without cough or pneumonia, also has been identified. This type sometimes has been associated with rapid spread of the bacteria from air conditioning towers. However, there also have been outbreaks of the disease in hospitals, particularly among individuals whose immunity is depressed, in which contaminated air conditioners do not appear to be involved. Extensive efforts are being made to determine how the bacteria are spread under such conditions.

Treatment with the right antibiotics is successful if begun early in the course of the illness, and prevention can take place if contaminated sources of water are treated with germicides. It is not known where the organism resides in nature, but it has been isolated from certain samples of soil and water.

There remains much to be learned about Legionnaires' disease. Already it is clear that there are many different types of Legionella and that other organisms resembling it also cause pneumonia and related infection.

Legionella is not contagious from one person to another. No vaccine is available, although research is progressing.

Tuberculosis

As recently as 1950 tuberculosis was one of the most common causes of death in industrialized nations. Since then, improved hygiene, housing, and nutrition have eliminated the spread of the bacteria and effective drugs for treatment have been developed. Nevertheless, in slums and pockets of poverty in the United States and in other countries, tuberculosis is still a significant cause of disease and death.

Tuberculosis produces a chronic infection in many people. Others carry the tubercle bacillus in their bodies for long periods and do not become sick or show any evidence of tuberculosis. Nevertheless, at some time these men and women may suffer decreased resistance, allowing the bacteria to multiply aggressively and invade the tissues, producing active disease.

Evidence of pulmonary tuberculosis includes persistence of fever over many weeks, night sweats, loss of weight, and cough, sometimes producing blood-streaked sputum. The bacteria can spread from the lungs to kidneys, bones, brain, intestines, and throughout the body. That is why signs and symptoms of the disease can arise from almost anywhere.

Persons who have been exposed to tubercle bacilli develop sensitivity to tuberculin, the highly purified protein extracted from the microorganisms. Because resistance has developed, they will react positively when a small amount of tuberculin is injected into the skin. A red spot will develop at the site of the injection two or three days later. In many parts of the country there are common infections not caused by tuberculosis but by organisms similar to the tubercle bacillus, so the skin test does not always mean that the individual has been exposed to tuberculosis. The meaning of a positive skin test must be carefully evaluated by physicians, especially in those regions.

Even when the positive skin test indicates exposure to tuberculosis, it does not mean active tuberculosis, only that the tubercle bacillus has at some time multiplied in the person's body. A chest X ray, sputum analysis, and other tests may be necessary to determine whether there is active disease or whether the disease is under control.

Tuberculosis is a completely treatable disease, with several drugs effective in killing tubercle bacilli. However, such drugs must be given for months or years to ensure that the bacteria are eradicated. If the drugs are stopped early, a relapse can occur, and bacteria that were not killed sometimes become resistant to the drugs. That resistance makes it more difficult to eradicate the infection with subsequent treatment.

Patients with active tuberculosis sometimes spread the germs to others. Therefore, when a case is discovered, it is customary to test the family and others in close contact with the infected person. In general, only someone who is coughing can spread the microbes, although other body fluids can spread the disease. However, a patient who has been properly treated usually becomes noninfectious quickly and can be in full contact with others.

A vaccine known as BCG has been developed from the tubercle bacillus. It has its greatest use in individuals who face a high risk of developing the disease. It is not needed for most people in the United States. Individuals who have received the BCG vaccine react to the skin test as though they have active disease.

GASTROINTESTINAL INFECTIONS

Gastrointestinal infections are those that affect either the stomach (gastro) or the intestines. When the stomach is irritated, there is usually nausea and vomiting, sometimes known as gastritis. When the intestines are irritated, there is usually diarrhea and cramping pains, sometimes known as enteritis. Commonly, there will be a combination of the two, generally called gastroenteritis.

Gastroenteritis

Gastroenteritis usually lasts only one or two days. It can be caused by a large number of infectious and toxic agents. These include contamination of food by excesses of metal, such as foods that have been stored in tin containers too long; or toxins that appear naturally in foods, such as toxic mushrooms; or toxins that are released into sprouted potatoes. Most commonly, however, bacteria and viruses account for gastroenteritis.

The most common toxin comes from food contaminated with certain staphylococci that multiply in the food. Eating the food leads to feelings of illness within a few hours. The person may notice increased amounts of saliva, nausea, vomiting, abdominal cramps, and mild diarrhea. Fever is uncommon. If vomiting is severe, particularly in a small child, dehydration can occur, a particular problem in hot weather. In these cases, medical help should be obtained promptly.

Staphylococci that cause this type of food poisoning are particularly likely to multiply in foods containing dairy products, such as salad dressings and cream-filled desserts, but they also multiply in certain meats and meat products. If the food is refrigerated properly, the staphylococci do not multiply and the toxins do not accumulate. No specific treatment is needed, except to correct dehydration by giving fluids.

In recent years researchers have discovered that a large number of viruses also cause gastroenteritis. The virus-caused variety has many names, such as "winter vomiting disease" and "intestinal flu." A group of viruses known as rotaviruses are particularly involved, although others can be responsible. Usually, there is diarrhea with nausea and vomiting. The illness lasts a few days, then slowly goes away. There is no specific treatment except to watch for dehydration and to correct it if severe. The method of spread of the virus is probably hand to mouth, or hand to food to mouth, via contact with infected people. Those who have symptoms should not prepare food for others.

Diarrhea

Diarrhea is difficult to define, but it is best described as more and looser bowel movements than usual. In the more severe forms, movements are quite watery, with blood or pus and a great deal of mucus. Most people normally have no more than one to three bowel movements a day, and many move their bowels only every two or three days, so the true definition of diarrhea is based on individual habits. Because so many different bacteria, viruses, protozoa, worms, and toxic materials can cause diarrhea, each episode must be looked at carefully to determine the cause, particularly if the episode affects many people and is severe.

Among the most important bacterial causes of diarrhea are the bacteria known as *Salmonella*, *Shigella*, certain types of *E. coli*, *Yersinia*, and *Vibrio cholera*. The most important protozoal causes are amoeba and *Giardia*. Any of the worms that infect the intestines can cause diarrhea, the most common being hookworms, whipworms, schistosomes, strongyloides, and tapeworms. Probably the most common chemical cause of diarrhea is alcohol.

Diarrhea usually disappears in a few days. However, in infants, small children, elderly people, or those already dehydrated or sick from another cause, diarrhea can be particularly severe, and medical attention should be sought promptly. Medical help is also required if the diarrhea lasts more than one to two days, if it is accompanied by fever and severe abdominal cramps, if it is severe and frequent or accompanied by blood, pus, or mucus in the stools, or if it is accompanied by rashes, jaundice (yellowing of the skin or whites of the eyes), or extreme weakness. All these symptoms should be treated as danger signals.

Cholera is the most severe form of diarrhea. Fortunately, it is now largely limited to tropical and subtropical countries. Victims of cholera may put out a huge amount of fluid from the intestinal tract. As many as 10 gallons a day have been recorded. It is easy to see how victims can become terribly dehydrated. Research has shown that if there is rapid replacement of the water and the salts excreted with it, the person recovers quickly. Certain antibiotics are effective in killing the bacteria that produce some types of diarrhea, including cholera, which helps shorten the course of the disease.

Whatever the cause, the major complication of diarrhea is dehydration. To offset it, persons who are not vomiting a great deal can drink fluids. Fluids that contain salts and small amounts of sugar are particularly beneficial. A good homemade mixture is a quart of water with a teaspoon of sugar and a pinch of salt. However, fluids should not be forced on persons who feel that they will only vomit them immediately. Severely dehydrated individuals can be given fluids intravenously.

Certain organisms that cause diarrhea can spread to other parts of the body. For example, amoebas may settle in the liver and cause abscesses. Typhoid fever is accompanied by the spread of the bacteria to other organs in many cases. Sometimes the diarrhea is misjudged: infectious hepatitis sometimes starts as a mild diarrhea, but then jaundice appears, indicating that it is not food poisoning.

The methods of spread vary, but the organisms usually enter the body through the mouth. Infected persons who contaminate the food and food that comes from animal sources that carry these organisms are major sources of spread. (Most meats and poultry contain many of the bacteria that cause food poisoning, but the bacteria are killed if the foods are cooked adequately.) Contaminated water is a common source of organisms causing diarrhea, particularly in areas where the sewage disposal system is inadequate. Sometimes animals die and spread bacteria into the water. Homosexual activity has also been implicated in spreading the unwanted bacteria from person to person. Epidemics of amebiasis, giardiasis, infectious hepatitis, bacillary dysentery, and typhoid fever have all been traced to contamination of food or water spread from individual to individual.

Typhoid Fever

Typhoid fever is a particularly severe form of salmonella infection caused by the strain known as *Salmonella typhi*. Symptoms include sustained high fever often lasting for several weeks, severe headache, constipation, a feeling of severe illness, and sometimes cough. Small red spots may appear on the abdomen. The major complications are intestinal hemorrhages. The intestines may be perforated by the bacteria, a serious problem indeed.

In contrast to other *Salmonella* strains that are widely found in domestic and wild animals, the typhoid bacillus lives only in humans. Because the bacillus is cast off from the body through bowel movements, it can contaminate food and water unless sanitary precautions are taken. In the past typhoid fever occurred in widespread epidemics because drinking water systems were contaminated by sewage. Today the water supplies are safe in most developed countries. When an outbreak of typhoid fever occurs, it is usually because a typhoid carrier (a person who is carrying the typhoid bacilli but shows no obvious symptoms) unknowingly contaminates food before it is eaten by others.

Persons who have recently recovered from typhoid fever sometimes continue to shed germs in the stool for weeks, months, or even for a lifetime. Many are not aware that they are typhoid carriers, although they are aware that they had the disease. Such carriers should observe special sanitary precautions. After

---

Precautions to Prevent Gastroenteritis and Diarrhea

- Infected persons should not handle food others will eat.
- Wash hands after using the toilet and before preparation of food.
- Prepared food should be refrigerated if not eaten promptly.
- Meat and meat products should be cooked. Avoid rare and raw foods.
- Never eat pork and poultry when they are pink (not thoroughly cooked).
- A frozen turkey or large fowl should be completely thawed before being stuffed and roasted. If the interior of the turkey is not completely thawed, it may not cook thoroughly. Bacteria will multiply and gastroenteritis will spread.

---

using a toilet, they should spray the seat and bowl with disinfectant. They should wash their hands carefully afterwards, and wash before handling foods. Known carriers should not be involved in the preparation or handling of food in restaurants.

Typhoid fever can be treated with antibacterial drugs, and a vaccine is available that lowers the risk of contracting the disease. A person traveling into areas where typhoid fever still occurs should be vaccinated as a precaution (see page 697). The vaccine is not effective if the person receives a large dose of typhoid bacilli in food or water, but it is effective against smaller doses. The vaccine itself often causes some swelling and pain of the arm and even a mild fever.

Hepatitis

Research over the past few years has uncovered several different types of hepatitis. Two main forms have been definitely identified. A third form and perhaps additional ones are being recognized.

Type A hepatitis. "Infectious hepatitis" and "serum hepatitis" are the traditional names for the most common types. Infectious hepatitis is more precisely called type A hepatitis. The virus causing this disease usually spreads through bowel movements after being ingested much like the viruses of food poisoning. Within two to five weeks, susceptible persons who have acquired the virus will develop nausea, vomiting, loss of appetite, and loss of taste for cigarettes and many foods.

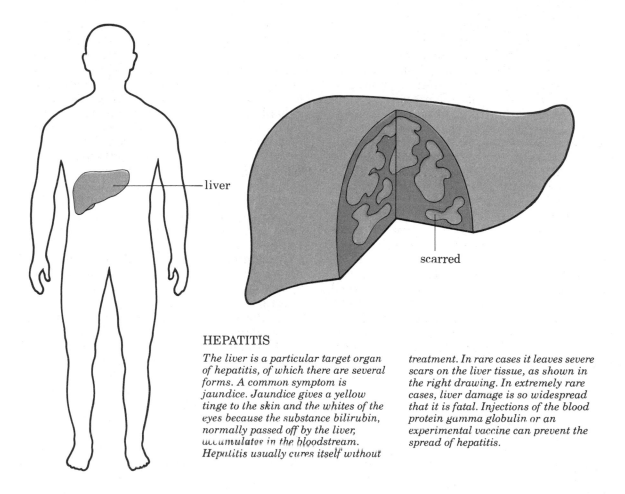

liver

scarred

HEPATITIS

The liver is a particular target organ of hepatitis, of which there are several forms. A common symptom is jaundice. Jaundice gives a yellow tinge to the skin and the whites of the eyes because the substance bilirubin, normally passed off by the liver, accumulates in the bloodstream. Hepatitis usually cures itself without

treatment. In rare cases it leaves severe scars on the liver tissue, as shown in the right drawing. In extremely rare cases, liver damage is so widespread that it is fatal. Injections of the blood protein gamma globulin or an experimental vaccine can prevent the spread of hepatitis.

They often develop intense feelings of fatigue and muscle and joint aches. The urine may become dark, the color of the stools more like clay, and jaundice may appear (yellowing of the skin and whites of the eyes). Sometimes there is mild fever. Children often have a milder illness and do not always develop jaundice, but they still spread the virus to others.

Type A hepatitis usually clears up within a week or two, but in some instances continues for several months. In a few relatively rare instances the disease progresses to cause severe scarring of the liver, known as cirrhosis. Convalescence needs vary. Some persons feel fit within a few days or weeks, while others require months to return to normal. Occasionally, those who have resumed full activity suffer a relapse. The illness sometimes reappears, although generally in a milder form. A rare complication of type A hepatitis is infection so severe that the liver is destroyed, causing death in less than a week.

There is no specific treatment for type A hepatitis except bed rest. Precautions similar to those for gastroenteritis and typhoid fever should be taken to avoid spreading the virus to others. Individuals with type A hepatitis are not likely to spread the disease to other members of their family or to those with whom they are in close contact. Nevertheless it is a good idea to have ill persons use separate dishes and to wash them separately in a dishwasher or in strong detergents to minimize any possibility of spread.

Type B hepatitis is often more severe than type A. The virus is most commonly spread from the blood of an infected individual to others, but it can be ingested in food or water, too. Type B hepatitis is a particular problem among homosexuals because it is spread by certain forms of sexual contact. Type B hepatitis usually takes longer to incubate. The disease often does not appear for six months after someone has acquired the virus. It is often slower to heal than type A, and is more likely to leave the person with scarring of the liver. A few persons retain type B virus in the blood for many years. Like type A, there is no specific treatment except bed rest.

Both types of hepatitis are accompanied by virus in feces, saliva, tears, and blood. In both instances unsanitary conditions can aggravate spread of the disease. Untreated sewage often contains hepatitis virus because so many people pass the virus out in their feces. Hepatitis outbreaks have been traced to shellfish taken from waters contaminated by untreated sewage. Narcotics addicts who share needles without sterilizing them are also particularly likely to pass type B virus to one another. Carriers of type B hepatitis virus should never be permitted to give blood for transfusions. Carriers can be detected by a simple blood test.

Protection against the spread of hepatitis, particularly type A hepatitis, can be achieved by injections of human gamma globulin, a blood protein that carries antibodies against the virus and that can neutralize the infectious particles before they spread. In recent years scientists have developed a vaccine against type B hepatitis. Still in the experimental stage, the vaccine appears to be effective, although it takes two or three months after injection for the effect to be fully realized.

Blood tests can distinguish type A and type B hepatitis. The use of the tests has disclosed another form of hepatitis that is transmitted by blood products and is neither A nor B. It has been termed "non-A/non-B hepatitis," but in fact it may represent a group of infections. Research in non-A/non-B hepatitis has been helped by the discovery that this form of hepatitis can be produced in chimpanzees.

Many viruses other than the ones usually associated with hepatitis can spread to the liver and produce jaundice. Infectious mononucleosis (see page 690) is often associated with jaundice, as is a disease called cytomegalic inclusion disease. In fact, any severe infection can produce some degree of jaundice.

URINARY INFECTIONS

Urinary infections are among the most common of all infections, occurring in 10 to 20 percent of women and in about one-half of one percent of men at some time in their lives. The infections are often present without causing symptoms, so specific tests have been developed to detect them.

Infections of the urinary system are usually caused by the common bacteria found in the intestinal tract. These bacteria find their way to the urethra, the conduit from the bladder that leads outside the body. The female urethra is quite short, opening near the vagina. The bacteria ascend along the urethra into the bladder and multiply in urine. The cells lining the urethra inhibit bacteria to some degree, so the greater length of the urethra in males probably explains why infections in men are much less common than in females.

No one knows why some women develop urinary tract infections although the majority do not. Sometimes the bacteria are introduced by the use of catheters or other instruments, but this accounts for only a minority of infections in women. Instruments and surgery account for the overwhelming majority of infections in men.

The symptoms of cystitis (bladder infection) consist of a frequent urge to urinate, awakening at night with this urge, painful urination, and pain in the lower abdomen. The kidney is often infected, too, also without symptoms. When symptoms are produced, they usually are the same as those of bladder infection, but there also can be fever and pain over the kidney area.

Infections of the urinary tract are found in about one percent of grade-school girls and rise by about one percent for each 10 years of life, so that at any given time about seven to eight percent of women over 70 have a urinary infection. Many urinary infections disappear spontaneously only to return later, so that the total number of women in each age group who have had urinary infections is three to four times the number infected at any one time. These figures suggest that there is a common pattern through which women get their infections, but no one knows why, except for the minority of infections in which an instrument is directly involved.

Although bladder infections in men usually follow instrumentation, in older men they may result from enlargement of the prostate gland. The prostate is located just below the neck of the bladder through which the urine is discharged. Enlargement of the prostate, common in men over 50, can impede complete emptying of the bladder. If bacteria are present and if not all of the urine can be emptied, the bacteria will multiply within the bladder and can spread to the kidney. This is why it is difficult to eradicate infections in the presence of obstruction or any other abnormality that interferes with the free drainage of urine.

The diagnosis of urinary tract infection is made by finding numerous bacteria in the urine, often accompanied by evidence of pus or blood. A great variety of antimicrobial drugs can be given, and the discomfort is usually relieved in a day or two.

Because the symptoms are not specific, a person can have one or more of them, but examination of the urine reveals no evidence of infection. For instance, many people have backaches, but infections of the kidney account for only a small percentage of backaches. Similarly, there are many reasons why the urine might burn on passage, including infections limited to the urethra, injury, and even various types of neuralgic pains. Accordingly, cultures of the urine are necessary to determine whether a urinary infection is present.

In cases of infection, the urine sometimes looks cloudy, as though it contained pus. Sometimes blood is passed. But cloudy urine does not always mean pus. Urine is often cloudy just after a meal because the urine becomes more alkaline as acid is pumped into the stomach for digestion. An alkaline urine causes some salts to become insoluble, making the urine appear cloudy. All of this means that only careful examination of the urine by skilled practitioners can determine whether a urinary tract infection is present.

It is often said that sexual intercourse produces urinary infection, and women are often advised to wipe from front to back after urinating or after a bowel movement in order to prevent the spread of bacteria toward the urethra. Neither of these ideas has any scientific evidence of support. Although folklore and even medical literature suggest a link between sexual activity and urinary infection, and terms such as "honeymoon cystitis" are popular, in fact the rate of infection in women who have frequent sexual intercourse is the same as in women who have intercourse infrequently. For people in whom infections recur often, it is wise to give an antibacterial drug for several months as a way of permitting the urinary tract to heal itself without new infections. The tendency of urinary infections to recur is high, which can be troublesome unless steps are taken.

Drinking plenty of water probably helps prevent urinary infections by causing the bladder to be emptied often. Bacteria that have entered the bladder have no opportunity to multiply before being passed out. This is a preventive method only, however. Antimicrobial drugs are still the most effective way to deal with urinary infections once they occur.

When a woman has repeated infections, or when infections occur in very young children, it is customary to X-ray the kidneys to be certain that there is no correctable anatomic defect and to assess the degree of damage. Many obstructions can be corrected surgically, although it is a matter for careful judgment and requires consultation among skilled physicians.

If bacteria have invaded the kidney and produce symptoms that are more severe, the kidney could be seriously damaged. Accordingly, kidney infections should be looked for even when there are no symptoms, and should be treated promptly if discovered. Any obstruction must be relieved promptly. Occasionally, kidney infections spread into the bloodstream and become quite serious, or they break out of the kidney and produce abscesses around it that require surgical treatment. Sometimes an infection will lead to formation of a kidney stone, or a stone forms for other reasons and produces obstruction, which in turn makes it difficult for an infection to be cured.

Cultures should be taken before treatment of a kidney infection because the bacteria responsible may be resistant to a particular antibiotic or may persist without causing symptoms after the infection apparently has subsided. Many physicians urge patients with histories of urinary infections to have cultures several times a year even when there are no symptoms, because even an infection with no symptoms can produce continued low-grade damage in some persons.

INFECTIONS OF THE NERVOUS SYSTEM

Meningitis

Meningitis, which is inflammation of the meninges, the membranes that cover the brain and the spinal cord, is a most serious infection when caused by bacteria, although usually somewhat less serious when caused by viruses. Fortunately, bacterial meningitis is rare, and effective antibiotics are available, so the likelihood of death or of severe brain damage is much less than it was decades ago.

Bacterial meningitis occurs in epidemics and as isolated single cases. The symptoms are fever, sleepiness to the point of inability to wake up, confusion, irritability, stiffness, and pain in the neck. Often there is pain in the muscles of the back and legs. There may be an associated rash, with tiny, dark red spots all over the body. Before antibiotics, untreated meningitis was almost always fatal. Even with the best of treatment, a few cases are still fatal. Because the infection produces inflammation of the brain and spinal cord, muscle weakness or brain damage may occur afterwards. Of course, the earlier and the more effective the treatment, the less the likelihood of severe damage.

The bacteria most commonly involved in bacterial meningitis are the meningococcus, pneumococcus, and *Hemophilus influenzae.* All are spread from person to person by cough or sneezing. The meningococcus is the most likely of the three to occur in outbreaks and most commonly affects children and young adults, although older persons do get the disease. Meningococcal meningitis is a particular problem in military installations and other places where a large number of people are close together. Many people harbor the bacteria in the nose and throat without becoming ill, so the organism spreads readily. Most people are immune to the meningococcus, and it is not clear why a few people do not have this immunity. What is known is that in susceptible persons, the organism is acquired through inhalation, resides in the nose and throat, and spreads through the bloodstream to the central nervous system. It often attacks other organs as well. The meningococcus often causes small hemorrhages in the skin, in the joints, and elsewhere in the body, and there is a tendency for small blood vessels to plug up. The organism can be identified by bacterial cultures of the nose and throat, blood, or spinal fluid.

The pneumococcus, the organism responsible for bacterial pneumonia, is the most common bacteria to produce meningitis in older adults. Often it will spread to the central nervous system through the bloodstream when a person already has lobar pneumonia, but in some instances, pneumococcus appears in the spinal fluid without an associated pneumonia.

Hemophilus influenzae is an organism that is also found in the noses and throats of most people. Certain types are particularly likely to produce bacterial meningitis. The bacterial meningitis produced by hemophilus is most common in children aged 18 months to four years, but it can occur in older and younger individuals. As children grow older, most de-velop antibody to hemophilus, but younger children do not have it. Infants tend to be protected by the antibody passed from the mother during pregnancy. The period between the disappearance of this fetal immunity and the acquisition of new immunity is the period of highest risk.

To determine which bacteria are producing meningitis, it is necessary to examine the spinal fluid. The sample is usually obtained by inserting a small needle between the vertebrae into the spinal cord. It is essential that the test be performed, because different antimicrobial drugs act differently on various bacteria, and a drug that is effective against one type of meningitis does not always help against another. The kinds of bacteria that produce meningitis are not limited to meningococcus, pneumococcus, and hemophilus, although they are the most common. Other microorganisms that can produce meningitis include various types of streptococci, various organisms of the group called "gram-negative rods" such as *E. coli,* and organisms of the Listeria group.

Preventing the spread of meningitis is not critical except for the meningococcal form, in which it is customary to isolate ill persons and to examine members of the family and close contacts to determine whether they have acquired the bacteria. Frequently, all members of an affected family are asked to take a drug to prevent infection. Similarly, when meningitis appears in a military installation or an institution in which there is close contact among individuals, a preventive drug may be used in an effort to halt the spread. Such steps are not necessary in meningitis caused by pneumococcus, hemophilus, or the other types of bacteria.

It is almost impossible to take care of victims of meningitis at home. The disease presents an acute medical emergency and requires treatment in a hospital. Patients with meningitis are extremely uncomfortable and need maximum comfort to relieve their symptoms. They usually prefer a quiet room without bright light and often will be unwilling or unable to communicate for days even after the acute infection has begun to subside. Nevertheless, complete recovery is the rule, although death or disability occurs in a few cases.

Vaccines have been developed against some types of meningococcal meningitis, but they are not widely used because the risk of acquiring the disease is so low. However, in high-risk populations, the vaccine is commonly used.

The present vaccine, however, does not protect against all types of meningococci, and efforts are being made to develop vaccines that will be widely effective.

Viral meningitis produces symptoms similar to those of bacterial meningitis, but in general they are milder. There is headache and pain in the neck muscles. The eyes may be sore, and the person often wants to avoid bright lights. There is usually a fever and often a rash. The person may be unresponsive, confused, and delirious. Most viral meningitis cases resolve spontaneously in a week to 10 days without treatment, and rarely cause nerve damage. A few types of viral meningitis are more likely to have a serious aftermath than others.

Viral meningitis cases usually occur in clusters in midsummer, and the viruses involved are probably spread by respiratory or gastrointestinal routes. A variety of viruses are responsible. These usually can be identified by cultures or blood and spinal fluid tests. Another reason for the tests is that viral meningitis cannot be distinguished from bacterial meningitis by symptoms alone.

Encephalitis means an inflammation of the nerve cells of the brain rather than inflammation of the brain coverings, as in meningitis. A variety of viruses can infect the brain, including herpes, measles, mumps, and chickenpox. The spread of these viruses to the brain is rare, but when encephalitis occurs, brain damage can result.

Poliomyelitis

Until the mid-1960s, poliomyelitis was a dreaded disease that occurred in outbreaks each summer, affecting large numbers of children and often leaving a few of them with muscle paralysis. Two types of vaccines have been developed, one using a killed virus and the other a live, weakened organism. Both vaccines have been effective, and their use has almost completely eradicated "polio" from the United States and from other countries in which they are widely used. The only cases seen now are in individuals who have not been immunized because they refused or missed immunization through oversight.

Poliomyelitis produces fever, headache, vomiting, sore throat, and later produces pain in the muscles, followed by paralysis. The virus is probably swallowed, and multiplies in the intestinal tract, spreading to the nervous system in a small percentage of persons. Before the vaccine, it was estimated that about 100 cases of mild and inapparent poliomyelitis occurred for each one that caused paralysis.

The vaccine has become so valuable that it is virtually useless to describe the symptoms of acute poliomyelitis.

The most widely used vaccine is the live virus form. The attenuated virus grows in the intestinal tract and induces immunity. It is easily swallowed in a liquid preparation and has been incorporated into various types of sweets. There is about one chance in a million that a person who swallows the virus will prove so susceptible that true poliomyelitis will emerge. After a child has been immunized and the virus is multiplying in the body, persons in close contact with the child receive a certain amount of exposure, too, so their immunity may be boosted as well. In rare instances the virus mutates into a more invasive form, and persons who have been in contact with immunized children have become infected with the invasive virus. To prevent this, parents and family members also should be given vaccine if they have not been vaccinated within the preceding 10 years.

The killed virus vaccine appears to be slightly less protective and is not as widely used in the United States, although some countries continue to use it exclusively. Those who receive the killed vaccine by injection occasionally have mild local pain or swelling at the injection site, but they rarely have other side effects. The vaccine can be mixed with other childhood vaccines, such as those for diphtheria, tetanus, and pertussis (whooping cough).

One problem with the poliomyelitis vaccine is that many parents have not been as careful to see that their children are immunized as they were in the past when polio was feared. The live attenuated virus vaccine has the advantage that a certain amount of immunity is conferred in a population by spread from an immunized person to others. Ideally, however, each child should receive proper immunizations, and failure to do so increases the risk of developing the disease.

Rabies

Rabies is a viral disease of the central nervous system that many years ago was one of the most feared of all diseases. There are many "mad dog" stories describing how the animal acts irrationally, has jerking movement, and runs wildly in circles with saliva dripping from the mouth and jaws. This saliva contains the virus. A bite introduces it under the skin of a susceptible person, and then it spreads to the central nervous system.

Once rabies appears in human beings, recovery is exceedingly rare. Fortunately, however, the incubation period between the time of the bite and the time the disease begins to produce its severe effects is several weeks, so there is time to immunize the bite victim against the disease. Rabies now is so rare in the United States that there are usually fewer than five cases per year in the entire country. This is partly due to rabies control programs and laws or advice to dog owners to have pets immunized regularly. Most cases of rabies now result from the bites of wild animals or bites of dogs that have been bitten by wild animals. Among the animals that have spread the viruses to humans are bats, skunks, foxes, and horses.

When an animal bites a person, particularly if the behavior is odd and the bite is unprovoked, it is important to catch the animal, check its vaccination history (if it is a domestic animal), examine it for illness, and if necessary sacrifice it and examine the brain for evidence of rabies virus. If the bitten person has been exposed to rabies, treatment must begin promptly. The bitten area should be flushed with large amounts of soap and water and scrubbed briskly to wash out the virus and prevent it from spreading to the central nervous system. An antiserum also prevents spread of the virus to the nervous system, and vaccines can be given to build up antibody. There is evidence that rabies in animals is increasing, which could lead to more cases in people. That is why it is important that any animal bite be investigated carefully.

Tetanus (Lockjaw)

Tetanus is a serious disease that need never occur. The organism that causes lockjaw, *Clostridium tetani*, produces spores that act as tiny seeds. They can be found in the soil and in the intestinal tracts of man and animals. The spores transform themselves into multiplying bacteria only if little or no oxygen is present. Spores commonly enter all of our bodies through cuts, burns, scratches, and other wounds. Only when there is dead tissue or when the tissue has closed over a wound and excludes oxygen can the microorganisms develop. They then produce tetanus toxin, a powerful nerve poison that travels along the nerves to produce damage to the central nervous system.

The interval between the time of a wound and the appearance of symptoms ranges from a few days to months. Severe cases usually appear quickly. The onset of tetanus causes restlessness, irritability, stiffness of some muscle groups, and sometimes difficulty in swallowing. Muscle spasm in a limb or jaws is sometimes the first evidence of the disease, hence the name "lockjaw."

Treatment of tetanus consists of giving victims oxygen and assisting their breathing if the paralysis has affected the muscles of respiration. Although antibiotics kill the bacteria, they do not neutralize the toxin that has already been released. Accordingly, antitoxin is widely used as a neutralizing agent.

Tetanus toxoid has been even more useful in preventing the disease. This material has been produced from tetanus toxin by chemically changing it to make it nonpoisonous but still able to cause the body to produce antitoxin. Such toxoid, given to children at monthly intervals for three injections, will confer immunity for ten years or longer. When a person has been injured and there is concern about tetanus, however, it is customary to give another dose of toxoid which immediately restimulates the immunity. Because of widespread use of this approach, tetanus has been an exceedingly rare disease in recent wars even though millions of men were wounded.

When it appears, tetanus may be limited to one limb and can be quite painful. Those with this limited form generally recover with proper treatment. Generalized tetanus can be severe and often leads to death.

Botulism

Botulism results from eating canned foods that have been inadequately sterilized, allowing the organism *Clostridium botulinum*, common in soil and in feces, to multiply and produce its toxin. As in tetanus, the organism multiples only in the absence of oxygen, which is why it is a particular problem in canned foods. The toxin it produces is one of the most powerful poisons known. Even tiny traces can be fatal. Great care must be taken in the sterilization of home canned foods and of preserved meats. The toxin does not produce a bad taste or foul odor, and often there are no obvious signs of spoilage. However, boiling for 30 minutes destroys the toxin. Thus, if there is the slightest suspicion about home canned foods, they should be thoroughly boiled before use and should not be tasted before boiling.

Most recently it has been discovered that these bacteria will grow in an infected wound or even in the intestinal tracts of young infants and cause severe symptoms and death. It is not known how the bacteria are introduced there.

Persons who develop botulism usually complain first of blurred vision and double vision. The mouth becomes dry, the eyes are dilated, and there may be difficulty in speaking and ultimately in breathing. These symptoms sometimes appear within hours after eating, or up to three days later.

Antitoxins counter the lethal effect and are valuable in protecting persons in whom symptoms have not yet appeared but who have eaten food that has caused botulism in others. Strictly speaking, botulism is not a bacterial infection but is an intoxication (poisoning by a toxin). In most instances the toxin is preformed in the food.

EAR INFECTIONS (OTITIS)

Infections of the ear are called otitis. An infection of the outer ear is called external otitis, and infection of the middle ear is otitis media. External otitis is a common disorder of the ear lobe skin or of the ear canal. It has a variety of causes, including bacteria, viruses, and fungi. External infections even follow allergies, but scratches and injury appear to be the most common inciting factors, with bacteria commonly invading the injured area. Most injuries are caused when foreign objects such as pencils or matches are inserted to clean the ear. These often scratch the skin, which then becomes infected. That is why we have the ancient and only slightly exaggerated rule: Don't put anything in your ear smaller than your elbow.

External ear infection is more common in tropical climates, where heat and moisture make it easier for bacteria and fungi to multiply. It is common in swimmers for the same reason. Treatment is aimed at keeping the area clean and dry, and treating the inflammation with drugs. When the infected organism has been identified it is usually possible to apply topical medication to stop its growth. Occasionally, the infection becomes severe and spreads. Systemic treatment is then required.

Internal ear infection, usually otitis media, represents infection of the space behind the eardrum and is a common disorder of children. The middle ear is a chamber containing the small bones that pick up sounds and transmit them to the nerves. This chamber is connected with the throat through a small tube called the eustachian tube. When viruses or bacteria colonize the interior of the nose and mouth and produce disease, they often spread along the eustachian tube into the middle ear. Ordinarily, the eustachian tube drains the middle ear, so bacteria and accumulated secretions pass out readily. But in infants, the opening is small and the tube becomes blocked easily, either through swelling and inflammation or because the adenoids, situated at the back of the throat adjoining the tube, swell in response to infection and block the tube. Without proper drainage, bacteria multiply within the middle ear and invade the tissues behind the eardrum.

The usual sequence is for the infant to have a cold followed five to ten days later by crying, a reddened ear, and some degree of pawing or striking at the ear. Older children who can describe the problem complain of pain in the ears and a sense of fullness and difficulty in hearing. These symptoms may be accompanied by fever. Antibiotics are usually effective, but sometimes it is necessary to continue them up to two weeks. Occasionally, the inflammation is so severe that it is necessary to puncture the eardrum to allow the pus to drain. Middle ear infection must be treated promptly to prevent hearing loss. In rare cases the infection spreads to the central nervous system.

Some physicians feel that middle ear infection is more common in allergic children (see chapter 21, "Allergy and the Immune System") and will prescribe allergic desensitization in an attempt to forestall repeated infection.

MEASLES, MUMPS, AND GERMAN MEASLES

Along with chickenpox, doctors consider measles, mumps, and German measles (rubella) to be the common childhood diseases. Vaccination against these viral infections began about 15 years ago and has greatly decreased their incidence (see chapter 27, "Taking Care of Your Child"). When one of the diseases does appear, it is more likely to strike an older person who has never received immunization. In the 1970s outbreaks of these diseases occurred in high schools, colleges, and military bases.

Adults who develop these infections can be affected more severely than children. Measles, best known for the skin rash it produces, sometimes spreads to the lungs or brain, producing an inflammation of the brain membranes that is usually troublesome but rarely fatal and that seldom causes later consequences.

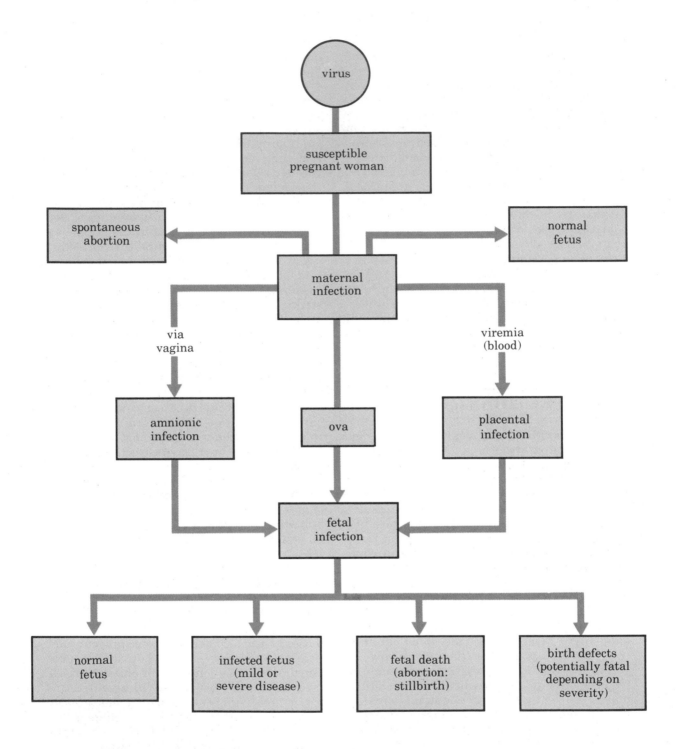

PREGNANCY AND DISEASE

Most viral infections of pregnant women have no effect on the developing child. However, among those that do spread to the infant are rubella (German measles), cytomegalovirus, herpes virus, and toxoplasmosis, caused by a protozoon. The chart depicts possible outcomes of maternal infection. A virus disease in a pregnant woman can cause miscarriage or fetal infection, or it might have no effect on the fetus, *which is the most common result. If infection does reach the fetus, it is by one of three routes: via the ova (egg cells); via an infected birth canal (amnionic infection), the common course in cytomegalovirus and herpes virus; or through the bloodstream and placenta, as in rubella. If the child is infected, one of four outcomes can occur (bottom), but the usual result is a normal birth.*

Similarly, mumps, an infection of the salivary glands, can spread to different parts of the body. Some persons with mumps develop meningitis or aches in the abdomen because various internal organs become involved. Sometimes the testes are attacked. In rare cases males become sterile afterward.

German measles (rubella) tends to produce not only a rash but also joint pain and swelling, and sometimes spreads to the lungs. If it strikes a woman during the first three months of pregnancy, it can spread to the developing infant and cause birth defects. A pregnant woman who develops rubella must receive medical care.

It is important that all children be vaccinated against these diseases. The inoculations usually are given at 15 months of age. Adults at risk, such as young women who expect later to be pregnant, would be wise to be vaccinated for their own protection and to prevent spread of these diseases in the community.

BONE AND JOINT
INFECTIONS

Osteomyelitis. Bones can become infected after an accident in which a bone breaks and fragments pierce the skin. Bone infections also occur when a wound infection spreads to the bone beneath, and when bacteria are carried to the bone through the blood. The condition is called osteomyelitis. Bone infections usually are caused by staphylococci, but many other bacteria can be involved.

Bone infections can be painful and interfere with function. They have the potential to cause scarring and chronic infection that lasts for a lifetime. Bone infections must be treated promptly and vigorously with antibiotics.

Septic arthritis. Joint infection, known as septic arthritis, can develop after an accident in which the joint is opened and bacteria are introduced, or when bacteria from the blood spread to the joint, where they settle and multiply. One blood-borne bacterium particularly likely to infect joints is the gonococcus, the organism of gonorrhea. Other organisms, such as staphylococci, also attack joints.

When infected, the joints become hot, painful, swollen, and tender. A small amount of joint fluid can be removed through a needle and examined for bacteria. Sometimes the joint must be drained surgically to release the pus and bacteria. Prompt treatment with antibiotics is necessary because the joint is likely to become scarred and nonfunctional.

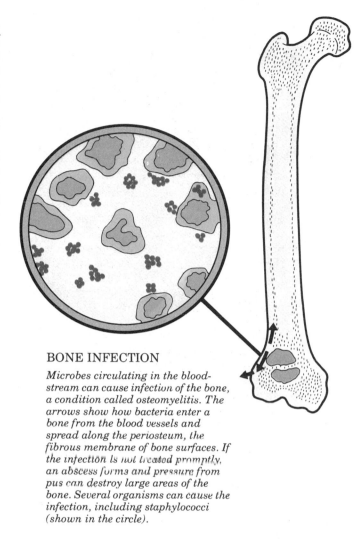

BONE INFECTION

Microbes circulating in the bloodstream can cause infection of the bone, a condition called osteomyelitis. The arrows show how bacteria enter a bone from the blood vessels and spread along the periosteum, the fibrous membrane of bone surfaces. If the infection is not treated promptly, an abscess forms and pressure from pus can destroy large areas of the bone. Several organisms can cause the infection, including staphylococci (shown in the circle).

BLOOD POISONING

The term blood poisoning generally means that bacteria have invaded the bloodstream. The scientific terms are bacteremia and septicemia. These terms are often used interchangeably, but in a strict sense the term septicemia is used when bacteria are multiplying in the bloodstream, and bacteremia is used when bacteria are in the bloodstream but not multiplying. The distinction is difficult to make. Almost all kinds of harmful bacteria can enter the blood at one time or another, often as a result of an infected wound. In general, bacteria in the blood means that the infection is serious. Certain bacteria may seed themselves throughout the body and set up secondary areas of infection in any of the organs. Intensive treatment is necessary, including drugs, and sometimes surgery is needed to drain areas of pus.

Toxic-Shock Syndrome

In 1980, toxic-shock syndrome, a rare illness, was noticed with increasing frequency in women of menstrual age. This infection produces high fever, diarrhea, muscular aches, dizziness, and a sunburn-like rash that eventually peels. Up to 10 percent of those affected died. Many of the women who became ill used a particular brand of menstrual tampon that has since been withdrawn from the market. Toxic shock begins during or immediately after a menstrual period, but only women using tampons become ill. The syndrome appears to be caused by a bacterium, *Staphylococcus aureus,* that is present in the genitals of a small number of women.

Toxic-shock syndrome is rare. Only three in every 100,000 menstruating women acquire this disease each year. The chance of death from toxic shock in a year is about one in 350,000, compared with a death risk from driving a car of one in 6,000. To prevent toxic shock, women should change tampons frequently. Substitute a napkin if collection of menstrual fluids will continue for many hours without an opportunity to change tampons, such as overnight.

SKIN DISEASES

Boils and Carbuncles

Boils (furuncles) are areas of inflammation with pus in the center. They occur on the skin and in surrounding tissues. The infection usually originates in a hair follicle. Sometimes many boils come together to form a carbuncle, which represents a kind of "super boil." These in turn may extend deeper into surrounding tissues.

Boils and carbuncles are usually caused by staphylococcus organisms and occur most commonly in areas of the body that the hand can reach and scratch, such as the face, back of the neck, buttocks, chest, armpits, and other places with hair and sweat glands. Furuncles and carbuncles also follow minor scratches brought about by irritation from clothes, straps, and belts. People who repeatedly have boils commonly carry staphylococci in their noses and throats, as well as on their skin, making it easy for a scratching finger to transfer the staphlylococci beneath the surface, where they can multiply.

The treatment for most boils is conservative. Warm packs help the body fight the bacteria. The pus that forms represents the breakdown of body tissues, bacterial cells, and the white blood cells that gather around the bacteria to destroy them. Boils should not be squeezed or lanced unless they have become contained with no sign of spreading inflammation and unless they have begun to form a point with clearly discernible pus. If the boils are broken, the bacteria can spread throughout the skin, so the area and the entire skin should be thoroughly cleansed with soap and water followed by a simple antiseptic solution such as hexachlorophene.

Bacteria can enter the bloodstream from carbuncles and furuncles, particularly if they have been lanced or squeezed before the bacteria have been contained within the lesion. This kind of "blood poisoning" can be serious, because the bacteria can spread throughout the body and set up abscesses in many places. Treatment calls for antibiotics and surgical drainage, if necessary, to remove as much of the pus as possible.

Chickenpox and Shingles

Chickenpox (varicella) and herpes zoster, commonly called shingles, are caused by closely related or perhaps identical viruses. When children are first exposed to the virus of chickenpox, a certain percentage are already resistant and develop antibody without becoming ill. Others develop a rash over the entire skin, indicating that the virus has spread throughout the body. The symptoms of chickenpox are fever and a feeling of illness, followed by a rash that begins as red, raised, fiercely itchy spots. Tiny blisters later develop in the center of each spot. The blisters appear to be filled with pus, although they usually are not. The blisters develop crusts and heal, and usually leave no scars unless they become infected with bacteria as a result of scratching. The entire process takes about two weeks to run its course. Occasionally, the virus spreads to the lungs or to the central nervous system, even in children or adults who develop typical chickenpox. Pneumonia in adults caused by the chickenpox virus can be a serious disease.

After the rash heals, the varicella virus apparently is able to persist in nerve cells for many years and reappear decades later as "shingles." Under these conditions the virus multiplies in nerve cells involving a particular area of the spinal cord. The virus spreads along the nerve pathways and becomes distributed along that specific nerve. The word "shingles" comes from the Latin word for girdle because the rash often appears to spread in a girdle-like fashion, usually along one side of the body. Occasionally, however, shingles occurs in a widespread form with a rash all over the body.

In contrast to chickenpox, shingles produces pain along the nerve. The pain usually precedes the appearance of the rash and may persist for months after the rash has cleared. Occasionally the muscles in the affected area remain weak. In some individuals who have severe illnesses that weaken the immune system, the virus spreads from the nerve cells to the skin more readily and even spreads throughout the body.

In both chickenpox and shingles, the virus is present in the blister fluid, so it can be spread by contact with the fluid or the dressings around the blisters. In addition, persons with chickenpox exhale viral particles into the air. The blister fluid, however, is infectious for only a day or two after the first blisters appear. Chickenpox is not as highly contagious as some of the other infections of this type, such as measles (see page 681). However, if it is feared that the infection might spread to a person already weakened, it is necessary to isolate the patients.

There is no specific treatment for either form of infection, except to make the person comfortable and use local soaks to help dry the rash and prevent secondary bacterial infection. Experimental drugs have been tried but are not ready for general use.

Herpes Simplex (Fever Blisters)

The herpes simplex virus causes an infection that is well known as cold sores or fever blisters. These sores occur particularly often at the junction between the lips and the skin. They also occur in the mouth and throat and on the genital organs. Just why some people have recurrent herpes outbreaks while others are resistant is not clear. However, there is evidence that persons in close contact with others who have recurrent cold sores, such as hospital workers or spouses, are also likely to acquire the infection, suggesting that the virus is not highly contagious but can spread. Occasionally, the virus spreads to scratches in the skin

and causes typical lesions on the fingers and hands, similar to those caused by chickenpox or herpes zoster. This is when the virus is most easily spread to others.

Herpes simplex is also known as *Herpes hominis,* and there are two types of the virus. One is particularly likely to be found around the mouth and face, the other around the genital organs, although either can occur throughout the body. Herpes occasionally spreads to the eye where it can produce a severe eye infection (see chapter 12, "The Eyes"). Drugs can be instilled into the eye to prevent growth of the virus there, but these drugs have little or no effect on skin rashes. Occasionally herpes spreads to the central nervous system and produces an inflammation of the brain known as encephalitis. Victims may become sleepy and comatose. There is strong evidence that antiviral drugs are effective in treating herpetic encephalitis, which is a serious but uncommon disease.

Smallpox

Smallpox is a severe disease that has been one of mankind's most dreaded plagues. The lesions break out all over the skin and mucous membranes in varying degrees of severity, accompanied by fever and general feelings of extreme illness. In earlier centuries, smallpox was one of the most frequent causes of death.

In the 18th century physicians began to realize that some people who had suffered a mild form of smallpox were protected from a recurrence. It became a widespread practice for individuals to take small amounts of the blister fluid from smallpox victims and inoculate themselves (by scratching the skin with a sharp instrument dipped in the infected fluid) in the hope of inducing a mild disease. These makeshift vaccinations usually were effective, although occasionally severe disease and even death occurred. Later it was recognized that milkmaids who contracted cowpox (a cattle disease) on their hands were immune to smallpox. The physician who made the most careful observations of this phenomenon, Dr. Edward Jenner, began to inoculate people with cowpox virus to prevent smallpox. The cowpox virus produced a rash resembling smallpox but always limited to one or two places on the skin. Gradually, the methods of producing this virus and of inoculating with it became standardized and a worldwide program of vaccination was started under the auspices of the World Health

Organization. The process was so successful that smallpox has been eradicated. The last known case occurred in northeastern Africa in the autumn of 1977. Some people feel that smallpox vaccination gradually will become unnecessary. The search goes on for evidence of new cases or for the appearance of a similar virus in animals, which might bring the disease back to an unvaccinated susceptible population. Because these uncertainties remain, it is still wise to vaccinate children for smallpox, although it is no longer legally required. However, children with eczema and other chronic skin conditions should not be vaccinated because of the possibility that the virus will spread to these lesions of the skin.

Leprosy

Leprosy is also known as Hansen's disease, after the Norwegian scientist who first identified the bacteria that cause it. Leprosy bacilli look somewhat like the bacteria that cause tuberculosis, but usually they do not multiply in artificial culture media, only in cells of the host. Like tuberculosis, leprosy probably infects many more people than those who develop its characteristic skin rash or nerve disorders. Because leprosy bacilli invade and damage the nervous tissues, certain areas of the body can lose the ability to feel temperature or pain. Mutilations and deformity may appear on the skin, arms, legs, or face because of injury caused by the lack of sensation.

Biblical references to lepers probably described deforming skin diseases other than leprosy as it is known today. Worldwide, about 12 million persons suffer from leprosy. Most of them live in tropical countries, but the disease still occurs (although rarely) in Hawaii, Puerto Rico, and in the southern United States. Leprosy still causes deformity. Patients whose disease primarily affects the nerves may develop discolored areas of the skin because the nerves are deadened. Ultimately, the fingers or toes may shrivel. On the other hand, patients whose leprosy is primarily in the skin itself may develop thick knobby growths that distort the features. Sometimes people with this form of leprosy are said to have faces like lions.

Certain drugs cure leprosy, but successful treatment can take years. Some persons must take drugs the rest of their lives. Occasionally, symptoms worsen after treatment with drugs, but the relapse is temporary. It occurs because the killed bacteria release products that lead to reactions by the body. However, the disease, if recognized, is not nearly as dangerous now as it once was.

How leprosy germs spread from person to person is not known. The bacteria probably are found in cells of the nasal secretions and in cells of individuals with severe skin disease. These are inhaled by others. However, the disease is not highly communicable and it takes prolonged contact over many years to acquire it. Even spouses of persons with leprosy remain healthy after living together for many years.

Lepers probably were isolated in the past both from fear of spread and revulsion at their appearance. The leper colonies that still exist primarily provide occupational and physical therapy for those so badly disfigured that society rejects them.

VENEREAL DISEASE

Venereal disease has been known almost from the beginning of recorded history. However, careful records of venereal disease rates are available only for the past 70 or 80 years. Of the infections that are spread by sexual contact, the most common have been syphilis and gonorrhea. Less common are chancroid, granuloma inguinale, and lymphogranuloma venereum. Recently it has been demonstrated that infectious agents such as Chlamydia, mycoplasma, *Herpes hominis,* Trichomonas, and others can be spread by sexual activity. Homosexual and perhaps heterosexual activity may account for the spread of amoeba giardis, hepatitis, and dysentery, illnesses usually not sexually transmitted.

Since about 1960, there has been an enormous spread of venereal disease. About three or four million cases of gonorrhea and syphilis occur yearly in the United States, and many go unrecognized and untreated. Factors that account for the epidemic include greater sexual freedom, mobility of populations, widespread use of contraceptive methods that do not interfere with germ transmissions, an unwarranted belief that antibiotics give quick cures, a lack of awareness of the health complications, lack of awareness of safeguards, and the lack of foolproof chemical or mechanical means for preventing spread of infection. Teenagers and young adults account for more than half of all reported cases of venereal disease. Workers in venereal disease clinics are often astounded by how uninformed and misinformed many young people are.

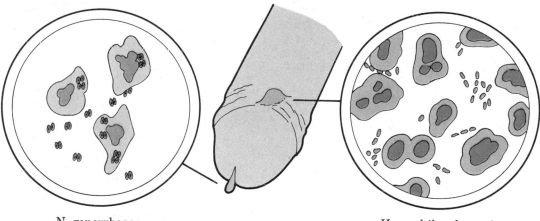

N. gonorrhoeae

Hemophilus ducreyi

VENEREAL DISEASE

The most common form of disease spread by sexual contact is gonorrhea, caused by the gonococcus bacterium, shown in the circle at left. Male symptoms are painful urination and discharge from the penis (center drawing), which occur one to seven days after exposure. Females sometimes have no symptoms, but repeated or continued infection can cause sterility. The circle at right shows Hemophilus ducreyi bacilli, which cause the venereal disease chancroid. Less common in the U.S. than in other areas, its first symptom is a small red lump on the genitals (as shown in center drawing) that may break down and form a painful ulcer. Another disease, nonspecific urethritis, also causes discharge and painful urination, but the organisms causing it are too small to be seen with a microscope.

Gonorrhea

The most common venereal disease is gonorrhea, caused by small round bacteria that come in pairs, *Neisseria gonorrhoeae.* This disease spreads principally by sexual contact, and acquisition of the disease by nonvenereal sources is rare, although newborn infants can be infected by passing through the birth canal of an infected mother. Immunity is produced slowly, if at all, by each attack, so a person can have gonorrhea repeatedly. After repeated episodes, the female pelvic organs become scarred, sometimes leaving the woman unable to become pregnant. In the male there may be local scarring that leads to sterility and difficulty in urination. In newborns, the organism can enter the eyes and produce infections that lead to blindness. Most states require that antibacterial drops be put into the eyes of all newborn babies as a precautionary measure.

Gonorrhea most commonly infects the genital organs, although the anus and the throat also harbor the germs. Initial symptoms occur within a day up to a week after exposure. The male has a burning sensation on urination followed soon by a discharge from the penis that drips small amounts of pus. On the other hand, many infected women notice no symptoms except painful urination and a slight increase in discharge. They continue sexual activity and spread the infection because they do not feel ill. In females, too, the infection can spread upward through the fallopian tubes to the ovaries and involve tissues along the womb, causing fever and severe abdominal pain, a form of pelvic inflammatory disease. Even with treatment, these organisms can scar and interfere with future pregnancy. In both sexes gonorrhea can spread to the joints, the nervous system, and the heart valves if not treated promptly.

Gonorrhea usually can be treated with antimicrobial drugs. It is important in preventing the spread of gonorrhea that sexual partners be treated simultaneously so that one is not reinfected after treatment. The patient should refrain from sex until the infection has been cured and should notify all persons with whom he or she has had sexual relations so they can be treated. Gonococci that are resistant to commonly used antibiotics have been found, particularly in Southeast Asia. Fortunately, the resistant organisms have not spread rapidly throughout the United States.

Syphilis

Syphilis is caused by a spiral shaped microorganism called *Treponema pallidum*. The disease is spread by direct contact, usually of a sexual nature. If pregnant woman is syphilitic, the infection can spread to her infant. The organisms that cause syphilis initially produce a hard painless sore called a chancre at the site where the germs have entered. Chancres usually appear on the genitals and occasionally on the lips, but they can appear anywhere on the body.

The chancre represents the primary stage of syphilis. It usually disappears even without treatment. In the secondary stage weeks or months later, the organism spreads throughout the body and a generalized rash typically appears, often accompanied by ulcers in the mouth that are infectious. The rash itself is full of microorganisms. The infected person may have swollen lymph nodes, and may develop signs that the organisms have spread to various organ systems. In the third stage, which may appear many years after the secondary stage, a variety of effects occur, so many that syphilis has been called "the great imitator." Almost any organ system of the body can be affected. Among the most widely known complications are general paresis, which leads to severe mental illness; tabes dorsalis, in which there may be loss of feeling and movement difficulties affecting the legs; and aortic aneurysm, in which the organisms of syphilis penetrate the body's main artery, which brings blood from the heart to the rest of the body. The artery can become dilated because of the weakness produced by the invasion of the organisms. The dilation may rupture, causing immediate death. Disease of the heart valves also occurs.

With proper treatment an infectious person can be made noninfectious to others in one or two days. Treatment is so effective that the tertiary forms of syphilis are now seen only rarely.

Syphilis is diagnosed by using a blood test. Most states require the test of both partners before a marriage license will be issued. It should also be performed on all pregnant women as part of prenatal care. A few immunologic diseases and a few infections such as malaria can produce false positive reactions to some tests for syphilis. A series of specialized blood tests can solve this problem.

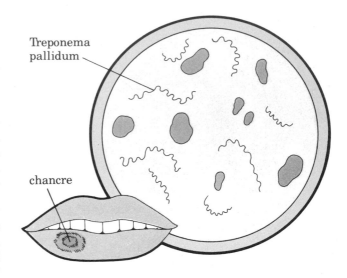

SYPHILIS

The organism that causes syphilis, Treponema pallidum, is colorless, so special techniques are necessary to make it visible under the microscope. The first sign of primary syphilis is usually a hard, painless sore at the site where the germ entered the body. The sore, called a chancre, most commonly occurs on the genitals, but can occur on any part of the body, including the lip. Infected women may never see the sore if it develops on the vagina.

Nonspecific Urethritis

This term was introduced to describe instances in which there was evidence of inflammation in the urethra, but gonorrhea was not present. Research indicates that a genus of tiny bacteria called *Chlamydia,* almost a virus in size, accounts for a substantial percentage of nongonococcal urethritis. Still other tiny bacteria called *Ureaplasma urealyticum* have been suggested as causes for some of these cases, and a protozoan, Trichomonas, also has been implicated. Certain common bacteria invading the urethra also have been suspected of causing the symptoms, so urethritis can stem from a variety of microorganisms.

The symptoms are similar to those of gonorrhea but usually are milder. There is pain on urination and often a watery or mucous discharge from the penis or the vagina. Women often have fewer symptoms than men and may feel well until the infection reaches the uterus or adjacent structures, when pain develops.

Antibiotics have been successful in treating these infections, but they are different from those used for gonorrhea. That is why it is necessary to distinguish gonorrhea from other causes of urethritis and to provide the correct drug. As with gonorrhea it is important to treat all sexual partners and to refrain from sexual activity until the infection is cured.

Lymphogranuloma Venereum

The organism that causes lymphogranuloma venereum is also a Chlamydia somewhat like the one involved in nongonococcal urethritis. Lymphogranuloma venereum is common in Asia, Africa, and South America but only about 500 cases are reported annually in the United States, mostly in males.

The disease is sexually transmitted. Any time from a few days to a few weeks after sexual contact with an infected person, a painless blister develops on the genitals. This heals rapidly and can go unnoticed. A few weeks later the lymph glands in the groin become painful and swell, and the individual develops fever, chills, loss of appetite, headache, and muscle and joint pains. If the swelling glands are not treated, they sometimes become still larger and break down, draining pus. It may take months for the lesion to heal. Occasionally the organisms spread throughout the body to the eyes, nerves, skin, and joints. Sometimes they spread to the rectum, causing scarring, strictures, and bloody discharge from the rectal area. When the disease is diagnosed, drugs can be given that bring rapid healing.

Chancroid

Chancroid is a sexually transmitted disease produced by the *Hemophilus ducreyi*. The disease is found all over the world and is particularly common in areas of poverty and poor hygiene. After exposure to an infected person, the individual, usually male, notices a little red lump on the genitals in two to 14 days. Pus drains from the lump in a few days and the skin breaks down, producing a painful, slow-healing ulcer that sometimes is confused with the primary stage of syphilis. Occasionally the lymph glands in the groin swell and abscesses form, leading to ulcers and scars in the genitals and groin. Drug treatment is successful if begun promptly. It is important to differentiate chancroid from syphilis, herpes, and other sexually transmitted diseases because each requires its own type of treatment.

Granuloma Inguinale

Granuloma inguinale is another common disease in many parts of the world such as Asia and the Caribbean, but fewer than 100 cases are reported annually in the United States. The disease begins as an ulcer that progresses slowly and remains chronic, often extending along the lower part of the pelvis and around the genitals. The ulcer usually appears within a week but can occur as late as two or three months after sexual exposure. Preceding the ulcer there may be a small raised area that breaks down into the ulcer. The ulcer is usually painless but bacteria can infect it, producing tenderness and unpleasant odors.

The ulcer may persist for many months because it does not cause much trouble, and the fact that it has persisted for so long is one of the diagnostic points suggesting that granuloma inguinale is present. The microorganism that causes this infection is not known, but by examining material taken from the ulcer, it is possible to see small bodies known as Donovan bodies, named after the scientist who first identified them. These appear as tiny bacteria surrounded by a clear space.

Antibiotics can treat granuloma inguinale, but the treatment should be extended until the lesion is completely healed, which can require many weeks.

Genital Herpes

Herpes infections have been discussed under *Herpes simplex*. *Herpes genitalis*, *Herpes hominis B*, and *Herpes hominis type 2* are all names for the same virus. This virus is common and is spread by sexual activity. Within a few days after contact, small exceedingly painful blisters occur on the genitals or on other areas of contact. After a few days the blisters dry and ulcerate, with crusts forming on the surfaces, and then healing follows in a week or two. After healing, the virus may become latent, which means that it remains in cells in the area but produces no symptoms. Weeks, months, or even years later the sores may return again, as happens with infections by the related virus that causes fever blisters or cold sores. In fact, the virus of fever blisters can infect the genitals and the virus of the genitals can infect the skin elsewhere (see page 685). There is no specific treatment for genital herpes infections. There is little to do but take mild analgesics or use surface anesthetics to lessen the pain, and wait for the infection to heal itself. Drugs under development may be useful in the future.

FEMALE GENITAL INFECTIONS

Vaginitis is a general term to describe a secretion of pus or excess mucus from the vagina. Several kinds of bacteria are normally present in the vagina, and do not produce disease. However, bacteria occasionally are acquired, sometimes through sexual contact and sometimes through no apparent mechanism, that produce local infection. The vagina becomes painful, the amount of discharge increases, and bacterial cultures demonstrate the presence of bacteria.

Candida albicans is a yeastlike microorganism that can produce vaginitis. A small number of yeast cells are normally present in the vagina, but occasionally the numbers increase and produce inflammation. Overgrowth of the yeasts occurs by the elimination of normal bacteria through the use of antibiotics, and is favored by changes in hormones during the menstrual cycle. Women using oral contraceptives seem to have more of these yeasts than other women. A number of drugs used in salves or rinses can control the yeast, although there is a high tendency for these infections to recur. Yeast infections are not sexually transmitted as a rule, although this can occur. In males, the yeasts can cause a rash on the penis, but usually do not produce other evidence of disease.

Trichomonas vaginalis is a small protozoan microorganism that produces vaginitis. The yellowish-green discharge has a distinct odor. The infection can pass from male to female sexual partners and back again. These organisms, which can be controlled by drugs, rarely produce any discomfort in males, only females.

In many instances vaginitis appears without any specific bacterial cause. In other instances certain bacteria are found in greater abundance than normal and many physicians regard these bacteria as causing the vaginitis. The judicious use of local drugs will sometimes help to determine the best treatment. In a few cases vaginitis persists for long periods and is difficult to cure. Doctors do not know why.

MISCELLANEOUS DISEASES

Infectious Mononucleosis

Persons who become ill with infectious mononucleosis (glandular fever) usually develop mild fever, sore throat, and headache. They notice that the lymph glands all over the body—in the armpits, groin, elbows, and around the neck—become swollen and somewhat tender. Occasionally, in severe cases, the liver is involved and jaundice develops. Sometimes there are central nervous system problems such as paralysis and difficulty in breathing. Most commonly, however, the disease makes people feel quite ill for a few days, then recovery occurs within days or weeks. Occasionally there are relapses, so that months pass before the victim feels entirely well. Although the virus that causes this illness may spread from child to child, when young children are infected they usually have a mild illness that does not resemble infectious mononucleosis. However, people age 15 to 30 develop a more severe form of the illness. The virus that causes the infection is found in saliva and respiratory secretions but does not readily spread from one individual to another without close contact. It is for this reason that the disease has been incorrectly called the "kissing disease." Any form of close contact will permit the virus to spread. Kissing is not the only method.

The virus that causes infectious mononucleosis is known as the E-B virus, named for the discoverers, Drs. Epstein and Barr. The virus infects some of the white cells in the body and particularly the lymph glands where certain white cells reside. The disease gets better by itself without specific treatment; indeed, no specific treatment is known. Most acutely ill persons want to remain in bed and to move around only when they feel better. In rare cases the spleen, an organ in the upper left side of the abdomen, becomes infected and ruptures, leading to the appearance of blood in the abdomen. If a mononucleosis patient develops sudden severe abdominal pain, he or she must be rushed to a hospital under emergency conditions. Because of fear of this complication, it is advised that patients with infectious mononucleosis avoid strenuous exercise such as vigorous body contact sports until at least three weeks after the onset of the disease.

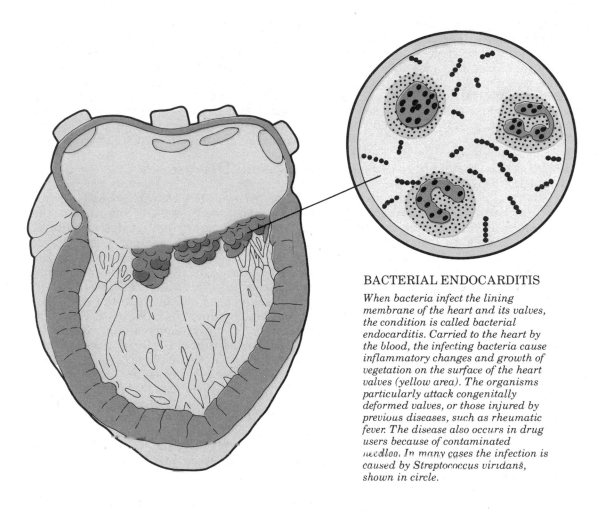

BACTERIAL ENDOCARDITIS

When bacteria infect the lining membrane of the heart and its valves, the condition is called bacterial endocarditis. Carried to the heart by the blood, the infecting bacteria cause inflammatory changes and growth of vegetation on the surface of the heart valves (yellow area). The organisms particularly attack congenitally deformed valves, or those injured by previous diseases, such as rheumatic fever. The disease also occurs in drug users because of contaminated needles. In many cases the infection is caused by Streptococcus viridans, shown in circle.

Bacterial Endocarditis

Bacteria that enter the blood through a variety of ways pass through the heart valves as the blood circulates. Occasionally some of these bacteria settle on a valve, particularly if the valve has been damaged. Such bacteria can quickly destroy a heart valve, with potentially fatal consequences.

Bacterial infection of the heart lining is called bacterial endocarditis. Some victims have a mild fever and fatigue for many weeks, some become severely and acutely ill, depending on the bacteria responsible. Bacterial endocarditis has been a particular problem in recent years because narcotics users inject themselves with contaminated preparations containing bacteria that attack the heart valves.

When the valve has been damaged, it is usually because of a previous attack of rheumatic fever, or arterial sclerotic disease of a heart valve. Sometimes a congenital defect of the valves is responsible. Surgery to replace damaged valves is now possible. Newly implanted heart valves also become infected, but only rarely. Bacterial infection of the heart valves requires vigorous treatment. Otherwise, the disease is virtually always fatal.

Many physicians note that bacteria from the mouth and teeth often enter the bloodstream after vigorous chewing or after dental work. That is why physicians and dentists advise patients to take antibiotics before dental work in an attempt to reduce the possibility of endocarditis. Although it is not certain that this approach is useful, it is widely recommended. Persons planning dental work should discuss the possibility with their dentists.

Toxoplasmosis

Toxoplasmosis is caused by a small protozoan known as *Toxoplasma gondii*. Toxoplasmas are common in the environment and can be isolated from virtually all domestic and farm animals. About one-fourth to one-half of American adults carry antibodies to toxoplasma, indicating that at some time they were infected with the organism. In adults the disease usually is mild, with swelling of the lymph nodes and minimal discomfort. However, if a pregnant woman acquires toxoplasmosis, the organism can spread to the developing fetus and cause serious defects involving the brain, heart, eyes, and other organs.

Toxoplasmas are spread among humans through infected raw meat, but heat kills the organisms quickly. However, the infection is also transmitted by the feces of young cats. Because of a peculiarity in the digestive system of cats, the parasites can remain in their intestinal tracts for a long time. This discovery alarmed many cat lovers, but it is not necessary to sacrifice the cat if sensible precautions are taken. A blood test for toxoplasmosis can be taken from any pregnant woman. If she has protective antibodies, there is no danger. If not, she should observe safeguards, such as eating only well-cooked meats (no rare food). Young kittens should not be allowed in the household. If there is a kitten, a veterinarian should test its feces for toxoplasmas. As a further precaution, a pet cat should be fed canned or commercial dry catfood, not rare meat or underdone table scraps. (However, cats can acquire toxoplasma from contact with other cats or by catching mice.)

An expectant mother should not have contact with the litter box, and litter boxes should be emptied daily, because it takes two to four days after excretion for feces to become infective. The litter should be incinerated or disposed of carefully. If it is buried in the garden, a pregnant woman should not dig in the same area. In general, it is wise for a pregnant woman to avoid close contact with cats unless it is known that the cats are free of toxoplasma.

Drugs have been developed to treat toxoplasmosis, but there is no treatment after the fetus becomes infected.

Cat Scratch Disease

The organism responsible for cat scratch disease is not known, but it is assumed to be a virus carried by cats. It is a more common disease than generally supposed. Following a scratch or a bite by a cat, the individual develops a scaly ulcer at the site. The ulcer heals slowly and then the lymph nodes nearest the ulcer begin to swell without producing pain.

The lymph nodes sometimes swell to the point at which they drain and heal spontaneously, but it may take many weeks to reach this point. When there is a suspiciously enlarged lymph node, doctors often recommend that the node be removed surgically and examined to be sure that the swelling stems from cat scratch disease rather than from a tumor. There is no treatment for cat scratch disease.

Kawasaki Disease

This disease, also known as mucotaneous lymph node syndrome, is named for the Japanese physician who first described it. It usually affects children under five years of age. Many cases have been recognized in the United States. The child develops fever, red eyes, red mouth and throat, rash, swollen legs or arms, and swollen glands in the neck that cannot be explained. The cause of Kawasaki disease is unknown. Some young victims develop abnormalities of the blood vessels of the heart, with serious complications. We do not know how to treat this disease.

The fever and rash usually last seven to ten days, then gradually resolve. Hospitalization is rarely necessary, although about one percent of the children who develop the disease die, primarily from the heart abnormalities. The rash occasionally is mistaken for measles, scarlet fever, or rubella.

Reyes Syndrome

Reyes syndrome was first recognized and described in 1963. Several days after a mild viral respiratory infection a young child vomits, becomes sleepy and delirious, may have convulsions, and finally lapses into coma. Some children have died and others are left with mental impairment. The illness is rare. News accounts have given the impression that the disease is more common than it is.

The cause of Reyes syndrome is not known. It affects children age 2 to 16 and is most common in association with influenza type B epidemics, but also occurs with influenza type A, chickenpox, and a variety of other viral infections. Reyes syndrome is associated with severe liver problems. Sometimes the liver fails, allowing substances to accumulate in the body that injure the brain. Why the liver fails is not understood. However, the liver failure and the other symptoms can be treated to help the child through the acute illness. Thus, mortality from Reyes syndrome has been falling, even while investigators attempt to discover the cause and ways to prevent the disease.

ACTINOMYCOSIS AND NOCARDIOSIS

Certain higher bacteria that are capable of branching (and therefore are somewhat closer to plants) cause disease. The two most common examples are the organisms *Actinomyces bovis* and *Nocardia asteroides*. Actinomycosis is a chronic infection that is most common around the mouth and jaws, but occasionally occurs in the lymph nodes of the neck and occasionally spreads to the lungs and elsewhere. The organisms are common in soils and hay, and often are introduced into the tissues by a puncture wound. Many cases have occurred when people chew on hay and have punctured the gums with a sharp fragment.

Treatment is effective with certain antibiotics, but surgery is sometimes necessary.

Nocardial infections are particularly common in individuals whose immunity has been suppressed. Nocardia can produce fevers, pneumonia, pleurisy, and other changes. These infections are usually susceptible to sulfonamids, so it is important that nocardiosis be accurately diagnosed and not treated with the wrong drug.

Pneumocystis carinii is a small organism that is common in nature and rarely produces disease. However, in people who are receiving drugs for treatment of tumors or to suppress tissue rejection after organ transplant, pneumocystis may cause fever and pneumonia. Because the organism cannot be cultivated but is identified only by special strains from the tissues, it may be necessary to take biopsies or try to remove small amounts of tissue or tissue fluid with a needle. These organisms can be readily controlled by some newer drugs, but are not affected by some of the most commonly used antibiotics. It is therefore important that they be recognized so that specific treatment can be instituted.

FUNGAL INFECTIONS

In addition to *Candida albicans,* also known as monilia, there are strains of Candida that produce infections. Other pathogenic yeasts are *Torulopsis glabrata* and *Cryptococcus.* Most of these are harmless but occasionally they are associated with a variety of disease states. A yeastlike organism called Blastomyces can produce ulcers of the skin and mucous membranes, particularly in diabetics. New antibiotics are often effective in controlling infections caused by these organisms.

Several molds also produce disease, particularly in individuals whose immunity has been depressed by drugs or by an underlying disease. Among the common molds that produce infections are organisms of several genera: *Aspergillus, Penicillium, Rhizopus, Sporothrix, Fusarium,* and others. All of these infections, however, are relatively uncommon.

Histoplasma, coccidioidomycosis, and blastomyces are three fungi that cause lung infections in certain parts of the United States. Coccidioidomycosis is limited to the Southwest and California. Histoplasma is found in the Midwest, particularly around the major river basins such as the Ohio and Mississippi, but occasionally it can be found as far east as the Hudson River Valley. Blastomyces is limited to the South and Southwest. Infection by these fungi normally produce only symptoms of a mild cold, but in rare individuals the infection can severely damage the lung and spread throughout the body.

WORMS

Worms are the largest organisms that infect humans. Tapeworms can grow to a length of 10 feet. Worms are a problem in warm climates and where hygiene and sanitation are poor. Worldwide, hundreds of millions of people are infected with hookworm, roundworm, whipworm, and a variety of other parasites. In poverty-stricken areas in the United States, particularly in the Southern states, worm infestations are frequent. Pinworm is the most common in the United States. It spreads rapidly among small children in play groups and at school.

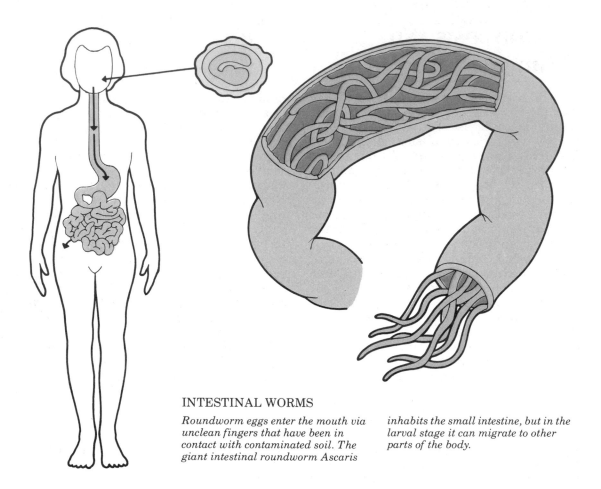

INTESTINAL WORMS

Roundworm eggs enter the mouth via unclean fingers that have been in contact with contaminated soil. The giant intestinal roundworm Ascaris

inhabits the small intestine, but in the larval stage it can migrate to other parts of the body.

Most worms reside in the intestine or in the blood vessels around the intestine. A few types are found in other areas of the body. For example, the worm that causes trichinosis burrows into muscles, and the longworm into the lung. Pinworms sometimes leave the intestine and burrow into the skin around the anus, where they deposit eggs that a child might pick up under the fingernails. Worms can live for many years inside the body. Most commonly the person carrying them shows no symptoms unless the infection is severe. Worms usually do not multiply in the body, so an infection with one or two worms will not worsen unless there is repeated exposure to more worms. Most infected people have a small number of worms and are not ill. In most instances the worms die and the infection resolves unless the person acquires new ones.

Intestinal worms, such as tapeworms, whipworms, roundworms, hookworms, and threadworms, produce mild abdominal cramping and diarrhea if the infection is severe enough. In the most severe forms there is anemia, bowel obstruction, and possible malnutrition. Schistosomes, also known as bilharzia, are worms that live in the bloodstream around the intestines. They sometimes spread to the liver, producing jaundice, or to the kidneys, producing blood in the urine. Although rare in the United States, schistosomiasis is a common infestation in much of the world. It does not produce severe difficulties unless the infection is heavy. In severe cases, however, there can be disease of the liver and other organs.

Worms spread from person to person by several methods. One source is eating poorly washed or uncooked foods or foods that have been washed with contaminated water or contaminated with feces. Another source is eating beef or pork that has been inadequately cooked. In a few instances, an individual who walks barefoot on ground contaminated with human feces may pick up worms such as hookworm and Strongyloides. These worms hatch from eggs in the ground and burrow into the skin of a passerby. They migrate through the skin, move throughout the body, and finally pass into the intestine.

Pinworm infection is acquired by another means. The worms spread to the anus, producing itching in the adjoining skin. The person scratches the area and picks up the eggs on his or her fingers. The eggs then are transferred to other people if the hands and fingernails are not clean. Usually, if there is pinworm infection in a family, it is advisable to treat all family members. Worms also can be acquired by swimming in water contaminated with human feces. Schistosomes have a stage in their life cycle when they live in fresh-water snails. The individual who swims in this water acquires the worms when they burrow into the skin and move to blood vessels, from which they spread throughout the body.

Trichinosis is named for the worm that causes it, *Trichinella spiralis*. In its development in humans, the worm lives for a short time in the intestines, then spreads throughout the body. It invades the muscles and forms small cysts that sometimes cause pain but most often are painless. The worms produce the same cysts in pork. Fortunately, the worms are killed if the pork is thoroughly cooked or is kept frozen for at least 48 hours. Trichinosis usually produces no symptoms, but if the infestation is severe the person develops diarrhea, muscle pains, weakness, fever, puffiness around the eyes, and sometimes evidence of kidney disorder.

All of the common worms can be eliminated with drugs. However, the best way to avoid these infections is to follow rules of hygiene.

INSECT-BORNE INFECTIONS

Infections transmitted by insects are particularly common in countries with warm and moist climates. They are less common in the United States because of successful programs to control mosquitoes and other disease-carrying insects.

Viral encephalitis

Among the most severe of insect-borne infections is viral encephalitis. The illness is caused by a virus spread by the bite of a mosquito. The mosquito first bites an animal that carries the virus, then transfers it when biting a human. Therefore most encephalitis occurs during the mosquito season, from late spring until frost. A person who develops encephalitis may become confused, feverish, sleepy, develop headache, vomiting, staggered walk, difficulty in talking, talk nonsense, or seem to be in a perpetual state of nightmare. Some of the viruses that cause viral encephalitis can destroy parts of the brain. Depending on the amount of invasion, the infected person might return to normal or might be left with brain damage. There is no specific treatment for the viral encephalitis carried by mosquitoes. Other types, most of them limited to tropical areas, can now be treated by drugs and there is hope that treatments will be developed for the mosquito-borne variety. In recent years vaccines have been developed for some types. Individuals traveling to high-risk areas should inquire about the vaccines.

Effective preventive measures include spraying the environment to stop mosquitoes from breeding, quarantine of infected animals, and discouraging mosquito bites by using household screens and insect repellents.

Varieties of encephalitis found in the United States include western equine encephalitis and eastern equine encephalitis, both spread from horses, and St. Louis encephalitis.

Plague

Throughout history plague, spread by the bites of fleas, has been one of the worst killers of all known infections. The disease is now rare in the United States, occurring primarily in the West, where flea-carrying ground squirrels and other small rodents are still a reservoir of the infection. Every year a small number of cases occur in remote areas of southern California, Arizona, and New Mexico, where ground squirrels and small rodents live near homes. Fleas then spread from rodents (usually as they are dying of the plague) to the human host. Most people who develop plague have recently handled a dead or dying rodent. The bite of the infected flea injects the plague bacteria into the tissues. Symptoms are high fever and swollen, enlarged lymph glands near the bite. These enlarged glands were known as buboes, accounting for the term bubonic plague. Because the flea bites most commonly occur in the legs, the glands of the groin are most likely to show buboes.

The germ of plague can spread to the lungs, causing pneumonia. This form, commonly known as pneumonic plague, is dangerous because coughing can spread the germ to others and the infection itself can be severe and life-threatening. This germ was responsible for the great plagues of history. Several antibiotics now are effective in treating plague, and vaccines have been developed for persons in high-risk situations. Prevention primarily involves decreasing the rodent population near where people live. Individuals should avoid ground squirrels, gophers, prairie dogs, and other rodents, and should not pick up dead animals.

In epidemic areas the black rat carries the infection and the rodent flea passes it along. There is some evidence that the human flea transmits the disease, too. Fortunately, fleas are uncommon as human parasites these days, although in the days of the Black Death they were extremely common. However, control of the rat population is still important. Plague has diminished because of rat control, because of cleanliness that has led to the disappearance of fleas from humans, and because of the absence of an insect in most parts of the United States that can readily bite both man and infected small rodents.

Rocky Mountain Spotted Fever

Rocky Mountain spotted fever is caused by a species of *Rickettsia,* one-celled microbes that fall between viruses and bacteria, and that usually grow only in living cells. The disease gets its name from the Rocky Mountain area where it is most common. However, cases have been found in fairly large numbers throughout the New England states and on islands such as Martha's Vineyard and Nantucket, as well as in the mid-Atlantic area. The disease probably can be found throughout the United States but is relatively uncommon. The wood tick carries rickettsia in the west and a dog tick carries it in the east. The rickettsia probably is found in common rodents and is transmitted to the tick when the tick bites the animal. The tick then transmits the rickettsia to its descendants.

The disease generally occurs in late spring and summer when ticks are abundant. Victims frequently are children who play in woods or wet grass. The child develops chills, fever, severe pains in bones and muscles, and a spotted rash that may become bloody after a few days.

The rash appears first on the wrists, ankles, and back, then spreads over the body. Fortunately, there are antibiotics that are completely effective. If the disease is recognized early, and if the child or parents recall that it was preceded by a tick bite, antibiotics can be given promptly and a cure usually follows. If the disease is exceedingly severe, however, it may be fatal. Before antibiotics the fatality rate was about 20 percent.

It is important to know that all wood ticks and dog ticks are potential carriers of the disease. It is advisable to inspect your body for ticks after walking in tick-infested areas or in woods or tall grass. Children who play in such areas should be inspected regularly for the presence of ticks. A tick should be removed using a piece of tissue to avoid touching it directly and to avoid crushing the animal, which should be flushed down a toilet (see chapter 35, "First Aid"). Parents who examine children should remember that ticks can crawl into the ear canals or hide in the hair.

Lyme Arthritis

This illness, identified only in the late 1970s, was first described in Old Lyme, Connecticut, hence its name. Cases have since been recognized in other parts of New England and New York. A child becomes sick with fever and develops a peculiar blotchy rash, with swelling and pain in one or two large joints. The cause of this disease is unknown, and recovery may take several months. Many victims remember having been bitten by ticks before symptoms occurred, and the illness occurs only in areas where there are large numbers of ticks, so a relationship with tick bites is suspected. The precautions for Rocky Mountain spotted fever should be used to prevent Lyme arthritis. No specific treatment is known.

Tips for Travelers

If you are traveling to an area in which there are substantial changes in lifestyle from yours, have a medical checkup before departure and after return. Carry your optical lens prescription with you. If you have diabetes, are allergic to drugs, or have any other condition that could require emergency care, carry a tag, bracelet, or card describing the condition on your person at all times. Assemble a small medical kit in consultation with your doctor. The kit could include laxatives and antidiarrheal drugs, a medicine to control pain, an antihistaminic, adhesive bandages, a thermometer, and selected antibiotics based on the area in which you will be traveling.

Travelers with chronic illnesses should restrict their visits to areas where competent advice and drugs are available. They should carry a doctor's statement of their health condition and any advice about drugs and dosage in the event of a flareup.

Outside Europe, Western nations, and countries in which sanitary facilities are well developed, precautions should be taken. Raw foods should not be eaten. Vegetables should be hot and freshly prepared, and not warmed over. Breads are usually safe, but if there is doubt, ask to have the bread toasted. Fruits can be eaten if the skins are carefully washed or if the fruit is peeled with a clean dry knife and if the fruit has no breaks in the skin. Alcoholic beverages and beer are safe. Local soft drinks are usually safe. Local tap water should not be used for brushing teeth unless you are assured of safety. Many places will provide bottled boiled water. Hot tea, coffee, cocoa, or other hot drinks are safe.

Requirements for immunization for foreign travel have been liberalized, but many countries still have specific rules. Consult the local office of the U.S. Public Health Service for information about specific countries. The Public Health Service can indicate whether there are outbreaks in the country you plan to visit.

Required vaccinations must be recorded on an international certificate of vaccination provided by the U.S. Public Health Service. It must be properly stamped and executed. Your own physician can give all of the vaccinations except that for yellow fever. It is useful to have a booster with tetanus toxoid if none has been given in the past 10 years. If you are entering an area where infectious hepatitis is prevalent, many doctors will offer an injection of gamma globulin, which can provide protection for three to five months.

All visitors who are entering malarial areas should consult their physicians about precautions and about the possible need for antimalarial drugs. Weekly tablets can prevent the disease. The tablets should begin two weeks before departure and should be continued for four weeks after return. Some strains of malaria are resistant to certain drugs. Your physician or the U.S. Public Health Service will provide information about resistant malaria and suggest alternative drugs.

Cholera is spread through contaminated water and food (see page 665). Cholera vaccine has only slight value in preventing the disease, but hygienic rules about food and water are most important. Antibiotics provide rapid treatment. The replacement of the water and salts lost when cholera appears is essential.

Yellow fever remains widespread in many parts of Africa and in South and Central America. Therefore, many countries in these areas require that travelers be vaccinated against the disease. A booster must be given every 10 years.

Typhoid and paratyphoid fever are less common than they once were, but they are still a source of concern in tropical areas. The vaccine has some effectiveness, and a booster should be taken every four to five years.

Smallpox immunization is no longer required.

Typhus immunization is not recommended except for travelers going into the interiors of northern India, Burma, Indonesia, Taiwan, Peru, Vietnam, and western Asia. Typhus can be treated with antibiotics.

Plague vaccination is unnecessary unless there is specific advice from local health officers. Vietnam is one country where plague is endemic.

CHAPTER 29   MICHAEL B. SHIMKIN, M.D.

CANCER

Cancer. The very word drives fear into the hearts of many. Although this disease of proliferating cell growth does not claim as many lives as heart disease or stroke, nor cripple as many as arthritis or diabetes, the seemingly random way it strikes and the universality with which it seems to touch every family make it the most feared of human afflictions, as public opinion polls repeatedly attest. Moreover, for all the money and efforts that have been poured into cancer research, the disease still refuses to yield its secrets, refuses to give in to surefire or simple treatment. The last half century has seen many strides against cancer, yet many central mysteries remain.

Cancer can arise in any part of the human body. In earlier chapters of this book the authors have discussed its origin and ravages in relation to their medical specialties, because diagnosis and treatment are different for different forms of cancer, according to where it occurs. Indeed, it differs for individual patients. Thus, a full discussion of lung cancer including treatment methods will be found in Chapter 8, "The Lungs," leukemia in Chapter 6, "The Blood," colon cancer in Chapter 20, "The Digestive System," and so on. This chapter concerns general aspects of cancer, its development and spread, the need for fuller use of prevention and treatment methods to reduce cancer's toll, and the basis for research that leads to better methods of treatment, prevention, and control.

Cancer can be fatal unless recognized promptly and treated effectively. But it is not inevitably fatal, and some types can be prevented. With present methods of surgery, radiation, and chemotherapy, the overall salvage rate is approaching 40 percent. Those results can be improved through earlier diagnosis and treatment, and incidence of some forms of cancer could be significantly reduced if people followed known preventive measures. Medical guidance is essential, but the primary responsibility rests with the individual and his or her own choices. Such choices should be based on correct, up-to-date information.

IS CANCER INCREASING?

Cancer is not a single disease, but more than 100 different diseases with a common characteristic: abnormal growth, division, and proliferation of cells, which spread from their site of origin to other parts of the body, invading and destroying normal organs and tissues as they spread. In all its forms, cancer is the second leading cause of death in the United States, trailing only heart disease. In recent years, there have been more than 800,000 new cases of cancer annually (excluding skin cancer) and 400,000 deaths in a population of more than 220 million. That means that 313 of every 100,000 Americans will be diagnosed as having cancer this year, and 165 of every 100,000 will die.

Cancer occurs most frequently among older people. The fact that Americans live longer, thanks to better living conditions and the conquest of many infectious diseases, is the primary reason. More people are surviving to the age at which cancer has always been most prevalent. When the figures are adjusted to reflect this shift in age distribution of the population, it can be seen that incidence and death from most forms of cancer have changed little. The exceptions are the tragic increase in lung cancer, particularly among men, and the steady decrease in stomach cancer in both sexes.

Pathologists classify cancer by the body tissue in which it originates. Cancer of the skin or other surfaces is called carcinoma. If the surface is composed of glands, such as in the stomach or the breast ducts, it is called adenocarcinoma. Cancer that arises from connective tissue is called sarcoma. Sarcoma cases are further classified by the cell type involved.

CANCER INCIDENCE RATES BY SEX AND AGE:

United States, all races combined, all sites (except skin and carcinoma-in-situ).

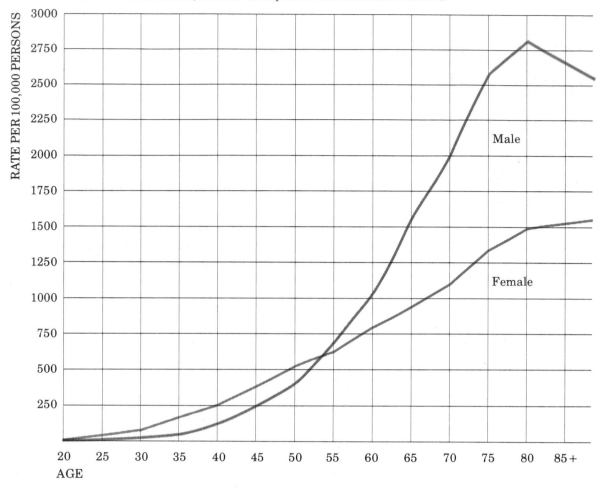

AGE AND CANCER

The incidence of cancer rises steadily with age in both sexes, but the increase is sharper among males after age 50, primarily because of cigarette smoking. The increase among women is more gradual. Although cancer is more common among women under 55, it is more likely to strike men after middle age. The rate of incidence begins to decline at about 75.

Hence the term lymphosarcoma refers to cancer arising within lymphatic cells, and osteosarcoma means cancer in bone cells. Melanoma is a "black" cancer arising from pigment cells of the skin or eye, and leukemia is a group of cancers of the blood cells. A still further form of classification refers to the appearance of the cells under the microscope. Examples include small-cell carcinoma of the lung and clear-cell carcinoma of the kidney.

WHAT IS CANCER?

Human beings begin with the union of a male and female sex cell, each containing half the genetic material that will shape the new being. Cells that form by divisions of this initial fertilized cell orient themselves and assume different shapes and functions. Through this process, known as differentiation, the single original cell evolves by a precoded plan into a complex, closely integrated community of some 100 billion cells that make up the adult human body. Each cell contains the genetic

CANCER INCIDENCE BY SITE AND SEX:

United States (age-adjusted to 1970 U.S. population).

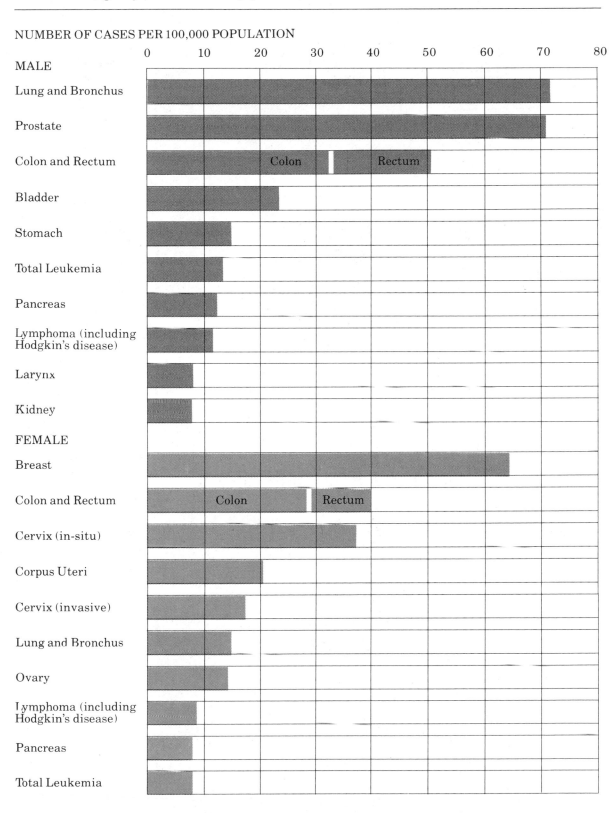

NUMBER OF CASES PER 100,000 POPULATION

THE PROGRESSION OF CANCER

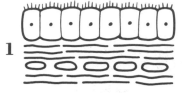

1 NORMAL LINING
OF A LUNG AND BRONCHUS

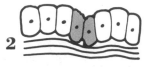

2 METAPLASIA
(changes)

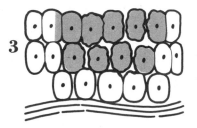

3 CARCINOMA-IN-SITU
(no penetration)

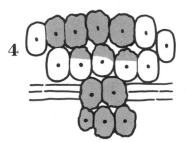

4 INVASIVE CANCER

There are six stages in the development from normal cells to widely spread disease, as shown in this example of the progression of lung cancer. The No. 1 drawing shows the normal lining of the small tubes of the lung—a single layer of cells with a brush-like border (cilia) on a connective tissue base called a basement membrane. Blood, lymph channels, and nerves are beneath the membrane. In drawing 2 chronic injury from smoking has damaged the cells. They are disorganized, have lost their cilia, and are piled up in more than one layer in some places. This stage is called metaplasia. In drawing 3 the cells are visibly changed, with many layers piled up. However, they have not penetrated the basement membrane. The stage is called carcinoma-in-situ, meaning "in place." In drawing 4 the abnormal cells have broken through the basement membrane into underlying tissue, the stage known as invasive cancer. Drawing 5 shows the stage called regional metastasis. In this stage the cancer has reached the lymph channel, and a colony has been established in a lymph node. In the final drawing at lower right, the bloodstream has carried cancer cells to the brain and liver and set up additional colonies. This final stage is called distant metastasis.

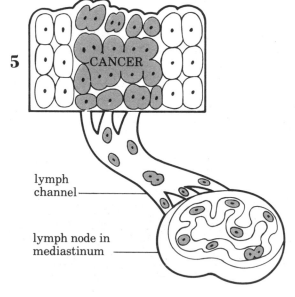

5 CANCER

lymph channel

lymph node in mediastinum

REGIONAL SPREAD
OF CANCER

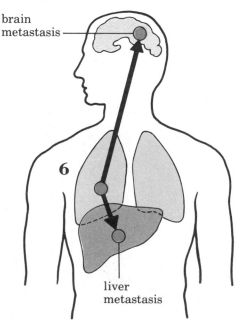

brain metastasis

6

liver metastasis

DISTANT SPREAD OF CANCER

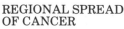

identity of the individual, yet the functions of cells forming different organs and tissues are restricted to those needed for the whole organism. Repair and healing by cell division also are strictly controlled.

Cancer is an abnormality of body cells that have escaped from these controlled behavior patterns. How and why this escape occurs is one of science's major mysteries. It could be caused by a loss of "repressor" substances that presumably limit the activities of normal cells. Or it could be caused by the introduction of some outside substance such as a virus. It might be that a virus already present is activated by some other event. We do know that the transformation of normal cells to cancer cells is then transmitted to succeeding cell generations, suggesting that the change involves DNA (deoxyribonucleic acid), the genetic mechanism of the cell.

The transformation of normal cells to cancer cells resembles a mutation, the sudden permanent change in cell composition caused by some force from outside that affects the cell. In cancer probably more than one sudden change is involved. But whether the change is caused by one event or several, the altered cell must then survive and divide successfully to form a mass of abnormal cells. Possibly this progression is promoted by the addition of other substances or stimuli not in themselves cancer-producing, or by a drop in the defense mechanisms that normally protect the body against change. There is evidence that the abnormal cells sometimes reverse their behavior and return to normal, so the process may not be inevitably and invariably one-directional. (And the change may follow a different timetable in different persons, often halting completely for a time, an event called remission.)

A mass of cells growing rapidly and independently and no longer contributing to normal organ function is called a tumor, or neoplasm. Not all tumors are cancerous. Some, which grow within a capsule and do not recur after removal, are called benign, although this does not mean they are always harmless. If they occur in vital organs or where there is limited space for expansion, such as within the skull, benign tumors can be life-threatening. Cancer, however, is said to be malignant because it always carries the capacity to kill. It can invade or squeeze nearby tissue, drain vital resources of the body, spread to distant parts of the organism, and totally disrupt and destroy normal function.

Cancer's spread, called metastasis, is its distinctive and dangerous feature. As cancer cells multiply and grow, they invade the channels of the lymphatic system and lodge in the lymph nodes, such as those under the arm, which are frequent targets in breast cancer. They also may penetrate blood vessels. The bloodstream or lymphatic system carries the cells to distant parts of the body, so that secondary colonies (metastases) may be established in vital organs such as the liver or brain. Since "curing" cancer means removing every last cancerous cell, a metastasized cancer is virtually impossible to eradicate.

We usually speak of three stages of cancer: (1) localized, when the cancer is limited to its original site; (2) regional, when it has reached adjacent organs or nearby lymph nodes; (3) and distant, or disseminated, when the cancer cells have been carried to other parts of the body. Although we think of cancer as a localized solid tumor initially, it can occur in non-solid structures, as it does in leukemia, a cancer of the bloodstream.

THE CAUSES OF CANCER

Although precisely what happens to change a normal cell into a cancerous one remains unclear, we know of several events and substances that can lead to cancer in man, animals, and in cells grown on artificial nutrients in glass flasks (in vitro carcinogenesis). The list of carcinogens, or cancer-producers, includes chemicals, viruses, and physical events.

Although hundreds of chemicals have been reported to produce cancers in experimental animals, only about two dozen have been verified as causes of cancer in man. The table on page 704 lists some of them. Most of these are limited to industrial or medicinal exposures. Three are of general importance: (1) tobacco smoke products, especially of cigarettes, which produce chemicals called polycyclic aromatic hydrocarbons; (2) asbestos, especially combined with tobacco smoking; (3) excessive use of estrogens, the female sex hormones.

Tobacco smoking has caused widespread lung cancer and is associated with cancer of

SOME CHEMICALS THAT CAUSE CANCER IN HUMANS

Substance	Site of cancer
Polycyclic hydrocarbons	
Soot, tar, oil	Skin
Tobacco smoke	Lung
Aromatic amines	
2-naphthylamine, benzidine and derivatives	Bladder
Alkylating agents	
Mustard gas and derivatives	Lung
Melphalan and related chemicals	Bone marrow
Asbestos	Pleura, lung
Arsenic	Skin, lung
Benzene	Bone marrow
Vinyl chloride	Liver
Chrome ores	Lung
Nickel ores	Lung, nasal sinus
Isopropyl oil	Nasal sinus
Estrogens	Uterus, vagina
Phenacetin	Kidney, pelvis
Immunosuppressive drugs	Lymphatic system

the mouth and esophagus, especially when combined with heavy drinking. Estrogens have been implicated in cancer of the uterus in women. Asbestos induces a high rate of cancer among those who work with it, especially if they are also smokers, but its effect on persons less heavily exposed is unclear.

Among industrial carcinogens, aromatic amines—used by dye manufacturers and by other industries—produce bladder cancer. Vinyl chloride induces a rare type of liver cancer among heavily exposed workers. Alkylating chemicals, which are drugs used to treat advanced cancer, can also cause cancer. One of the most potent carcinogens, aflatoxin, is produced by a fungus, and is related to liver cancers in the tropics. A group of reactive chemicals called nitrosamines produce cancer in animals. Their role is undetermined in human disease.

Two important physical agents that can cause cancer are X rays or other forms of ionizing radiation, and sunlight or actinic radiation. Ionizing radiation induces leukemia, thyroid cancer, and, when the source is radium or plutonium, cancer of the bone. Sunlight induces skin cancer in people of light complexion.

The production of cancer by these chemicals or physical agents is dose-dependent, which means that the greater or longer the exposure, the greater the risk of cancer. The more time a blond spends in the sunshine, the greater the chance of developing skin cancer. The more cigarettes smoked, the higher the cancer risk.

Viruses have been demonstrated to cause cancers in many animals, from frogs to monkeys. Although conclusive evidence of virus-induced cancers in humans is still lacking, there appears to be little doubt that man eventually will be included on the list.

Cancer-causing (oncogenic) viruses consist of DNA or RNA, the nucleic acids that are the components of the genetic mechanism of all forms of life. In some way, these viruses become part of the structure of the cell, altering it in such a way that it has cancerous properties. It also has been demonstrated that such viruses may be present in the cell, yet latent and undetectable until aroused to activity by some precipitating event.

There are several viruses suspected of causing certain types of human cancer. The Epstein-Barr virus is associated with a jaw cancer among African children, as well as cancer of the nasopharynx among southern Chinese. The hepatitis B virus is associated with liver cancer, and a herpes virus (HSV2) is associated with cancer of the cervix. If it can be established that a virus causes cancer, the door would be opened to cancer vaccination or protection.

REACTIONS TO CANCER

Cancer, like any disease, occurs when some outside stimulus interacts with the body's disease-fighting immune system. The strength of our defenses is largely determined by genetic makeup—what we inherit from mother and father.

There are a number of genetically determined cancers, all rather rare. One is cancer of the eye (retinoblastoma), which can be transmitted to offspring by two parents who carry the gene but are not affected themselves. Two other examples are multiple polyps of the colon that become cancerous, and xeroderma pigmentosum, a skin disease that develops into cancer. We also know that some families experience aggregations of cancers. Genetic factors are not easily separated from environmental ones. Nevertheless, a history of cancers in your family should alert you to increased risk that requires closer surveillance. Women whose close female relatives have had breast cancer represent one such higher-risk group.

Cancer cells require nutrients just as normal cells do. Therefore, diet must play a role in the development of cancer. In experimental animals, restricting food to levels that keep them lean but nutritionally well-fed not only reduces the occurrence of cancers, but lengthens the life-span. Excess calories probably stimulate cancerous growth in human be-

ings as well, so limiting one's food intake is sound advice, and it may protect against heart disease as well as cancer.

The body's immune system plays a role against cancer, as it does against any invader recognized as foreign. Individuals in whom the immune system is deficient or depressed are especially prone to develop cancers of the blood and lymph tissues. Agammaglobulinemia, the inability to produce immune antibodies, is an example of a genetic immune deficiency that leaves the body vulnerable to blood and lymphatic cancers. Suppression of immune response may be produced by drugs given to transplant surgery patients to prevent rejection of the new organ, and it may be produced among patients treated successfully for cancer with similar drugs. A promising area of research involves stimulating the immune mechanisms that may help to prevent cancer or kill individual cancer cells before they can gain a foothold. Interferons, proteins made by cells to fight viruses, are being tried against cancer. The research is in its early stages, however.

CAN WE PREVENT CANCER?

There are two types of disease prevention. Primary prevention aims to block the disease from occurring, and secondary prevention strives to halt its consequences at the earliest possible moment.

Primary Prevention

A significant proportion of cancers can be prevented. Cancer of the lung is the No. 1 cancer killer among men, and second among women only to breast cancer. Three-fourths of the cases of lung cancer are caused by smoking cigarettes.

Tobacco smoking also is involved in cancers of the mouth, pharynx, larynx, and esophagus, especially when combined with alcohol consumption and poor nutrition. And smoking is involved in cancer of the bladder. Alcohol, although not considered a primary carcinogen, is related to cancer of the liver. The elimination of tobacco smoking and of alcohol consumption, combined with proper nutrition, could reduce cancer cases by at least 15 percent and perhaps as much as 30 percent. This is the enviable rate recorded by religious groups whose members follow a restricted diet and do not smoke or drink.

Avoidance of unnecessary X-ray exposure and of too much sun are preventive steps individuals may take. X-ray exposure of children, even for dental work, and of pregnant women should be used only when no alternative methods will do. Control over industrial chemicals such as asbestos, beryllium, beta-naphthylamine, and related aromatic amines require government action.

Cancer prevention is best practiced as part of general health protection, a cooperative effort between the individual and his medical advisor. The two components in health protection are: (1) life-style, in which temperate food habits and personal safety measures are particularly important, along with avoidance of tobacco, alcohol, and drugs, and (2) body awareness, in which the individual becomes better acquainted with his or her body and its functions, and thus is alert to changes requiring medical attention. These recommendations extend beyond the individual to the family unit, with parents particularly influential in establishing the behavior patterns of the children.

Secondary Prevention

There is no single test for cancer. Recognizing cancer depends on being alert to certain signs and symptoms that may or may not mean that the disease is present. A high "index of suspicion" and quick response can promote early discovery of cancer with a higher prospect of cure. The American Cancer Society lists these seven warning signals:
- Change in bowel or bladder habits.
- A sore that does not heal.
- Unusual bleeding or discharge.
- Thickening or lump in breast or elsewhere.
- Indigestion or difficulty in swallowing.
- Obvious change in wart or mole.
- Nagging cough or hoarseness.

If these or other signs of abnormality or illness persist or progress for a few weeks, seek medical advice immediately.

Regular physical examinations are important, too. The American Cancer Society recommends that women between 20 and 40 should have a breast examination by a physician every three years. They should examine their own breasts for lumps or changes every month, and have a baseline breast X ray between ages 35 and 40. The cancer society also recommends a pelvic examination for uterine cancer every three years in this age group (and for sexually active teenagers), and regular "Pap" tests for cervical cancer—two initial tests a year apart, then a test at least every three years. After age 40, a woman should have an annual breast examination by a physician, continue monthly self-examinations, and have yearly X rays after 50. She should have a yearly pelvic exam, a Pap test every three years if two previous tests have been negative, and an examination of the tissue of the lining of the womb, or endometrium, after menopause. The society recommends that both sexes should have annual rectal and stool tests for colon-rectal cancer, and visual examination by proctoscope every three to five years. Persons in high-risk groups, such as women with a family history of breast cancer, should have more frequent examinations.

These tests, of course, are conducted only for screening purposes, not for diagnosis.

Detection of pre-cancerous abnormalities (those that eventually may develop into cancer) is one of the benefits of regular medical checkups and of being alert to symptoms. Many potentially cancerous abnormalities are readily recognized by doctors. Prompt treatment will often prevent them from developing into cancer.

TREATING CANCER

It is generally recognized within the medical profession that there are three effective forms of cancer treatment:
- Surgery, removal of all or as much as possible of a cancer, and often of lymphatic structures through which cancer might spread.
- X ray and other controlled forms of radiation to destroy malignant cells.
- Chemotherapy, which is treatment with drugs or combinations of drugs.

Choice of treatment requires expert medical evaluation of a particular form of cancer in a particular patient. Specialists in cancer treatment (oncologists) often make this judgment. Some cancers are treatable by X rays; other forms are not, at least not in doses that can be tolerated by the patient. Forms of treatments may be combined or given in sequence. Radiation or chemotherapy may precede or follow breast cancer surgery.

**DRUGS
THAT AFFECT
ADVANCED
CANCERS**

Type of cancer	Drugs (usually combinations)
Choriocarcinoma (women)	Methotrexate, dactinomycin, vinblastine
Childhood leukemia (lymphocytic)	Daunorubicin, prednisone, vincristine, 6-mercaptopurine, methotrexate, BCNU, L-asparaginase
Hodgkin's disease	HN2, vincristine, prednisone, procarbazine, bleomycin, adriamycin, vinblastine
Testicular cancer	Dactinomycin, methotrexate, chlorambucin, cis-platinum dd
Wilms' tumor	Dactinomycin with surgery and radiotherapy, vincristine
Neuroblastoma	Cyclophosphamide, adriamycin, vincristine, procarbazine
Prostate	Estrogens
Breast	Androgens, estrogens, 5-fluorouracil, vincristine, prednisone, methotrexate, adriamycin, tamoxifen
Chronic lymphocytic leukemia	Alkylating agents, prednisone
Osteogenic sarcoma	Methotrexate, adriamycin

Surgical techniques used in cancer treatment are described in chapter 31, "Understanding Your Operation." Radiotherapy is described in chapter 32, "X Rays and Radiology," and in chapter 25, "Breast Cancer."

Chemotherapy alone is used only for a few widely disseminated cancers that cannot be reached by other means. It has a high success rate in choriocarcinoma, a rare cancer in women, and in acute lymphocytic leukemia, a blood cancer of children. In combination with radiation, it has improved the cure rate against Hodgkin's disease, a cancer of the lymphatic system. For many types of cancers of other sites, drugs may help to prolong life and alleviate symptoms.

Some prostate and breast cancers depend on hormones for growth. Antagonistic hormones may help in treatment of these cancers. Immunotherapy, a means of turning the body's natural defense systems against cancer, has been used in combination with chemotherapy but results thus far have been disappointing. Newer and better chemical agents against cancer can be confidently predicted. The table above lists some effective chemotherapies.

Unorthodox Treatments

Some persons who have cancer, or think they have, turn in hope or desperation to unorthodox treatments. Some of these treatments are offered in goodwill, but others are quackery. They are usually harmless but useless. The tragedy is that precious time is lost during which recognized treatment might bring the disease under control.

FIVE-YEAR CANCER SURVIVAL RATES
FOR SELECTED SITES

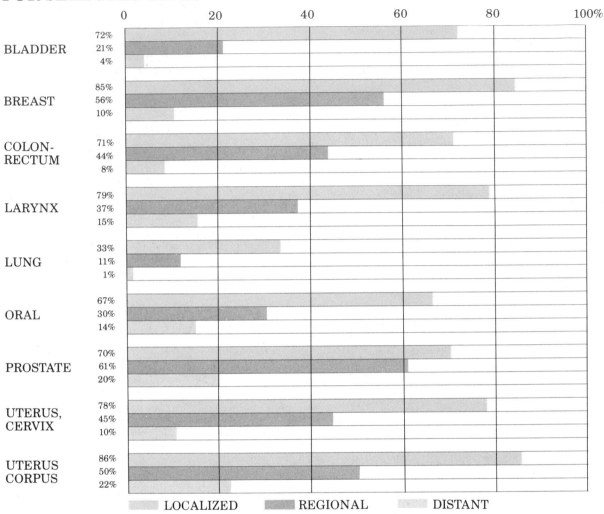

The Cure Rate for Cancer

In recent years, some of these treatments have been allowed for use in certain states. One of these is laetrile, a substance obtained from apricot pits. Despite prolonged scientific investigation, no benefits have been shown to stem from its use. Clinics offering laetrile and other unorthodox treatments have become established on the Mexican side of the U.S.-Mexican border, where licensing regulations are different. Although these clinics have received considerable publicity, their results are unsubstantiated.

The outcome of a cancer case depends on the type of cancer and the stage at which it is treated. For every type of cancer, the outlook, or prognosis, is much better if the tumor is removed or treated while still localized. The outlook becomes less favorable when the cancer has spread, usually to the nearest lymph nodes draining the area. With cancers that are widely spread through the body, the outlook is unfortunately quite grim.

Doctors consider a cancer "cured" when the patient survives five years or longer after treatment, without recurrence of the disease.

Cure rate by these standards is best for cancers of the uterus, cervix, and breast, where the figure is more than 50 percent. For cancer of the colon and rectum, prostate, bladder, and Hodgkin's disease, the survival rate is between 30 and 50 percent. When the disease is treated while still localized, these figures nearly can be doubled. But for cancer of the esophagus, pancreas, and lungs, the percentage of cures is dismally low. The chart on page 708 summarizes the cure rate at various stages of cancer and at various sites in the body.

Effective treatment of cancer, is, unfortunately, strenuous, and side effects can be severe. Cancer surgery is usually radical, meaning that extensive tissue must be removed in an effort to be sure that all the cancer has been excised. Radiation treatment must be carried out over a period of time in order to deliver doses that are lethal to cancer cells yet tolerable to the patient. Drugs used against cancer often have serious side effects on the blood-forming tissues and the immune system, as well as unpleasant symptoms.

As more cancer patients are cured, rehabilitation becomes increasingly important. Removal of the rectum with a permanent colostomy, or artificial anus on the abdominal wall, removal of the voice box for cancer of the larynx, as well as amputations of the breast or limbs require not only prosthetic devices and retraining, but social and employment acceptance. Radiation and many anticancer chemicals can produce other forms of cancer. The occurrence of leukemia is increased among patients cured of cancer at other sites by these treatments, although the risk usually is outweighed by the benefits. One of the prime goals of cancer research is to find not only more effective but gentler therapies.

More than half of all cancer patients die of or with their disease. The care of terminally ill patients is another serious medical and social problem. Facilities developed in England called hospices attempt to combine such care with emphasis on spiritual support and death with dignity. Increasingly, terminally ill cancer patients are allowed to live out their lives at home in familiar surroundings with loved ones nearby.

LOOKING TO THE FUTURE

In 1937 the United States passed the National Cancer Act, a national commitment to solving the problem of cancer. The legislation was broadened in 1972. Public support of the fight against cancer is demonstrated by the annual contributions to the American Cancer Society and by the expanded efforts evident in other countries of the world.

The scientific consensus is that cancer is a problem that can be solved, and that progress is being achieved. The progress is steady but slow. The slow pace is easily understood when the complexities of the problem are realized. In cancer we are dealing with the very nature of biologic matter, and the wondrous mechanisms through which it programs the hereditary integrity and diversity of each animal and plant species. The science of molecular biology has yielded knowledge of the chemical components and structure of the DNA molecule. Transfer of DNA segments between cells of different species makes it possible to examine the functions of such segments. It is there, in the heart of the cell, that the secret of cancer lies.

Although we don't know "the answer to cancer," we are learning what external stimuli cause cells to become malignant, how to strengthen the human body against such aberrant cells, and how to combat their ravages with drugs. Progress is unmistakable.

It is simplistic to expect to discover one "cause" or one "cure" for all the diseases we call cancer. It is likely that the mechanisms by which chemicals and viruses produce cancerous changes are significantly different. And, more certainly, the cell types of different cancers are affected differently by different drugs and varying methods of therapy. New drugs undoubtedly will replace many of those we now use. A promising area of treatment research is among synthesized natural substances that act against viruses.

Future prevention of cancer, now limited to avoidance of identified carcinogens, may include vaccinations against specific forms of cancer with defined viral or other antigens. Strengthening an individual's resistance to cancer by chemical means is already an active research approach.

Virology, immunology, and chemotherapy may well stand for the first three letters spelling *vic*tory over cancer. The day is not yet here, and we shall experience many disappointments before it dawns. But with patience and perseverance, the problem will be solved.

CHAPTER 30   PATTI TIGHE, M.D.
DANIEL X. FREEDMAN, M.D.

EMOTIONAL AND MENTAL HEALTH

When a person is psychologically healthy, he or she enjoys an inner sense of well-being and an ability to function well in the world. A healthy person can cope with the problems of everyday living, feel emotion, love others, work successfully, play with enjoyment, and be reasonably optimistic about the future. When stress comes along, he or she can react flexibly, according to the needs of the situation, not in an inflexible, rigid way. Psychological health enables a person to balance his or her own interests and needs for self-expression with responsibilities to family and community.

The symptoms of psychological illness are not clear-cut. No sharp line divides normal and abnormal feelings and behavior. Rather, the pattern, intensity, and especially the duration of a particular mode of behavior or feeling mark the border between illness and the simple fluctuations of reaction to everyday living. Of course, some severe emotional disorders produce unusual behavior apparent to everybody.

This chapter will deal with syndromes whose symptoms are so prolonged and pronounced that they require medical attention. These disorders include unusual feelings of distress or emotional pain; impairment of function in one or more areas—interpersonal, occupational, or sexual; and the serious inability to fully use one's potential. All stem from psychological, biological, or social roots, or more commonly from a combination of the three. As in all areas of medicine, classification is incomplete and changes frequently as we gain knowledge.

Twenty million Americans currently require treatment for emotional difficulties. One-third of all hospital beds are occupied by people with mental illnesses. Their disorders account for more days of hospitalization than any other cause. Including lost productivity, the cost of their hospitalization is about $20 billion a year. Yet for each patient under care, the amount of federal and private money spent for mental-illness research is one-tenth of what our society allocates to other disabling disorders such as heart disease and cancer.

Psychological illness continues to bear the stigma it has carried through the ages, subjecting individuals with emotional disorders to misunderstanding, shame, and guilt. Society still looks on their problems with a moralistic and secretive attitude rather than understanding them to be the legitimate medical problems they are.

THE ORIGINS OF EMOTIONS AND BEHAVIOR

Why do we feel the way we feel? What makes us behave the way we behave? Those who study the subject conclude that a complex interweaving of psychological, biological, and social factors determines each individual's pattern of feelings and behavior. The process begins early in life, even before birth.

Psychological Factors

A long-standing psychological explanation for behavior is based on the idea of unconscious conflict. According to this theory, we all enter life with a certain set of basic drives and wishes. These include the drive to have what we want when we want it, to experience pleasure rather than pain, to be unconditionally approved and supported, and to be angry and retaliate when we are frustrated or deprived. We also develop an inner sense of prohibition against these drives and wishes, producing potential for conflict. Because everyone has a similar set of drives, society has established taboos and regulations to make for order, further increasing the likelihood of a clash. That is why we all must learn to control our feelings, to delay gratification, and, in general, to follow the rules instead of the drives. Because this is a compromise solution, the price paid by everyone is the potential for conflict, which generally remains unconscious. The psychologically healthy person is one who can work out ways to balance these two opposing pulls.

Another ingredient in healthy psychological growth is freedom from truly excessive stress or deprivation. A child whose life situation is too disadvantaged and whose minimal survival needs are not met may not develop healthy ways of coping with life. He may develop a pattern of self-defeating behavior and psychiatric symptoms. This is not universally true, as we know. Some children have a combination of perceptions, ingenuity, talents, and resources that enables them to rise above an early life of unfortunate circumstances.

The interaction between a child and the most significant caretaking person (in our culture, usually the mother) is another major determinant of early development. The ideal caretaker embodies qualities that facilitate optimum psychological growth in the child. These include three abilities: to strike a balance between unqualified loving and limit-setting, to encourage the development of innate skills and talents, and to gradually help the child enter and master the larger world of the community while still providing his or her basic needs for nurture, attachment, and closeness within the family. The parents' own personalities significantly influence their capacity for and style of effective child-rearing. Parents obviously are less effective if they are immature and self-centered, depressed, chronically resentful of the burden of the child, obsessed with their own occupation, or more seriously emotionally ill. Marital strain, open quarreling, and a general atmosphere of unhappiness and discontent also can take their toll on a child's development.

Relatives, neighbors, teachers, brothers, and sisters can compensate for parental deficiencies and for other deprivations. This wider network is always necessary to broaden a child's perspective and to serve as models in adapting to life situations. These people can help to bring out individual potential during these important years.

According to these notions of personality development, basic habits are learned early in life. If learning has been faulty, the resulting habits can be self-destructive and impede further learning. But in advantageous circumstances, early self-destructive habits can be modified and replaced by better ones, even after adolescence.

Social Factors

A person's mental health and his or her social environment are intricately interwoven. Abnormal behavior as well as overt psychiatric symptoms can be brought on or changed by social and cultural conditions. Undesirable circumstances (low social class, poverty, sexism, racism, discrimination, and lack of family support) correlate with poor psychological adjustment (stress, anxiety, depression, role confusion, a sense of helplessness, and failure to achieve potential). Of course, the fact that these frequently occur together does not necessarily mean that one always causes the other. A great many mentally ill persons have never experienced these adverse conditions.

Overall, there is a direct relationship between economic position and mental health. Greater numbers of poor people suffer from the more serious psychological disorders, especially psychoses, addictions, and alcoholism. This is particularly true when poverty is linked with low social mobility, general social instability, fragmented family ties, and community disharmony. A sense of hopelessness and a perception of inability to improve one's life are undoubtedly factors that contribute to psychological problems. Still, many people respond to social instability and precarious life situations creatively and constructively, so the poor are not inevitably vulnerable to psychological problems, nor are the rich immune from them.

Second-class status can be a powerful determinant of how people adjust. Our society defines "nonwhiteness" as inferior. Because many people define themselves by the way others react to them, nonwhites may develop a self image of inferiority. If there are no strong countervailing family traditions or personal resources to draw upon, the child may grow up with a poorly formed identity or sense of self, and low self-esteem. Our society remains pervaded by institutional racism, with its systematic barriers to the acquisition of power by nonwhites. Reactions to such limitations can be lowered self-esteem, rage, chronic stress, and anxiety. These are debilitating symptoms in themselves but they also may lead to more severe disorders.

Social attitudes and institutions communicate the same message of inferiority to women. As more women have begun to work outside the home in recent years, they have come into closer contact with overt discrimination. This problem has been compounded by the expectation that employed women also will handle the full burden of responsibility for child-rearing and running a household. Society's acceptance of role change for women has been slow. For many women this period of transition and upheaval frequently brings frustration, guilt, a sense of inadequacy, and particularly lowered self-esteem. Such role conflict also may increase the likelihood of developing more serious psychiatric symptoms.

The full-time mother who does not work outside the home runs different risks. Her self-esteem may be too dependent on the success of her children and her husband. She also faces a paradoxical situation. Having fulfilled the idealized role of full-time mother, she nevertheless receives a major portion of blame if her child does not develop well. Even if she enjoys her role, she sometimes fears that employed women will scorn her.

The social institution of the family has a powerful impact upon all of its members. The extended family—a network of aunts, uncles, grandparents, cousins, close friends, and neighbors—is an invaluable resource for development and growth. The recent decline of the extended family has been accompanied by the predominance of the nuclear family—two parents and their children—that is relatively isolated from the informal presence of relatives and others. Also, divorce and single-parent households have come to be much more acceptable social patterns. Households composed of several adults and children have been shown to be as effective as the husband-wife nuclear family in fostering psychological growth in children. But a full understanding of the effects of changing household patterns on mental health remains incomplete.

Evidence does exist that social change of any kind produces strain for all involved. We also know that individuals with more supportive social contacts, such as marriage, frequent visits with relatives and friends, church participation, and group participation, tend to live longer, experience fewer illnesses, and cope better with minor and major life stresses.

Biological Factors

The body regulates itself through a vast network of interdependent biological systems that operate with chemical and electrical responses to signals from the environment or other body systems. Automatic feedback allows these systems to work together for smooth functioning physically, emotionally, and behaviorally. Each system is regulated much as a thermostat regulates temperature in a room. Malfunction of any of these regulating mechanisms can lead to an exaggeration or a deficit in chemical and electrical events in the body. Automatic smooth function is then disrupted. High blood pressure is an example of a normal biological system out of control. Drug addiction and anxiety states may prove to be examples of the body misperceiving signals and failing to monitor appropriately a chemical reaction in some body system.

The brain is the organ in closest touch with the environment. It is also the major organ regulating the responses of other body systems. Since the 1970s, sophisticated and delicate research techniques have made it possible to measure changes in brain function so that brain activity can be experimentally altered and then correlated with behavior. Resulting theories propose that electrical and chemical abnormalities in brain function significantly contribute to psychiatric illnesses and other disorders of feeling and behavior.

The brain is composed of billions of cells called neurons (see chapter 9, "The Brain and Nervous System"). The circuit construction of the brain consists of an astronomical number of connections among these neurons. The neurons communicate bits of information to each other by transferring minuscule amounts of chemicals (neurotransmitters) across tiny spaces (synapses) between the cells. The transfer occurs because an impulse is generated in certain specialized parts of the cell. The information passed from cell to cell in this system is the physical basis for thinking, moving, perceiving, remembering, and virtually every other human dimension.

Research into the human brain is primarily focused on identifying these chemicals, relating feelings, functions, and behaviors to each, and understanding how environmental events trigger their transmissions. Researchers also are seeking to identify which brain areas deal with specific functions, behaviors, and feelings.

For human beings to function best, nerve cells and circuits must develop normally and be maintained in good working order. Prenatal events can seriously change later behavior and emotions. Maternal psychological well-being, nutrition, environmental toxins, and drugs can affect brain development of the unborn child. Scientists cannot yet even begin to visualize how factors of early childhood such as maternal attention or hours spent watching television can influence the development of the brain systems that control behavior and feelings. Fortunately, there is increasing evidence that injured child and adult brains can compensate for impairments and learn new ways to accomplish lost functions.

Each new discovery about biological events within the brain is greeted (by the press and scientists alike) with great hope and the expectation that it will constitute the definitive breakthrough in the understanding and treatment of psychiatric illness. In fact, this research is in an early stage, comparable to the period in medical history when it was first becoming apparent that microorganisms (viruses and bacteria) were responsible for infectious diseases. A full scientific understanding of the biological bases of psychiatric illness is a hope for the future. As with infectious disease, precise and effective drug treatment can be expected to follow.

In explaining individual qualities and tendencies, the ancient division between heredity (that with which one is born) and environment (that which is shaped by upbringing and life experience) is as significant today as it has been for centuries. Two people may grow up with apparently similar histories of childhood adversity and deprivation, yet one will develop serious psychiatric disorder and the other become a well-functioning citizen. More and more, we are learning that genetic endowment contributes significantly to both human vulnerabilities and potentials.

Preliminary studies indicate that the basis of individual temperament may be partially genetically determined. Each person has relatively fixed and enduring personality traits and predictable emotional and behavioral responses to life situations. It is now clear that each infant is born with qualities of temperament that persist into childhood and beyond. These significantly influence how active or passive the child is, the regularity or irregularity of habits, how he or she responds to stimulation, and the length of his or her attention span.

Clearly then, the quality of the relationship between an infant and parent is not determined entirely by the parents' personality or "parenting ability." A parent will respond quite differently to a naturally quiet, receptive, predictable baby than to an irritable, jittery, unsmiling one. This is an example of the complex interplay between heredity and environment and of the difficulty of isolating biological and psychological factors.

Studies of many generations in one family, of twins raised together and raised apart, and of foster children have shown that behavioral tendencies and some psychiatric illnesses run in families. In these families, some individual members will develop a given hereditary disorder; others are only predisposed to it. That is, subsequent experiences can interact with the inherited tendencies to trigger inappropriate behavior or mental illness. For other family members not exposed to the same experiences, the predisposition will lie dormant and never show itself.

Many psychiatric abnormalities presumably involve an inherited predisposition. They include schizophrenia, manic-depressive disease, certain other types of depression, obsessive-compulsive personality disorder, and phobic personality disorder, all of which are discussed later.

DISORDERS OF EMOTION AND BEHAVIOR

Development and Adjustment

Personality development continues beyond childhood. The personality can grow and mature throughout the adult years. Each new stage of life necessitates coping with a different set of "crises." At each level, we must reexamine our sense of identity (who we are), interpersonal relationships, career and other goals, values, and our perspective on life and death.

When a person moves from adolescence to adulthood, the time comes to alter the image of parents as all-knowing guides and ever-available sources of support, to acquire adult values and ethics, to solidify gender identity, and to make vocational choices. In early adulthood, one must go on to explore alternatives in many areas, making decisions about career, marriage, parenthood, and a life-style. Those who make these transitions in their early twenties are in the position, by their mid-thirties, to reassess whether the earlier decisions are appropriate for their current life. Commitments are reexamined and are either altered or strengthened.

Middle life typically is characterized either by achievement of stability, with continuing productivity and contributions to the future, or by stagnation, leading to early decline. For both men and women, many important changes in biological function occur. Inevitable experiences require significant adjustment. They include success or failure of career and other activities, illness and death of parents, and the independence of children. There is an increasing awareness of the passing of generations.

The later years also can be marked by difficult circumstances—the waning of intellectual and physical capacities, the loss of a spouse, declining energy and activity, occupational retirement, a decreasing sense of usefulness, and impending death.

Some stress may accompany each of these transitions. Because stress normally contributes to the continuing development and growth of the personality, management of these transitional states brings the opportunity to move toward either more effective or more disorganized functioning. In the process of adapting to change, we can learn more innovative problem-solving techniques and develop more creative and mature modes of coping. Or, if the necessary adjustment is greater than the person can accomplish, adaptation fails, and inappropriate, less-mature styles reemerge. Occasionally, severe and long-standing emotional disorders can result. The actual outcome depends on the stability of the person's personality, the extent of his or her social support network, and the presence of circumstances of deprivation. But it is probably safe to say that almost everyone who goes through the transitional phases of life experiences some degree of stress.

Transient adjustment reaction is the psychiatric term for poor response of short duration to these transitional stresses. The severity of the maladjustment can range from mild anxiety to serious physical or emotional symptoms. An adolescent who was too dependent on his parents as a child may develop physical illness on leaving for college, so that departure is postponed. An intelligent, competent woman who neglected her own personal development after marriage to stay home may begin to experience anxiety attacks after the birth of a third child. A work-oriented, 50-year-old businessman may develop depression and back pain soon after he fails to get an anticipated promotion.

All these situations may also involve underlying psychiatric problems. But the symptoms that develop at the time of the life-stage transition can be considered a separate disorder if the person soon returns to his or her previous behavior after the milestone is passed.

The diagnosis of transient adjustment reaction also applies to a poor response to inordinate stress in other situations. Again, the symptoms can be mild to severe but recede as the situation improves. A man who dropped out of high school, drifts from job to job, and has no stable, intimate relationship may experience the symptoms of a classical depression when fired by his employer if he has no savings and is refused state aid. But if his financial status is stabilized, he returns to his own characteristic level of functioning. Clearly, he has long-standing problems of psychological maladjustment, but his depression is a separate, temporary disorder, induced by the situation and abated with elimination of the stress.

Divorce, severe marital discord, serious illness, lawsuits, and other life crises also can precipitate transient adjustment reactions. But these problems of living usually do not become chronically disabling. Family, friends, clergy, social agencies, and family physicians can provide adequate support to help the person through the crisis. When a sufficiently supportive environment is lacking, however, or when the personality is not sufficiently flexible, the symptoms may become chronic, and the diagnosis of transient adjustment reaction would not apply.

Character Disturbances and Neuroses

Everyone has a fairly constant personality style—predictable ways of perceiving the world and coping with opportunities, challenges, and misfortunes. Different individuals tend to be anxious, compulsive, depressed, passive and dependent, withdrawn, given to physical complaints, or flighty. This is simply "the way they are." It is the way a person knows himself or herself to be. Under stress, these modes of behavior or particular coping styles become exaggerated: the flighty person becomes flightier, and the withdrawn person pulls further into a shell. But these remain simply extreme forms of the individual's usual traits. This persistent pattern of response, as individual as one's fingerprints, is a person's character (or personality) style.

In some persons, however, the collection of traits is so pronounced that it interferes with normal functioning. Their responses are maladaptive, counterproductive, and are not adjusted to fit the situation.

People whose persistent behavior patterns fit this description fall into one of two categories—those with character disorders (also known as personality disorders) and those with neuroses. Although the two overlap in many ways, there is increasing agreement among doctors that character disorders and neuroses are distinct entities.

Character disorders range from mild to severe. When the disorder is mild, the person's behavior resembles normal functioning. A person with a moderate disorder is usually viewed as eccentric. Severe disorders can be genuinely disabling. The style traits are so exaggerated that normal functioning is seriously interfered with.

The significant feature of a character disorder is that the persons are seldom made uncomfortable by its existence. Their behavior is not accompanied by anxiety, unlike neurotics, and they do not view themselves as ill. In fact, they may deny that the behavior pattern exists. If they admit that it does exist, they may deny that it is abnormal. For this reason they do not respond well to psychotherapy.

There are many types of character disorders, too many to describe here. A few of the more common follow.

The obsessive-compulsive personality is perfectionistic and competitive. He or she is preoccupied with punctuality, orderliness, cleanliness, and doing things just right. Commonly, the person engages in repetitive rituals, like incessantly checking gas jets, or always touching or arranging objects in a certain, unvarying order. Obsessive-compulsive people crave work, whether exalted or trivial. They are ambitious, and need to control everything. Often they cannot express feelings, and, indeed, may even lack the ability to experience them. They may fall into depression when they cannot meet their own unrealistically high standards.

The passive-aggressive personality expresses anger in disguised ways. Procrastination, stubbornness, inefficiency, "forgetting," and negativism characterize these people. While appearing to comply, they, in fact, manage subtly to defy authority. By seeming to be helpless and needy, they actually provocatively manipulate the surroundings toward their own ends.

Hysterical or histrionic personalities are emotionally overreactive and dramatic. They need to be the center of attention and are preoccupied with their appearance and the impression they make on people. They may seem to be sexually preoccupied, but they simply wish to be taken care of and treated as special. They seem to others to be seductive but are actually selfish and self-centered.

Schizoid personalities are loners. They have few friends and little social life. They are shy and reclusive and avoid intimacy. They seem aloof, cold, detached, and sometimes bland.

Antisocial personalities are impulsive, untrustworthy, and irresponsible toward persons and property. Some, such as the confidence man, are experts at mobilizing people and manipulating them to their own ends. They transgress rules and regulations, but they experience little guilt and do not respond to punishment. They do not appear to distinguish right from wrong. A history of school truancy and juvenile delinquency is common in these individuals, though by no means do all truants and delinquents develop this character. Adult antisocial behavior can occur in "rebels" who are responsible and capable of trust, but find satisfaction in opposing society.

The cause of personality disorders is poorly understood. There is some evidence that genetically determined traits may contribute. Faulty learning patterns and defective problem-solving techniques may be involved, too.

Grossly disturbed family settings tend to produce individuals with personality disorders more often than do smoothly functioning families. The former include families where one parent controls and dominates, families in which the child is scapegoated so parents can avoid facing marital difficulties, and settings in which the child is taught that the world is not to be trusted, or that other people must be outsmarted and cheated if one is to get ahead. Undoubtedly the role of social and economic deprivation is also important. Nevertheless, all the components necessary for healthy personality development are not understood. Even the best environment does not guarantee the best outcome in some cases.

Neuroses also are defined by specific, persistent patterns of responses to life events. Unlike those with character disorders, however, people with neuroses experience uncomfortable symptoms that are thought to be related to unconscious conflict. Neurotic symptoms result in impairment of normal functioning and usually are accompanied by feelings of anxiety. Three prominent forms of neurosis are anxiety neurosis, phobic neurosis, and obsessive-compulsive neurosis.

Anxiety neurosis exists in 2 to 5 percent of the U.S. population. Anxiety in response to an unpleasant memory or the anticipation of an unpleasant experience is common, normal, and necessary. It is even a powerful motivating force to stimulate people to seek relief from a threatening situation. But a diffuse feeling of anxiety not related to a specific cause is not normal. This state, known as free-floating anxiety, is characterized by a sense of dread or panic and a feeling that something terrible is about to happen. Physical symptoms are common—tensed muscles, chest pain, fast heart rate, abdominal cramps, and light-headedness. The attacks may come several times daily to once every few months. Normal life can be mildly to severely restricted. Anxiety neurosis sometimes shows a strong family history, and possibly is genetically determined. In these cases, the neurosis often begins in early adolescence. Because the physical symptoms resemble those of a wide variety of physical illnesses, a thorough medical evaluation is essential.

Phobic neurosis is characterized by irrational fear in the presence or anticipation of harmless objects or situations. Phobic persons may fear insects, enclosed spaces, open spaces, high places, or driving in an automobile. Phobias can develop suddenly or gradually, and can appear intermittently or so continuously that the person is virtually incapacitated. It is estimated that up to 15 million Americans suffer from phobias severe enough to interfere with functioning. About one million are so disabled that they cannot work outside the home or manage even common household tasks. For example, some are so fearful of injury or impending death that a magazine picture of an accident or the sound of a siren in the distance can trigger a severe panic attack.

Phobics are aware that their fears are irrational, yet the sensations of panic or losing control are so intolerable that the precipitating situations or objects must be avoided at all costs, and they develop elaborate measures to ward them off. Avoidance attempts may be as restrictive as the panic itself. A person with a phobic fear of water may walk several blocks out of his way to avoid passing a building with a fountain in the lobby. Most phobics are ashamed of their irrational fear, judge it to be a sign of cowardice, and hide it from all but close friends or family.

Frequently a phobia is a disguised way of expressing anxiety originating in unconscious conflict by displacing it onto a specific object or situation. The object can be avoided, and thereby the anxiety is avoided, too. Some phobias may be a learned response caused by an early exposure to a frightening situation: a person's fear of high places may date from a long-forgotten fall. However, for many adults, experiences of sudden overwhelming panic and impending doom, without any forgotten unconscious or conscious cause, lead to the development of phobic avoidance rituals simply to ward off the attacks.

Obsessive-compulsive neurosis, unlike the obsessive-compulsive personality disorder, is characterized by conscious anxiety at the time of the obsessive thoughts and compulsive acts. Patients with this disorder can be severely disabled. An example of a typical obsession is the persistent intrusion of an unwanted thought or urge over which the person has no control. The obsession may be a single word or idea or a very complex notion. Intrusive swear words, sexual images, or something as simple as a fragment of a song are common. The consequence of the symptom may be that the patient is unable to concentrate on anything else or even to hold a conversation.

Compulsive rituals vary from simple actions to complex behavioral patterns. Extreme compulsions also can be seriously disabling. Repeated handwashing, one of the more common compulsive rituals, is usually associated with overwhelming fear of dirt and contaminants. The practice can lead to inflammation or even ulceration of the hands and arms. Often the normal activities of living are impeded because the ritual occupies so much time. Compulsions this severe also restrict a patient's family. The family of a compulsive handwasher may have to adhere to a very rigid set of rules and restrictions to maintain a setting of meticulous cleanliness.

One view of the cause of obsessive-compulsive neurosis is that, as with phobias, the thoughts or actions serve to prevent anxiety that may be related to unconscious frightening or forbidden impulses. Another theory suggests that a biochemical malfunction in the brain is involved.

Psychosis

Psychosis is not a specific clinical diagnosis, but rather a descriptive term. It denotes extreme loss of contact with reality. Psychotic states are characterized by serious personality disorganization, disruption of most areas of adaptation, the experience of unrealistic thoughts and feelings, and odd, inappropriate behavior. The current definition of psychosis corresponds to such earlier terms as "madness" or "lunacy."

Schizophrenic patients are psychotic only during the periods in which symptoms are severe. Patients with mania, depression, paranoid states, and organic brain syndromes can be intermittently psychotic. Many diseases, injuries, and drug reactions can produce temporary psychological illness of psychotic proportions.

Schizophrenia

Schizophrenia is a group of diseases that is among the most severe and disabling of mental illnesses. These diseases are characterized by disorders of thinking, perception, feeling, behavior, and social relationships.

A schizophrenic's thinking tends to be illogical or controlled by a private logic that others do not understand. Connections between one thought and the next are not apparent, and rapid shifts in content occur. Thoughts may come very slowly and with great difficulty or may seem to be interrupted suddenly, especially thoughts associated with intense feelings such as anger or fear. The capacity for abstract thinking frequently is impaired. Schizophrenics may experience delusions, strongly held false beliefs that cannot be changed despite reason or evidence to the contrary. They may be certain that others control them or their thoughts, or that they are being harassed, followed, or tortured. Delusional thinking may reflect a self-perception of exceptional importance. The voice on the radio is talking directly to him, he has a direct communication with God, or he can unrealistically influence another person.

The most common schizophrenic perceptual distortions are hallucinations, sensory experiences occurring in the absence of an actual stimulus. Auditory hallucinations, in which the person "hears" a voice talking to or about him, or voices talking to each other, are the most frequent type. A schizophrenic may experience imaginary smells and tastes, too. The schizophrenic's use of language is marked by private symbolism. Or he may misuse words, construct new words, or speak in peculiar phraseology.

The expression of feelings in schizophrenia tends to be reduced in intensity and frequency. Emotional response is shallow, and the experience of pleasure rare. He or she may react inappropriately, such as laughing on hearing sad news. The extremes of response are frenzy (extreme agitation, continuous movement, and loud talking) or catatonia (absolute silence and inhibition of all movement).

Schizophrenics have difficulty establishing close relationships, and tend to withdraw into a world of their own. The range of isolation includes simple shyness to total reclusiveness. As the condition gradually worsens, patients may ignore personal cleanliness, appearance, and social decorum, and may assume bizarre habits and life-styles.

About two million Americans (one percent of the population) are schizophrenic. Among some groups of urban poor, the incidence may be as high as six percent.

One-half of all psychiatric hospital beds in the United States are occupied by schizophrenics. Most must be rehospitalized periodically. Only one-fifth of discharged schizophrenics hold jobs. Since schizophrenia usually begins in the career-forming years of late adolescence or early adulthood, schizophrenics belatedly enter the job market and thus tend to hold low-paying jobs. (Thus, conditions of poverty may not produce more schizophrenics. Rather, schizophrenics may sink into the lower-income ranks.) Education also may be interrupted, and marriage and successful family life are infrequent. As schizophrenics' psychiatric history tends to follow them, they live with pessimism, shame, social ostracism, and perpetual fear of rehospitalization. An estimated 10 percent of schizophrenics commit suicide.

Most experts now agree that schizophrenia is actually several different diseases. Some patients pursue a relentless downhill course. They experience frequent psychotic episodes with general personality deterioration between episodes. Other patients have intermittent psychotic periods, but function fairly normally between those periods. They do not deteriorate with time.

There are many theories about the cause of schizophrenia. Heredity undoubtedly plays an important predisposing role. Current research implicates a genetic component in as many as 40 percent of cases. The significance of psychological and social factors—parent-child interaction, family relationships, and environmental stress—has not been reliably assessed. But there is no doubt that biological, psychological, and social factors interact in complex ways to produce the clinical syndrome.

Interestingly, symptoms resembling those of schizophrenia can be caused by circulatory diseases (hardening of the arteries), endocrine diseases (thyroid dysfunction), nutritional deficiencies, drug abuse (LSD, amphetamines, and alcohol), and other psychiatric illnesses. That is why a thorough medical evaluation is the necessary first step in management of a person with these symptoms.

Affective Disorders

Depression. It is estimated that one-fifth of all Americans will suffer from depression at some time in their lives. Depression is the psychiatric disorder for which the greatest number of people seek medical help and from which they suffer the most without seeking help. It occurs most frequently in the middle years of life, the time of highest job productivity and greatest family responsibility. The most serious consequence is suicide.

Virtually everyone experiences occasional periods of depression—times of sadness or depressed mood, with a reduction of usual enthusiasm and interest in life. These episodes usually are precipitated by a stressful event, most commonly a loss. The loss can be real or symbolic, and of any kind—loss of health, a relationship, financial security, attention, or self-esteem. The most predictable depression is grief following the loss of a loved one. These depressions are appropriate for the situation. They usually are short-lived, moderate in intensity, and only mildly and temporarily disruptive of normal activities and enjoyment. How quickly the person recovers depends on his or her personality strengths and network of support systems.

The psychiatric disorder known as depression is a constellation of more serious signs and symptoms involving changes in mood, perception and thinking, and bodily function. The patient feels sad, discouraged, and sometimes irritable. Crying spells are frequent. He or she may be beset by inappropriate feelings of guilt, a decreased sense of self-worth, helplessness, hopelessness, and a loss of interest in and pleasure from usual activities. Thoughts of suicide are common. The most frequent changes in body function are decreased appetite, weight loss, constipation, and sleep disturbances (usually early awakening). Thinking is slowed, and is characterized by difficulty in concentrating and by indecisiveness. Energy is decreased. The depressed person usually moves slowly, or, conversely, may be agitated, pacing the floor and wringing his or her hands. Some have multiple physical complaints. Loss of interest in sex is prominent. In psychotic depression, delusions and hallucinations frequently occur. Any of these symptoms alone may be the first indication of a serious depression and should signal an investigation for other symptoms and signs.

One form of depression seems to involve no perception of depressed mood by the patient. Rather, he or she describes only a physical problem, related to any organ system, for which no cause can be found. This form of "masked" depression is particularly common in the elderly.

Researchers disagree on the number and types of depressions and the best way to classify them. There may be several distinct diseases resembling one another but characterized by different causes, courses, and degrees of responsiveness to treatment.

One current hypothesis suggests a possible difference between depressions triggered by an event and those apparently unrelated to any specific happening. A given experience can have great significance to one person and very little to someone else. The meaning of the event or loss to the individual seems to be the important factor. Another group of patients has a depressive disease with episodes appearing "to come out of the blue."

Depression can be characterized by recurrence at intervals varying between every few months to two or three in a lifetime. Some forms of depression appear to run in families.

Mania is characterized by a general speeding up of most functions. The person's mood is elevated, expansive, fluctuating, or irritable. Speech is rapid; rhyming and punning are common. Thinking is easily distracted, with rapid shifting from one topic to another. The need for sleep is markedly reduced, energy level is very high, and self-esteem is inflated.

The person demonstrates poor judgment without insight. He may engage in unrealistic business deals or extravagant spending of money. Delusions are common at the peak of the episode. Mania is usually a recurrent disease, with intervals between episodes varying from months to years. A triggering event is usually not apparent.

Manic-depressive disease is characterized by intermittent episodes of both mania and depression. (The American Psychiatric Association now officially uses the classification, "Major Affective Disorder, Bipolar" for mania and manic-depressive disease, and "Major Affective Disorder, Depression," for depression.)

Evidence indicates that at least some forms of affective disorders probably run in families. A higher incidence also has been demonstrated in persons or families with a history of alcoholism. Scientists have noted changes in the chemical functioning of the brain that point toward a biological basis for some depressions and for mania. The symptoms of depression can be caused and mimicked by numerous physical illnesses, including diabetes, thyroid disease, and cancer, and by many drugs used for medical problems, especially those for high blood pressure.

Suicide is a serious problem in depression and mania. It is estimated that between 5 and 15 percent of depressed patients succeed in killing themselves. Although they frequently make explicit reference to their suicidal impulses, families and physicians tend to minimize them. Subtle clues include talking about taking a long trip, suddenly making a will and putting affairs in order, preoccupation with death or with suicide of a friend, a profound sense of hopelessness and despair about the future, or a sudden sense of calm and resignation in a person who previously had been complaining and feeling bad.

Family and friends should be alert for depression and suicidal thinking in persons who are isolated and alone, who have experienced a recent loss, or who are chronically ill. It is essential that others intervene, since the patient's depressed mood, general slowing of thought, and hopeless outlook tend to keep him from calling a doctor.

Disorders With Prominent Physical Symptoms

Stress. Stress is a way of describing what happens to an organism that must cope with change. Psychological and physiological mechanisms aim to maintain stability while simultaneously adjusting to stressful events in the environment. The reasonable and healthy pressures of life are necessary for best physical and psychological functioning. How a person responds to the ordinary pressures of life is a highly individual matter. A person's individual habits also help to cope with overload or extraordinary experiences. If too much change or adaptation is required, the demands produce physical and psychological consequences.

Some people cope; others do not. Response depends on a variety of factors: how the demand of the situation is perceived, habit, early life experiences, temperament, personality and the range of coping responses, the capacity to learn new habits, and the social support system.

Poor adaptation to stress can lead to a wide range of undesirable consequences: excessive anxiety, increased dependency, irritability, depression, a lowered threshold for anger and frustration, and even criminal behavior.

However, it seems that any disruption of the steady state takes its toll on the human body and psyche. The simple experience of normal life events, positive and negative, has a cumulative effect on physiological and psychological health even when a person adapts well. The mere experience of change, regardless of its psychological significance to the individual, correlates remarkably with increased likelihood of illness. The greater the magnitude and number of life changes during a given time period, the greater the likelihood a person will develop physical and psychiatric symptoms.

Life events range from the serious to the trivial. Forty-three life events have been extensively studied and rated in terms of relative importance. The most significant in contributing to risk of illness appear to be death of a spouse, divorce, or marital separation. Others in decreasing order of importance include: death of a family member, personal injury, marriage, retirement, pregnancy, a business change of any kind, a large mortgage, a child leaving home or beginning or ending school, a change in social activities, a change in sleeping and eating habits, and vacations. Even apparently positive changes such as occupational advancement and a move to a bigger house can contribute to increased risk of illness.

Individuals who experience two to three times the expected number of life changes in a year are at much greater than average risk of developing a fatal heart attack within a year or two. The principle applies to virtually all medical problems: tuberculosis, diabetes, depression, the common cold, and even athletic injuries. Undoubtedly many factors affect the actual appearance of symptoms. But it is now clear that excessive life change over a short period of time significantly increases the risk of development or worsening of physical and psychological disease and accidents.

In our complex society, it is helpful to recognize and plan for life changes and, where possible, to pace them. For instance, during a year in which a parent has died and a child has left home, it would be ill-advised to move or change jobs.

Psychophysiological disorders. The bodily mechanisms that operate to maintain a steady state account for the close association between emotional states and physical changes. It is well known that experiences of embarrassment, guilt, anger, or rejection can lead to blushing, rapid breathing, an increase in heart rate and blood pressure, nausea, diarrhea, and stomach pain. About one-third of patients seeking medical help have physical complaints that are intertwined with psychological and social distress.

According to one theory, psychophysiological disorders are the physical expression of emotional states kept out of awareness. Instead of being felt (consciously experiencing an emotion), these emotions are "somatized"—the person is unaware of the psychological upset and instead develops a backache, headache, nausea, or other physical symptoms. According to this notion, a person cannot tolerate an unpleasant emotion, but is unable to alter circumstances to eliminate the source of stress. A physical symptom develops rather than psychological symptoms such as a phobia or a compulsion.

LIFE EVENTS AND STRESS

Rank	Life Event	Mean Value
1	Death of spouse	100
2	Divorce	73
3	Marital separation	65
4	Jail term	63
5	Death of close family member	63
6	Personal injury or illness	53
7	Marriage	50
8	Fired at work	47
9	Marital reconciliation	45
10	Retirement	45
11	Change in health of family member	44
12	Pregnancy	40
13	Sex difficulties	39
14	Gain of new family member	39
15	Business adjustment	39
16	Change in financial state	38
17	Death of close friend	37
18	Change to different line of work	36
19	Change in number of arguments with spouse	35
20	Mortgage over $10,000	31
21	Foreclosure of mortgage or loan	30
22	Change in responsibilities at work	29
23	Son or daughter leaving home	29
24	Trouble with in-laws	29
25	Outstanding personal achievement	28
26	Wife begins or stops work	26
27	Beginning or ending of school	26
28	Change in living conditions	25
29	Revision of personal habits	24
30	Trouble with boss	23
31	Change in work hours or conditions	20
32	Change in residence	20
33	Change in schools	20
34	Change in recreation	19
35	Change in church activities	19
36	Change in social activities	18
37	Mortgage or loan less than $10,000	17
38	Change in sleeping habits	16
39	Change in number of family get-togethers	15
40	Change in eating habits	15
41	Vacation	13
42	Christmas	12
43	Minor violations of the law	11

The stress events can trigger medical illness. Some are more likely to do so than others. The Social Readjustment Rating Scale, compiled by Drs. Thomas Holmes and Richard Rahe of the University of Washington, rates 43 events in terms of their impact on health. The effects of these are cumulative—the more such events experienced in a single year, the greater the likelihood that the person will become ill. A total of 150 to 199 points in a year on this scale carries moderate risk of health problems. Accumulating 200 to 299 points carries medium risk, and 300 points or more brings severe risk. Although many events are "positive," it is the experience of change that provides the stress.

A specific event appears to act as a trigger. A patient may be admonished by an employer or experience a rejection (actual or perceived) from an important or respected person. Or it may be the anniversary of a death or other significant loss. The reaction to the event is unpleasant emotion—rage, helplessness, loss of self-esteem—but the ultimate response is physiological, such as pain, diarrhea, or chest tightness. An event can produce indifference in one person but have important psychological meaning to someone else. The brain "tags" each perception and experience with a specific emotional charge.

Repeated occurrence of the same pattern can result in exaggerated and sustained physiological changes. Traditionally asthma, ulcerative colitis, peptic ulcer, essential hypertension, and some skin diseases have at times been referred to as "psychosomatic" disease. More recent understanding suggests that serious tissue changes can occur in any organ system that has a built-in vulnerability.

The automatic physical response to stress itself can be adaptive or maladaptive. The body normally reacts to stress with shifts in blood pressure, blood sugar levels, and hormone levels, with increased blood supply to the brain and muscles, and with hypervigilance. This "fight or flight" response is appropriate as long as the stress lasts. But for some people, the body responds as though the stress signals continue after the event is over, as though an emergency were present all the time. Clearly, the physical and probably the psychological mechanisms involved in stress response can overshoot or respond to the wrong signals and produce serious tissue damage and physiological malfunction.

The mechanisms by which psychological experiences are translated into physical malfunction and by which the stress response maintains itself chronically out of control are not clearly understood. As described earlier, personality structure can render one susceptible to a physical response to stresses. Probably in some persons, a particular organ system is vulnerable by heredity, so that in an emotionally charged situation one person is susceptible to respiratory problems, another to skin reactions. Frequently entire families react to stress in similar ways.

Researchers are trying to discover the bodily mechanisms by which emotions prolong, worsen, and possibly even initiate nonmental medical symptoms. Investigation of the interplay among physical factors, psychological factors, and the environment is focused on the influences of heredity, upbringing, learning, chronic stress and deprivation, and environmental factors such as toxins, food substances, pollution, and health habits. The extent to which "automatic" bodily activities such as pulse and blood pressure can be brought under voluntary control is not known.

Nonetheless, there is evidence that for some persons, learning to recognize, accept, and express unpleasant feelings can lead to a remarkable decrease in physical symptoms.

Hypochondriasis. "Hypochondriac" is a term commonly applied to people with many long-standing physical complaints. Hypochondriasis superficially can resemble a psychophysiological disorder but is very different in origin and response. True hypochondriacs are characterized by a remarkable preoccupation with physical symptoms, actually organizing their lives around their presumed illness. They insist that they are very sick and seem more content when viewed that way. No amount of testing or consulting with doctors will convince them otherwise. The more the doctor attempts to reassure them, the worse they feel. Frequently, they switch from doctor to doctor in search of confirmation of their illness.

It is clear that hypochondriacs genuinely suffer, yet the reasons that they experience pain and other physical discomforts with such excess sensitivity, and remain so preoccupied with their symptoms, are not clear.

Hypochondriasis can serve many unconscious psychological aims. It is most commonly a face-saving device for people who want to be taken care of. Some may have had deprived childhoods, or may have had to function as caretakers for siblings or parents. The "physical" illness serves as a ticket of admission to doctor and hospital care, and a legitimate reason for being dependent on others and being unable to carry out responsibilities. They may become attached to medications, since these "prove" to the world that the patient is sick.

The appropriate approach by both physician and family is to acknowledge the hypochondriac's symptoms and discomfort, not to struggle and argue. Once accepted, some patients can make accommodations sufficient for reasonable functioning.

Organic disease. Many patients with psychiatric problems are misdiagnosed as having organic disease, and treated incorrectly with vitamins, hormones, and drugs. Conversely, many physical illnesses masquerade as psychiatric disorders, with emotional symptoms among the most noticeable features. Physicians and patients alike can be distracted by these complaints and fail to thoroughly investigate a possible underlying organic illness. Patients with previous psychiatric histories are most vulnerable. Between 10 and 30 percent of patients admitted to psychiatric clinics have a physical illness that accounts for their psychiatric distress.

Disease of virtually every organ and metabolic system can have psychological symptoms. Disorders of the endocrine glands frequently produce changes in emotions and behavior. Thyroid disease, for instance, can produce weight gain, lethargy, apathy, fatigue, and depression, or alternately, weight loss, irritability, anxiety, and hyperactivity. Adrenal disease is sometimes characterized by suspiciousness and apathy, or emotional instability and even delusions. Benign and malignant brain tumors, cancer of the pancreas and lung, and diabetes can first show themselves with personality changes, apathy, intermittent anxiety attacks, and depression. In fact, depression is the most common emotional symptom caused by a physical disease.

Anyone who experiences emotional or behavioral changes should have a thorough physical evaluation before assuming a psychiatric cause is responsible for the symptoms.

Disorders of Aging

Organic brain syndromes are characterized by the gradual onset of disordered thinking, perception, and behavior. Patients lose recent memory, forget names, and become disoriented, especially to time, day, and year. They become less alert, seem mildly confused, and have difficulty paying attention and learning new information. Mood can change rapidly with little or no provocation, and crying, anger, agitation, and belligerence are common. Occasionally these changes occur suddenly over a short time.

When seen in the elderly, organic brain syndromes are commonly attributed to the presumably inevitable effects of senility. In fact, the normal processes of aging do result in disruption of brain functions in a fairly characteristic way. However, many other treatable factors account for identical changes. Less than five percent of people over 65 actually manifest senile dementia.

Correctable physical conditions that may cause organic brain syndrome include heart failure, infection, low blood sugar, thyroid disease, dehydration, and poor nutrition. Social and psychological stress also can induce the condition temporarily in some older people. The syndrome is also a side effect of many prescription and nonprescription drugs. These include digitalis, blood thinners, cortisone, high blood pressure medication, sleeping pills, and anti-anxiety agents. Mental and intellectual changes in the elderly therefore should not be dismissed as the normal consequence of aging. It is important to look first for a treatable condition.

Depression. Mild to serious depression also is common among the elderly. The incidence of severe but untreated depression is highest in this stage of life. Only 11 percent of the U.S. population is over 65 years of age, yet 25 percent of successful suicides are in this age group. This high incidence of depression is related to the complex interplay between medical, psychological, and social factors. The lives of the elderly are routinely characterized by stressful situations: physical illness, multiple deaths of family and friends, loss of productivity, loss of status and financial independence, and loss of control of property and finances. There is much time to brood. Feelings of helplessness, uselessness, and wishing to give up develop easily. Declining vision and hearing may further isolate older people and increase their dependency, while the social support network tends to withdraw.

Depression in the elderly often shows the classical clinical symptoms described earlier, the feelings of worthlessness, fatigue, loss of appetite, withdrawal, irritability, and sleep disturbance. Very commonly, though, the depression is masked (see page 719), presenting itself in the form of multiple physical complaints or vague physical decline. Patients with chronic organic illness may fail to recover or regain normal functioning because of an underlying depression and the wish to give up. These masked depressions can cause the patient to withdraw, and the patient's family to respond by paying him or her less attention. Such physical and social isolation can lead to malnutrition, vitamin deficiency, and dehydration. This worsens the depression and establishes a vicious cycle.

The most seriously misdiagnosed depression of the elderly is the very common type that mimics organic brain syndrome. Memory loss, forgetfulness, and confusion are actually signs of depression in these cases, but are dismissed as senile changes.

Clearly, depression in the elderly is difficult to diagnose, frequently is completely overlooked, and consequently goes untreated. Most of these disorders respond to drug treatment and psychotherapy, but they must be identified before they can be treated.

Sexual Dysfunction

Only recently has society been able to tolerate open discussion of sex and its role in life. However, sexual dysfunction is common and is both a cause and a result of marital discord. Many couples spend years, if not lifetimes, with mild to serious sexual unhappiness. Frequently they do not even discuss the problem between themselves. Only a minority seek professional help. Patients who do approach physicians often come with disguised symptoms—headaches, backaches, vague discomforts—because the real problem is either unrecognized or too embarrassing to talk about.

The most common sexual problems among men are impotence and premature ejaculation. Impotence is the inability to experience an erection or to maintain an erection long enough for successful intercourse. Premature ejaculation is that which occurs before both partners are ready. The most frequent sexual problems for women are dyspareunia, vaginismus, and anorgasmia. Dyspareunia is pain during intercourse. Vaginismus is pelvic muscle spasm that makes entry difficult or impossible. Anorgasmia is inability to experience orgasm, with some degree of sexual arousal or none at all.

Because these conditions occasionally are caused by physical problems or are side effects of medication, the doctor first prescribes a thorough physical evaluation. Loss of interest in sex also is a common early symptom of depression. Frequently, however, the origin of sexual dysfunction is a psychological problem whose cause may be unrelated to sex. For instance, conscious or unconscious fears about the ability to succeed occupationally or socially may be translated into sexual dysfunction.

The most common cause of sexual dysfunction is marital discord. The symptoms can have many explanations. People who feel misunderstood by, are afraid of, or cannot trust a spouse may manifest their feelings indirectly through sex. When a spouse feels uncertain about the other's commitment and faithfulness, or when the relationship is built on overt or hidden competition, sexual functioning may be impeded, too. If a spouse does not live up to the other's wishes and fantasies, disappointment and resentment can be expressed through the sexual relationship.

Cultural restrictions on sexual expression and enjoyment, directed especially toward women, also inhibit full development of healthy sexuality. Simple ignorance about the anatomy of the genital system, the physiology of sex, and sexual technique frequently lead to poor adjustment. Often sexual symptoms arise from a combination of causes.

Treatment of sexual dysfunction depends on its cause. Biological problems require medical management. Psychological problems respond best to individual psychotherapy. For marital maladjustment, psychotherapy of the couple together is appropriate (see page 726). If there appears to be no substantial psychological maladjustment, short-term sexual therapy which focuses on actual sexual methods may be successful. Couples are educated in sexual techniques and are helped to overcome their fears and inhibitions about performance. General communication is enhanced. Instruction includes exercises to help couples become more aware of touch, sight, and smell. The importance of foreplay for sexual pleasure is emphasized, and techniques of stimulation and positions for intercourse are taught. At each session, the couple discusses problems and progress since the last session, and new instructions are given.

PSYCHIATRIC TREATMENT

All treatments for psychiatric disorders have four goals: (1) to prevent or eliminate symptoms, (2) to maintain or restore the capacity to perform at work, in personal social relationships, in school, and in the family, (3) to achieve the self-regulation and self-control necessary to reach fulfilling goals, and (4) to develop the capacity to recognize and correct counterproductive behavior patterns.

To benefit from any form of psychotherapy, a patient must be well-motivated with a strong wish to get better. Reliability and trust are essential. No psychotherapy provides an automatic transformation; the patient has to work at it. The process usually involves transient ill feelings as old habits are changed and feelings about unconscious conflicts are resurrected.

Many activities (perhaps as many as 200) have been given names and called therapies. Those that are genuine medical treatments can be understood on the basis of a few fundamental principles.

Psychological Therapies

Psychological therapies aim to modify undesirable personal characteristics—feelings, attitudes, responses, and behaviors. These therapies incorporate two basic notions about most psychiatric disorders, particularly neurosis and character disorder. The first is that unconscious conflict, while originating in childhood, is alive and active in the adult personality. The second is that stressful interpersonal and environmental factors interact with the personality to exceed a person's flexibility of response and capacity to cope. A number of therapies are based on this philosophy.

Psychoanalysis. In psychoanalysis, patient and analyst work together to understand how troublesome feelings and behaviors relate to earlier life events. The goal is to rework unconscious conflicts by using the treatment relationship. Previous response patterns are changed and symptoms are relieved because core components of the personality are changed. Psychoanalysis requires several sessions weekly and lasts from two to five years or more. Patients must have relatively mature personalities at the start, possess adequate financial resources, and be able to tolerate the lengthy process. Although widely publicized, this psychiatric treatment is not appropriate for most patients.

Insight therapy, or psychoanalytically oriented therapy, is more limited. Its aim is understanding and elimination of certain psychological conflicts to bring about symptom relief. Attention is directed toward current interpersonal difficulties. Therapy takes place one to three times weekly, and lasts one or two weeks to several years.

Relationship therapy aims to help a relatively immature or underdeveloped personality to grow. The treatment deals with current issues and provides a period of stability in a relationship that is different from the patient's previous relationships, which tended to impede growth. Patient and physician focus on new techniques of problem solving. The patient gains control of his or her life by more accurately perceiving the environment and eliminating long-standing patterns of distortion. Family contacts and medication are employed as necessary. Although this once- or twice-weekly therapy can last from a month to several years, it tends to be shorter than other forms of therapy.

Supportive therapy does not aim at major symptom relief. Rather, the goal is to provide support during difficult and stressful situations and to help a patient "return to normal." The physician offers advice and actively helps the patient organize and focus his or her life. Occasional hospitalization, family sessions, and medication are used. Supportive therapy ranges from a few sessions centering on a crisis to many years.

Behavioral Therapy

The theory of behavioral therapy is that maladaptive responses are undesirable habits that have been learned over a period of time, and that new and more adaptive habits can be learned to replace them. Reasons for the symptoms are less important, and the notion of unconscious conflict is of minor significance. Behavioral therapies focus on what the patient does and says, and what the therapist can observe about the behavior.

Each response or symptom is described by the patient as explicitly and objectively as possible. What else was happening at the time is noted, too. The patient may keep a careful diary, detailing each occasion of response and the surrounding events. Once the connection between events and response becomes clear, an attempt is made to learn new ways of reacting to the triggering situation. Much as with programmed learning, mastery is achieved by understanding and change proceeding at the individual's own pace.

Stuttering is a typical symptom treated by behavioral techniques. For example, a seven-year-old experiences loss of parental attention when a new baby is born. Until the baby's arrival the child's fluent speech was taken for granted and elicited no response from the parents. But when the child suddenly begins to stutter, it attracts a flurry of attention. Parents may unwittingly reinforce the child's stuttering in their wish for their child to develop normally. In a behavioral approach to the treatment of stuttering, environmental antecedents (the shift of parental attention away from the child to the newborn) and behavioral consequences (loss of the previously developed level of speech) are the focus. Treatment is aimed at fostering and learning new responses. Parents and others are taught not to respond to or punish the child for the stuttering, but rather to reward normal speech with attention and praise. The child then speaks normally again because attention is restored.

This form of treatment is based on the relationship of the behavior of the patient to environmental events. The most common behavioral therapies use various principles of learning theory to modify behavior and repetitive response patterns. These techniques have had some success in the treatment of phobias, severe obsessions and compulsions, intense anxiety states, and sexual dysfunction. They are frequently employed for addictive disorders such as alcoholism, drug abuse, obesity, and smoking.

Social learning therapy, a form of behavior therapy, can be helpful for chronic schizophrenic patients with limited social and occupational skills. They learn the simple functions needed for normal living, such as shopping, managing finances, social behavior, and holding a job.

Biofeedback is a recently developed form of behavior therapy that offers promise for the future. With this treatment, the mind is trained to control bodily reactions. Biofeedback has shown some success in the amelioration of symptoms based on stress, such as tension headaches, and for the hard-driving, compulsive behavior characteristics of some personality disorders. It is also being explored as a treatment for disorders such as irritable or spastic colon (abdominal pain and constipation or diarrhea related to stress).

Group Therapy

Group therapy encompasses a wide range of treatment rationales and goals.

Supportive or counseling groups aim to maintain and strengthen healthy parts of an individual personality. Participants focus on the skills of interacting with others, and on conscious problems of living. Patients learn from each other and are reinforced by the group members in developing more adaptive behaviors. Insight-oriented groups try to make participants aware of their unconscious feelings and thoughts that produce symptoms. Interactions within the group are used to understand underlying meanings of behavior and to foster more basic changes. Some groups aim at overcoming a mutual problem, such as a phobia or a sexual difficulty, using behavioral learning techniques.

In general, anyone who can benefit from individual therapy also can benefit from group sessions. Patients with all types of neuroses respond well, but particularly those who have difficulty dealing with others, who are competitive, or who feel uncomfortable in close relationships. Group therapy is one of the most effective treatments for people suffering from personality disorder. Since these persons often are unaware that they have a problem, or acknowledge the behavior but deny its effects, group interactions help them to understand the effects of their present behavior as well as to learn new patterns of response. Schizophrenic patients, who have poorly developed interpersonal skills, tendencies toward isolation, and difficulty trusting others, frequently do well in group treatment, especially in combination with medication.

Severely depressed patients, who must always be considered suicide risks, should enter group therapy only after thorough psychiatric evaluation. All patients face some risk on entering group therapy, because direct confrontation temporarily can worsen symptoms for almost everyone.

Marital Therapy

Marital therapy aims to help relatively stable couples who have conflicts with emotional, sexual, social, financial, or child-rearing problems. This form of treatment has become more important in recent years with changes in the family, more open relationships and alternatives to marriage, and with the decline in previously supportive institutions such as the extended family and the church. These changes have placed demands on couples to fulfill functions and assume roles once left to other institutions.

Marital therapy aims to help the individual partners as well as the couple as a unit, because the relationship itself can maintain and worsen individual problems. Many approaches are used. The most common aim is to understand the unconscious basis for feelings and expectations, and to use specific techniques to analyze and change behavior patterns. Treatment frequently begins by focusing on a specific complaint, then moves ahead to explore the nature of the relationship, and finally seeks to change poor behavior patterns between the partners and to encourage personality growth and development in each. Partners learn to take responsibility for understanding the personality, needs, and hopes of the spouse as well as his or her own, and to face the consequences that each individual's behavior brings to the relationship.

The five most frequent complaints of couples who seek marital therapy are lack of communication, continuous arguing, unfulfilled emotional needs, sexual dissatisfaction, and financial disagreements. Problems in communication are the most frequently described symptoms. One partner may be intimidated by the other, may be unable to express thoughts and feelings, or may have unrealistic, infantile expectations of the relationship.

Marital therapy can succeed only if both partners have a genuine motivation to explore and change the relationship. If one participates only to please or pacify the other, results usually are poor.

Marital therapy sometimes results in a decision to divorce. This possibility can frighten couples into avoiding treatment and maintaining an unsatisfactory relationship. Those who do divorce usually describe a feeling of having done everything possible to save the relationship. This reduces the likelihood of subsequent guilt about not having tried hard enough and also minimizes unrealistic fantasies about what might have been. Divorce in these circumstances is sometimes the best solution.

Family Therapy

Family therapy focuses not only on the individual's personality and past development but also on each person as a member of the family.

Emphasis is on understanding how individual behavior originates in the family's needs and expectations, and how the behavior then feeds back into the family to further influence the interactions. This can shed light on the origin and development of the family's patterns of interacting, as well as insight into the individual's unconscious conflicts.

From this perspective, a problem can be seen in several different ways. For instance, a child may feel anxious about going to school. From the point of view of mother–child interaction, excessive closeness and dependency may be fostered if the child is allowed to stay home. From the point of view of the marriage, the couple may be quite antagonistic toward each other and come together only to discuss the child's problem. Clearly one function of the child's symptom is to maintain the marriage in a special state of tension. In a sense, the child's unhappiness has some benefit because it provides a basis for communication between the parents as well as an excuse to avoid discussing the problems in their own relationship.

Many psychiatric problems are best approached, at least initially, by involvement of the entire family. In the above example, focusing only on the child would leave the other contributing family difficulties unsolved.

Drug Treatment

Treatment of psychiatric disorders has been revolutionized in the decades since 1950 by the introduction and widespread use of effective medications that improve emotional and behavioral responses by affecting brain activity and function. They help the mind and the body return to normal.

Antipsychotic agents can be effective in the treatment of some aspects of all psychotic states including schizophrenia, severe manic-depressive illness, psychotic depressions, and paranoid states. In acute psychosis, the drugs reduce agitation and calm the person's emotions. They also diminish hyperactivity, disturbances of thinking, hallucinations, and delusions. Secondarily, withdrawal and social isolation are lessened.

Most schizophrenic patients who improve with these agents require continued outpatient drug treatment to prevent relapse. Others can discontinue the medication, but require close medical monitoring so treatment can be reinstituted at the earliest reappearance of symptoms. Severely manic or profoundly depressed patients, especially those with hallucinations and delusions, respond to antipsychotic drugs during the initial phase of treatment until more specific slower-acting drugs begin to work.

Antipsychotic medications are used with caution. The side effects, including muscle spasms, involuntary shaking of the limbs, and low blood pressure, occasionally can be severe but usually are treatable. However, long-term neurological side effects have been reported and research is under way to discover the cause and management of these symptoms.

Drug treatment of psychotic disorders has dramatically reduced psychiatric hospitalizations. Additionally, patients on medication are emotionally calmer, so they respond better to psychotherapy. Drugs cannot change unfavorable life situations, but can reduce their impact on a patient's capacity to cope. However, all these drugs interact extensively with other kinds of medication, and careful medical monitoring is essential.

Antidepressant drugs recently have come into widespread use. They are quite successful for some patients. Their greatest effect seems to be in depressions which include problems of physical functioning—difficulties of sleeping and eating, constipation, and slow movement. Patients with intermittent recurrent depression who respond to medication often continue the drug for some time after the symptoms have subsided to avoid a relapse.

Some depressed persons experience only partial improvement of their symptoms. This variability of response probably reflects the variety of forms of depression. Patients with low-grade continuous depression actually respond better to psychotherapy than drugs. For patients who do respond to antidepressants, a combination of drugs and psychotherapy is often used.

There are two main classes of antidepressant drugs. Tricyclic antidepressants are most commonly used. They must be administered for approximately three weeks to produce a change in mood. Side effects include sedation, dry mouth, constipation, and blurred vision; these do not, however, appear in everyone. In the elderly, tricyclic antidepressants may have cardiac and urinary side effects. Tricyclics are continued in decreasing dosages for several months after the symptoms have subsided to ensure complete remission.

For very severe depressions of psychotic proportion, both antipsychotic agents and antidepressants are administered simultaneously during the first few weeks for control of delusions and hallucinations. Antidepressant medications also have been shown to be effective for some phobias and for anxiety states with panic attacks.

Lithium is the drug most effective for the treatment of mania. It usually controls the acute episode within two weeks. Continued indefinitely, lithium can prevent future manic episodes or reduce their intensity and length. There is some indication that lithium also may help to prevent future episodes of depression in some patients with manic-depressive disease, and perhaps in some cases of recurrent depressive disease as well. Side effects include lightheadedness, dizziness, sleepiness, staggering and numbness, and nausea and vomiting. These can be significant, especially for patients with dietary restrictions, so close medical monitoring is essential.

Anti-anxiety agents (tranquilizers) are the most commonly used prescription drugs of any type. While most doctors and patients use them wisely, overuse has been a matter of public concern. Patients most vulnerable to misuse are those who misuse alcohol.

When a patient reports nervousness to a doctor, both parties frequently find it easier to use a pill rather than to investigate the source of anxiety. Patients who are temporarily under unusual stress are frequently given a drug. So are those with mild character disorders that lead to a response of anxiety to the normal stresses of life. In actual fact, these people probably could control and reduce their anxiety simply by taking some time with their doctor to explore and understand the circumstances causing the upset, and then planning ways to deal with it. Also, patients with more severe disorders who actually require psychiatric referral are sometimes given medication instead. The misuse of anti-anxiety medication deprives patients of the opportunity to gain control of difficult situations and to obtain referral for proper treatment.

Some patients improve simply because they are taking a pill and are in contact with a caring authority figure, the doctor. So the actual benefits of these drugs are difficult to measure. When correctly used, however, they can alleviate symptoms quickly, enabling the patient to adapt and learn alternative approaches to a problem.

Contrary to popular notions, tranquilizers can be addicting. Serious withdrawal problems may occur when a person tries to discontinue the drug after a long period of use. Depression is worsened by these drugs, but they are sometimes prescribed for the anxiety that accompanies or masks depression, so careful evaluation by the physician is essential.

Electroconvulsive Treatment

Electroconvulsive therapy is a safe, effective treatment for several kinds of depression and the most effective treatment for some depressions. It retains an ominous stigma based on its use in the early part of the century. Electroconvulsive therapy does not result in shock in the surgical or psychological sense, nor does it result in the experience of a convulsion. Patients are in the hospital, receive a sedative to induce sleep and a muscle-relaxing drug to avoid convulsive movements, and feel no pain. One or two electrodes are applied to the temples with salt water or electrojelly, similar to the technique used for electrocardiograms. A mild electrical current is passed through the electrodes, but the person feels no pain. He or she is awake in a matter of minutes. Current techniques result in minimal side effects, the most common being short-term memory loss.

Electroconvulsive therapy is the most effective treatment for psychotic depressions. It is also very effective for severe depressions with physical symptoms, the psychotic phase of depression in manic-depressive disease, and some depressions that accompany the aging process. Many depressed patients who do not respond to drug treatment experience relief of symptoms with electroconvulsive therapy.

Hospitalization

As noted, the number of persons hospitalized for psychiatric treatment has decreased dramatically since the mid 1950s. Hospitalization today is reserved primarily for short-term treatment of acute episodes of psychiatric illness. For chronic illnesses, intermittent hospitalization in combination with drug treatment after discharge results in shorter hospital stays and fewer episodes of rehospitalization. Nevertheless, certain patients with disorders difficult to treat, primarily schizophrenics, require long-term or frequent hospitalization. Hospitalization also remains important for evaluation of persisting problems that are difficult to diagnose.

The concept of partial hospitalization developed as a response to problems with the traditional long-term hospital stay. Hospitalized patients are deprived of the support of family, friends, and job. This can increase the severity and the length of their illness.

Day hospitalization provides a structured program, usually in a community mental health center or an outpatient clinic, from nine to five. Patients return home for the evening. The professional staff serves a therapeutic role, and the setting aims to reinforce independent functioning. Vocational and social rehabilitation play a prominent part, particularly job training in preparation for specific occupations. Patients also are coached in skills such as personal grooming, housekeeping, consumer buying, and social interaction.

Some inpatient units encourage improved patients to pursue work, school, or housekeeping during the day, and return to the hospital for the night.

Other Treatments

Recent technical advances have led to increased claims of psychiatric cures, especially for schizophrenia. As these new "treatments" appear, they tend to capture public attention and unrealistically raise expectations about significant breakthroughs. Treatment of schizophrenia with huge doses of vitamins or with hemodialysis is a recent example. Little systematic research on these approaches has been done and there is no scientific evidence that they are effective. These and other techniques are undergoing systematic evaluation.

"Experiences" designed to help symptom-free people achieve greater individual potential and self-actualization are sometimes referred to as therapies. These groups aim to increase a person's general self-awareness and understanding of others and to foster warmer, more significant personal relationships. Encounter groups, sensitivity groups, and T groups are examples.

While the goals are laudable and the experiences helpful for many, problems can arise for disturbed or psychotic people. These are not therapy settings conducted by trained professionals, and the seriousness of a person's problem can be minimized or overlooked. In some cases, the "process" worsens the psychological symptoms. A person who is seriously troubled or symptomatic, as opposed to one simply seeking greater fulfillment, should be evaluated by a psychiatrist before joining one of these groups.

Finding Treatment

It is important for state licensing agencies and mental health associations to protect the public against incompetent and unscrupulous "practitioners." Many who present themselves as "therapists" have no training or inadequate training.

Strain and distress from the problems of everyday life require encouragement from one's physician as well as help in using the available social network. Some people seek help directly from specialized social agencies, such as vocational training centers or senior citizen services.

However, true disorders of emotion and behavior initially should be assessed by a physician (M.D.). These evaluations can be by psychiatrists (who are medical doctors with specialty training in disorders of emotion and behavior), by other medical specialists such as internists, gynecologists, and pediatricians, or by family physicians.

Referral to nonmedical professionals is appropriate for many patients. Psychologists are an important part of the total treatment team. Those referred to as "doctor" hold a Ph.D. in psychology. Many are experts in psychological testing, which can be a diagnostic tool for the physician in cases that are not clear-cut. Other psychologists have extensive clinical experience (as opposed to research or experimental training) as the core of their education. They often work in specialized areas of therapy. Social workers have professional training in case work. They are expert at assessing and devising ways to handle social problems (housing, education, job, and money). Psychiatric social workers acquire advanced training, providing expertise in some forms of psychotherapy.

UNDER-STANDING YOUR OPERATION

"My operation" has long been a favorite topic of human conversation, almost as popular as the weather. It is easy to understand why. Most of us undergo an operation only two or three times in our lives, so that these moments are landmark, not to say unforgettable, occasions. They also help to remind us of our mortal nature.

But an operation is just one event in the treatment of disease or injury. The procedure itself stands out as a dramatic, mysterious, and perhaps even dangerous event, but of equal importance are the diagnosis of the problem, the preoperative preparation, and the care of the patient after the operation for return to a full and healthy life. Helping the patient understand what is involved in surgery is important, too, so that he or she can approach the event with confidence and a positive attitude toward eventual recovery. The more a person knows and understands about an illness, the better he or she is able to participate in maintaining health.

UNDERSTANDING SURGERY

Surgery is defined as the science of medicine in which operations are used as part of the treatment. Thus surgeons perform operations, which generally are carried out in operating rooms, although an increasing amount of surgery takes place on an outpatient basis, in clinics, or in surgicenters. But the term surgery refers not merely to the operative event but to the entire field and care of the patient. Sometimes people speak of "major" and "minor" operations. In the strict sense, all operations are major, because if complications develop, the results may not be satisfactory or the procedure may be life-threatening. In common usage, however, an operation is considered minor if done with the use of local anesthesia while the patient is awake, or if it is performed for diagnostic purposes with the patient asleep under general anesthesia.

Operations also are classified as elective, urgent, or emergency procedures. An elective operation is one carried out for a disease or abnormality that is not life-threatening or one in which a delay would not harm the patient. An example is a patient with gallstones who has had several previous attacks of pain but does not have symptoms now. The operation could be performed this week, this month, or later. An operation is indeed recommended, because future attacks are probable, but speed is not the primary consideration. An urgent operation is one in which delay could produce serious problems or life-threatening complications if not carried out in a few days or weeks. An example is a cancer in which the malignancy could spread to other organs if not removed promptly. An emergency operation is one required immediately, within minutes or hours. In cases of appendicitis, the operation usually should be done within a few hours. In a ruptured abdominal aortic aneurysm, a defect in the main blood vessel in the abdomen, an operation may have to be carried out within a few minutes to save the patient's life.

By and large, operations are recommended or indicated for medical problems that cannot be treated in any other way. The general categories include:

(1) Drainage of infections such as abscesses.

(2) Removal of organs suffering from disease or damage, including:
• Inflammations such as appendicitis.
• Metabolic abnormalities producing stones, as in the gallbladder.
• Arteriosclerosis or hardening of the arteries producing blocks in blood vessels and gangrene in limbs or other areas.
• Malignant diseases (cancer).
• Degenerative disease processes such as enlargement of the prostate gland.

(3) Correction of anatomic abnormalities such as hernias in the groin, and other congenital and acquired abnormalities.

(4) Repair of injuries to structures, including bones, tendons, skin, and muscles.

(5) Improvement of functional abnormalities such as replacement of the hip joint because of severe disabling arthritis.

(6) Improvement of blood supply to an organ damaged by disease in the arteries supplying the organ. An example is the coronary bypass graft operation for arteriosclerosis of the coronary arteries supplying the heart muscle.

(7) Replacement of organs that have been destroyed or no longer function satisfactorily. The kidney, of course, is transplanted routinely. Heart and liver transplants and combined heart-lung transplants have been successful in a few patients. Joints and bone can be transplanted or replaced. Transplants of the pancreas and sections of intestine are being studied.

(8) Cosmetic surgery to improve appearance or self-image.

The Surgical Vocabulary

Basic definitions help to explain surgery. The suffix *otomy* means to cut into. Thus an exploratory operation in the abdomen is called a laparotomy or celiotomy. An incision into the chest or thoracic cavity is called a thoracotomy. An incision through the skull exposing the brain is called a craniotomy. An incision in the eardrum to drain a middle ear infection is called myringotomy.

The suffix *ectomy* means to remove. Thus a colectomy is removal of part or all of the colon. Removal of part of the stomach is called a gastrectomy and removal of the gallbladder is a cholecystectomy. Removal of the kidney is a nephrectomy.

The suffix *ostomy* means to bring out or create an opening to the surface. Creating an opening for the colon on the abdominal wall is called a colostomy. If the end of the small intestine is brought out through the abdominal wall for drainage of intestinal contents, the procedure is called an ileostomy. An opening in the stomach to the abdominal wall is called a gastrostomy.

Reconstruction of an organ or area is described by the suffix *plasty*. Opening the outlet of the stomach is a pyloroplasty. The suffix *itis* means inflammation, as in appendicitis. Other commonly used surgical terms include ligation, anastomosis, and ischemia. Ligation means to tie off or close with a tie or ligature. Anastomosis means to join together the ends of two hollow tubes, such as intestines or blood vessels. Ischemia means decreased blood flow to an organ or tissue. Most people already know that a suture is the "stitch" a surgeon takes in closing up a wound.

The surgeon uses many specialized instruments. The scalpel for making incisions in the body is familiar to most of us, and so is the forceps, but there are many others, some of which originated far back in history. More recently electricity and electronics, high-frequency sound, and laser beams have been developed for use during operations. A new generation of miniaturized instruments has been developed for use under a microscope in delicate operations.

Although some of the surgeon's education is gained in the classroom, most of what he must learn about technique comes from working with experienced surgeons as they practice their art and craft. It is frequently easier to understand an operation if you can see it rather than merely read about it. For that reason this chapter will rely heavily on step-by-step illustrations of many procedures.

Choosing a Surgeon: Specialties and Specialists

An operation may be recommended by your family physician or another consultant. You may consider it because of an abnormality or a disease of which you are aware, or it may be thrust upon you in an emergency situation with injury or sudden, life-threatening disease. Your family physician, internist, or pediatrician may recommend a surgeon to you, you may know a surgeon, or someone in your family or a friend may know a surgeon. Regardless of how a surgeon is located you want to be sure that he or she is a capable, well-trained specialist. Your best assurance of this training and capability is that the doctor is board certified in the particular specialty.

Some years ago groups of surgeons established boards of their peers to define the amount of training and experience required for someone to be a safe, capable surgeon in that specialty. These requirements specify a period of hospital residency and clinical training, after which the applicant must pass an examination to establish competence and be certified by the board. It is perfectly reasonable to ask your surgeon if he is board certified. Such documentation is on display in most surgeons' offices.

The trained general surgeon is certified by the American Board of Surgery, indicating that he or she has had five years of residency following four years of medical school, has had independent responsibility as a surgeon, has carried out a large number of operations, and has passed an examination verifying surgical knowledge. The general surgeon is trained in diseases of the abdomen and gastrointestinal tract including the liver, gallbladder, pancreas, intestines, hernia, the endocrine glands (thyroid), problems of the head and neck, and other areas. The general surgeon also may be trained to carry out operations for fractures and operations involving other organ systems such as the kidney, bladder, prostate, and the female organs.

Among other specialists, orthopedists or orthopedic surgeons specialize in diseases and surgery of the skeletal system, bones, joints, ligaments, and tendons. Urologists or urological surgeons specialize in diseases of the kidney, ureter, bladder, and prostate gland.

Otorhinolaryngologists specialize in diseases of the ears, nose, throat, and larynx. Ophthalmologists are expert in diseases of the eye. Neurosurgeons specialize in diseases of the central nervous system, including the brain, spinal cord, and peripheral nerves.

Some specialties require additional training and experience beyond the five years of general surgical training. This is true of cardiothoracic surgery, in which a qualified general surgeon is trained by several years of additional preparation in surgery on the heart, lungs, and esophagus, with board certification by the American Board of Thoracic Surgery. The plastic surgeon usually has had two years of additional training following general surgical training and is certified by the American Board of Plastic and Reconstructive Surgery. Pediatric surgery has a certificate of special competence to indicate special training and experience in the field of surgery on children. Some surgeons limit practice to a certain area of special interest and develop expertise in fields such as transplantation of organs, oncology (cancer treatment), colon and rectal surgery, hand surgery, and other highly technical areas.

There are several ways to locate a trained, board-certified surgeon. The county medical society in your area will provide the names of specialists and verify board certification. A teaching hospital or a hospital associated with a medical school can furnish names of its surgical staff. A medical school faculty will have highly trained surgeons. From these sources it should be possible to locate a trained surgeon in whom you can have confidence.

Diagnostic Studies

Your illness or injury may require certain studies to diagnose the problem, to determine the extent of disease, and to determine which type of treatment might be best. It is important to understand the nature of such studies, the information they can provide, and their limitations. Many such diagnostic studies will determine without surgery that there is something wrong, that there is a lump or a shadow or an abnormality in an organ. Usually, however, the exact nature of the abnormality cannot be determined without an operation to obtain a specimen or piece of tissue by biopsy for microscopic examination.

The most common diagnostic tests use X ray. Chest X rays will show structural abnormalities of the lung, the ribs, and the heart. Swallowed barium, an opaque white liquid, will allow X ray to show abnormalities or obstructions of the esophagus, stomach, duodenum, and small intestine, a procedure known as an upper gastrointestinal series. Barium put into the colon through the rectum will detect tumors, inflammations, and obstructions of the colon. The CAT scan (computerized axial tomography), which combines X ray and a computer, provides better definition of a lump, a mass, fluid in the body cavities, the chest, the abdomen, and the brain. Ultrasound, or sonography, developed originally for submarine detection, has demonstrated its usefulness in the detection of fluid, abnormal masses, lesions, or stones in the organs by passing high-frequency sound waves into the body and charting their echoes.

The science of fiberoptics, which is the transmission of light along fine glass fibers that can be bent and curved, allows the surgeon to look inside most body cavities and hollow organs. The fiberoptic bronchoscope permits visual inspection of the inside of the tracheobronchial tree as far out as the small bronchi within the lung, so that lung tumors can be diagnosed at an early stage. Fiberoptic examination of the upper gastrointestinal tract allows visualization of the lining of the esophagus, the stomach, and the duodenum. A small tube (catheter) can be threaded through the fiberoptic scope into the common bile duct and pancreatic duct to allow injection of dye and permit visualization of those organs. This technique is called ERCP, or endoscopic retrograde cholangiopancreatography. A straight, lighted tube called a sigmoidoscope is used for visualization of the lower 25 centimeters of the colon and rectum. The fiberoptic colonoscope is used to inspect the lining of the entire colon. The urologist relies upon cystoscopy, inserting a small lighted instrument inside the bladder to view the inner surfaces. Small catheters can be passed within the cystoscope up the ureters into the kidney, permitting the injection of dye and X-ray examination. This procedure is called retrograde pyelography.

The fiberoptic laparoscope allows inspection inside the abdominal cavity, and allows small operative procedures to be carried out at the same time. In this case, air or gas is introduced into the cavity to separate the peritoneum, the shiny membrane that covers the organs, from the organs themselves. The laparoscope is inserted through a small incision in the abdomen. Tiny blades, forceps, or an electrical cautery can be fitted on the end of the scope, enabling the surgeon to carry out small surgical procedures under direct observation. The female sterilization procedure, in which the fallopian tubes are ligated or tied off, is often carried out in this way.

Cardiac catheterization is the diagnostic study of the heart and the great vessels, the body's main arteries and veins. In this procedure, a catheter is threaded through an artery or vein in the arm or groin and passed through the circulation until it reaches the chambers of the heart. Dye can then be injected to show by X ray the movement of blood within the heart or in the coronary arteries that supply blood to the heart muscle. This allows precise diagnosis of congenital defects in the heart, abnormalities of the valves, obstructions in the coronary arteries, and other problems.

By using these methods, it usually is possible to make a precise diagnosis of the disease and its extent before an operation is contemplated or recommended. The diagnostic studies are not always conclusive, however, and an exploratory operation may be required to establish the exact nature of the problem. The initial operation may be a biopsy, a minor surgical procedure to obtain a bit of tissue for pathological examination. After special preparation of the sample, the pathologist uses a microscope to determine the exact cell structure and type of lesion. This can be done while an operation is in progress and is called a frozen section diagnosis.

The Cost of Surgery

For most common operations, surgeons in a particular region charge standard fees. The amount usually is based on the time and effort involved in the total care of the patient. It covers ordering and reviewing the preoperative diagnostic studies or work-up, preoperative visits, preparation for the operation, the procedure itself, postoperative care until time of discharge from the hospital, and initial postoperative office visits. It is not limited to the operation itself. Fees may vary depending on the complexity and length of the operation, and on whether complications develop. Patients should feel free to discuss fees with their surgeon before an operation. The surgeon's fee is usually only part of the total cost of hospitalization and the operative procedure. Most patients now have insurance coverage that includes the cost of hospitalization, diagnostic tests, and operation, but insurance coverage can vary substantially, and it is worthwhile to be sure your coverage is adequate beforehand, rather than be surprised afterwards.

Second Opinions

When an operation has been recommended, do you need a second qualified opinion? In most cases, a patient already has it. Normally, the family physician, internist, or pediatrician recommends an operation and sends the patient to a surgeon. The surgeon either confirms the need for an operation or advises against it—a second opinion. If he or she is well trained, experienced, and board certified, the surgeon's opinion should be reasonable and probably most surgeons would agree with it.

All of us have read in the news media about operations or surgery said to be unnecessary. It is true that differences of opinion exist about whether certain elective operations should be performed. The greatest controversy centers on tonsillectomy, removal of diseased tonsils in children, and operations of the female reproduction system, particularly the uterus. In either case, operations may be carried out that are not strictly necessary for reasons of health. But in these cases, the patient often has a key voice in the decision. For example, a woman with painful or copious menstruation may have no anatomic abnormality of the uterus but rather a functional problem related to her hormonal balance. If she has no wish to bear more children, she may request that her uterus be removed (hysterectomy) to stop the bleeding problem and to eliminate the small potential risk of later malignancy. A reputable surgeon may agree to remove the uterus, even though it may be normal. Other physicians or surgeons may consider the operation unnecessary because the woman could have been treated with hormones or by other nonsurgical means.

Before any operation, the patient should ask, "Why should I have this operation? What are the alternatives?" And he or she should discuss them openly and in detail with the surgeon beforehand. If the patient is still uncertain, a second opinion can be sought. Programs that make a second opinion mandatory may produce more problems than they solve and only lead to confusion. Who is to determine that the second opinion is more reliable than the first? The best way to eliminate unnecessary operations is to insist that all operations be done by trained, board-certified surgeons.

Different Operations for the Same Disease

For certain diseases a standard operation is done by all surgeons in almost exactly the same manner. For inflammation of the appendix (appendicitis), there is really only one treatment: removal of the appendix. But removal can be performed with slight technical variations. Some surgeons tie the stump of the appendix where the base enters the wall of the cecum, a portion of the large intestine, so that the contents of the cecum do not escape. Others tie and invert the stump with sutures in the cecal wall, burying the stump inside. The reason for these differences in technique is that no single approach is foolproof. For example, if the stump of the appendix simply is tied, the ligature may work loose later, producing leakage and an abscess. This occurs extremely rarely, but remains a possibility. On the other hand, burying the stump may allow a small abscess to develop within the cecal wall, another rare but not unheard of possibility. The surgeon usually makes his choice on the basis of the particular case and his experience.

In the treatment of such conditions as hiatus hernia and reflux esophagitis (see page 741) or duodenal ulcers (see page 742), different operations may be recommended by different surgeons. The difference may be much more than just a minor detail of technique, but a completely different approach that even includes a different location for the incision. Why these big differences in approach to a common problem? Is the best technique a matter of opinion among surgeons? Is it because no one really has the complete answer? None of these is the case. The truth is that the basic principles of all surgical approaches are practically identical and each approach has specific advantages and drawbacks under certain circumstances.

In any operation, complications may occur. To try to minimize them, different methods are constantly being developed to improve the safety of the operation, to decrease side effects, and to improve the long-term result. For example, the underlying principle in the treatment of duodenal ulcer disease is to reduce gastric acidity and allow the ulcerative process to heal. This can be done in several different ways, all of which are effective in certain circumstances. Differences in the patient,

in the disease process, and in the circumstance may dictate that one operation is better than another. Here again the judgment of the trained surgeon is best, rather than insistence on a single standard procedure. The three basic types of operations for sliding hiatus hernias all are quite satisfactory. In skilled hands the success rate can be 90 to 95 percent with any of them. The important thing is that the surgeon know one of these operations well, be able to carry it out well, and thus be able to assure the patient of a good result. The differences in technique may be confusing or of concern to patients, however, and should be discussed openly with a surgeon beforehand.

BEFORE THE OPERATION

After an abnormality has been diagnosed and an operation recommended, the surgeon usually carries out an overall evaluation of the patient. This requires a detailed history of previous illnesses, operations, and family history. Of particular importance is information about allergies to certain drugs and medications, and about prior problems of bleeding, which must be recognized before an operation is undertaken. A family history of bleeding problems and other matters may require special study. Previous illnesses, particularly of the heart and lungs, must be recognized. A complete physical examination must be carried out to detect any other abnormalities. Basic laboratory studies will be necessary either before or shortly after admission to the hospital. These include a chest X ray to be sure there is no active disease in the lungs that would produce problems with a general anesthetic. An electrocardiogram is usually recommended, particularly for patients over 40 who are having a major operation. Basic examination is carried out on urine and blood, to discover the oxygen-carrying capacity of the blood and whether the patient has anemia or chronic blood loss. The white blood cells are counted. Depending on the patient's history and particularly upon the nature of the operation, other tests may be ordered. These could include more detailed examination of heart capability, such as testing the heart during exercise, or measurement of pulmonary function and the gas pressures in the arterial blood to indicate the capabilities of the lungs.

From these findings, the surgeon can make a reasonable estimate of the risk of operation. Any operative procedure requiring an anesthetic carries some degree of risk. Untoward and unpredicted events can occur that may be beyond the control of the surgeon and his team. From experience a trained surgeon can estimate the potential risk in most circumstances, and discuss this risk with the patient.

Obviously, before any operation the patient should be told the details of the procedure, the hazards and possible complications. For example, a 35-year-old woman who is to have her gallbladder removed but is otherwise completely normal has a better than 99 percent chance of surviving and being well afterward. The chances that she will not survive are only about one in 500. If, however, the patient is 65, has had two coronary attacks, and is diabetic, the risk of the same operation rises to about five percent. There are certain emergency problems, such as a ruptured abdominal aneurysm, where the chances of survival may only be 50 percent with an operation. However, the alternative is that without an operation all such patients would die. Thus the consideration of risk must be balanced with the need for the operation. A life-threatening condition requires the acceptance of higher risk. An elective operation is not recommended if the risk seems excessive.

Preparing a patient immediately before the operation has certain routine requirements. Usually a laxative or enema is given to empty the colon of its contents. Often only liquids are given by mouth the night before the operation. The patient may not be allowed to drink or eat anything after midnight to guarantee that the stomach is empty in the morning. This enforced fast is necessary so that anesthesia may be given safely, because vomiting can occur during anesthesia and contents of the stomach may be aspirated into the lungs. A sleeping medication is often prescribed the night before, too, since many patients understandably have difficulty sleeping because of concern about the next day's events. Just before the operation an injection is usually given to decrease secretions of saliva and to help the patient relax. Other preparation may be necessary for particular operations. For operations where the risk of infection is high, antibiotics are given before and during the operation.

ANESTHESIA

An important part of an operation is the participation of specialists in anesthesia. An anesthesiologist is a physician with special training and board certification in anesthesiology. An anesthetist is often a trained nurse who has specialized in anesthesia and possesses documented capablity for giving anesthetics. Anesthetics are divided into those producing general anesthesia, in which the patient is asleep or anesthetized, and local anesthetics, which are injected to block the sensation of pain in a particular region of the body. General anesthetic agents are divided into two categories—those that are inhaled, such as the various gases (nitrous oxide, ether, halothane, ethrane), and those injected into the vein, particularly the barbiturates, the rapidly acting barbiturate Pentothal,® and various paralytic agents such as curare. The choice usually depends on the nature of the operation, the condition of the patient, and the patient's preference.

In preparing for anesthesia, the anesthesiologist will talk with the patient the night before an elective operation, review the history, examination, and studies, and make a recommendation about the safest and best anesthetic agent and approach to be used, in consultation with the surgeon. The method of administering anesthesia will be discussed and the patient should ask questions about anesthetic agents and other concerns.

With a general anesthetic, it is usually safest to wait until the patient is asleep, then insert a tube through the mouth, between the vocal cords and into the windpipe (trachea). This tube is equipped with an inflatable cuff to help prevent gastric juices from coming up the esophagus into the throat and passing into the lungs. The patient may be helped to breathe with a mechanical ventilator. Before the anesthetic is administered, the anesthesiologist or anesthetist inserts several small tubes (cannulae) into veins in the arms or legs. These allow administration of fluids to replace body fluids lost during the operation and to maintain urine flow and kidney function. The tubes are also available should it be necessary to administer blood during the operation.

It has become common to use other monitoring devices in the operating room. Small electrodes are placed on the patient's chest and extremities to record the heart action continuously during many operative procedures. A small cannula may be placed in the radial artery of the wrist or elsewhere to measure arterial blood pressure continuously. A catheter may be inserted in the neck down through the right side of the heart and out into the pulmonary artery to the lung in order to measure pressures there and give a better estimate of the adequacy of heart action. For operations on the heart, such continuous monitoring is critical. For an inguinal hernia repair most monitoring would not be necessary except in an elderly, poor-risk patient.

THE OPERATION

The operating room is a special environment in which absolute cleanliness and protection of the patient are the guiding principles. The rooms are bright, well-lighted, and functional in decor. They are designed to be clean and easy to keep that way. They require constant air flow, with the air filtered to remove bacteria. Medical personnel must wear special clothing. This means "scrub suits," masks, head coverings, gloves, and even coverings for shoes, in order to maintain cleanest possible surroundings. Before the operation begins, the surgical team scrubs for about ten minutes, washing and brushing the hands, fingernails, and arms with a bacteria-killing soap. Special "scrub nurses" aid in the preparation.

We sometimes speak of an operation as performed by a surgeon, as though he or she were working alone, but in fact, most operations require a surgical team. In addition to the anesthesiologist and assistants, the surgeon usually will be aided by one or more assistant surgeons, and there will be a corps of trained operating-room nurses. Sometimes the operating-room crew includes a number of technicians assigned to monitor certain equipment, such as an electrocardiograph.

The operation begins with the anesthetic. After it has been administered, the patient is positioned on the table so that the site where the incision is to be made is exposed. The skin is then prepared by careful washing, often with an antibacterial agent to decrease contamination. Next, drapes are placed around the area of the incision to maintain a sterile environment. The incision is made, usually with a scalpel, through the skin, through the subcutaneous tissue (the fat beneath the skin), down to the fascia and muscle if the incision is in the abdomen, to the joint, or to the ribs if an incision is being made in the chest. Small clamps called hemostats are placed on the ends of the vessels to control bleeding. Vessels are then closed either by a ligature or tie of catgut, silk, or other material, or by the use of electrocautery, an electric current that produces heat and burns the tip of the vessel to close it. The body cavity is then opened and a general exploration carried out to confirm the presence of the suspected disease process, its extent, and other abnormalities. With an incision through the abdominal wall into the peritoneal cavity, the surgeon can explore the liver, gallbladder, stomach, duodenum, small intestine, large intestine, kidneys, and bladder. The "operation" is then performed. Diagnostic information may be obtained during the operation by removal of small portions of tissue as a biopsy for frozen section diagnosis by the pathologist or by X rays "on the table."

During the operation the anesthesiologist is responsible (with the surgeon) for supporting and maintaining the vital processes of the patient. While the surgeon is busy with the operation itself, the anesthesiologist maintains anesthesia and supports and assists breathing, often by way of a tube for the mouth into the trachea—an endotracheal tube. He or she monitors heart action, blood pressure, adequacy of ventilation, kidney function in some patients, and the general state of the patient. The anesthesiologist gives intravenous fluids to maintain the circulation and blood transfusion if blood is lost in sufficient quantities to require it. In all major operations, it is customary to have blood that has been matched with the patient available in the blood bank. Some operations always result in blood loss sufficient to require transfusions. Others, such as removal of a gallbladder, do not, but blood should be available if unexpected bleeding occurs.

Following completion of the operative procedure, the incision is closed by sutures ("stitches") in each layer of tissue. Then a dressing is applied, anesthesia is stopped, and the patient is allowed to awaken. The endotracheal tube may be removed then or later.

During or after the operation a number of tubes or drains may be inserted. With many abdominal operations, a nasogastric tube is used. This is a small rubber or plastic catheter inserted through the nose, down the esophagus, and into the stomach to drain gastric contents and decrease the amount of swallowed air that enters the intestine. The tube is often inserted in the operating room after the patient is anesthetized. Placing it through the nose is more comfortable than through the mouth, and the patient is less likely to gag. Operations in the lower abdomen often require a Foley catheter with a small balloon on the end to drain the bladder. Foley catheters are used routinely to measure urine output during and after the operation, and to ensure kidney function. After an operation on the chest, tubes must be brought out through the chest wall for two to three days in order to remove accumulated air, blood, or fluid. These are called thoracostomy tubes or chest tubes, and must be attached to an underwater seal apparatus and suction in order to maintain the negative pressure in the chest needed for breathing. Exploration of the common bile duct is often followed by insertion of a chest tube for a week or so to drain bile and assure healing of the duct. In other operations various drains may be left in place, coming out through the incision or from the body cavities in order to allow fluids, blood, or other materials to come out and avoid hematoma (a swelling filled with blood), abscess, or infection.

The patient is taken from the operating room to a recovery room for close observation and care as he or she awakens from the anesthetic. Here, nurses with special training monitor vital signs, heart rate, blood pressure, breathing, and urine output until the patient is awake and responsive and can be safely returned to a hospital room. This may require one to four hours. If the patient has had a potentially life-threatening operation such as an open-heart operation, he or she may be taken directly to a surgical intensive-care unit and remain there for several days or longer. Such a unit can provide sophisticated monitoring of vital signs, specialized nursing care, and fail-safe systems to support vital processes such as breathing and circulation. When a patient can breathe satisfactorily without assistance, when the circulation is stable, when kidneys are functioning normally, and if there are no other immediate threats to life, he or she may be discharged from intensive care to a regular hospital room for further convalescence.

Convalescence

There is a normal response to injury that man and all biologic organisms have. The nervous system, the endocrine system, and the metabolism all react to injury in order to help us survive and proceed through the healing process. The body goes through a specific sequence of events devoted to healing the wound and repairing the injury. These events are much the same whether the person has been hit by a car or operated on for cancer of the rectum.

The initial phase of recovery begins with the operation or injury and lasts for two to three days if the injury is relatively minor and if there are no complications. During this period the patient prefers to remain quiet, wishes not to be disturbed, is not interested in food, and is not particularly concerned with surroundings or such activities as combing hair, applying makeup, reading, or other everyday matters.

At first the patient will have pain from the incision. Pain medication, often a narcotic such as Demerol, morphine, or codeine, may be required every three or four hours to help relieve it. Unfortunately not all pain can be relieved, because too much medication will depress vital functions. The patient must take deep breaths and cough to keep the lungs functioning normally and prevent the lung collapse that can occur after operation.

It is important that the patient be helped to sit up, move about, and talk soon after the operation. He may need to wear a catheter because of difficulty in passing urine, and intravenous infusion of fluids, water, salt, and glucose may be necessary until he can take things by mouth.

After two to five days, if there are no complications, the patient arrives at a turning point. The injury phase stops, and he or she begins to feel a bit better, and becomes interested in life again. He may feel like eating again if the gastrointestinal tract is intact, and may want to get up and move about. Interest in personal appearance and in the surrounding world returns.

The third period begins after the turning point. It involves the slow gain in strength and replacement of the losses that occurred during the injury phase. People feel weak after an operation because much of the metabolism is concentrated on repairing the wound or the injury. This period requires replacement of protein that has been broken down, which may take six weeks or longer, depending on the severity of injury and age of the patient.

The fourth or final phase is that in which weight lost during the injury or operation is replaced. It may cover several months. The actual length of convalescence until the patient feels himself again depends on a number of other psychological and socioeconomic factors. The average, well-adjusted patient should feel close to normal and be back to full activity one month to six weeks following a major operation. Some people may be able to return to work earlier, and for others convalescence can be prolonged.

Complications

Unfavorable events occur even in the best of hands and in the best of circumstances. Complications after an operation can be classified into two categories: general complications that may follow any operation and specific complications after a particular operation.

General complications can affect almost any organ of the body. One general complication is bleeding, which can occur after any operation, but is more common after those on the vascular system. Pulmonary problems can occur, producing what has been called pneumonia but is more exactly termed atelectasis, the collapse of portions of the lung after a general anesthetic. Infection also may occur, or the wound may break down and fail to heal properly. Clots can develop in the legs, particularly in the veins of the calves, during and after an operation. If the clots break off and go to the lungs, they produce pulmonary emboli. These, on rare occasions, can be fatal. A patient who has had a heart attack may have clots form inside one of the ventricles of the heart. These, too, can break loose, pass into the circulation and block a blood vessel, producing symptoms of diminished blood supply to an organ. It can involve the leg, brain, or any area of the body.

If an organ has been damaged or diseased before an operation, the stress may overwhelm it and cause it to fail. A heavy smoker who has chronic lung disease may have lung failure. A patient whose heart previously has been damaged by valvular or coronary artery disease may have heart failure. Stroke may occur in someone with poor circulation to the brain which was not evident before the operation. Kidney failure occurs for a variety of reasons.

Fortunately, by close attention to detail, with detailed knowledge of each patient's overall health, and by a carefully planned and executed operative procedure, complications usually can be kept to a minimum. Precautions can be taken when the risk of a particular complication is increased. Finally, if complications do occur they often can be taken care of speedily. Transfusion can help restore blood lost by continued bleeding, for instance. When this is done, the patient can survive and eventually recover completely.

Specific complications occur in the area of the operation itself. For example, if it is necessary to remove a segment of the colon because of a cancer, the severed ends of the colon must be reunited in an anastomosis. Occasionally, because of reduced blood supply or local infection, this anastomosis will leak during the postoperative period. Fecal material may pass into the peritoneal cavity, causing infection (peritonitis). Fortunately, this serious problem usually can be treated successfully. Following removal of a breast for a malignant tumor, fluid may accumulate underneath the skin, or portions of the skin edges that are sutured fail to heal. This problem can be successfully treated, too.

Will the Operation Be Successful?

Results of an operation can be predicted in general terms and the possibilities discussed with the patient before the operation is decided on and performed.

Generally speaking, the results of any operation depend upon the severity of the disease process, its duration, how much of the organ is involved, and the general health of the patient. Removal of an inflamed appendix should allow an individual a completely normal life-span without further difficulties. Removal of a diseased gallbladder should produce excellent results in practically all patients. Removal of a diseased organ because of a benign tumor also should produce an excellent outcome. However, if the organ has been removed because of a malignant tumor, the results vary. The most important factor is the organ involved. Cancer of the sigmoid colon, if found early before the tumor has spread, can be cured in a high percentage of patients. A cancer of the pancreas, however, a different disease process, can be cured in only a small percentage of cases. The location, type, and extent of the malignancy at the time of diagnosis are critical factors. A small, well-differentiated tumor, discovered early before spread to other organs or lymph nodes, may have a good possibility of cure. If the tumor has spread to other organs, however, it is not likely to be completely cured. Removal can at best bring hope for relief of symptoms for a time.

Results of operations carried out to repair such abnormalities as hernia can be excellent, but a small number will recur nonetheless. The recurrence rate for an adequately repaired inguinal hernia is about two or three percent.

ABDOMINAL OPERATIONS

The abdominal cavity contains the organs of digestion (see chapter 20, "The Digestive System"). It is separated from the chest cavity above by the diaphragms and at the lower boundary by the pelvis. Within the abdominal cavity are the stomach, duodenum, small intestine, large intestine, liver, spleen, and pancreas, and in women the uterus, fallopian tubes, and ovaries. The kidneys lie against the back, covered by the lining of the abdominal cavity, the peritoneum.

Any operation within the abdomen requires an incision through the abdominal wall or through the flank muscles. This means cutting through the skin, through a layer of fat under the skin called the subcutaneous tissue, and through a thick fibrous band overlying the muscles of the abdominal wall called the fascia. Under these three layers, forming an envelope or sac for the contents of the abdomen, is the thin shiny membrane called the peritoneum.

Location of the incision depends on the operation and the location of the organ to be removed or repaired. The incision must be long enough to enable the surgeon and his team to see the organs inside clearly, and give them room to insert their instruments or their hands through the incision to carry out the procedure.

After the operation is completed, the incision must be closed. Several techniques are used. The basic principle is to close each layer with sutures or stitches. The peritoneum is often closed with a running suture of a material called chromic catgut, which will dissolve after two to three weeks. The muscles and fascia are then brought together, usually with a nonabsorbable suture of silk, cotton, plastic, or nylon, which will remain in place permanently. The subcutaneous tissue is brought together next, often with sutures that will be absorbed later. Finally the wound in the skin is closed, using fine sutures of silk or other nonabsorbable material, metal clips, or staples. Although this is the part we can see, sutures or clips on the surface are the least important in closing an incision. The main strength comes from sutures in the fascia. Depending on the location of the incision, skin sutures are usually left in place for a week to 10 days before being removed. During the first few weeks after an operation the incision is held together by the sutures while the healing process is taking place through formation of scar tissue by the laying down of fibrous tissue called collagen. As this material is deposited by the body cells and matures, it gains in strength. After four to six weeks the scar tissue is strong enough that the sutures are no longer relied on.

The most common complication of an incision is infection. In spite of all attempts to maintain sterility, it is simply impossible to remove all bacteria from the skin of the patient and from the various crypts in the skin, such as hair follicles and sebaceous glands. An incision may permit bacteria from these locations to enter the body. In addition, even the cleanest operating room may contain a few bacteria that can lodge in the incision.

An infection in a healing incision is usually not evident until about the fifth day after operation. It may produce a result as simple as slight redness around the sutures, or an abscess may form, requiring removal of the skin sutures and drainage. Rarely, an incision will fail to heal and will break open, a condition called wound dehiscence. If the entire wound separates it is necessary to return the patient to the operating room for resuturing. If this occurs, it is usually during the first week after the operation, not after the patient has been discharged from the hospital.

Exploratory Operations

A laparotomy or a celiotomy is an incision into the abdominal cavity to allow exploration of the organs inside. The procedure usually is used when an abnormality is suspected but precise diagnosis cannot be made. These occasions include recurrent or persistent fever without apparent cause, persistent and recurrent pain in the abdomen similarly unexplained, crampy abdominal pain and distention with episodes of partial intestinal obstruction, and possible tumors of such organs as liver, pancreas, and small intestine.

Your surgeon may recommend an exploratory operation if diagnostic tests have failed to reveal a cause for your problem. An exploratory operation, although never entered into lightly, is a recognized and acceptable approach to diagnose an illness that persists and is bothersome for the patient. Occasionally a patient undergoing such an exploration for vague or undefined symptoms is found to have a malignancy that is widespread within the peritoneal cavity or abdomen and cannot be removed. Patients and their families may wonder why the problem can go undiagnosed, then be untreatable when first diagnosed by an exploratory operation. The expression has been used, "The patient was just opened and closed." The reason for this unfortunate circumstance is that some cancers originating in the pancreas, the ovary, the small intestine, and perhaps other organs, even when very small, spread on the surface throughout the peritoneal cavity and implant on other organs such as the peritoneum itself, on the liver, on the layer of fat over the intestine called the omentum, or elsewhere. It has been part of folklore that such a patient, after an exploratory operation revealing widespread cancer that cannot be removed, seems to go from apparently good health before the operation to rapid deterioration and death in a few weeks or months. In such cases the operation may indeed contribute to the patient's deteriorating condition. This is true in part because of the effects of anesthetic and the operation, and because the body's internal balance may be altered, allowing the tumor to grow and spread more rapidly.

Operations on the Stomach and Duodenum

Hiatus hernia. Protrusions or bulges of abdominal organs through the diaphragm into the chest are called diaphragmatic hernias. Several types occur in newborn infants because of failure of the diaphragm to form properly and thus separate the chest and abdominal cavities. The most common herniation through the diaphragm in an adult is through the esophageal hiatus, the oval opening through which the esophagus passes into the stomach (see chapter 20, "The Digestive System").

Normally the junction of esophagus and stomach lies several centimeters below the diaphragm in the abdominal cavity. Due to a number of factors including straining, coughing, obesity, and pregnancy, the opening can become stretched or enlarged. A portion of the stomach then pushes up into the chest, so that it lies behind the heart. The displacement itself would produce little difficulty beyond some fullness after eating or when gas is swallowed, except that the abnormality interferes with the valve mechanism at the junction of the esophagus and stomach. Normally, this valve mechanism, a sphincter muscle in the lower part of the esophagus, prevents stomach acid from refluxing up into the esophagus. When acid does enter the esophagus and bathes its lining, called the mucosa, it produces a burning sensation, the typical heartburn of indigestion. Frequent acid reflux will cause esophagitis, or inflammation of the mucosa. There may be choking, coughing, and recurrent lung infections as acid and gastric juices are aspirated into the lungs. If such a process continues, the wall of the esophagus will become scarred and thickened and the esophageal canal narrowed. The patient will experience problems swallowing, a condition called dysphagia, and may not be able to eat solid food, being reduced progressively to a liquid diet.

The repair of a hiatus hernia includes restoring the stomach to its normal position in the abdominal cavity and repairing the valve mechanism to prevent acid reflux and allow the inflammatory process in the esophagus to heal. The operation can be carried out through an abdominal incision or through an incision in the left side of the chest to allow work on the problem from above. The original valve mechanism, the muscle of the lower esophagus, cannot be repaired, but can be strengthened by wrapping a portion of the stomach around the esophagus and suturing it in place. This reinforcement actually produces a flap-valve type of mechanism. This is the principle of all modern repairs of hiatus hernias. The valve mechanism must be constructed so that reflux of acid is prevented but the patient can swallow normally and can also belch and vomit, if necessary.

The three types of operations, all of which are satisfactory if done properly, are named for the surgeons who developed them—the Nissen operation and the Hill operation, performed through an abdominal incision, and the Belsey operation, performed through a thoracic incision. If the patient's disease has progressed to formation of a stricture (narrowing) of the esophagus, then a more complex reconstruction procedure becomes necessary.

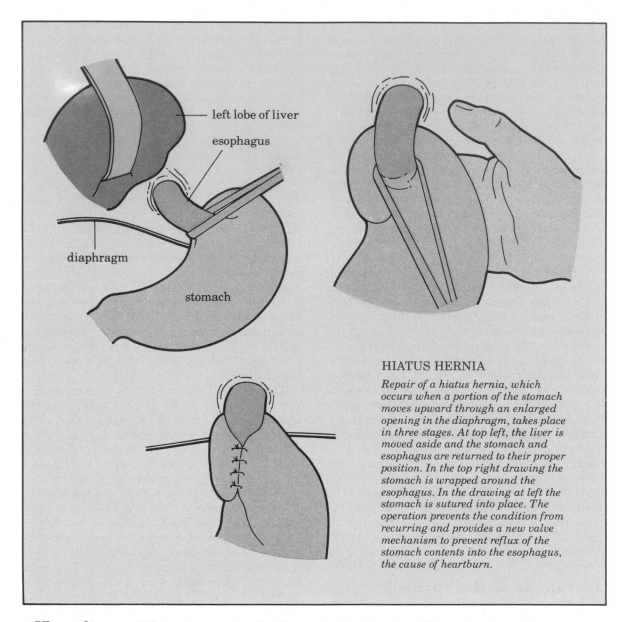

left lobe of liver

esophagus

diaphragm

stomach

HIATUS HERNIA

Repair of a hiatus hernia, which occurs when a portion of the stomach moves upward through an enlarged opening in the diaphragm, takes place in three stages. At top left, the liver is moved aside and the stomach and esophagus are returned to their proper position. In the top right drawing the stomach is wrapped around the esophagus. In the drawing at left the stomach is sutured into place. The operation prevents the condition from recurring and provides a new valve mechanism to prevent reflux of the stomach contents into the esophagus, the cause of heartburn.

Ulcer disease. Ulcers commonly develop in the duodenum, the intestinal area just below the pylorus or outlet of the stomach, because the lining of the duodenum is bathed with acid from the stomach. Basically, the cause of ulceration of the duodenum is excess gastric acid production. Treatment requires the use of antacids to neutralize the acid, sedation to decrease tension and the production of acid, and various blocking agents to decrease or block the formation of acid. Most ulcers will respond to such medical treatment. However, certain problems require an operation. They include bleeding, perforation, obstruction, and "intractable" ulcers.

Bleeding. The ulcer may extend through the wall of the duodenum, involving a vessel in the wall or behind it.

Perforation. If the ulcer is on the outer surface of the duodenum, it may erode through the wall and allow gastric and duodenal contents to escape into the peritoneal cavity, a sudden and serious problem.

Obstruction. As the ulcerated inflammatory process continues, scar tissue may be formed that obstructs the duodenum, usually at the pylorus.

Intractability. Certain patients have ulcer disease that responds to treatment initially, only to recur and persist, and an operation may be recommended.

Operations for complications of ulcer disease require correction of the complication and some procedure to reduce the production of gastric acid to prevent recurrence.

For a bleeding ulcer, the first step obviously is to stop the bleeding. This can be done most simply by opening the duodenum or stomach, exposing the ulcer, and suturing the bleeding vessel. Following this the ulcer may be removed if it is in a location where removal is possible, along with an additional procedure to reduce gastric acidity (see below).

When a perforation occurs, the first requirement is to close the perforation by suturing, or by bringing a portion of the fatty tissue called the omentum over the hole and suturing it into place, which will allow the opening to seal. The contents of the stomach that have spilled throughout the abdominal cavity are removed and the surface of the peritoneum cleaned with warm salt water. Further surgery may then be carried out to reduce gastric acid as well.

For obstruction caused by scar tissue, it is necessary either to remove the scarred area by what is called a resection, eliminating that portion of the stomach and closing it off with sutures, or to bypass it by building a connection (anastomosis) between the stomach above the obstruction and the intestine below it.

For intractable ulcers that do not heal or do not stay healed, the primary objective is to reduce acid formation and prevent recurrence.

Operations to reduce gastric acidity fall into several types and combinations. One approach is to remove the lower two-thirds of the stomach. This is called a gastric resection, or subtotal gastrectomy. It eliminates the major acid-producing portion of the stomach, particularly the lower part called the antrum. The upper third of the stomach is then connected directly to the intestinal tract. This is usually done by bringing a loop of the jejunum, the part of the small intestine just beyond the duodenum, up over the colon and suturing to form an anastomosis of the stomach. The procedure is called a gastrojejunostomy. The duodenum, which has been divided just below the stomach, is closed into a blind pouch. Secretions from the pancreas, gallbladder and bile duct, which normally feed into the duodenum, now pass down into the duodenum and around through the gastrojejunostomy.

A second major approach to reducing gastric acid production is to cut the vagus nerves, which stimulate the stomach to produce acid.

These nerves, which regulate many internal functions, pass along the esophagus to the stomach and on to the other portions of the gastrointestinal tract. The branches to the stomach are severed in an operation called a vagotomy. There are a number of specialized ways of making the division. In a truncal vagotomy both nerves are entirely divided. In a selective vagotomy only the nerves to the stomach itself are cut.

Because vagotomy reduces the tone of the stomach so that it does not empty well, a procedure to promote drainage is likely to be carried out at the same time. The thickened muscle of the pylorus or outlet of the stomach may be divided (pyloromyotomy), or the entire wall divided and sutured to increase the size of the pyloric opening (pyloroplasty). Another procedure, which removes the lower third of the stomach including the outlet of the stomach and the pylorus, is called an antrectomy. It is followed by gastrojejunostomy or gastroduodenostomy to reconstruct the stomach. Still a third type of drainage procedure bypasses the pylorus area by bringing a loop of jejunum up to the outer curvature of the stomach to form a gastrojejunostomy. Thus a vagotomy is usually combined with a drainage procedure, either a pyloroplasty, antrectomy, or gastrojejunostomy.

The most common operation for ulcer disease is a vagotomy plus antral resection or antrectomy. In this operation the ulcer is removed, particularly if it lies in the first portion of the duodenum. If the ulcer occurs further down in the duodenum it becomes impossible to remove because it lies close to where the common bile duct or the ducts from the pancreas come in. Then the ulcer is left in place, the duodenum is closed above it, and a gastrojejunostomy is constructed. The ulcer should heal, once the acid no longer comes into the duodenum.

Ulcers occur in the stomach as well as the duodenum. Called gastric ulcers, they account for about one in five cases of ulcer disease. Gastric ulcers are related to increased acid production but may be produced in part by failure of the stomach to empty properly. The primary concern with a gastric ulcer is to be sure that it is benign, either by viewing the ulcer through a diagnostic instrument called a gastroscope, or by obtaining tissue for review and study by a pathologist. A benign gastric ulcer may also heal without surgery. If an operation is required, the ulcer and the affected portion of the stomach usually are removed in a procedure similar to that for duodenal ulcers.

ULCER SURGERY

There are several operations for gastric ulcer, one of which is depicted here. Top drawing shows the relationship of internal organs involved in the operation. The dotted line is an incision at the midline, a common incision for abdominal operations. At bottom left, an ulcer in the lower stomach is to be treated by removing a portion of the stomach, a procedure known as a gastric resection. At bottom right, the ulcerated segment of stomach has been removed, a loop of the jejunum has been brought up and joined to the upper stomach, and the duodenum has been closed off. The entire operation is known as a gastrojejunostomy.

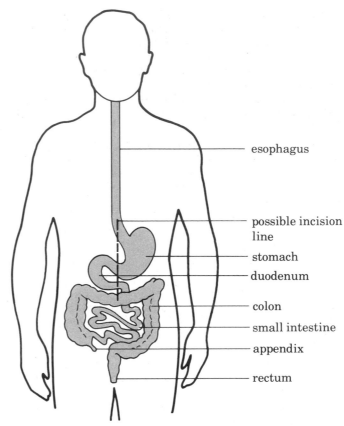

esophagus

possible incision line

stomach

duodenum

colon

small intestine

appendix

rectum

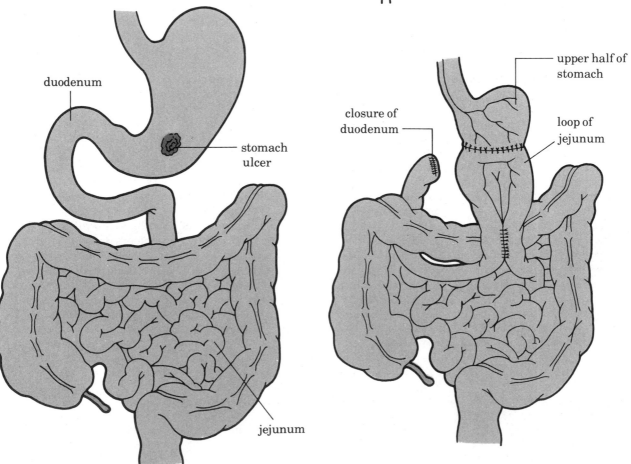

duodenum

stomach ulcer

jejunum

closure of duodenum

upper half of stomach

loop of jejunum

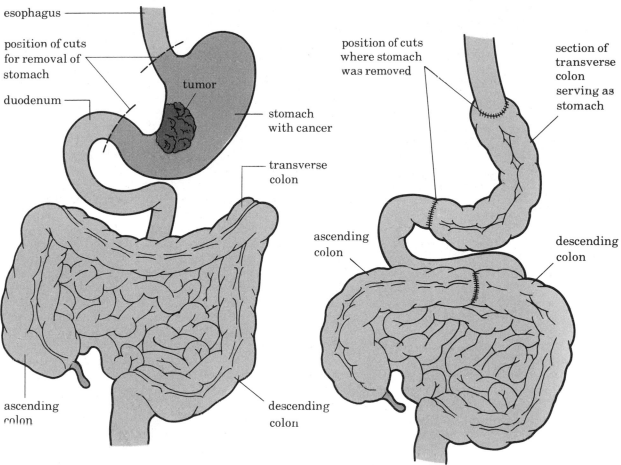

esophagus

position of cuts
for removal of
stomach

duodenum

tumor

stomach
with cancer

transverse
colon

ascending
colon

descending
colon

position of cuts
where stomach
was removed

section of
transverse
colon
serving as
stomach

ascending
colon

descending
colon

REMOVAL OF THE STOMACH

*For a cancer of the stomach, it is
sometimes necessary to remove the
entire organ and use a section of the
colon as a substitute. The procedure is
known as a total gastrectomy. At left,
the dotted lines show where the
stomach is to be divided from the
esophagus above and the duodenum
below. The shaded area represents the*
*tumor. A segment of transverse colon
will replace the stomach. At right, the
stomach has been removed and the
segment of colon joined to the
esophagus and duodenum. The ends
of the colon are then brought together
(crosshatched line), completing the
reconstruction.*

Tumors. Both benign and malignant
tumors are found in the stomach. Fortunately
cancer of the stomach seems to be decreasing
in frequency. Although it still occurs, it is
much less common than in the past. The cancer
may begin as an ulcer, with all the initial ulcer
symptoms including bleeding, pain, perforation, and obstruction. This is why accurate
diagnosis of presumed ulcer disease is important. If a cancer is confirmed by biopsy or
gastroscopy, the affected portion of the
stomach is removed, along with a portion of
normal stomach surrounding it and the adjoining lymph nodes. The remaining portion of the
stomach is joined with the small intestine by
gastrojejunostomy. It is seldom necessary to
remove the entire stomach, although in rare

cases this may be done, as shown above. A section of small intestine is then brought up to
form an anastomosis, or a section of the transverse colon is used as a conduit between the
esophagus and the duodenum.

A major function of the stomach is to serve as
a reservoir for food. If the upper one-third to
one-fourth of the stomach can be left in place, it
will function satisfactorily and allow patients
to eat fairly normally. At first, they may be
unable to eat a full or normal meal and must
eat smaller amounts more frequently. Gradually, however, the gastric pouch adjusts and patients may return to a normal diet and normal
quantities. Patients usually lose weight during and after a gastric operation. Normal postoperative loss is 10 to 15 pounds.

Operations on the Small Intestine

The small intestine is the portion of the gastrointestinal or digestive tract that runs from the stomach to the colon. It is about 20 feet long. Although it is continuous, it is usually classified as having three sections—the duodenum (just beyond the stomach), the lengthy jejunum, and the ileum, which joins it to the colon. Intimately associated with it is an apronlike skirt called the mesentery, from which the intestine hangs, as though it were the skirt's hem. The mesentery provides the intestine's blood supply.

The task of the small intestine is the absorption of nutritive materials from the food digested by the stomach, so any disease that affects it generally must be treated promptly or the whole body suffers. Surgery is frequently performed because disease of the small intestine usually affects only a portion of the organ. The diseased section can be removed, and the severed ends joined together into a shorter but still functional organ. A smooth union is possible because the intestine is of uniform diameter, and its great length allows for removal without the section being missed. When the section is cut out, a pie-shaped wedge of the mesentery is usually removed with it. The usual procedure is to clamp off the target area, remove it, then suture the ends and mesentery back together. The blood vessels of the mesentery are tied off, too.

Most of the intestinal complaints, whether of the small or large intestine, that bring a person to a surgeon produce a similar group of symptoms. These include blood in the stool, abdominal pain that is sometimes sharp and severe, nausea and vomiting, bloating, and the inability to pass gas or stool. It is not always easy to differentiate the cause of the complaint, so if the symptoms do not subside, an exploratory operation may be necessary. In many cases, however, the treatment is similar, calling for removal of the affected area.

Adhesions are the most common surgical problem involving the small intestine. Adhesions are fibrous connections or bonds between segments of intestine, abdominal wall, or omentum, a fatty apron hanging from the stomach and tranverse colon. Adhesions develop from areas of injury or inflammation following previous operations, when segments of intestine adhere to one another or to the undersurface of the incision. Adhesions can produce kinks or twists of the small intestine, which then result in partial or complete obstruction. The condition is heralded by crampy abdominal pain and bloating, followed by nausea and vomiting, with inability to pass gas or stool. The twists or kinks may cut off the blood supply to the intestine, producing infarction or gangrene (called strangulation). This process is a threat to life. Gangrenous intestine turns black and eventually will perforate, producing peritonitis. Adhesions occur to some extent after all abdominal operations. They cannot be prevented but usually do not produce problems. They usually are not present in someone who has not had an abdominal operation.

To correct adhesions, it is necessary to open the abdomen, find the site of the adhesions and obstruction, and divide the adhesions, a procedure called lysis of adhesions. If a portion of the intestine is twisted and infarcted or gangrenous, the portion must be removed and the divided ends above and below the gangrenous segment sutured together to form an anastomosis. Much of the small intestine can be removed without producing any particular difficulty. If, however, all of the small intestine must be removed, a serious problem of malnutrition occurs.

Tumors of the small intestine, both benign and malignant, various inflammatory diseases such as Crohn's disease or regional enteritis, and diseases of the blood supply to the small intestine also may require removal of a portion of the intestine and anastomosis.

Intussusception, a condition found most commonly in children, occurs when one portion of the small intestine telescopes inside another, producing pain and obstruction. In children the telescoping can often be reduced with a barium enema, an X-ray procedure in which barium is put into the colon and passed backward to build up pressure and push back the misplaced intestine.

The blood supply to the intestine can be interfered with in several ways. A heart attack or diseases of the heart valves may produce blood clots that break loose and go on to block the mesentery vessels of the intestine. Atherosclerosis or hardening of the arteries can involve these vessels as well.

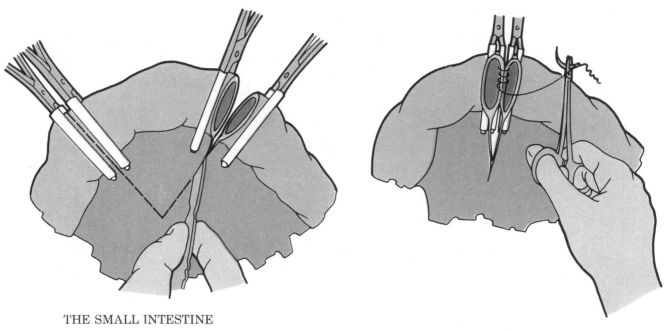

THE SMALL INTESTINE

A common operation for disorders of the small intestine is to remove the diseased section and shorten the bowel's length, as shown in these drawings. At left, the portion of bowel has been clamped off on both sides of the diseased area. The surgeon then cuts across the bowel between the clamps and also removes a wedge from the mesentery, the apron-like sheet of tissue that provides blood to the intestine. The blood vessels are divided and tied off and the two ends of the bowel are sewn together (right drawing) to restore continuity.

Appendectomy

The appendix is a vestigial or rudimentary organ. It is a short, hollow blind tube of intestine attached to the cecum, the first portion of the large intestine lying just below its junction with the small intestine at the so-called ileocecal valve. Inflammation of the appendix (appendicitis) occurs when fecal material gets into the lumen or hollow channel of the appendix and obstructs it. The appendix cannot rid itself of this obstruction and it contracts and becomes inflamed. At first a localized phenomenon, the infectious process moves through the wall of the appendix to adjoining organs. If the appendix perforates or becomes gangrenous, fecal material may leak into the peritoneal cavity. If not quickly treated, the condition can go on to form generalized peritonitis (inflammation of the peritoneum) or an abscess. It usually takes 12 to 24 hours for an acutely inflamed appendix to develop gangrene or perforation.

Removal of an inflamed appendix (appendectomy) is generally uneventful. The procedure requires a small diagonal or oblique incision in the lower right portion of the abdomen. The few small blood vessels that supply the appendix are divided. The base of the appendix is divided where it joins the cecum, then tied off by a suture. As discussed on page 735, the stump of the appendix may be either tied or buried in the cecal wall to hold in the cecal contents. The procedure also aims to prevent a common complication after appendectomy, an abscess or infection of the incision, the result of bacteria seeping through the wall during inflammation. It is difficult to eliminate contamination totally from such a highly infective organ.

Inflammation of the appendix (appendicitis) is a great mimic of other diseases. The reason is that the appendix can occupy various locations in the abdomen. Normally only about three inches long, it may be far longer in some persons and extend from the cecum into the pelvis alongside the colon or uterus. It may lie underneath the cecum and ascending colon, in which case it is called a retrocecal appendix. It may extend into the left side of the abdomen and produce pain on the left side instead of the right, as it normally does. Thus the diagnosis of appendicitis in its early stages can be extremely difficult. For this reason it is impor-

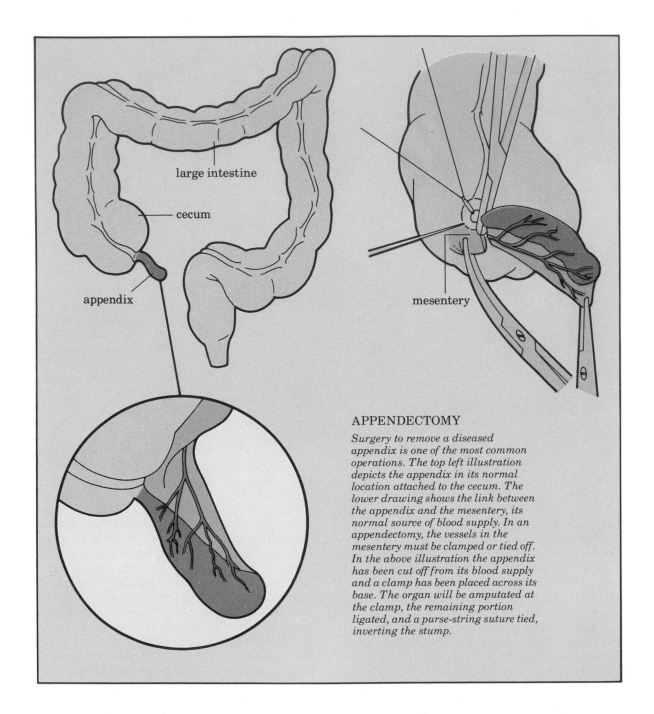

large intestine

cecum

appendix

mesentery

APPENDECTOMY

Surgery to remove a diseased appendix is one of the most common operations. The top left illustration depicts the appendix in its normal location attached to the cecum. The lower drawing shows the link between the appendix and the mesentery, its normal source of blood supply. In an appendectomy, the vessels in the mesentery must be clamped or tied off. In the above illustration the appendix has been cut off from its blood supply and a clamp has been placed across its base. The organ will be amputated at the clamp, the remaining portion ligated, and a purse-string suture tied, inverting the stump.

tant to seek medical aid when an episode of abdominal pain does not subside rapidly.

If appendicitis has progressed to gangrene, perforation, or rupture with localized contamination by bacteria and the beginning of an abscess, the difficulty of the operation is increased. It may not be possible to remove the appendix because of the severity of the inflammatory process. Instead, the surgeon may drain the area of infection and advise the patient to have the appendix removed later after inflammation and infection subside.

Operations on the Colon

The primary disease processes involving the colon (large intestine) that may require an operation include cancer, diverticulitis, ulcerative colitis, and inflammatory bowel disease or granulomatous colitis. Polyps of the colon and bleeding from blood vessel abnormalities within the colon walls also may call for surgical care.

Cancer. Cancer of the colon usually announces itself by a change in bowel habits. The warning signs are increasing constipation, blood in the stool, crampy abdominal pain, weight loss, feeling poorly, loss of appetite, and anemia. If a person has one or more of these signs, the surgeon usually will order diagnostic studies. The first step usually is a test of the stool to see whether blood is present, which could indicate intestinal bleeding from a tumor. The inside of the colon may then be inspected, either by a sigmoidoscope, which allows the surgeon to inspect the lower 10 inches of the intestine where most cancers develop, or by colonoscope, the flexible device that permits examination of the colon's entire length. A barium enema also may be given. The barium outlines the contours of the colon to be visualized by X ray.

If cancer is found, the type of surgery performed will depend on its site. Regardless of location, however, it is always necessary to remove the cancerous portion of the bowel surgically unless the patient is too ill for the operation. The procedure is called colectomy. Besides the cancerous portion, a segment of colon above and below the tumor is cut out to ensure that the cancer has been removed completely. The surgeon also takes out the mesentery, the fatty tissue surrounding the blood vessels to the colon, and the lymph nodes. Cancer of the colon spreads primarily and initially to lymph nodes along the blood supply to and from the colon. After these portions have been removed, the severed ends of the colon are reunited.

Sometimes, the first clue to a colon cancer is bowel obstruction or perforation, which can lead to peritonitis. An emergency operation is then necessary. It may be necessary to perform a colostomy, in which a portion of the colon is brought through the abdominal wall outside the body to form a stoma. This artificially created sac allows contents of the colon to collect outside the body so they do not produce obstruction or contamination of the peritoneal cavity in the event of perforation. The arrangement may be temporary or permanent. If it is permanent, the patient may be fitted with a collecting bag, depending on the location of the colostomy in the colon. Its contents may be disposed of at the patient's convenience, or the patient may be taught to irrigate the colostomy each day with a catheter in order to have bowel movements through the colostomy stoma.

If a cancer of the colon is located in the rectum or close to the anus, it may be necessary to remove the entire rectum and anus. The colon above the site of the tumor is then brought out through an incision in the abdominal wall to form a permanent end-colostomy. The operation is called an abdominoperineal resection, and also requires a bag for colon contents. The colostomy is covered only by a small gauze dressing. Irrigation once a day usually will allow emptying of the colon and good control of the colostomy without spillage.

Polyps, which are small outpouchings on stalks, may develop in the mucosa, the lining cells of the walls of the colon. Polyps are generally benign growths, but may be malignant or become malignant. Formerly it was necessary to remove polyps by operation, making an incision through the abdominal wall and then into the colon. Polyps can now be removed by colonoscopy. The lighted sighting device is fitted with tiny retractable blades or with an electric cautery that can sear off the growths.

Diverticulitis. A diverticulum is an outpouching in the colon wall. The most common location for diverticula is in the sigmoid colon on the left side, just above the rectum. The reason may be the angulation of the colon at this location, plus pressure in the lower segment as the colon fills. The outpouchings in themselves do not produce difficulty, but may start an inflammatory process called diverticulitis. Diverticulitis can lead to swelling and obstruction, and to perforation producing peritonitis or bleeding. These complications can be life-threatening.

Operation for diverticulitis depends on the stage and extent of the disease. If a person has had recurrent attacks of abdominal pain due to diverticulitis, a barium enema is given to determine by X ray the exact location and extent of the diverticula. An elective operation is then carried out to remove the affected segment. The operation requires careful preparation, because the colon normally is filled with massive amounts of bacteria. This material, if it escapes into the peritoneal cavity, can cause serious infection. Laxatives and a low-residue or liquid diet are given beforehand to eliminate stool in the colon, and antibiotics are administered to decrease the number of bacteria.

Complications of diverticulitis require more specialized care. An initial colostomy may be performed, or the diseased segment may be removed with a temporary colostomy to allow the inflammatory process to subside. Afterwards the two ends of the severed intestine will be brought together to restore continuity and rid the patient of the inconvenience of a colostomy. It is hazardous to bring together two divided ends of colon to form an anastomosis if there is inflammation of the colon or peritonitis and if the colon has not previously been prepared by cleansing.

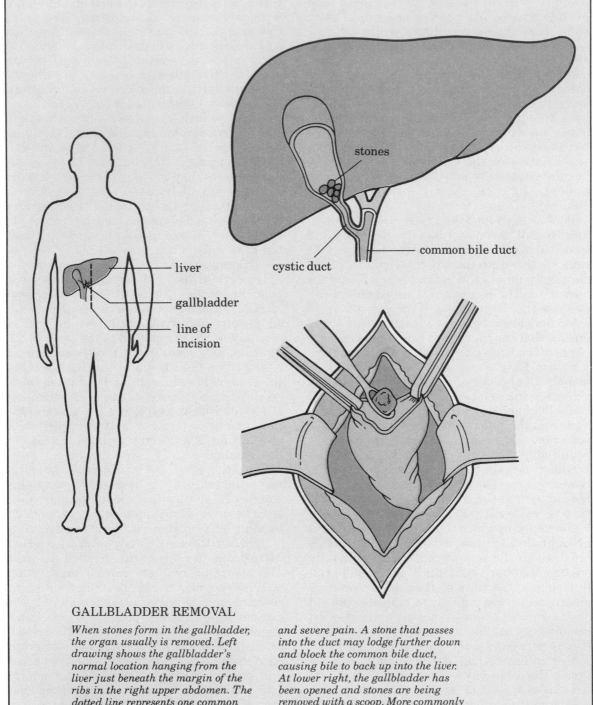

stones

common bile duct

cystic duct

liver

gallbladder

line of
incision

GALLBLADDER REMOVAL

*When stones form in the gallbladder,
the organ usually is removed. Left
drawing shows the gallbladder's
normal location hanging from the
liver just beneath the margin of the
ribs in the right upper abdomen. The
dotted line represents one common
incision. Stones at the outlet to the
cystic duct (upper right) can obstruct
the gallbladder or cause inflammation
and severe pain. A stone that passes
into the duct may lodge further down
and block the common bile duct,
causing bile to back up into the liver.
At lower right, the gallbladder has
been opened and stones are being
removed with a scoop. More commonly
the gallbladder is removed entirely
and the cystic duct is tied off at its
junction with the common bile duct.*

Ulcerative colitis and inflammatory bowel disease (granulomatous colitis) are quite different diseases, but produce somewhat similar symptoms. These include inflammation of the lining of the intestine, diarrhea, weight loss, crampy abdominal pain, and bleeding. Both diseases may be treated by medication for long periods. However, many patients ultimately have difficulty because of repeated or acute attacks. In addition, ulcerative colitis that persists for a number of years increases the risks of cancer. Ultimately both diseases may require an operation to remove the affected portion of the colon. Sometimes the entire colon, rectum, and anus are involved. Removal of the entire colon (total colectomy) is followed by creation of an opening for the small intestine to come out through the abdominal wall. This is called an ileostomy, and is done by turning the wall of the intestine back on itself and sewing it to the skin in a region where the patient can wear a bag over the stoma. Stool coming from the ileum is liquid, so some container is necessary. Despite this arrangement, the patient can be totally rehabilitated and lead a relatively normal life afterwards.

The Biliary Tract, Bile Ducts, and Gallbladder

The biliary tree or tract is a system to drain bile from the liver into the intestine. Small bile ducts within the liver merge into the two hepatic ducts from the right and left lobes of the liver, and these come together to form the common bile duct. The common bile duct runs down to and enters the duodenum, along with ducts bringing secretions from the pancreas. Coming off the common bile duct is a sac called the gallbladder. This is a reservoir for the storage of bile, filling between meals, then emptying after eating to send bile to the intestine to aid in digestion.

Gallstones. Among the constituents of bile are calcium and cholesterol. Both tend to precipitate out and form solid material, which then goes on to form a stone. Stones (cholelithiasis) are the most common disease of the biliary system. The stones may produce symptoms in themselves, cause inflammation of the gallbladder (cholecystitis), obstruct the gallbladder, or pass through the cystic duct leading from the gallbladder and obstruct the common bile duct, so that bile backs up into the liver and causes jaundice. The treatment is to remove the gallbladder, a procedure called a cholecystectomy, as shown on page 750. An incision is made, usually on the right side of the abdomen but sometimes at the midline. The gallbladder is removed from the enveloping capsule that holds it to the underside of the liver. The cystic duct is followed down to its junction with the common bile duct and is divided and tied off. If stones have passed into the common bile duct, it may be necessary to open the duct and remove the stones, a procedure called a choledochostomy. Subsequently, surgeons commonly leave a small T-shaped tube in the common bile duct for about a week. The tube prevents scarring, which might produce a stricture or narrowing that would obstruct bile. Often during an operation the surgeon will obtain an X ray of the common bile duct while the patient is on the operating table, using an injection of dye through the cystic duct called a cholangiogram. This is to determine whether there are abnormalities of the duct and to see whether bile can flow easily into the duodenum.

If stones are found it is always best to remove the gallbladder rather than simply empty out the stones, because the gallbladder is diseased and stones will form again. Sometimes, however, as an emergency procedure in a very sick patient, it may be the surgeon's best judgment simply to make an incision in the gallbladder, remove the stones, and insert a drainage tube. This can be a life-saving procedure. Later, however, the gallbladder should be removed when the patient's condition improves. Loss of the gallbladder is not a serious handicap. Most persons can live normal lives (and eat normal diets) without it.

Operations on the Pancreas

The pancreas is an organ of digestion that lies behind the stomach and extends from the curve of the duodenum over to the left side of the abdomen to the spleen. Two primary types of disease affect it, pancreatitis and cancer.

Pancreatitis, or inflammation of the pancreas, is sometimes produced by gallstones, which obstruct the duct draining the pancreas. The condition also is associated with heavy drinking. The inflammatory process can be so extensive that it extends through the wall of the pancreas (because of the potent enzymes produced by the organ) to liquefy or digest tissue. The treatment of acute pancreatitis is by means other than an operation, usually medication and abstinence from alcohol. However, many of the complications of pancreatitis may require an operation, particularly an abscess or a pseudocyst. Pancreatitis can become a chronic debilitating process with frequent recurrences and continuous pain. An operation may then be recommended to drain the obstructed pancreatic duct into a loop or segment of small intestine sewn to the pancreatic duct. All or practically all of the pancreas also may be removed (pancreatectomy). Pancreatic hormones and insulin, which is produced in the pancreas, are given afterwards.

Cancer of the pancreas has been increasing gradually for several decades. The reasons are not known. Unfortunately, because of the location of the pancreas, such cancers can grow extensively before they produce symptoms and are discovered. Diagnosis of pancreatic cancer in time to do something about it is extremely difficult. Techniques are being developed to try to detect malignancy earlier and more accurately.

Cancers of the pancreas most commonly occur in the head of the pancreas, where the pancreatic duct drains into the duodenum. Such a tumor may block the confluence of the pancreatic duct and the common bile duct and produce jaundice as an early symptom. If cancer of the pancreas is diagnosed, an operation is recommended. If the tumor has not spread from the pancreas to adjoining lymph nodes or to the liver, removal of a portion of the pancreas and the duodenum is required. This is called a pancreaticoduodenectomy or Whipple operation. It is not possible to remove the head of the pancreas without removing the duodenum, which lies snugly around it and shares its blood supply. The entire pancreas often is removed because there may be microscopic extension of the cancer into the rest of the pancreas. This is called a total pancreatectomy. Loss of the pancreas produces digestive difficulties and brings on diabetes because the cells (islets of Langerhans) that produce insulin are in the pancreas. The digestive process can be improved, however, by giving the patient pancreatic enzymes, and the diabetes can be controlled by insulin injections, allowing a patient to live a reasonably normal life after total pancreatectomy. If a cancer of the pancreas cannot be removed, a bypass operation may be done in which bile from the gallbladder is drained into the jejunum by creating a connection between those two organs.

Other tumors may develop in the pancreatic cells that produce hormones. A tumor of the islet cells that produce insulin is called an insulinoma. The islet cells may have to be removed, which can be done by removing the tumor with that portion of the pancreas. Other tumors may stimulate the production of the hormone gastrin, which regulates acid production in the stomach and is associated with severe ulcer disease.

The Liver

Two types of problems may require operations on the liver. Injury is the most common. It is usually caused by an accident in a fast moving vehicle such as an automobile or motorcycle, or by a fall. The impact cracks or ruptures the liver, and the normally firm tissue breaks up into pieces, producing severe hemorrhage. An immediate operation is needed to control the bleeding, either by suturing the liver or by removing a portion if it has been destroyed (partial hepatectomy). A large portion of the liver can be removed with eventual recovery of the patient because the remaining liver will increase in size to carry on the functions required. Some liver injuries, however, can be immediately fatal if large cracks reach the major blood vessels.

Tumors of the liver, either benign or malignant, are quite rare. One type that has been increasing is the hepatic adenoma, associated with the use of birth control pills. These benign tumors cause discomfort mainly because of their large size, and they may rupture and hemorrhage. Malignant tumors also originate in the liver. If the tumor is limited to one lobe, it may be possible to remove the cancerous lobe. These are extensive operations that involve considerable risk for the patient. The liver is also a common target organ for spread of cancer from other parts of the body.

Cirrhosis is a common disease of the liver, sometimes caused by chronic infection of the liver (hepatitis), but more often by alcoholism. The disease causes the production of fibrous tissue that gradually destroys liver cells and interferes with the flow of blood into the liver from the intestines. Normally, blood coming from the intestine carrying the products of digestion flows through the portal venous system, the collecting veins that bring blood to the liver by way of the portal vein. This blood passes through the liver to deliver nutrients for processing, then returns to the heart by way of the hepatic veins. In cirrhosis, the fibrous tissue prevents the blood from flowing easily, and pressure in the portal venous system increases. As the pressure increases, a condition called portal hypertension, the blood tries to find its way back to the heart by other circuits and connections through the venous system, and large dilated veins develop.

A primary target is the veins of the lower esophagus, where the portal venous system of the liver connects with the systemic venous system returning blood to the heart. Large dilated veins in this area are called esophageal varices. They are thin-walled, and under high pressure they may break and produce severe hemorrhage. An immediate operation may be required to stop the bleeding and obliterate these veins or reduce the pressure so that they do not bleed again. Even if bleeding is controlled without an operation, surgery may be necessary later to reduce pressure and prevent future bleeding.

Operations for esophageal varices all use the principle of forming a connection (anastomosis) between one of these veins and a normal vein returning blood to the right side of the heart. These shunting procedures come in several types. The portocaval shunt joins the portal vein directly to the inferior vena cava, one of the body's principal veins. A splenorenal shunt joins the splenic vein, part of the portal system, with a renal vein draining from the kidney into the inferior vena cava.

The Spleen

The spleen is a specialized organ lying beneath the diaphragm on the left side of the abdomen. It is part of the lymphatic and reticuloendothelial system, which helps remove various materials from the blood, including broken down or old red blood cells, debris, and bacteria, and contributes to the immune system.

Injury is the most common problem of the spleen. In bicycle, sledding, or vehicular accidents, direct injury to the left chest and left flank may tear or rupture the spleen or its capsule, producing hemorrhage. Formerly, any sign of rupture or injury to the spleen led to immediate operation and removal of the spleen (splenectomy). Recently it has been recognized that the possibility of infection is increased after splenectomy, particularly in young children. Therefore, surgeons try to save the spleen if the injury is not extensive. A small tear or a small laceration of the spleen can be repaired safely if hemorrhage can be controlled. Otherwise a splenectomy is still required. Adults can function normally without a spleen because its functions are assumed by other organs of the lymphatic system. Children require special safeguards against life-threatening infection.

Tumors of the spleen also may require splenectomy. There are several other abnormalities of the spleen in which blood platelets that play a role in blood clotting may be destroyed in excess numbers, or the spleen may be involved in a disease of the blood in which red blood cells are broken down (see chapter 6, "The Blood"). These may require removal of the spleen. Removal is also done for Hodgkin's disease, a cancer of the lymph nodes. An exploration of the abdomen (staging laparotomy) is conducted to determine the stage of the disease and involvement of lymph nodes, spleen, and liver, so that accurate therapy with X ray and drugs can be started.

HERNIA

A hernia is a protrusion of the contents of a body cavity through its enveloping wall because of a defect in the tissues. Although a hernia can occur within the skull and brain or within the chest, most commonly we consider hernia as a protrusion of contents of the abdomen or the peritoneal cavity through a defect in the abdominal wall, through the diaphragm into the chest, or through the floor of the pelvis in the region of the anus or vagina. Hiatus hernia, protrusion of part of the stomach through the diaphragm, is described on page 741.

Inguinal hernia in the male is the most common hernia. It occurs frequently in newborn or young males, when it is called an indirect inguinal (groin) hernia. The condition is related to prenatal development of the testicles, which form within the abdomen. At birth the testicle, with its attached blood vessels and the drainage tube for sperm (the spermatic cord), migrates through an opening in the abdominal wall (the internal inguinal ring) down a canal in the groin into its final position in the scrotum. If the opening is somewhat large, or if a portion of the lining of the peritoneal cavity descends with the testicle, a sac of the lining tissue is formed. A portion of the wall or a loop of small intestine may be pushed into this sac. This will create a bulge in the groin, often painful and usually uncomfortable.

Indirect inguinal hernias may not be apparent at birth. They may be found or develop later, even in adult life, when a small sac which

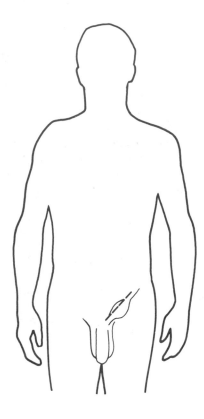

INGUINAL HERNIA

The common hernia of males occurs when the inguinal ring opening to the scrotum weakens and enlarges, allowing a portion of intestine to push through the opening and producing a bulge in the groin, as shown above. The stages of hernia repair are shown in the succession of drawings. (1) An incision has been made through the skin, exposing the fatty layer and the fascia overlying the inguinal canal. (2) The fascia and muscle fibers have been separated, showing the hernia beneath. (3) The hernia sac, which has been protruding through the inguinal ring, is freed from surrounding tissue. The spermatic cord carrying blood to the testicles and sperm from the testicles can be seen below it. (4) The hernia sac is opened, inspected, and emptied. Fat or bowel is pushed back into the peritoneal cavity and the base of the hernia sac is sutured (arrow). Poupart's ligament is used as an anchor for sutures, which close the weakened area behind the spermatic cord and narrow the opening through which the cord passes. (5) The sutures have been tied, closing the muscle, fascia, and back wall of the inguinal canal but allowing the cord to pass through it. The outer layers then will be closed over the cord.

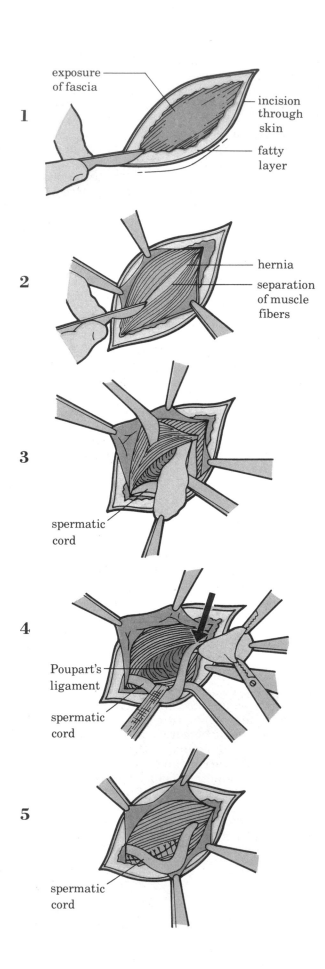

was initially of no consequence enlarges, allowing the intestine to enter or go down into the scrotum.

In older men the stresses of life, particularly coughing, sneezing, straining during bowel movements, physical exercise, and lifting may combine with the weakening of the tissues with age to produce a weakness in the inguinal region allowing the abdominal contents to push through the back of the inguinal canal. This is called a direct inguinal hernia. It, too, produces an uncomfortable bulge and may involve other organs, including the bladder.

Inguinal hernias are much less frequent in the female because the inguinal canal contains only a vestigial cord of fibrous tissue. A hernia can occur in females, however, in which the protrusion and the sac are below the groin itself and extend into the upper portion of the thigh alongside the blood vessels supplying the leg (the femoral vessels). There is a small opening in this region through which herniation can occur. This condition is called a femoral hernia.

The presence of either inguinal or femoral hernia requires an operation. Both types only grow larger with time and produce more difficulty. Part of the problem, of course, is their mere presence, plus the discomfort and size. A more serious possiblity is that segments of large or small intestine can enter the sac and cannot be pushed back into the abdomen. This is called an incarcerated inguinal hernia, and when it occurs acutely an urgent operation is recommended. That is because the ring through which the bowel has herniated may constrict the intestine, blocking its blood supply and producing gangrene. This is called strangulation of the bowel. The intestine may be obstructed, too. It is then necessary to remove the strangulated portion of the intestine and bring the severed ends together in an anastomosis. This additional surgery increases risk.

The repair of an ordinary inguinal hernia requires elimination of the emptied hernia sac by dissecting it free from the adjoining tissues, ligating or closing the neck of the sac where it protrudes from the abdomen, then repairing the tissues of the inguinal canal so that herniation does not occur again. The fascia or fibrous tissue and the muscles are brought together over the defect to close it permanently (as shown on page 754). The operation is usually successful, and the hernia does not often return. However, there is always the possibility of a recurrence, for two reasons. First, in the young male particularly, the spermatic cord still must come through the orifice in the abdominal wall and run in the inguinal canal to the testicle. Thus the orifice or internal ring cannot be closed so tightly that it obstructs the blood supply to the testicle or blocks the flow of sperm from the testicle. And it may enlarge in the future and herniate again. In addition, the tissues of an older man can break down with wear and tear, also contributing to recurrence.

The period of recuperation after hernia surgery is much shorter than it once was. Most patients are discharged from the hospital within a day or two, and can return to work within a week. The surgeon usually recommends that the patient abstain from heavy lifting for about six weeks to prevent the wound from separating, but afterwards there is no need to favor the herniated side or to curtail physical activity.

Herniations elsewhere in the abdominal wall are extremely infrequent other than at the site of previous incisions. After an incision in the abdominal wall has been closed and the healing process takes place, there should be no defect through which intestine may protrude. However, the incision may break down or sutures may separate because of stress immediately after the operation, allowing a noticeable herniation later. These incisional hernias can reach enormous size if neglected. They should be repaired when discovered if the patient's health is otherwise satisfactory. Repair consists of reopening the previous incision, dissecting out the edges of the fibrous tissue and muscle of the defect, removing the hernia sac, and closing the abdominal wall.

BREAST OPERATIONS

The chief reason a woman comes to a surgeon is that she has a lump or mass in her breast (see chapter 25, "Breast Cancer"). This condition can arise from a number of causes, including a cyst, chronic cystitic disease, a benign tumor, or breast cancer. Any of these calls for further investigation, which may begin with an X ray of the breast (mammography) and often will require a biopsy. Biopsy means removal of all or part of the lump to determine its composition by microscopic study. The operation may be performed with local or general anesthesia, depending on its location and the preference of the patient and surgeon. At one

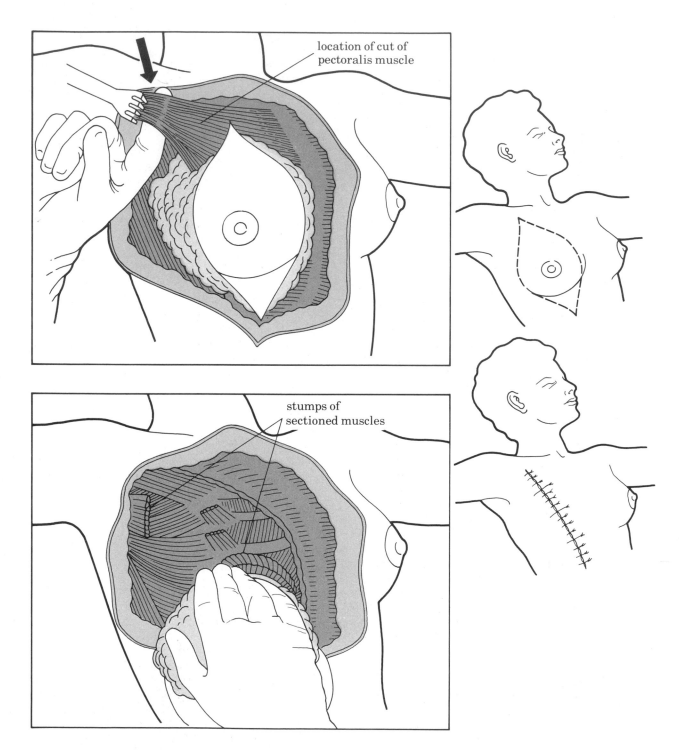

location of cut of
pectoralis muscle

stumps of
sectioned muscles

RADICAL MASTECTOMY

Radical mastectomy for breast cancer removes the entire breast, underlying muscles and lymph nodes, and tissue in the armpit. The drawing at upper right outlines the normal incision. At upper left the skin and breast tissue have been cut free. The pectoralis major and minor muscles leading to the arm will be divided at the arrow to expose the armpit, or axilla, where lymph nodes and tissue overlying the lymphatic vessels will be excised. The muscles then will be removed, as shown at the lower left. The skin is then closed (lower right). Sometimes a skin graft is used to bring the two sides of the wound together.

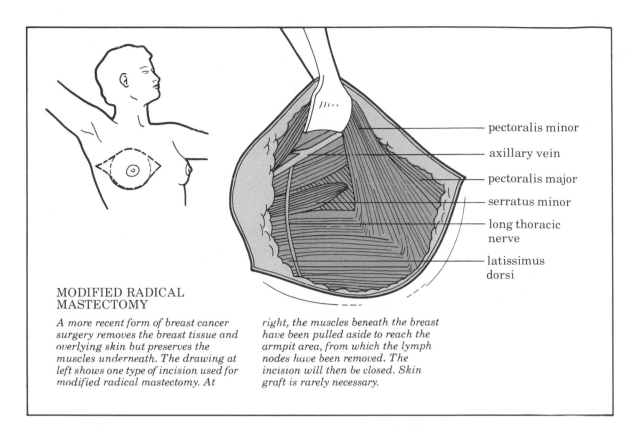

MODIFIED RADICAL MASTECTOMY

pectoralis minor
axillary vein
pectoralis major
serratus minor
long thoracic nerve
latissimus dorsi

A more recent form of breast cancer surgery removes the breast tissue and overlying skin but preserves the muscles underneath. The drawing at left shows one type of incision used for modified radical mastectomy. At

right, the muscles beneath the breast have been pulled aside to reach the armpit area, from which the lymph nodes have been removed. The incision will then be closed. Skin graft is rarely necessary.

time, the microscopic study often was conducted while the woman was still anesthetized. If it was found to be malignant, surgery was performed immediately. Today, the initial operation often is performed for diagnostic purposes only. If the lump is benign, no treatment is necessary. A malignancy calls for treatment, but not always surgery.

There are different types of breast cancer that develop and spread in different ways. The treatment must be based upon the type of cancer, as well as other factors. Treatment of cancer of the breast is changing rapidly, and no single approach is ideal. Modifications of operations and improved irradiation and chemotherapy (drugs) are being developed. Under certain circumstances, any of several approaches may be used.

The standard operation for many years has been the radical mastectomy. This operation requires removal of the entire breast including the site of previous biopsy and all of the skin overlying the breast. The breast tissue itself is completely removed, along with the two sets of underlying muscles from the chest wall to the arm, the pectoralis major and pectoralis minor.

All of the lymphatic tissue draining the breast, and the lymph nodes and lymphatic tissue underneath the arm (the axilla) and along and overlying the nerves and vessels to the arm are removed. The skin of the chest wall is then closed. A skin graft may be used to help close the wound. Radical mastectomy removes the entire tumor plus any potential tumor sites in the remainder of the breast, as well as the lymph nodes draining the breast, which are often the first place for cancer spread.

More recently, the modified radical mastectomy has been used. This operation also removes the entire breast tissue and skin, but the pectoralis major and minor muscles are preserved (after being pulled out of the way temporarily to remove the lymphatic tissue under the arm).

Simple mastectomy involves removing the entire breast tissue and the lymphatic tissue under the arm. The underlying muscles are left in place. Radiation treatment usually follows if the tumor is malignant.

Recently, surgeons have been using another approach, that of wedge excision, or "lumpectomy." The primary tumor itself is taken in a wide removal, but most of the breast is left intact and is reconstructed afterwards. The operation is followed by X-ray treatment of the

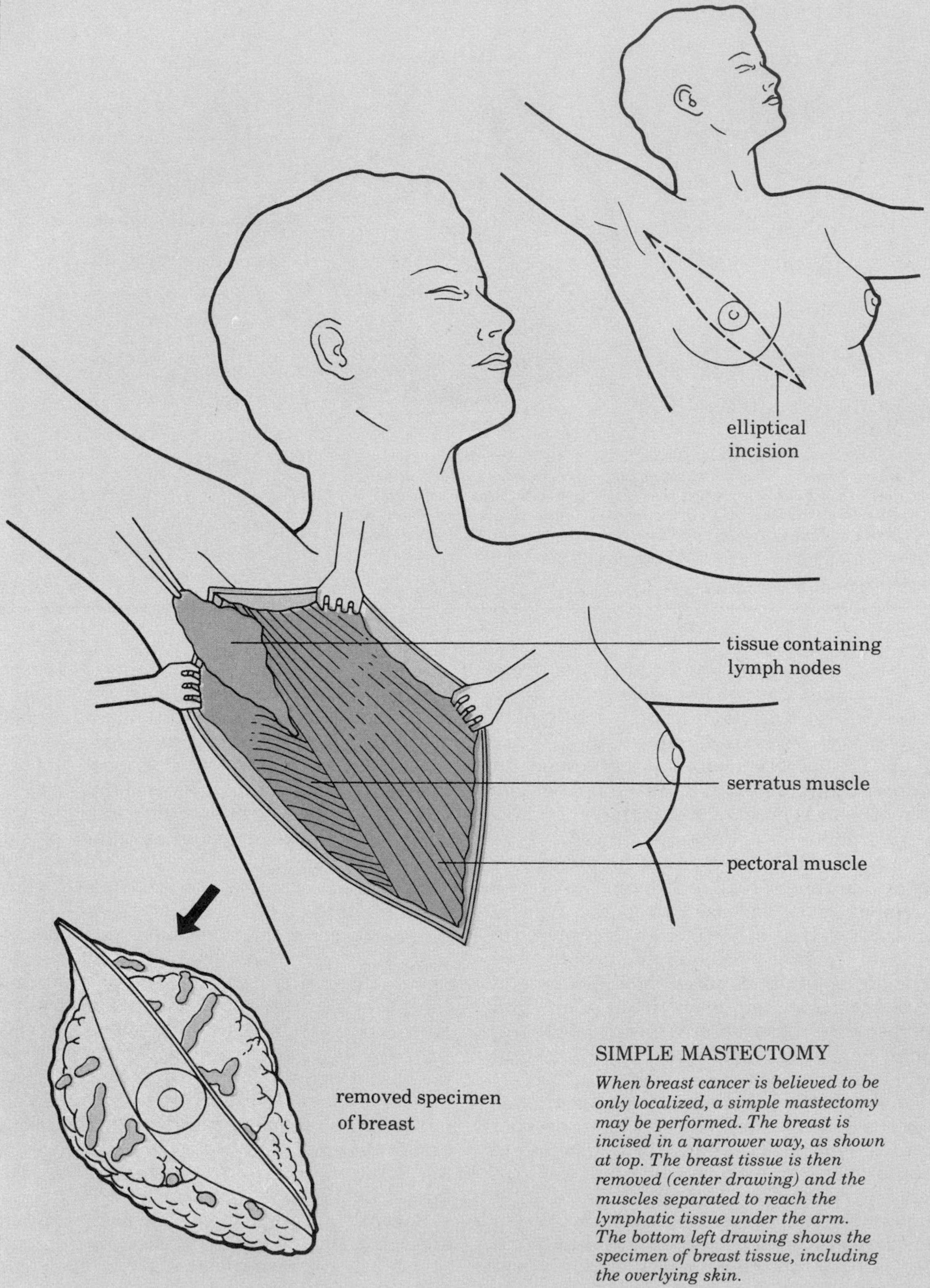

elliptical incision

tissue containing lymph nodes

serratus muscle

pectoral muscle

removed specimen of breast

SIMPLE MASTECTOMY

When breast cancer is believed to be only localized, a simple mastectomy may be performed. The breast is incised in a narrower way, as shown at top. The breast tissue is then removed (center drawing) and the muscles separated to reach the lymphatic tissue under the arm. The bottom left drawing shows the specimen of breast tissue, including the overlying skin.

breast, underarm, and neck. Chemotherapy (drug therapy) may be added. In "lumpectomy" the underarm lymph nodes may be biopsied, or a few removed to determine whether they contain malignancies.

No matter which operation is performed, the decision to use chemotherapy afterward may be made on the basis of whether the lymph nodes in the armpit region (axilla) contain tumor. If the tumor is not discovered until it has spread beyond the breast to the lung, bones, or liver, radiation, chemotherapy, or both are usually recommended instead of surgery.

If the tumor returns after initial treatment or recurs elsewhere in the body, chemotherapy or radiation may be used. Other operations may be recommended if cancer reappears, depending on the age of the patient and the location and problems with the tumor. Sometimes removal of the ovaries (oophorectomy) can be helpful in suppressing the growth of a recurrent tumor. Removal of the adrenal glands or the pituitary gland also can be beneficial.

After mastectomy, some women may elect to have reconstruction of the missing breast by plastic surgery. A Silastic capsule is implanted to form the substance for a new breast. The success of this operation depends on the type of tumor and the amount of tissue removed. Sometimes skin grafts are performed to cover the implanted capsule.

OPERATIONS ON THE
HEAD AND NECK

The thyroid gland. A nodule or lump within the thyroid gland may be a cyst, a benign tumor, or cancer. Often it is necessary to remove the nodule and adjoining thyroid tissue to determine whether the nodule is benign or malignant.

The normal thyroid gland has two lobes that lie on either side of the windpipe. They are joined across the middle by the isthmus of the thyroid. To operate on the thyroid gland, a transverse incision is made in the neck just above the clavicles or collarbones. The overlying neck muscles are then divided in the middle and held to the sides to expose the thyroid

gland. The gland and nodule can then be inspected. Usually a nodule is found on only one side of the gland and that lobe is removed (lobectomy). With a benign tumor and certain forms of cancer, lobectomy may be sufficient. For other forms of cancer it may be necessary to remove the thyroid totally (thyroidectomy). Afterwards, the patient must take thyroid hormone by mouth.

Goiter, another form of thyroid disease, is decreasing in frequency. A goiter is enlargement of the thyroid gland, often to massive size. The extraordinary growth usually is caused by lack of iodine in the diet, but may arise from other causes. Although relatively painless, the bulge on the neck can become so huge that it is unsightly, uncomfortable, and may hamper breathing. The goiter then must be removed surgically. A small portion of the thyroid tissue is left on either side of the trachea to provide thyroid hormone. This procedure is called a subtotal thyroidectomy.

Overactivity of the thyroid gland is called hyperthyroidism. It usually causes enlargement of the gland, too, but not to such large proportions as goiter. Hyperthyroidism produces other symptoms, however, including nervousness, loss of weight, and bulging of the eyes. In the past hyperthyroidism was almost always treated by removal of much of the thyroid gland (subtotal thyroidectomy) after preparation of the patient with antithyroid drugs and iodine compounds. More recently, many patients with hyperthyroidism have been treated with radioactive iodine or other drugs. An operation is still necessary, however, in some cases, particularly in young patients in whom the risk posed by the radioactivity may be of concern. The operation for hyperthyroidism removes all of the thyroid gland except for two small fragments on both sides of the neck, enough for normal thyroid function. A hazard of any thyroid gland operation is the possibility of injuring the nearby laryngeal nerves. These small nerves run underneath the thyroid gland into the larynx and control the vocal cords. Damage to one of these nerves can paralyze one of the vocal cords and produce a hoarse or husky voice.

The parathyroid glands. The parathyroids are small endocrine organs adjoining the thyroid gland, two on either side, usually just above and below the thyroid lobes. These glands secrete a hormone called parathormone, which controls calcium metabolism. There are several diseases of the parathyroid glands that mandate an operation. Overactivity of the parathyroid glands produces a disorder of calcium metabolism. Stones may form in

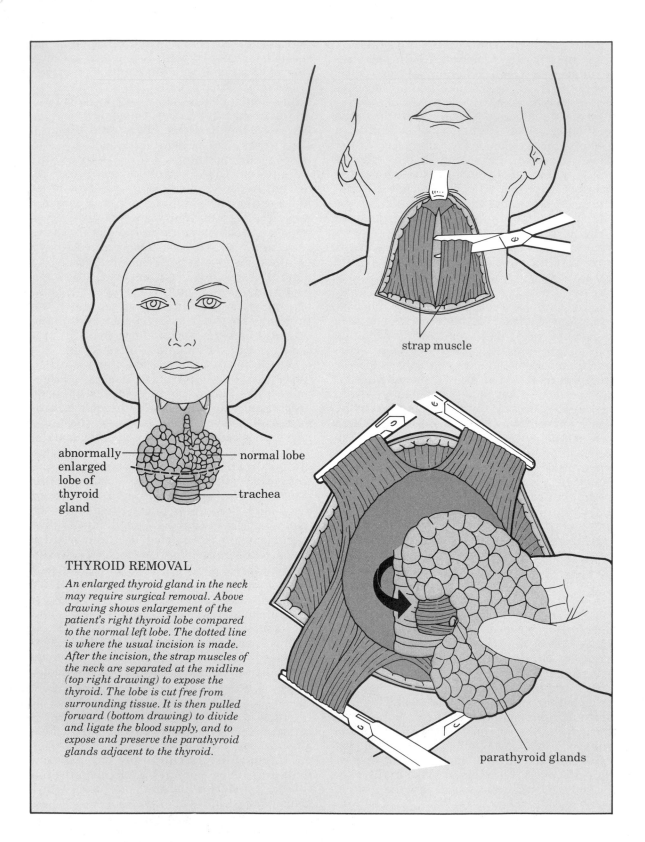

abnormally enlarged lobe of thyroid gland

normal lobe

trachea

strap muscle

parathyroid glands

THYROID REMOVAL

An enlarged thyroid gland in the neck may require surgical removal. Above drawing shows enlargement of the patient's right thyroid lobe compared to the normal left lobe. The dotted line is where the usual incision is made. After the incision, the strap muscles of the neck are separated at the midline (top right drawing) to expose the thyroid. The lobe is cut free from surrounding tissue. It is then pulled forward (bottom drawing) to divide and ligate the blood supply, and to expose and preserve the parathyroid glands adjacent to the thyroid.

the kidneys (see chapter 22) or the amount of calcium in the bones may decrease. This overactivity may stem from enlargement of all of the parathyroid glands, called hyperplasia, or from a benign tumor of one or more of them, called an adenoma. Either one calls for an exploratory operation to inspect the glands and perhaps to perform a biopsy. It may be necessary to remove one or more of the glands.

A number of diseases other than those of the thyroid gland may produce a lump in the neck. Certain congenital problems are found in young children. The most common cause of a lump in the neck of an adult is enlargement of a lymph gland or node. It may be benign, it may be associated with inflammation of the nose, throat, or ears, it may be caused by spread of a malignancy from somewhere in the nose or throat, or it may be a primary process or malignancy arising in a lymph node, as in Hodgkin's disease or lymphoma. Such lumps may require removal by operation to determine their exact nature.

Tumors in the mouth, on the tongue, throat, or lip are most commonly squamous-cell carcinomas, a form of skin cancer arising from the surface of the mucous membranes of the mouth (see chapter 7, "The Skin"). Many are readily visible, and usually are detected promptly. To remove them while still superficial is a simple office procedure under local anesthesia. This is particularly true of tumors of the lip or face. However, tumors of the tongue and mouth require more extensive removal. If the tumor has spread to the lymph nodes in the neck, removal of the primary tumor must be followed by what is called a radical neck dissection. An incision is made in the neck. The subcutaneous tissue, the sternocleidomastoid muscle (one of the major muscles in the neck), and all of the lymph nodes overlying the main blood vessels are removed. This operation is designed to remove all lymph nodes involved with the cancer and to prevent its recurrence.

OPERATIONS ON THE RECTUM AND ANUS

The last short segment of the colon above the anus is the site of the most common type of cancer in both men and women. It is also the location of benign but painful conditions that sometimes call for the surgeon's attention. The rectal area is a series of pockets, pleats, and tucks, the natural result of the gathering effects of the purse-string muscle that closes the natural opening. Inflammation, swelling, and infection can occur in these areas, and surgery may be necessary to correct it.

An anal fissure is a tear in the lining of the anal canal or its mucous membranes. The result is bleeding and pain during a bowel movement. It usually is caused by constipation or straining at stool. The doctor usually tries first to treat a fissure with stool softeners, changes in diet, medication to stimulate regular bowel movements, or sitz baths. If the fissure does not heal, it may be necessary to operate and remove it. The sphincter muscle may be dilated to keep pressure off the site until it heals.

A fistula occurs when one of the glandular crevices of the anus, called a crypt, becomes inflamed or infected. The infection may burrow through the soft flesh and produce an abnormal opening to the outside a tiny distance from the natural opening. The initial treatment is the same as for a fissure, but if preliminary treatment is not successful, an operation may be necessary. The procedure opens the fistula or excises it and dilates the anal sphincter to allow healing.

Hemorrhoids are dilated veins covered by folds of skin just within or outside the anal canal. They result from inflammation in the anal canal, aggravated by pressure such as straining during a bowel movement. They are often classified as internal, arising inside the rectum and sometimes extending to the outside, or external, when the vein dilates outside the anal opening. Hemorrhoids frequently exist without symptoms, but occasionally they may bleed or cause pain during bowel movements.

Hemorrhoids can be prevented by careful attention to diet to achieve regular, soft bowel movements without straining, and by scrupulous cleansing of the anal region, including washing within the external portion of the anal opening. Hemorrhoids should be treated initially by exactly the same approach as for a fistula or fissure. Medication applied externally also may be helpful to soothe the inflammation. Sometimes a blood clot may form in a hemorrhoid, or a ring of hemorrhoids around the anus may become so large and bulky that they cause painful bowel movements. These may be removed in a simple office procedure called a hemorrhoidectomy, with the aid of a local anesthetic. Islands of mucosa and skin are left between the hemorrhoids to hasten healing.

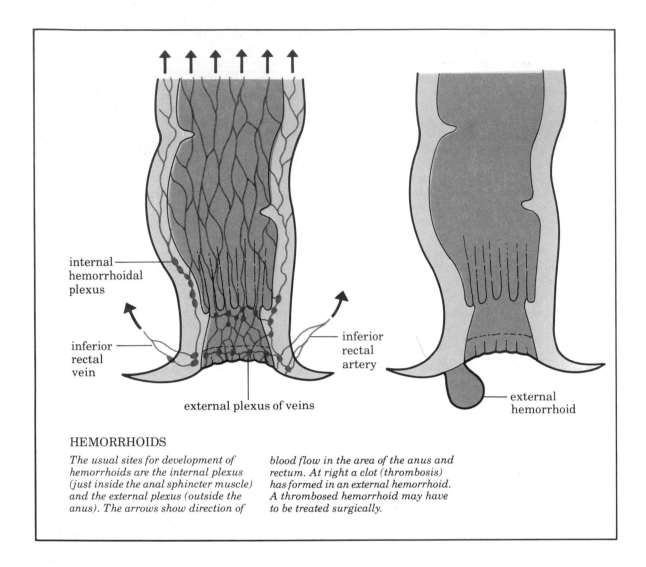

internal
hemorrhoidal
plexus

inferior
rectal
vein

inferior
rectal
artery

external plexus of veins

external
hemorrhoid

HEMORRHOIDS

*The usual sites for development of
hemorrhoids are the internal plexus
(just inside the anal sphincter muscle)
and the external plexus (outside the
anus). The arrows show direction of*
*blood flow in the area of the anus and
rectum. At right a clot (thrombosis)
has formed in an external hemorrhoid.
A thrombosed hemorrhoid may have
to be treated surgically.*

AMPUTATIONS

Amputations of injured limbs and appendages have been one of the historic roles of surgeons. In the past it often was necessary to remove an arm, leg, finger, or toe because it had been so badly damaged or crushed in a farm or industrial accident that repair was impossible. In addition, the injury threatened to spread infection to the rest of the body so that the limb had to be sacrificed to save a life. This is the reason amputations were such a common consequence of war. More recently, however, the development of antibiotics has lessened the risks of infection, and improved surgical techniques have enabled surgeons to save many limbs that previously might have been lost. Indeed, it is now sometimes possible to restore a limb that has been cleanly severed.

Reimplantation surgery is the name given to the reattachment of a severed body part. It is a delicate, difficult, and prolonged procedure, requiring specialized equipment. Much of the work must be done under magnification, using tiny instruments. The first step is to reconnect the severed blood vessels by anastomosis. The major arteries and veins are brought together using suture material finer than a human hair. Severed muscles and tendons must be reattached, then the bony structures, where this is possible. Nerves may be reunited during the initial operation, or nerve repair may be delayed until the skin has been closed and allowed to heal. Functional results for reimplantation of fingers and hands have been better than for entire arms and legs because nerve repair has not been as successful in larger parts. Nonetheless, results have been encouraging enough that surgeons now urge that when a part is amputated cleanly, it should be preserved on ice until the person and the part can be transported to a hospital for possible reimplantation.

Amputation itself is still necessary for particularly extensive or crushing injuries and for the effects of certain diseases. Tumors of the bone, tendon, soft tissue, or skin may force amputation to prevent spread of the disease. Arteriosclerosis or diabetes also may make amputation necessary. In the case of arteriosclerosis, arterial hardening may gradually reduce or block blood flow to the legs, causing damage to the tissues supplied by these arteries, and perhaps causing gangrene. Reduced blood supply and reduced sensation in the legs and feet because of nerve damage are consequences of long-term diabetes, which can ultimately lead to gangrene.

Amputation of any part for whatever cause is a relatively straightforward procedure. The exact steps depend on the part and the extent of the damage. In most cases, the entire damaged area of bone is cut away, the blood vessels and nerves tied off, and a flap of skin sewn over the stump of the part to allow for better fitting of an artificial part, or prosthesis. Where possible, the surgeon will attempt to save the joint. If arteriosclerosis has damaged a foot and ankle, the surgeon will prefer to amputate below the knee rather than above it. In some cases, however, above-the-knee amputation is required.

Prostheses used following amputation are another area of recent advance. It is now possible to fit an amputee with an artificial limb or appendage that allows him or her to function virtually normally, not only to walk without a limp but to run and even engage in sports.

OPERATIONS ON BLOOD VESSELS

Injuries to blood vessels are common and may require repair by operation, either joining the ends of the severed blood vessels by anastomosis or replacing the damaged vessel by a graft. Injury may produce an abnormal connection between an artery and a vein (an arteriovenous fistula) which must be corrected. Congenital abnormalities of blood vessels also require correction.

Arteriosclerosis, or hardening of the arteries, and its consequences are a more frequent cause for surgery on the blood vessels. This degenerative disease, common in older persons, leads to thickening of the arterial walls. Fatty material is deposited on the wall,

first narrowing the inner channel or lumen (stenosis), and finally producing an occlusion or complete block so that blood supply is reduced to tissues served by the artery.

In addition, blood pressure may be elevated, causing a blood vessel wall to become thin and bulge. This outpouching is called an aneurysm. When it reaches a certain size, the aneurysm may rupture and bleed. Although aneurysm can occur anywhere, the most common site is the abdominal aorta, the main artery below the diaphragm. There an aneurysm may form a large pulsating mass, which the patient or a physician can feel. As it expands, it may cause pain in the back, the abdomen, or the flanks. Severe pain usually means that the aneurysm is expanding rapidly or beginning to leak or rupture.

A ruptured aneurysm, even when treated promptly, is associated with a high mortality rate because so much blood is lost before the hemorrhage can be stopped. If the aneurysm is discovered before it ruptures, however, it can be treated quite satisfactorily by an operation. The ballooned portion of the vessel is removed. The section of the artery is replaced with a synthetic or plastic graft, usually of woven or knitted Dacron.

Narrowing and occlusion of blood vessels occur most commonly where blood vessels branch. A common site is in the carotid arteries in the neck, which supply blood to the brain. Narrowing in the internal carotid branch may result initially in attacks of dizziness, light-headedness, loss of memory, and other symptoms that together are called transient ischemic attacks. A stroke may occur at the onset or with persistence of symptoms, with temporary or permanent damage to the brain tissue caused by the loss of blood supply. If transient ischemic attacks bring attention to the narrowing before a stroke occurs, an operation can be performed to remove the inner lining of the thickened portion of the artery and restore normal blood flow to the brain. This operation is called a carotid thromboendarterectomy (see chapter 11, "Stroke"). Results to date have been good with extremely low risk and few complications.

The next most common site for arteriosclerotic narrowing is in the blood vessels supplying the legs. This often occurs in the superficial femoral artery, which passes from the groin through the thigh to the lower leg behind the knee. Blockage of this major artery initially causes pain in the calf muscles while walking. The condition is termed intermittent claudication (see chapter 5, "Blood Vessel Disorders"). The pain will often go away completely if the person stops or sits for a few minutes. Eventually the disease may narrow other blood vessels, too, with pain in the foot or leg even at rest. There also may be numbness and tingling. If the process becomes even more extensive it may lead to gangrene of the foot, ankle, and lower leg, requiring amputation.

To determine the location and extent of vascular disease, arteriography is performed. A needle is inserted into the artery, dye injected, and X rays obtained. If the person's legs hurt while resting, an operation should be considered. If pain only occurs with exercise, but is severe and limits the patient, an operation may depend on the findings and general health of the patient.

The customary operation for diminished blood supply to the legs is a bypass graft. A conduit is brought from above the block in the artery to a vessel below it. If the block or narrowing is in the abdominal aorta or its major branches coming down to the groin, the bypass is made with a plastic prosthetic graft called an aortic bifurcation graft. A Y graft is put in, with the stem of the Y coming from the aorta and each limb of the Y going down in the groin to the femoral artery in either leg. When a bypass graft is to be carried out from the femoral artery at the groin down to the popliteal artery entering the lower leg behind the knee, the surgeon usually will use one of the patient's veins. The choice is usually the saphenous vein, which lies near the surface in the thigh and calf. It is big enough and experience has shown that it will serve as a conduit for many years. The saphenous vein, however, has valves to help blood move against the flow of gravity from the foot back toward the heart. The vein must therefore be reversed in a bypass so that blood flows to open the valves rather than against the valves, which would close them and lead to an occlusion.

A narrowed vessel sometimes may develop a blood clot in the narrowed segment. This is a thrombosis which can cause acute life-threatening or limb-threatening changes requiring immediate treatment.

A common problem after any operation is the formation of blood clots in leg veins. This is because the patient must lie flat during the operation. Normal muscle action, which squeezes the veins of the calf and moves the blood back to the heart, does not take place. Circulation may be sluggish and coagulation heightened. One consequence may be thrombophlebitis, with pain in the calves or swelling in the legs. The gravest threat, however, is the possibility that the clot will break off and migrate to the lung, where it lodges and blocks a blood vessel. This is called a pulmonary embolism, and can produce serious difficulty or be immediately fatal if the clot is large.

OPERATIONS ON THE LUNGS AND ESOPHAGUS

The Lungs

Surgical treatment may be needed for several problems of the lungs, including chest injury, infection that does not clear up, abscesses, birth defects, and tumors.

Pneumothorax occurs when air finds its way outside the lung and into the thoracic cavity, compressing the lung, interfering with breathing, and producing chest pain. This is most commonly caused by rupture of a bleb, a small ballooned area at the top of the lung. To treat pneumothorax, a tube is inserted into the chest or pleural cavity. The tube is connected to a drain that terminates under water. As the patient breathes in, water rises in the tube; as the patient exhales, air is forced out of the pleural space and bubbles through the water as it is released. This water seal allows the ruptured area eventually to seal, the lung to expand, and the air to be eliminated from the chest space. The same method is used after any chest operation to remove blood, fluid, or air. This is necessary because during breathing, negative pressure is generated within the chest by expansion of the chest wall and movement of the diaphragms, which allows air to flow through the mouth or nose, through the trachea into the lungs, and then out again.

Tumors of the lung may be benign, called adenomas, or malignant (see chapter 8, "The Lungs"). There are a number of different types of lung cancers, each requiring individual and separate approaches to treatment. Commonly, the suspicion of tumor is raised when the patient begins to cough up blood (hemoptysis), leading to a chest X ray, or has a routine screening examination in which a mass or shadow is detected. Diagnostic tests are then undertaken to determine whether the mass or shadow is an inflammatory process, such as pneumonia, or a benign or malignant tumor.

An early step is usually bronchoscopy, visual inspection of the trachea and bronchi. The new generation of fiberoptic instruments allows the physician to look down into very small bronchi and obtain biopsies of tissue or scrapings using a small brush. Often the exact nature of the lesion can be determined by this technique. But it is not always possible to identify the precise cause of the shadow. It then becomes necessary to perform an exploratory thoracotomy, with an incision in the chest and separation of the ribs. A small nodule on the surface of the lung may be removed by excising only that portion of the lung (wedge excision) and repairing the adjoining portion with sutures or by using a stapling device that fires a small row of staples across the tissue. Stapling devices are helpful in operations on the lung because the tissue is thin and easily broken or pulverized. Any portion of the lung that is cut leaks air, which can be stopped with such a device. If the nodule is larger but is still thought to be benign, the surgeon may remove a portion of the affected lobe of lung, called a segmental resection. If the suspicious shadow represents a benign or malignant tumor limited to one lobe of the lung, only that lobe is removed (lobectomy).

However, if the tumor is extensive or involves the origin of the main bronchus to a lung, it may be necessary to remove the entire lung (pneumonectomy). In this procedure, the pulmonary artery, which runs from the heart to the lungs, is ligated and divided, as are the pulmonary veins, which run from the lungs to the heart. Then the bronchus is divided close to the trachea and the lung removed. The stump of the bronchus is closed by sutures or a stapling device. The cavity in the chest where the lung was gradually fills with fluid after the operation and later becomes fibrous tissue. Removal of a lung can be well tolerated if the other lung is healthy enough. Patients live normally for many years afterwards.

Esophagus

Hiatus hernia (see page 741) is the most common problem of the esophagus requiring an operation. The organ also may develop benign tumors, which can be removed easily, or abnormalities of motion such as achalasia, which can be treated by operation.

Cancer may develop in any portion of the esophagus, but is most common in the lower third, nearest the stomach. Unfortunately many esophageal cancers are quite extensive when discovered, because the cancer must be large before it interferes with swallowing, the usual initial symptom. By then, the cancer already may have invaded adjoining structures, including the back, the heart, the diaphragm,

and the lungs. If the cancer has not spread, it should be removed promptly. The operation may require an incision in the abdomen to free the stomach from its attachments, after which an incision is made in the chest. The tumor and much of the esophagus are then removed. Continuity is usually restored by joining the esophagus above the tumor to the stomach below the tumor, bringing the stomach up into the chest as a gastric tube.

HEART OPERATIONS

Probably no field of surgery has made such tremendous advances in recent decades as that of operations on the heart. There are two types of heart problems that may require an operation, congenital heart defects and acquired heart disease, and both have benefited from the strides in contemporary heart surgery.

The giant steps forward date from the development of the heart-lung machine. Abnormalities within the heart can be treated directly only by what is called an open-heart procedure, and in such circumstances it is necessary to use cardiopulmonary bypass. The heart-lung machine is designed to take over the work of the heart and the lungs temporarily, allowing the surgeon to work inside the heart without the heart beating. The apparatus has two basic components. Blood from the body passes through an oxygenator, where it receives oxygen and rids itself of carbon dioxide. The blood is filtered of debris and impurities and goes to the next basic component, the pump, to be sent back into the circulation. In some heart-lung machines, the blood is cooled during the operation to protect the organs. Blood from the operative field is brought back to the machine by a suction device so that it is conserved. During this procedure the patient must be given an anticoagulant drug to keep the blood from clotting.

Congenital heart defects usually are discovered in infancy or early childhood. These abnormalities may be as simple as a "hole" in the heart (in which a partition has failed to close), an atrial or ventricular septal defect, or failure of a valve to develop and open properly, producing a narrowing or stenosis, such as pulmonary valvular stenosis. Another defect occurs when an opening that was necessary in fetal life fails to close after birth (patent ductus arteriosus). Others include failure of the inner channel of a major blood vessel to develop, pro-

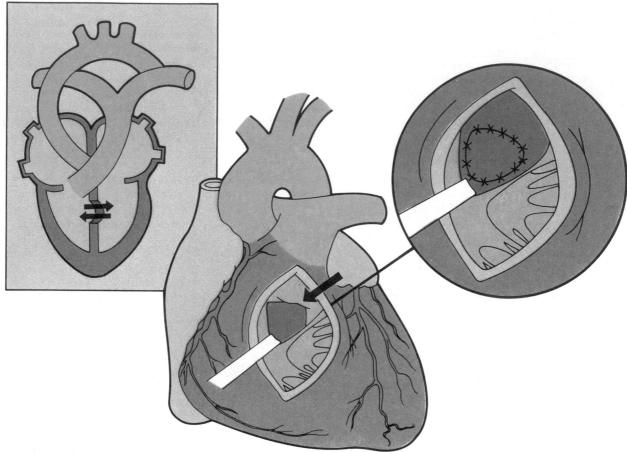

SEPTAL DEFECT

An abnormal opening in the wall between the heart's right and left ventricles, called an interventricular septal defect, allows oxygenated and unoxygenated blood to mix, as shown by the arrows in the inset drawing. The defect can be closed by inserting a patch of tissue during open-heart surgery. A heart-lung machine maintains circulation while the surgeon works on the bypassed heart. In the middle drawing a retractor exposes the opening (arrow) between the two ventricles. At right, the patch has been fitted into place with small interrupted sutures around its entire circumference.

ducing coarctation of the aorta, and narrowing of the aorta beyond the aortic arch.

Some of the more simple and straightforward congenital problems can be corrected shortly after birth or during early years of childhood. Patent ductus arteriosus can be eliminated by ligation or division of the ductus. The ductus arteriosus is a short tube connecting the aorta and the pulmonary artery, which, if it remains open after birth, carries blood to the lungs. Before birth, the lungs do not function and the ductus arteriosus allows blood to bypass them. It normally closes at birth. If it does not, it is said to be patent, and must be closed so that aortic blood does not pass into the lungs and increase pressure.

Coarctation of the aorta is corrected by cutting out the narrowed section of this important blood vessel and bringing the severed ends together. If the narrowed segment is long, it may be necessary to insert a graft.

In the past, some of the severe congenital cardiac defects required some procedure shortly after birth to help the infant get by until he or she grew a bit and a total correction could be carried out with the aid of the heart-lung machine. In recent years, however, even newborns have been operated on using the heart-lung machine. The procedure has been made safer by hypothermia, which means lowering the infant's temperature so organs will better tolerate a period without blood.

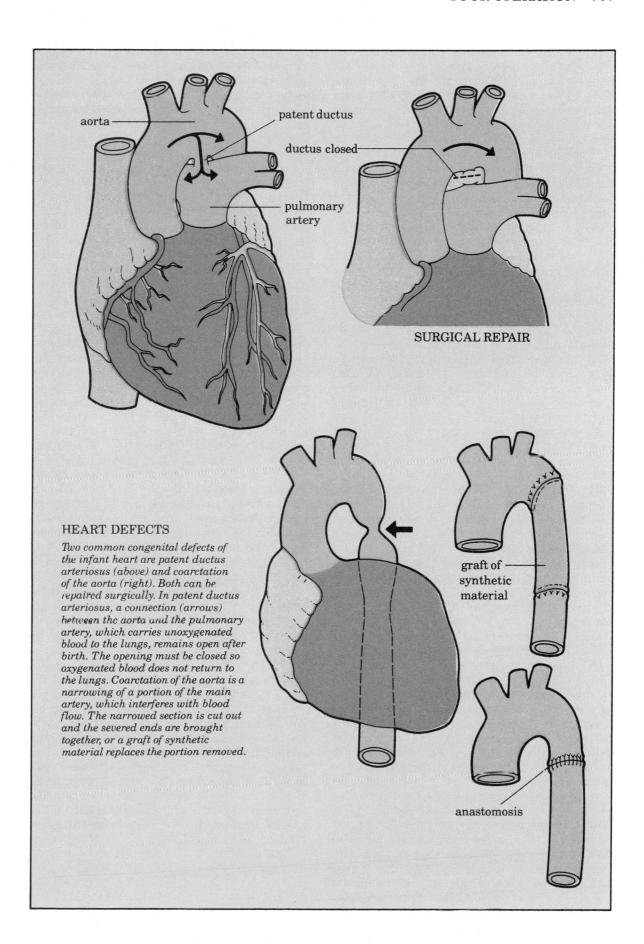

aorta

patent ductus

ductus closed

pulmonary artery

SURGICAL REPAIR

HEART DEFECTS

Two common congenital defects of the infant heart are patent ductus arteriosus (above) and coarctation of the aorta (right). Both can be repaired surgically. In patent ductus arteriosus, a connection (arrows) between the aorta and the pulmonary artery, which carries unoxygenated blood to the lungs, remains open after birth. The opening must be closed so oxygenated blood does not return to the lungs. Coarctation of the aorta is a narrowing of a portion of the main artery, which interferes with blood flow. The narrowed section is cut out and the severed ends are brought together, or a graft of synthetic material replaces the portion removed.

graft of synthetic material

anastomosis

Acquired heart diseases, disease of the cardiac valves, and coronary artery disease are usually considered separate entities. Ironically, however, as patients with valvular heart disease have been enabled to survive longer, many are developing combinations of valvular disease and coronary artery disease together.

Valvular heart disease in an adult usually occurs as the aftermath of rheumatic fever and rheumatic heart disease (see chapter 3, "The Heart and Circulation"). It primarily involves the mitral valve between the heart's two left chambers, the left atrium and the left ventricle, or the aortic valve at the outlet of the left ventricle to the aorta, where blood enters the general circulation. Sometimes aortic valve disease results from a birth defect. The valve normally has three leaflets, but some persons are born with a two-leaflet aortic valve, a bicuspid valve rather than the normal tricuspid valve. Later in life calcium deposits or other abnormalities may form in the defective valve, producing narrowing (stenosis) or leakage. A valve that becomes loose or dilated so that blood leaks back is called a regurgitant or insufficient valve.

Coronary artery disease, in which the vessels that bring blood to the heart are narrowed or blocked, may also produce abnormalities of the cardiac valves, particularly the mitral valve. And, as part of the aging process, the fibrous bands that hold the mitral valve (chordae tendinae) can rupture, producing mitral regurgitation. Disease of the pulmonary valve leading to the lungs is rare in adults. Disease of the tricuspid valve between the heart's right chambers is usually secondary to disease of the mitral valve, producing backup of blood through the lungs and into the right side of the heart.

The first operation to be performed on heart valves was a mitral commissurotomy, or mitral valvotomy, in which, with the heart beating, a finger was inserted through an appendage of the left atrium into the narrowed valve to push it open. The valve often would function satisfactorily thereafter. Gradually surgeons learned to use instruments for this purpose. This operation is still performed occasionally on patients who have only mitral stenosis and no complications.

In most cases, however, when valve disease produces symptoms or problems and interferes with the patient's normal life, the valve must be replaced. One of the more exciting areas of medicine is the development of artificial valves of the heart. There are a number of artificial valves, each with a slightly different purpose. The two basic types are a ball-and-cage valve and a flat or disk valve. Commonly, the replacement for an aortic valve is taken from the heart of a pig. The tissue is processed and preserved by fixing solutions, then attached to a ring, sterilized, and sewn into the heart. Such porcine valves have been in place for as long as ten years, and are being used more extensively. Plastic valves are also used and some appear to last indefinitely.

Replacement of an aortic or a mitral valve requires an open-heart procedure using the heart-lung machine. The incision is made in the midline of the chest dividing the sternum and approaching the forward surface of the heart. This is called a median sternotomy. The silent heart is opened, and the diseased valve removed. The replacement valve is sewn in place, using strong nonabsorbable sutures. Afterward the edges of the divided sternum are held together with wires, allowing it to heal.

Coronary artery disease is arteriosclerosis, or narrowing of the small arteries that bring blood from the aorta to the heart muscle, the myocardium. There are two main coronary arteries, right and left. The left artery divides into two major branches, the left anterior descending coronary artery and the circumflex artery. Any or all of these vessels can become narrowed or totally obstructed. The initial symptom usually is chest pain during exertion, called angina pectoris, caused by inadequate blood supply to the heart. Angina itself does not usually produce heart damage. Unfortunately many men and women have as their first symptom sudden severe chest pain followed by myocardial infarction ("heart attack") or death of a portion of the heart muscle. The lucky patient recovers. Many die.

A great step forward was taken when it became possible to study obstructed coronary blood vessels by coronary arteriography. In this technique a small tube (catheter) is inserted into the femoral artery in the groin or into the brachial artery at the elbow, threaded up into the aorta, and then into each of the coronary arteries. A dye is injected that can be seen on X ray. A moving picture is taken before, during, and after injection of the dye to watch the blood flow in the coronary arteries and identify the areas of narrowing.

The coronary bypass operation developed from arteriography. The bypass most commonly uses the large superficial veins of the thighs and legs, the saphenous veins, to build a conduit around the obstruction in an artery.

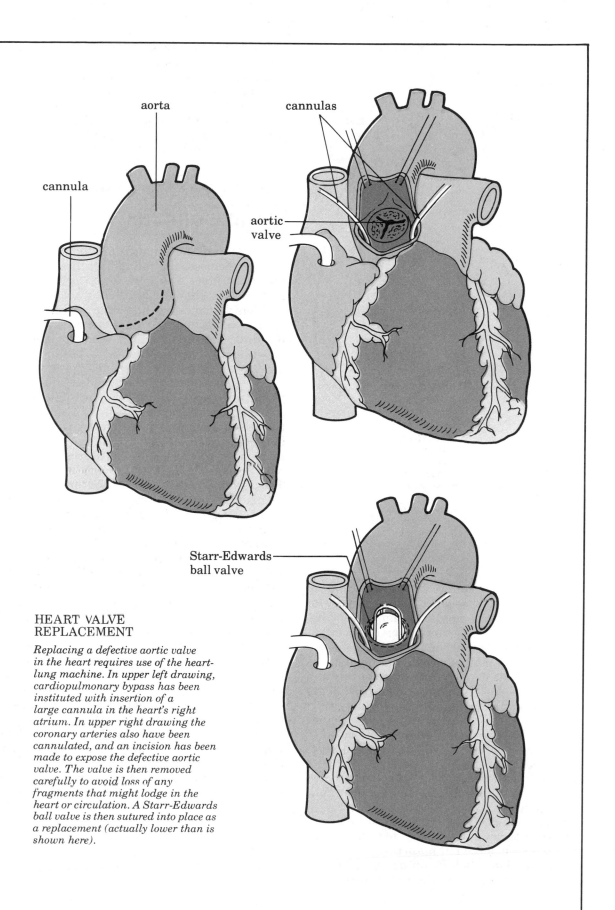

aorta

cannula

cannulas

aortic
valve

Starr-Edwards
ball valve

HEART VALVE REPLACEMENT

Replacing a defective aortic valve in the heart requires use of the heart-lung machine. In upper left drawing, cardiopulmonary bypass has been instituted with insertion of a large cannula in the heart's right atrium. In upper right drawing the coronary arteries also have been cannulated, and an incision has been made to expose the defective aortic valve. The valve is then removed carefully to avoid loss of any fragments that might lodge in the heart or circulation. A Starr-Edwards ball valve is then sutured into place as a replacement (actually lower than is shown here).

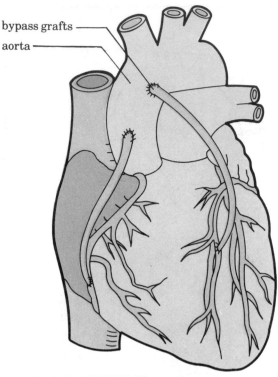

bypass grafts
aorta

CORONARY BYPASS

The technique of bypassing a blocked coronary artery uses a saphenous vein from the leg. Above, grafts have been made from the aorta to the right coronary artery (left side of drawing) and the left anterior descending artery. Because the saphenous veins contain valves, they must be reversed so that blood flow is not restricted.

The bypass graft comes from the ascending aorta just above the heart and runs with an anastomosis to the small coronary artery beyond the point of narrowing or obstruction. The internal mammary artery lying along the chest wall also may be used for a conduit.

Bypass grafts usually are carried out around any vessel more than 50 percent obstructed. As many as six grafts may be carried out in an individual patient, depending on the circumstances. The operation cannot be performed in every case, however, The indications for coronary bypass grafting are:
• Severe angina pectoris with activity, which interferes with the patient's livelihood or ability to enjoy life.
• Certain types of obstruction frequently associated with severe difficulty and death, such as obstruction of the left main coronary artery.
• Complications such as an aneurysm of the ventricle or disorders of the mitral valve.

There has been debate about whether a patient's life expectancy is increased by a bypass operation. The experience of many surgeons now indicates that this is indeed the case. More time is necessary, however, to evaluate the long-term effects. However, a bypass can be done safely, it relieves symptoms, and many patients are enthusiastic about the result.

OPERATIONS ON THE
FEMALE ORGANS

Disorders of the female reproductive system (uterus, ovaries, the fallopian tubes, and vagina) may involve only one organ, or the entire system (see chapter 24). The most common problem is abnormal bleeding, which can be excessive bleeding during menstrual periods, bleeding between periods, and spotting or bleeding after menopause. These abnormalities, if persistent, are investigated by the most common operation for women, dilatation and curettage, or "D and C." The dilatation is to open the mouth of the uterus, the cervix, and the cervical canal with the passage of dilators of gradually larger size. Curettage consists of scraping the interior of the uterus or womb with a long-handled, spoon-like instrument. The tissue obtained is submitted for pathological examination. A biopsy of the cervix may be taken. "D and C" is usually performed with general anesthesia but seldom requires more than an overnight stay in a hospital.

A common abnormality of the uterus is development of a benign tumor called a fibroid. Fibroid tumors can reach the size of a grapefruit. A number of them may develop in the uterus simultaneously. After menopause they usually decrease in size. Fibroids seldom present great difficulty for a woman. An operation is not often necessary to remove them, nor is surgery frequently needed for abnormal bleeding before menopause. Occasionally, however, either problem may lead to a recommendation for total removal of the uterus (hysterectomy), which could be accepted by the patient. Thus removal of the uterus may be necessary even though the condition is benign.

Hysterectomy for whatever reason is carried out by an incision in the lower abdomen, as shown on page 771. The incision can be ver-

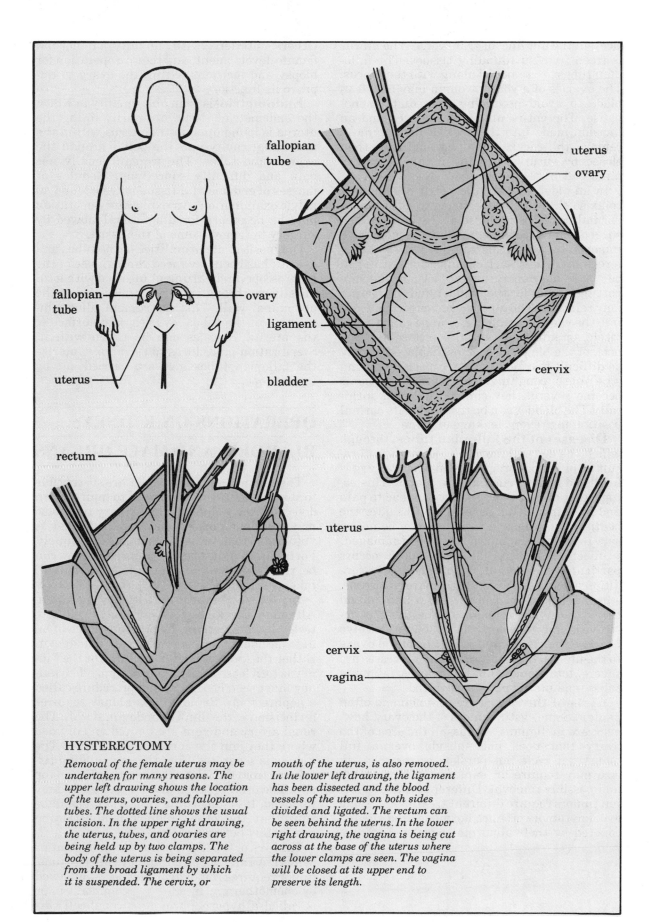

fallopian tube

ovary

uterus

fallopian tube

uterus

ovary

ligament

cervix

bladder

rectum

uterus

uterus

cervix

vagina

HYSTERECTOMY

Removal of the female uterus may be undertaken for many reasons. The upper left drawing shows the location of the uterus, ovaries, and fallopian tubes. The dotted line shows the usual incision. In the upper right drawing, the uterus, tubes, and ovaries are being held up by two clamps. The body of the uterus is being separated from the broad ligament by which it is suspended. The cervix, or

mouth of the uterus, is also removed. In the lower left drawing, the ligament has been dissected and the blood vessels of the uterus on both sides divided and ligated. The rectum can be seen behind the uterus. In the lower right drawing, the vagina is being cut across at the base of the uterus where the lower clamps are seen. The vagina will be closed at its upper end to preserve its length.

tical, in the midline, or transverse. The uterus is freed from surrounding tissues. The fallopian tubes are removed along with the uterus. The ovaries of a young woman may be left in place to avoid producing immediate menopause. The entire uterus is removed and an incision made into the apex of the vagina to remove the cervix, too. The vagina is then closed by sutures, making it into a kind of blind pouch.

In an older woman, the pelvic organs may relax so that the uterus tends to fall from its normal position (prolapse of the uterus). The surgeon may recommend that the uterus be removed by way of the vagina, a vaginal hysterectomy. Under such circumstances, this can be a safe, easy operation. Sometimes the supporting tissues for the bladder and the rectum may relax too. The bladder may protrude down into the vagina, producing a bulge called a cystocele, or into the rectum, a rectocele. If the neck of the bladder becomes displaced, it may be difficult to control urine, especially during straining or coughing. If any of these problems become severe, they can be corrected surgically. The bladder can be restored to its normal position to prevent leakage of urine.

Diseases of the fallopian tubes, through which the egg cell normally descends, can result from a tubal pregnancy in which an egg is fertilized before reaching the uterus. This ectopic (out-of-place) pregnancy can lead to pain and bleeding within several months after the beginning of the pregnancy. It may be necessary to remove the tube if it has been damaged.

Infection in the fallopian tubes occurs particularly as a result of gonorrhea. The condition is called pelvic inflammatory disease. Abscesses may form in the tubes and around the ovaries. The function of the tubes is destroyed, and the woman is unable to conceive because the egg cannot travel from the ovary to the uterus. If the infection and abscesses are severe, total removal of the ovaries, fallopian tubes, and uterus may be required.

Cysts of the ovary are common and often benign. Some cystic tumors of the ovary, however, are malignant. A mass in the area of the ovary that does not subside over a full menstrual cycle but persists or increases in size may require an exploratory laparotomy and possibly removal. Different types of ovarian tumors require different treatments. Some ovarian tumors produce hormones and are discovered by their abnormal hormonal effects.

Others interfere with fertility or normal female development, and require operation for biopsy and incisions within the ovary to improve its function.

Endometriosis is an abnormality in which the endometrial tissue ordinarily lining the uterus is found outside the uterus within the abdominal cavity and the pelvis around the ovaries and tubes. The woman usually has pain and difficulty conceiving. Nodules or masses of endometrial tissue may be found on pelvic examination. An exploratory operation may be necessary for diagnosis, followed by surgery to remove some of the tissue.

Diagnosis of abnormalities of the tubes and ovaries has been advanced through use of the laparoscope, an instrument inserted with local anesthesia through a very tiny incision in the abdominal wall. This instrument allows inspection of the tubes, ovaries, and surface of the uterus. Biopsies can be taken with it. Sterilization procedures to tie off or cauterize the fallopian tubes also are carried out by laparoscope.

OPERATIONS ON KIDNEYS, BLADDER, AND MALE ORGANS

The kidneys and the bladder are susceptible to stones and tumors as well as to injury. Birth defects of the kidney or the urinary tract also may call for an operation. And the kidney is vulnerable to interruptions in its blood supply. Fortunately, a diseased or injured kidney can be removed and the remaining kidney will take over its functions.

Injury is one reason for a kidney operation. Although the kidney is normally well protected by its location, the crushing force of an auto accident, for example, can damage it. Either the kidney itself is ruptured or the kidney is torn loose from its blood supply. The kidney must then be removed, a procedure called a nephrectomy. Removal of a kidney requires an incision in the flank or abdominal wall. The renal artery and vein are ligated and divided where they join the aorta and vena cava. The kidney is separated from the surrounding tissue and from the adrenal gland that lies on top of it. The ureter is then divided and the kidney removed. It is important for the surgeon to be sure that the other kidney is functioning adequately before removal.

Tumors of the kidney may be malignant or benign. A rare tumor of infancy called Wilms' tumor requires removal of the kidney followed by chemotherapy. In adults, a common tumor is called a hypernephroma or renal-cell carcinoma. This tumor may announce itself by blood in the urine or pain in the flank. If the kidney is removed promptly before the tumor has spread elsewhere, the outlook is promising.

Kidney stones frequently are small and may pass unnoticed down the drainage ducts of the kidney, through the ureters, into the bladder, and then outside via the urethra. Sometimes, however, a stone will obstruct the ureter, causing urine to back up into the kidney and causing severe pain. An operation will then be necessary to open the ureter and extract the stone. Stones also can develop within the kidney and reach such size that they fill the interior of the organ. These stones, nicknamed "staghorn" calculi for the shape they take, require that the kidney be gently split open and the stone lifted out. The two halves of the organ then can be reunited with sutures.

The blood supply on which the kidney depends can be compromised by a number of causes, including arteriosclerosis and a disease called fibromuscular hyperplasia. In either case, the renal artery supplying the kidney may be narrowed. The narrowed portion can be bypassed, using a synthetic graft to link the normal portions on either side. Or a procedure called angioplasty can be used. A balloon is carefully threaded into the narrowed area and then suddenly inflated under strong pressure. The narrowed artery is consequently forced open, and it usually remains open.

Bladder problems requiring a surgeon's attention include stones, tumors, and infection. The latter problem is more common in females because the very short urethra allows organisms to migrate from the vagina into the bladder. Bladder stones, like those elsewhere in the urinary system, may be passed without incident. Or they may collect within the bladder and require operative removal.

A removal technique called fulguration allows tumors to be burned off with a miniature electric cautery fitted on the end of the scope. Sometimes, however, a bladder tumor is not detected until it has reached such large size that the entire organ must be removed.

When the bladder is removed, a way must be provided for the collection and disposal of urine. A procedure called a Bricker or ileal pouch has proved most satisfactory. It uses a section of small intestine to construct a conduit and reservoir. A length of the intestine is removed and the divided ends rejoined by anastomosis to provide continuity. The segment is then sewn closed at one end, and the two ureters are attached to either side of it. The open end of the intestinal segment is brought out through the abdominal wall through a hole in the skin to form a dimple. A bag is worn over the dimple for collection of urine.

Prostate gland disease is the most common abnormality of the male urogenital system. This gland surrounds the base of the bladder and the urethra and provides prostatic fluid, which combines with sperm to make up semen or male ejaculate. The prostate often enlarges in older men, a condition called benign prostatic hypertrophy, and tends to squeeze the urethra and produce difficulty in emptying the bladder (see chapter 23, "The Male Reproductive System"). Early symptoms are slowing of the stream during urination, and necessity to get up frequently at night to urinate. Eventually complete obstruction can occur. With bothersome symptoms or obstruction, it may be necessary to remove part or all of the prostate. If the gland has become extremely large the entire gland may be removed by an open operation through the bladder or around the base of the bladder via an incision in the abdomen. The technique is called suprapubic prostatectomy or retropubic prostatectomy. The entire prostate gland is "shelled out" of its capsule and removed. A simpler operation is called a transurethral resection. Because it does not remove the entire gland, symptoms can recur. This operation is performed through the urethra in the penis by insertion of an instrument called a resectoscope. Diathermy or cautery is used to cut out the inside of the prostate gland, to open the outlet of the bladder and allow for freer flow of urine. A large amount of prostate tissue can be removed in this way.

Cancer of the prostate gland is said to occur in more than 60,000 men annually, most of them past 60. It may be an incidental finding after a transurethral resection or after a prostatectomy. It may produce symptoms of obstruction or make its presence known by pain in the surrounding bone. The treatment of prostate cancer is improving rapidly. It consists of irradiation, orchiectomy, or a radical perineal prostatectomy, and combined hormone therapy to suppress the prostate gland and spread of the cancer. A radical operation is done only if the tumor is small and confined to the prostate gland. If the tumor has spread, removal of the testicles and administration of female hormones (estrogens) may decrease the hormonal stimulation of the tumor.

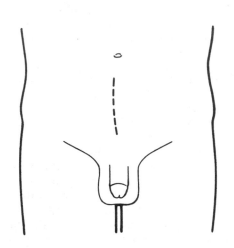

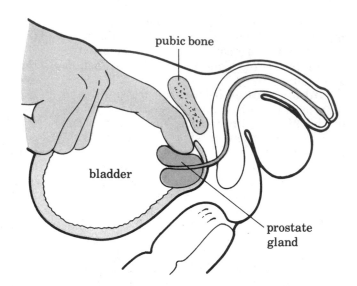

PROSTATE SURGERY

Suprapubic prostatectomy is one operation for removal of the prostate gland. An incision is made on the line shown on the left. The bladder is entered by an incision and the prostate is shelled out, or enucleated, by the finger, as shown at right. The procedure removes the entire prostate gland.

Testicle abnormalities may require operation. Torsion or twisting can occur if the testicle does not become well positioned as it descends from the abdominal cavity into the scrotum shortly after birth. It may twist later and obstruct the blood supply with sudden, severe pain and a mass in the scrotum or the testicle. An emergency operation is required to untwist the spermatic cord before gangrene sets in. Large cystic swellings can occur, producing a painless soft mass around the testicle called a hydrocele. The hydrocele can be treated by removal of the sac. A hard and painful mass, on the other hand, requires further investigation because of the possibility of a cancer. This usually requires an incision in the groin to bring the testicle up from the scrotum for inspection. If a malignancy is found, a radical removal of the testicle and the spermatic cord is required, called an orchiectomy. Follow-up treatment depends on the type of tumor. In certain tumors removal of the lymph nodes in the abdomen is necessary. In other tumors irradiation of the lymph nodes in the abdomen and chest may help.

ORTHOPEDIC SURGERY

Operations on the skeletal system (orthopedic surgery) are sometimes required to correct structural abnormalities or deformities caused by disease. More often, the problem that brings a person to an orthopedic surgeon is an injury, either to the bones or to the ligaments, tendons, or muscles supporting them. The most publicized orthopedic surgery, of course, is that performed on athletes. But as more and more people take up sports, an increasing number of athletic injuries come to the orthopedist's attention.

Fractures of the bones are a common injury. They do not always require surgery, although they do require medical attention. Fractures can be classified in several ways. A closed fracture is one in which the skin is intact. In an open fracture the ends of the bone protrude through the skin. Contamination of the exposed ends can lead to infection of the bone, called osteomyelitis. A fracture may be undisplaced, in which the bone is cracked but the ends of the bone remain together and are lined up properly, or displaced, with the fragments separated and the ends angulated, twisted, or otherwise abnormally aligned. An undisplaced fracture requires support while the fracture heals, either by plaster cast or another method to preserve alignment of the bone. Displaced fractures, however, often require surgery, either a closed procedure in which the fracture site is manipulated to align the bones or an open operation necessary to bring the fracture edges together. It may be necessary to support the fracture site by what is called internal fixation. In its simplest form, internal fixation means insertion of a screw into a broken segment of bone to hold the segment in place. A more extensive fixation fastens a metal plate across a fracture site, holding it by screws on either side of the fracture. Internal fixation also can be provided by a metal rod inserted within a bone such as the femur, the large bone of the thigh. A fracture of the hip joint often requires the insertion of a nail across the fracture site and a plate as well, as illustrated at right.

Injuries to joints also may require operation. An ordinary dislocation does not require surgery, but severe dislocations may. Recurrent dislocation of the shoulder calls for operation, too, because the tissues around the joint have become so lax that the shoulder joint can slip in and out with minimal cause. Other injuries to a joint include the tearing of structures around it, such as the four ligaments supporting the knee joint and the cartilage (meniscus) cushioning the two bones within the joint. This is a common injury among football players. The violent force of a tackle can tear loose the ligaments and shear off bits of cartilage. The ligaments must be reattached to the bone. Cartilage does not heal itself and fragments must be removed or they will float loose in the joint and interfere with joint motion. This may require an operation, but sometimes it can be done with an arthroscope.

Arthritis. A rapidly expanding field of orthopedic surgery is treatment of the effects of arthritis. The disease itself is treated by medical means, of course, but the arthritic changes in the joints, which produce pain, disability, and limitation of motion, may be treated much more satisfactorily by an operation. Total replacement of joints crippled by arthritis has become one such method. Replacement of virtually every joint has been attempted, but results are better for some than for others.

Hip joint replacement can be done safely and with excellent results. The patient may be almost completely rehabilitated. Even those

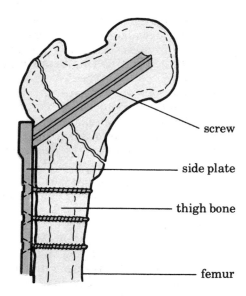

screw

side plate

thigh bone

femur

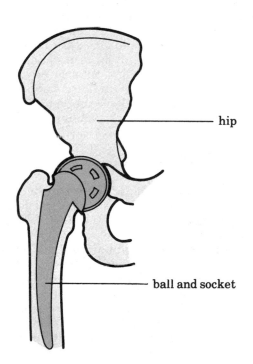

hip

ball and socket

HIP REPAIR

A broken hip, which is really a fracture of the neck of the thighbone (femur), often requires surgery to hold bone fragments together. At top, a long nail has been inserted across the fracture site into the broken femoral head. The nail is anchored to a side plate, which in turn is secured by screws into the shaft of the femur. In the lower drawing, the stainless-steel ball has been cemented in place to replace a worn femoral head. Such an operation is increasingly used for arthritics, who are often returned to near-normal mobility.

who have been immobilized before the operation may be able to walk afterward. The socket (acetabulum) is frequently deformed in arthritis. The ball, or head of the thighbone, may be worn so that it slips from the socket, or may have developed bone spurs that limit motion. The socket usually is replaced with an acrylic substance shaped into socket form and glued into place. The ball, or femoral head, is made of stainless steel cemented into the thighbone.

In finger joint replacement, a Dacron or Silastic prosthesis is used to restore mobility to the hands. A knee joint has also been used in a number of cases.

Tumors of the bone may require removal of a portion of the skeletal system. Malignant tumors include two types, osteogenic sarcoma and Ewing's sarcoma. The treatment of malignant tumors of bone is rapidly advancing. In the past it was felt that all tumors could be treated only by radical amputation of the limb, if the tumor had not spread to the lung or other sites. Other approaches are now used. Chemotherapy may contribute to saving an affected limb. For benign tumors or locally malignant tumors involving large amounts of bone, it is possible to replace the damaged area with a large bone graft or even a joint.

NEUROSURGERY

Among problems of the nervous system calling for a surgeon's skill are congenital defects, injury, tumor, and blood vessel disease within the brain.

Hydrocephalus, an abnormality of formation and removal of fluids of the central nervous system, is present in some children at birth. The fluid collects in the brain, causing pressure, enlargement of the skull, and stretching of the brain tissue. This abnormality may be treated surgically by attaching a valved conduit from the ventricular system of the brain to the abdomen or kidney to allow removal of the fluid.

Brain injury usually results from a fall or auto accident. If the skull is fractured and presses on the brain, an operation may be required to remove pressure. More often the skull is not fractured, but blood collects under the skull and compresses the brain. Such accumulations require exact diagnosis to locate the blood and remove it. An incision is made in the skull directly over the site. Then a small burr hole is drilled through the bone, or a small circle of bone is removed with an instrument called a trephine. The clot can then be lifted from outside the lining of the skull (the dura mater), or the lining can be opened to remove

the clot. A larger hole can be created if necessary by elevating or removing a flap of bone.

Brain tumors occur in many different forms. A variety called a glioblastoma multiforme is extremely malignant. It may require an operation for diagnosis but treatment is difficult because it is difficult to remove the entire tumor. Benign brain tumors, however, often develop within an enclosed capsule and can be removed in their entirety if near the surface. A portion of the cranium or skull is removed to expose the tumor, as shown on page 777, after which it is removed. Tumors deeper in the brain, while benign, are more difficult to remove. These may occur in young people.

Operations in or on the brain require meticulous technique to prevent injury to the soft nervous tissue and to eliminate bleeding, which would compress and further damage the brain. If certain portions of the brain are involved by a tumor and must be removed, permanent deficiencies such as weakness, paralysis, or loss of sensation may result.

Blood vessel problems involving the brain also may require an operation. An aneurysm, which is a bulge in the vessel wall, may develop in the small blood vessels of the brain. These cerebral aneurysms may blow out, producing hemorrhage into the brain and sudden loss of consciousness. If the condition can be determined before a rapid increase in blood pressure causes stroke, a tiny clip can be placed to seal off the aneurysm. This involves a delicate operation on the surface of the brain.

Arteriosclerosis and hypertension in older persons can cause a vessel to blow out, so that blood collects within the brain tissue and must be removed. Arteriosclerosis can cause narrowing or obstructions of some of the small blood vessels supplying blood to the brain, and stroke may result. If the abnormality is detected before stroke occurs, a bypass graft can be performed to route blood around the blockage. Vessels in the neck are joined through the skull to the small vessels in the brain beyond the point of obstruction (see chapter 11, "Stroke").

Spinal cord injury occurs most commonly with a fracture of the cervical spine (broken neck). The spinal cord may be compressed or divided, causing total paralysis below the point of injury. It is usually irreversible because the spinal cord does not regenerate itself. Partial injury, however, may be helped by an operation to take the pressure off the cord.

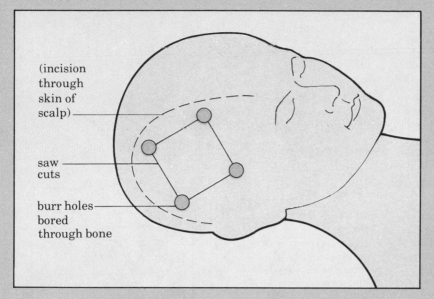

(incision through skin of scalp)

saw cuts

burr holes bored through bone

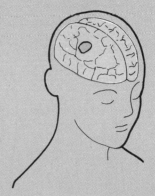

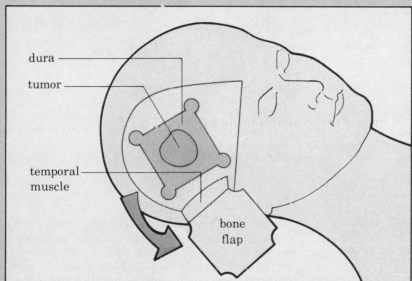

dura

tumor

temporal muscle

bone flap

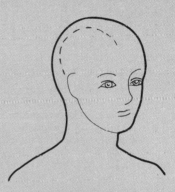

tumor

bed of tumor in brain tissue

BRAIN SURGERY

To remove a tumor on the surface of the brain (top right), the skull must be opened, a procedure called craniotomy. The usual incision is marked by the dotted line in the upper left drawing. Four holes are drilled as shown, connected, and the flap of bone turned back, exposing the tumor and the brain covering (dura). The tumor is lifted from its bed in the brain tissue, keeping the tissue itself intact. The bone and skin flaps are replaced and the incision closed, as shown in the lower right drawing.

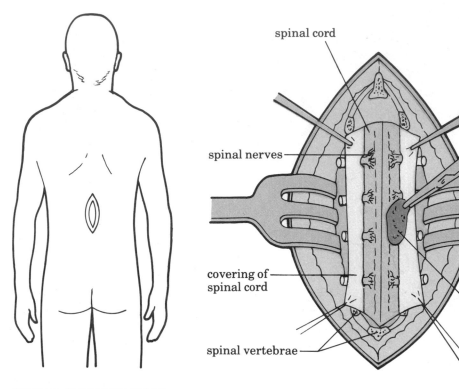

spinal cord

spinal nerves

covering of
spinal cord

spinal vertebrae

tumor

SPINAL CORD SURGERY

An operation to expose the spinal cord to remove a tumor, or for a ruptured intervertebral disk, is called a laminectomy. An incision is made in the back, exposing the spinal nerves running from the cord, the covering of the cord, and the vertebrae. In the drawing above, a tumor is being removed from the cord. A similar incision is made for disk removal.

A ruptured intervertebral disk is a common abnormality of the human spine. Disks are small elliptical sections of fibrous cartilaginous tissue. They serve as cushions between the bony vertebral bodies of the spine, held in place by ligaments. By degeneration of tissues, by pressure, and perhaps by forward bending of the spine, the tissues may give way, allowing a disk to be pushed out from between the vertebrae. The result is pressure on the nerve roots coming from the spinal cord or on the terminal nerves coming off the spinal cord. This pressure can then produce severe pain in the back extending down the legs and can interfere with nerve supply to the foot and leg, limiting movement of the muscles.

Often the symptoms of a ruptured disk are fairly straightforward. If a disk appears to be ruptured, initial treatment is often bed rest. Recurrent problems may require an X-ray study (myelogram) to determine whether there is pressure in the region of the nerves and spinal cord. If the myelogram discloses a ruptured disk and the patient's symptoms are not relieved by rest and treatment, or if they recur frequently, removal of the disk may be required in a procedure called a laminectomy. An incision is made over the back and a portion of bone is removed over the spinal cord and its distal nerves. These are then retracted gently and the disk pulled from its site behind the nerve roots.

The primary problem involving nerves of the arms and legs is injury by laceration or amputation. This may require suturing the nerves together carefully. A divided nerve will degenerate all the way back to the spinal cord to its parent nerve cell. A sutured nerve may gradually regenerate itself, with sensation and muscular function returning, but this may take many months to develop.

OPERATIONS ON THE EARS, NOSE, AND THROAT

Tonsillectomy. The single most common operation performed in the United States has been the tonsillectomy—removal of the tonsils from the throat of a child. Tonsillectomy is often combined with an adenoidectomy, removal of the adenoid tissue at the back of the nose, so the operation is nicknamed "T and A." At one time it was felt that a "T and A" should be done routinely on all children at about the time they enter school to decrease likelihood of throat infections, tonsillitis, and particularly of streptococcal infections, which could lead later to rheumatic fever and rheumatic heart disease. It has been increasingly recognized in recent years, however, that routine removal of tonsils and adenoids is not necessary and may be inadvisable for some children. There is always a small risk with any operation requiring anesthesia, and complications can occur.

It is natural, in any case, for children's tonsils to be large and active. The tonsils are a part of the lymphatic and infection fighting immune system. As the growing child encounters new sources of infection, the entire lymphatic system is kept busy producing antibodies. After childhood, tonsillar tissue gradually decreases in size and eventually disappears. Simply having enlarged tonsils is not a reason for operation. A tonsillectomy should be carried out only if the child's tonsils are so enlarged that he or she has shortness of breath, difficulty swallowing, repeated severe bouts of tonsillitis, ear infections, abscesses, or serious enlargement of lymph nodes.

A tonsillectomy should be done with the child admitted to the hospital, at least overnight. The procedure calls for a surgeon expert in this operation, and careful anesthesia. As shown on page 780, the tonsils are dissected from the surrounding throat tissue and a snare or ligature or cautery applied at the base of the tonsil, where the blood supply enters. With a careful dissection and careful control of bleeding there should be a minimal risk of hemorrhage later. The adenoids are hidden above the palate and therefore are hard to visualize without general anesthesia. Whether they should be removed at the same time depends upon their enlargement.

The larynx. Diseases of the larynx that may require surgical treatment include benign and malignant tumors. Benign polyps or papillomas can develop on the vocal cords.

These can be removed with an instrument called a laryngoscope inserted down the throat with local anesthesia. Laryngeal cancer, if confined to the midportion of one vocal cord, can be treated best by radiotherapy. This is preferable because it leaves the patient with a good voice. If a cancer is more extensive, reaching the junction of the cords, it is best treated by removing a portion of the larynx (hemilaryngectomy). An even more extensive tumor calls for a total laryngectomy, removal of the entire larynx. The trachea or windpipe then must be brought out through the skin and sutured to the neck. Without a larynx, the patient must learn substitute methods of speech. There are several rehabilitative approaches. One is to learn esophageal speech, in which air is aspirated into the upper third of the esophagus, then belched out to produce sound through articulation with the mouth. Another approach is to use an electrical amplifying device as a vocal substitute, holding the electrolarynx over the opening in the throat to produce sound. Communication can be effective with either method. Training programs are available to teach both.

Tracheostomy. The trachea, or windpipe, runs from the bottom of the larynx into the chest where it divides into two tubes, one into each of the lungs. These two major tubes are called the main bronchi. The trachea is composed of cartilaginous rings with muscle behind. The rings support the airway so it does not collapse when we breathe. Injuries, obstruction, or other problems may require opening the trachea below the larynx. A small incision is made in the skin of the neck overlying the trachea. The muscles are separated in the midline. The isthmus or connecting portion of the thyroid gland is pulled upward. An incision is then made in the larynx, usually removing a small circle of one of the tracheal rings. Through this incision a cannula, or tracheostomy tube, can be inserted so it lies easily in the trachea, comes to the outside, and allows breathing. If the patient requires assistance for breathing, a small cuff can be placed around the tracheostomy tube to seal it so that a machine used to push air into the patient's lungs will not leak. A tracheostomy is usually temporary, and when it is no longer needed, the tube can be removed. Over the next few days the hole will close and heal.

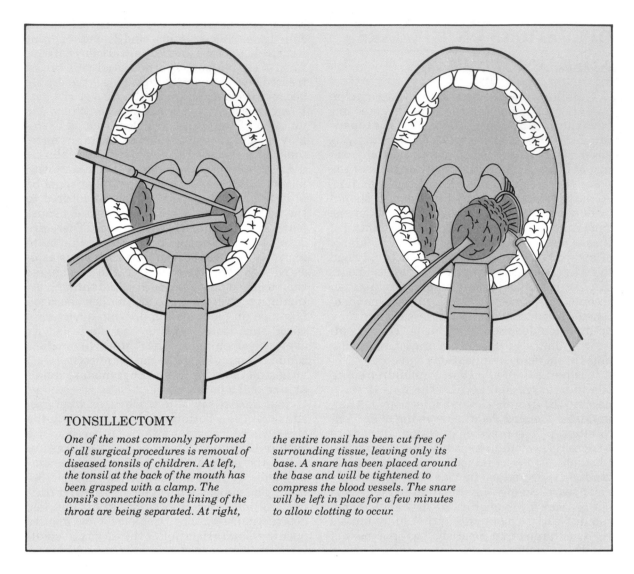

TONSILLECTOMY

One of the most commonly performed of all surgical procedures is removal of diseased tonsils of children. At left, the tonsil at the back of the mouth has been grasped with a clamp. The tonsil's connections to the lining of the throat are being separated. At right, *the entire tonsil has been cut free of surrounding tissue, leaving only its base. A snare has been placed around the base and will be tightened to compress the blood vessels. The snare will be left in place for a few minutes to allow clotting to occur.*

The ear. Infection in the ear is particularly common in childhood. Middle ear infection, called serous otitis media, may require an operation to drain fluid collected behind the eardrum. In an acute infection an incision is made in the eardrum when it is bulging to drain the fluid. This is called myringotomy, an office procedure done with local anesthesia. For chronic infections it may be necessary to leave a tiny drainage tube in place through the eardrum. The placement of tubes, called tympanostomy, usually is temporary and usually requires hospitalization. Extensive infection can spread into the mastoid bone cells just behind the ear, causing pain and tenderness. An abscess may form within the mastoid bone cells. A mastoidectomy may then be necessary. An incision is made behind the ear to remove all of the bone containing the mastoid air cell. With early antibiotic treatment for ear infections, mastoidectomy is required only rarely.

A common cause of hearing loss is otosclerosis, which produces fixation and immobility of the small bones of the middle ear. These bones transmit sound from the eardrum through the middle ear (see chapter 13, "Ear, Nose, and Throat"). One of these bones, the stapes, becomes fixed so it does not move or transmit sound. It is possible to operate on patients with otosclerosis. The preferred procedure is to remove the stapes and replace it with an artificial bone made of a stainless steel wire and cellulose sponge.

OPERATIONS ON THE EYE

A cataract is clouding of the normally transparent lens of the eye. The most common cause is aging, as the protein in the lens gradually hardens and yellows. The hardening interferes with the transmission of light through the lens onto the retina at the back of the eye.

In the past it was necessary to delay an operation to remove cataracts until the entire lens had hardened. Then the lens could be separated from its capsule without leaving particles behind that could become opaque and interfere with vision later. Recent techniques allow the entire lens and capsule to be removed, so the patient need not tolerate a long period of declining vision. However, some surgeons still postpone removal of a cataract from one eye if the other eye retains good vision. That is because the eyeglasses used for a patient after a single cataract removal cause a difference in magnification, and the two eyes see objects in different magnification, resulting in double vision. In such a situation the good eye, being the stronger, would dominate.

The operation is carried out by an incision at the junction of the clear portion of the eye (the cornea). The upper portion of the cornea is turned back and a small opening is made in the iris, which is the colored part of the eye. The lens usually is removed with a freezing probe (cryoprobe). The incision is then closed with fine sutures or tiny clips. In some cases an artificial lens replaces the natural lens.

The clear central outer portion of the eye is called the cornea. The cornea can become cloudy as a result of injury, infection, or genetic predisposition to progressive deterioration. When clouding occurs, light is blocked from passing through the lens to the retina. The condition is treated by transplanting a healthy cornea from a human donor, one of the most successful of transplant operations. If a scar does not extend deeper than the outer layers of the cornea, it can be replaced with a corneal graft of the same thickness. However, with the advent of very fine sutures and the operating microscope, full thickness corneal transplants can be carried out. The entire defective cornea is removed and a graft cornea of the same size and shape is fitted exactly into the hole and sutured to the remaining rim of the patient's cornea.

Glaucoma is a disease in which fluid pressure within the eyes rises so high that it damages the optic nerve. This is the leading cause of blindness in the United States. Often glaucoma can be controlled by the use of drugs to reduce the amount of fluid. If not, an operation may be required. The simplest operation is an iridectomy, performed in cases of acute angle closure glaucoma, the least common form of the disease, in which rapid and severe blockage develops in the channels that normally allow fluid to drain from the eye. Part of the iris is cut loose to deepen the channels for draining and to relieve the pressure.

Filtering operations are used for chronic glaucoma, in which there is damage to the sponge-like drainage system of the eye. This type of operation is often performed after medications have failed and damage to the optic nerve at the back of the eye has occurred, causing a reduction in vision. The purpose of this operation is to promote drainage through a trough to the outer coat of the eye. In these procedures a hole is created so there is a connection from the anterior chamber, where the aqueous fluid circulates, to the outer coats of the eye. The hole is covered by the conjunctiva, a thin veil that lines the eyelids and the eye and covers the sclera, the white part of the eye. Sometimes a piece of iris is also cut so that it will be drawn into the hole where it functions as a stopper. In severe chronic glaucoma an operation may be carried out to decrease the formation of the fluid that circulates in the eye. This fluid is produced by the ciliary body just behind the iris. The ciliary body may be frozen or superheated to destroy its ability to make the fluid.

The retina is the specialized tissue lining the inside of the back of the eye. It is light receptive, perceiving images and transmitting them through the optic nerve to the brain. This thin layer of tissue is held against the back of the eyeball by the pressure of the fluid within the eyeball. When a break or a hole in the retina permits fluid to accumulate between layers, the retina is detached from the back of the eyeball and vision is destroyed.

There are several surgical techniques to correct a detached retina. Using local anesthesia behind the eyeball, a hollow needle can be inserted into the eye to drain the fluid that is between the retina and vascular layer. The retina and the vascular layer can then be frozen together with a freezing rod or seared with a laser beam or heating needle. Sometimes it is necessary to put a "buckle" on the outer layer of the eyeball in the detached area to push the blood vessel layer (choroid) against the retina. The "buckle" remains on the outer coat of the eyeball permanently.

Diabetic retinopathy, a consequence of long-continued diabetes, is a common form of blindness. In proliferative retinopathy, new blood vessels develop on the retina and cause blurred vision or blank spaces in the visual field. A laser beam seals off the vessels and reduces the risk of hemorrhage.

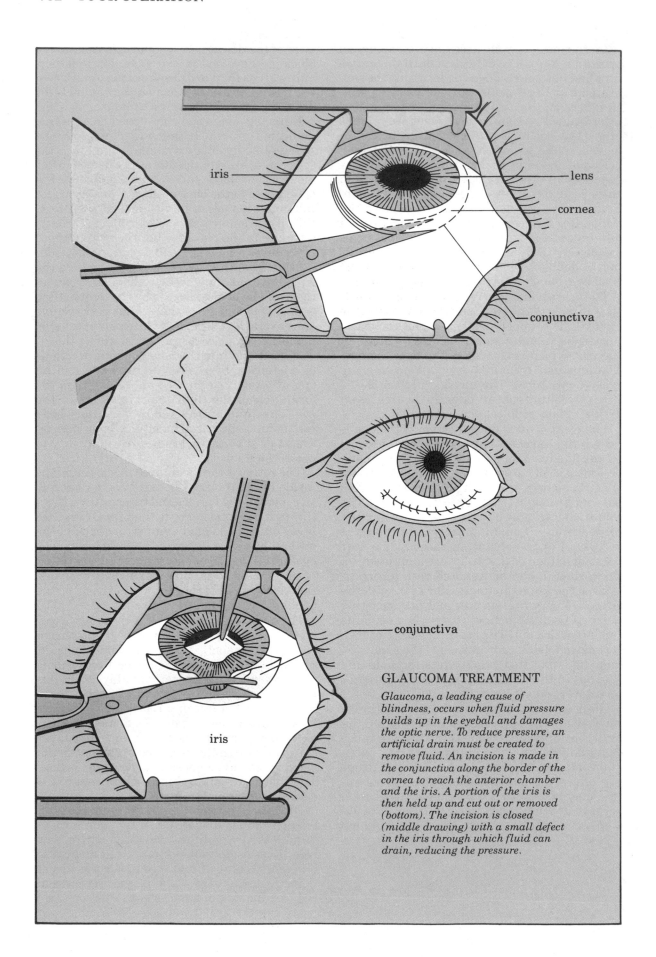

iris

lens

cornea

conjunctiva

conjunctiva

iris

GLAUCOMA TREATMENT

Glaucoma, a leading cause of blindness, occurs when fluid pressure builds up in the eyeball and damages the optic nerve. To reduce pressure, an artificial drain must be created to remove fluid. An incision is made in the conjunctiva along the border of the cornea to reach the anterior chamber and the iris. A portion of the iris is then held up and cut out or removed (bottom). The incision is closed (middle drawing) with a small defect in the iris through which fluid can drain, reducing the pressure.

PEDIATRIC SURGERY

Complex or serious birth defects that produce problems in the newborn and require an operation are best taken care of by a specialist in such abnormalities, the pediatric surgeon. Such men and women have had five years of training in general surgery followed by an additional one or two years in pediatric surgery. They develop the expertise to carry out major operations in newborn infants weighing only a few pounds. Such abnormalities are not frequent but do require special expertise for proper care. Some of the more common congenital problems that are life-threatening and require operations in the newborn period include esophageal atresia, in which a portion of the esophagus fails to develop an inner channel, and a tracheoesophageal fistula, in which the esophagus connects to the trachea so that everything the infant swallows enters the lungs. In an imperforate anus, the opening does not develop, and a passage from the colon or rectum must be made surgically.

A common abnormality, particularly in male infants, is a thickening of the pylorus, the muscle in the outlet of the stomach. This condition, called hypertrophic pyloric stenosis, results in vomiting at about six weeks of age. It can be corrected by dividing the muscle. Atresia of the biliary system occurs when the external bile ducts do not form, so the infant is jaundiced at birth. In certain forms of biliary atresia a bypass operation can be carried out to drain bile into the intestine. Hirschsprung's disease is a malady of the newborn in which a segment of the colon does not relax and must be removed.

The most common problem in infancy, of course, is that of inguinal hernia. A herniation of the bowel through the diaphragm of the newborn is called a Bochdalek hernia and is immediately life-threatening. In this situation the lung on the herniated side may not have developed because of the pressure of the intestine pushing through the diaphragm.

TRANSPLANTATION SURGERY

An organ transplanted from one person to another is totally accepted by the body only when donor and recipient are identical twins. In all other individuals, even close relatives, a transplanted organ will be rejected by the recipient unless the body's immune system is depressed and maintained in a depressed state. In organ transplants, the chemical agent most commonly used is called azathioprine. Adrenal steroid hormones are also used, and in certain circumstances a serum that destroys white blood cells is given. Transplantation of the kidney is now done commonly and transplant surgeons believe it is the treatment of choice for most patients with end-stage kidney failure.

The five-year success rate using a kidney from a living relative averages about 75 percent. The other source is a person whose kidneys were normal and who has died from some cause such as head injury. In these cases, the five-year success rate is slightly better than 50 percent. The major problem limiting the number of kidney transplants is the short supply of cadaver kidneys.

Tissue typing is the technique used to determine similarity or disparity of genetic makeup between the donor and the recipient. This tissue typing consists of what are called histocompatibility tests (see chapter 21, "Allergy and the Immune System"). When recipient and donor are closely matched, as in transplants between living relatives, graft survival is better. There is controversy about survival of transplants from a cadaver to an unrelated person. As techniques for better typing and matching are developed, it appears likely that survival rates will improve.

Liver transplants are by no means as common as kidney transplants. They number in the hundreds rather than thousands. Survival beyond five years has been rare. However, the technique is rapidly improving.

Undoubtedly the transplant operation that has most captured the public imagination is that of the human heart. Performed by only a few specialized teams, heart transplants also occur in limited numbers. Most patients die within the first few years, but one survived for nearly seven years. Certainly, no patient should be considered for a heart transplant if any other approach might help. But results continue to improve and if better methods of rejection control can be achieved, heart transplants could become an acceptable treatment for end-stage heart disease.

CHAPTER 32   A. EVERETTE JAMES JR., SC. M., J.D., M.D.

X RAYS
AND
RADIOLOGY

The first step in treating any illness is to identify it accurately. Physicians call this diagnosis. To establish a diagnosis, physicians often seek specialized help. To learn more precisely what is happening inside your body and what changes are taking place, they sometimes call upon the sophisticated equipment and trained personnel in the field of radiology.

X rays, radionuclides (isotopes), CAT scans, and ultrasound—all methods of obtaining images of what's inside the body—are a major part of your doctor's diagnostic capabilities. Application of these methods to assess your health depends on the skills of a group of physicians called radiologists. Like all other physicians, the radiologist must be graduated from a college or university and then a medical school with an M.D. degree. To become proficient in the use of X rays and other imaging methods, the radiologist must spend at least four additional years in specialized training.

The power to explore within the human body without surgery began unceremoniously in 1895 in Wurzburg, Germany, when a bearded, laconic physicist named Wilhelm Conrad Roentgen was conducting experiments in his laboratory. Attempting to pass electrical currents through tubes containing rarefied gases, he accidentally discovered an electromagnetic ray of very short wavelength. The ray could penetrate the body and record on sensitized film shadowy images of interior organs and bones. Roentgen named his discovery X ray, using the algebraic designation "X" for something unknown.

Only four years later, Pierre and Marie Curie in Paris isolated the radioactive chemical element radium, which gives off rays as it decays. The specialty of radiology had its genesis in these two scientific discoveries. In the decades since there has been continuous development of instrumentation, growth of sophistication of electronics, and use of these techniques in the care of the sick.

About half of the U.S. population receives some type of diagnostic X ray, nuclear medicine, or ultrasonic study each year. A child who has suffered a fractured arm falling from a bicycle, a pregnant woman who experiences problems with the unborn fetus, an automobile accident victim, a patient with a serious heart problem, someone who needs an operation—the list is almost infinite. Radiology is a science of perception. It allows doctors to "see" inside the body and make more accurate judgments of health and disease.

RADIATION SAFEGUARDS

Properly chosen and carefully performed radiographic (X-ray) examinations are an indispensable part of modern medicine. In this nuclear age, however, most of us are aware of the possible harmful effects of cumulative exposure to radiation. People are concerned about the short-term and long-term consequences of X-ray exposure, both to themselves and to their unborn children.

Radiologists must always consider the problem of X-ray exposure when determining a particular course of action for a patient, balancing the benefits and the potential risks of radiation.

Radiation exposure that does not contribute to the examination can largely be avoided by reasonable measures. If an X-ray examination is not medically essential for the patient's care, it should not be performed. According to guidelines written by the American College of Radiology, the radiologist should not recommend an examination if it is not medically essential and is encouraged to dissuade your physician from requesting it. In the consultation process a more appropriate examination might be chosen, or your clinical care team may decide it is in your best health interests not to have any radiographic study. Knowing the hazards and limitations as well as the virtues of these procedures is part of the radiologist's extra four years of training.

The American College of Radiology is a professional society that represents physicians who specialize in radiology. It and other societies that exchange research findings and ideas, such as the Association of University Radiologists, and societies for education and re-education of practitioners, such as the Radiological Society of North America and the American Roentgen Ray Society, continually develop and publish guidelines and recommendations for the use of X rays. For example, after studying the use of X rays to examine pregnant and possibly pregnant women, radiological scientists have issued the following statement:

"There is no period, including the 10 to 14 days following the onset of menses, during which a radiological examination of the pelvis or abdomen of a woman of childbearing potential can be conducted with no biological risk to the real or potential embryo or fetus. Research suggests that this risk is about the same from some time before conception to birth, although the predominant biological factors vary with the stage of pregnancy during which irradiation occurs."

On the basis of extensive research, the American College of Radiology adopted the following policy:

• Abdominal radiological examinations should be requested only after full consideration of the clinical status of the patient, including the possibility of pregnancy. These studies may be postponed or selectively scheduled, in those infrequent instances where the examination could be deferred, if necessary, until the establishment of or the end of pregnancy without risk.

• Termination of pregnancy is rarely justified because of the potential radiation risk to the embryo or fetus from a diagnostic X-ray examination.

Radiation is not the only hazardous agent in the human environment. There are many other hazards to life and health, both natural and man-made, and many are similar to radiation in their effects. However, the spectacular manner in which atomic energy first came to public notice resulted in much greater public anxiety than has been associated with many other technological advances. Extensive investigations of the biological effects of radiation have been performed, and more is probably known about injury from radiation than about other toxic agents such as atmospheric nitrous oxides or the hydrocarbons that pollute the air we breathe.

Risks are often an unavoidable part of the advances in medicine and technology that bring comfort and prolong life. Human life has always involved calculating risks and weighing them against the potential benefits. Drugs that save many lives can, in certain circumstances, cause injury or death. In the same way, ionizing radiation used in the diagnosis of disease occasionally leads to injury or malignant change. However, there is no firm evidence that significant harmful effects result from radiation exposures of a few rads or less, the amount in a diagnostic X ray. Nevertheless, it is prudent for radiologists to assume the possibility of harmful effects and to minimize X-ray exposure.

Measuring radiation. Various measurements have been devised for X-ray exposure. The first, adopted in 1928, was called the Roentgen. It is a measure of exposure only, without reference to absorbed dose or the effect in humans. More pertinent are two units that have been adopted to describe the potential implications of the radiation exposure.

One is the rad (radiation absorbed dose), the unit of absorbed dose of radiation. Another is the rem (Roentgen equivalent man), the unit of dose of ionizing radiation weighted for its effectiveness in a given case. Care must be taken in using this unit because it is not subject to precise physical measurement.

As a reference point, the National Council on Radiation Protection and Measurements has said that a single dose of 450 rads to the entire body would be lethal to most persons, while a dose of 200 rads probably would not require medical care. For comparison, the average person's yearly radiation dose from all sources is 55 millirads (or 55/1000ths of a rad). Relatively minute doses of a few millirads are delivered during the average X-ray examination Therefore, the implications of an individual X-ray exposure are minor, but must always be balanced by a positive expected patient benefit.

DISCOVERING HIDDEN INJURIES

The complex world we live in is often a traumatic one. Injuries and the sudden development of an acute disease process, such as a heart attack, stroke, or a bleeding ulcer, are some of the causes that send patients into emergency departments of hospitals. In the past it was sufficient for physicians to repair the more obvious and spectacular injuries, such as external bleeding or fractured bones, and later transfer the patient to a hospital bed or elsewhere for more therapy. However, for modern medicine, this is not always sufficient.

One patient in the emergency room might have obvious external damage, while another might have no external signs of illness. Yet both (or neither) could be perilously close to death from trauma, or experiencing a crisis because of a disease that is not evident. Doctors must determine as rapidly as possible what the problem is. In recent years many hospitals have developed a section of the radiology department that is in or close to the emergency department to supply X rays to emergency patients when they need it most.

If an accident victim with a ruptured major artery or grave but unknown brain damage reaches the emergency room, an accurate diagnosis must be established rapidly.

As a part of the emergency medical team, the radiologist can help discover the so-called "hidden injuries," can confirm the emergency physician's clinical suspicion, or perhaps provide the answer for a difficult diagnostic problem. Better X-ray machines, image intensification, production of more sensitive X-ray films, and rapid processing can produce images in 90 seconds or less, saving lives in acute trauma and disease processes.

Many of the developments in diagnostic radiology help to investigate the blood vessels and lymphatic system. In these procedures, the radiologist injects a contrast material into the vessels to make them opaque so that X rays will not pass through them. That makes these vessels identifiable on the exposed X-ray film. Most of these examinations are performed on hospitalized patients, often on an elective basis. Those performed in emergency circumstances will identify vessels that have been injured, filled with blood clots, or that are about to rupture. Bleeding can be decreased or even stopped by placing substances in the vessels under X-ray guidance. Obstructed vessels can be opened and dilated to allow passage of blood by inserting small balloons or removing clots. The dramatic lifesaving procedures can be accomplished by insertion of the catheter by the radiologist into the vessel without a surgical operation. This development has given doctors the potential to treat a bleeding ulcer as well as to open the main artery to the leg if it has become narrowed to the point of preventing blood flow. This procedure has been used successfully in the emergency treatment of a condition called intestinal angina, in which patients have acute abdominal pain because the bowel is not receiving enough blood. Substances injected into the abdominal vessels cause the vessels to dilate and improve the flow of blood to the wall and lining of the intestines. While clots (thrombi or emboli) may be mechanically compressed or extracted from the blood vessels by this technique, they also can be dissolved by using drugs.

Emergency radiology is a well-established practice that formerly was concerned with routine examinations such as X rays for broken bones. These studies can be performed by a technologist but must be interpreted by a radiologist. Other emergency procedures, such as fluoroscopy, which allows immediate visualization of the shadows of body structures on a screen, must be performed by a radiologist.

For victims of automobile accidents, violent acts, or natural disasters, it is important to have a correct assessment of the extent of injuries as quickly as possible. For some, such as those with fractured bones, the simplest X-ray examinations will often suffice. In other patients, detailed X-ray examinations, particularly of the vascular (blood vessel) system, are required. The injury, bleeding, and distortion of surrounding tissues can prevent assessment of the injury by routine physical examination. That is when the information acquired by the so-called "special radiographic procedures," especially vascular X-ray studies, becomes necessary. Through a development called digital radiology, the artery can be rendered opaque by injecting the contrast media in the vein rather than having to place a catheter in the artery. With improved diagnostic radiologic studies providing more accurate information, these patients have a better chance of recovery.

Problems other than injury. It is not necessary to be injured to require treatment in an emergency center. Other equally serious problems occur as a result of disease processes. These patients often pose a greater diagnostic dilemma than the accident victim because the cause of their acute symptoms is often not clear. In these cases diagnostic radiology procedures can be critically important.

Among the most frequent of such problems are perforation of the abdominal cavity, intestinal obstruction, spontaneous rupture of the wall of the principal artery of the body (the aorta), and massive bleeding from the stomach or other parts of the gastrointestinal tract.

THE USES OF RADIOLOGY

There are many facets to the specialty of radiology. One way to understand their use is to begin with an explanation of the most common examinations and progress to the more unusual and sophisticated ones.

Chest X Ray

The chest radiograph (chest X ray) is the radiological examination you are most likely to have. For this procedure the patient stands with the chest pressed against a panel that holds an X-ray film in a cassette. The organs and structures of the body absorb some of the X rays, preventing them from reaching the film. The amount of absorption depends on the organ's density and other properties. The degree of exposure, much like in photography, will be represented on the film by varying shades of gray. Those areas with the least tendency to absorb the X rays appear dark, and dense structures such as bones, which absorb most of the X-ray beams, appear whiter.

CHEST X RAY

The chest X ray is the most common and basic radiographic examination. It is often obtained for diagnostic purposes and to evaluate the respiratory system before anesthesia. The patient stands with chin upraised and chest pressed against a metal panel containing the film. Rays generated by the X-ray tube pass through the body, and images of the internal structures are projected on the film (lower drawing). The intensity of the image depends on the amount of X rays absorbed by each part of the body.

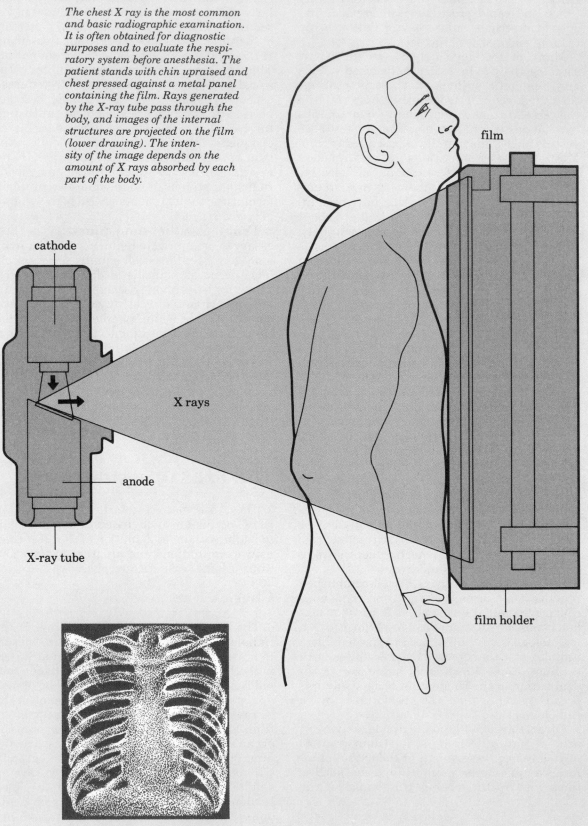

film

cathode

X rays

anode

X-ray tube

film holder

UPPER GI SERIES

To inspect the digestive system, the radiologist relies on a contrast material that will absorb X rays, creating an image of the organs it passes through. The patient swallows barium while the radiologist watches its progress by using a fluoroscope. The upper GI series allows the doctor to observe the structure of the affected organs and how they work. It is often used in patients suspected of having an ulcer or tumor.

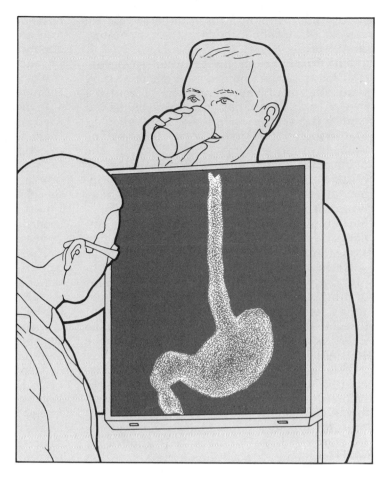

The routine chest X ray can show a great deal about your general health. The radiologist can evaluate the size and shape of your heart, the condition of your lungs, and the condition of the bones that make up your thoracic cage. He or she can also detect enlargement of the great vessels (such as the aorta), enlargement of a heart chamber (cardiomegaly), and whether there is a shadow within the lung that might represent an infection or a tumor.

Not only can the anatomy be depicted, but by interpreting the anatomical changes the radiologist is often able to determine how well a structure or organ is working. This process is known as "reading" the X ray. A radiologist can detect and define the abnormality, and decide the significance of the findings.

Contrast Examinations

The radiologist also uses specialized studies called contrast examinations. The simple radiographic studies such as the chest X ray often require only that you stand before a screen or lie on a table, without any preparation. In the contrast examination you may have to swallow a substance, have the contrast material injected into a vein, or have the contrast medium instilled directly into a particular structure or organ.

The "upper GI series." For a gastrointestinal examination, often called an "upper GI series" or "barium meal," the patient swallows a glass of a substance called barium. He or she stands before an instrument called a fluoroscope while the radiologist observes the passage of the barium through the gastrointestinal tract. This substance is opaque to the X rays, so the radiologist can follow its course through the digestive system. This allows the radiologist to inspect areas not normally visible on X ray. The observations can be recorded on conventional radiographs, which act as "stop-action" pictures, or can be placed on videotape or moving film.

Barium enema is another commonly performed X-ray examination. For this procedure the patient must prepare 24 hours in advance by following a liquid diet and using laxatives and cleansing water enemas. The radiologist will instill barium through a rectal tube into the colon. The barium enema is a way to determine the status of the muscular wall and the lining of the large bowel. Gastrointestinal studies are often used to detect ulcers, tumors, or any abnormality of the gastrointestinal tract.

The intravenous urogram or pyelogram (IVP) is the most common example of a study requiring intravenous injection of contrast media. In this examination a contrast material containing iodine is injected intravenously, and is then concentrated by the kidneys. The concentration and movement through the urinary tract show kidney function and show collection and drainage structures of the kidney, ureters, and bladder. An intravenous urogram is used in screening patients for a particular kind of hypertension. It is also important in the evaluation of infections and stones in the urinary tract.

Arthrography. Contrast media occasionally are placed directly into one of the organs or joints. Injection into joints, called arthrography, is important in evaluation of joint disease. Damage to cartilage, especially in the knees as well as shoulder and hip joints, can be evaluated by this method.

The gallbladder series is another common study using contrast media. The night before the examination the patient must swallow a number of pills or a liquid that will concentrate in the gallbladder if that organ is functioning properly. This concentration of the contrast media will be seen on the X-ray film. From this simple procedure the radiologist can determine gallbladder function and may be able to see the connections (ducts) of gallbladder, liver, and duodenum. Stones in the gallbladder are readily detected, too. Nuclear medicine and ultrasound (see pages 791 and 795) also are used to study the gallbladder.

Interventional Radiology

Angiography. An even more complex examination your physician may request is an angiogram. The radiologist inserts a catheter into one of your blood vessels, usually by threading into a vessel in the thigh, then moving it gradually to the target area. By careful placement of the catheter an injection of contrast material can determine the position and configuration of the blood vessels serving a particular organ or part of the body. This technique has been used successfully in the heart as well as in the cerebral (intracranial) circulation. A procedure that outlines the vessels supplying the heart muscle, known as coronary angiography, has been used extensively to identify persons who face high risk of heart attack or to evaluate those suspected of having

had a heart attack (myocardial infarction). Before an operation involving the vessels that supply the extremities, particularly the legs, an angiogram is obtained to determine the status of the vessel itself and the blood flow through the vessel.

In more recent times, angiography has been used not only to diagnose diseases but to treat them, using catheters, balloons, and the direct injection of materials. This has been particularly useful in an instance in which there is profuse bleeding. By placing a catheter into the blood vessel, bleeding can be stopped by injecting a form of clotting agent or by simple occlusion (blocking) of the bleeding vessel or vessels.

The ability to pass balloons through blocked or narrowed blood vessels has resulted in the use of angiography to treat occlusive vascular disease (blockage of vessels), particularly in the legs. The balloon is moved into position via catheter, then inflated under pressure to open the blockage or widen the channel. The method can be used in patients who cannot be treated by surgery because of other health risks. Recently, radiologists have also used balloon dilation to open blocked coronary arteries (see chapter 3, "The Heart and Circulation"). Drugs and other agents also can be delivered to selected areas of the body by catheters. This field of "intraventive angiography" is in its infancy and probably will represent an important alternative treatment for certain diseases in the future. It is not difficult to understand the advantages of being able to open narrowed vessels or to stop critical bleeding without a major operation.

Mammography

One in 14 American women develops breast cancer, with the risk increasing substantially after ages 30 to 35 (see chapter 25, "Breast Cancer"). Breast cancer is the leading cause of cancer death among women. A way to save the lives and improve the quality of life of these women is to detect the disease early when it is curable.

Mammography, a specialized type of breast X ray, is the most accurate way to detect early breast cancer. A mammogram often will show a cancer even before it can be felt by a woman or her physician. In screening centers nation-

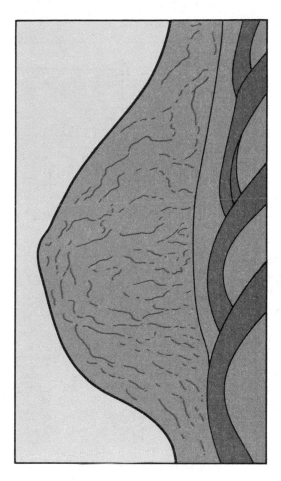

MAMMOGRAM

A xeroradiographic mammogram discloses the internal structure of the breast. This specialized X ray can detect abnormal growths even before they can be felt by the woman or her physician. Some doctors advise women to have a baseline mammogram between ages 35 and 40, then mammograms at regular intervals thereafter. If detected early, breast cancer is usually curable.

wide, which have examined hundreds of thousands of women, many breast cancers have been found by mammography that were not detected by physical examination.

When to consider mammography. Women with a breast condition requiring medical attention (lumps, pain, discharge) sometimes have mammography before treatment begins. Many physicians and cancer specialists believe that women should have a first (baseline) mammogram between the ages of 35 and 40, even if there is no indication of breast disease. This exam provides a basis for comparison to detect any change that may occur later. How often repeat mammograms should

be obtained depends on the woman's age, her personal likelihood of developing breast cancer, and the appearance of the breasts on the baseline mammogram.

The risk of developing breast cancer is higher for women who:
• have had cancer in one breast.
• have a close relative who has had breast cancer.
• have not borne children.
• had their first child when they were over 35.
• began menstruation at age 11 or younger.

Mammography has been controversial, but in this well-defined use it appears to be a valuable procedure. Ultrasound and other techniques of cancer detection are being evaluated.

Nuclear Medicine

Nuclear medicine uses radioactive compounds called isotopes to determine the structure and function of organs or areas of the body. In diagnostic X-ray procedures radiation passes through the body from an external source, the X-ray tube. In nuclear medicine minute amounts of radioactive substances are introduced directly into the body, usually by injection into a vein. An instrument then detects the radiation and translates this energy into spots of light that expose a conventional X-ray film. The developed image on the film, which is often called a scan or scintigram, shows the distribution of radioactivity in the organ being evaluated. The image or scan is examined by the radiologist.

Following injection, the radioactive compounds circulate through your body to the areas in which your doctor is interested. Compounds are chosen that will concentrate in the target area. As they circulate, the compounds might be altered or might become attached to certain tissues. The radiologist, by observing how and where the radioactive compounds pass and concentrate, is able to acquire information about changes in the body.

Two principal types of instruments are used in nuclear medicine. One is the scanner, in which the recording device moves back and forth in straight lines, recording images of the emitted radiation as the detector passes over the body. The other instrument is a camera in which there is a large surface (interface) between the recording device and the patient. This instrument is able to record the radiation emitted from the body without the patient or the instrument having to move. Through sophisticated electronics, these instruments are able to reconstruct the internal configuration of the body.

NUCLEAR MEDICINE

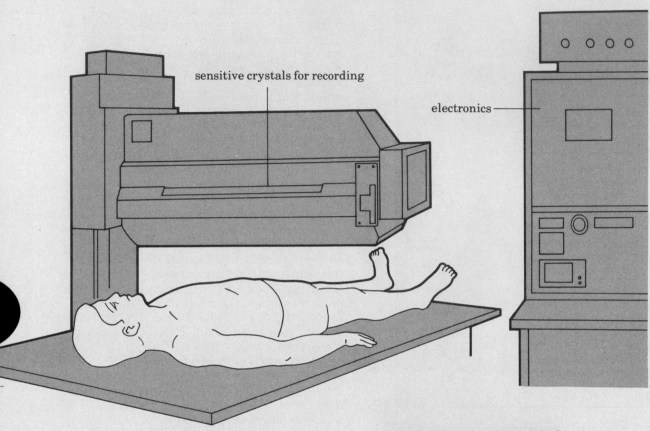

sensitive crystals for recording

electronics

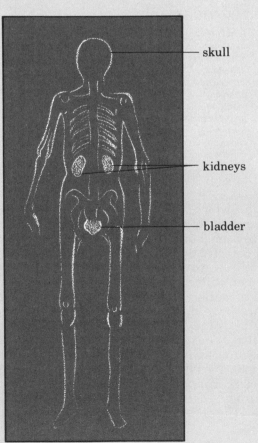

skull

kidneys

bladder

THE BODY SCAN

By placing minute amounts of radioactive compounds selectively into particular organs or parts of the body, the specialist in nuclear medicine can make an internal examination. While the patient lies on a table, the movable instrument containing sensitive crystals passes back and forth over the body, recording radiation emitting from organs and structures where the compounds have accumulated. The images then are translated electronically into spots of light that are recorded on film. At right is the result of the study. The radioactive substance has concentrated in the kidneys and bladder, disclosing that their function is normal in this case.

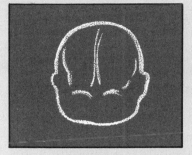

ANTERIOR IMAGE

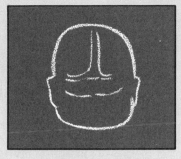

POSTERIOR IMAGE

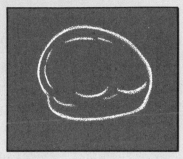

RIGHT LATERAL IMAGE

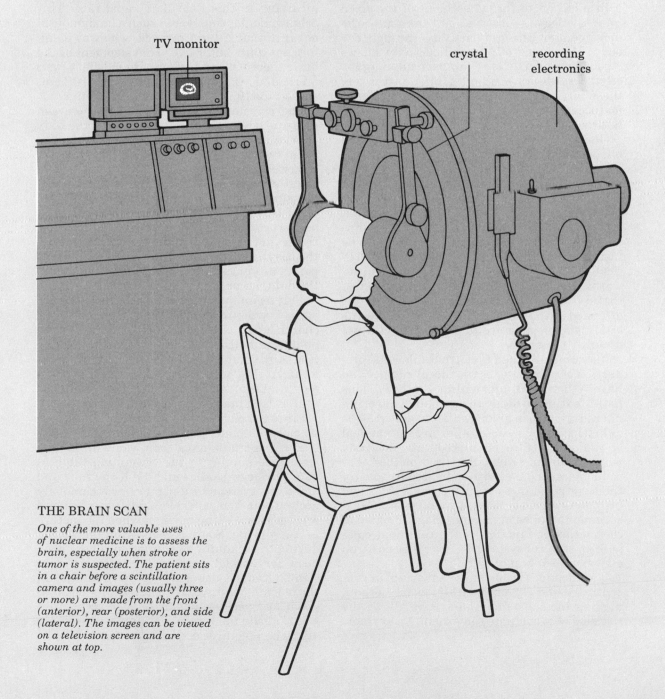

TV monitor

crystal

recording electronics

THE BRAIN SCAN

One of the more valuable uses of nuclear medicine is to assess the brain, especially when stroke or tumor is suspected. The patient sits in a chair before a scintillation camera and images (usually three or more) are made from the front (anterior), rear (posterior), and side (lateral). The images can be viewed on a television screen and are shown at top.

A variety of radioactive compounds are used to travel to different parts of the body because of their specific properties. By choosing the appropriate compounds a radiologist can selectively investigate the heart, brain, liver, thyroid gland, bones, lungs, and many other organs or body systems. When the radioactivity is concentrated in a region, it is recorded by the camera or scanner as dots on an X-ray film. Regions with a high concentration of radioactivity appear dense, with closely placed dots, while regions of lower activity have fewer dots. A physician trained in nuclear medicine can recognize abnormal patterns of dot distribution, and interpret the pattern accordingly.

In addition to the assessment of the fixed images, doctors observe and measure the movement of the radioactivity through the body. Movement of the radioactivity shows blood flow and indicates how particular organs or structures are working. Motion pictures of these observations allow diagnosis of abnormalities even before anatomical changes can be detected.

One of the most exciting developments in nuclear medicine has been the ability to create images of the heart muscle. Using selected isotopes and a gamma or scintillation camera, a radiologist can assess whether a patient has had a heart attack, whether he faces a great risk of one, and whether a heart attack has damaged the heart's ability to pump blood. The instrumentation for cardiac imaging is sophisticated and somewhat expensive but the rewards are great. To have a noninvasive test that requires little patient cooperation and is attended with minimal discomfort represents a tremendous advance in evaluation of heart disease and stroke.

Instruments called cyclotrons allow the production of radioisotopes that decay rapidly and have a brief half-life within the body. This half-life (time to decay to one-half of the original radiation) of a given radiation dose may be as brief as a few seconds, allowing a great deal of radioactivity to be placed into the body without undue risk. By this method the radiologist can label with radioactivity some of the basic substances (such as amino acids and nitrogen) used by cells in metabolism. Measurements can be made and images created of the metabolic function of the cells that compose an organ or system. This is called positron emission tomography (PET).

If a substance is normally "taken up" or concentrated mostly or entirely in one organ, making the substance radioactive allows the radiologist to evaluate that organ. An example is iodine, used by the thyroid gland to make the hormone thyroxin. Radioactive iodine injected in small amounts into the veins concentrates in the thyroid and shows its anatomy. The amount concentrated during a limited time indicates how the thyroid is working.

Computerized Tomography (CAT Scanning)

The CAT scan (computerized tomography) is a diagnostic technique developed in England in the early 1970s and used clinically in the United States since 1973. Developments are occurring in this field at a rapid rate. This achievement is considered such a fundamental advance that Allan Cormack, who was a significant contributor to the development of the basic theories, and Godfrey Houndsfield, who fabricated the first working instrument, shared the 1979 Nobel Prize for medicine.

The principle of CAT scan is that we can measure how organs and structures of the body change the properties of an X-ray beam. The beam (whose characteristics are well known) is passed through the body at many angles and the alterations of the beam from each angle are measured and stored in the memory of a computer (see page 796). By examining the internal structure of the body from enough angles, the scanner builds a picture of the density of the tissue at a particular point. If enough points are placed on a later reconstruction of the data, an image can be formed.

This technique was first used to produce images of structures in the brain. The brain was chosen because there was little motion and the anatomical structures are confined to a space (the skull) that varies little from patient to patient. At first only a single X-ray source and a single detector were employed. Later multiple sources and many detectors were used.

From the patient's viewpoint, a CAT scan is no more discomforting than any routine X-ray study. If you undergo a scan, you will lie on a small bed similar to the examining table in your physician's office and the X-ray tube and detector system will move continuously around you. You experience no discomfort and are not aware of the moment when the picture is being made. Some persons even fall asleep during the scanning examination. There is no need for special preparation, although patients often are asked not to eat breakfast on the morning of the study. They wear a hospital gown to avoid buttons or brass buckles that would shield the X rays. Patients must remain still when pictures are being generated.

Sometimes it is necessary to inject contrast media to enhance certain parts of the body on the computed tomographic picture. In this case, the patient is given an injection into a vein, and sometimes swallows a liquid contrast medium to outline the gastrointestinal tract. The contrast material is denser than body tissues, which diminishes the X-ray beam and enhances the visibility of the structure or organ.

Because the computed tomographic scan is an X-ray procedure, patients do receive radiation exposure. The amount of exposure is about the same as in other X-ray studies, and less than some. The tube that produces the X rays is heavily shielded so that only the area of the body being examined is exposed. Highly sensitive electronic X-ray detectors are used to do the measurements so that only a small amount of radiation must pass through the body.

During the scan and other X-ray procedures, the technologist stands behind a wall and other personnel in the room wear protective aprons. This is not because of a large amount of radiation in a single scan, but because the technologists who work in the area every day face repeated exposure. Therefore, they need to protect themselves from even the small amount of radiation they might receive during only one test.

Immediately after the CAT scan examination, the pictures and images produced and stored in the computer are evaluated by the radiologist. If additional images are needed, they will be obtained before you leave. The images or pictures produced by the data stored and retrieved from the computer show your body in cross sections. That is, your body appears to the radiologist as if you had been sectioned in half, and the bottom half removed, with the radiologist looking up at the top half (see page 797). The radiologist can see the organs lying within the body and their relationship to each other. Diseases change the normal appearance of these organs by changing their shape or by altering their ability to absorb the X rays. Because a single picture only demonstrates the cross section of those organs where the body was X-rayed, several images are made to visualize the total extent of the areas in question. This is based on the same principle as the radiographic tomograms (*tomo* meaning "cut" or "slice" and *graph* meaning "picture").

For a test that normally takes less than one hour to complete, the computed tomographic scan might appear to be expensive. The technology is complex and the cost of producing these instruments is high. However, with this machine your doctor can be certain that you are receiving one of the most advanced diagnostic tests available. In many cases the CAT scan can eliminate other examinations that are more expensive, time-consuming, and uncomfortable for the patient. Moreover, a CAT scan can be performed on an outpatient basis, while other tests might require hospitalization. Because of the high costs of CAT scanners (as much as $1,200,000), federal and state agencies limit their distribution.

Recently, a technique has been developed using radio frequency waves rather than X rays to make images in much the same manner as CAT scans. This process is called nuclear magnetic resonance (NMR). In NMR, a patient sits inside a huge magnet. The chemistry of tissues inside his body is analyzed by a camera and a computer that record how hydrogen atoms in the tissues react to powerful magnetic fields. Ultimately, researchers hope they will be able to distinguish diseased from normal tissue through NMR.

Ultrasound

Ultrasound is the medical use of sonar, which has been used by bats and dolphins for millions of years. High-frequency sound waves reflected from surfaces of different densities (interfaces) within the body can be used to form diagnostic images. This method of evaluation is becoming an important subspecialty in medicine. Ultrasound or sonographic technique has the capability to portray anatomical structures in detail by a noninvasive method that apparently has no significant side effects. The basic principle involves making an image from sound waves that are passed into the body and reflected back when two tissues of different sound transmission quality are encountered. Sonar used in navigation is a familiar nonmedical form of this technology.

The sound waves are generated from a device called a transducer, which is placed in contact with the skin. A gel or oily substance such as mineral oil ensures uniform contact of the transducer surface with the skin. The same transducer that generates the sound wave acts as a receiver to record the wave's reflections. The sound is generated by placing an electric signal on the crystal of the transducer, causing it to change shape in a minute fashion. Although the change occurs immediately against the skin, the patient does not feel the compression it produces. The sound wave passes into the body until it is reflected back or until its energy is spent.

COMPUTERIZED AXIAL TOMOGRAPHY (CAT SCAN)

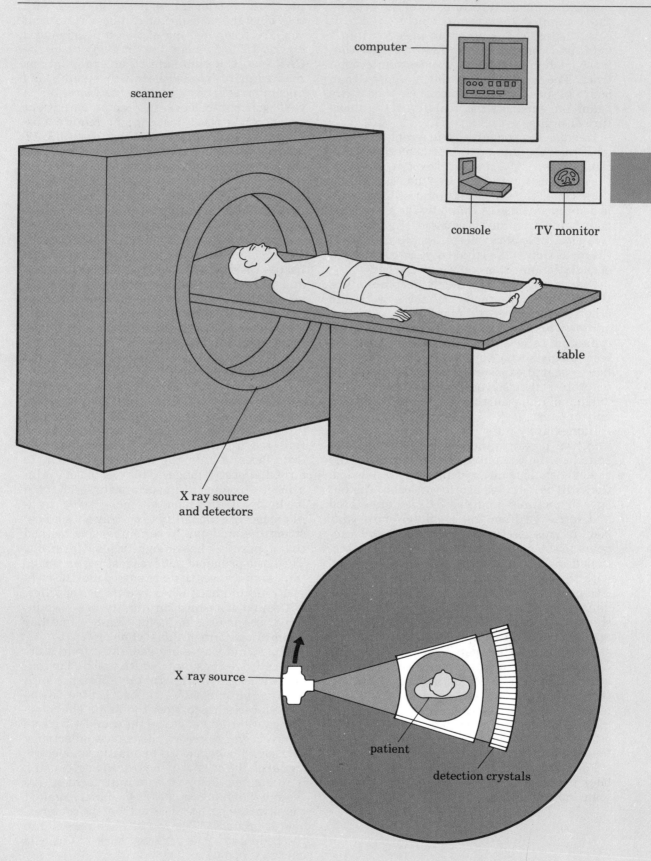

computer

scanner

console   TV monitor

table

X ray source
and detectors

X ray source

patient

detection crystals

film with body scans

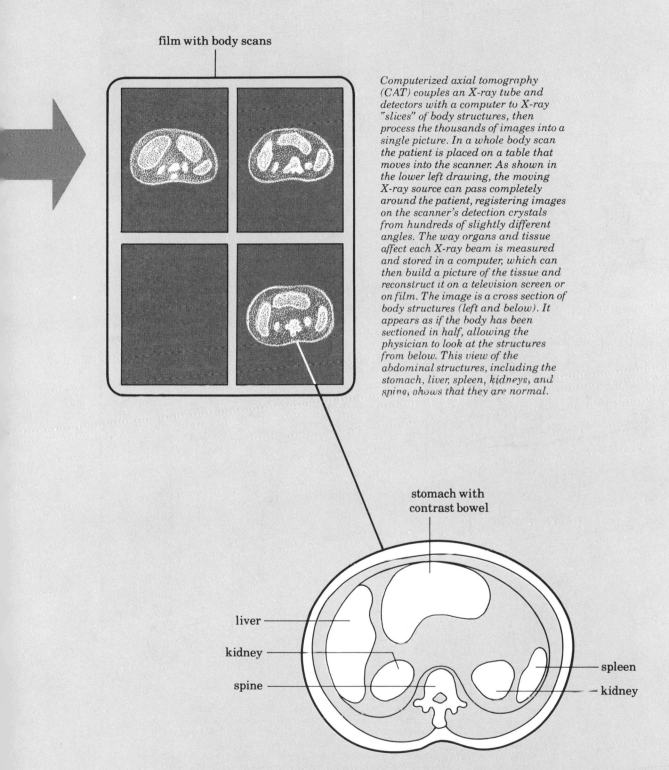

Computerized axial tomography (CAT) couples an X-ray tube and detectors with a computer to X-ray "slices" of body structures, then process the thousands of images into a single picture. In a whole body scan the patient is placed on a table that moves into the scanner. As shown in the lower left drawing, the moving X-ray source can pass completely around the patient, registering images on the scanner's detection crystals from hundreds of slightly different angles. The way organs and tissue affect each X-ray beam is measured and stored in a computer, which can then build a picture of the tissue and reconstruct it on a television screen or on film. The image is a cross section of body structures (left and below). It appears as if the body has been sectioned in half, allowing the physician to look at the structures from below. This view of the abdominal structures, including the stomach, liver, spleen, kidneys, and spine, shows that they are normal.

stomach with contrast bowel

liver

kidney

spine

spleen

kidney

NORMAL ABDOMINAL CAT

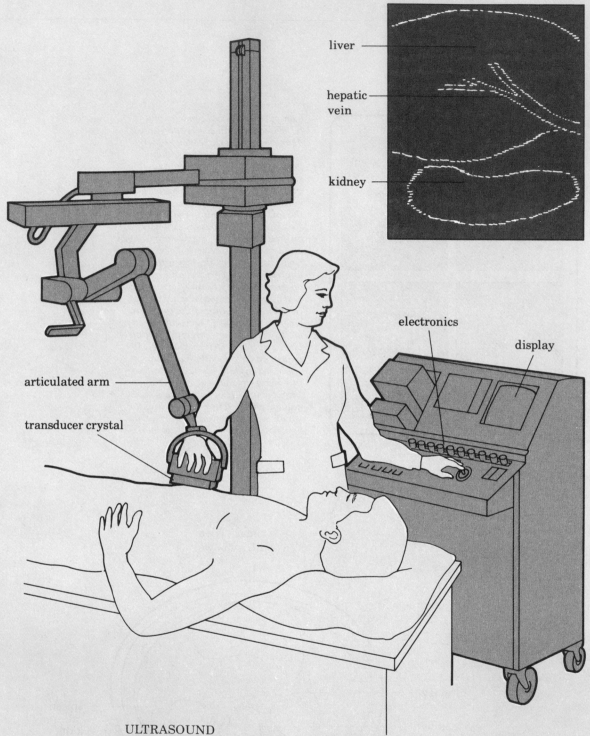

liver

hepatic vein

kidney

electronics

display

articulated arm

transducer crystal

ULTRASOUND

The ultrasound machine uses the principle of sonar to measure the reflection of high-frequency sound waves from interior body surfaces. While the patient lies on a table, an electronic device beams a high-frequency wave into the body, then detects the "echo" that occurs when the wave encounters an interface between tissues. When the reflected wave reaches the transducer surface, it is converted electronically into dots of light, which are displayed on a television screen. The inset at top shows the ultrasound image of the abdominal structures of liver, kidney, and hepatic vein.

The distance that a sound wave travels in the body depends on the frequency and length of the wave and the density of the tissues it encounters. Dense tissues that consist of large particles transmit sound slowly. Air does not transmit at all. There is little difference in the velocity of sound waves traveling through liquids but enough difference within the various parts of the body to be detected when the sound waves are reflected back to the transducer.

When the sound wave is reflected back to the transducer, the crystal again changes shape. This change is converted into an electrical pulse that eventually produces a light dot on a screen much like a television screen. The distribution and intensity of the dots as they build up create a picture that can then be recorded by a camera or on videotape (see page 798).

The property of the body that allows sound to be transmitted as an energy form through tissue is called acoustical impedance. If two adjacent parts of the body have the same acoustical impedance, an ultrasound wave that passes into their tissues will be transmitted through them. If the parts have different acoustical impedance, the sound will be reflected from the interface, the area where their surfaces adjoin. For example, sound waves that encounter an interface between soft tissue and air will be totally reflected. This is why ultrasound is not effective in investigating problems of the chest if it is necessary to pass through the lungs. As sound passes through tissue it is also absorbed. The rate of absorption can be measured. This is a measure of the relative loss of the intensity of the sound beam in a tissue per unit of length that the sound beam travels in that tissue.

The amount of information obtained from an ultrasound scan has increased markedly in the past several years because of two improvements in instrumentation. Formerly, the light dot intensity (generated from the echoes that are converted into electric signals) was recorded as an "all or none" phenomenon. Now the intensity of the echo can be expressed as shades of gray. This gives the radiologist better resolution and anatomical detail, recording not just the outlines of the organs, but the internal structures as well.

The second basic improvement is the use of multiple transducer crystals. Multiple-crystal devices allow a number of sound beams to be emitted in very short sequences and the reflections recorded at extremely frequent intervals. This creates a motion picture of the body organs and their movement. Multiple-crystal devices are known as "real time" machines because they are capable of creating images of movement as they occur. Heart motion and the propulsion activity of the bowel can be seen.

With these instruments diagnostic sonography can be performed at the bedside, in the emergency room, or in the nursery.

The use of ultrasound in medicine has developed rapidly since 1970, but man has used sound waves to determine position and structure for several decades. Since World War II the military has used echo-receiving devices (sonar) to locate submarines. A similar technique of penetrating objects with sound waves is used to examine the internal structure of industrial products, to locate schools of fish, and to explore layers of rock beneath the earth for geological purposes.

In ultrasound, frequencies are hundreds of times higher than those the human ear can detect. With the newer devices doctors not only see the outline of the organs but can look at their internal characteristics because the sound waves penetrate the organ. This, coupled with the ability to observe movement of the body organs and structures in a non-invasive manner, has made ultrasound an effective diagnostic technique. With increasing public concern about exposure to ionizing radiation, ultrasound offers an alternative.

RADIATION THERAPY

Radiation therapy is the use of high-energy X rays to treat diseases, especially cancer. Ionizing radiation, which emanates from cobalt electrons and other sources, penetrates cells and kills them by inhibiting their division. All tissues, noncancerous as well as cancerous, are affected by radiation, but cancer cells usually are more susceptible.

There are many types of cancer and they act in different ways. Radiation therapy is one of the major methods available to treat cancer. It can be used alone or in combination with surgery or drugs (chemotherapy). Radiation therapy is the preferred treatment for most cancers of the cervix, lymphomas such as Hodgkin's disease, and many head and neck tumors. Many other tumors can be treated effectively by surgery or irradiation, but the organ will be better preserved with irradiation. Some cancers do not respond to irradiation, so surgery and chemotherapy are used in these cases, if feasible. Because each patient's health is individual, a thorough understanding of the problem is needed to decide the best treatment. This requires a doctor's examination, a review of previous hospital records,

X rays and pathology studies, and sometimes special examinations. These steps help determine whether radiation treatments are needed and the best way of delivering them.

The radiation therapist or cancer specialist in charge of treatments is a physician who has had specialized training in the use of radiation and other methods to treat disease. Although the radiotherapist is responsible for determining whether a patient could benefit from X-ray therapy, the family physician, surgeon, cancer specialist, pathologist, and other specialists also have joint responsibility to see that all treatment options are considered.

Because radiation affects all cells, both normal and abnormal, treatments must be planned so that most normal tissue is spared as much exposure as possible. This requires that the cancer area be accurately located. Because many cancers are deep inside the body, their exact location in relation to the outside surface must be found. This can involve taking a number of X-ray studies of the cancer area with a special X-ray unit of the treatment machine, or the use of radioactive isotopes, ultrasound equipment, or CAT scanning.

Calculations are made, usually by computer, to determine the best method of administering radiation. In order to treat only the abnormal tissues and leave most normal cells undamaged, the cancer sometimes is treated from several directions. That is why a patient may receive radiation from opposite sides of the body or from varying angles. In some instances, devices hold the patient immobile during treatment.

Patients who receive radiation therapy are treated with either curative or palliative intent. If cure is not possible, then improving the quality of life for several years is the goal. Patients receive palliative radiation therapy to relieve pain, bleeding, starvation, etc. An estimated 50 to 70 percent of all cancer patients require radiation therapy at some time during the course of the disease.

Radiation therapy patients usually receive treatments four or five times per week for three to eight weeks. For example, a patient may receive a dose of 5,000 rads in 25 treatments over five weeks. (A rad is a measure of the radiation absorbed by the tissue.) However, the treatment can be as short as one day. Patients are not made radioactive by external treatment techniques.

There are three general categories of external radiation therapy equipment, classified mainly by their energy range:
• Superficial X-ray machines with an energy range of 85 to 180 kilovolts are used to treat only lesions on the skin or just below it.

• Orthovoltage equipment, formerly called deep X rays, historically has been used for deep-seated tumors, but now is in less common use. With these machines, the maximum radiation dose occurs at the skin surface. Thus, the dose that can be delivered to a deep tumor is limited to the skin's tolerance of radiation. Orthovoltage equipment is relatively inexpensive and requires only a few millimeters of lead shielding in the treatment room wall for adequate protection. Although it is simple and reliable in operation, the beam it generates has limited depth penetration and it irritates the skin. Most doctors believe it should no longer be used in the treatment of deep-seated cancers.
• Megavoltage, introduced in the 1950s, has overcome many of the problems associated with orthovoltage equipment. The physical characteristics of the higher energy megavoltage beam make it an effective treatment for deep-seated tumors.

In megavoltage X ray the maximum dose occurs appreciably beneath the skin surface and usually there is modest or no skin reaction. The margins of the beam are better defined than those of an orthovoltage X ray, making it easier to minimize the doses of radiation received by vital nearby organs. The greater penetration of megavoltage irradiation makes it possible to deliver large doses deep within the body. With radiation of low energy, bones absorb considerably larger doses of radiation than do soft tissues (muscles, connecting tissue, etc.). Bone absorption is minimized in the high-energy range.

The History and Future of Radiation Therapy

Radiation therapy (or radiation oncology) is a relatively young field. The medical use of radiation dates back only to the 1890s when X rays and radium were first discovered and when radiation was thought to be the "cure" for many previously incurable diseases.

In its early days, radiation therapy was a poorly understood adjunct to surgery. Irradiation often was delivered in single, massive doses using unsophisticated equipment.

By the 1920s and 30s, however, patients were receiving irradiation in smaller doses over several weeks. Splitting the dose, known as fractionation, was found to improve radiation's effectiveness against tumors while significantly reducing damage to normal tissues. Over the next few years, as units and measures for radiation were developed, treatment improved.

But radiation therapy, even as it became a more exacting clinical science, did not immediately find its own niche as a medical specialty. As recently as 1955, radiation therapy generally was practiced by radiologists who usually devoted most of their time to diagnostic work.

In recent years therapy has become recognized as a specialty distinct from diagnostic radiology and nuclear medicine. Separate training programs for radiation therapists and radiation therapy technologists are now standard and the specialty boards now examine in both diagnosis and therapy.

With the development of megavoltage equipment, more effective radiation therapy techniques have become available. More advances in radiation therapy are expected in the next few years as techniques perfected through clinical research are put into practice. Much research and clinical attention has been given to radiobiology, the study of how cells, organ systems, and tumors respond to radiant energy. Because of lessons learned through this research, the future of radiation therapy probably will bring the increased application of techniques using oxygen (oxygen increases the responsiveness of cells to radiation), hypothermia, and other new methods.

Cancer continues to claim the lives of thousands of Americans annually, and as long as the methods to prevent cancer remain unknown, radiation therapy will continue to make a substantial contribution to the care of cancer patients.

THE EFFECTS OF RADIATION

One of the questions that patients often ask is, "What do the effects of radiation feel like and is the use of radiation and other energy forms in medicine safe?" There is no sensation when X rays or gamma rays are administered. With diagnostic levels of radiation, there are no changes in body function noticed by the patient. After two or three weeks of radiation therapy, the skin in the area of treatment can appear red. This is technically termed "erythema" and is often equated with sunburn. The skin reaction is a natural consequence of the treatment and will gradually disappear. Occasionally, patients receiving radiation treatment complain of nausea and loss of energy. Medication can control the symptoms of this "radiation sickness," which often disappear shortly after treatments are completed.

A major risk of excessive radiation exposure is the mutation of genes. These traits could be transmitted to children as hereditary characteristics. Gene mutation can result from exposure of the reproductive organs to radiation. That is why these organs are shielded from the radiation beam whenever possible.

When genetic injury does occur, it can be permanent. X-ray dosage is cumulative. For this reason, not only are patients protected, but so are the people who work in the radiological field. This is the reason for the film badges and measuring devices worn by radiation workers. Lead aprons are worn and the technologist steps behind a protective panel or shield during the exposure.

Lead is used to absorb the X rays in the doors, control booths, floors, and ceiling of the X-ray room so that radiation does not escape to nearby locations and expose other people.

Some X-ray procedures have been changed because of the potential damage from the dose received by patients. Fluoroscopic examination of the chest, once a routine procedure, is only performed when a patient's symptoms definitely warrant it. The use of routine photofluorographs in the detection of tuberculosis by mobile chest units has been abandoned.

During a patient's examination the technologist will determine the area of radiation exposure by shining a light through the same aperture from which the radiation will be emitted. This helps pinpoint the area to be exposed during the study. Cones and diaphragms regulate the size of the X-ray beam and focus it only on the appropriate area. Aluminum filters are placed in the radiation beam to eliminate low-level radiation that is unnecessary to the image. Much more sensitive X-ray film and detectors are used in radiological studies than previously, allowing exposure levels only a fraction of those formerly needed to gain the same amount of information. During fluoroscopy, a technique known as image intensification allows lower doses of radiation.

The consultation that occurs between the physician and the radiologist safeguards the patient. The consulting physician will often describe the patient's symptoms and consult with the radiologist about the best way to find their cause. The radiologist often recommends an alternative or an additional study.

The use of ionizing radiation by persons without specialized knowledge is not recommended. The radiologist and radiological science team are the only persons who should routinely be allowed to use these energy sources in the diagnosis and treatment of human diseases. The safeguards are in their educational experience and background.

CHAPTER 33   LESTER F. SOYKA, M.D.

DRUGS
AND
MEDICINES

Man has been described as the only drug-taking animal, a characteristic as unique as his opposable thumb. Man's desire to take drugs predates recorded history. For centuries drugs were consumed in the form of dried leaves, plants, and concoctions of berries, roots, and herbs, although most of today's new drugs are synthetic organic molecules. Man has always looked for ways to relieve pain and a variety of other complaints. Moreover, drug-taking frequently has been incorporated into religious ceremonies and festivals.

RATIONAL AND IRRATIONAL DRUG USE

Man's mind is both rational and irrational, and so is his drug-taking behavior. The wide use of drugs and medicines for therapeutic purposes is covered in other chapters in this book. Man has used his rational mind to select and invent remedies designed to provide relief from a variety of symptoms such as pain, inflammation, cough, and vomiting. Perhaps even more rational is the use of drugs to cure disease, which is different from using them to relieve symptoms. Historical uses of drugs (such as quinine, which can cure malaria) were identified in folk medicine. However, in those days people were not able to identify such treatment as curative. The development of salvarsan by Paul Ehrlich in 1907 heralded an era of discovery based on the principle of selective toxicity, in which a particular drug is directed toward a particular illness. Ehrlich used an empirical approach in which he found that the 606th compound of arsenic that he studied was effective in the treatment of syphilis. The highest level achieved in the use of drugs to cure disease is to be found in the use of antibiotics and associated chemotherapeutic agents. Few drugs are more dramatic in their power to cure than penicillin.

The next step down the ladder of rationality is the use of drugs for symptoms that are not easily or objectively measured. In recent decades, drug therapy has been used most extensively for symptoms of anxiety. Anxiety is not easily defined nor measured, so it is difficult to assess a drug's success scientifically. Moreover, a "gray zone" of rationality arises from a basic conflict: using part of the brain for a decision that involves the brain itself, the organ affected by the disorder. This is a question often raised about man's ultimate ability to understand mental illness.

Also in the "gray zone" of rationality is the overuse of a drug that has a sound therapeutic basis but which becomes overused because the treatment lasts too long, too much of the drug is used, or the drug is used more frequently than needed. Overuse is not only irrational but possibly destructive (see page 809). Such behavior frequently is associated with drugs that alter mental state, even though their therapeutic use is for a completely different purpose. For example, corticosteroids (cortisone and others) are used to suppress an inflammatory condition such as rheumatoid arthritis, but because of the altered mental state produced by these drugs, they sometimes are used too long, or too often.

Yet another form of drug-taking behavior belonging to the "gray zone" is the use of drugs for recreation. Beginning with the ancient Bacchanalian festivals, we can trace through history a multitude of alcohol-containing beverages and mood-altering drugs found in plants and mushrooms to today's multifaceted use of 100 or more drugs and chemicals for recreation. Drug use has been defended as an integral part of individual and social needs, accepted as normal in many contemporary circles. Nevertheless, such use can be harmful to an individual, friends and family, or society. Alcohol remains the cornerstone of recreational drug use worldwide, but cultural considerations influence which drug people use. Smoking marijuana is predominant for many persons. Chewing coca leaves predominates in some South American countries, and hashish is used in certain Moslem groups where alcoholic beverages are prohibited.

Yet another facet of recreational drug use, often considered trivial or incidental, involves substances whose usage has become so ingrained that they are no longer recognized as drugs. An example is caffeine, a mild central nervous system stimulant found in coffee, tea, and cola beverages. Because it can cause mild degrees of tolerance, withdrawal symptoms, and psychological dependence, and because of worldwide popularity, caffeine has been termed the most common drug of abuse.

THE MODERN ERA:

MIRACLE DRUGS

Although some useful agents such as opium, cinchona bark, digitalis leaf, and salicylates came to us from previous centuries, the discovery of penicillin ushered in the modern era of drug therapy. For the first time a few doses of a drug would provide not just symptomatic relief, but a true cure, by killing the bacteria causing the disorder. In fact, the mode of its discovery—progressing from serendipitous laboratory observations through isolation and identification and then clinical trials in patients—set a pattern for drug development that is largely followed today.

Three distinct phases led to the development of penicillin. First, Dr. Alexander Fleming, a British scientist, observed in 1928 that colonies of certain bacteria died when their culture dish became contaminated with the common bread mold *Penicillium notatum*. He did not extend this observation nor did he see it as having any relevance to human disease.

The second phase began with the work of Drs. Howard Florey and Ernst Chain in 1939 that resulted in extraction and purification of penicillin. Its first administration to patients produced "miraculous" effects. The work of Dr. Florey and his group was disrupted by World War II and the German bombing of London. Nevertheless, by 1941 they had successfully treated four of six patients with infections resistant to sulfa drugs, the only available chemotherapy then available. Florey came to the United States in 1941 to explore the possibility of mass production of penicillin. It happened that Florey had met Dr. John F. Fulton, a reknowned neurophysiologist at Yale. That is why the first patient to be treated in the United States was Mrs. Ogden Miller, the 33-year-old wife of Yale's athletic director. She had developed blood poisoning after a miscarriage and was near death with fever ranging from 103 to 106 degrees for more than four weeks. The penicillin arrived from England by airmail on a Saturday morning and a small trial dose was given at 3:30 Saturday afternoon. Larger doses were then begun every four hours. By 9 a.m. Sunday Mrs. Miller's temperature had dropped to normal and she began to eat for the first time in four weeks. This singular event aroused excitement and initiated a full scale effort by the Merck company to produce penicillin.

The treatment of the second patient at Yale was almost as dramatic. A 60-year-old man had been near death for more than a week with a high temperature and a count of 150 bacteria per milliliter in his blood. He was given penicillin at 4 p.m. and by midnight his temperature had returned to normal. He recovered consciousness and the next morning the blood contained only one bacterium per milliliter.

Commercial production of penicillin was undertaken first in small flasks and later in huge vats containing thousands of gallons of fermentation broth. Production was so successful that by D-Day in Normandy, 1944, there was enough penicillin to treat all severe casualties, both British and American. The 1945 Nobel prize for medicine and physiology was given to Florey, Fleming, and Chain.

The idea of the "miracle" drug has excited the imagination of both scientists and laymen so much that it has taken more than three decades to establish a balanced and rational drug concept, that of risk versus benefit. We now appreciate that *no* drug is without potentially severe and even fatal adverse effects. For example, although penicillin can cure certain bacterial infections, a few rare allergic individuals suffer a fatal anaphylactic reaction from a single dose (see chapter 21, "Allergy and The Immune System"). Usually, adverse effects are less dramatic but still damaging. Thus, the careful physician and the prudent patient will compare the potential benefits of a drug with the possible hazards.

Although hundreds of millions of dollars are spent annually by the federal government and the pharmaceutical industry in new drug research and development, only about six to 10 new drugs reach the market in a year. Of these, perhaps only one-half represent important new discoveries. The others are modifications of existing molecules, so-called "me-too" drugs. Although we now have other "miracle drugs" besides penicillin, the discovery of new additions is a slow and expensive process.

MAJOR CLASSES OF DRUGS

Drugs are usually classified according to the organ that is their principal site of action or target, or according to the microbe or parasite that they act against. Other drugs are classified by indication, that is, by their use for a particular condition or disease. Names of these drugs often contain the prefix *anti-*, antihypertensive, antiarrhythmic, anticonvulsant.

However, it must be recognized that a drug can act on an organ other than the one that is diseased. For example, a diuretic, which acts on the kidney, can be used to lighten the burden on the heart by ridding the body of excessive fluid. In that case the site of action is a healthy, normal kidney, while the therapeutic goal is to improve the function of the diseased or damaged heart. Conversely, the digitalis glycosides (digoxin and digitoxin) act directly on the heart to increase its strength of contraction, thereby improving the functions of the kidney and resulting in an increase in urine flow. That is why they appear to have the same effect as a diuretic. It is important to understand where and how the prescribed drug acts, because this information will provide a basis for understanding both desirable and adverse drug effects.

Another way to categorize drugs is to divide them according to the therapeutic goal or intent. Here we identify five goals. First and foremost is the goal of producing cure. Unfortunately, we have only a handful of drugs capable of producing cures. Like penicillin, many of these are in the class of antibiotics.

The second category includes drugs used for palliation. Palliation means lessening severity of the disease, and thereby improving the quality of life. Drugs such as corticosteroids are administered to patients with rheumatoid arthritis to lessen the severity of the disorder without any hope of curing it. Another major field for palliation is that of cancer chemotherapy. Certain drugs used in combination, or in conjuction with surgery or radiation therapy, result in a significant number of cancer cures. More often, however, the physician prescribes drugs to lessen the severity of the malignant disease, to relieve pain, to improve the patient's day-to-day life, and to increase the survival time, without any expectation of a cure.

A third category of drugs includes those used for symptomatic relief, most often of a minor, self-limited illness. Common examples are cough mixtures, cold medicines, and aspirin for the ordinary upper respiratory tract infections or the common cold. Often these medications are obtained over the counter (without a prescription). Symptomatic relief remains an important part of the practice of medicine and a goal of the use of prescription drugs, but often the well-informed patient can use inexpensive over-the-counter products to relieve symptoms. This saves time and money, and the patient avoids a more potent, expensive, and potentially toxic drug.

Pharmacist, Pharmacologist, Physician: Who Does What?

Several classes of professionals are involved in evaluating drugs. A pharmacologist is a scientist, usually holding a Ph.D. degree, who is concerned with the ways in which chemicals influence biologic systems and in turn are altered by the user. When such individuals also have medical training, they are called clinical pharmacologists. Both the pharmacologist and the clinical pharmacologist should be differentiated from pharmacists, who are trained to prepare and dispense drugs on the order of a physician. Pharmacists also dispense medicines that can be sold without a prescription (over the counter). Recently, the impact of specialization has spread from medicine to pharmacy, and some persons now receive training in a hospital setting during two or three years of post-pharmacy training. These individuals are called clinical pharmacists and do not have medical training. All these must be differentiated from those able to write prescriptions for drugs: the physician (M.D.), the osteopath (D.O.), the dentist (D.D.S.), and veterinarian (D.V.M.).

A fourth category includes drugs used to prevent disease. Prime examples are vitamins, particularly the water soluble vitamins, C and B complex, for which there is a daily requirement. Immunizations with killed or weakened live bacteria, such as vaccines for diphtheria, tetanus, and pertussis (DPT), and immunizations with killed or weakened viruses, such as for the prevention of polio, influenza, and measles, also fall into this group. The prevention of disease is by far the most cost-effective and desirable approach to health care.

The fifth category includes medications used to obtain an effect believed by the consumer to be desirable, yet not related to a disease. The outstanding example is the oral contraceptive—"the pill." This medication, of which there are several forms sold, has had a tremendous impact on the United States and the world. The arrival of "the pill" caused scientific medicine to reevaluate considerations of risk versus benefit, because these must be calculated with the awareness that millions of healthy young women take a medication that has serious and even fatal adverse effects.

HOW YOUR DOCTOR
LOOKS AT DRUGS

The term pharmacokinetics was first used in 1953 by Professor F. H. Dost of Giessen, West Germany, to describe the mathematical study of the behavior of drugs in the body. Although this field appears to be abstract, it is clear that the application of pharmacokinetics has led to considerable advances in our understanding of the way drugs act in man. The pharmacokinetic phases are absorption, distribution, metabolism, and excretion.

Absorption: entry into the body. A drug usually must travel across several tissue barriers to its target. In the topical form of therapy, in which the drug is applied directly to the skin or mucous membranes of the nose, mouth, vagina, etc., the approach is direct. However, drugs are usually taken orally, undergoing changes in the stomach and intestine before passing through the bloodstream to the target organ. During hospitalization a more direct route is often needed, so drugs are administered directly into the bloodstream (intravenous), or deposited below the skin (subcutaneous) or into a muscle mass (intramuscular) to achieve rapid and complete absorption. The parenteral (other than oral) route is sometimes employed outside the hospital for drugs that would be destroyed in the stomach. Insulin, for example, is injected beneath the skin to treat diabetes mellitus. Many drugs can be administered parenterally, but the general dislike of patients for injections and their discomfort, plus the need to maintain sterility, stimulate drug manufacturers to develop products that can be taken orally whenever possible.

Distribution: where the drug goes. In most cases the drug finds its way into the bloodstream and is carried throughout the body. Many drugs are distributed to one of the major fluid compartments of the body, most often the total body water or the extracellular fluid. In contrast, some drugs have highly specialized distribution and concentrate in particular organs. If the concentration is selective for the target organ, there is therapeutic advantage. For example, the digitalis glycosides, such as digoxin, are highly bound to the heart, where they improve the heart's ability to contract and stabilize abnormal rhythms. If, however, high concentrations of a drug are found in organs that are not the therapeutic target, there can be toxic effects. Because many drugs are eliminated from the body by the liver or kidneys, high concentrations and thus toxicity may occur in these organs.

Despite its general distribution, a drug must achieve sufficient concentrations at its molecular site of action, termed the receptor (see page 807). Special aspects of distribution are the limited penetration of drugs into some areas. One important example is the so-called "blood-brain barrier." This means that certain drugs do not readily pass into the brain. This is an advantage when it limits adverse effects of a drug intended to act on another organ. Conversely, poor penetration is a disadvantage if the drug's target is the brain, such as in the treatment of tumors or leukemia affecting the central nervous system.

Another special case is the placenta. For many years doctors believed that the placenta was a barrier to the passage of drugs, thus protecting the fetus from drugs and chemicals in the mother's circulation. Although this is true for a few substances, most drugs do pass across the placenta and achieve concentrations comparable to those in the mother. In general it is prudent to assume that anything in the mother's blood will reach the fetus.

Special problems of limited distribution lead the physician to administer a drug directly into an area. Examples are injections into the spinal fluid to reach the brain and spinal cord (intrathecal), into an abscess or wound, or into a joint (intraarticular).

Elimination: ridding the body. The principal routes for elimination of a drug from the body are via the liver and biliary system (and from there into the gastrointestinal tract), or via the kidney, in which case the drug or its metabolites appear in the urine. The balance between these major routes of elimination ranges widely. Drugs such as penicillin undergo little if any metabolism and are rapidly excreted unchanged in the urine. Other drugs are extensively metabolized and appear almost exclusively in bowel movements, having been excreted via the bile. Another mechanism leading to elimination of the drug results from incomplete absorption from the gastrointestinal tract. Other routes of elimination are less important overall, including the breath via the lungs, perspiration and other body secretions, and breast milk. Although these routes usually contribute only to a trivial degree in the overall elimination of a drug fom the body, distribution into such fluids as semen accounts for action of the drug far removed from its more concentrated or conspicuous sites.

PHARMACODYNAMICS
(HOW A DRUG ACTS)

Pharmacodynamics refers to how drugs exert their actions in the body. In general, the drug combines with a receptor in a reversible manner, according to the law of mass action. That law decrees that enough drug molecules must be present in the vicinity of the receptors on the cells to occupy sufficient numbers of receptor sites and cause a particular response. The more drug molecules added to this system (the larger the dose) the higher the probability that the molecules of the drug will interact with the receptors.

Drug-Receptor Interactions: The Basis of Drug Effects

Modern pharmacologic theory is based on the concept of a drug molecule effecting a unique relationship with a receptor molecule on the surface of a cell or within it. This combination in turn leads to a biochemical event or events which change the structure or function of the cell or group of cells within a tissue.

The effects of the combination of a drug molecule with a receptor vary widely and depend on the site of the receptor. A common site for drug receptors is the cell membrane. Interaction with cell surface receptors is involved in immediate type allergic responses. They occur when the allergen molecule interacts with an immunoglobin E (IgE) antibody attached to the membrane of certain cells, particularly mast cells (see chapter 21, "Allergy and the Immune System"). The precision fit of the allergen to the antibody is remarkable. Individuals sensitive to a food or drug respond to only one of the many thousands of molecules to which they are exposed.

Another fundamental effect of the drug-receptor interaction is a change in the property of the cell membrane to act as a conductor of an electrical current, called an action potential, which is responsible for transmission of impulses along nerves and all excitable tissues. Blocking nerve transmission by drugs produces local anesthesia useful for dental and surgical procedures.

The drug receptor can be a specific enzyme on the cell surface. A change in enzyme activity leads to a cascade of events within the cell.

Another mechanism of action on cell surface receptors is to change permeability of the membrane. This can change the electrical properties of the membrane or bring about a number of other actions on metabolic events inside the cell.

Drugs and receptors also interact within the cell. Here the drug alters enzyme activity, or combines with a receptor in the fluid part of the cell (cytoplasm) to form a complex, which then is translocated to the nucleus of the cell, where it may interact with the genetic material. Some drugs enter the nucleus directly, without combining with a receptor, and interact with DNA, RNA, and proteins within the nucleus.

All of these effects on target cells can result in a quantitative change (an increase or decrease in cellular activities) or in a qualitative change (the cell stops an activity or starts a new one). The activities sometimes are confined to a single enzyme function, and sometimes include a number of activities, even leading to the ultimate effect of a drug: causing the death of a cell.

Adverse Drug Reactions

Ideally, relatively few cells of a particular type in an organ would be affected by a drug, leading to a highly specific, limited, direct action. Unfortunately, few if any drugs are that specific. Most affect a large number of cell types in most organs of the body. Therefore, drugs result in both desired therapeutic effects and undesired adverse reactions.

Adverse reactions fall into three categories. First are those that are extensions of the direct actions of the drugs. These make up the majority of adverse drug reactions. The second group of adverse effects results from unusual, highly individualized responses or from allergic reactions. These are not directly related to the recognized pharmacologic activities of the drug and are not dependent on the dose or duration of use. A third type results from individual differences in rates at which the drugs are used by the body and their products released. In any individual these differences may produce a significant amount of a toxic product that occurs only in minor amounts in most people.

An important concept in understanding adverse drug reactions is that the time course of drug action on different organs varies widely. Moreover, actions by the drug can continue long after most of the administered dose has been eliminated, because a few drug molecules remain attached to receptors or because the drug has set into motion a series of complex, biochemical events that continues after the drug has been eliminated from the body.

Altered Responses to Drugs

While we can understand how a drug acts when administered in average doses to the average person, many factors can change the expected response. One of the most prominent, seen with the drugs most subject to overuse, is called tolerance. One form, called metabolic or dispositional tolerance, results from an increase in the activity of enzymes, primarily in the liver, that change the drug to inactive metabolites. This phenomenon, called enzyme induction, occurs in response to a large number of prescription drugs, as well as to chemicals contained in food (such as charcoal broiled meats) and environmental pollutants (such as cigarette smoke). In addition to dispositional tolerance, which mainly emphasizes changes in the drugs, there is change in the response of the target cells themselves.

Another prominent form of tolerance, termed behavioral tolerance, changes the response to a dose of a drug. For example, when a person is anxious, drinking coffee may accentuate the anxiety, yet a cup or two after a meal can be pleasantly relaxing.

GETTING THE MOST FROM YOUR PRESCRIPTION

To avoid toxicity, including the threat of misuse and abuse, you should be aware of ways to obtain the most benefit at the least risk from a doctor's prescription. The person receiving a prescription should inquire about the desired effect and obtain simple but clear directions for the drug's use, length of treatment, and the side effects to be expected. A few drug products include a printed circular called a patient product insert. Patients should read the insert, which provides detailed medical and scientific information about the drug, although it is written in technical language. Many package inserts are published in the *Physician's Desk Reference,* which is available at many bookstores.

Generic vs. trade names. Considerable controversy and confusion exists about the cost savings of prescriptions written by the generic name. The savings vary widely from product to product, ranging from trivial to substantial. In most instances the generic drug will be therapeutically equivalent to the trade name product if both are marketed by reputable firms. It is clear that some generic drugs are below standards, just as it is true that the presence of a brand name does not ensure that a product is without flaws, or even that it is

made by the company whose name appears on the label. If a medication is to be taken for a long time, you can usually save by buying a large package, say 1,000 or even 5,000 tablets. This saves the dispensing fee, which in some cases exceeds the cost of the medication itself. Many newer products are protected by trade name and there is no generic equivalent available. Substantial cost savings also can be gained by your selection of a pharmacy.

Despite the emphasis of some consumer activitist groups, the major cost saving in drugs comes from limiting prescription drugs to strict medical need and from the avoidance of new, generally expensive drugs, which may offer little or no advantage over tried and true drugs. For example, for many patients the new nonsteroidal anti-inflammatory agents used for arthritis offer no advantage over aspirin, but some physicians feel compelled to prescribe them instead of aspirin because the patient expects something new and expensive, which carries the magical connotation of being better. Both physician and patient must exhibit trust in one another's judgment, and confusion usually can be avoided by a frank discussion.

What to ask the pharmacist. Pharmacy education has undergone a remarkable development during the past few decades. Modern pharmacists are well educated and can provide a considerable amount of information about drugs. The patient should try to make maximum use of their expertise. Particular questions to ask the pharmacist have to do with proper dose, timing and duration of medication, and special storage conditions.

Compliance. One of the most vexing problems facing doctors is the failure of patients to carry out directions. Study after study has shown that even when patients understand the need, many will fail to complete a course of therapy as simple as taking one penicillin tablet three times a day for 10 days. Perhaps because of embarrassment, patients rarely volunteer that they have failed to take the required number of tablets each day or to report interruptions in therapy. The physician, unaware of why the drug didn't work, then prescribes another drug, increases the dose, or considers other approaches, such as surgery. Every patient should report clearly any deviation from the prescribed therapy. If questions arise about the wisdom of continuing therapy in the face of side effects, the physician should be contacted.

Length of treatment. Following the doctor's orders is particularly important in regard to length of treatment. There is a natural tendency to discontinue medication once symptoms disappear. This can result in failure to eradicate an infection, or it may mean that an underlying problem is not resolved, such as the constriction that causes bronchial asthma. Other reasons are more complex and perhaps seem mysterious or unnecessary to a patient. For example, the treatment of "strep" throat must be continued for 10 days to prevent delayed consequences such as rheumatic fever, not because the infection itself requires 10 days of therapy. It is especially difficult for patients to comply when the disorder produces no symptoms, such as in mild hypertension (high blood pressure), yet compliance is important.

Drug interactions. An important factor in the effects of a drug is its interaction with other drugs or with chemicals in foods, beverages, or the environment. The interactions can enhance side effects, diminish the drug's effectiveness, or cause other responses that interfere with the desired effect. Two drugs administered at the same time may interefere with the absorption of one another. Similarly, a drug can act as an inducer to enhance the activity of liver drug-metabolizing enzymes, which then more rapidly degrade the drug. Some drugs enhance or retard the elimination of another drug, often by altering its distribution. As we will see with drugs of the sedative-hypnotic family (see page 810), drugs whose chemical structures and names appear quite different may produce cumulative pharmacologic effects (synergism) or even more strongly enhance the effects of one another (potentiation). It is important to inform your doctor of all drugs you are taking. Some pharmacists establish patient indexes to alert them to the possibility of drug interactions with each new prescription.

DRUG ABUSE

Although the term "drug abuse" has become part of our everyday language, a more accurate term is "substance abuse." This definition includes not only abuse of prescription and over-the-counter drugs, but excessive caloric intake, alcohol consumption, use of tobacco, and the use of illicit drugs. When substance abuse becomes extreme, the behavior is labeled addiction. Less extreme behavior is termed dependence and applied to cigarette smoking, excessive coffee drinking, or overeating. It is not clear whether addiction and de-

pendence represent the same basic disorder modified by socioeconomic and other factors, or whether individual personality differences determine the exact choice of a substance to be abused.

In 1964 the World Health Organization (WHO) defined drug dependence as consisting of three aspects: tolerance, physical dependence, and compulsive abuse (psychic craving). Most workers in the field would add self-administration and destructive consequences to the user as characteristics of drug dependence.

Tolerance means that repeated administration of the same dose leads to a lessened effect. The substance's original effect becomes diminished after repeated doses of the same size, but can be reinstated by increasing the dose. Tolerance is believed to underlie drug dependence and can be demonstrated with all of the common drugs of abuse.

Dependence is sometimes divided into psychic and physical categories. Psychic dependence exists when stopping use of the drug does not produce physical reactions but results in drug-seeking behavior or "craving." Habituation is another term often used but it is poorly defined. It generally indicates lesser degrees of dependence. Physical dependence is manifested by obvious signs of drug withdrawal, such as when narcotics or barbiturates are abruptly discontinued after long-term, high-dose use. Perhaps the distinctions between psychic and physical dependence exist more in theory than reality, and derive from the outmoded concept of a division between mind and body.

Tolerance is related to dependence in part because as the initial effects diminish with repeated use, the person must employ larger or more frequent doses to attain the original effect. The diminished response to the original dose may lead to withdrawal symptoms. The development of tolerance, therefore, contributes to the dependence process by requiring ever-increasing doses to attain the desired effects.

Compulsive abuse. Another aspect of drug dependence is called compulsive abuse, psychic craving, or drug-seeking behavior. Controversy exists about whether there are certain personalities for whom drug-taking indicates an underlying psychological disorder. Some believe that if we are given the opportunity, a conducive social setting, and peer acceptance, we all seek chemical relief from anxiety, fear, boredom, or pain in one form or another. For many of us the drug-taking behavior is limited to socially acceptable medication, or to trivial sorts of over-the-counter products, such as headache remedies, laxatives, or cough drops. Even the current food faddism and the megavitamin craze could be expressions of drug-taking behavior.

Next in frequency, and ingrained in 20th century social life, is a widespread acceptance of use of alcoholic beverages. The cocktail has become integrated into the daily activities of a large segment of our society. Wine, beer, and liquor are served at most social, family, fraternal, and other gatherings.

Perhaps the next step is the overuse of prescription drugs, particularly those of the sedative-hypnotic class, such as benzodiazepines. The two most popular members of this group of drugs, Librium® and Valium,® have been the two most prescribed drugs in the United States for several years. Beyond this lies the wide range of illicit drugs, of which marijuana is by far the most commonly used. Within this spectrum many compulsive abusers use individual substances interchangeably. Nevertheless, some people settle on a single agent for persistent abuse, such as alcohol or heroin.

Genetics is an important aspect of compulsive abuse. Although it is often difficult to separate genetic from environmental influences, certain forms of drug abuse, particularly alcoholism, appear to have a strong genetic foundation. Epidemiologic studies indicate that Irish and Swedish males, whether they reside in their native country or emigrate to the United States, have the highest rates of alcoholism. In other population groups, such as in Iceland and isolated communities in northern Canada and Alaska, environmental influences appear to be responsible for the high incidence of alcoholism. Laboratory experiments indicate that certain strains of mice show a preference for drinking alcohol-containing solutions. Most inbred mouse strains, like other species, do not voluntarily ingest alcohol, even if the taste is masked. Apparently they do not like the effect. However, mice of some strains prefer drinking alcoholic solutions, and maintain a high blood level over extended periods, presumably because it is pleasurable for them. This suggests that certain gene pools (nationalities) have a genetic, biochemically determined predisposition to seek the effects of alcohol.

DRUGS COMMONLY ABUSED

Sedative-Hypnotic Drugs

Although there are important differences among the substances categorized as sedative-hypnotic, the similarities are even more impressive. All of them except marijuana show varying degrees of dispositional and functional tolerance (see page 808). Abrupt withdrawal following chronic, high-dose abuse can result in a severe, sometimes fatal, abstinence syndrome. In fact, it is often said that no one has died from the decidedly uncomfortable but relatively safe withdrawal from heroin or narcotic abuse, known as "going cold turkey," but deaths have resulted from acute withdrawal from barbiturates, pentobarbital (Nembutal®) and secobarbital (Seconal®). The withdrawal from abuse of alcohol, barbiturates, benzodiazepines, and meprobamate can bring on hallucinations, seizures, lowered body temperature, and other life-threatening conditions.

Alcohol. Ethyl alcohol (ethanol) is a simple organic molecule usually obtained by the fermentation of sugars or starches by a yeast, which results in the conversion of the sugar to ethanol and water. This fermentation and the use of flavorings and associated products are an important part of the cultures of most races.

Different responses to alcohol. Tolerance for alcohol has both a dispositional and a functional basis (see page 808). Functional tolerance can be illustrated by comparing figures for blood-alcohol levels. One basis for the diagnosis of alcoholism used by the National Council on Alcoholism is the lack of behavioral impairment at a blood-alcohol concentration of 150 milligrams per deciliter (mg/dl) or above. Yet, a concentration of only 100 mg/dl (0.10%) is considered clear evidence in almost all states of driving while intoxicated. In studies performed by Drs. N. K. Mello and J. H. Mendelson at the Alcohol and Drug Abuse Research Center of Harvard Medical School, chronic alcoholics allowed to follow their own drinking schedule while performing a simple task maintained blood levels of 200 to 300 mg/dl and were able to perform complex tasks accurately even when blood alcohol levels exceeded 250 mg/dl. The lethal concentration of alcohol in the blood is about 550 mg/dl, indicating that in an alcoholic, only a slim margin exists between apparently normal behavior and death.

Cross-tolerance. Another characteristic of the alcohol abuser is cross-tolerance. Tolerance for alcohol is associated with a tolerance for other drugs of the sedative-hypnotic family. Nonetheless, the absolute ceiling for a lethal dose remains unchanged, resulting in truly dangerous potential when members of this class (alcohol and barbiturates, for example) are combined.

Effects on the unborn. It has become clear in recent years that a woman's heavy drinking during pregnancy has detrimental effects on the growth and development of her fetus. This condition is termed the fetal alcohol syndrome. Even small amounts of alcohol during pregnancy (greater than one drink per day) can detectably affect the fetus. Since having several drinks per day is considered normal "social" drinking by many, a reevaluation of what should be considered appropriate drinking during pregnancy is clearly needed. In addition, studies in animals indicate that high alcohol consumption by males before mating with untreated females results in adverse effects on the offspring. Whether such studies, which include narcotics, will prove applicable to humans remains to be seen.

Alcohol and the nursing mother. In contrast to our recent awareness of the dangers of alcohol during pregnancy, long-standing concern about drinking by nursing mothers appears to have been unnecessary. Although alcohol appears in breast milk at a concentration similar to that in the mother's blood, few reports have surfaced of intoxication or other effects on the nursing infant. Many writers refer to a single case of a nursing infant who became intoxicated after the mother drank a bottle of port wine. Since that 1936 report there has been only one other, a case of an infant who developed a rare condition (pseudo Cushing's syndrome) and whose mother was a heavy drinker. Even assuming a sustained blood concentration in the mother of 200 mg/dl, which is unlikely to continue for many days, the maximum amount excreted in a quart of breast milk would not be more than the equivalent of a teaspoon of 100 proof bourbon. Recognizing that even small amounts might affect an infant during development, it remains highly unlikely that the extremely low levels contained in the breast milk of a woman who is an occasional social drinker will have a detrimental effect. Moreover, by drinking immediately after a feeding, a woman can minimize the alcohol in the breast milk.

Barbiturates. Drugs of this class are used for the management of anxiety and insomnia, and to prevent epileptic seizures. Their use as sleeping pills has diminished because use leads to the loss of the rapid eye movement

Who Is an Alcoholic?

The identification of who is an alcoholic and who is a social drinker remains controversial because of overlap in the behaviors and because of the derogatory implications of the word "alcoholic." Society is still debating whether alcoholism is a medical illness or a social disease or a moral handicap. The National Council on Alcoholism has developed extensive, precise criteria to establish the diagnosis of alcoholism. In brief, the major criteria include:

- Physiological dependency as shown by evidence of a withdrawal syndrome—tremors, hallucinations, seizures, or delirium tremens (DTs).
- Evidence of tolerance for the effects of alcohol. One example is a blood alcohol concentration of more than 150 mg/dl without gross evidence of intoxication. Another is the daily consumption of a fifth of a gallon of whiskey or the equivalent amount of wine or beer.
- Medical findings indicating a major alcohol-associated illness.
- Drinking despite strong medical and social recommendations, or the patient's own recognition of loss of control over alcohol consumption.

Of great importance is the recognition of early signs of alcoholism. These include: gulping drinks; surreptitious drinking; early morning drinking; medical absences from work for a variety of reasons; shifting from one alcoholic beverage to another; preference for drinking companions, bars, and taverns; a loss of interest in activities not directly associated with drinking; drinking more than the peer group; unexplained changes in family, social, and business relationships; complaints about wife, job, and friends; major family disruptions; loss or frequent change of jobs; and financial difficulties.

(REM) phase of sleep. As a consequence, barbiturate users suffer lethargy, confusion, anxiety, and worsened insomnia.

As with alcohol, relatively small doses of barbiturates initially produce excitation and exhilaration, while large doses cause drowsiness and sleep. Overdoses cause coma and death. With alcohol, however, man has learned to modify the dose, time of ingestion, occasion, and setting to achieve exhilaration and relief from anxiety without undue sedation. Still, speaking of an alcoholic beverage as a "nightcap" recognizes its sedative properties.

Dosage rather than blood concentration indicates the degree of tolerance that develops from overuse of barbiturates. For example, the usual sedative dose of pentobarbital (Nembutal®) is one-tenth of a gram. Some abusers use 10 to 12 times that dose to attain the desired mental state, whereas the lethal dose remains at about two grams (twenty 100 mg capsules). A lethal dose can be achieved easily by combining the usual daily dose with modest amounts of other sedative-hypnotic drugs, commonly alcohol. Frequent newspaper reports of deaths of celebrities from such combinations point to the slim margin of safety. The United States appears to be following the lead of the United Kingdom and European countries by phasing out the use of barbiturates as nighttime sedatives because of their abuse potential, their frequency of use for suicide, and the serious consequences of accidental overdose.

Benzodiazepines. Two of the prominent members of this family of drugs, chlordiazepoxide (Librium®) and diazepam (Valium®), have been the leading prescription drugs for the past decade, each accounting for sales of hundreds of millions of dollars annually. While these drugs have extremely useful properties, they have many similarities to the barbiturates. One major advantage is that the lethal dose is extremely high, making it virtually impossible to take a suicidal dose. However, if the abuser combines one or more benzodiazepines with other sedative-hypnotic drugs, particularly barbiturates and alcohol, the result can be fatal. Certain of the benzodiazepines, flurazepam (Dalmane®), for example, have virtually replaced barbiturates as nighttime sedatives, largely because of their lesser inhibition of REM sleep, relatively low addiction potential, and high therapeutic index (the ratio between an effective and a lethal dose).

Chronic, high-dose use of benzodiazepines produces marked physical dependency, probably to an even greater extent than barbiturates. The dose of Librium® or Valium® that can be taken by the abuser is much greater (compared to the standard dose) than the escalation of doses that can be taken by the barbiturate abuser, partly because of the sharp upper limit to the tolerance for barbiturates. A major convulsive seizure often occurs after abrupt withdrawal from benzodiazepines. Because of cross-tolerance and their anticonvulsant properties, barbiturates are frequently substituted for benzodiazepines during controlled withdrawal.

Meprobamate, marketed as Equanil,® Miltown,® and Meprospan,® was once one of the most frequently employed tranquilizers, but was eclipsed by the benzodiazepines. It was introduced as a muscle relaxant and was believed to have little abuse potential. In fact, abuse does lead to tolerance and a severe withdrawal syndrome, including insomnia, tremors, a staggering gait, and vomiting. The syndrome can progress to an acute psychotic reaction, major convulsive seizures, coma, and death. Unlike the benzodiazepines, which are eliminated slowly so that the gradual fall in blood concentration tends to modify or completely avoid acute withdrawal symptoms, the rapid excretion of meprobamate leads to acute withdrawal symptoms one to two days after discontinuation. As long as the dose is limited to two or three tablets a day, withdrawal reactions are extremely uncommon. The mild sedative effect and relative lack of effects on other areas of the brain yield certain advantages and cause meprobamate to be retained in medical usage. Clearly, it has been overprescribed and overused in the past.

Marijuana. The history of the use of marijuana can be traced to ancient Eastern writings. Its use throughout the Western world, which has spread with explosive rapidity, has exceeded our understanding of its effects and hazards. The pharmacology of this drug is complex, because the active principles of marijuana plants are altered by the way the drug is used. Many studies suggest that the major active constituent is delta-9-tetrahydrocannabinol (THC). This chemical is supposedly available "on the street," but what is sold is actually several other drugs, frequently phencyclidine. It is unclear whether data obtained from studies of ingestion of pure THC accurately represent the effects of smoking marijuana or hashish.

The breadth of marijuana use in the United States is astounding, with literally millions of individuals, ranging from pre-teens through the elderly, having experimented. There are frequent users in every social class. Needless to say, considerable controversy exists about its properties. Recent evidence that marijuana combats the nausea and vomiting associated with many anti-cancer drugs, and helps in the management of glaucoma, has led to state laws allowing strictly controlled medical use.

What is marijuana? In the United States, the term marijuana refers to any part or extract of the plant, but the most active compounds are concentrated in the exudate of the female flower clusters. This resin is found in preparations called "hashish" and "charas." The potency, and perhaps exact makeup, of any marijuana preparation varies tremendously, depending on the plant strain, growth conditions, and method of harvest. Further confusion arises because the natural material is sometimes diluted with a variety of substances, including other drugs.

Pharmacologic properties. Marijuana possesses the properties frequently found in the sedative-hypnotic drugs, but also causes euphoria and hallucinations. Although physical dependence does not develop, whether tolerance develops is unclear. Some investigators believe that tolerance does develop within a week. Marijuana appears to be generally well tolerated.

Serious adverse reactions to unadulterated preparations are rare, but include acute paranoia and psychotic reactions. As with other drug reactions, adverse effects are more common with high doses, such as hashish, and are highly individualized. Increased heart rate and dilation of the blood vessels of the eye are common. One important effect is the impairment of driving ability and other fine motor and coordination skills. Another is a distorted perception of the passage of time. Impaired driving performance is sharply aggravated by using alcohol at the same time, an important point because many people smoke marijuana and drink alcoholic beverages together. In addition, damage to the respiratory tract can occur after heavy hashish smoking, which can cause bronchitis, asthma, laryngitis, and sinusitis.

Heavy smoking several times a day results in a chronic intoxicated state and produces such symptoms as apathy, mental dullness, lethargy, and mild to severe impairment of judgment, concentration, and memory. However, a month of heavy consumption of hashish would be the equivalent of smoking hundreds of ordinary American marijuana cigarettes.

Marijuana and motivation. Another hotly debated issue is whether regular use of marijuana results in a feeling of apathy, the "amotivation syndrome." This is a particular concern because marijuana is used regularly by some teenagers and college students, many of whom appear to experience difficulties in psychosocial adjustments. Frequently, the appearance and performance of teenagers is less than that expected by their parents, and

marijuana smoking is blamed. Obviously, it is difficult to separate a youth's diminished drive and ambition from the disruption of the family structure and general social unrest of these turbulent times.

Dr. Mendelson and coworkers (see page 810) have also examined this question. They studied patterns in casual users and heavy users who worked at a task for 21 days, for which they were rewarded either with marijuana or money. All subjects smoked marijuana every day. Casual smokers smoked an average of 2.6 cigarettes per day, heavy users smoked an average of 5.7. Both groups increased the amount they smoked over the 21-day period, with casual users ending the period at an average of 5.8 cigarettes daily, and heavy users 14.3 per day. Nonetheless, productivity remained constant while marijuana use increased, arguing against a clear relationship between marijuana effects and motivation, at least as defined in this artificial setting. The same studies found that when allowed access to both alcohol and marijuana, there was a significant decrease in alcohol consumption compared to a period when only alcohol was available. Fourteen of 16 subjects decreased alcohol use when marijuana was permitted. Tobacco use also accompanied alcohol and marijuana, and it is known that there is a significant positive correlation between the use of alcohol and tobacco and a correlation between the use of marijuana and tobacco. Although it is unclear how these research results apply to the question of motivation, it is clear that simultaneous availability of marijuana and alcohol did not lead to a significant increase in the use of both drugs. On the other hand, it is probable that easy access to marijuana, which would occur if it were legalized, would lead to a substantial increase in use by both casual and heavy smokers. Moreover, modest degrees of intellectual impairment and lack of drive may be more apparent in a competitive intellectual setting, such as in high school or college, than in a research ward.

Concerns about marijuana. Despite the lack of clear evidence linking marijuana to harmful physical effects, a number of health care professionals have observed that heavy marijuana use by adolescents does have detrimental effects on motivation, school performance, and family relationships. These effects are difficult to document and perhaps occur in the absence of any demonstrable physical damage. These observations are alarming because of a marked increase in marijuana use by children of junior high school age and even younger. The conclusion that occasional marijuana use by an adult has little detrimental effect on health does not rule out harmful effects from frequent use by young children and adolescents.

Clearly, marijuana use affects driving performance, a particular concern because automobile accidents are the major cause of death and disability in teenagers and young adults.

Detrimental effects on memory and learning, which have been demonstrated in the laboratory, are also of concern when the drug is used by students. It is not known whether interference with learning can be reversed later in life.

One of the most alarming recent developments has been the tremendous growth and exploitation by the drug paraphernalia industry. Several slick magazines and comic books laud the supposed virtues of drug use and instruct persons in use of drugs. The paraphernalia industry glamorizes the use of marijuana and attempts to make it fashionable, producing advertising of the same caliber that induces young people to smoke cigarettes or purchase expensive merchandise. Parents should be aware of such paraphernalia and drug-oriented literature because of their potential effects on children.

Central Nervous System Stimulants

Drugs of this class cause elevation of mood and psyche, producing excitation rather than sedation. Nonetheless, they have many of the same characteristics of the sedative-hypnotics, such as physical tolerance, serious and even fatal adverse reactions, and compulsive drug-seeking behavior.

Amphetamines. The amphetamines rose to prominence in part through their alleged usefulness in the management of obesity. Although this diet use has been limited by the U.S. Food and Drug Administration (FDA) to four weeks, many individuals, particularly young and middle-aged women, were introduced to amphetamines through a prescription given by a doctor for management of appetite. Because of government controls on production and sale, perhaps the largest source of amphetamines in the United States is illicit. The most prominent drugs in this class are dextroamphetamine (Dexedrine®), benzadrine, and methamphetamine (Methedrine® and

Desoxyn®). Other drugs in this class are used primarily for appetite control, but are closely related. Examples are phenmetrazine (Preludin®), phentermine (Ionamine®), and diethylpropionhydrochloride (Tenuate®).

Little if any physical dependence develops with amphetamines, although abrupt withdrawal can result in changes in sleep patterns, lethargy, somnolence, and in rare cases, severe depression. The question of physical dependence is complicated because many amphetamines and amphetamine-like drug preparations contain another drug, usually a barbiturate. Tolerance for the amphetamines develops slowly but can become substantial. As with barbiturates, in the individual with a high level of tolerance, the margin between the dose required to produce euphoria and the dose that will cause toxic psychosis is very narrow. Intravenous use is most prominent with abuse of methamphetamine (nicknamed "speed"). The high doses that are possible and the severe adverse effects have led to the warning "speed kills."

Small doses of amphetamines administered to a nondependent person can result in an increased sense of well-being, an apparent sharpening of wits, and decreased fatigue. These properties have led to misuse by students, housewives, truck drivers, and night workers. High doses have been shown to reduce mental sharpness and to impair performance even when the person is not fatigued. Irrational behavior, sight and sound hallucinations, and paranoid delusions occur. Long-term chronic use leads to impaired brain function, which may be permanent despite discontinuation of the drug.

In contrast to these effects, small doses of amphetamines and methylphenidate (Ritalin®) are widely and successfully used to manage children whose behavior is characterized as hyperkinetic. Because of lack of euphoria in such children, and perhaps for other reasons as well, there is no tendency to escalate dosage. There have been no reports of increased use of stimulants or other drugs later in life, and no reports of drug dependence of any sort.

Cocaine. Like marijuana, cocaine is a naturally occurring product found in the leaves of the coca plant, which grows in Peru and Bolivia. The local Indians combine the leaves with a clay-like material and keep a wad in the cheek, possibly as an adaptation to their difficult life in the high Andes Mountains. The use of cocaine at parties, usually after intranasal administration (sniffing), started in the 1920s and was popularized in the 1970s by Hollywood stars and the disco scene. Cocaine's high price and limited availability have restricted its use.

Cocaine is also used intravenously, which produces a fleeting effect requiring repeated doses at 5- to 15-minute intervals. With high doses, toxic signs occur, such as rapid heart rate, palpitations, hallucinations, and paranoid delusions. In the height of a hyperexcited paranoid state, some users become belligerent and assaultive. Prolonged "sniffing" of cocaine leads to perforation of the nasal septum because of intense and prolonged constriction of the blood vessels. Following its introduction into medical use by Sigmund Freud, cocaine has been used as a local anesthetic and to constrict blood vessels. Other effects of high doses include fever, dilated pupils, rapid heart, irregular respiration, abdominal pain, vomiting, and convulsions. Following stimulation, a depression may develop that, with acute poisoning, can result in death from paralysis of the respiratory center.

Neither physical dependence nor tolerance develops with prolonged use of cocaine.

Hallucinogens

Drugs in the hallucinogen class are characterized by lack of recognized medical usefulness and are taken primarily for their psychedelic effects. All are illicit. The psychic effects are prominent even with low doses that produce relatively minor physiologic changes.

An important characteristic is that the effects are not predictable because they are highly individualized and greatly influenced by the user's state of mind, companions, and a number of other conditions. A dose might produce little or no effect, might be a stimulant, or might be a sedative, all depending on the person's mental state and surroundings.

LSD. The synthetic compound LSD (D-lysergic acid diethylamide tartrate) is related to the alkaloids of ergot, a fungus that infests rye and other grains in Europe and North America. Although synthesized in 1938, LSD's remarkable central nervous system effects were not discovered until the drug was accidentally ingested by a researcher in 1943. Tolerance but no physical dependence develops extremely rapidly, and is lost as rapidly after use is discontinued. An initial dose of 200 to 400 micrograms can be raised to several thousand micrograms after a few days of continuous use of LSD.

The LSD "trip" is characterized by exciting feelings of strangeness and newness of experience, including vividly colored and changing hallucinations and insights. Unpleasant experiences are frequent, however, and include confusion, acute panic, reliving of prior events, and depressive and terrifying experiences. These acute effects sometimes appear to disrupt long established behavior patterns, and effects sometimes linger after use of the drug is stopped. The drug removes the usual restraints on intensity of emotions, which may be pleasurable or may lead to feelings of fear, sadness, and despair that overwhelm the user.

One of the strangest of the drug's effects has been termed "flashback." At intervals after LSD use, symptoms recur unpredictably, even months after a single dose. These vary from gentle alterations in mood to severe feelings of disruption. In some cases the flashback appears to be brought on voluntarily, but frequently it is triggered by emotional stress or by the administration of another drug with hallucinogenic properties. The ultimate flashback is said to occur when, after many trips, the user is able to feel the same continually without taking the drug.

LSD has been studied extensively because of its remarkable properties, which include its status as one of the most potent drugs ever discovered. This implies that its reaction with the receptor must be highly specific, because so little of this odorless, colorless, tasteless drug can produce remarkable central nervous system effects.

Phencyclidine. An agent similar to LSD, phencyclidine hydrochloride (Sernylan,® angel dust, PCP) has become a common and extremely dangerous drug. Introduced into veterinary medicine as a potent animal anesthetic, it was diverted into street traffic, where it was substituted for other drugs or used to increase the effects of diluted drugs such as LSD. In addition to central nervous system effects such as convulsions, hallucinations, toxic psychosis, sedation, and vivid, frightening dreams, phencyclidine can cause a severe elevation of blood pressure which can rupture small blood vessels in the brain and cause death.

Miscellaneous. A variety of other chemically related agents also produce LSD-type effects. Other diverse hallucinogenic compounds are found in morning glory seeds.

Mescaline is found in the peyote cactus indigenous to the Rio Grande Valley and used in traditional Indian ceremonies by tribes of the Southwestern United States. Mushrooms containing hallucinogens are psilocybin and psilocin. Native cults in Mexico consume these mushrooms as part of a religious experience. The effects are similar to those of LSD.

Jimsonweed is another native plant that produces hallucinations. Because of its pronounced effects in blocking nerve impulses, large doses are characterized by fever, agitation, and confusion, with severe intoxication resulting in convulsions, paralysis, coma, and death. Other effects are dilation of the pupils, rapid heart rate, decreased sweating and salivation, inability to urinate, and a warm, flushed skin. These effects also occur with many anticholinergic drugs, such as atropine and scopolamine. (These drugs are used therapeutically but in large doses can cause hallucinations, particularly in susceptible individuals, typically children and the elderly.)

Ingestion of Jimsonweed (stinkweed, thorn apple, locoweed) illustrates the evolving nature of drug abuse in the United States. Recognition of Jimsonweed intoxication did not appear in medical literature until 1975. It has been used for many years as a hallucinogen by Indian tribes in the Southwest. They brew the plant and use the resultant drink in coming-of-manhood and religious rites. The bizarre behavior of animals that have eaten the plant, which is common in the southwestern United States, led to the nickname "locoweed." Animals learn to avoid the plant. The usual name is a corruption of Jamestown weed, because the first recorded consumption by man occurred at Jamestown, Virginia, when soldiers under Captain John Smith ate the plant as part of a salad.

Narcotic Analgesics and Analogues

In many statutes, the word narcotic has achieved a legal definition that includes a variety of drugs, including marijuana and cocaine. Pharmacologically, the term narcotic refers only to drugs having both a sedative and analgesic (pain-reducing) effect, and is limited to opiate and opiate-like drugs. Categories include the naturally occurring alkaloids and semisynthetic derivatives, primarily morphine, codeine, and heroin; the synthetic compounds, including meperidine (Demerol®) and its derivatives; and methadone and its close relative propoxyphene (Darvon®). The benzomorphans, primarily pentazocine (Talwin®), have both a pain-reducing effect and a narcotic blocking effect.

Morphine is obtained from opium, which is the dry juice of the poppy plant. Opium contains 10 percent morphine and one-half percent codeine. Morphine elevates the pain threshold and alters the user's reaction to pain. It produces drowsiness and euphoria in some individuals, but anxiety and nausea in others. Constriction of the pupils, constipation, and slowed breathing occur in all patients. Large doses lead to severe respiratory depression, which is the cause of death in poisoning by morphine or any of the narcotic analgesics. Constriction of the pupil is the best indication that the drug has been used. Addicts do not develop tolerance to this effect, nor to its constipating effect. During withdrawal from the drug, the pupils of addicts become widely dilated.

Morphine provides one of the most remarkable examples of tolerance. The usual dose for a patient in pain is one one-hundredth gram of morphine sulfate twice a day, but addicts have been known to take as much as four grams in a day, a 400-fold increase. Such doses would be enough to kill several nontolerant persons. Following discontinuation of morphine, tolerance returns to normal in one to two weeks, after which the individual again responds to a small dose. Thus, after a period of abstinence during which tolerance has been lost, an addict can easily overdose from taking the accustomed injection.

The state of tolerance is immediately reversed by the administration of the narcotic antagonist naloxone. When done under carefully controlled conditions, this is a valuable diagnostic test, but it can produce a severe withdrawal syndrome. Morphine itself is not commonly abused.

Heroin. The agent of choice for narcotic addicts is heroin, which differs from morphine only by a small chemical modification. What appears to be a trivial difference in structure produces a compound that rapidly enters the brain and produces the euphoria. Addicts prefer heroin even though eventually it is almost entirely metabolized to morphine. Indeed, "blind" studies have demonstrated that addicts cannot differentiate between heroin, morphine, and related narcotic analgesic drugs. This is another example of nonpharmacologic factors influencing not only the effects of the drug, but its role in the spectrum of dependency and abuse. Heroin was once marketed as a safe, nonprescription drug, but under today's laws it cannot be legally manufactured or imported into the United States because of its high addiction potential.

There is no evidence that opiates damage the brain or other organs, even after years of continuous use, if other aspects of the individual's life are controlled. However, complications of illicit drug use and intravenous injection include infections of the liver and other organs, and damage to the kidneys, lungs, nerves, and muscles. Heroin abuse carries the constant risk of death from overdose, and additional dangers arise because foreign substances are added to heroin as adulterants. The major form of toxicity results from the social consequences of narcotic addiction, including crime, joblessness, and personal and family neglect. Most heroin users turn to crime to support the high cost of procuring enough to achieve a "high" and to avoid withdrawal.

Heroin withdrawal symptoms first appear about eight hours after the last dose, and peak within three days. Tearing, nasal stuffiness, yawning, and sweating appear first, followed by restless sleep, goose flesh, dilated pupils, agitation, and tremors. At the peak, the addict exhibits weakness, insomnia, chills, stomach cramps, nausea, vomiting, diarrhea, and severe muscle aches in the legs and back. The course of withdrawal lasts one to two weeks. Administration of small doses of an opiate, barbiturate, or benzodiazepine will alleviate the symptoms. However, restitution of tolerance does not eliminate craving for the drug, which appears to explain the low success rate achieved even in long-term, drug-free maintenance programs.

Codeine differs from morphine only slightly. In the body it is slowly and incompletely converted to morphine. Codeine is less sedative and less analgesic than morphine, and is less addictive because tolerance develops slowly. Unlike morphine, codeine can reach effective blood levels when taken by mouth. It is commonly used for management of mild pain and as a cough depressant. Because codeine will suppress the withdrawal syndrome, theft of samples from physician's offices and clinics is not uncommon. Similarly, paregoric (camphorated tincture of opium) can be diverted from its normal use as a diarrhea treatment in order to maintain a low level of addiction.

Meperidine (Demerol®) is a synthetic, orally effective compound that possesses essentially the same properties as morphine. Because of its availability and because it is effective when taken orally, it has been the most widely abused narcotic among physicians, nurses, and other health professionals.

Drugs closely related to meperidine are alphaprodine (Nisentil®), frequently used by anesthesiologists, and diphenoxylate, which is used to control diarrhea. Diphenoxylate is addictive and overdose causes severe but reversible respiratory depression.

Methadone was developed by German scientists during World War II and called Dolophine in honor of Adolf Hitler. Although the chemical structure does not resemble that of morphine, its properties are similar, except that methadone is effective orally and has a much longer duration of action. Its primary use is as an aid in the rehabilitation of heroin addicts.

Methadone blocks the euphoric action of other narcotic analgesics, but it must be taken daily and it continues rather than cures addiction. Methadone maintenance programs substitute one addiction (to methadone) for another (to heroin). Diversion to street use is extensive, and constitutes a major drug source for other addicts. The so-called Methadone Maintenance Program was initially developed by Drs. Vincent P. Dole and Marie E. Nyswander in New York City in the mid-1960s and continues to be controversial. From their single program the number of clinics has increased across the United States so that an estimated 80,000 patients have been maintained on methadone in recent years. Methadone maintenance programs are extremely expensive and success is largely dependent upon the educational and social development of the addict. The most optimistic statistics indicate that about one-half of the addicts will continue in a program for a year, and that after one to three years of methadone maintenance, withdrawal of methadone will lead to a 50 percent or greater return to narcotic use (recidivism).

Propoxyphene (Darvon®). This derivative of methadone has become one of the most widely used pain-reducing drugs. Some estimate its potency to be between that of aspirin and codeine. However, some studies have indicated that the usual doses of propoxyphene alone have little effect, or are inferior to two tablets of aspirin. Nonetheless, the drug is widely prescribed. Its availability, in part, has led to frequent abuse, particularly in conjunction with abuse of other drugs. In 1977 the U.S. Food and Drug Administration listed propoxyphene in Schedule IV of the Controlled Substances Act. Schedule IV drugs are those that "may lead to limited physical dependence or psychological dependence," but which may still be prescribed by physicians.

Because of continued problems with propoxyphene abuse, the package insert labeling was revised in 1979 to reflect the risks associated with improper use. The change recognized that Darvon® had become a major cause of drug-related deaths, particularly when involved with excessive use of alcohol, tranquilizers, or sedatives. Because of the rapid onset of action in large overdoses (20 percent of deaths occur within the first hour), propoxyphene should not be prescribed for patients with a history of emotional disturbances, suicidal impulses, or drug abuse. Moreover, the label indicates that when taken in higher than recommended doses over long periods, propoxyphene can produce drug dependence, characterized by psychological dependence and less frequently by physical dependence and tolerance. It was estimated that the abuse potential of propoxyphene was similar to that of codeine.

These problems do not mean that propoxyphene cannot be used safely for minor pain, such as after dental procedures or minor injuries, especially when used with aspirin, local cold or heat (depending on the time between injury and treatment), and rest.

Pentazocine (Talwin®). This synthetic drug has pain-reducing properties but is also a weak narcotic antagonist and thus not strictly comparable to drugs such as heroin, codeine, methadone, and propoxyphene. Although believed to have low addiction liability, it has become, like propoxyphene, a widely abused drug, frequently diverted from legitimate medical channels or abused after legitimate prescription for pain.

PREVENTION OF DRUG ABUSE

The adage relating the sixteen-fold advantage that an ounce of prevention has over a pound of cure is never more true than in the prevention of drug abuse. Although the average person may think of prevention in terms of ghetto populations, drug abuse involves individuals of all ages, social classes, and geographic areas. Clearly much needs to be done to assure proper housing, living standards, adequate nutritional and health care services, and educational facilities, but possibly of greater importance in dealing with drug abuse is what can be achieved at the personal level and within the family.

Here are some commonsense guidelines for avoiding drug abuse.

• Do not use any drugs, except when absolutely necessary, for the relief of psychological problems such as stress and anxiety. Many solutions are available other than drugs, including recreation, exercise, group interaction, and learning to deal with the individuals who

provoke stress, particularly spouse, children, and employers.

• Recognize that availability of drugs in the home can lead to temptations for adolescents and others. Moreover, availability may lead to use of the drug for an improper reason or provide a source of accidental poisoning for the curious toddler. Discard unused prescription drugs promptly following completion of a course of therapy. Be prudent about the availability of alcoholic beverages when teenagers are in the house.

• If drugs are needed or used, particularly in chronic illness, practice moderation and learn to recognize the early warning signs of abuse. This is not to say that pain relief should not be sought when it becomes debilitating or limits activity. Nonetheless, a variety of methods have been developed to relieve pain, even severe pain such as that suffered by patients with cancer. Recognition and acceptance of early warning signs are absolutely essential to avoid being deluded and "hooked." Not only are psychological "blinders" put on by those who abuse drugs, but the effect of centrally acting drugs that blur consciousness and distort reality further hinders an individual's ability to accept a diagnosis of drug abuse.

• Learn about and be wary of drugs that are prescribed. The busy, harassed physician can become an unwitting accomplice by prescribing a drug and inadvertently contributing to the development or maintenance of an abuse problem. This is particularly true with the sedative-hypnotic and tranquilizer drugs.

• Emphasize the traditional values of family structure by giving attention to children and being aware of their activities and companions. Boredom, lack of supervision, and absence of role models within the family are fundamental causes of experimentation with and recreational use of drugs by children and teenagers.

EARLY RECOGNITION OF DRUG USE AND ABUSE

It is distressing that increased numbers of teenagers have serious problems with alcohol, marijuana, and multi-drug use and abuse. In fact, it appears that initiation into the use of alcoholic beverages and the smoking of marijuana currently occurs during elementary and junior high school. While parents need not respond in an excessive or hysterical manner when they discover occasional use of alcoholic beverages, marijuana, or tobacco, one cannot assume that the child will "outgrow" it. It must be recognized that daily use can lead to a habit and to extensive experimentation. Many adult abusers can trace their problem to their early teen years. Particularly if practiced alone, daily, in large amounts, or if use corresponds with school, recreation, or work activities, the problem must be recognized. Recognition is the first step toward dealing squarely with the problem.

Certain early warning signs can alert parents or friends to drug use.

(1) Physical evidence of drug availability. The individual may almost deliberately leave drugs around the house, in his or her room, clothes, or school locker, perhaps unconsciously wanting to be discovered. This is a significant gesture on the part of the young person seeking relief from the guilt associated with clandestine drug use.

(2) Specific signs of particular drugs should be known by parents, and are easily recognizable if one is able to accept the fact that one's child, friend, or companion is using drugs.
• *Alcohol:* odor on breath, or the inappropriate use of breath mints or candy, garrulous talking, loud speech, excited and then sedated behavior, oversleeping in the morning.
• *Marijuana:* the distinctive odor after smoking, the presence of fragments of dried leaves in the clothing, giggling, bloodshot eyes, skipping from subject to subject when talking.
• *Amphetamine:* excitation, hyperactivity, depression, inappropriate fits of temper, difficulty concentrating, belligerent attitude.
• *Barbiturates and other hypnotic-sedatives:* excitation, users are unsteady on their feet, clumsy, and appear to have ingested alcohol.

(3) It should be general policy to discuss from time to time the use of drugs with children by gently probing about drug use among their friends, classmates, and other children in the neighborhood. If such questioning is done in a nonaccusatory manner, parents can establish a condition of trust in which the child can keep parents abreast of trends in school and community. The child or teenager who talks very much about drugs, or not at all about drug use, and is embarrassed or expresses an overly vigorous denial when asked about personal experimentation with drugs, is highly suspect.

(4) Poor school performance, especially inability to get assignments done on time, sloppy work, deterioration in handwriting, tardiness, and unexplained absences, and trumped-up or forged excuses from school are warning signs.

(5) A general lack of motivation and withdrawal from academic and extracurricular activities, particularly by an individual who previously has engaged in them.

(6) The individual who is frequently out of the house, particularly when his or her friends are members of the community suspected of drug use. Similarly, someone who is fascinated with the drug culture or counterculture segment of society will almost certainly be subject to peer pressure to experiment with drugs.

(7) A deterioration in appearance, unkempt and untidy clothing, and generally poor personal hygiene.

It is difficult at times to distinguish some of these characteristics from common teenage behavior, and such signs may be more obvious and meaningful in older persons, although older teenagers and adults are often more secretive and devious. Drug abuse can be hidden easily and the possibility of drug use should not be dismissed because of a lack of signs. Many times alcoholics have long years of abuse before it is obvious even to their family, close friends, or business associates.

TREATMENT OF DRUG ABUSE

Treatment of drug abuse depends on the nature and duration of the abuse, but certain common features can be identified. The recognized failure of most short-term detoxification programs for alcohol, barbiturate, and narcotic abuse has led to the recognition that long-term rehabilitation, including psychological support, physical reconditioning, job training, and counseling, is necessary to obtain good results. For some a drug-based approach is useful, as in the use of methadone in maintenance programs. For others a group living situation is more effective.

Treatment of the alcoholic remains a frustrating and controversial problem. A pharmacologic approach that has proven useful for some is the use of disulfiram (Antabuse®), a drug that prevents the further metabolism of acetaldehyde, the immediate metabolite of ethanol. The accumulation of acetaldehyde produces extremely unpleasant effects, such as flushing, nausea, and vomiting if the patient drinks alcohol while taking disulfiram. A variety of similar negative conditioning methods have been employed, but the most effective treatment appears to be mutual support groups, best exemplified by Alcoholics Anonymous. These groups provide the support and education needed to rehabilitate the drug abuser. Most believe that once "dried out" an alcoholic must forever abstain from alcoholic beverages, although rare individuals return to responsible social drinking.

CHAPTER 34   PHILIP W. BRICKNER, M.D., F.A.C.P.

CARING FOR THE ILL PATIENT AT HOME

Not too many years ago, most people who were ill or injured remained in their homes and a doctor came to their bedside. House calls are uncommon these days. The usual course is to hospitalize the ill and injured because the resources for their treatment are in one place. Moreover, many of the illnesses that once required prolonged care at home have declined dramatically in incidence. Tuberculosis and rheumatic fever are two examples.

But there are still occasions when home care is important. Children and adults alike still get acute, short-term illnesses such as chickenpox or influenza that confine them to bed for days or weeks. Recuperation after injury or surgery is another occasion for home care. The chronically ill, those with disabling arthritis, for instance, usually benefit from remaining at home. So do the terminally ill, who often prefer to live out their lives in familiar surroundings.

There is one important reason to care for patients at home: Except for those few instances where hospitalization or long-term placement in a nursing home is required, people fare better at home. Comfort is more easily found, surroundings are friendlier, personal needs are fulfilled more promptly, and costs are lower. The effect on people of being forced to meet the routine requirements of any institution is often unhappy. Whenever possible, try to keep ill or injured patients at home.

THE HOMEBOUND AGED

Home care is especially important for older people. If an aged man or woman develops chronic health problems, a choice should be available. Simply forcing a person into an institution is barbarous. To remain independent at home should be a jealously guarded option.

Organized, long-term home health care programs for the aged are gradually becoming available across the country. Legislators and others who set policy and are responsible for public tax money have begun to realize that home health care programs for the aged serve two major purposes: The often desperate wishes of the older people themselves are fulfilled, and the interest of the public is served as well, because care at home is significantly cheaper than nursing home costs.

Many agencies offer services designed to help the aged stay at home. These include visiting nurse agencies, which provide professional and homemaker staffs, plus meals-on-wheels programs, friendly visitor programs, and telephone reassurance programs. Local offices for the aging are good sources of information about these programs.

For older people who are seriously disabled, the problems are more complex, especially if they live alone. Hospital-based teams of doctor, nurse, and social worker must be formed to work with patients in their own homes. Information on programs for the seriously disabled can be obtained by writing to Chelsea-Village Program, 153 W. 11th St., New York, N.Y. 10011.

Aged people should understand that they need not be manipulated into a nursing home or other chronic care institution. When the patient has no family, it is the responsibility of community agencies to create a network of services for care at home. When relatives or friends are available, they can help.

ILL PEOPLE AT HOME

When people are ill at home, paying attention to the practical details of their care makes the difference between comfort and misery for the patient, and often the difference between success and failure of treatment. You needn't make elaborate plans for the care of a person with a routine or self-limiting illness. But if you must provide extended care to a member of your family, talk the plan over with the doctor. Of course, you'll want to discuss it with the patient, too, and with other members of the family. The care duties should not fall on a single member of the family, but should be a shared responsibility. Even children can help.

If it appears that care will continue for a long time, it might be wise for one or more members of the family to take a course in home nursing. Such courses are offered by local Red Cross chapters and other community agencies.

Your program should stress independence, not dependence. Remember, the basic goal of all treatment is to return the patient to active life as quickly as possible. Even during acute stages of illness and after surgery or injury, patients should be encouraged to carry out some normal activities of daily living, such as washing, eating, combing hair, or brushing teeth. Muscles should be used as soon as possible. Stretching in bed, moving arms and legs deliberately, graduating from bed to chair and from chair to walking all should be urged upon the patient. Otherwise muscles become weak, joints stiffen, and full recovery is delayed.

Good Nursing Habits

Regardless of the nature of the patient's illness, certain nursing practices should always be followed. These practices are for your benefit as well as the patient's. Their intent is to prevent transferring the patient's illness, and to avoid carrying infections to him or her.

Hand washing. Wash your hands with soap and running water before and after attending the patient. Keep your fingernails trimmed closely. Wash above your wrists. Rinse well. Rinse the bar of soap after each use. Dry your hands with a clean towel or paper towel.

Waste disposal. Flush away the patient's bowel and bladder wastes immediately. Provide a covered container for soiled tissues and bandages. Line it with a paper or plastic bag that can be closed without touching the contents. Place the bag where the patient can reach it. Pick up soiled materials through a fold of newspaper or use tongs. Provide paper tissues for nasal and throat discharges. Keep them within the patient's reach.

Dishes. Depending on the illness, it may be a good idea for the patient to have dishes and eating utensils separate from the family's. Ask your doctor. You may wish to consider disposable dishes and cutlery. However, hot water and detergent, plus hot water rinsing and drying, remove or destroy most infectious agents. Your usual dishwashing methods will be adequate unless the patient's illness requires special precautions. A dishwasher is ideal. It uses water at temperatures higher than human hands can tolerate.

Linen. Collect soiled sickroom linens in a bag or newspaper and wash them in your usual way, but separate from other laundry. The linens may be dried with the rest of the family laundry unless other directions are given.

Medications

Follow the doctor's directions in giving medicines to a patient cared for at home. It is particularly important, of course, that prescription medicines be given at the proper time and in proper dosage. Make sure you understand what that means. Some medicines should be given before meals on an empty stomach in order to be absorbed properly. Some need to be taken with food, others should follow a meal.

Certain drugs, such as antibiotics, are commonly used only for the length of the illness. Others must be taken for prolonged periods, some for a lifetime. Insulin for diabetes mellitus is an example.

Be sparing with pain medication. Here the doctor's directions are particularly important. No one likes to see a loved one in pain, but improper use of pain-killers can be dangerous.

Caution should also be used with nonprescription drugs such as aspirin or laxatives.

If the Patient Has a Communicable Disease

Illnesses that spread from person to person require extra precautions. Widespread immunization has substantially decreased many of these, including the childhood diseases of measles (rubeola), german measles (rubella), mumps, and whooping cough (pertussis). But chickenpox, influenza, the common cold, and hepatitis are still with us.

People assigned to care for a patient with an infectious illness should have had the disease, making them less vulnerable, or should be immunized (when immunization is available).

If the patient has a respiratory disease that can be spread by coughing or sneezing, both patient and home nurse may wish to wear a mask covering nose and mouth. These can be bought at a pharmacy or fashioned from gauze or cloth.

For a disease such as hepatitis, which is transmitted through blood, stool, and bodily secretions, care must be taken in disposing of the patient's wastes. If the person is bedfast and requires a bedpan, the wastes should be flushed away immediately and the utensil thoroughly rinsed. The helper should scrub his or her hands thoroughly afterwards. An ambulatory patient who can use the bathroom should be reminded to flush promptly and to wash thoroughly.

A thorough review of precautions should be undertaken with the doctor at the beginning of the illness.

The "Sickroom"

The old-fashioned idea of a "sickroom" is seldom necessary for short-term illnesses, but you may wish to make special provisions for long-term care. The ideal location is a cheery, well-lighted room. It should be quiet, well-ventilated, and on the first floor near the bathroom. It should be arranged for efficiency, but not stripped down like a hospital ward. The basics are the patient's bed, a night table that he or she can easily reach, chairs for the patient and visitors, a waste can lined with a paper or plastic bag, and a table for supplies and for you to use when changing the linens or giving a bath. A table on wheels is a good idea. A bed table for meals or reading is handy, too. You'll probably want a television or radio.

If the room is near the living quarters of the house, the patient can call you when needed. But if the only available room is upstairs or isolated from the mainstream of the household, he or she will need a way to attract attention. A bell or buzzer is suitable, or even a tin pan.

Keep medicines and other supplies together and easy for you to reach. Keep the room clean without being fanatic about it. Dust the room with a damp cloth and use a vacuum sweeper so that you do not stir up dust.

The Patient's Bed

For a brief illness, the patient's own bed is usually satisfactory. For extended home care, choose a bed that saves the nurse's energy. A single or twin bed is easier to make than a double bed, and the patient is more accessible. If the patient is completely bedridden and likely to require care for a long time, it may be wise to rent a hospital bed from a supply company or a rental agency. Equipment is sometimes loaned by community agencies.

The mattress should be firm and resilient. If bedsprings sag, a piece of plywood between mattress and springs will give support.

Ordinary beds are lower than hospital beds. This makes little difference if the patient is out of bed frequently, sits in a chair, and goes to the bathroom. But a little extra bed height saves wear and tear on the home nurse by reducing stressful bending and reaching. Height can be added by putting a second mattress on top of the first. Or the legs of the bed can be raised by putting them in tin cans filled about two-thirds full with sand or gravel. Place the cutout end of the can or something else flat and firm on top of the sand. Cement blocks, wood blocks, or firmly tied stacks of newspapers can serve the same purpose.

Position the bed so that neither the foot nor the sides are against a wall.

The usual sequence of bedding, from the mattress up, is as follows: Mattress pad, bottom sheet, waterproof pad (if necessary), drawsheet, top sheet, blanket, and spread.

It is convenient to use a fitted sheet as the bottom sheet. It fits snugly at the corners of the mattress and leaves few wrinkles. The top sheet should be wide and long enough to be tucked under the mattress to hold the sheet smoothly and firmly. Make sure the top sheet is generous enough for the patient to move freely and to accommodate pillows, footrests, or other appliances under the covers. Use enough blankets for comfort.

Making the bed with the patient in it is tricky, but it can be mastered after a few attempts. Follow the steps on page 825. Fitted sheets simplify the process.

If the patient needs bedpan care, is incontinent, or perspires profusely, a pad of moisture-resistant material may be needed under him or her. But it is best omitted if possible. Rubber sheets and similar materials tend to make a person feel uncomfortably warm. Washable waterproof materials with a cloth covering can be purchased. Oilcloth or old shower curtains are serviceable substitutes. You may even use a large plastic garbage bag.

A drawsheet may or may not be needed. This is simply a short sheet immediately under the patient, extending from the head to the knee region. Smooth the drawsheet and tuck the ends under the mattress sides to hold it securely. A drawsheet is often helpful when turning or moving the patient, and it gives a little extra mattress protection.

Use pillows and backrests imaginatively and in quantity for patient comfort. Besides providing support in the sitting position, pillows can hold people on their sides, elevate the feet, or keep the knees flexed. An upholstered backrest with arms is worthwhile.

Footrests are used to keep bedclothes from pressing on the toes and to give a firm surface to exercise against.

Moving the Patient in Bed

Urge the patient to move himself or herself if possible. If this is not possible, explain what you are going to do before you do it. Remove or pull down top bedding for freedom of movement. Roll and slide the patient gently; do not lift unnecessarily. Think of the hips and shoulders as "pivots" of the body. The patient should be close to the edge of the bed so the nurse doesn't have to bend awkwardly.

If the patient is to get into a chair brought to the bedside, help him or her sit up and provide support while you swing the legs around to hang over the bed. Keep giving support until any momentary dizziness passes. A patient's chair should be sturdy and should have arms that can be grasped to help himself or herself out of bed. If the patient cannot help, you may need another person's assistance.

CARE OF THE BEDRIDDEN PATIENT

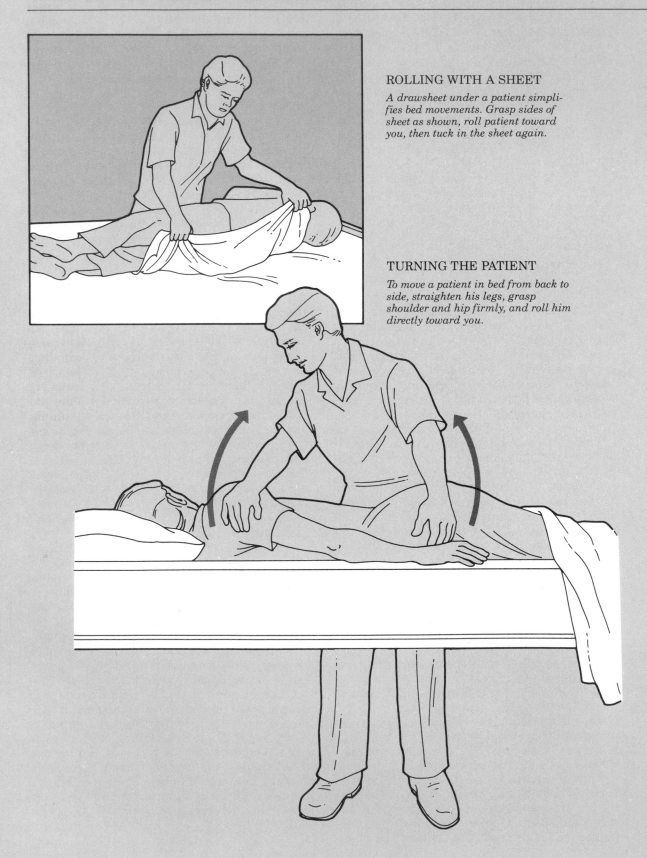

ROLLING WITH A SHEET

A drawsheet under a patient simpli-fies bed movements. Grasp sides of sheet as shown, roll patient toward you, then tuck in the sheet again.

TURNING THE PATIENT

To move a patient in bed from back to side, straighten his legs, grasp shoulder and hip firmly, and roll him directly toward you.

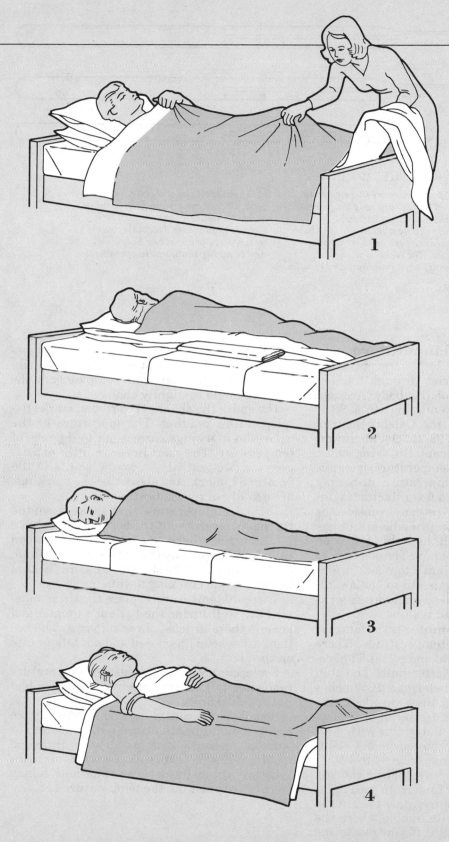

MAKING AN OCCUPIED BED

There are four steps in making a bed with the patient in it: (1) While patient holds the blanket, pull top sheet from beneath it. (2) Roll the blanket-covered patient to one side of the bed. Loosen bottom sheet and drawsheet on unoccupied side and tuck along the patient's back. Tuck in clean bottom sheet and drawsheet on unoccupied side. (3) Roll patient over the soiled linen to clean side of bed. Strip off soiled bottom sheet and drawsheet. Pull exposed edge of clean bottom sheet and drawsheet toward you and make the rest of the bed. (4) Tuck in top sheet and blanket at foot of bed.

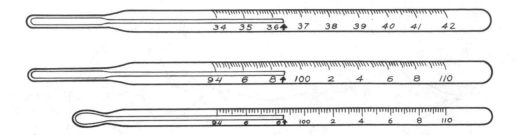

CLINICAL THERMOMETERS

Two types of mercury thermometers are used to measure body temperature. Oral thermometers (top two drawings) have a relatively long bulb that holds the red or silver measuring material. The rectal type, most commonly used in infants and certain *older patients, has a shorter, fatter bulb. Thermometers are graduated in either Fahrenheit (bottom two) or Celsius (top) scales. Normal rectal temperature is about one Fahrenheit degree higher than oral temperature.*

How to Take the Temperature

Body temperature varies through the day and in different parts of the body. Average normal temperature taken by mouth is 98.6° Fahrenheit. (Normal in the Celsius [metric] system is 37°.) A range of 98° to 99° Fahrenheit is not particularly significant. But fever, which means excessively high temperature, is significant. A subnormal temperature also may have meaning. Whether a fever fluctuates, increases, disappears and returns, subsides or does not subside after taking medicines, or has other characteristics—all these things may be important for a doctor to know. The doctor may ask you to take the patient's temperature at certain times or intervals. If so, follow directions faithfully and keep an accurate written record of the time and reading.

The clinical thermometer is the familiar instrument for taking temperatures. There are two general types, oral and rectal. The rectal type has a shorter, fatter bulb. The thin glass tube of the thermometer, about 3½ inches long, has short and long lines that look like ruler markings on one side, and figures usually beginning with "94" and ending with "110" on the opposite end. Figures on a Celsius thermometer usually range from 34 to 42.

Read the thermometer by holding the end opposite the bulb in your fingers. In good light, look through the peak of the glass toward the flat base. There is a little bubble where the clear glass joins the bulb. If you rotate the thermometer slowly, the bubble appears to widen. Above it you should see a flat silver or red ribbon. If you don't, rotate the thermometer slightly one way or the other until the ribbon appears. It disappears completely if the viewing angle is slightly changed.

The end of the silver or red ribbon marks the temperature reading. The long lines of the ruler-like markings correspond to degrees of temperature. The short lines are fifths of a degree (or two-tenths). An arrow points to the 98.6° or 37° mark, and above this the markings are usually in red, indicating fever.

To take a temperature, first shake down the thermometer to about the 95° mark. To shake it, hold the thermometer firmly between thumb and fingers by the end opposite the bulb and give two or three sharp downward flicks of the wrist, like cracking a whip.

To record temperature, place the thermometer bulb well under the patient's tongue and keep it there at least three minutes. The patient must keep lips closed and not talk or bite on the stem.

For accuracy, do not measure temperature immediately after the patient has eaten or had hot or cold drinks.

Rectal temperature is about one degree Fahrenheit higher than oral temperature. For various reasons, such as dry or inflamed mouth, nasal congestion with mouth-breathing, or an uncooperative patient, it may be necessary to take the temperature rectally.

The thermometer bulb should be lubricated with cold cream, petroleum jelly, or oil and inserted about one inch into the rectum. It should be kept in place three minutes.

After use, clean the thermometer with cool or tepid water and soap. Hold the thermometer by the top, wet a cotton wipe, wrap it around the stem, and wriggle it downward with firm finger pressure. Rinse with clean, tepid water. Repeat the same operation, dry the thermometer, and put it in its container. It is not necessary to use powerful antiseptics. Do not hold the thermometer under hot running tap water or in a basin of hot water. This may break the instrument.

If you cannot read the thermometer, put it away without shaking it until someone else can read it.

What happens if a clinical thermometer breaks in the mouth and some of the contents are swallowed? Nothing much, but to be safe, call your doctor.

Bathroom Functions

A bedpan is an uncomfortable, inefficient device in which people are expected to urinate and defecate. However, if a patient cannot get out of bed, there may be no alternative. Obtain a plastic lightweight bedpan of the smallest useful size. The larger it is, the more difficult for the patient to use.

Graduate the patient to a bedside commode as quickly as possible. This is a chair with a hole in the seat and a bucket or pan underneath which can be withdrawn for cleaning.

Finally, allowing the patient to go into the bathroom and use the toilet, when the doctor permits, is often a moment of great joy, with important psychological benefits in addition to physical ease.

Always remember that patients value privacy, especially in these circumstances, and respect this need when possible.

Skin Care

Basic cleanliness of the patient is of high importance. It is common sense, good hygiene, important for morale, and necessary to avoid complications such as inflammations and infections of the skin. If patients who are incontinent soil themselves, careful and prompt cleaning is required. Permitting the patient to lie in wet sheets is undignified, uncomfortable, and leads to skin breakdown.

Bedsores (decubitus ulcers) are skin erosions that, when not dealt with aggressively, lead to destruction of underlying tissue such as muscles and tendons, extending down to bone. These ulcers tend to occur over areas where pressure is applied to the skin by the body's position in bed. The heels, lower back, elbows, shoulder blades, and the back of the skull are vulnerable.

Earliest sign of a bedsore is tender, warm, and slightly reddened skin. Watch for this when caring for a patient, and call it to the doctor's attention. In later stages the skin is purplish, broken, and raw, circulation is impaired, and treatment is difficult.

The best treatment of bedsores is prevention. Here the home nurse is very important. When bathing the patient, inspect the skin for any unusual redness, breaks, or discoloration.

Cleanliness is vital. Moisture from discharges predisposes to skin breakdown. Keep the patient's skin dry. Be prompt in attending incontinent patients.

Don't rub reddened, tender skin areas vigorously. Wash the area gently with warm soapy water, rinse, pat dry, sponge with rubbing alcohol (unless the skin is broken), and cover with large cotton pads unless the doctor advises other measures.

Patients who face the highest likelihood of bedsores are those who cannot move freely in bed. Frequent turning of the patient is essential, as is the use of foam rubber "doughnuts" to keep skin away from sheets.

Once skin has broken down, healing is slow and difficult, requiring assiduous professional attention from doctor and nurse.

Bathing the Patient

A quick bath stimulates circulation, is refreshing, and of course cleansing. A daily bath for the patient is customary, but use judgment. More frequent baths may be necessary if there is too much soiling. On the other hand, too frequent or prolonged baths can be fatiguing and may cause softening of the skin. If the patient has a skin rash or sore areas, ask the doctor about bath precautions.

For bed baths, protect bedding with towels or blankets. Wash each part of the body quickly. Rinse off the soap, dry thoroughly, cover, and proceed to the next area. Dry skin creases and folds particularly well. Let the patient help if he or she is able.

Measuring Pulse and Respiratory Rates

The doctor may ask you to count the patient's pulse and respiratory rate. If so, keep a written record of the reading, the date, and the hour. You will need a watch or clock that is graduated in seconds.

The pulse is usually counted at the wrist. A little below the base of the thumb, just inside the point where a projection of the wristbone can be felt on the thumb side, an artery runs under the skin of the inner surface of the wrist. Place your fingertips (not your thumb) on this part of the patient's wrist. Press just hard enough for pulsations to be felt. Count for 60 seconds. Take the pulse when the patient is quiet.

The average adult has a pulse rate of 70 to 72 per minute, but this can vary considerably in either direction and still be normal. Activity and excitement as well as illness can cause changes in the pulse rate.

The pulse also can be taken in other areas where an artery crosses bone near the skin surface, such as at the temples or between the

TAKING THE PULSE

To take a person's pulse, place index and middle fingers on the inside of the wrist just below the base of the thumb. Press gently until you can count the beats. Average pulse rate is 70 to 72 per minute. The pulse also can be measured at the throat or at the ankle.

ankle bone and heel on the inner side of the foot. Under certain circumstances, the doctor may suggest checking the pulse at one of these spots.

Respiration (the breathing rate) is best counted when the patient is not aware of what you are doing, because mere observation may change the rate. Breathing is affected by apprehension, exertion, and other factors. The breathing rate of adults at rest ranges between 14 and 18 per minute. It is faster in children and faster still in infants.

Use of Heat and Cold

The use of heat and cold is important for the patient's comfort and in some cases is part of treatment. In using them, however, it is vital that you understand the purpose and that you follow the physician's directions. Too much heat or cold can cause injury or make the person's disease worse.

Heat is soothing, eases muscle spasm, and decreases some forms of pain. Heat may be applied dry (by electric pad, hot water bottle, or lamp) or moist (by compresses).

Too much heat can burn. Don't apply anything to the patient's body that is too hot to hold in your hands, or that feels too warm to the skin of your inner forearm. Check electrical heating devices for broken wires and be sure to follow the manufacturer's directions. Check a hot water bag for leaks.

Never apply heat for more than one hour at a time without the doctor's permission.

Remember that a comatose or disoriented patient or a baby can't tell you that a hot water bag is too hot. Be careful when applying heat to an infant or a patient who is sedated, semiconscious, or who can't move. Also, be careful with persons who have diabetes mellitus or circulatory or neurological problems. They may have reduced sensations in the extremities.

A hot compress furnishes moist heat. Use folded gauze, flannel, or soft woolen fabrics. Dip into water, then squeeze out excess moisture. Test the compress on your own skin. Apply loosely to the affected part. A strip of plastic sheeting can be laid over the compress to keep moisture in. Cover with a towel or soft cloth, or use a hot water bag to maintain heat and hold the compress in place. Replace the compress with a warm one when the first begins to cool. Continue as long and repeat as often as the doctor recommends.

Steam inhalation is soothing to congested breathing passages. Inhaled steam helps to soften thick secretions, and eases coughing, hoarseness, and sore throat. Technically, what

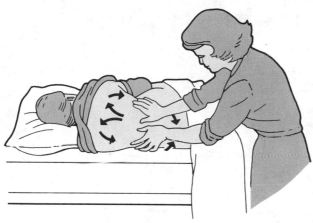

THE BACK RUB

Massaging the back can relieve numbness, stimulate circulation, and improve the patient's spirits. Move hands in the directions shown by arrows. Use firm, long, gentle strokes with a kneading motion. Do not remove your hands between strokes. Lubricating the hands before beginning is helpful.

the patient inhales is not live steam, but water vapor. But this vapor can be hot enough to burn, or a wobbly container of scalding water may be tipped over, so take precautions.

An electric vaporizer is a worthwhile investment. Follow the manufacturer's directions. Vaporizers should be placed close enough to the patient so that vapor is concentrated in the air that is breathed. Length of treatment and time of day for use should be decided by the physician.

Satisfactory steam inhalation also can be obtained from simple household equipment. Pour steaming water into a broad-mouthed pitcher or container placed in a pan on a table low enough for the seated patient to lean over it. Drape a blanket or towel over the patient's head and shoulders and above the pitcher in such a way that steamy vapor is concentrated for inhalation.

Cold compresses or soaks are used for comfort, to reduce swelling or bruises, and for other purposes.

Soak folded gauze, flannel, or soft cloth in a basin of ice water. Wring thoroughly so water doesn't drip. Apply to the affected part. Re-

place with a freshly wrung compress when the first becomes warm. Stop if the person shows signs of becoming chilled.

If you can fit the part of the body to be soaked into a tub or basin of cold water, do so. Soaking is more efficient than a compress.

Sponge baths to reduce fever may be needed. Rubbing alcohol mixed with water is an efficient coolant because alcohol evaporates quickly and evaporation is a cooling process. (Alcohol may be inadvisable if the skin is broken.) Use cool but not ice-cold water. Dip cloths in water, squeeze out excess moisture, and bathe the body, including armpits and groin. Measure the patient's temperature intermittently. Stop the bath when the temperature has fallen sufficiently.

Equipment

Some items of sickroom equipment make it easier to give care or make the patient more comfortable and contented.

A bed table is a flat surface on which meals are served and which the patient can use for writing, drawing, and other activities while sitting or propped up in bed. Simple U-shaped tables with long feet that slide under the bed and a top that projects above the bedclothes can be bought and used for many purposes. The tops can be tilted and adjusted for height. An ironing board can be used in a similar way, or a folding ironing board or padded board can be supported by the backs of chairs pushed against the sides of the bed. With a little cutting, taping, and ingenuity, a stout paperboard carton can be made into a serviceable bed table. Cut holes in opposite sides of the carton for the patient's legs to fit under.

A bed cradle is a means of keeping the weight of bedclothing off the patient's body. Here, too, a paperboard carton cut with holes that arch over the patient's outstretched body is serviceable. Often, firm cushions or pillows strategically placed beside the patient will support sheets and blankets enough to provide comfort.

A bed rope gives the patient something to pull on to help himself sit up or turn in bed. Tie a strong rope, strap, or nylon clothesline securely to the foot of the bed, with the loose end within reach of the patient.

Safety devices. Simple modifications may ease life at home for disabled or frail people. In a house with stairs, moving the bedroom to the ground floor can help. Install guard rails around the bathtub, or a grab-bar in the shower. An elevated toilet seat can solve the problem of getting up for those whose muscular strength is limited.

CHAPTER 35   MICHAEL ELIASTAM, M.D., M.P.P., M.P.A.

FIRST AID

First aid is *first* aid—the immediate care that you provide in an emergency, before someone with more medical training arrives to take over, or before the victim can reach medical help. First aid covers all kinds of care for all kinds of injuries, from the simple minor scrapes and bruises that do not require a doctor's attention to the care provided in an emergency, while waiting for an ambulance or speeding to a hospital.

Every family member should be prepared to provide first aid, because there is no time to learn in the crucial seconds after an accident strikes. That requires both training and equipment. A good beginning is for one or more family members to take a first-aid course, as well as one in cardiopulmonary resuscitation (CPR), the technique for maintaining or restoring a victim's heartbeat and respiration. Both types of courses are offered by local Red Cross chapters, heart associations, YMCAs, Boy Scout troops, and other community groups. It is important to keep up your skills, too. CPR requires yearly certification because with lack of practice, one quickly forgets the technique, and poorly administered CPR is worthless.

An even more basic step is to educate every member of the family, children included, in the kind of emergency service provided in your community and how to summon it. That may mean a paramedic ambulance provided by the fire department, a private ambulance service, or a volunteer emergency crew. In some communities, physicians prefer to be called directly in all but the most dire emergencies, so they can decide whether the person should be seen at home, at the physician's office, or in a hospital emergency department. In large cities and their suburbs, the preferred course usually is to dial the emergency number and have the emergency ambulance system come to you and transport the ill or injured person to the hospital.

To find out how the system works where you live, ask your physician, phone your police or fire department, or call your municipal or county offices and ask about emergency services.

The information section at the front of your telephone directory usually lists emergency numbers. Some communities have a single number, usually 911, to be called in any kind of emergency. Others have their own numbers. You should record the emergency number or numbers directly on your telephone. Listing it inside the telephone directory is a good idea, too, but it is not always possible to locate the directory in the excitement of an emergency.

Taping the number onto the telephone guarantees that it will be in the right place when you need it. But don't merely record the number. Try it first, to be sure it is correct and to find out how a call will be handled. No agency truly committed to emergency care would take such a call amiss.

Having your own physician (or a relationship with a clinic, group practice, or local hospital) is part of emergency preparation, too. Then your medical history will be recorded in one place. That makes it easier for a physician on the scene during an emergency to learn about your previous illnesses, drug allergies, and medications, and thus provide better care.

Another telephone number you should record is that of the local poison control center. These centers provide immediate information about how to deal with the effects of almost every known drug or chemical that people may take either accidentally or intentionally. In some communities, you may call the central emergency number and the dispatcher will put you in touch with the poison control center, or provide the necessary information.

A list of first-aid supplies that should be in every home is provided on page 833. But don't limit them just to the home medicine chest. Be sure to carry a similar first aid kit in your car, recreational vehicle, boat, and anywhere else you might need it in an emergency.

WHAT TO DO
IN AN EMERGENCY

In emergencies, minutes count. Follow these steps to make the most of the time:
● Don't get hurt yourself. You can't help the victim if you're injured in a foolhardy attempt at rescue. If you cannot reach an injured person without risking injury, wait for assistance.
● Do not move the victim unless he is at risk of further injury. Spinal cord damage can result. Keep him lying flat on his back, or if he is already on his side, leave him that way but see that he is able to breathe properly. Do not sit or stand him up.
● If the patient appears unconscious, make sure that he is breathing. If not, give mouth-to-mouth resuscitation (see page 834).

• Make sure that the mouth and throat are free of blood, secretions, or vomit. Wipe them out with a finger or handkerchief. Pull the tongue forward if it appears to have slipped into the back of the throat.

• If the patient has suffered a fall, try to avoid moving the neck. Attempt to open the airway to ease breathing by lifting the jaw. This is done by putting the hands on either side of the jaw and lifting the jaw up and away from the back of the throat (see page 834).

• Check for a pulse by feeling in the neck over the carotid artery (see page 837).

• If no pulse is present, begin external cardiac compression (cardiac massage).

• Stop serious bleeding. Apply pressure directly on the wound with any clean cloth, gauze, or handkerchief. Push hard. If the bleeding is from an arm or leg wound, elevate the limb above the level of the body. Do not use a tourniquet unless other measures fail to stop the bleeding, and then only if it continues to be serious.

• Treat shock (see page 844).

• If the patient appears cold, pale, and clammy, lay him down, cover him with a light blanket, and provide reassurance. Avoid giving anything by mouth if the person is unconscious or semiconscious. A good rule of thumb is to give water only if the patient can hold the container himself and does not have chest or abdominal wounds.

THE TWO-MINUTE

PATIENT EVALUATION

Sometimes you do not actually witness an accident, but simply come upon a person who has been involved in one or who appears seriously ill. You need to make quick assessment of the condition. Do this in two steps, the primary survey and the secondary survey.

The Primary Survey

First, check airway breathing and circulation ("ABC" is a good way to remember it). Look for any obvious bleeding that is contributing to the emergency. Immediately take care of the airway breathing and circulation as outlined on page 834 and following what you have learned in a CPR course. Stop any significant bleeding by direct pressure.

The Secondary Survey

The secondary survey is conducted only after airway breathing and circulation have been treated. Start at the head and work down if the person is unconscious. If conscious, start at the wrist by checking the pulse. At the same time, talk to the person and establish if the brain is functioning by asking him simple questions about himself and his surroundings, or asking him to follow simple commands.

• Quickly look at the person's eyes to see whether the pupils are equal and whether they respond to light. A difference in pupil size may indicate head injury or brain damage in an unconscious patient. Feel the scalp and the sides of the head and the neck for evidence of blood, injuries, or pain to help localize the problem. If the person appears to have fallen, be careful about moving the head and neck to prevent spinal damage. Protect the neck with rolled towels or clothing to immobilize it if moving is necessary. Note whether the person is bleeding from the ears or nose, and whether a clear fluid resembling water is draining from the ears or nose. This can represent cerebrospinal fluid, which normally surrounds the brain. Its presence may indicate a fracture of the skull under the brain. Examine the mouth for injuries. Remove any dentures or loose teeth if the patient is not fully conscious, or if he appears likely to become unconscious.

• Check the neck for tenderness, and gently palpate (feel with your hands) the shoulders from both sides, checking for tenderness that could indicate fracture of the shoulder girdle and collarbones. Compress the chest by pushing on both sides and then from front to back. If you produce pain, a fracture somewhere in the chest is indicated. Ask a conscious person to take a deep breath. Pain on breathing also may indicate rib fractures.

• Remove enough clothing to look at the chest and abdomen for evidence of injury. Seat belt marks, bruises, or tire tread imprints and similar marks may indicate possible internal bleeding. Think of the abdomen as a clock with twelve o'clock located at the midpoint of the ribs and six o'clock pointing down the pelvis. Push moderately at each of the clock's four quadrants to check whether pressure at any point produces pain. Any pain at all may indicate an internal injury.

• Compress the pelvis from side to side. Pain

FIRST-AID SUPPLIES

You can buy a fairly complete first-aid kit at a pharmacy or department store, but a prepared kit isn't necessary. Your own medicine cabinet already may be amply stocked. Always keep your supplies together, so you won't have to hunt for them in an emergency. Check them regularly to see whether they need to be replenished. Never keep them locked, because you don't want to be forced to search for a key in an emergency.

You may wish to store the supplies in a moistureproof container so they can be taken along on family outings. Better yet, keep a duplicate kit in the family car. Remember that there should be a complete kit in every car, boat, or recreational vehicle.

Quantity	Item
20	Paper cups, for giving fluids.
1	Flashlight and spare batteries.
1	Blanket.
1	Pillow (or inflatable cushion).
	Newspapers (to place under the person on cold or wet ground or for use as emergency splint).
10 of each	Individual adhesive bandages in ½-inch, ¾-inch, 1-inch, and "round" spot sizes.
Box of 12	2x2-inch sterile first-aid dressings, individually packaged, for open wounds or burns.
Box of 12	4x4-inch sterile first-aid dressings.
1 roll	Roller gauze bandage, 1 inch by 5 yards.
1 roll	Roller gauze bandage, 2 inches by 5 yards.
1 roll each	Adhesive tape, 1- and 2-inch widths.
2	Triangular bandages, 36x36 inches, folded diagonally, for use as a sling or to hold dressings.
6	Safety pins, 1½-inch size.
1 bar	Mild white soap, for cleaning wounds, scratches, etc.
1 pair	Scissors with blunt tips, for cutting bandages and tape.
1 pair	Tweezers, for removing splinters.
1	Tourniquet—a wide strip of cloth, at least 3 to 4 inches by 20 inches, for use when bleeding can be controlled in no other way.
1 container	Syrup of ipecac, for use in cases of suspected poisoning.
1 3- to 4-ounce bottle	Rubbing alcohol.
1 pair	Nail clippers.
1 container	Aspirin or aspirin substitute (acetaminophen), adult strength.
1 container	Aspirin or aspirin substitute (acetaminophen), children's strength.
1 bottle	Calamine lotion, for insect bites.

or tenderness may suggest pelvic fractures. Check the legs and thighs for pain, tenderness, or blood, which may indicate fractures or significant cuts or bruises. Ask the person to move the feet and check whether he or she can feel your touch. Do the same for the arms, having the person move the hands and feel your touch.

• Always remember to examine the back of the patient, including the buttocks and upper thighs. Often, because patients are lying on their backs or because they are clothed, important injuries are overlooked that later can produce shock and even death. If a spinal injury is suspected, do not move the patient. Insert your hands under the back to feel for blood, deformity, or pain.

Two minutes spent in evaluation can be invaluable in pinpointing the right first-aid measures to take, or in enabling you to report the extent of injury to medical personnel who arrive on the scene. Evaluation should be practiced ahead of time, and learned as part of any first-aid course you take. You should never do your first two-minute assessment on a real victim under emergency conditions.

CARDIOPULMONARY
RESUSCITATION

Any time an adult or child stops breathing, artificial respiration, or mouth-to-mouth resuscitation, may become necessary. This is a method of breathing for the victim by blowing your breath into his or her lungs. It can be life-saving, and it has the advantage of needing no special equipment or preparation time. Speed is important, because irreversible brain damage can occur if breathing stops for more than four to six minutes. CPR cannot be learned on a crash basis, with the victim in front of you. You should take instruction beforehand and keep your skills up to date. The drawings at right illustrate the basic technique, and should be reviewed regularly. One way to stay proficient is to become a volunteer instructor and teach CPR to others.

MOUTH-TO-MOUTH RESUSCITATION

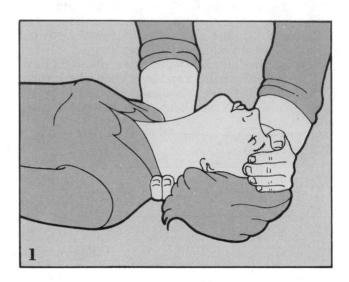

Place the victim on his back. Clean any visible foreign matter from the mouth with your fingers or with a cloth wrapped around your fingers. Tilt the person's head toward the ceiling by placing one hand under the neck and the other on the forehead. This provides a clear airway.

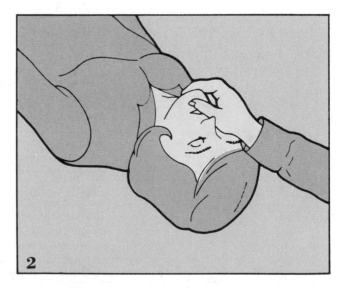

Listen for air outflow from mouth, and watch chest for movement indicating breathing. If air does not move in and out of the chest easily, pull or push the person's jaw from behind into a jutting-out position, preventing the tongue from falling back into the throat. Check to see whether breathing is occurring.

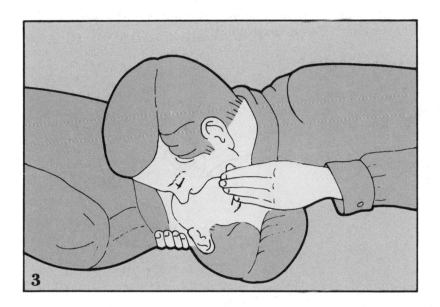

Place your mouth completely over the victim's mouth. Keep one hand under the neck to maintain a straight airway, and pinch off the nostrils with the other hand. Breathe into an adult victim's mouth at a rate of 12 breaths per minute.

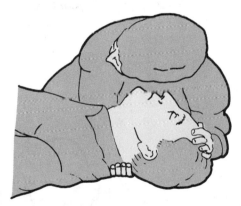

After four quick breaths, remove your mouth and listen for outflow from the victim's lungs. If you do not feel him exhale, see the chest rise and fall, or feel resistance to your own breath, recheck the head and mouth positions.

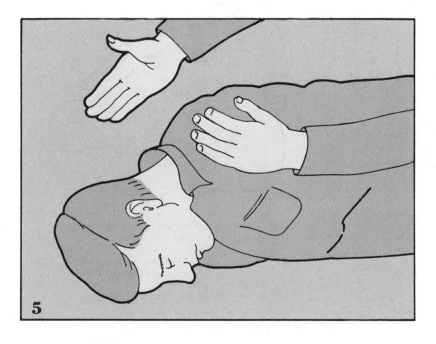

If there is still no air exchange, turn the victim on his side and give him several sharp whacks between the shoulder blades to dislodge obstructions in the throat. Resume mouth-to-mouth breathing and continue until help arrives, or until you are convinced there is no reason to continue the procedure.

MOUTH-TO-MOUTH RESUSCITATION OF SMALL CHILDREN

An infant or small child who has stopped breathing requires mouth-to-mouth resuscitative techniques different from the techniques used for an adult.

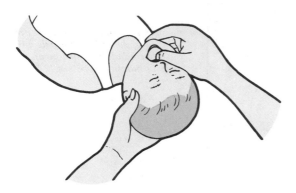

1 *Place the child on his back, clean foreign matter from his mouth.*

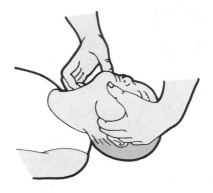

2 *Move the child's jaw into a jutting-out position, as with adults.*

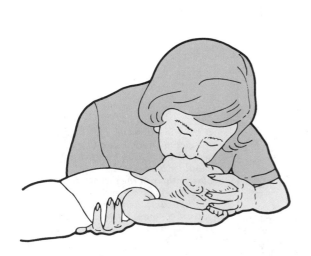

3 *Put your mouth over both mouth and nose to make a leakproof seal. Breathe at a rate of about 20 breaths per minute—about once every three seconds, compared to the adult rate of once every five seconds.*

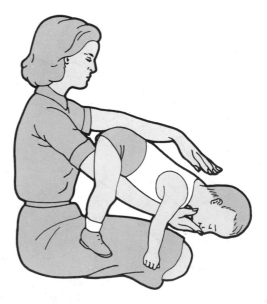

4 *Check to see if you are getting an air exchange. If not, check the jaw position to be sure the airway is clear, or hold the child headdown over one of your arms and whack between the shoulder blades.*

ARTIFICIAL CIRCULATION (CARDIAC COMPRESSION)

If a person has stopped breathing, the heart also may have stopped. If no pulse can be felt, emergency measures must be taken to stimulate the heart and restore circulation. Compressing the victim's chest can start the heart beating as follows:

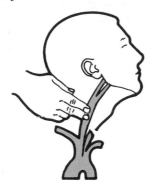

Check for a pulse. The most sensitive pulse is in the carotid artery of the neck, between the windpipe and the neck muscle. It often can be felt when other pulse beats have ceased. Feel gently with your fingers to avoid damage to the windpipe.

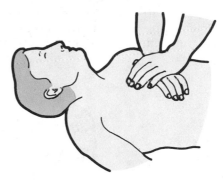

If no pulse can be felt, place both hands on the lower breastbone two inches above the "V" of the ribs and compress the chest vigorously, at the rate of at least once per second (60 to 80 compressions per minute). The area of compression should be 1½ to 2 inches in an adult, half that in a child.

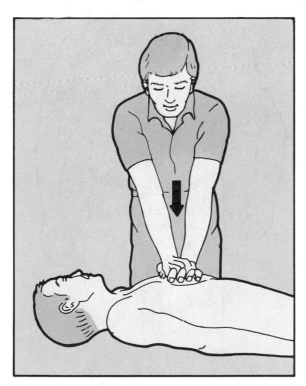

If you are alone, provide both artificial breathing and cardiac compression. Give two quick breaths and compress the chest 15 times (a rate of 80 per minute). Then give two more quick breaths, followed by 15 more compressions.

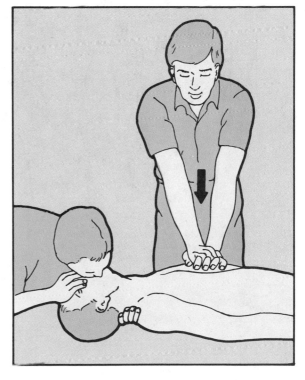

If two persons are present, one can provide breathing, the other chest compression. They should take positions on either side of the victim, and may change off. The chest should be compressed 60 times per minute, or once every second. For every five compressions, there should be one breath.

CHOKING

Adults or children can choke to death on small objects that become lodged in the windpipe. In adults, the offending object is often a bit of food. With children, toys, parts of toys, or other small objects are more often responsible. Choking on food often occurs in a restaurant and happens so suddenly that it may be mistaken for a heart attack, hence the nickname "cafe coronary."

The best way for a person to rid himself of an obstruction in the windpipe is by coughing it out. In a choking incident, one should not jump too soon. If a person is choking but appears able to talk (or to cry normally, in the case of a

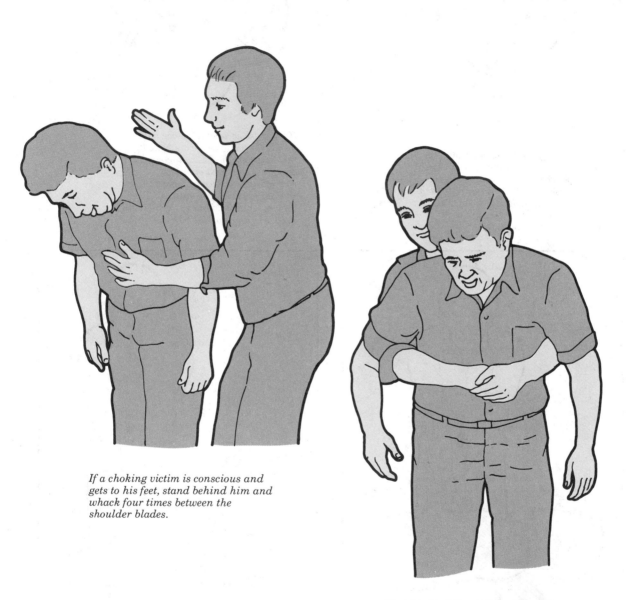

If a choking victim is conscious and gets to his feet, stand behind him and whack four times between the shoulder blades.

Stand behind the victim, slip your arms around his waist, lock your hands under his ribs in the solar plexus area, and rapidly squeeze his abdomen four times. Air will be forced out of the lungs against the obstruction, propelling it into the mouth. Repeat the sequence of backslaps and abdominal thrusts until the airway is clear.

baby), it is probably unnecessary to do anything initially. A person who can talk has an adequate airway and should generate enough pressure to push out the obstruction.

If a person cannot talk, if the cry sounds as if the airway is partially obstructed, or if the person loses consciousness, emergency steps must be taken immediately. These procedures are known as the obstructed airway maneuver, the abdominal thrust, or the Heimlich maneuver. Like CPR, they should be learned in a training course. Most first-aid courses provide instruction in dealing with choking victims, whether conscious or unconscious.

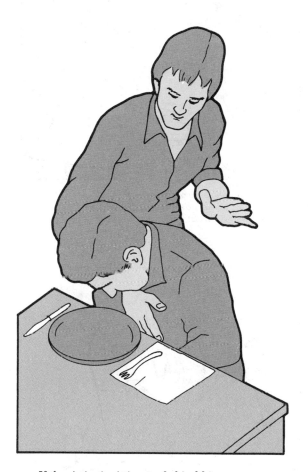

If the victim is sitting, go behind his chair and lean him forward. Give the same four back slaps between the shoulder blades.

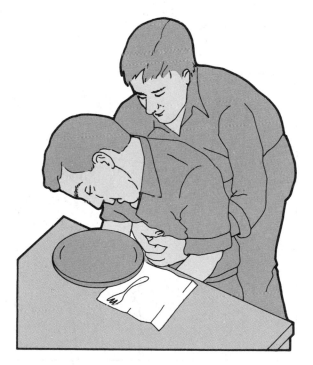

Encircle his body with your arms. Locking your hands under his ribs as above, squeeze the abdomen.

UNCONSCIOUS CHOKING VICTIM

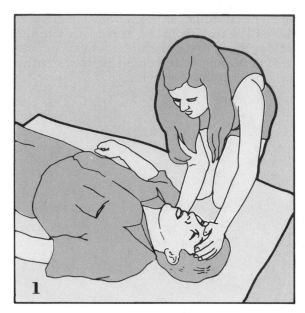

An unconscious victim should be placed on his back, with his jaw jutting upward to provide an airway (see page 834).

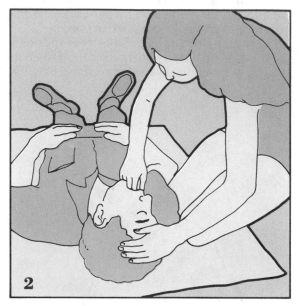

Kneel on one side of the victim, turn his head to the side, and clear out his mouth and throat with your fingers.

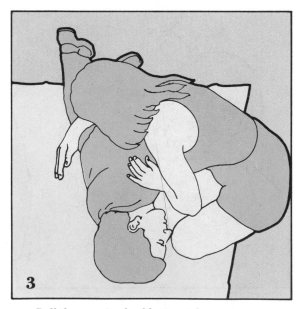

Pull the opposite shoulder toward you and give four vigorous slaps between the shoulder blades.

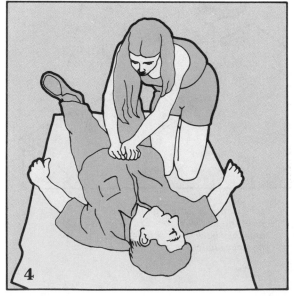

Compress the lower part of his chest four times to force air out of his lungs and into the windpipe. Immediately turn his head to one side and clear his mouth of secretions (second drawing), then repeat the maneuver.

DROWNING

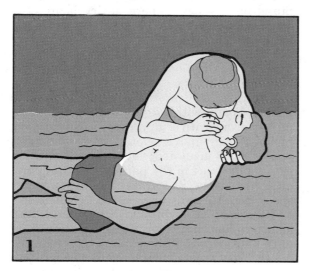

In a suspected drowning, start
artificial respiration while still in the
water (as soon as you can support the
victim's head and shoulders).
Continue as you wade toward shore.

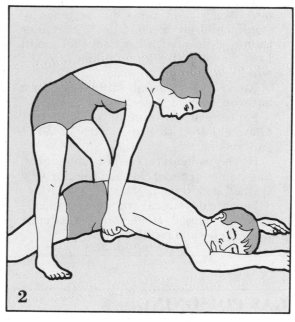

Make only one attempt to empty water
from the lungs by rolling the victim on
his or her face for a few seconds.

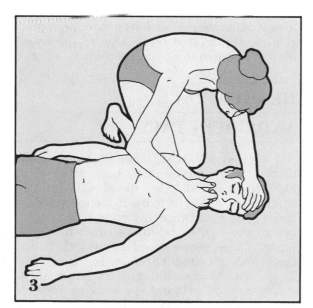

Return the victim to his or her back,
clear the mouth, and continue
mouth-to-mouth resuscitation and
checking for pulse. If there is no pulse,
use cardiac compression.

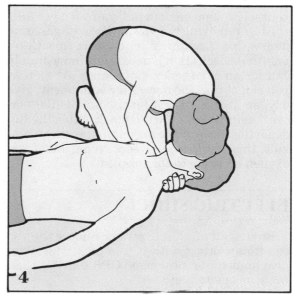

Continue mouth-to-mouth breathing
and cardiac compression until an
emergency ambulance arrives. Do not
give up early or stop to clear water from
the lungs. Apparent drowning victims,
especially those who have been in cold
water, often can be saved after long
periods of cardiopulmonary
resuscitation.

Preventing Asphyxiation and Drowning

Keep beans, peanuts, fruit pits, buttons, pins, beads, and coins out of reach of small children. Permit no toy smaller than a child's fist. Check toys for small loose parts that may be taken into the windpipe.

Never leave a small child alone in a bathtub, even for a second.

Fence your swimming pool; do not allow children to use it without adult supervision.

Have gas heaters, ranges, appliances, and home furnaces checked regularly by trained servicemen.

Never run your car engine with the garage door closed. Have your car exhaust system checked regularly.

GAS POISONING

First and most important, get the victim to fresh air. Be sure to protect yourself when entering the gas-filled area. Use an efficient mask if you can, or at least tie a rope around yourself so someone can pull you out if you fall.

After removing the victim from the gas area, assess his breathing and start mouth-to-mouth resuscitation if necessary. Immediately call for an emergency ambulance. As soon as you can obtain the necessary equipment, give oxygen at the highest level possible (100 percent) using a tight-fitting mask. Often the fire department or emergency ambulance can provide this assistance. Keep giving high-flow oxygen en route to the hospital.

ELECTRIC SHOCK

First, shut off the current or remove the victim from contact with it (see page 843), then give immediate, prolonged CPR until you can get someone to help.

Serious electric shock paralyzes breathing centers and causes unconsciousness. Ordinary house current can cause fatal shock under some circumstances.

Don't touch the victim until current is turned off or the victim is free of contact with current. You may be risking your life by electrocution.

Insulate yourself from the earth and from the victim with dry, nonconducting materials. Never use anything metallic, wet, or damp.

Then pull the wire away from the victim. Stand on dry newspapers, a dry board, the dry rubber floor mat of your car, or a dry folded coat.

Use a dry stick, a dry board, dry rolled newspapers, or a dry floor mat to pull or push the wire from contact with the victim.

If the victim lies on the wire, he may be pushed from it with a dry board. Or he may be pulled away with a dry rope. Insulate your hands with dry gloves, cloth, or newspapers. If your hand is insulated, you may with caution grasp a dry part of the patient's clothing and drag him away. Be careful not to touch his shoes, because nails may conduct electricity.

After contact is broken, give immediate mouth-to-mouth resuscitation and continue until help arrives. If the victim's body has stiffened, do not assume that he cannot be revived. Breathing centers paralyzed by electric shock take a long time to recover—victims have recovered after eight hours of artificial respiration. Don't get discouraged and give up.

Lightning. Use the same first aid as for electric shock, except that you may touch the victim immediately and begin artificial respiration at once.

To avoid danger from lightning, seek the lowest point nearby, such as a ditch or depression. Avoid isolated trees. One of the safest places to be in a lightning storm is in a car.

HEART ATTACK

AND CHEST PAIN

A heart attack occurs when the blood supply to the heart muscle has been blocked or abruptly reduced. The usual cause is an obstruction in one or more of the coronary arteries. The result in many persons is sudden, severe chest pain and almost immediate collapse. These people need instant CPR and emergency treatment if they are to survive. They should be brought to a hospital emergency department as soon as possible (with CPR administered en route), or have CPR administered until emergency equipment can be brought to them.

A second group of heart attack victims develops chest pain following exercise, although sometimes it occurs while doing nothing very active. The pain is often in the center of the chest behind the breastbone and sometimes radiates down the left arm. It may be accompanied by nausea, vomiting, and sweating.

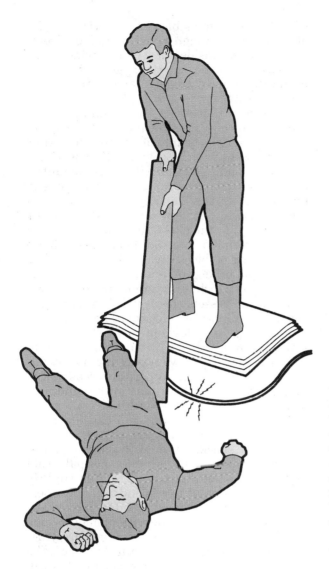

ELECTRIC SHOCK

Turn off electric current before attempting a rescue. If it cannot be turned off, insulate yourself by standing on dry, nonmetallic materials that will not conduct electricity, such as piled newspapers. Use a dry board, rope, or rubber car mat to push or pull the victim from contact with the wire. Do not use anything even slightly damp. Begin CPR immediately, as soon as the victim is free from the wire.

Preventing Electrical Accidents

Locate all switches and appliances where they can't be touched from the bath, shower, or sink.

Don't touch electrical appliances or outlets while standing on wet floors or in puddles.

Use three-prong grounding plugs or have equipment permanently grounded.

Shut off electricity at the fuse box or circuit breaker before making electrical repairs.

Replace all frayed electric cords. Cover unused wall sockets with protective plates, adhesive tape, or blank plugs. Never touch a dangling wire; call the utility company. Don't use metal ladders close to electricity.

For these persons, it is most important that the patient's physician be notified and the emergency ambulance be summoned. Sometimes this chest pain indicates a condition called angina pectoris due to a temporary decrease in blood to the heart. It will soon go away without serious effect. But when the pain does not disappear soon after onset, the patient must be evaluated by an appropriately trained physician. Therefore, he should be taken to an emergency department, preferably by a paramedic emergency ambulance in communication with the doctors at the hospital, or, if an ambulance is not available, by family car. Transportation should be rapid and efficient but should not frighten the patient and unnecessarily worsen his anxiety and cardiac condition.

The immediate care for this patient involves reassurance, while allowing him to sit in the most comfortable position. Sometimes sitting is more comfortable than lying down. If a physician has prescribed medications for the chest pain, they should be administered.

STROKE

Stroke usually occurs in older people and is caused by bleeding in the brain, or by a blockage in a blood vessel, cutting off the blood supply to a portion of the brain. The person usually complains of weakness, loss of sensation, or inability to use one side of the body. Sometimes speech is slurred, or the person has difficulty speaking, even though conscious. He may seem confused and unable to understand what is said. The face may be paralyzed on the same side of the body and the corner of the mouth may droop.

The treatment is to keep the patient quiet and reassured, and not to give anything by mouth because of difficulty in swallowing. An emergency ambulance should be summoned and the patient should be transported to a hospital emergency department. Unless an ambulance is unavailable, it is best not to transport the victim by family car lest he collapse en route with only the driver present.

UNCONSCIOUSNESS

A person who is breathing but is hard to arouse or appears unable to respond to simple commands may be stuporous or unconscious. Regardless of its cause, this is a serious condition calling for immediate measures. The first and most important step is to make sure that the person can breathe properly. If he or she is lying on the back and you are not sure whether there is head or neck injury, leave the person in that position but perform the jaw lift shown on page 834 to ensure an adequate airway. If the head or neck seems unhurt, turn the person on his side with his head slightly downward. That way, if he vomits, the material will run out of his mouth rather than being sucked into his lungs. Carry out a quick examination (see page 832) for obvious external bleeding or visible major injuries.

The odor of alcohol on the breath should not be taken to mean that the victim is drunk. Some diseases produce strange odors on the breath. Or, the person who has been drinking may have fallen and suffered a head injury, which might be the cause of the unconsciousness. A careful search for identification and information regarding possible medical causes such as diabetes should be conducted. Do not try to give a semiconscious patient anything by mouth. Call for an emergency ambulance, carefully observe the airway, protect the patient from further injury, and transport him promptly to a hospital emergency department.

SHOCK

Shock is the medical condition that occurs when body tissues do not receive enough oxygen-carrying blood. It can arise from a number of causes. The basic components of the system involved in preventing shock are the heart, which pumps blood to the tissues; the blood vessels through which the blood flows; and the blood inside the vessels, which contains red cells that carry oxygen, as well as proteins, white blood cells, and nutrients for the tissues.

Conditions that affect the pump are heart attacks, which weaken the pump by damaging the heart muscle, or injuries to the chest that damage the heart and prevent it from working properly. Conditions that affect the amount of blood flow are injuries (such as stab wounds or bullet wounds) that damage blood vessels and allow blood to pour out, either externally or internally into the chest, abdomen, pelvis, or thigh. External or internal blood loss reduces the amount of blood available for carrying oxygen and other nutrients to the tissues. A third way in which this system can break down is when the vessels themselves are damaged because of allergy or infection. The vessels dilate, enlarge, and develop tiny holes in their walls. Fluid then leaks through the walls into the tissues, causing severe swelling. The swelling can occur in such important areas as the tongue, the back of the throat, or the windpipe, and can interfere with breathing.

Any of these conditions can cause a catastrophic drop in blood pressure, the chief indication of shock. In mild shock, the pulse becomes very fast, the skin becomes pale, cold and clammy, and the patient is often slightly confused and unable to respond to simple questions because of reduced blood supply to the brain. In severe shock, the patient may become unconscious and the pulse may be barely detectable. In anaphylactic or allergic shock, the pulse is fast but the skin is warm and flushed.

Treatment

Shock can be fatal and should be treated promptly. The first step is to check airway breathing and circulation. Start mouth-to-mouth resuscitation if the patient is not breathing properly, and begin cardiac compression if the pulse cannot be felt.

The patient should be placed flat if conscious, or on his side if unconscious. The head should be level or lower than the rest of the body. External bleeding should be stopped immediately by direct pressure. The legs may be elevated by flexing them at the hips. If it appears likely that the patient will need surgery, nothing should be given by mouth, because this might interfere with the administration of the anesthetic.

INTERNAL BLEEDING

Internal bleeding is extremely dangerous because the blood loss cannot be seen. Large volumes of blood may be lost before the condition is discovered. It may happen in the abdomen following injury to the spleen, the liver, or the kidneys; in the pelvis following fractures or damage to the bladder or the large blood vessels; in the thigh following fracture to the thighbone; or in the chest following damage to the heart, the lungs, or the large vessels. Often the first indication of internal bleeding occurs when the patient starts going into shock.

Internal bleeding always should be suspected when a person has been involved in a major fall or accident with a violent impact. A driver who is thrown against the steering wheel, or a passenger or driver who was not wearing a seat belt and is thrown from the car is a possible victim. A motorcyclist who has fallen off the vehicle at high speed also should be evaluated for internal bleeding.

A careful examination may show certain telltale signs of possible internal bleeding, such as bruising and abrasions of the skin over the chest. The victim may complain of pain and tenderness over the chest. Similarly, tenderness over the upper abdomen may indicate damage and bleeding of the internal organs. Abrasions, bruises, or even the imprint of a seat belt over the upper abdomen are other clues.

Internal bleeding is not always caused by injuries. It can result from ulcers, ruptured veins, tumors, and drugs, such as alcohol.

The first and only sign of internal bleeding may be shock. Other signs can be:
• In a stomach injury, vomited material is black-brown, resembling coffee grounds.
• In an injury to the upper intestine, the stools may be black and tarry. (This is because blood that has been digested by acid from the stomach turns black.)
• An injury to the lungs and chest may produce coughed-up blood that is either frothy or that contains dark lumps of blood.

If there are signs of internal bleeding, leave the person in position, without moving him. Do *not* give any liquids or anything by mouth. Treat shock if it develops (see page 844) Keep the person covered with a light blanket. Provide reassurance. Transport immediately to a hospital, preferably by emergency ambulance.

BLEEDING

Serious bleeding. For deep cuts, severed blood vessels, and spurting or oozing blood, press a clean cloth firmly against the wound.

Remove enough clothing to see the wound clearly. Cover the wound with a sterile compress and apply firm hand pressure directly over the wound. Exert steady, not intermittent, pressure using your finger, hand, or the heel of your hand. Continue until bleeding stops.

Use clean materials, such as sterile gauze, folded clean handkerchiefs, freshly laundered towels, or strips from sheets to cover the bleeding point.

If no sterile items are available, do not hesitate to use clothing, soiled materials, or your bare hand. Blood loss is more dangerous than an immediate risk of infection.

Bleeding from legs and arms. If a wound is in an arm or leg, elevate the limb and support it with pillows or similar padding. The wound should be higher than the level of the heart. Do not elevate the limb if bones are broken or if a fracture is suspected. Firm, sustained pressure and elevation of the arm or leg usually will control the bleeding

Pressure dressing. When bleeding stops, apply a pressure dressing. Put a gauze compress or folded layers of clean cloth over the bleeding point (do not use fluffy absorbent cotton in direct contact with the wound). Press the compress with your fingers and apply a suitable bandage to fix the dressing in place. You can make a gauze compress bandage from a strip of cloth with a thick layer of gauze in the center and tails for wrapping and tying. Almost every bleeding wound can be controlled by pressure dressings alone.

The bandage must not be too tight because the wound area may swell. Inspect the bandage occasionally. If an edge of the bandage cuts into flesh, loosen the bandage a little. Otherwise, do not disturb or remove the bandage after it has been applied. If blood oozes into the bandage, cover it with another protective folded layer of bandaging material.

General measures. Do not apply salves, ointments, or medicines to deep wounds unless instructed by a doctor. Covering a wound with sterile gauze or clean cloth protects against further contamination.

Do not try to cleanse a deep or seriously bleeding wound (bleeding cleanses it internally) unless medical help is long delayed or there is gross contamination.

If essential, cleanse the skin around the wound with clean (tap or boiled) water stirred with soap to make a sudsy solution. First scrub your hands with soap and water.

Cover the wound and a small area of surrounding skin with sterile gauze. Dip a tuft of sterile absorbent cotton into the soapy solution and apply it gently to the exposed skin, stroking away from the wound. Use a fresh cotton tuft for each stroke. Greases and oils may be removed with kerosene, naphtha, or rubbing alcohol. Always wash away from the wound, and keep the patient lying down.

Treating suspected shock. Some degree of shock is imminent in all cases of serious bleeding. Have the shock victim lie flat on his back. Cover him and keep him comfortable, but not overheated. Loosen any tight clothing. If necessary, cut clothing away to avoid twisting, turning, or manipulating the patient.

Do not give stimulants, and do not give anything by mouth if the patient has an abdominal wound or if internal bleeding is suspected.

Tourniquets

A tourniquet is a dangerous instrument. It is a constricting band around a limb that shuts off blood to all points beyond it. Tissues die of gangrene if deprived of blood too long.

A tourniquet is of value as a first-aid tool only when there is risk of losing a limb. To stop the bleeding, always try direct pressure first. If this fails, and a tourniquet must be used, there must always be unbroken skin between the bleeding wound and the tourniquet.

Massive bleeding from arm or leg. Always position the tourniquet between the wound and the heart. For arm bleeding, position it about a hand's width below the armpit. For leg or thigh bleeding, position it about a hand's width below the groin.

Place the tourniquet as close to the wound as possible but not at its edge or directly over the wound.

A tourniquet may be fashioned from any fairly wide (about 2 inches) material long enough to go twice around the limb with ends left for tying. A belt, stocking, scarf, or a strip torn from clothing will serve. Some first-aid kits contain a tourniquet. Do not use wire, rope, cord, or anything else that could cut into the flesh, except in a dire emergency.

How to apply a tourniquet. Wrap the band around the limb twice and tie a half-knot. Place a stick over the knot, and tie a tight knot over the stick. Twist the stick to tighten the band just enough to stop the blood flow. Tie the free end of the tightened stick with another bandage to hold it in position.

Do not loosen or remove the tourniquet once it has been carefully applied. Fatal blood loss can result from intermittent loosening. The tourniquet can stay on safely for 30 to 45 minutes. Get the person to medical help as soon as possible.

Leave the tourniquet in plain sight. Do not hide it with a bandage or clothing. Also note the time when it was applied, so it can be loosened on schedule. If you do not accompany the person to the hospital, pin a note or tie a label on his clothing to notify others of the tourniquet. Tell the ambulance personnel about the tourniquet.

Abrasions

Skinned knees, scraped elbows, and other children's injuries can bleed or ooze blood. If coarse bits of dirt are in the wound, pick them out with small tweezers sterilized by passing them through a match or a gas flame. Rub the wound gently with a bar of plain mild soap under running water, or wash it lavishly with soap and water and a clean cloth or pieces of sterile gauze or cotton (use a fresh piece for each swabbing). Rinse under running tap water. Cover with sterile dressing or an adhesive bandage. If dirt is ground into the wound, get medical attention.

Blisters

Water blisters or blood blisters are caused by itching, rubbing, or chafing of the skin. If the blister is small and unbroken, wash it gently with soap and water, and cover it with sterile gauze or an adhesive compress. Leave it undisturbed until fluids are absorbed naturally.

A large blister is likely to be bumped and broken, or to rupture spontaneously. Cover with a sterile dressing or adhesive bandage.

If blistered skin has been rubbed off, exposing the raw skin surface, clean the area with warm soap and water and sterile cotton swabs. Cover with a sterile dressing. Watch for signs of infection (spreading redness, radiating red lines, or pus). At such signs, seek medical help.

Bleeding from Bruises

Bruises, or contusions, are caused by blows or falls that break small vessels under the skin without breaking the skin surface. The injury is first red, and then discolored (a "black eye" is a typical bruise). Minor bruises need little first aid. But internal bleeding may accompany bruises of the abdomen. Other severe bruises may involve broken bones and thus require medical help. If the skin is broken, treat the bruise as an open wound.

For minor bruises, apply something cold—ice, an ice bag, or cloths wrung out in very cold water—to relieve pain and limit discoloration. After a day or so, heat may be applied.

WOUNDS, CUTS, AND BRUISES

The first and most important step in treating a wound in a conscious victim is to stop the bleeding; cleansing the wound may be done later. For minor wounds, it is seldom necessary to use antiseptics unless specifically instructed by a doctor. The area around the wound generally may be cleansed with warm water, mild soap, and a clean cloth.

Cuts and Scratches

For small, minor cuts, wash the area well with a mild soap and a clean cloth or with cotton swabs that have been dipped into warm soapy water. Rinse under running water from a faucet or poured from a pitcher.

Cover the wound with an adhesive bandage or sterile gauze held in place by adhesive tape.

For deep or extensive cuts, don't apply medicines. Control bleeding by hand pressure over a gauze pad, clean cloth, or handkerchief until a doctor arrives. Tie a bandage over sterile dressing if help is delayed.

If the skin around the wound is grossly dirty and the patient is far from medical help, clean the area gently with soap and water after bleeding stops, washing away from the wound.

In cases involving deep cuts, which may need stitches to minimize scars, always get medical aid.

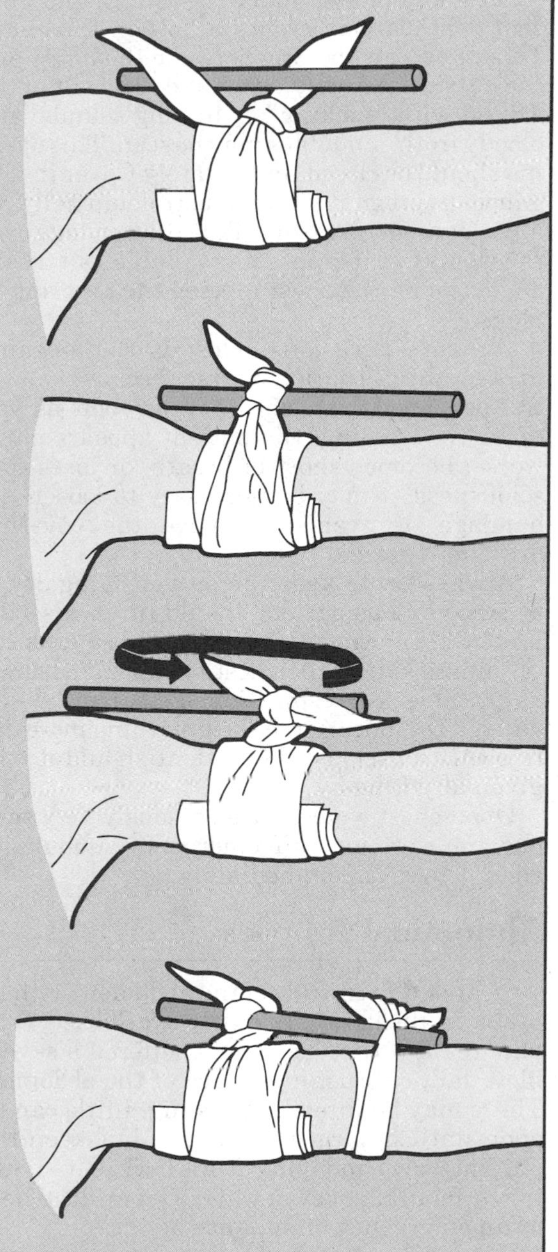

THE FOUR STEPS IN APPLYING A TOURNIQUET

To apply a tourniquet, wr... band of cloth ... between the w... a half-knot (a... a stick on the h... with the secon... the stick to incr... enough to stop t... stick in place by... bandage below t...

Chest Wounds (Sucking Injuries)

Crushing blows, punctures, stabs, and gunshot wounds may create a hole in the chest. This allows an opening between the lungs and the outside. Air may enter and blow out of the wound with "sucking" or hissing sounds, and bloody froth or bubbles may be seen. This opening should be closed immediately. Cover it with gauze impregnated with petroleum jelly, or any clean, soft dressing. Tape the bandage over the wound, or if tape is unavailable, put a bandage around the chest to keep the covering in place.

On rare occasions, closing the opening makes the situation worse because air is trapped inside the chest. If, as soon as you cover the opening, the patient appears much worse, becomes short of breath, or loses consciousness, it may be necessary to loosen the bandage or even to remove the covering dressing.

Always try to keep the patient lying down; an unconscious patient should lie on his side, preferably on the injured side. This allows the uninjured side of the chest to expand as much as possible for respiration. Legs can be elevated if this does not make breathing more difficult. If conscious, the patient should not be given anything by mouth.

Open chest wounds are obviously very serious injuries, and an emergency ambulance should be called immediately.

Abdominal Injuries

"Closed" wounds of the abdomen (with no break in the skin) are easily overlooked. Suspect them if the victim has suffered a severe blow, fall, or crushing injury of the abdomen. There may be internal bleeding. Little can be done until a surgeon explores, but keep the patient warm and lying on his back. Give nothing by mouth, not even water. Get medical help or an emergency ambulance at once.

"Open" wounds of the abdomen—deep wounds, cuts, stabs, or shots—require a sterile dressing or clean cloth over the wound to draw the edges together, and pressure to stop bleeding. There may be internal bleeding. Keep the patient lying flat on his back and warm until an ambulance arrives. See "Puncture Wounds," at right.

Protruding intestines must not be allowed to dry out. This could be fatal. Cover them immediately with a large sterile dressing and a

> ### Preventing Cuts, Scratches, and Penetrating Injuries
> Teach children not to run with or throw sharp objects.
> Keep cutlery or sharp-edged tools in storage compartments with edges shielded, or in cutlery racks.
> Keep your home workshop power tools disconnected. Lock switches and power supply so children can't turn them on.
> If guns are kept in the house, keep them unloaded and in a locked cabinet.
> Keep a clean yard, free of bottles, cans, broken glass, boards, nails, and wire.

bandage (or a clean cloth in an emergency), and keep the dressing constantly moist. Use warm salt water to moisten the dressing, preferably boiled water with one teaspoonful of salt to each pint. In an emergency, use the cleanest water you can get; intestines must not be dry for an instant. Do not try to put the intestines back in place. Give nothing by mouth. Keep the patient warm, on his back, and with his knees bent over a rolled blanket or coat. Call an emergency ambulance immediately.

Puncture Wounds

Penetrating, perforating injuries are inflicted by relatively small objects driven under the skin, sometimes deeply, or entirely through body, leaving entrance and exit wounds (perforating wounds). They may be caused by stepping on a nail; bullets or shot; wood, glass, or metal splinters; and particles driven by firecrackers, firearms, or other types of explosions.

A small puncture wound may be washed with soap and water and rinsed under running water. Cover with a dressing or adhesive bandage. The entrance point of a puncture wound is usually small and bleeds little. It cannot be cleaned in depth, and so it is useless to try to force antiseptics into the wound.

Treat like other wounds according to the immediate emergency (shock, fracture, etc.). If you are sure it will not cause further injury, encourage bleeding to "wash out" the wound by pressing gently around its edges.

Always see a doctor for treatment of puncture wounds. There is danger of tetanus (lockjaw) from organisms that may be carried into the body.

FISHHOOK IN THE FLESH

If the fishhook is caught in the flesh and cannot easily be removed, and if it is not embedded in a critical area such as that around the eye, follow these steps:

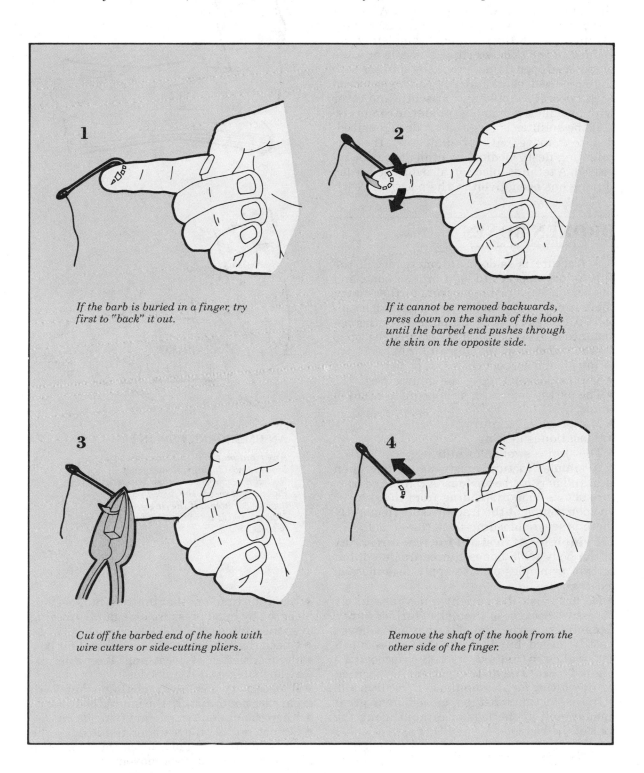

1 *If the barb is buried in a finger, try first to "back" it out.*

2 *If it cannot be removed backwards, press down on the shank of the hook until the barbed end pushes through the skin on the opposite side.*

3 *Cut off the barbed end of the hook with wire cutters or side-cutting pliers.*

4 *Remove the shaft of the hook from the other side of the finger.*

Splinters

If one end of a splinter or thorn protrudes above the surface of the skin, it may be grasped with tweezers or the fingers and pulled out at the same angle at which it entered. Wash afterwards with warm, soapy water, and apply an antiseptic. If the splinter is completely embedded in the skin, sterilize a needle or knife blade in an open flame. Probe the splinter with the sterilized point until it can be removed with tweezers. Apply an antiseptic and cover with an adhesive bandage or sterile compress.

If the splinter is large or too deeply embedded to remove without damaging the surrounding flesh, medical treatment may be required. A tetanus injection also may be needed if none has been given in the past five years.

BROKEN BONES

A fracture is seldom an emergency. If the only injury appears to be a broken bone, and the person is not in danger from further injury, there is no need to hurry the victim to a hospital. Call an emergency ambulance or other assistance (the ski patrol if the injured person is a skier, for example) and wait for help.

You should suspect a broken bone if:
● The victim can't move the injured part.
● The part is deformed, or appears to be out of shape.
● Movement is painful.
● Sensation is lacking.
● The skin is swollen or blue.

A simple fracture exists under unbroken skin and may not be obvious. A compound fracture shows bone protruding from the skin, or an open wound at the fracture site; frequently there is severe bleeding from the wound.

Principles of first aid for fractures. Any of the body's 206 bones can be fractured, but certain principles of care apply regardless of location.
● Do not move the patient unless absolutely necessary because of the risk of further injury. Great harm can be done if the patient is moved hastily, pulled, bundled into the back seat of a car, or allowed to stand or sit up, or to move the injured part. Leave the patient in position while waiting for an ambulance or medical aid.
● If the victim must be moved from great danger, pull at the legs or armpits along the axis of the body.

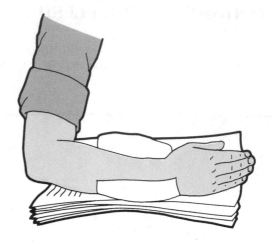

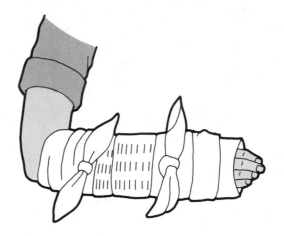

AN EMERGENCY SPLINT

Any rigid material will immobilize a broken limb during an emergency. Rolled newspapers are often handiest. Place a pad inside the folded paper, then tie as shown. If the fingers turn blue, the splint is too tight and should be loosened.

● Examine first for other injuries. Stop serious bleeding by hand pressure or a gauze dressing over the wound.
● Check the victim's mouth and throat for possible obstruction of breathing. Keep the airway open. Give CPR if needed.
● If necessary, cut away clothing, but with great care not to disturb the injured body part.
● Keep the patient warm and lying down.
● Do not put a pillow under the head if the neck is injured. Instead, block the head with padding to prevent neck movement.

If medical help will be delayed and the patient must be transported:

• Do not try to set bones.

• Always apply splints before moving or transporting the patient. Splint the patient where he lies.

• Apply a clean dressing and bandage (no antiseptic) if a bone protrudes through the skin or the skin is broken.

• See page 875 for information on how to transport an injury victim.

Splinting materials. The purpose of a splint is to give the broken body part constant support and to immobilize it so that the broken bone ends will not grind together. Almost anything that is rigid enough will serve to hold the limb in position—boards, sticks, a rifle barrel, an umbrella, a cane, a jack handle, or a tightly rolled magazine or floor mat. The splint must be long enough to extend above and below adjacent joints in order to prevent motion. Hard objects must be well padded with cotton, cloth, or soft materials before placing them in contact with the injured part.

Broken arm, forearm, or wrist. Have the patient lie on his back. Gently place the forearm across his chest at a right angle to the upper arm, with palm flat on the chest. Prepare two padded splints: an inside splint from the elbow to the palm, and an outside splint from the elbow to the back of the fingers. Tie the splint in place with two bandages, one above and one below the fracture. Adjust a necktie sling to hold the fingertips three or four inches above the level of the elbow unless the forearm is more comfortable at a different level (see illustration at right).

To make a newspaper splint, cover the fracture site with a thick gauze bandage and roll folded newspapers over it, then tie.

Upper arm. Place the arm gently at the side in as natural a position as possible with the forearm at right angles and lying across the chest, palm side in. Make a splint longer than the bone it supports. Place one padded splint outside the arm, from slightly below the elbow to slightly above the shoulder. Tie with two cloth strips, one above and one below the fracture site. Support the forearm with a necktie sling. Bandage the arm to the body.

If splint materials are unavailable, bind the arm firmly to the side with cloth strips wrapped around the chest. Support the arm with a sling.

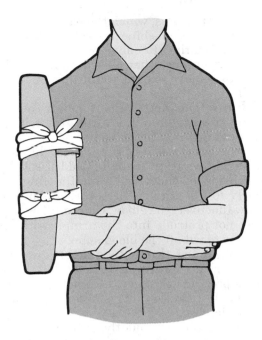

UPPER ARM SPLINT

Make an upper arm splint longer than the bone it supports, and tie in two places near armpit and elbow.

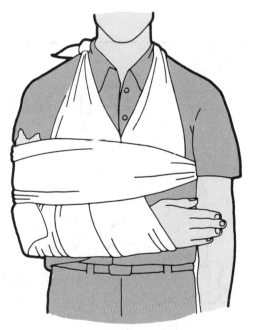

NECKTIE SLING

A sling made from a triangular bandage supports a splinted forearm or upper arm. A bandage holding the upper arm to the chest will minimize jolting movements.

In arm fractures, watch the patient's fingertips. If they become blue or swollen, loosen the splint slightly. Remove rings, bracelets, wristwatches, or other objects that would be hard to remove should the arm and fingers swell.

Elbow. If an injured elbow appears bent, do not try to straighten it. Put the arm in a sling and bind it firmly to the body.

If the arm and elbow are straight, leave them that way. Put a single padded splint on the inside of the arm, from the fingertips nearly to the armpit. Tie securely above and below (not over) the elbow. Caution: The splint must not protrude into the armpit with such force as to cut off the blood supply.

Broken leg (knee to ankle). Lower leg fractures are easily jostled, so that broken bones protrude through the skin or cut blood vessels. Use caution if it is necessary to move the patient.

Remove the shoe gently, cutting laces and the shoe itself, if necessary. Grasp the foot firmly and pull slowly to straighten the leg and foot to a normal position. If working alone, tie the feet together after the leg is in a normal position. If someone is available to help you, hold the leg in position while your helper prepares the splints.

Pillow splint: Slide a folded blanket, robe, or firm pillow under the injured leg. Lift the leg no more than necessary while supporting the broken bones. Tie a pillow splint around the leg in five places. Use a stick or any rigid object for added stiffness.

Board splints: Use two padded boards, about four inches wide, that reach from just above the knee to just beyond the heel. Pad them especially well at the ankle. Put a splint on each side of the leg; tie as shown.

If no splints are available, put a blanket, folded towels, or soft cloth between the patient's legs and tie the injured leg to the sound leg (but not if the break is near the ankle).

Broken thigh (upper leg, hip). Fracture of the femur, the body's largest bone, can be serious. Shock may follow. Call an emergency ambulance quickly. The injury may be obvious: the injured leg may appear shorter. The foot may flop, or the person may be unable to raise his heel from the ground when lying with knees flat. But there may be no deformity, and the injury may look only like a bruise. When in doubt, treat the injury as a fracture. Put one hand under the heel and the other over the instep; steady the limb and pull it gently into a normal position. If working alone, tie the feet together temporarily.

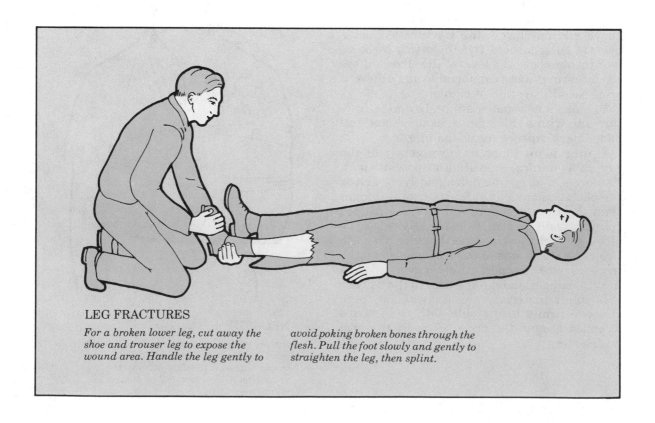

LEG FRACTURES

For a broken lower leg, cut away the shoe and trouser leg to expose the wound area. Handle the leg gently to avoid poking broken bones through the flesh. Pull the foot slowly and gently to straighten the leg, then splint.

Prepare seven broad long bandages or cloth strips. Use a small stick to push them under the hollows beneath the knees and back.

Use two board splints, four to six inches wide and well padded. The outer splint should reach from the armpit to the heel; the inner splint from the crotch to heel. Tie the splints.

Broken kneecap. Straighten the leg gently. Rest leg on a four-inch-wide board splint underneath the leg. Pad the splint, adding extra padding under the knee and ankle, and tie. Leave the kneecap exposed. Watch for swelling; loosen ties if necessary. Caution: If the knee joint is fractured, or if you're in doubt, do not try to straighten the leg.

Broken ankle. Use a pillow splint or rolled blanket that extends well beyond the heel.

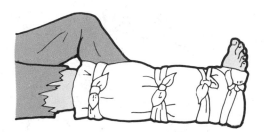

BROKEN ANKLE

Splint a broken ankle with a pillow or rolled blanket that immobilizes the foot as well as the leg.

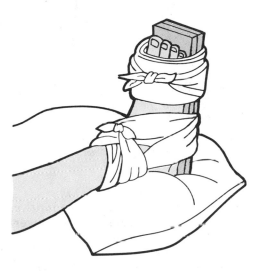

BROKEN FOOT

For foot fractures, place a padded splint under the sole. Rest the foot on a pillow.

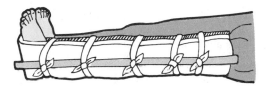

PILLOW SPLINT

A pillow splint can be tied around a broken leg in five places. A stick or other rigid object may be added to give stiffness.

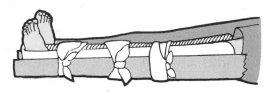

BOARD SPLINT

Board splints go on either side of the leg. Pad well between the boards and legs. Tie above and below the break.

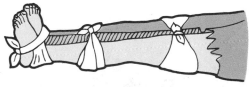

TIE LEGS TOGETHER

If no splint materials are available, tie the broken leg to the uninjured leg as shown to prevent movement. Tie with strips of cloth (you can use the patient's shirt). Put padding between the two legs.

Broken foot or toes. Place a padded splint under the sole of the foot and tie, but not too tightly.

Trunk fractures (ribs). A broken rib is indicated by pain on breathing or coughing. The person may take shallow breaths to lessen the pain or hold his hand over the break to limit chest motion when he breathes. Bandaging may restrict the person's breathing, so bandage only if necessary to relieve severe pain. Put a broad pad over the break then a broad cloth strip around the chest. Tie a single knot over the pad. Tighten a second knot. Tie two similar bandages in place to give firm support.

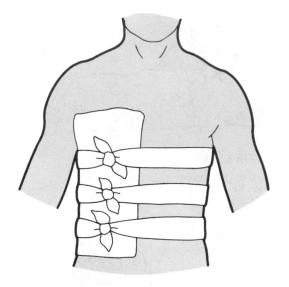

FRACTURED RIBS

Bandage possible fractured ribs lightly to avoid restricting breathing. Place a broad pad over the suspected break and tie it in place with cloth strips. Do not bandage ribs if victim coughs blood.

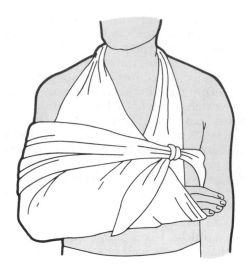

BANDAGE SLING

Put the arm in a triangular bandage sling with fingertips exposed. Adjust the height to the most comfortable position. Tie the arm to the body with a towel or cloth over the sling.

Broken ribs should not be bandaged with great force and tightness because of the danger of a rib end puncturing a lung.

Alternative: Make a tight chest binder from a pillowcase, sheet strip, or any large cloth. Wrap tightly around the chest when the patient exhales; fasten the chest binder securely with safety pins.

Caution: If the patient coughs up bloody froth or bright red blood (lung puncture), do not apply tight bandages. Get medical aid immediately. Give first aid for shock until a doctor takes over.

Collarbone fracture. Fractured collarbone ends usually can be felt by passing the fingers over the curved bone above the top ribs. The patient usually cannot raise his arm above the shoulder. The injured shoulder will be lower than the other when the arms hang.

Pelvis fracture. Pelvis fracture is a very serious injury. Broken bones of the pelvis (the basin-shaped structure between the spine and the lower limbs) may damage important abdominal organs. Automobile accidents and squeezing, crushing hip injuries are among the causes. Watch for great pain in the lower abdomen and possible difficulty in urination. If in doubt, treat as a fracture. Be extremely careful in handling a person with a possible fractured pelvis. Do not move unless absolutely necessary.

Don't move the patient if medical help is on the way. Keep him lying down. Bandage ankles and knees together, with legs straight or

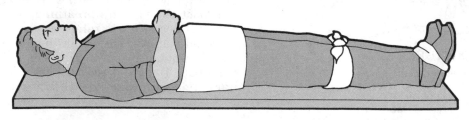

BROKEN PELVIS

For this extreme injury, bandage the ankles and knees together; work a broad bandage under the hips and tie if absolutely necessary to move the victim. Minimize movement to prevent broken bones from damaging or penetrating internal organs.

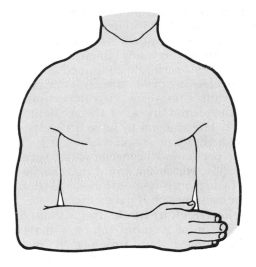

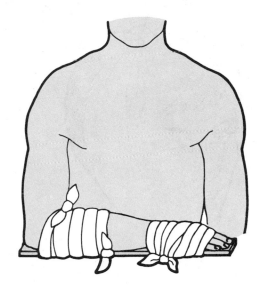

HAND FRACTURES

(1) Three steps are used in splinting hand fractures. First, place the hand laterally across the body.

(2) Using a board longer than the forearm, splint the injured arm palm down and tie at the wrist and elbow.

knees bent—whichever is most comfortable.

If the patient must be moved, slide a broad bandage under the hollow of the back, work it under the hips, and tie snugly but not tightly or fasten with safety pins. Transport the patient face up on a board or stretcher (see page 875 for instructions).

Fractured jaw (lower). A broken lower jaw is indicated by saliva trickling from the mouth or loosened or damaged teeth. There may be bleeding from the mouth. Raise the lower jaw gently to a normal position, and support it with a broad bandage under the chin tied at the top of the head (see page 856).

If the patient vomits or bleeds from the mouth, remove the bandage at once. Turn the head to one side, support the jaw gently with your hand, and replace the bandage when vomiting stops.

Fractured nose. A broken nose may result from an athletic event, a bicycle accident, or a hard fall. Misalignment and swelling are the chief clues. It is not necessary to splint a broken nose. Gauze may be inserted into the nostrils if not forced in an upward direction, but pushed gently straight back. If the nose bleeds, press the nostrils together between the thumb and index finger for several minutes. Press cold cloths over the nose. Have the patient hold his head back slightly and breathe through his mouth. Apply a sterile dressing if it is an open wound. A broken nose is not a dire emergency, but get prompt medical attention for the patient to prevent deformity.

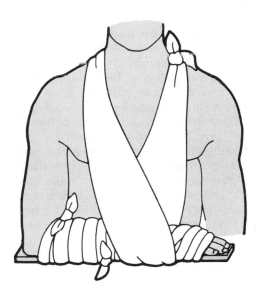

(3) Use a cravat or triangular bandage for a sling, keeping the splinted arm parallel to the ground.

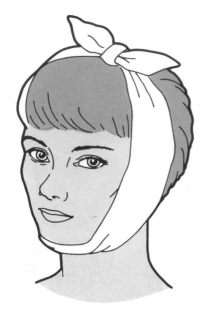

JAW FRACTURE

If a broken jaw is suspected, raise the lower jaw gently to a normal position, then hold it in place with a broad bandage tied to the top of the head.

Skull fracture or concussion. Assume that any severe blow to the head, even if the patient does not become unconscious, is a skull fracture or concussion (a bruise of the brain). Any person who has suffered head injury should be kept quiet and be seen by a doctor as soon as possible, even if he seems to have "recovered." Symptoms may be delayed.

For immediate first aid, keep the person lying down and warm. Do not let him sit up or walk. Observe him closely and make simple tests for possible brain injury: Ask simple questions or give simple directions for him to follow. It is important to note his responses so you will be aware of any change later.

A very important sign of serious brain damage may be found by directing a flashlight beam at the eyes. Normally the pupils will react to light by constricting. Both pupils should react equally. If one pupil is large and fails to respond to light, while the other is smaller and constricts normally, the person may be bleeding around the brain or into the brain and should be taken to an emergency department as quickly as possible. While waiting for the ambulance, pay careful attention to the breathing. It may be necessary to give mouth-to-mouth resuscitation or even cardiopulmonary resuscitation.

Watch, too, for a change in the level of consciousness. If a head-injury patient becomes stuporous or sleepy, or if he develops slurred speech, cannot carry on a simple conversation, or cannot follow simple commands, this may indicate bleeding inside the skull and possibly in the brain. This is especially important if the patient appeared fine after the accident or injury, but later begins to have difficulty with speech, memory, or simple tasks.

If the person loses consciousness, turn him on his side, watch for vomiting, and be prepared to do mouth-to-mouth resuscitation and cardiac compression if necessary.

Broken neck or back. Tragedy can result if the victim of a spinal injury is moved by well-intentioned but uninformed persons. Even a slight movement of the head or back may sever nerves and cause paralysis or death. What you don't do in the first few minutes is more important than what you do.

DO NOT move or lift patient from where he lies until medical help arrives.

DO NOT bend or twist his head or body in any direction.

DO NOT put a pillow under his head or give a drink of water.

DO NOT pull him out if he is imprisoned in a wrecked car unless there is danger of fire. Wait for medical help.

DO NOT jackknife him into the back seat of a car and rush to a hospital (see page 875).

What to do. Suspect a broken back or neck and treat it as a fracture if the patient has had a bad fall, a "whiplash" neck injury, a crushing or impact injury, or, in fact, has been involved in any accident in which the back or neck is bent or struck.

If the patient is conscious, ask him to move his hands and fingers. If he cannot, suspect a neck fracture. If he cannot move his feet and toes, suspect a back fracture. He may complain of pain in the neck or back. There may be no other sign. Consider the circumstances of the injury.

Summon an ambulance at once. While waiting, keep the patient warm and covered. Do not move or lift him.

If the patient must be transported to a hospital, see page 875.

BURNS

Burns require prompt treatment for several reasons. First, an infected burn can produce a severe scar that takes a very long time to heal. Second, burns caused by chemical smoke can seriously damage the throat, the windpipe, and the lungs. Third, burns affecting certain structures such as the hands and the elbows can heal with scars that can severely limit the movement of these joints. The result can be serious disability.

Classification of Burns

Burns may be classified in one of two ways. One way is to classify them as first-degree, second-degree, or third-degree burns.

First-degree burns cause only redness of the skin. Sunburn is a first-degree burn, and often can involve extensive areas of the whole body. Widespread sunburn, which can be accompanied by swelling and fluid collection under the skin, is often called sunstroke. It may be accompanied by heatstroke (see page 872), a much more serious condition.

Second-degree burns result in redness of the skin plus blistering. These areas can be large as well, and the blistered areas can become infected and result in serious scar formation.

Third-degree burns are those in which the superficial skin and fat are burned and deep structures such as muscle, nerves, and blood vessels are visible or even damaged. These are the most serious burns, although they may not be painful because nerve endings have been destroyed.

Another way of classifying burns is by calling them partial- or complete-thickness burns.

Partial-thickness burns are those in which only the skin and part of the underlying tissue are red and blistered and damage goes no deeper. These are very painful because the nerve endings are not destroyed.

Full-thickness burns involve the whole skin and subcutaneous tissue down to muscle or fat. They are often not painful because the nerve endings have been destroyed.

Burns acquired in a closed space such as a room with little ventilation are dangerous because hot smoke containing chemicals may have been inhaled. Often these burns do not show their dangerous effects for 12 to 24 hours. Anyone who has burns around the mouth or inside the mouth or who coughs up sooty sputum should be examined by a doctor for burns of the lungs.

Preventing Burns

Keep handles of pots and frying pans turned away from the edge of the kitchen range.

Don't put hot tea, coffee, or other liquids on a tablecloth or scarf hanging over the sides of a table. A child may pull the cloth or run into it and tip over steaming liquids.

Never leave a small child alone in a bathtub. He or she may turn on the hot water faucet. Place the child in the tub facing the faucet so he or she won't back into the hot metal.

Don't hold a child in your lap while you drink or pass hot beverages.

Cover hot pipes and radiators.

Keep matches and cigarette lighters out of reach until a child is old enough to be taught their safe use.

Never leave children alone around a bonfire, outdoor grill, fireplace, glowing coals, or an open flame.

Treatment of Burns

Burns that cover less than five percent of the skin area and are not on the face or the hands can be treated at home. Immediate care is to place the burn under cold running water to relieve pain. Then cover with a clean, dry dressing. Gauze impregnated with petroleum jelly sometimes can be used if the burn is small. Cover with a clean dressing, and change it daily. The burn can be washed with soap and water while healing. If signs of infection such as an increase in pain, swelling, fever, or the appearance of pus occur, the patient should see a physician.

Burns that cover more than five percent of the skin area and burns of the face and hands require prompt examination in a doctor's office or emergency facility. The larger the burn, the more necessary that the patient go to an emergency department. Meanwhile, immediate treatment can be given by placing the burned area under cold running water, or by covering it with cloths soaked in cold water. Cover the area with a dry, clean dressing before transporting the patient.

If the face has been burned or the victim is coughing up sooty sputum, it is important that he be given oxygen, and be transported rapidly to an emergency department. Burns of the airway can result in the swelling and eventual narrowing of the airway, causing breathing difficulty. In major burns involving more than 20 percent of the body surface, shock can occur because the injury "burns off" water from the body, and the body oozes fluids through the burn. The victim needs intravenous fluids to replace those lost through the burn site.

Home care. For superficial burns of between 5 and 10 percent of the body and not involving the face or hands, follow these simple steps:
• Don't open intact blisters.
• If blisters are ruptured, carefully trim the edges of the broken flesh.
• Wash the burns with soap and water.
• Keep the burns covered with a dry, clean dressing.
• Watch carefully for signs of infection such as increased redness, pain, swelling, or draining.

Special burns. If the person appears to have been burned by chemicals, immediately drench the involved area with clean water. Place the victim in a shower, if available, and forcefully spray the burned areas. Remove the victim's clothing while under the shower. Summon an emergency ambulance, and transport the patient to an emergency room.

Infection. To guard against tetanus, a burn victim's inoculation record should be checked and antitetanus shots given if needed. In addition, antibiotic treatment may be needed to prevent infection by organisms already present in the area of the burn.

BANDAGES AND BANDAGING

In an emergency, do not try to apply bandages in complex, precise, professional ways unless you have had special training. The first-aider's bandages will be replaced by a doctor. Elastic bandages, types that conform to body contours, and adhesive compresses all help to make bandaging simpler.

In bandaging, first apply a sterile gauze compress large enough to cover the wound. Then apply a bandage over the compress.

Bind the bandage firmly but not too tightly. Use just enough pressure to stop the flow of blood. The wound may swell and make the bandage so tight that it shuts off circulation. Watch the wound for swelling and blueness, and for edges cutting into flesh.

COMMON BANDAGES

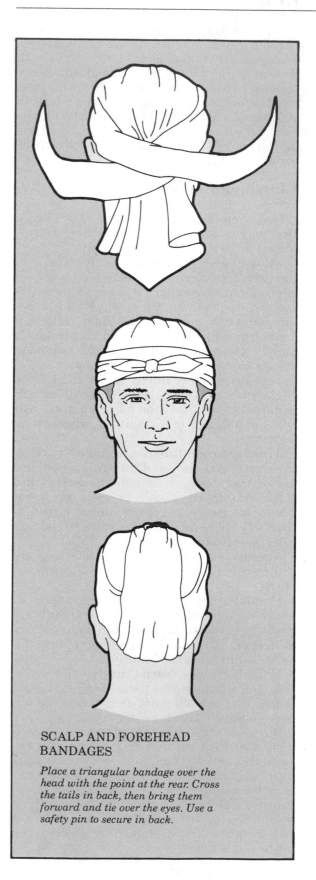

SCALP AND FOREHEAD BANDAGES

Place a triangular bandage over the head with the point at the rear. Cross the tails in back, then bring them forward and tie over the eyes. Use a safety pin to secure in back.

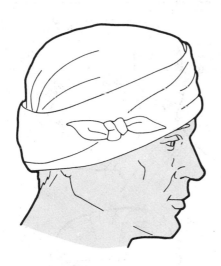

EAR AND HEAD BANDAGES

Fold a triangular bandage into a cravat shape. Tie it over a compress that covers the wound.

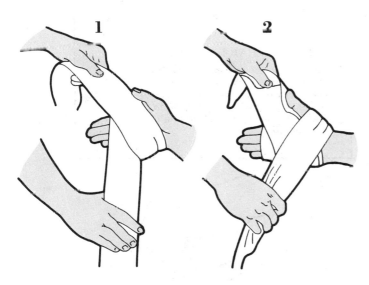

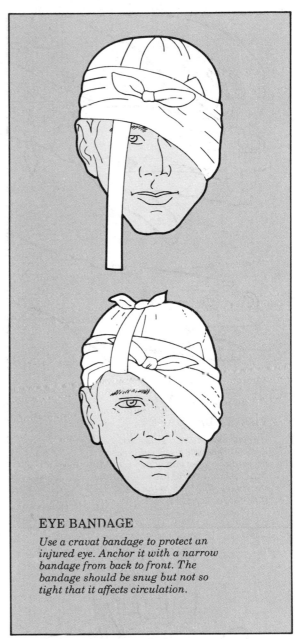

EYE BANDAGE

Use a cravat bandage to protect an injured eye. Anchor it with a narrow bandage from back to front. The bandage should be snug but not so tight that it affects circulation.

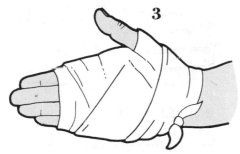

BANDAGING THE PALM

Bandaging a hand injury is a three-step procedure. (1) Wrap a cravat around the hand, leaving the thumb out. (2) Carry the lower end of the bandage in back of the hand around the thumb. (3) Wrap the remaining ends of the bandage around the hand and fingers, and tie.

COMMON BANDAGES continued

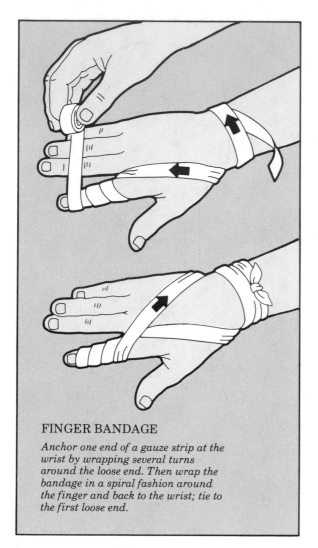

FINGER BANDAGE

Anchor one end of a gauze strip at the wrist by wrapping several turns around the loose end. Then wrap the bandage in a spiral fashion around the finger and back to the wrist; tie to the first loose end.

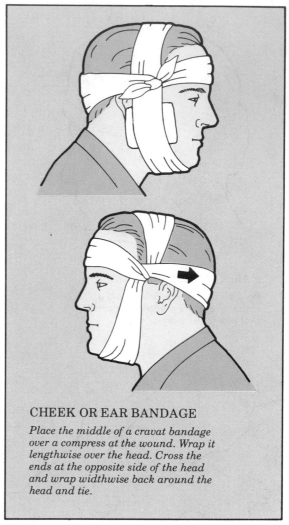

CHEEK OR EAR BANDAGE

Place the middle of a cravat bandage over a compress at the wound. Wrap it lengthwise over the head. Cross the ends at the opposite side of the head and wrap widthwise back around the head and tie.

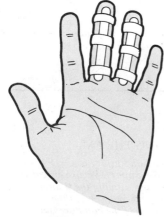

BROKEN FINGER

Place small splints (ice-cream sticks or coffee stirrers may be used) along the length of the finger(s). Tape in place in three places.

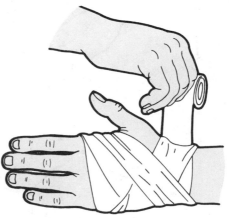

INJURED HAND OR WRIST

Wrap a wide bandage in figure-eight fashion to protect the hand or wrist.

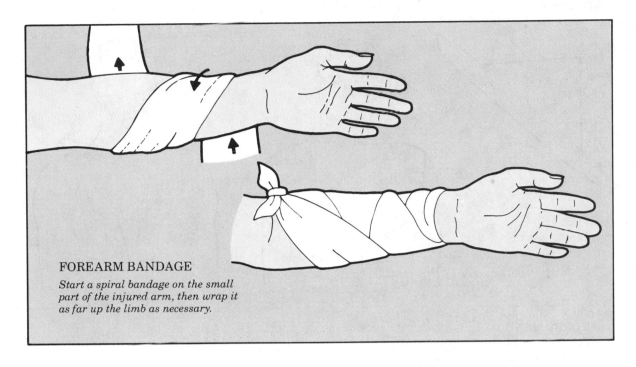

FOREARM BANDAGE

Start a spiral bandage on the small part of the injured arm, then wrap it as far up the limb as necessary.

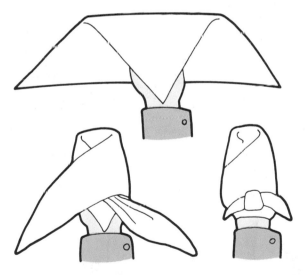

HAND OR FOOT BANDAGE

Use a triangular bandage. Fold it back over the injured hand or foot, wrap as shown, and tie.

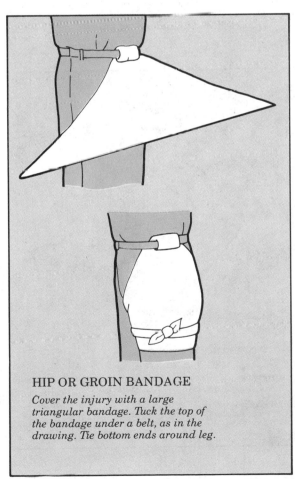

HIP OR GROIN BANDAGE

Cover the injury with a large triangular bandage. Tuck the top of the bandage under a belt, as in the drawing. Tie bottom ends around leg.

COMMON BANDAGES continued

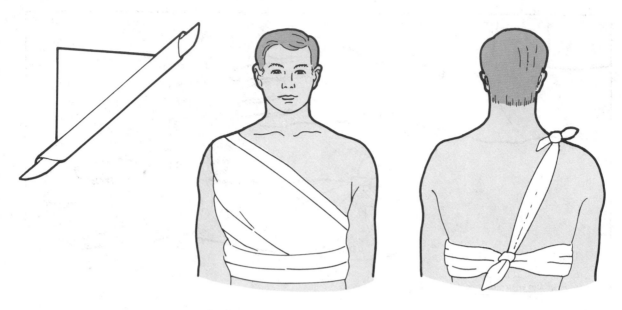

TORSO BANDAGE

Roll the base of a large triangular bandage partway, as shown. Tie the rolled part of the bandage around the victim's waist. Place the point of the triangle over the shoulder and adjust *the bandage to cover the wound. Use a second cravat or length of cloth to link the triangle end to the portion at the waist. Tie or pin the ends.*

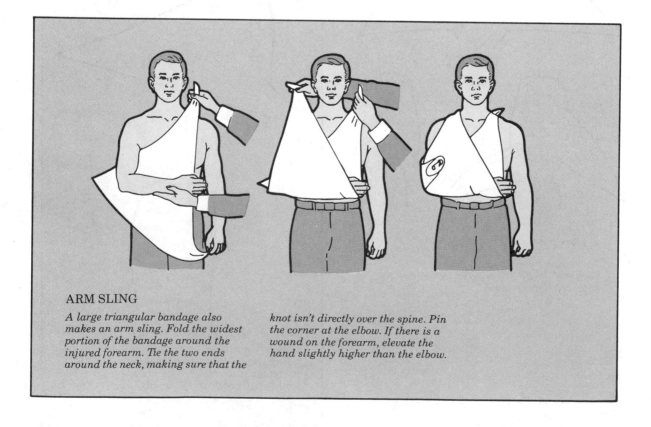

ARM SLING

A large triangular bandage also makes an arm sling. Fold the widest portion of the bandage around the injured forearm. Tie the two ends around the neck, making sure that the *knot isn't directly over the spine. Pin the corner at the elbow. If there is a wound on the forearm, elevate the hand slightly higher than the elbow.*

Materials. Sterile packaged materials in many sizes should be parts of every first-aid kit: roller gauze bandages (which can be folded to make compresses), adhesive bandages, bandage compresses, sterile gauze compresses (available in various sizes), and cotton rolls (never use a fluffy cotton bandage in direct contact with a bleeding wound).

Freshly laundered and ironed sheets, handkerchiefs, napkins, pillowcases, and towels make suitable dressings in an emergency. Just use the cleanest cloth available.

Triangular bandages are useful. They can be made from muslin, a bed sheet, or clean cloth, about 40 inches square; cut them diagonally to make two bandages. (Boy Scouts are taught to use their neckerchiefs.) Fold to make strong, long bandages (cravat bandage) of the desired width.

A universal protective dressing covers and protects limb wounds, or can be used as a splint in fractures, or for pressure treatment of burns until medical aid arrives. Follow these steps:

Apply a layer of sterile gauze (a covering compress for open wounds). Then, apply a one-inch layer of absorbent cotton.

Wrap with several layers of muslin or clean cloth and cover with waterproof plastic.

POISONING

Poisons can enter the body in different ways. These include swallowing, breathing (inhalation), absorption through the skin, and by injection or envenomation. Injected poisons include abused drugs such as heroin and "speed" (amphetamines); envenomation refers to bites by snakes or insects.

To treat a poisoning victim, follow these steps:
• Remove the patient from any further exposure to the poison.
• Ensure that the airway breathing and circulation are adequate.
• Reduce the chance of further absorption of the poison. Depending on how the poison was taken in, this may be done by washing the skin with water, by giving a lot of water to drink, by causing vomiting, by giving a laxative or cathartic, or in rare cases by using a specific antidote.
• Phone your local poison control center.

• Provide the following information:
Your name.
Your address.
Your telephone number.
The patient's name and age.
What the poison is.
When it was taken.
What symptoms have occurred up to now.
What steps you have taken to treat the poisoning.
• Follow the instructions given to you by the poison control center.

Swallowed Poisons

If you are unable to contact the poison control center or other emergency facility for instructions, take these steps for treatment of swallowed poisons:
• If the patient is conscious and is able to talk to you or to hold a glass, give as much water as he or she can drink. Large amounts of fluids may cause vomiting, and vomiting should be encouraged for all swallowed poisons except those that are caustic. This is usually easy to determine because caustic substances burn the mouth, tongue, and throat. Or, information on the poison's container may state that the contents are caustic.
• Give the victim syrup of ipecac—two tablespoonfuls for an adult, one tablespoonful for a

---

Preventing Poisonings

Keep household chemicals out of reach of small children. A high shelf or locked cabinet should be used for disinfectants, lye, ammonia, flammable and noninflammable cleaning fluids, insecticides, bleaches, rat poisons, moth balls, kerosene, gasoline, turpentine, and paint thinners.

Never put chemicals into a soft drink bottle or a container associated with food—a sip can be swallowed before it can be spit out.

Never put anything on food shelves except food. Keep drugs, both prescription and nonprescription, locked up.

Do not leave pills in a purse, pocket, or bedside table where children may find them.

Never tell a child that a pill is candy or "tastes like candy."

Never take a medicine until you have read the label. If the label is gone or is illegible, discard the bottle.

child. As noted on page 833, this substance should be part of every family's first-aid supplies. It is available in drugstores without prescription. After giving the ipecac, have the victim drink six to eight glasses of water. If vomiting has not occurred in 20 to 30 minutes, the dosage may be repeated, in the same quantity. Do not repeat the dosage more than once.

Ipecac should *not* be given and vomiting should *not* be induced if the offending substance is caustic or corrosive, such as lye, disinfectant, ammonia, or toilet-bowl cleaner, because substances that burn on the way down may also burn on the way up. Nor should ipecac be used for swallowed kerosene, gasoline, or turpentine. In these cases, the physician or poison control center may administer special medication to offset the effects and speed transit through the system.

A so-called universal antidote for swallowed poisons, available in some drugstores, should *not* be used. Even if the poison container carries instructions, it is best to follow directions from the poison control center. In general, antidotes are not very useful in treating poisonings. Most are no better than swallowing plain water or milk, and some actually may be harmful. In addition, they may provide a false sense of security.

After the person has vomited and if he or she appears wide awake, alert, and unharmed, you may give activated charcoal, also available in drugstores, in a quantity of about one teaspoon to a glass of water. Follow the charcoal with a large dose of Epsom salts or any other common laxative. This should only be done in consultation with the poison control center.

Transport the patient to a hospital emergency department or your doctor's office. Take the bottle, box, or container from which the poison came, including the remaining liquids, tablets, powders, or particles, and the label if it contains information. For prescription drugs, take the container with the pharmacist's name and the prescription number. If the person has vomited, recover the vomited material and take it, too.

Poisoned Unconscious Victims

If the patient is not fully conscious and is unable to hold a glass of water in his hand, lay him on his stomach or on his side and ensure that breathing is adequate. Keep his mouth free of secretions by wiping it with a handkerchief or finger. Keep the airway open by using the techniques described on page 834. Call an emergency ambulance.

If breathing appears inadequate, start mouth-to-mouth resuscitation, and if the pulse disappears, start cardiac compression.

Keep the patient covered, but not too warm. Do not give stimulants of any kind. Give nothing by mouth to a semiconscious or unconscious patient. Fluids will go into the lungs and can cause pneumonia.

Food Poisoning

Do not assume that all severe intestinal upsets which occur after eating are caused by food poisoning. Appendicitis and other illnesses may cause similar symptoms. The chief clue to food poisoning is when more than one person becomes ill after eating the same foods that were spoiled or improperly prepared.

The most common forms of food poisoning are infections caused by bacteria or their toxins in contaminated foods. Symptoms may be very mild, lasting only a few hours, or very severe and urgently needing medical aid. Most bacterial food poisonings are caused by staphylococci (a germ family that causes boils and abscesses) or salmonella organisms.

Staphylococcal food poisoning may cause symptoms almost immediately, commonly within two to four hours after eating. Symptoms of salmonella poisoning usually are longer delayed—from six hours after eating to a day or even two days later.

Symptoms. Nausea, vomiting, diarrhea, and cramps are the primary symptoms of food poisoning. There also may be considerable abdominal pain and distress; the abdomen feels soft, rather than rigid. In salmonella poisoning, there may be chills and fever, too. A doctor should be consulted promptly.

Do not give laxatives, cathartics, or anything by mouth as long as there is persistent nausea and vomiting.

Put the patient to bed and keep him or her warm.

After nausea and vomiting subside, give large quantities of water or soft drinks.

Preventing Food Poisoning

In sanitary food handling, lack of refrigeration (keeping foods at room temperature or warmer for several hours) underlies most cases of food poisoning. Food handlers with cut fingers, colds, and boils may introduce germs that can multiply rapidly in foods that are not thoroughly cooked or that are heated very little, such as salads, meringues, salad dressings, creamed dishes, custard fillings, and cold cuts.

Refrigeration retards growth of germs. If no refrigeration is available, consume foods soon after preparation; discard leftovers. On picnics, car trips, and camping trips, keep food in a portable icebox.

Botulinus Poisoning

Botulinus poisoning is caused by powerful toxins of organisms that may be in improperly home-canned foods, especially low-acid foods. Commercially canned foods and home-canned foods canned by the pressure method are safe. Boil home-canned foods for 30 minutes before eating to ensure their safety.

Symptoms commonly begin 18 to 24 hours after eating contaminated food, but may not appear for several days. Nausea and vomiting may not occur. More common symptoms include: great fatigue, dizziness, headache, blurred or double vision, difficulty in breathing, swallowing, or speaking, and muscular weakness. The body temperature may be subnormal.

Botulinus poisoning can be fatal. Medical attention should be obtained *at once*.

Mushroom Poisoning

The best first aid is prevention. No test can prove unknown mushrooms safe to eat. Avoid all wild mushrooms.

If mushroom poisoning occurs, call an emergency ambulance immediately. Keep the person quiet and lying down until help arrives. If the symptoms occur in the woods or far from medical aid, get the person to a hospital emergency department immediately.

Symptoms of mushroom poisoning may appear within a few minutes to two to three hours after eating, but some varieties do not cause symptoms for up to 48 hours.

Common symptoms include abdominal pain, diarrhea, dizziness, blurred or double vision, cold sweating, and cramps in the arms or legs.

If possible, keep a sample of the mushroom for identification.

Weed and Plant Poisoning

Leaves, roots, berries, seeds, and other parts of many weeds, wild plants, and garden plants (foxglove, monkshood, rhubarb leaves, lilies, and others) may be toxic if eaten. Teach children not to eat strange berries, fruits, or plant parts; avoid them yourself. Check your garden for poisonous plants. Ask your local nursery for advice. Symptoms of plant poisoning vary. They usually include abdominal pain, cramps, nausea, and vomiting (juice stains may be visible around the mouth).

Induce vomiting immediately.

Treatment. Give large amounts of water or milk, as well as the standard dose of ipecac.

After the person has vomited, give activated charcoal.

Call the poison control center and an emergency ambulance. Save a specimen of the plant or part thought to have caused the poisoning.

Street Drugs

Certain illegal drugs (and some prescription drugs) can cause a medical emergency because of overdose, contamination of the substance (especially if obtained on the street from a "pusher"), or the so-called "bad trip." Symptoms of overdose or reaction to a contaminated drug can be loss of consciousness, sweating, confusion, or dizziness. The victim of a "bad trip" may retain consciousness but may be overcome by terror, see or hear frightening things, become violent, or behave in a bizarre manner.

Treatment. Try to keep the atmosphere as calm as possible and attempt to reassure the person. Place him or her in a quiet room, dim the lights, and remain nearby.

If breathing appears to have stopped or you cannot detect a pulse, begin CPR and call for an emergency ambulance immediately.

Unless instructed by a doctor or medical aide, do not give any medication, including tranquilizers or sedatives.

By continual voice and hand contact try to "talk the person down" and carry him through the bad experience.

If a conscious person seems to be deteriorating, becoming violent, having trouble with breathing, or going into shock, call for an emergency ambulance immediately. Bring with you any drugs or material that the patient has used or taken.

BITES

Poisonous snakebites. Not everyone who claims to have been bitten by a snake actually has been bitten. Often, simply seeing a snake nearby convinces a frightened person that he or she has been bitten, when in fact no bite has occurred. When a bite does occur, the skin is not always broken. Even if it is broken, the snake's venom may not have been injected into the wound. Thus, only a minority of snakebite victims are in danger of poisoning. (Remember, however, that venom may enter the body through an existing break in the skin.)

Signs that indicate that a venomous snakebite has occurred include:
• Two small puncture marks comprising the wound.
• Severe, immediate pain at the site.
• Severe swelling and blistering at the site of the bite.
• Progressive swelling of the entire leg or arm.

(Bites very rarely occur on the face or body, but when they do, they are more serious and require immediate medical attention.)

Treatment. General treatment for snakebite victims is as follows:
• Help the victim to lie down, reassure him, and keep him quiet.
• Do not give alcohol or any stimulants to the victim.
• Elevate the limb and apply a cold compress to the bite. Do not apply ice. Apply a constricting band, or a *loose* tourniquet, above the bite. The tourniquet should not cut off blood flow; you should be able to feel a pulse beyond it. It is only intended to stop flow from the lymphatic vessels. Loosen every 15 minutes.

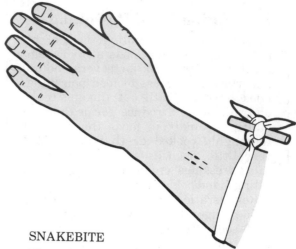

SNAKEBITE

First-aid treatment of snakebite should be attempted only within 30 minutes of the time of the bite. Place a loose tourniquet above the bite area, but don't tie it so tight that it constricts the blood flow. Check for a pulse below the bite to be certain. With a sharp knife, cut two parallel incisions through the fang marks, each about three-eighths inch deep. Suck venom from the wound with your mouth, spitting out each time, or use the suction cup furnished in most snakebite kits.

• If you are not in deep woods or far from medical help, call an emergency ambulance or take the person immediately to an emergency department. (If possible, phone first to be sure the hospital is prepared, or to learn if another nearby hospital specializes in such treatment.) Carry the victim if possible, otherwise walk him slowly to medical assistance.
• Do not use snakebite kits containing antivenom except under a physician's instructions, or unless medical help cannot be obtained quickly. Antivenom is a dangerous substance. Because it contains horse serum, humans may react against it and it should only be used when the danger of an adverse reaction is less than the danger of the snakebite.
• If the bite has occurred within 30 minutes, or if you are far from a hospital, it may be advisable to incise the wound and suck out the venom (see above). Using a sharp knife, cut through the bite three-eighths inch deep in two parallel lines, one through each bite mark. Actual cutting of the flesh should be minimized. Do not cut over nerves or tendons. Suck the venom out

either with a suction cup (provided in most snakebite kits) or by mouth, spitting out the venom each time.

• If possible, kill the snake with a long stick, and carry it on the stick or in a bag. Bring it to the hospital for identification. This is helpful when the doctor has to decide whether to use antivenom.

• Do not move the victim unless absolutely necessary.

Insect bites. For relief of pain and itching from mosquito, flea, and other insect bites, apply ice or wet dressings; hold under cold water. Apply a paste of baking soda moistened with water, or apply diluted household ammonia to the bite and surrounding skin. Calamine lotion and rubbing alcohol or lotions containing alcohol also help to relieve itching. Do not scratch an insect bite. Scratching may result in infection.

Tick bites. Ticks are small insects that burrow into the skin and can cause such serious diseases as Rocky Mountain spotted fever, tularemia, and relapsing fever. A tick often can be felt before it starts to burrow under the skin, but usually not after it begins to suck. Ticks often are picked up in areas of damp grass or woodlands, but they are sometimes brought indoors by domestic animals, or may be found in suburban gardens. Children are especially vulnerable. Examine their clothing, skin, and hair after playing in "tick territory," especially in the spring.

The head of a tick tenaciously resists removal from skin. Don't try to remove ticks with unprotected fingers or allow crushed parts or juices to contact the skin. It may help to make ticks "let go" if you coat them with nail polish, petroleum jelly, or grease, or smother them with kerosene, turpentine, or gasoline. Remove them carefully with tweezers.

Afterward, wash the site thoroughly with soap and water.

Wear high shoes with trouser ends tied around the tops when hiking in tick country.

Stings. Bee, wasp, hornet, or yellow jacket stings may be relieved by cold packs containing baking soda. Ice cubes and ice bags also give comfort.

Preventing Bites and Stings

Teach children not to maul or torment pets and not to approach stray animals.

Wear calf-high boots in snake country; watch your step in the woods; probe the underbrush with a stick before trampling on it (75 percent of snakebites occur near the ankle; most of the rest in wrist or hand areas).

Tie shut the open ends of sleeves and trouser legs when strolling through tick-infested grasses and weeds.

Wear light-colored clothing. Bees and stinging insects are attracted to dark colors, tweeds, flannels, sweaty clothing, hair oils, and perfumes. If "attacked" by a hostile bee, move slowly, don't make jerky movements, slap, or run, unless a whole hive is after you.

Wear gloves when cleaning out a garage to protect against a possible bite from a black widow spider.

If you upset a nest of insects and suffer a "massive dose" of many separate stings, get into a tepid tub bath with a package or more of baking soda stirred into it.

Bees often leave their "stinger" in the center of the sting. The stinging apparatus can be seen as a tiny dark object. It continues to pump venom into the wound after the bee is gone. Pinch the stinger between two fingernails or grasp it with tweezers and remove it gently. Do not remove the stinger with an outward scraping motion of a fingernail. That forces more venom out.

A few people become so extremely sensitized to insect venom that a sting can cause a serious, even fatal, allergy-like reaction known as anaphylaxis (see page 869).

Spider bites. Two common American spiders can inflict serious bites—the small brown (recluse) spider and the black widow. The latter is a coal-black spider with a pea-size abdomen marked with a reddish hourglass design.

The black widow's bite causes intense pain, muscle spasm, and a weak pulse. The pain moves gradually from the wound and concentrates in the abdomen. The brown spider's bite may not be immediately painful, but if not treated it causes tissue breakdown in the area of the wound.

Get to a doctor or hospital emergency department immediately. Save the dead spider for identification, if possible. Meanwhile, wash the wound with soapy water and watch for signs of shock.

Animal bites. Immediate first-aid treatment of animal bites is the same as for other common wounds, except for the possibility of rabies (see below). Bite injuries range from barely perceptible tooth marks to severe injuries that must be treated as major wounds.

Most bites inflicted by dogs, cats, squirrels, rats, mice, and small animals are local soft-tissue injuries. Immediate first aid aims to prevent infection and promote healing.

Cleanse the wound thoroughly with soap and water. Preferably, wash it under running water with soap. Paint with antiseptic.

Cover the bite wound with a sterile dressing and bandage.

See a doctor. Always see a doctor if the bite, no matter how trivial, is on the face, hands, head, or neck area.

Human bites. A human bite may be a real bite or it may be inflicted by teeth that stop the blow of a fist. The human mouth commonly contains varied and virulent bacteria, and serious, undermining, spreading infections often follow human bite wounds.

Give first aid as for an animal bite, then have a doctor take over.

Rabies

Rabies is a very rare disease in humans. It is often fatal, although recently a few people have survived because of advances in hospital treatment. The disease results from an infection of the nervous system by the rabies virus, transmitted by an infected animal either through a bite or through licking the damaged human skin. The offending animal is usually a wild species, such as a skunk, fox, raccoon, or bat, but it also may be a domestic animal, such as a dog or cat that has been infected by a wild animal.

Treatment of possible rabies cases involves use of a vaccine that can be very painful and that must be given frequently. If possible, the animal should be captured, observed, and examined. Weeks or even months may pass before symptoms appear. For these reasons and because of the high mortality rate, it is important to have a trained physician evaluate every potential infection as quickly as possible in order to begin treatment if it is necessary.

Treatment. Whenever the possibility of infection with rabies is being considered, the following factors must be examined:

Species of biting animals. Foxes, skunks, coyotes, bats, raccoons, dogs, cats, and bears are the animals most commonly infected with rabies. Bites of rats, hamsters, guinea pigs, gerbils, chipmunks, squirrels, rabbits, mice, and other rodents have never caused rabies in humans in the United States.

How the bite occurred. The most important factor is the "unprovoked attack." Many animals bite people when teased, cornered, or otherwise provoked. If an attack occurs for no such reason, one should assume that the animal is potentially rabid, especially if the animal bit a person attempting to feed or handle it.

Bite or lick. The rabies virus is transmitted in the saliva of the biting animal. Therefore, it is important to check whether the skin has been broken by the teeth during the bite. If the suspected animal did not bite, but licked skin that is scratched, abraded, or has open wounds, or if the animal licked mucous membranes such as the inside of the mouth, these should be considered nonbite exposures, and just as serious as bite exposures.

Is the biting animal vaccinated? Properly vaccinated and immunized domestic animals very rarely get rabies, and therefore very rarely transmit the rabies virus to humans.

Treatment of bites or scratches. The most important action to be taken immediately is to clean the bite or scratch aggressively. Soap and water should be used to thoroughly wash out the wound. You should contact your physician or go to an emergency department for evaluation and treatment. The physician should consider the need for tetanus prophylaxis, additional cleaning of the wound, and the use of antibiotics to control infection.

What to do with the animal. In the United States, it is common for the local health authority to investigate the immunization status of a domestic animal that has bitten a human. These animals should be confined and observed by a veterinarian for ten days, and any illness in the animal should be reported immediately to the health department. The department will usually sacrifice the animal and arrange for the brain to be examined for rabies virus. Stray or unwanted dogs or cats should be immediately sacrificed and their brains examined for rabies virus.

Because of the difficulty in evaluating wild animals for rabies, a wild animal that bites or scratches a person should be killed at once and its brain examined, if at all possible.

ANAPHYLAXIS

Anaphylaxis is the condition resulting from an allergy to a foreign substance such as pollen, fish, penicillin, or bee or wasp stings. It sometimes follows massive stings. It is a much more severe form of allergy than hay fever. A person can be allergic to almost any substance, and he or she may not necessarily have been exposed to the substance before.

Usually the reaction begins soon after the person is exposed to the substance (an injection of penicillin, or a bite by a wasp) and the major serious effects are breathing difficulty and shock. Early signs include skin rashes, blebs on the skin, swelling of the tongue, and itching in the back of the throat. These may progress to severe wheezing, difficulty with breathing, confusion, and collapse. Swelling of the face, eyelids, and extremities may occur, and the patient may collapse, or, in some cases, suffer cardiac arrest.

The treatment involves calling an emergency ambulance immediately. Persons who are known to suffer serious allergic reactions should receive an epinephrine injection to counteract the effects. Often these people carry epinephrine in their purses or pockets, and wear an identification "Medic-Alert" tag. It may be necessary for you to administer the epinephrine (adrenalin) if they are not able to do so.

You should lay the patient down and be prepared to give mouth-to-mouth resuscitation and even cardiopulmonary resuscitation.

Mild cases in which there is no shock or difficulty in breathing, but just skin itchiness and a skin rash, may be treated with an antihistamine such as Benadryl. However, any patient with a new reaction should communicate with his or her physician relatively soon, even if an emergency ambulance is not called.

THE EYES

Chemical burns. There is only one thing to remember when dangerous chemicals get into the eyes: Wash them immediately with large amounts of cool water. Chemicals continue to burn as long as they remain in the eye.

Immediate flushing of the chemical minimizes eye damage and may prevent it entirely. Don't waste time trying to find out whether the chemical is an acid or an alkali. It makes no difference.

Hold the head under a faucet with the eye in the running stream of cool water. The stream should have good flushing force but not high pressure. Turn the head so the stream flows over the affected eye and away from the unaffected eye. If both eyes are contaminated, direct water on both eyes simultaneously or in rapid alternation. Flush the eyes thoroughly before you take time to call a doctor.

You can't use too much water. Keep on irrigating the eyes with water for 5 or 10 minutes or until you are very sure that all dangerous chemical material has been washed out. Remember, powder particles may be trapped under the eyelids. Separate the lids gently so water can reach all parts.

If there's no faucet handy, seize any source of water or any bland fluid you can lay your hands on quickly—a carton of milk will serve in an emergency. Put the patient on the floor, flat on his back, and pour water from a pitcher, tumbler, or any container, into the corner of the eye next to the nose so the fluid streams over the eyeball and under the eyelids. Repeat, repeat, repeat!

Or, the eye may be held in a stream of water bubbling from a drinking fountain. Or, the eyes may be submerged in a bowl of water while the patient repeatedly blinks them.

After all chemical materials are washed from the eyes, call a doctor. What you do in the first few seconds and the next few minutes to wash acids or alkalis from the eyes is more important than anything the doctor can do later. Cover both eyes with a sterile gauze compress (even if only one has been affected) and take the patient to a doctor, or call for an emergency ambulance.

Contusions of the eyeball. Hard blows that do not cut or penetrate the eye may "bruise" it internally and can be serious, even though the injury may not "look bad." Delayed damage may result from slow hemorrhage or injury to internal eye structures. Take no chances if the eye has suffered a severe blunt blow. You may apply cold compresses (do not use hot compresses) but don't rely on first-aid measures alone. Arrange for prompt examination by an eye physician.

Foreign bodies in the eye. It is safe to use simple first-aid measures to remove cinders, eyelashes, or specks that rest loosely on the surface of the eyelid or eyeball. Do not attempt to remove embedded particles that resist simple first-aid procedures. Never rub or scratch an eye that "has something in it." This may cause scars, or drive particles farther into the eyeball. Always wash your hands before touching the eyes.

Pull the upper eyelid out and down over the lower lid, or shut both eyes for a few minutes to cause a flow of tears that may wash out the particle.

If this does not work, fill a clean medicine dropper with warm water or a boric acid solution to "flood" the eye and flush out the foreign body.

If the speck is visible, gently pull the lower eyelid out and downward for inspection. Use a moistened cotton applicator or the corner of a clean cotton cloth to lift out the speck. If the speck is not visible, lift the upper lid and look for it. Remove with applicator or clean cloth.

Do not use more vigorous methods to remove particles embedded in lids or eyes. Cover with a sterile gauze compress held or gently taped in place, and see a doctor immediately.

Penetrating eye wounds. All perforating wounds of the eye are serious, no matter how small, and call for immediate medical help. A

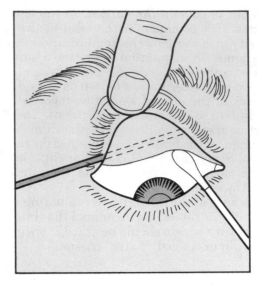

SPECK IN THE EYE

A dust particle or small object, seen when the upper eyelid is turned back over a stick, may be removed with a moistened cotton-tipped applicator. Do not rub a speck embedded in the eye because you may scratch the eyeball.

tiny speck buried deep inside the eye may leave little outward trace. Do not apply oils or ointments. Instead, cover both eyes with a sterile compress (to lessen harmful eye movements) and bandage lightly in place (do not use hard pressure). Go to a doctor at once, transporting the victim flat on his back on a stretcher, if possible.

Some penetrating eye wounds, such as stabs from pointed objects, are obvious and terrifying, but equally serious injuries may look less frightening. A tiny piece of steel hurled off from tool-grinding or nail-pounding may be lodged in an eye that looks normal. Anyone who has felt something strike his eye should be examined by a doctor promptly. Glass splinters, sand, and transparent sharp articles that become lodged in the eye may not be visible on ordinary observation.

Black eye. An "ordinary" black eye is a bruise. For immediate first aid, apply pressure to the involved area, preferably with cold compresses or cloths wrung out in cold water. If done at once, this helps to minimize discoloration. A severe black eye may involve deeper injury and need more intensive attention.

LODGED, INHALED,
OR SWALLOWED OBJECTS

Ear. Children may insert small objects into the ear canal. Peas, beans, and popcorn swell when wet and are hard to remove.

Do not dig at the object with a toothpick, hairpin, or wire, which risks grave danger of injuring the ear canal or eardrum, and may push the object further in.

Rarely is there any immediate danger. If the object appears loose, gently pull the earlobe backward and tilt the child's head so the object can fall out. If this fails, take the patient to a doctor who has instruments to remove the foreign body. If the object is a bean or seed, a little olive oil or mineral oil can be dropped in the child's ear to lessen the swelling.

Insect in the ear. If an insect crawls into the ear, turn head to one side and drop in some warm olive oil or mineral oil to suffocate the insect. If no oil is available, use warm water. The dead insect may float out. Try turning out the lights and shining a flashlight into the ear to attract the insect. If this approach does not work, have a doctor remove the insect.

Nose. Children sometimes slip beans, grains, and small objects into their nose. There usually is no immediate danger, but great harm can be done trying to remove the object with crude instruments. Drop olive oil into the nostril to soothe tissues and prevent swelling. The child may blow his nose gently (both nostrils open), never forcibly, after oil is instilled. If this does not dislodge the object, take the child to a doctor.

Stomach. Tacks, open safety pins, needles, and other small sharp objects are frequently swallowed by children. Do not administer a laxative. Go to a doctor. Most foreign objects that reach the stomach pass through the bowel harmlessly, but the doctor may follow the progress with a fluoroscope and intervene if the object becomes lodged or penetrates tissues. Never force a child who has swallowed a sharp object to vomit.

How to Prevent Swallowing Accidents

Never give popcorn, candy, nuts, or cookies that contain nuts to infants who can't chew them and may inhale them.

Don't let small children play with dry beans, peas, buttons, coins, nails, or screws. Check stuffed animals and other toys for easily removable small parts that a child may remove and swallow or stuff into body openings.

Make a habit of closing safety pins. Don't hold tacks, pins, or nails in your mouth while doing chores, or let children see you doing so.

Be sure that all bone fragments are removed from foods for small children.

FREEZING INJURIES

Frostbite. Skiers, snowmobilers, children who play outdoors in cold weather, and those who work outdoors are all susceptible to frostbite. Exposed parts of the body, especially the face or ears and the extremities, may appear bluish, or white with a grayish-yellow cast, and feel numb.

Do not rub the frozen part with snow or anything else. Frozen tissue is fragile and is easily damaged.

Do not expose the frozen part to intense direct heat, such as that from a hot stove, radiator, or heat lamp.

If outdoors, thaw the frozen part by using the patient's body or the body of another as a warmer. Place a frozen hand under an armpit or between the thighs. Place a warm hand over a frozen ear or nose.

Indoors, immerse the frozen part in tepid (not hot) water, warmed to about 100 degrees. Or, cover the part with warmed (not hot) towels or blankets. See a doctor for aftercare. If the part is deeply frozen, the condition is serious and requires immediate medical aid.

Prolonged exposure. Chilling of the entire body, from mild chilling to numbness, can be serious. Drowsiness can be a symptom and death can result.

For a mild chill, put the patient to bed in a warm room, cover well, and give hot drinks.

For serious freezing exposure, get the victim to a warm place. It this is not possible, two or three persons may warm him with their bodies, under blankets, or in a sleeping bag. If breathing is imperceptible or stopped, give mouth-to-mouth resuscitation.

Rewarm the victim rapidly by immersing in a tub of water at 78 to 82 degrees. Then wrap the victim in warm blankets and put him to bed. Give warm drinks, and summon help.

HEAT ILLNESSES

Heat cramps are painful spasms of abdominal, leg, or arm muscles caused by loss of body salt through profuse, prolonged sweating. They are most common in persons who do very hard physical labor in extremely hot surroundings for long periods. Cramps usually respond to firm hand pressure, warm wet towels, or a hot water bottle. Give the patient sips of slightly salted water.

Heat exhaustion occurs because body fluids and the salts they contain have been passed off from the body. The patient's skin is pallid, clammy, and moist; he may sweat profusely. Body temperature may be about normal, or perhaps slightly lowered or slightly elevated. The patient may exhibit nausea, scant urine, dizziness, and may faint.

Remove the patient to circulating air. Have him lie down and rest. Loosen his clothing. Give sips of slightly salted water (1 teaspoonful of salt to each pint of water), or coffee or tea as stimulants.

If symptoms of heat exhaustion do not subside readily, call a physician or an emergency ambulance.

Heatstroke is a grave emergency and can be fatal. Act quickly to cool the victim.

Symptoms include very hot, absolutely dry skin and no sweating. Body temperature is very high, from 104 degrees up to an incredible 110 degrees. The victim may exhibit weakness, dizziness, rapid breathing, nausea, unconsciousness, and sometimes mental confusion. Onset is often dramatically sudden.

Cool the victim rapidly. Apply an ice bag, crushed ice wrapped in a cloth, or cold cloths to the head. If the victim can't be moved to shelter, drench his clothes with warm water, poured on or sprayed from a hose.

Preferably, strip the victim's clothing, wrap him in a sheet, and keep the sheet wet with cold water. Place electric fans to blow on the cold sheet, and keep cloths or ice on the victim's head. At the same time, rub the victim's arms and legs toward the heart through the sheet.

Check body temperature every 10 minutes or so, preferably by thermometer, but if none is available, by feeling the skin. Keep repeating the cooling procedures until body temperature drops to between 101 and 102 degrees. If the temperature rises again, repeat the cooling procedures.

Fainting. The most common form of pallid unconsciousness, fainting is usually caused by temporary insufficiency of the blood supply to the brain. Correct this condition by positioning the head level with or lower than the trunk.

If you feel faint or about to "pass out," lie down if possible. If not, bend forward at the waist from a sitting position and put your head between your knees. If you can't lie or sit, kneel on one knee as if tying a shoe, to position your head lower than your heart.

In a crowded place, if someone feels faint, don't try to walk him out. Bend his head forward between his knees until he feels better. The best first aid for fainting is to keep the patient lying down, with head lowered or legs and hips elevated. Sprinkle cold water on his face to speed recovery.

After consciousness is regained, coffee or tea may be given. Recovery should be rapid—within five minutes. If unconsciousness is prolonged, or if fainting spells recur, call a physician or an emergency ambulance.

SPRAINS, STRAINS, AND DISLOCATIONS

Sprains result from tearing or stretching of ligaments that link the bones at joints and allow movement. They have become increasingly common because of weekend athletics. It may be difficult to distinguish between a sprain and a fracture—both may result from the same injury. If in any doubt, handle the injury as a fracture (see page 850). X rays are usually necessary to make the distinction. Many injuries assumed to be sprains by laymen are actually strains.

The symptoms of a sprain are: Pain in the joint which increases on movement, tenderness to the touch, difficulty in using the joint without pain, rapid swelling, and black and blue discoloration (which might not appear for several hours).

Immediate aid. These are not emergencies. Except for minor injuries, have the injury examined by a doctor within 6 to 12 hours. In skiing injuries, summon the ski patrol.

Relieve pain by resting the joint. Movement may complicate the injury.

Elevate the sprained joint higher than the rest of the body so it gets less blood and therefore will have less swelling. Support it with a pillow or padded clothing.

Bandage the joint to prevent unnecessary motion if the accident occurs far from medical help. Loosen the bandage if swelling increases.

For the first few hours after injury, apply an ice bag or cold compresses. This contracts vessels, minimizes swelling, and eases pain. Do not apply heat immediately after the injury.

Sprained ankle. If the injury occurs far from help or if it is absolutely essential for a sprained ankle to bear weight, a snug ankle bandage gives support for walking. Never walk with a sprained ankle (it might be broken) unless in a serious emergency.

Follow the illustrations at right to support a sprained ankle. Leave the shoe on, but loosen laces. Place a long bandage under the shoe in front of the heel. Bring bandage ends behind and above the heel, cross, bring them forward, and cross them over the instep. On each side of the foot, tuck the ends under the loops formed by the first step of bandaging. Pull the ends together and tie over the instep. For a sprained knee, wrist, or elbow, wrap well with an elastic bandage. Use a sling for a sprain of the wrist or elbow.

Strains. A strain is caused by overstretching or "pulling" muscles or tendons. Back strain ("crick in the back") is common.

Symptoms include a sharp pain or "stitch" at the time of injury, stiffness and soreness that get worse in a few hours, and pain on movement.

How to help. Put the injured part at rest. Sit or lie in the most comfortable position.

Apply heat in any form—hot water bottle, lamp, or heating pad.

Give a gentle massage with warm rubbing alcohol.

If the pain eases sufficiently, rub more forcefully or knead gently to help loosen stiffened muscles.

See a doctor if back strain is severe. Back strains frequently need strapping.

Dislocations. A blow, fall, or sudden twist may force a bone out of place at a joint, causing a dislocation. Some persons are prone to repeated dislocation of certain joints.

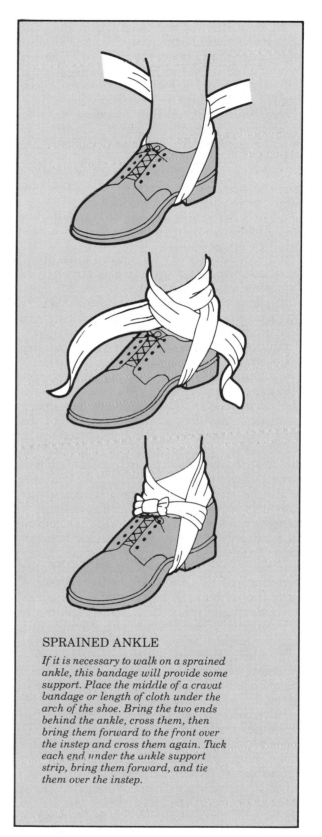

SPRAINED ANKLE

If it is necessary to walk on a sprained ankle, this bandage will provide some support. Place the middle of a cravat bandage or length of cloth under the arch of the shoe. Bring the two ends behind the ankle, cross them, then bring them forward to the front over the instep and cross them again. Tuck each end under the ankle support strip, bring them forward, and tie them over the instep.

An indication of a dislocation is that the joint looks out of shape compared to a similar joint. Swelling is usually rapid, and there is pain and tenderness at the injury site. The patient can't move the joint or motion is limited and the patient may be in shock.

Immediate first aid. Call an emergency ambulance or transport the person to a hospital emergency department if it can be done without risk.

Do not try to straighten the joint or force the bone back into place (except for a knee, jaw, finger, or toe dislocation; see below).

Suspect that bones may be fractured. In general, handle the injury as if the part were fractured (see page 850).

Put the patient in a comfortable position. Keep weight off the injured part. Give gentle support to the injured part.

Apply an ice bag or cloths wrung out of very cold water to the injured part to ease pain and minimize swelling.

Dislocation of the knee. Athletic injury is the usual cause of a dislocation of the knee. The dislocation is usually evident because the lower leg is out of alignment at the knee, displaced either forward or backward. The injury requires immediate attention because of the danger that the artery supplying blood to the lower leg may be stretched or trapped and the flow interrupted. Treatment requires two persons. One holds the victim at the shoulders while the other grasps the foot on the dislocated leg and pulls down as hard as possible to relocate the knee in a normal position. Splint as for thigh fracture. Transport to hospital immediately.

Finger or toe dislocation. Grasp the area with one hand on each side of the dislocated joint. Slowly pull the free end of the finger or toe in a straight line until it snaps in place. Do not use great force. If one or two attempts fail, wait for medical help. Do not try to reduce the large joint at the base of the thumb or the great toe joint. Don't pull a dislocated finger or toe if an open wound is near the dislocated joint. Dress the wound and get medical aid.

Jaw dislocation. In an emergency, a first-aider may try to correct a dislocated jaw.

Suspect a dislocated jaw if the lower jaw sags and the patient cannot close his mouth.

Treatment. Wrap your thumbs with cloth to protect them. Face the patient, put your thumbs in his mouth on his lower back teeth and your fingers under his chin. Press down

Preventing Back Strain

Low back strain is most often caused by improper lifting technique, or attempting to lift objects that are too heavy. The most important lifting rule is never to let the lower back arch forward. Do not bend from the waist, stiff-legged, to lift an object from the floor. Place your feet close to the object, crouch with your back straight and feet flat on the floor, and grasp the object firmly; lift slowly, using your thigh muscles.

Don't lean over a projection such as a radiator to lift a stuck window. Don't reach to pick up something when one arm is loaded with packages. Get help if the object to be lifted is heavy.

Don't lift if your footing is insecure—a slip or twist may wrench your back.

Sudden, quick lifting of heavy objects is dangerous, especially if you are unaccustomed to it. Do not continue trying to lift an object if you feel a slight discomfort in your back. Rest frequently when carrying heavy objects.

firmly and back with your thumbs, and upward with your fingers under his chin. Remove your thumbs quickly to prevent injury when the jaw snaps back in place.

Shoulder dislocation. Dislocation of the shoulder often occurs in young people, and less commonly in older age groups. The injury usually results when the arm is pulled backward and outward.

The awake patient experiences pain and complains of being unable to move the arm. Examination of the shoulder reveals that the normal shape of the shoulder is changed, and in certain kinds of dislocations the head of the humerus (the upper arm bone) can be felt below the collarbone. The shoulder tip is not rounded, and drops off sharply.

First-aid treatment is to place the upper arm in a splint, but not to force movement. It may be necessary to place bandages or a pillow in the armpit to support the arm and then lightly bind the arm against the side of the body. Shoulder dislocation is not a true emergency unless the patient complains of tingling or numbness in the hand on the injured side, or unless it is difficult to feel the pulse at the elbow or in the wrist. Absence of the pulse means that the injury may have interfered with the circulation, and the patient should be seen by a physician immediately.

TRANSPORTING
THE INJURED

If medical help or an ambulance will soon arrive, do not move a seriously injured person from where he lies unless absolutely imperative for his safety. Haste is rarely necessary and may do grave damage. Begin first aid while help is on the way. If the victim must be transported, do any necessary splinting where he lies.

Broken neck. A broken neck or back victim should be moved *only* if it is absolutely unavoidable. Put a rigid "stretcher" such as a door alongside the victim. One person kneels at the head, grasps the victim's head firmly between both hands, and steadies it so it does not twist in any direction. Helpers grasp the victim at the hips and shoulders and roll him onto his side. Place stretcher under patient and then roll the patient onto the stretcher. Move the entire body as if the patient were stiff as a log and unable to bend.

If the broken-neck victim is lying on his face or is crumpled, follow a different procedure. One person kneels and grasps the victim's head at the jaw angles, and exerts traction so the head does not turn or move. Then a helper gently straightens and supports the legs. One or two other helpers gently turn the body onto the stretcher, with the head and neck turning in unison.

Put a rolled cloth, sweater, or pads around the sides of the head to prevent rolling. Immobilize the head using tape or bandage. Don't place a pillow under the head. Fold the victim's arms and tie the body to the board stretcher.

If you're not sure whether the victim has a broken neck or a broken back, treat the injury as a broken neck.

Broken back. Handle a broken-back victim the same as a broken-neck victim. If he is lying facedown, he may be left that way if he can breathe adequately, and moved in facedown position for transportation. Keep the broken-back victim facedown if he is transferred to an ordinary stretcher. Make sure he can breathe easily.

Vehicle. If an ambulance is not available and the patient must be transported some distance, try to get a truck or station wagon with a flat bed, padded to ease jolts. If a passenger car must be used, remove the rear cushion or use a board or padding material to make a bed on which the patient lies full-length.

Carrying without a stretcher. When the victim need not be carried in a lying-down position, you may carry him without a stretcher. Consider the nature of the injury, and never try this with a broken-neck or a broken-back patient.

Three people should kneel on the same side, slide their hands under the victim's body, lift him to their knees in unison, then rise to their feet while turning the victim toward their chests. Work as a unit and coordinate movements.

If you must move a person alone, put one arm under the victim's knees, your other arm around his neck, lean back slightly, and lift the victim to a carrying position.

Don't "jackknife" the patient into the seat unless you are certain that his injuries are slight. Jolts, bumps, and sudden stops are dangerous; drive cautiously. Such transportation should be only a last resort. Helicopter ambulance service in some areas allows for transportation of the injured from even the most inaccessible places.

Blanket stretcher. An improvised stretcher can be used for patients (except those with a broken neck or back) who must be lifted or carried in lying-down position. If the patient has broken bones, splint them before moving. A blanket with edges rolled (or a rug or other stout fabric) is usually the simplest stretcher to improvise for carrying or lifting the patient.

Tuck a folded blanket edge against the patient. Turn him gently on his side, then very carefully push the blanket under him as far as possible. Turn him back to the center of the blanket, and pull the edge through.

Roll both edges of the blanket toward the patient in the center. Rolled edges give a firm grasp for carrying or lifting. A blanket stretcher can be carried by two bearers on each side, but three per side is preferable because it allows for more stable transportation.

INDEX

Page numbers in **Boldface** refer to illustrations or illustrated text.